HEALTH PSYCHOLOGY

Richard O. Straub

University of Michigan, Dearborn

Worth Publishers

Health Psychology

Printed in the United States of America.

ISBN: 1-57259-786-0

First printing, 2001

Senior Sponsoring Editor: Jessica Bayne
Development Editor: Betty Probert
Executive Marketing Manager: Renée Altier
Associate Managing Editor: Tracey Kuehn
Production Manager: Sarah Segal
Art Director: Barbara Reingold
Cover and Text Designer: Lissi Sigillo
Photo Editor: Meg Kuhta
Photo Researcher: Debbie Goodsite
Senior Illustration Coordinator: Bill Page
Illustrations: Todd Buck
Composition: Progressive Information Technologies
Printing and Binding: R. R. Donnelley and Sons—Harrisonburg
Cover Art/Part Opener Art: *Spiral Man* by Nicholas Wilton

Library of Congress Cataloging-in-Publication Data

Straub, Richard O. (Richard Otto)
    Health psychology / Richard O. Straub.
        p.   cm.
    Includes bibliographical references and index.
    1. Clinical health psychology. 2. Health behavior. 3. Social medicine. I. Title.

R726.5 .S783 2001
616′.001′9–dc21

                                                          2001046904

Grateful acknowlegement is made for permission to use the photos at the beginnings of the
following chapters: CH1: Bachmann/The Image Works; CH2: Serena Siqueland/Digital
Imagery/PhotoDisc; CH3: Michael Freeman/Corbis; CH4: Greg Kuchik/Digital
Imagery/PhotoDisc; CH5: Reuters NewMedia Inc./Corbis; CH6: Tony Arruza/Corbis; CH7:
Donna Day/Stone; CH8: Anna Lundgren/SuperStock; CH9: John Greim/Mira; CH10: AP/Wide
World Photos; CH11: Bruce Ayres/Stone; CH12: Will & Deni McIntyre/Photo Researchers, Inc.;
CH13: Photo Kishimoto; CH14: Sam Pellissier/SuperStock; CH15: Andy Caulfield/The Image
Bank; Epilogue: Zefa/Photonica.

Worth Publishers
41 Madison Avenue
New York, New York 10010
www.worthpublishers.com

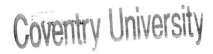

HEALTH PSYCHOLOGY

To Pam

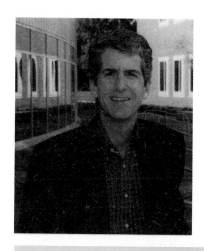

About the Author

Richard O. Straub is Professor of Psychology at the University of Michigan, Dearborn and is beginning his seventh year as Chair of the Behavioral Sciences Department. After receiving his Ph.D. in experimental psychology from Columbia University and serving as a National Institute of Mental Health/ Social Science Research Council Fellow at the University of California, Irvine neurobiology training institute, he joined the University of Michigan faculty in 1979. Since then, he has focused on research in health psychology, especially personality traits as risk factors for physical illness, mind–body issues in stress, and the effects of exercise on physical and psychological health. Professor Straub's research has been published in such journals as *Health Psychology,* the *Journal of Applied Social Psychology,* and the *Journal of the Experimental Analysis of Behavior.* A recipient of the University of Michigan's Distinguished Teaching Award, Professor Straub has written and hosted an introductory psychology course on the local college cable network and has produced print materials for several nationally published distance learning courses. His interest in enhancing student learning is further reflected in the study guides, instructor's manuals, and critical thinking materials he has developed to accompany well-known introductory and developmental psychology texts. This text allows Professor Straub to combine his interest in health psychology with his desire to teach young people.

Brief Contents

PART 5

Seeking Treatment 500

PART 6

Developmental Factors 636

Contents

PART SIX
Developmental Factors 636

Preface

"Your cancer is advanced. Inoperable. Try for whatever quality of life you can maintain. You have eleven weeks to live." Irv Kingston refused to believe this prognosis and instead mobilized every psychological, social, and environmental resource he could think of to battle his illness. With his positive, upbeat attitude, he insisted on undergoing a grueling (and useless, according to his doctor) regimen of cancer treatment. And his bravery worked: in January 1998, he received a clean bill of health and resumed his normal life.

Unfortunately, not all sufferers of life-threatening diseases such as cancer are so lucky. Some diseases take their toll, no matter what biological, psychological, or social interventions you try. However, in Irv's case, a healthy, constructive attitude helped him win the battle against cancer. More and more people are proving that illness and health are more than physiological states. In addition, people today are living longer and better—and that's what this book is all about.

Just 25 years ago, health and psychology were separate disciplines, each aware of the other but unable to connect in any meaningful way. Then, in 1978, health psychology was born. Since then, the field has grown steadily, with new research advances coming at a more rapid pace with each ensuing year. From the earliest research linking Type A behavior to increased risk for cardiovascular disease to the most current discoveries regarding the behavioral epidemiology of HIV, the "early years" of the field have been a time of great accomplishment.

More important than individual research findings has been the ongoing refinement of the *biopsychosocial (mind–body) model* as an interdisciplinary template for the study of health issues. Increasingly, researchers are able to pinpoint the physiological mechanisms by which anger, loneliness, and other psychosocial factors adversely affect health, and by which optimism, social connectedness, and a strong sense of self-empowerment exert their beneficial effects.

This textbook was conceived at the end of the initial, rapid growth period of health psychology. Understanding human behavior and teaching students are my two professional passions. Nowhere do these passions come together more directly for me than in the study of how psychology and health are interconnected. And nowhere can this connection be more clearly seen than in a textbook. My goal has been to write an introduction to health psychology that presents an up-to-date summary of the main ideas of the field, the evidence that supports these ideas, and how these ideas relate to students' interests and experiences in a manner that reveals the field to be the exciting and vitally important discipline I myself find it to be.

In an effort to communicate the excitement and value of the field, I have tried to keep my focus on ways to ensure that students understand—rather than just memorize—the concepts that make health psychology. The features I have concentrated on are:

- *Overarching theme.* The book follows the biopsychosocial (mind–body) model as the basic organizing template. Throughout, I have strived to convey how the components of this model interact dynamically in influencing the well being of the *whole* person. Each chapter dealing with a specific health problem—on AIDS, cardiovascular disease, cancer, and substance abuse, for example—presents a critical analysis of what we know to be the underlying biological, psychological, and social factors in the onset of the health problem, as well as how these factors affect the course of the disease and the outcome. My commitment to this interdisciplinary *systems* perspective on behavior stems from my eclectic graduate training (some would say, inability to make up my mind as to which career path I would follow!) as a student of learning theorist Herbert Terrace, physiological psychologist Richard Thompson, and social psychologist (and health psychology pioneer) Stanley Schachter.

- *Language and level.* Because the typical health psychology course draws students from many college majors, I have written the book so students need only a minimal background in psychology, including research methods in psychology (which are covered in a separate chapter). At the top of my list of priorities has been to forge a personal voice in the narrative—to help students make meaningful connections between the material and their own lives—while remaining true to the scientific integrity of the field.

- *Up-to-date coverage.* Few psychological disciplines generate more research each year—from a variety of related fields—than does health psychology. While retaining the field's classic studies and concepts, the book also presents the discipline's most important recent developments. More than 25 percent of its references are from research published since 1998.

- *Fully integrated gender and cultural diversity coverage.* One of my major goals has been to promote understanding of, and respect for, differences among groups of people and how these differences contribute to health and illness. But this effort extends far beyond merely cataloging ethnic, cultural, and gender differences in disease, health beliefs, and behaviors to an in-depth effort to stimulate students' critical thinking regarding the origins of these differences. For example, many differences in health-related behaviors are the product of restrictive social stereotypes and norms, economic forces, and other overarching ecological processes. Whenever possible, the text digs deeply into diversity issues by considering the origins of these behaviors and their implications for health-promoting treatments and interventions.

Examples of this integrated coverage can be found on the pages provided in the charts on pages xx–xxii.

- *Global perspective.* Mindful of the fact that we are all citizens of a shrinking world, and that the central health concerns and issues of various geographical regions are not the same, the book strives to offer a world-based health psychology that includes research findings, art, photos, and text examples that extend beyond North America and Europe.

- The *life-course perspective* in health psychology is introduced in a special chapter not found in other texts. Here, the student will learn about the special needs and health challenges of people in every season of life. As with gender and diversity, my approach is to teach students to think critically about aging and health. Increasingly, researchers are realizing that much of what was once considered normal aging is actually disease. Many older people who have made healthy lifestyle choices are rewriting the book on successful aging. In addition, because the choices people make as children and adolescents determine their fates in the later years, we begin our coverage with the problems of childhood and adolescence.

- *Coverage of complementary and alternative medicine.* According to a recent *Journal of the American Medical Association* report, four out of ten Americans use acupuncture, massage therapy, naturopathy, or some other form of nontraditional medicine. The question of whether these are valid new ways to health or merely snake oil is discussed in a special chapter.

- *High-interest boxes.* Throughout the book, three types of boxes are presented to supplement the surrounding narrative.

    Reality Check. These "self-tests" encourage students to examine their own health beliefs and behaviors. For example, students may fill out questionnaires concerned with identifying stress, controlling anger, evaluating high-risk health behaviors, trying to cognitively restructure headache pain, and many others. Each box also gives specific tips that encourage students to more actively manage their own health.

    Byline Health. Actual newspaper, magazine, or Internet articles address high-interest health topics currently being profiled in the popular media. Included among these are news clippings concerned with gender and smoking, women and AIDS, ethnicity and longevity, and the "French Paradox," to name a few. Each article is followed by questions designed to help students think critically about the issue or about the article itself.

    Diversity and Healthy Living. This feature expands the text's integrated coverage of gender and multicultural issues by highlighting specific health issues. For example, students will explore differences in how women and men cope with a grave national crisis, why hypertension is so prevalent among African-Americans, and the role of sociocultural factors in AIDS prevention.

- *Critical thinking exercises.* The text has two major goals: to help students acquire a thorough understanding of health psychology's knowledge base, and to help students learn to think like health psychologists. The second goal—learning to think like psychologists—involves critical thinking. To directly support this goal, each chapter includes a complete exercise designed to stimulate students' critical-thinking skills. These skills include asking questions, observing carefully, seeing connections among ideas, and analyzing arguments and the evidence on which they are based. Each exercise emphasizes one of six categories of critical thinking: *scientific problem solving, psychological reasoning, perspective taking, pattern recognition, creative problem solving,* and *practical problem solving.* Sample answers to each exercise, and an essay on using critical thinking in everyday reasoning, appear in the Instructor's Resources that accompanies this text.

- *Other pedagogical features.* The book includes a number of features designed to bring health psychology alive and reinforce learning at every step. Among these are the book's tremendous student-friendly visual appeal, which is enhanced by numerous graphs of research findings as well as useful and exciting photographs and artwork that illustrate anatomical structures as well as important concepts and processes. In addition, each chapter includes the following learning aids:

  An engaging case study or vignette at the beginning of each chapter gives an overview of the material, connects the world of health psychology to some concrete experience, and weaves a "thread" of human interest throughout the chapter. Many of these describe real situations. For example, Chapter 10 describes Lance Armstrong's heroic battle against cancer and his third Tour de France victory in July 2001.

  All important terms, which are boldfaced in the body of the text, are defined concisely and clearly in the margins to enhance students' study efforts. They are also listed, with their page numbers, at the end of each chapter.

  End-of-chapter summaries distill the important points, concepts, theories, and terms discussed in the chapters.

  List of Web sites that directs students to authoritative Internet resources for the most up-to-date online health information are included at the end of each chapter.

- *Epilogue.* The book ends with a brief chapter that reviews the broad lessons about which most health psychologists would agree and several of the most important unresolved questions.

Coverage of Culture and Multicultural Experience

Coverage of culture and multicultural experience can be found on the following pages:

Acculturation and immigrant stress, pp. 148–149

African Diaspora and health, p. 52

AIDS prevention, pp. 488–489

Antismoking campaigns, p. 352

Body mass and hypertension among African-Americans, pp. 51–53

Cancer,
and diet, pp. 428–429
prevalence worldwide, pp. 416–419
screening interventions, pp. 444, 446–447

Cardiovascular disease
global differences in, pp. 373–374
racial and ethnic differences in, 378–379

Community barriers to wellness, p. 230

Eating disorders, pp. 299, 302–303

Environmental stress, pp. 137–141

Gender roles and cultural values, p. 144

Health care use, pp. 514–515

Health discrepancies among ethnic groups, pp. 20–21

Health insurance, p. 229

Health system barriers, pp. 229–230

HIV transmission and AIDS, pp. 466–467

Obesity, pp. 284–286

Pain, pp. 571–573

Racial discrimination and cardiovascular reactivity, p. 381

Smoking cessation programs, pp. 356–360

Sociocultural perspective in health psychology, p. 28

Socioeconomic status
and cardiovascular disease, pp. 378–379
and health care use, p. 513
and obesity, pp. 284–286
and stress, pp. 170–171

Substance abuse, pp. 328–329

Symptom interpretation, pp. 509–510

Tobacco use, pp. 344–345

Coverage of Life-Span Issues

In addition to the coverage found in Chapter 15, life-span issues are discussed on the following pages:

Adolescence and
gradient of reinforcement, p. 228
invincibility fable, p. 236
optimistic bias, pp. 235–236
perceived vulnerability to risky behaviors, pp. 250–251
tobacco use, pp. 344–345

Age differences in sick-role behavior, pp. 511–512

Ageism and compliance, p. 237

Age-pain relationship, pp. 567–569

AIDS, p. 465

Asthma and childhood, pp. 100–101

Average life expectancy, pp. 22–23

Cancer and age, p. 425

Children coping with pain and medical procedures, pp. 536–537

Cigarette advertising and children, pp. 347–348

Diabetes and age, pp. 401–402

Disability-adjusted life expectancy, pp. 66–67, 224

Eating disorders, treatment of, pp. 303–308

Life course perspective, pp. 27–28

Life expectancy, calculating, pp. 222–223

Longevity and lifestyle, p. 222

Obesity-health relationship and age, p. 280

Research methods, pp. 55–59

Resilience in children, pp. 178–179

Retirement and health, p. 147

Shaping pain behavior in children, pp. 573–574

Smoking and aging, pp. 346–347

Social support and aging, p. 195

Space travel and aging, pp. 48–49

Stamina among the elderly, p. 179

Coverage of the Psychology of Women and Men

Coverage of the psychology of women and men can be found on the following pages:

AIDS and HIV transmission, pp. 465–466

Alcohol
and dating behavior, pp. 331–333
gender, and drinking contexts, pp. 337–338

Cancer, pp. 415–416, 441

Cardiovascular disease, pp. 375–378

Coping styles, pp. 172–173

Emotional reactivity, p. 170

Food behaviors and attitudes, pp. 278–279

Gender bias in medicine, pp. 29–30

Gender perspective, pp. 28–29

Gender, stress, and taste, p. 284

Hostility and anger, pp. 388–391

Job stress, p. 144

Male-pattern and female-pattern obesity, pp. 276–277

Medical compliance and gender, pp. 232–233

Pain, pp. 570–571

Reproductive system, pp. 108–111

Retirement and health, p. 147

Role overload and conflict, pp. 142–144

Sexism in health care, pp. 527–528

Sick-role behavior, pp. 512–513

Smoking-cessation programs, pp. 356–361

Social support, pp. 194–195

Stress response, pp. 149, 169–170

Substance abuse, p. 328

Type A behavior, p. 387

Use of health care services, pp. 512–513

Coverage of Women's Health

Coverage of women's health can be found on the following pages:

AIDS, pp. 468–469

Alcohol and pregnancy, p. 330

Body image and the media, pp. 299–301

Body image dissatisfaction, pp. 301–303

Breast cancer
choosing to test for the breast cancer gene, pp. 442–443
coping with, pp. 450–451
and emotional disclosure, pp. 453–454

and heredity, pp. 431–432
and Nurses Health Study, p. 429
and social support, pp. 453–454

Caregiving role and stress, p. 147

Eating disorders, pp. 295–299
treatment of, pp. 303–308

Employment and health, p. 142

Fertilization, pp. 111–112

Gender harassment, p. 147

Gestational diabetes, p. 402

HIV transmission during pregnancy, p. 476

Lung cancer, p. 426

Modifying delay behavior (mammography), pp. 446–447

Self-efficacy and high-risk sexual behaviors, pp. 481–482

Sociocultural factors in women's risk-related sexual behavior, pp. 488–489

Workplace violence against women, p. 141

Coverage of Positive Health Psychology

Coverage of positive health psychology can be found on the following pages:

Alcohol abuse prevention programs, pp. 342–343

Behavioral control, pp. 544–545

Behavioral immunogens, pp. 220–221

Cancer-fighting foods, pp. 428–429

Cancer-promoting behaviors, modification of, pp. 437–439

Daily uplifts and stress, pp. 136–137

Education programs, pp. 253–255

Emotional disclosure and health, pp. 54–55

Exercise, pp. 197–201

Explanatory style, pp. 179, 181–184

Hardiness, stress, and health, pp. 175–178

Health psychology interventions, defined, pp. 35–36

Healthy outlook on life, pp. 180–181

Heart and healthy diets, pp. 383–386

Hostility and anger, control of, pp. 399–400

Hypertension, control of, pp. 396–397

Hospitalization, increasing perceived control prior to, pp. 539–544

Nutrition, pp. 265–268

Optimism and immune system health, pp. 182–183

Optimum level of arousal, pp. 128–129

Personal control and self-efficacy, pp. 184–185

Self-efficacy beliefs in safer sex behaviors, pp. 478–479, 482–483

Reducing cholesterol, p. 397

Relaxation, pp. 201–202

Resilience and stamina, pp. 178–179

Self-regulation, pp. 186–188

Smoking inoculation programs, pp. 351–354

Social support
and physiology, pp. 192–193
and health and mortality, pp. 190–191

Stress, beneficial effects of, p. 128

Weight and health, p. 294

Work site wellness programs, pp. 251–253

The Multimedia Supplements Package

As an instructor and supplements author, I know firsthand the importance to a textbook of a good, comprehensive teaching package. Fortunately, Worth Publishers has a well-deserved reputation for producing the best psychology supplements around, for both faculty and students. The supplements package includes

Instructor's Resources and *Test Bank*

The *Instructor's Resources* feature chapter-by-chapter previews and lectures, learning objectives and chapter teaching guides, suggestions for planning and teaching health psychology, ideas for term projects, and detailed suggestions for integrating audiovisual materials into the classroom—all based on my many years of teaching health psychology. The comprehensive *Test Bank*, also based on my classroom experience and testing, contains almost 1,000 multiple-choice and short-answer essay questions. The questions include a wide variety of applied, conceptual, and factual questions.

A Full-Featured Web site (www.worthpublishers.com/straub)

The Web site offers a variety of simulations, tutorials, and study aids organized by chapter with periodic updates, including:

- *Question Mark Online Quizzing*, which features multiple-choice quizzes tied to each of the book's chapters (not from the test bank).

- *Interactive Flashcard System,* which tutors students on all chapter and text terminology and then allows them to quiz themselves on terms.
- Key modules from *PsychQuest: Interactive Exercises for Psychology* by Thomas Ludwig, Hope College. With *PsychQuest,* students explore research topics, participate in experiments and simulations, and apply psychology to real-world issues.
- *Customized PowerPoint Slides,* which were created for use in my health psychology course and refined throughout the semester. These slides focus on key terms and themes from the text and feature Power Point–designed tables, graphs, and figures.

Scientific American Video Collection in Health Psychology

This videotape on health psychology includes selections from the *Scientific American* television program, *Scientific American Frontiers,* hosted by Alan Alda. Created especially for the health psychology course, it includes more than 15 clips, which provide instructors with excellent tools to show current events and classic research in health psychology. Examples of the exciting research topics covered are obesity, pain, the efficacy of complementary and alternative medicine, gene therapy, and jet lag.

Acknowledgments

Although as the author my name is on the cover of this book, I certainly did not write the book alone. Writing a textbook is a complex task involving the collaborative efforts of a large number of very talented people. Particular thanks are due to Development Editor Betty Probert, whose vast knowledge of psychology, limitless patience, attention to detail, and editorial expertise have once again shepherded a mutual project through to completion. Betty and I have been a successful team for many years and—as with our other projects— her influence can be seen on every page of this text. Betty also edited and produced the *Instructor's Manual* and *Test Bank.*

At Worth Publishers—a company that lets nothing stand in the way of producing the finest textbooks possible—a number of people played key roles. Chief among these are Publisher Catherine Woods, whose initial interest, vision, and unflagging support gave me the push needed to start the project and sustained me throughout; Sponsoring Editor Jessica Bayne, whose passion for excellence, persistence in making sure every page was grounded in effective pedagogy, and salvific humor kept the project afloat; Managing Editor Tracey Kuehn and Production Manager Sarah Segal who worked wonders throughout production to keep us on course; Art Director Barbara Reingold and Designer Lissi Sigillo, whose creative vision resulted in the distinctive design and beautiful art program that exceeded my expectations; Media and Supplements editor Graig Donini, who coordinated the production of an unparalleled supplements package and always had an affirming word; and Deborah Goodsite and Meg Kuhta, who supervised the photo research that helped give the book its tremendous visual appeal.

Many colleagues, too, played a major role in developing this text. I am indebted to the dozens of academic reviewers who read part or all of this book, providing constructive criticism, suggestions, or just an encouraging word. Their input made this a much better book, and I hope they forgive me for the few suggestions not followed. I thank the following reviewers:

David Abwender
State University of New York, Brockport

Christopher Agnew
Purdue University

Jean Ayers
Towson University

Joy Berrenberg
University of Colorado

Marion Cohn
Ohio Dominican College

Karen J. Coleman
University of Texas, El Paso

Eliot Friedman
Williams College

Sharon Gillespie
Andrews University

Arthur Gonchar
University of La Verne

Bonnie A. Gray
Mesa College

Carol Hayes
Delta State University

Robin Kowalski
Western Carolina University

Kristi Lane
Winona State University

Leslie Martin
La Sierra University

Julie Ann McIntyre
Russell Sage College

James P. Motiff
Hope College

Virginia Norris
South Dakota State University

Amy Posey
Benedictine College

Kathleen M. Schiaffino
Fordham University

Elisabeth Sherwin
Georgia Southern University

Gabriee B. Sweidel
Kutztown University

Diane C. Tucker
University of Alabama, Birmingham

Rebecca Warner
University of New Hampshire

Eric Wiertelak
Macalaster College

David M. Young
Indiana University-Purdue University at Fort Wayne

Diane Zelman
California School of Professional Psychology, Alameda

Finally, heartfelt thanks to Pam, for her sage advice and unwavering confidence; to Jeremy, Rebecca, and Melissa, for helping me keep things in perspective; and to the many students who studied health psychology with me and assisted in the class testing of this book. They are a constant reminder of the enormous privilege and responsibilities I have as a teacher; it is for them that I have done my best to bring the field of health psychology alive in this text.

To those of you who are about to teach using this book, I sincerely hope that you will share your experiences with me. Drop me a line and let me know what works, what doesn't, and how you would do it differently. This input will be vital in determining the book's success and in shaping its future.

Richard O. Straub
University of Michigan, Dearborn
Dearborn, Michigan 48128
rostraub@umich.edu

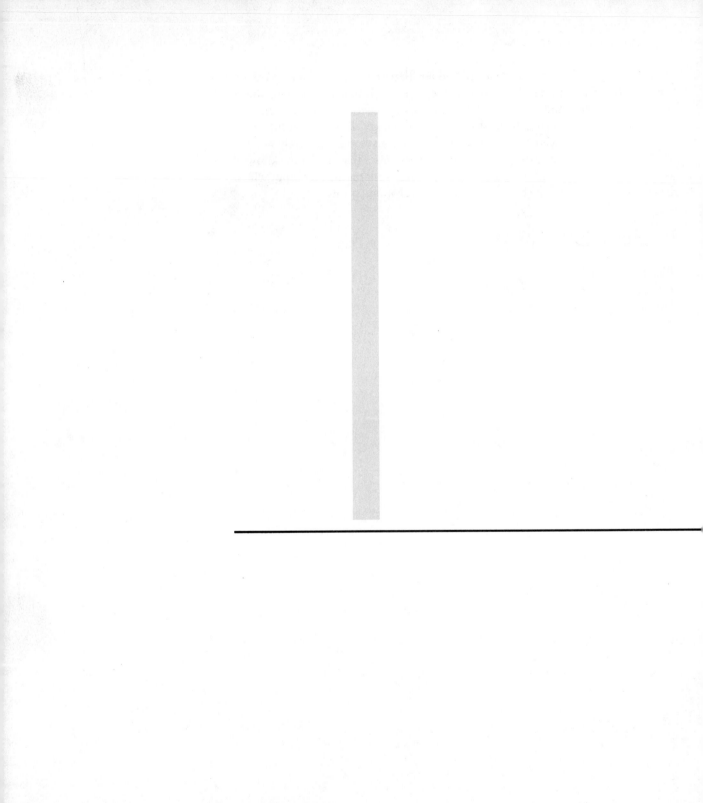

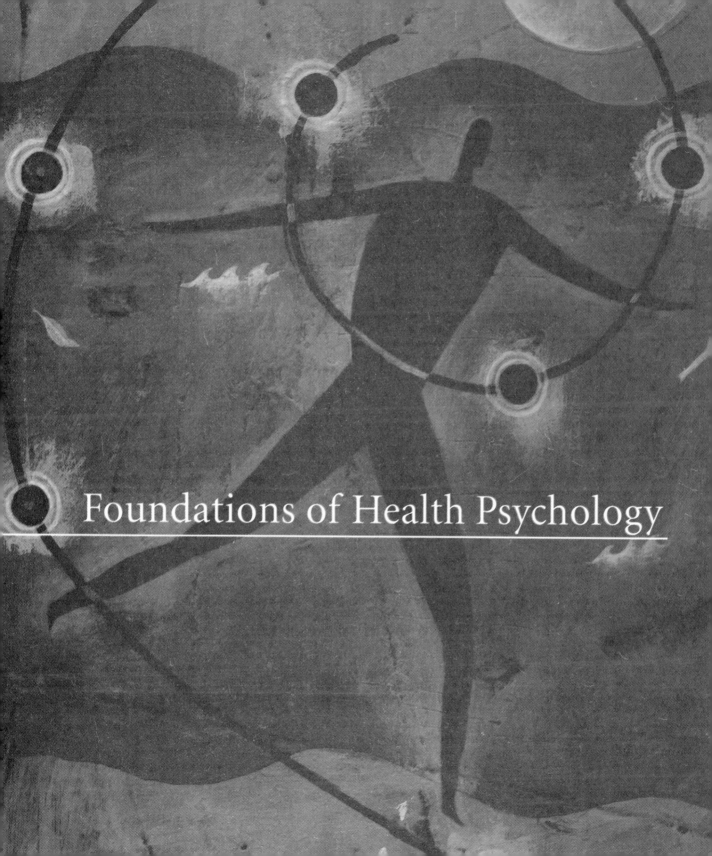

Foundations of Health Psychology

1

Introducing
Health Psychology

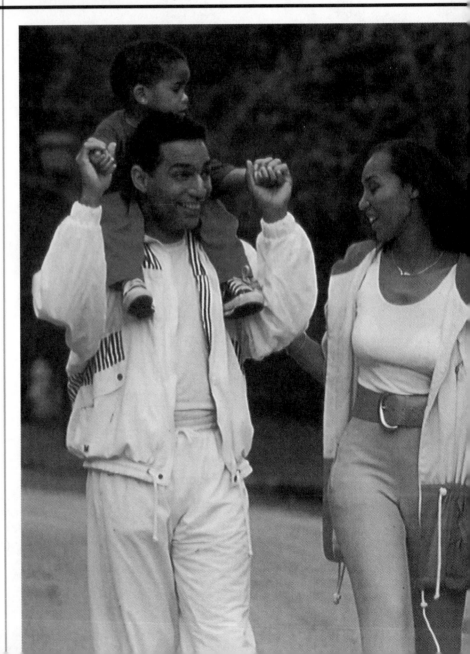

Kathleen's great-grandmother emigrated from Ireland to the United States in 1899. Hoping for a better life, she and her husband escaped the grinding poverty of their homeland and started a family. Things were better in her adopted country, but life was still hard. Doctors were expensive (and few in number), and she always had to guard against drinking impure water, eating contaminated foods, or becoming infected with typhoid fever, diphtheria, or one of the many other diseases that were prevalent in those days. Despite her vigilance, survival for herself, her husband, and her newborn baby (Kathleen's grandmother) remained uncertain. Life expectancy was less than 50 years, and one of every six babies died before his or her first birthday.

A century later, Kathleen smiles as she looks at the faded photograph of her great-grandmother, caught in a moment of laughter while playing with her daughter. She knows that her ancestor lived a long, productive life, dying at age 75 from a blood disorder that seems to run in the family. From her parents, she knows, too, that she has the same optimistic outlook and zest for life that fortified her great-grandmother against the hardships in her life. "How different things are now," Kathleen thinks, "but how much of her I still carry in me!"

Things are very different. For one thing, advances in hygiene, public health measures, and microbiology have virtually eradicated the infectious diseases Kathleen's ancestors feared most. For another, women born in the United States today enjoy a life expectancy of nearly 80 years, and men, although they have a shorter life expectancy than women, often reach the age of 72. Along with this gift of time, most people have become aware that health is much more than freedom from illness. More than ever before they are taking steps to ensure lifelong vitality by modifying their diets, exercising regularly, and remaining socially connected.

■ **health psychology** the application of psychological principles and research to the enhancement of health, and the prevention and treatment of illness

Health and Health Psychology

The story of Kathleen's family makes clear that many factors interact in determining health. This is a fundamental theme of **health psychology**, a subfield of psychology that applies psychological principles and research to the enhancement of health and the treatment and prevention of illness. Its concerns include social conditions (such as the availability of health care), biological factors (such as family longevity and inherited vulnerabilities to certain diseases), and even personality traits (such as optimism).

Like Kathleen, we are fortunate to live in a time when most of the world's citizens have the promise of a longer and better life, with far less disability and disease than ever before. However, these health benefits are not universally enjoyed. Consider:

■ The number of healthy years of life that can be expected on average equals or exceeds 70 years in 24 (mostly developed) countries of the world, but is estimated to be less than 40 years in 32 other (mostly developing) countries (World Health Organization, 2000).

■ Although average life expectancy continues to increase, white Americans consistently live 6 years longer than black Americans. Mortality rates for black infants continue to be more than twice those of white infants (Anderson, 1995).

■ Violence-, drug-, and alcohol-related deaths and injuries, and sexual hazards such as HIV, increasingly mark the transition from adolescence to adulthood, particularly among many ethnic minorities (Yee et al., 1995).

■ At every age, death rates vary by ethnic group. For instance, among American men and women aged 45–54, death rates are highest among non-Hispanic African-Americans (12 per thousand), followed by Native Americans (6.1 per thousand), non-Hispanic European Americans (5.0), Hispanic-Americans (4.9), and Asian- and Pacific Islander Americans (2.6) (National Center for Health Statistics, 1999).

■ During a seven-and-a-half-year study of 3,617 adults aged 25 and older, men who lived in urban areas were 62 percent more likely to die than men who lived in suburbs, small towns, or rural areas (House et al., 2000).

■ Although men are twice as likely as women to die of any cause, beginning in middle age women have higher disease and disability rates (National Center for Health Statistics, 1999).

■ Recent immigrants to the United States generally are healthier than longtime residents of the same ethnicity and age (Abraido-Lanza, Dohrenwend, Ng-Mak, & Turner, 1999).

- The United States spends a higher portion of its gross domestic product on health care than any other country but ranks only thirty-seventh out of 191 countries in terms of the overall performance of its health care system, as measured by its responsiveness, fairness of funding, accessibility by all individuals, and so forth (World Health Organization, 2000).

- More than 15 million adults worldwide between the ages of 20 and 64 die each year. Most of these deaths are premature and preventable (National Center for Health Statistics, 1999).

These statistics reveal some of the challenges to the quest for global wellness. These challenges include reducing the 30-year discrepancy in life expectancy between developed and developing countries; helping adolescents make a safe, healthy transition to adulthood; and achieving a deeper understanding of the relationships among gender, ethnicity, sociocultural status, and health.

This chapter introduces the relatively new field of health psychology, which will play a major role in meeting the world's health challenges in the new century and beyond. Consider a few of the questions that health psychologists seek to answer:

- How does your ability to relate well to others influence your health?

- How do your attitudes, beliefs, self-confidence, and overall personality affect your health?

- Do acupuncture, homeopathy, herbalism, and other forms of alternative medicine really work?

- To what extent are specific features of your environment, including architecture, noise level, and presence of sunlight, associated with your health?

- Can disease be caused by personal habits?

- What are the barriers to adopting a healthy lifestyle?

- Why are certain health problems more likely to occur among people of a particular age, gender, or ethnic group?

- What aspects of the typical adolescent lifestyle enhance or compromise health?

- Why is being poor a potentially serious threat to your health?

Health psychology is the science that seeks to answer these and many other questions about how your wellness is affected by how you think, feel, and act. We begin our exploration of this exciting field by taking a closer look at the concept of health and how it has changed over the course of history. Next, we'll examine the history and scope of health psychology, including how it draws on and supports other health-related fields. Finally, we'll take a look at

> The health of women is inextricably linked to their status in society. It benefits from equality, and suffers from discrimination.
> —World Health Organization, 2000

■ **health** a state of complete physical, mental, and social well-being

the kind of training needed to become a health psychologist and what you can do once you have obtained that training.

What Is Health?

The word *health* comes to us from an old German word that is represented, in English, by the words *hale* and *whole,* both of which refer to a state of "soundness of body." Linguists note that these words derive from the medieval battlefield, where loss of *haleness,* or health, was usually the result of grave bodily injury.

Today, we are more likely to think of health as the absence of disease rather than as the absence of a debilitating battlefield injury. Because this definition focuses only on the absence of a negative state, however, it is incomplete. Although it is true that healthy people are free of disease, most of us would agree that health involves much more. It is quite possible, even common, for a person to be free of disease but still not enjoy a vigorous, satisfying life. Health is not limited to our physical well-being.

The Three Domains of Health

Recognizing the inadequacy of the earlier limited definition of health, the United Nations established the World Health Organization (WHO). In its 1946 charter, the WHO defined **health** as "a state of complete physical, mental, and social well-being, and not merely the absence of disease or infirmity." This definition affirms that health is a positive, *multidimensional* state that involves three domains: *physical health, psychological health,* and *social health.*

Physical health, of course, involves having a sound, disease-free body with good cardiovascular performance, sharp senses, a vital immune system, and the ability to withstand physical injury. It also includes lifestyle habits that enhance physical health. Among these are eating a nutritious diet, exercising regularly, and sleeping well; avoiding use of tobacco and other drugs; practicing safe sex; and minimizing exposure to toxic chemicals.

Psychological health is being able to think clearly, having good self-esteem, and enjoying a general feeling of well-being. It includes creativity, problem-solving skills (such as seeking information on health-related issues), and emotional stability. It is also characterized by self-acceptance, openness to new ideas, and a general "hardiness" of personality.

Social health includes having good interpersonal skills, meaningful relationships with friends and family, and social support in times of crisis. It also relates to sociocultural factors in health, such as socioeconomic status, education, ethnicity, culture, and gender.

Each domain of health is, of course, influenced by the other two domains. For example, an emotionally stable person who has good problem-solving skills (psychological health) will probably have an easier time maintaining healthy social relationships (social health) than a depressed person who has trouble concentrating on the problem at hand. Conversely, poor physical health poses special challenges, both to a person's self-esteem (psychological health) and to relationships with his or her family and friends (social health).

Reality Check   *How's Your Health?*

As you'll learn in Chapter 2, health psychologists use a variety of methods to conduct research and guide their clinical interventions. These methods include laboratory experiments, field studies, and surveys such as this one. An applied health psychologist might use this type of questionnaire to gather background information for planning an intervention to help a person struggling with stress-related hypertension. For instance, the person's responses might reveal room for improvement in his or her physical health, perhaps through nutritional counseling or advice on starting an exercise program. As another example, a person who reports having difficulty managing stress may benefit from a cognitive intervention aimed at correcting his or her tendency to overreact to everyday hassles. Questionnaires such as this one are, of course, only starting points for research and clinical interventions. Once a potential area of health improvement has been identified, much more detailed and specific information must be gathered.

LIFESTYLE AND HABITS QUESTIONNAIRE

You can use this questionnaire to broadly examine your lifestyle and habits with respect to each of the dimensions of health and related health concerns, such as exercise and fitness and accident prevention. Read each of the following items. Write the number that best corresponds to your honest response. Add up your scores for each category. Then use the guidelines that follow to interpret your scores.

Rarely or Never	Sometimes	Usually	Always
1	2	3	4

Physical Health

— 1. I take care of my health.

— 2. I try to keep my body healthy and fit.

— 3. I am screened regularly for the health problems that are likely to affect people with my family history.

— 4. I am free of chronic or disabling diseases.

— 5. I feel I am basically in good health.

— 6. I am not bothered by allergies.

— 7. I do not lose much time at work or school because of illness.

— 8. I get at least 7 to 8 hours of sleep at night and wake up feeling rested and refreshed.

Physical health score _____

Exercise and Physical Fitness

— 1. I participate in moderately intense physical activity, like walking briskly or working around the house, for at least 30 minutes a day.

— 2. I participate in vigorous exercise like running, lap swimming, speed walking, or aerobics dance classes for at least 20 to 30 minutes a day at least three times a week.

— 3. I lead an active life.

— 4. I am about as physically fit as most people my age.

— 5. I spend much of leisure time involved in active sports or physical activities like bicycling, hiking, swimming, gardening, or playing competitive sports.

— 6. I have good physical endurance.

— 7. I participate in muscle-strengthening exercises at least several times a week.

___ 8. I have enough energy to get through the day without feeling fatigued.

Exercise and fitness score _____

Alcohol, Tobacco, and Other Drug Use

___ 1. I avoid smoking cigarettes

___ 2. I avoid all other tobacco use, including pipe smoking, cigar smoking, and smokeless tobacco.

___ 3. I avoid drinking beer or wine, or if I do, I avoid drinking more than 1 or 2 drinks a day.

___ 4. I avoid drinking in situations in which it would be unsafe to drink.

___ 5. I avoid binge drinking (drinking five or more drinks in a sitting).

___ 6. I avoid use of illicit drugs.

___ 7. I avoid socializing with people who use illicit drugs or drink to excess.

___ 8. I avoid using alcohol or other drugs to cope with problems or to make me feel more socially confident.

Alcohol, tobacco, and other drug use score _____

Preventive Health Practices

___ 1. I regularly visit my doctor for routine checkups.

___ 2. I have my blood pressure and blood cholesterol checked regularly.

___ 3. I practice monthly testicular/breast self-exams.

___ 4. If I engage in sexual intimacy, I practice safe sex.

___ 5. I avoid excessive exposure to the sun.

___ 6. I use sunscreen whenever I am out in the sun for more than a few minutes.

___ 7. I wash my hands after using the bathroom.

___ 8. I keep my vaccinations up to date.

Preventive health practices score _____

Accident Prevention

___ 1. I have a working smoke detector in my home.

___ 2. I have a working carbon monoxide detector in my home.

___ 3. I keep household chemicals safely stored.

___ 4. I wear seatbelts whenever I drive or ride in a car.

___ 5. I make sure that children are securely buckled in a car safety seat or seatbelt when riding in a car.

___ 6. I obey traffic rules when driving.

___ 7. I wear safety helmets and other recommended safety equipment when bicycling or rollerblading.

___ 8. I read and follow instructions for proper use of household cleansers, solvents, pesticides, and electrical devices.

Accident prevention score _____

Nutrition and Weight Control

___ 1. I limit my intake of fat, including saturated fat.

___ 2. I limit my intake of high-cholesterol foods such as eggs, liver, and meat.

___ 3. I follow a nutritionally balanced diet.

___ 4. I eat five or more servings of fruits and vegetables daily.

___ 5. I limit the amount of salt and sugar I consume.

___ 6. I eat food that is broiled or steamed, not fried or sautéed.

___ 7. I eat high-fiber foods several times a day.

___ 8. I am careful to keep my weight within a healthy range.

Nutrition and weight control score _____

Psychological Health

___ 1. I am able to concentrate on my work at school or on the job.

___ 2. I have a clear direction in life.

___ 3. I generally like myself.

___ 4. I am able to relax and unwind.

___ 5. I am hopeful about the future.

___ 6. I enjoy a challenge.

___ 7. I am able to express my feelings.

___ 8. I am able to manage the stress in my life.

Psychological health score _____

Spiritual Health

___ 1. I find meaning in life.

___ 2. I have a sense of connectedness to something larger than myself, whether it be organized religion, nature, or social causes.

___ 3. I believe every life has a purpose.

___ 4. I enjoy the arts—painting and sculpture, dance, music, or books.

___ 5. I believe that I have a worthwhile place in my community.

___ 6. I try to help people in need without expecting anything in return.

___ 7. I try to do things that will be of lasting value.

___ 8. I feel a need to make a difference in people's lives.

Spiritual health score ___

Social Health

___ 1. I have close friends.

___ 2. I am able to develop trusting relationships with others.

___ 3. I can express feelings of liking and love to other people as well as feelings of disappointment and anger.

___ 4. When there is a problem I can't handle on my own, I usually have or find someone to talk to about it.

___ 5. I have good relationships with family members.

___ 6. I am the kind of person who is there for people when I am needed.

___ 7. I am able to assert myself in a responsible way and not allow others to take advantage of me.

___ 8. I am respectful of the feelings of others.

Social health score ___

Environmental Health

___ 1. I keep informed about environmental issues such as the depletion of the ozone layer, the destruction of the rain forests, and acid rain.

___ 2. I recycle paper, bottles, and aluminum cans.

___ 3. I am aware of the safety and quality of the water I use.

___ 4. I participate in or contribute to environmental causes.

___ 5. I make sure any refuse I produce is properly disposed of.

___ 6. I avoid use of pesticide sprays in the house or yard, or if I do use them, I am careful to follow all safety instructions.

___ 7. I wash all fruits and vegetables before eating them.

___ 8. I make an effort to conserve water use and electricity.

Environmental health score ___

Interpreting Your Score

24 to 32—Congratulations! You appear to have adopted a healthy lifestyle with a minimum of health-compromising behaviors. Still, there may be room for improvement. What else can you do to optimize your health?

16 to 23—Although you clearly have established some healthy habits, you have a great deal of room for improvement. Examine responses that are less than "always," especially those that are "sometimes" or "rarely or never." Consider ways of changing your health behavior to improve your score.

Below 16—Based on these lifestyle factors, you appear to engage in far too many health-compromising behaviors. These behaviors could increase your risk of illness or accidents. What steps can you take to improve your score?

Source: Nevid, J. S., Rathus, S. A., & Rubenstein, H. R. (1998). *Health in the new millennium* (pp. 10–12). New York: Worth Publishers.

Health and Illness: Lessons from the Past

Although all human civilizations have been affected by disease, each has understood and treated it differently. At one time, our ancestors thought that disease was caused by demons. At another, they saw it as a form of punishment for moral weakness. Today, we wrestle with questions such as "Can disease be caused by an unhealthy personality?" Let us take a look at how views regarding health and illness have changed over the course of history. (You may want to refer to Figure 1.1 throughout the following discussion to get a sense of the chronology of changing views toward health and illness.)

Figure 1.1

A Timeline of Historical and Cultural Variations in Illness and Healing
From the ancient use of trephination to remove evil spirits to the current use of non-invasive brain scans to diagnose disease, the treatment of health problems has seen major advances over the centuries. A collection of treatments across the ages are shown below (from left to right): trephination (on an ancient Peruvian skull); acupuncture from China; early surgery in seventeenth century Europe; vaccination by the district vaccinator in nineteenth century London; and a CT (computed tomography) scan to observe brain activity in the twenty-first century.

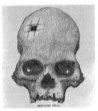

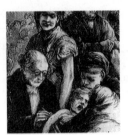

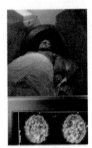

ANCIENT GREECE Illness caused by an imbalance of bodily humors; good diet and moderation in living would cure it.

PREHISTORIC PERIOD Illness caused by evil spirits and treated by trephination.

MIDDLE AGES (476–1450) Disease was divine punishment for sins, cured by miraculous intervention, invoking of saints, as well as bloodletting.

1800s Disease caused by microscopic organisms. Treatment was surgery and immunization.

TWENTY-FIRST CENTURY Biopsychosocial causes of disease. Modern flexible methods of treatment.

B.C. 10,000 · 5000 · 2000 · 1000 · A.D. 200 · 500 · 1000 · 1100 · 1400 · 1500 · 1600 · 1700 · 1800 · 1900 · 1960 · 1980 · 2000

ANCIENT EGYPT Demons and punishment by the gods caused illness. Sorcery and primitive forms of surgery and hygiene were treatments.

ANCIENT ROME (200 B.C.) "Pathogens" such as bad air and body humors caused illness. Treated by bloodletting, enemas, and baths.

1920s Disease influenced by mind and emotions and treated by psychoanalysis.

ANCIENT CHINA (1100–200 B.C.) Unbalanced forces of nature caused illness. Treated with herbal medicine and acupuncture.

RENAISSANCE Disease was a physical condition of the body, which was separate from the mind. Surgical techniques first used.

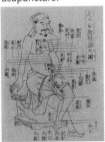

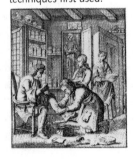

Credits (left to right): Trephinated skull engraving by English School (nineteenth century) published 1878 in "Incidents of Travel and Exploration in the Land of the Incas" by E. George Squier: private collection/Bridgeman Art Library; Illustration showing acupuncture: © Corbis; "The Surgeon," engraving by German School (seventeenth century): private collection/Bridgeman Art Library; "Vaccination" engraving, 1871: Hulton Getty/Liaison Agency; CT scan: © Premium Stock/Corbis.

Ancient Views

Prehistoric Medicine

Our ancestors' efforts at healing can be traced back 20,000 years. A cave painting in southern France, for example, which is believed to be 17,000 years old, depicts an Ice Age shaman wearing the animal mask of an ancient witch doctor. In religions based on a belief in good and evil spirits, only a shaman (priest or medicine man) can influence these spirits.

For preindustrial men and women, confronted with the often-hostile forces of their environment, survival was based on constant vigilance against these mysterious forces of evil. When a person became sick, there was no obvious physical reason for it: Rather, the stricken individual's condition was misattributed to weakness in the face of a stronger force, bewitchment, or possession by an evil spirit (Amundsen, 1996).

Treatment was harsh and consisted of rituals of sorcery, exorcism, and even a primitive form of surgery called *trephination*. Archaeologists have unearthed prehistoric human skulls containing irregularly shaped holes that were apparently drilled by early healers to allow disease-causing demons to leave patients' bodies. Trephination was practiced on both the living and the dead, suggesting that it played as important a role in cultural or religious ceremonies as it did in health care. Historical records indicate that trephination was a widely practiced form of treatment in Europe, Egypt, India, and Central and South America.

About 4000 years ago, some peoples realized that hygiene also played a role in health and disease, and they made attempts at improving public hygiene. The ancient Egyptians, for example, engaged in cleansing rites intended to discourage illness-causing worms from infesting the body. In Mesopotamia (a part of what is now Iraq), soap was manufactured, bathing facilities designed, and public sewage treatment systems constructed (Stone, Cohen, & Adler, 1979).

Greek and Roman Medicine

The most dramatic advances in public health and sanitation were made in Greece and Rome during the sixth and fifth centuries B.C. In Rome, a great drainage system, the *Cloaca Maxima,* was built to drain a swamp that later became the site of the Roman Forum. Over time, the *Cloaca* assumed the function of a modern sewage system. Public bathrooms, for which there was a small admission charge, were commonplace in Rome by the first century A.D. (Cartwright, 1972).

The first aqueduct brought pure water into Rome as early as 312 B.C., and cleaning of public roads was supervised by the *aediles,* a group of appointed officials who also controlled the food supply. The *aediles* passed regulations to ensure the freshness of meat and other perishable foods, and they arranged for the storage of vast quantities of grain, for example, in an effort to forestall famine (Cartwright, 1972).

■ **humoral theory** a concept of health proposed by Hippocrates that considered wellness a state of perfect equilibrium among four basic body fluids, called humors. Sickness was believed to be the result of disturbances in the balance of humors

In Greece, the Greek philosopher Hippocrates (c. 460–c. 377 B.C.) was establishing the roots of Western medicine when he rebelled against the ancient focus on mysticism and superstition. Hippocrates, who is often called the "father of modern medicine," was the first to argue that disease is a natural phenomenon and that the causes of disease (and therefore their treatment and prevention) are knowable and worthy of serious study. In this way, he built the earliest foundation for a scientific approach to healing.

Hippocrates proposed the first rational explanation of why people get sick. According to his **humoral theory,** a healthy body and mind resulted from equilibrium among four bodily fluids called humors: blood, yellow bile, black bile, and phlegm. To maintain a proper balance, a person had to follow a healthy lifestyle that included exercise, sufficient rest, a good diet, and the avoidance of excesses. When the humors were out of balance, however, both body and mind were affected in predictable ways, depending on which of the four humors was in excess. An excess of blood, for example, contributed to a *sanguine* (optimistic and cheerful) personality. Although a cheerful personality would seem desirable, Hippocrates believed otherwise: Too much blood, he said, increased the person's susceptibility to epilepsy, angina, dysentery, and arthritis. Treatment for excessive blood consisted of bloodletting (the opening of a vein to remove blood), cooling baths, and enemas. A *phlegmatic* person, who had an excess of phlegm, was listless, dull, and sluggish. Headaches, colds, and strokes were believed to be the result. Treatment consisted of hot baths, diuretics, and nausea-inducing herbs. The *choleric* person, who had an excess of yellow bile and a fiery temperament, was apt to require treatment for mouth ulcers, jaundice, and stomach ailments. Relief was found through bloodletting, liquid diets, enemas, and cooling baths. A *melancholic* person had too much black bile; a sad, brooding disposition (hence the term *melancholy*) was the likely result. Such a condition was also expected to contribute to ulcers and hepatitis that could be treated with a special diet, hot baths, emetics (drugs that induce vomiting), and the searing of body tissue with a hot iron (cautery).

Although humoral theory was discarded as advances were made in anatomy, physiology, and microbiology, the notion of personality traits being linked with body fluids still persists in the folk and alternative medicines of many cultures, including those of traditional Oriental and Native American medicine. Moreover, as we'll see in the next chapter, we now know that many diseases involve an imbalance (of sorts) among the brain's neurotransmitters, so Hippocrates was not too far off.

Hippocrates made many other notable contributions to a scientific approach to medicine. For example, to learn what personal habits contributed to gout, a disease caused by disturbances in the body's metabolism of uric acid, he conducted one of the earliest public health surveys of its sufferers' habits, as well as of their temperatures, heart rates, respiration, and other physical symptoms. He also pointed out the importance of each patient's emotions and thoughts regarding his or her health and treatment, and thus called attention to the psychological aspects of health and illness.

The next great figure in the history of Western medicine was the physician Claudius Galen (A.D c. 129–c. 200). A Greek by birth, Galen spent many years in Rome conducting dissection studies of animals and treating the severe injuries of Roman gladiators, from which he learned much that was previously unknown about health and disease. Galen wrote voluminously on anatomy, hygiene, and diet, building on the Hippocratic foundation of rational explanation and the careful description of each patient's physical symptoms.

Galen also expanded the humoral theory of disease by developing an elaborate system of pharmacology that physicians followed for almost fifteen hundred years. His system was based on the notion that each of the four bodily humors had its own elementary quality that determined the character of specific diseases. Blood, for example, was hot and moist. Galen believed that drugs, too, had elementary qualities; thus, a disease caused by an excess of a hot and moist humor could be cured only with drugs that were cold and dry. Although such views may seem archaic, Galen's pharmacology was logical, based on careful observation, and similar to the ancient systems of medicine that developed in China, India, and other non-Western cultures. Many forms of alternative medicine still use similar ideas today.

Non-Western Medicine

At the same time that Western medicine was emerging, traditions of healing were developing in other cultures as well. For example, more than 2000 years ago, the Chinese developed an integrated system of healing, which we know today as *traditional Oriental medicine (TOM)*. TOM is founded on the principle that internal harmony is essential for good health. Fundamental to this harmony is the concept of *qi* (sometimes spelled *chi*), a vital energy or life force that ebbs and flows with changes in each person's mental, physical, and emotional well-being. Acupuncture, herbal therapy, meditation, and other interventions supposedly restore health by correcting blockages and imbalances in *qi*.

Ayurveda is the oldest known medical system in the world, having originated in India around the sixth century B.C., coinciding roughly with the lifetime of the Buddha. The word *ayurveda* comes from the Sanskrit roots *ayuh*, which means longevity, and *veda*, meaning knowledge. Widely practiced in India, ayurveda is based on the belief that the human body represents the entire universe in a microcosm and that the key to health is maintaining a balance between the microcosmic body and the macrocosmic world. The key to this relationship is held in the balance of three bodily humors, or *doshas: vata, pitta,* and *kapha,* or, collectively, the *tridosha* (Fugh-Berman, 1997). We'll explore the history, traditions, and effectiveness of these and other non-Western forms of medicine in Chapter 14.

The Middle Ages and the Renaissance

The Middle Ages began with an outbreak of plague that originated in Egypt in A.D. 540 and quickly spread throughout the Roman Empire, killing as many as 10,000 people a day. So great in number were the corpses that gravediggers could not keep up. The solution was to load ships with the dead, row them out to sea, and abandon them.

The fall of the Roman Empire in the fifth century A.D. ushered in the Middle Ages (476–c. 1450), an era between ancient and modern times characterized by a return to supernatural explanations of health and disease. In a time when the church exerted a powerful influence over all areas of life, religious interpretations colored medieval scientists' ideas about health and disease. In the eyes of the medieval Christian Church, humans were regarded as creatures with free will who were not subject to the laws of nature. Because they had souls, both humans and animals were not considered to be appropriate objects of scientific scrutiny, and dissection of both was strictly prohibited. Illness was viewed as God's punishment for evildoing, and **epidemic** diseases, such as the two great outbursts of *plague* (a bacterial disease carried by rats and other rodents) that occurred during the Middle Ages, were believed to be a sign of God's wrath. The Church came to control the practice of medicine, and "treatment" frequently involved attempts to force evil spirits out of the bodies of sick people.

Although the loyal followers of Hippocrates and Galen continued to promote the scientific approach, most medieval physicians emphasized sorcery, demonology, and other mystical forms of treatment. And so there were few scientific advances in European medicine for the next fifteen hundred years.

In the late fifteenth century, a new age—the Renaissance—was born. Beginning with the reemergence of scientific inquiry, this period saw the revitalization of anatomical study and medical practice. The taboo on human dissection was lifted sufficiently that the Flemish anatomist and artist Andreas Vesalius (1514–1564) was able to publish a seven-volume study of the internal organs, musculature, and skeletal system of the human body. The son of a druggist, Vesalius was fascinated by nature, especially the anatomy of humans and animals. In the pursuit of knowledge, no stray dog, cat, or mouse was safe from his scalpel.

In medical school, Vesalius turned his dissection scalpel on human cadavers. What he found proved some of the medical writings of Galen and earlier physicians to be clearly inaccurate. How, he wondered, could an unquestionable authority such as Galen have made so many errors in describing the body? Then he realized why: Galen had never dissected a human body. Vesalius then realized that his purpose in life was to write the authoritative study of human anatomy. These volumes became the cornerstones of a new scientific medicine based on anatomy (Sigerist, 1958, 1971).

One of the most influential Renaissance thinkers was the French philosopher and mathematician René Descartes

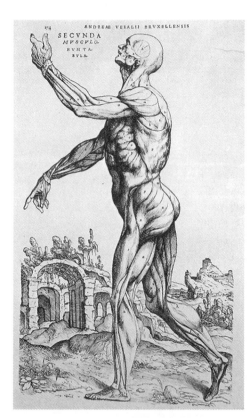

First Anatomical Drawings
By the sixteenth century, the taboo on human dissection had been lifted long enough that the Flemish anatomist and artist Andreas Vesalius (1514–1564) was able to publish a complete study of the internal organs, musculature, and skeletal system of the human body.
Musculature of a man by Andreas Vesalius, 1543. Fratelli Fabbri, Milan, Italy/Bridgeman Art Library.

(1596–1650), whose first innovation was the concept of the human body as a machine. He described all the basic reflexes of the body, in the process constructing elaborate mechanical models to demonstrate his principles. He believed that disease occurred when the machine broke down; the physician's task was to repair the machine.

Descartes is best known for his beliefs that the mind and body are separate and autonomous processes that interact minimally, and that each is subject to different laws of causality. This viewpoint, which is called **mind–body dualism** (or *Cartesian dualism*), is based on the doctrine that humans have two natures, mental and physical. Descartes and other great thinkers of the Renaissance, in an effort to break with the mysticism and superstitions of the past, vigorously rejected the notion that the mind influences the body. The (unscientific) study of the mind was relegated to religion and philosophy, while the (scientific) study of the body was reserved for medicine. This viewpoint ushered in a new age of medical research based on confidence in science and rational thinking.

Post-Renaissance Rationality

Following the Renaissance, physicians were expected to focus exclusively on the biological causes of disease. One hundred years after Vesalius, the Italian physician Giovanni Morgagni (1682–1771) published the first textbook of medical anatomy. Based on his findings from hundreds of human autopsies, Morgagni advanced the idea that the causes of many diseases reside in problems in the internal organs and in the muscular and skeletal systems of the body. At long last, Hippocrates' ancient humoral theory could be discarded in favor of this new **anatomical theory** of disease.

Science and medicine changed rapidly during the seventeenth and eighteenth centuries, spurred on by numerous advances in technology. Although Galileo had constructed an early thermometer in 1592, it had no scale of measurement and provided only crude indications of temperature variation. An important step forward in the science of measurement occurred in 1665 when Christian Huygens (1629–1695) proposed a fixed scale in which the freezing and boiling points of water were designated as "0" and "100," respectively—the origin of the centigrade system. By the end of the seventeenth century, *thermometry* (the measurement of temperature) was in widespread clinical use.

Perhaps the single most important invention in medicine during this period was the microscope. Although the use of a ground lens for magnification had been known in ancient times, it was a Dutch cloth merchant named Anton van Leeuwenhoek (1632–1723) who fashioned the first practical microscope. With a magnification power of 270 times, Leeuwenhoek's microscope was unsurpassed until the nineteenth century (Lyons & Petrucelli, 1978). Using his microscope, Leeuwenhoek was the first to observe blood cells and the structure of skeletal muscles. The English scientist Robert Hooke (1635–1703),

- **epidemic** literally, *among the people;* an epidemic disease that spreads rapidly among many individuals in a community at the same time. A *pandemic* disease affects people over a large geographical area

- **mind–body dualism** the philosophical viewpoint that mind and body are separate entities that do not interact

- **anatomical theory** the theory that the origins of specific diseases are found in the internal organs, musculature, and skeletal system of the human body

cellular theory formulated in the nineteenth century, the theory that disease is the result of abnormalities in body cells

germ theory the theory that disease is caused by viruses, bacteria, and other microorganisms that invade body cells

Leeuwenhoek's contemporary, constructed his own microscope and observed that plant tissues contain many small cavities separated by walls. Hooke named these cavities "cells," or "little rooms," and his observations became the basis of the nineteenth-century theory that the cell was the basic unit of all living organisms.

Discoveries of the Nineteenth Century

Once individual cells became visible, the stage was set for Rudolf Virchow (1821–1902) to outline the **cellular theory** of disease—the idea that disease results when body cells malfunction or die.

As is often the case in science, practical problems lead to an even deeper understanding of disease. In an elegant series of experiments, the French scientist Louis Pasteur (1822–1895) isolated the bacterium responsible for the spotted silk worm disease that threatened the French silk industry. And after proving that a microorganism caused rabies, he developed the first effective rabies vaccine. But Pasteur's most important contribution to medicine came in 1862, when he rocked the medical world with a series of meticulous experiments showing that life can only come from existing life. Until the nineteenth century, scholars believed in *spontaneous generation*—the idea that living organisms can be formed from nonliving matter. For example, maggots and flies were believed to emerge automatically from rotting meat. To test his hypothesis that life cannot be formed from nonlife, Pasteur filled two flasks with a porridge-like liquid, heating both to the boiling point to kill any microorganisms. One of the flasks had a wide mouth into which air could flow easily. The other flask was also open to air, but had a long curved neck that kept any airborne microbes from falling into the liquid. To the amazement of skeptics, no new growth appeared in the curved flasks. However, in the flasks with the ordinary necks, microorganisms contaminated the liquid and multiplied rapidly. By showing that a genuinely sterile solution remains lifeless, Pasteur set the stage for the later development of *aseptic (germ-free) surgical* procedures. Even more important, Pasteur's successful challenge of a 2000-year-old belief is a powerful demonstration of the importance of keeping an open mind in scientific inquiry.

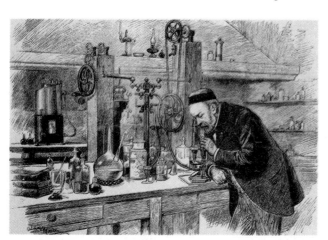

Louis Pasteur in His Laboratory
Pasteur's meticulous work in isolating bacteria in the laboratory, then showing that life can come only from existing life, paved the way for germ-free surgical procedures. © Bettmann/CORBIS

Pasteur's discoveries also helped shape the **germ theory** of disease—the theory that bacteria, viruses, and other microorganisms that invade body cells cause them to malfunction. The germ theory, which is basically a refinement of the cellular theory, forms the theoretical foundation of modern medicine.

Following Pasteur, medical knowledge and procedures developed rapidly. In 1846, William Morton (1819–1868), an American dentist, introduced the gas ether as an anesthetic. This great advance made it possible to operate on patients who experienced no pain and remained completely relaxed. Fifty years later, the German physicist Wilhelm Roentgen (1845–1943) discovered x-rays and for the first time, physicians were able to observe internal organs directly. Before the end of the century, researchers had identified the microorganisms that caused a variety of diseases, including malaria, pneumonia, diphtheria, leprosy, syphilis, bubonic plague, and typhoid. Armed with this information, medicine began to bring under control diseases that had plagued the world since antiquity.

The Twentieth Century and the Dawn of a New Era

As the field of medicine continued to advance during the early part of the twentieth century, it looked more and more to physiology and anatomy, rather than to the study of thoughts and emotions, in its search for a deeper understanding of health and illness. Thus was born the **biomedical model** of health, which maintains that illness always has a biological cause. Under the impetus of the *germ* and *cellular theories* of disease, this model first became widely accepted during the nineteenth century and continues to represent the dominant view in medicine today.

The biomedical model has three distinguishing features. First, it assumes that disease is the result of a **pathogen**—a virus, bacterium, or some other microorganism that invades the body. The model makes no provision for psychological, social, or behavioral variables in illness. In this sense the biomedical model embraces *reductionism,* the view that complex phenomena (such as health and disease) derive ultimately from a single primary factor. Second, the biomedical model is based on the Cartesian doctrine of *mind–body dualism* that, as we have seen, considers mind and body as separate and autonomous entities that do not interact. Finally, according to the biomedical model, health is nothing more than the absence of disease. Accordingly, those who work from this perspective focus on investigating the causes of physical illnesses rather than on those factors that promote physical, psychological, and social vitality.

Psychosomatic Medicine

The biomedical model advanced health care significantly through its focus on pathogens. However, it was unable to explain disorders that had no observable physical cause such as those uncovered by Sigmund Freud (1856–1939), who was initially trained as a physician. Freud's patients exhibited symptoms such as loss of speech, deafness, and even paralysis. One particularly intriguing case involved a patient who reported the complete loss of feeling in her right hand. Freud believed this malady, which he called "glove anesthesia," was caused by

■ **biomedical model** the dominant view of twentieth-century medicine that maintains that illness always has a physical cause

■ **pathogen** a virus, bacterium, or some other microorganism that causes a particular disease

psychosomatic medicine an outdated branch of medicine that focused on the diagnosis and treatment of physical diseases caused by faulty psychological processes

case study one of the oldest methods of observation, in which one person is studied in depth in the hope of uncovering universal principles

behavioral medicine an interdisciplinary field that integrates behavioral and biomedical science in promoting health and treating disease

unconscious emotional conflicts that had been "converted" into a physical form. Freud labeled such illnesses *conversion disorders,* and the medical community was forced to accept a new category of disease. A prolific writer, Freud's case histories of his patients' bizarre symptoms helped make *psychoanalysis* a dominant force during the first part of the twentieth century.

The idea that specific diseases could be caused by an individual's psychological conflicts was further advanced during the 1940s by the work of psychoanalyst Franz Alexander. When physicians could find no infectious agent or other direct cause for rheumatoid arthritis, Alexander became intrigued by the possibility that psychological factors might be involved. According to his *nuclear conflict* model, the presence of specific unconscious conflicts may lead to the presence of specific physical complaints (Alexander, 1950). That is, each physical disease is the outcome of a fundamental, or nuclear, psychological conflict. For example, individuals with a "rheumatoid personality," who tended to repress anger and were unable to express emotion, were believed to be prone to developing arthritis. By carefully describing a large number of physical disorders that were presumably caused by psychological conflicts, Alexander helped establish **psychosomatic medicine,** a reformist movement within medicine named from the root words *psyche,* which means mind, and *soma,* which means body. By definition, psychosomatic medicine is concerned with the diagnosis and treatment of physical diseases thought to be caused by faulty processes within the mind. The new field flourished, and soon the journal *Psychosomatic Medicine* was publishing psychoanalytic explanations of a range of health problems that included hypertension, migraine headaches, ulcers, hyperthyroidism, and bronchial asthma.

Psychosomatic medicine was intriguing and seemed to explain the unexplainable. However, it had several weaknesses that ultimately caused it to fall out of favor. Most significant was the fact that psychosomatic medicine was grounded in Freudian theory. As Freud's emphasis on unconscious, irrational urges in personality formation lost popularity, the field of psychosomatic medicine faltered. Second, psychosomatic medicine was questioned for the seemingly arbitrary categorization of some diseases as completely physical in nature, and others as psychological in nature. A third criticism of psychosomatic medicine was methodological; that is, the research was based primarily on **case studies** of individual patients, among the oldest but least reliable methods (see Chapter 2). Any individual case may be atypical and therefore misleading as the basis for a general theory. A final criticism is that psychosomatic medicine, like the biomedical model, was based on reductionism—in this case, the outmoded idea that a single psychological problem or personality flaw is sufficient to trigger disease. We now know that disease, like good health, is based on the combined interaction of multiple factors, including heredity, environment, and the individual's psychological makeup.

Although Freud's psychoanalysis and psychosomatic medicine were critically flawed, they laid the groundwork for a renewed appreciation of the connections between medicine and psychology. They started the contemporary trend toward viewing illness and health as *multifactorial*. That is, many diseases are caused by the *interaction* of several factors, rather than by a single, invading bacterial or viral agent. Among these are *host factors* (such as genetic vulnerability or resiliency), *environmental factors* (such as exposure to pollutants and hazardous chemicals), *behavioral factors* (such as diet, exercise, and smoking), and *psychological factors* (such as optimism and overall "hardiness").

Behavioral Medicine

During the first half of the twentieth century, the behaviorist movement, led by John Watson (1878–1958), Edward Thorndike (1874–1945), and B. F. Skinner (1904–1990), dominated American psychology. Recall from your introductory course that behaviorists define *psychology* as the scientific study of observable behavior. They further contend that only two types of learning account for most behaviors: classical conditioning (also called Pavlovian conditioning), or learning that takes place when we learn to associate two environmental stimuli that occur together in time; and operant conditioning, whereby behavior is strengthened if followed by a desirable consequence (reinforcement) or weakened if followed by an undesirable consequence (punishment).

By the early 1970s, practitioners conceived the idea of a field of **behavioral medicine** as a direct response to the behaviorist movement. Thus, the new field began to explore the role of classical and operant conditioning in health and disease. One of its early successes was the research of Neal Miller (1909–), who used operant conditioning techniques to teach laboratory animals (and later humans) to gain control over certain bodily functions. Miller demonstrated, for example, that people could gain some control over their blood pressure and resting heart rate when they were made aware of these physiological states. Miller's technique, called *biofeedback,* is discussed more fully in Chapter 4.

Although the wellspring for behavioral medicine was the behaviorist movement in psychology, a distinguishing feature of this field is its interdisciplinary nature. It draws its membership from such diverse academic fields as anthropology, sociology, molecular biology, genetics, biochemistry, and psychology, as well as the healing professions of nursing, medicine, and dentistry.

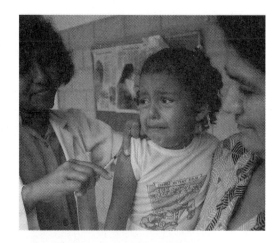

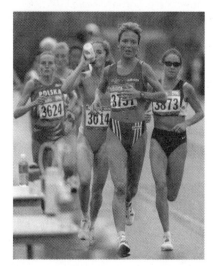

Classical and Operant Conditioning
(top) Classical conditioning: Not always painful, but it sticks with you! In this type of learning, we learn to associate two or more stimuli. A child learns, for example, that the sight of a hypodermic needle (an initially neutral stimulus) will soon be followed by a painful prick. © Jeremy Horner/Corbis

(bottom) Operant conditioning: The pause that refreshes. In this type of learning we associate a voluntary response with its consequence. The parched, fatigued runner, for example, learns that consuming a sports drink soon after a tough workout will quench thirst and help sore muscles recover faster. AP Photo/Thomas Kienzle

Diversity and Healthy Living

Health in the New Millennium

In 1991, the U.S. Department of Health and Human Services released *Healthy People 2000* (USDHHS, 1991), a report outlining the nation's highest priorities for promoting health and preventing disease among all Americans. The report was based on the best judgments of a large group of health experts from the scientific community, professional health organizations, and the corporate world. The report set 300 specific health objectives to be achieved by the year 2000. These were organized into three broad categories:

- *To increase the span of "healthy life" for all Americans.* Healthy life is a combination of average life expectancy and quality of life. Although the average life expectancy of all Americans is currently about 76 years, the average number of *healthy* years is much less: for instance, only 64 years for white Americans and 56 years for African-Americans. The goal was to reduce the number of "dysfunctional years" in which people survive in a state of declining health and poor quality of living.

- *To reduce the health discrepancies among Americans.* Historically, several measures of health have shown substantial differences among ethnic groups. For example, in 1997, average life expectancy was 74.3 years for white males but only 67.2 years for black males; 79.9 years for white females but only 74.7 years for black females (Centers for Disease Control and Prevention, 1999). The reasons for these discrepancies are undoubtedly complex but may include unequal access to health care, genetic susceptibility to specific diseases, and lifestyle differences.

- *To achieve access to preventive health care services for all Americans.* Many ethnic minorities have limited access to preventive health care. For this reason they tend to suffer more health problems and have a higher mortality rate. This goal seeks to understand and remove barriers that limit access to health care in these groups.

In 1998, a midcourse review demonstrated that the country was making significant progress toward about two-thirds of the objectives of *Healthy People 2000*. This progress included

- A decline in the three leading causes of death (heart disease, cancer, and stroke). Although this improvement was due in part to improved medical care, it also reflected a national decline in *health-compromising behaviors* (for example, 50 percent of adults smoked in 1955 compared with about 23 percent in 2000). At the same time, the nation has witnessed an increase in *health-enhancing behaviors* as people are exercising more, eating healthier diets that are lower in fat, and so forth.

- A decrease in the number of alcohol-related automobile deaths from 9.8 per 100,000 people to 6.8 per 100,000 people.

- A decrease in the number of suicides and work-related deaths.

- An increase in the percentage of Americans using seatbelts from 49.7 percent to 76 percent.

- A decline in marijuana and alcohol use among youth aged 12 to 17.

- A decline in the birth rate for unmarried women.

The Emergence of Health Psychology

In 1973, the American Psychological Association (APA) appointed a task force to explore psychology's role in the field of health, to determine whether psychology should remain only under the umbrella of behavioral medicine or establish a distinct field with its own goals and focus. Based on the task force's recommendations, in 1978 the APA created the division of health psychology (Division 38). Four years later, the first volume of its official journal, *Health Psychology*, was published. In this issue, Joseph Matarazzo, the first president of the division, laid down the four goals of the new field:

- Continued decline in the infant mortality rate.
- Continued increase in life expectancy.
- A leveling off in the death rate from AIDS.

Despite this progress, *Healthy People 2010* (USDHHS, 1998) notes that much work remains to be done. While the report continues to focus on eliminating health disparities among various sociocultural groups, it has a broader focus—to improve the health of all Americans. It also notes that use (and abuse) of certain drugs is once again on the rise, and nearly one million deaths in this country each year are preventable. On this last point, it is estimated that

- Control of underage and excess use of alcohol could prevent 100,000 deaths from automobile accidents and other alcohol-related injuries.
- Elimination of public possession of firearms could prevent 35,000 deaths.
- Elimination of all forms of tobacco use could prevent 400,000 deaths from cancer, stroke, and heart disease.
- Better nutrition and exercise programs could prevent 300,000 deaths from heart disease, diabetes, cancer, and stroke.
- A reduction in risky sexual behaviors could prevent 30,000 deaths from sexually transmitted diseases.
- Full access to immunizations for infectious diseases could prevent 100,000 deaths.

To confirm psychology's role in meeting the goals of *Healthy People 2010,* the American Psychological Association in collaboration with the National Institutes of Health and 21 other professional societies recently outlined a national research agenda related to health promotion. Published in 1995, *Doing the Right Thing: A Research Plan for Healthy Living* identified four priorities for research in the new millennium.

- Increasing the focus on the basic behavioral processes in the prevention, development, and treatment of chronic disease.
- Accelerating research related to health promotion and disease prevention.
- Extending research and health care to *traditionally underrepresented groups* such as women and minorities.
- Reshaping the health care system to bring more attention to health promotion and disease prevention.

The report also identified specific strategies for achieving a fuller understanding of the interaction of biological, psychological, and social factors in diseases such as AIDS, cancer, heart disease, arthritis, and obesity. These included the need for more research on early disease detection and screening programs, risk evaluation, and intervention programs to assist nonmedical caregivers in providing care for the physically ill.

Sources: Murphy, S. L. (2000). "Deaths: Final data for 1998." *National Vital Statistics Reports, 48*(11), Figure 3; Science Directorate of the American Psychological Association. (1995). *Doing the right thing: A research plan for healthy living.* Washington, DC: Author; U.S. Department of Health and Human Services. (1991). *Healthy people 2000: National health promotion and disease prevention objectives.* DHHS Publication No. (PHS) 91-50212. Washington, DC: U.S. Government Printing Office; U.S. Department of Health and Human Services. (1998). *Healthy people 2010.* Washington, DC: U.S. Government Printing Office.

- *To study scientifically the causes or origins of specific diseases, that is, their* **etiology.** Health psychologists are primarily interested in the psychological, behavioral, and social origins of disease. They investigate why people engage in *health-compromising behaviors,* such as smoking or unsafe sex.

  etiology the scientific study of the causes or origins of specific diseases

- To *promote health.* They are concerned with issues of how to get people to engage in *health-enhancing behaviors* such as exercising regularly and eating nutritious foods.

average life expectancy the number of years the average newborn is likely to live

- To *prevent and treat illness.* They design programs to help people stop smoking, lose weight, manage stress, and minimize other risk factors for poor health. They also assist those who are already ill in their efforts to adjust to their illnesses or comply with difficult treatment regimens.

- To *promote public health policy and the improvement of the health care system.* Health psychologists are very active in all facets of health education and consult frequently with government leaders who formulate public policy in an effort to improve the delivery of health care to all people.

A natural question from reading these goals would be, "How does health psychology differ from behavioral medicine?" The answer is, "Not very much." The distinction between the two fields has always been the source of considerable confusion. To cut through the confusion, we will refer to behavioral medicine as the interdisciplinary field that integrates behavioral and biomedical science in promoting health and treating disease. And, as we explained at the beginning of the chapter, *health psychology* is the subfield of psychology concerned with the enhancement of health and the prevention and treatment of illness using basic psychological principles.

Trends That Shaped Health Psychology

The challenge facing health psychologists in the twenty-first century is clear: how to help people adopt and maintain lifestyle changes that promote lifelong vitality. Ancient Greek philosophers stated this goal more succinctly: to help people to die young—as late in life as possible (Brody, 1996b). Four main trends in public health, psychology, and medicine combined to shape this challenge.

Increased Life Expectancy

Less than one hundred years ago, 15 percent of babies born in this country died before their first birthday (Figure 1.2). For those who survived, life expectancy was only slightly more than 50 years. With improved health care, today more than 90 percent of newborn babies survive to at least 1 year of age. In addition, **average life expectancy**—the number of years the average newborn is likely to live—has increased by more than 20 years. In the United States in 1999, the average life expectancy at birth was 79.7 years for women and 73.8 years for men (WHO, 2000). Despite this encouraging news, inequalities in life expectancy persist within countries, as well as around the world, and are strongly associated with socioeconomic class, even in countries with good health status on average (WHO, 2000).

Figure 1.2

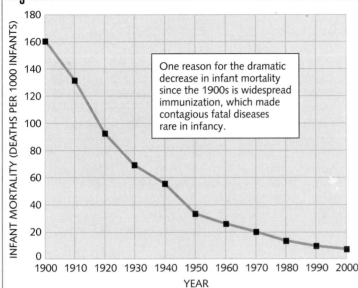

One reason for the dramatic decrease in infant mortality since the 1900s is widespread immunization, which made contagious fatal diseases rare in infancy.

Infant Mortality in the United States
Less than one hundred years ago, 15 percent of babies born in this country died before their first birthday. For those who survived, life expectancy was only slightly more than 50 years. With improved health care, today more than 90 percent of newborn babies survive to at least 1 year of age.

Sources: *Historical Statistics of the United States: Colonial Times to 1970*, by U.S. Bureau of the Census, 1975, Washington, DC: U.S. Government Printing Office p. 60; "Deaths: Final Data for 1998," by S. L. Murphy, 2000, *National Vital Statistics Reports, 48* (11), Table 27.

With people living longer lives, there is greater public awareness of health-related issues, and health has been redefined in broader, more positive terms. This new definition, which emphasizes lifelong physical, psychological, and social vitality, charts a clear role for psychology in health care.

The Rise of Lifestyle Disorders

During the seventeenth, eighteenth, and nineteenth centuries, people died chiefly from illnesses that were caused by impure drinking water, contaminated foods, or infection from sick people (Grob, 1983). It was not unusual for hundreds, or even thousands, of people to die in a single epidemic of smallpox, yellow fever, diphtheria, influenza, or measles. These diseases did not exist in the Americas before the arrival of European settlers. Smallpox, which was brought to the Americas by Europeans in the sixteenth century, killed nearly 90 percent of the population. The Native Americans died at an alarming rate for two reasons: First, they lacked immunity to the foreign microorganisms that caused these diseases, and second, their immune systems were weaker than the Europeans' due to a lower degree of variation in their gene pool.

Improvements in personal hygiene, nutrition, and public health (such as sewage treatment) during the nineteenth century led to a decrease in the number of deaths from infectious diseases. But it was not until Sir Alexander Fleming's discovery of penicillin in 1928 that public health took a truly dramatic turn upward. Before then, four of the top ten causes of death in the United

Table 1.1

The 10 Leading Causes of Death in the United States, 1900 and 1998

1900	Rate per 100,000	1998	Rate per 100,000
Heart disease and stroke	345	Heart disease	268.2
Influenza and pneumonia	202	Cancer	200.3
Tuberculosis	194	Stroke	58.6
Gastritis	143	Chronic obstructive pulmonary disease	41.7
Accidents	72	Accidents	36.2
Cancer	64	Pneumonia, influenza	34.0
Diphtheria	40	Adult-onset diabetes	24.0
Typhoid fever	31	Suicide	11.3
Measles	13	Nephritis and nephrosis (kidney disorders)	9.7

Sources: *Historical Statistics of the United States: Colonial Times to 1970, Pt. 1,* by U.S. Bureau of the Census, 1975, Washington, DC: U.S. Government Printing Office; "Deaths: Final Data for 1998," by S. L. Murphy, 2000, *National Vital Statistics Reports, 48*(11), p. 5.

States were infectious diseases such as *consumption* (tuberculosis), influenza, gastritis, and pneumonia (see Table 1.1, which compares death rates per disease in 1900 with those in 1998). In fact, the death rate from influenza and pneumonia alone was nearly four times greater than the death rate from all known forms of cancer. It is important to note that those of us who live in developed countries such as the United States benefit from a very privileged health care environment. In most of the developing countries in the world today, infectious diseases such as tuberculosis and pneumonia remain the leading causes of death.

The leading causes of death in developed countries today differ from those at the turn of the twentieth century in two important ways. First, unlike pneumonia, diphtheria, and the other diseases to which our ancestors more often succumbed, cancer, stroke, and heart disease are not the result of viral or bacterial infection. They are noncommunicable "lifestyle diseases" that are by and large preventable. In 1998, for example, more than one million of the deaths listed in Table 1.1 had *preventable cause,* as explained in Table 1.2.

Consider two lifestyle diseases: heart disease and cancer. An individual's risk of heart disease or lung, throat, or bladder cancer is greatly increased by smoking cigarettes, leading a sedentary life, and consuming a high-fat diet. Each of these behaviors is rooted, to varying degrees, in psychological and social factors. Refraining from smoking, sticking to an exercise program, and modifying one's diet require a tremendous psychological commitment that involves modifying long-held attitudes and habits.

A second change in the leading causes of death involves the pattern of illness. Prior to the twentieth century, the leading causes of illness and death were *acute disorders,* from which individuals either recovered within a matter of weeks or died swiftly. Today, people live with chronic diseases for many

Table 1.2

Preventable Deaths and Associated Costs

Cause of Death	Annual Number	Treatment	Cost per Patient ($)	Behavioral Factors
Heart disease	500,000	Bypass surgery	30,000	Smoking, lack of exercise, poor diet
Cancer	510,000	Radiation/chemotherapy	29,000	Smoking, lack of exercise, poor diet
Stroke	150,000	Rehabilitation	22,000	Smoking, lack of exercise, poor diet
Injuries	142,500	Treatment/rehabilitation	570,000	Alcohol use, failure to use seatbelts
Low birth weight	23,000	Neonatal care	10,000	Maternal behaviors
HIV infection	1–1.5 million	Pharmacology	75,000	Risky sexual activity, use of dirty needles

Source: *Healthy People 2000: National health promotion and disease prevention objectives.* DHHS Publication No. (PHS) 91-50212, by U.S. Department of Health and Human Services (USDHHS), 1991, Washington, DC: U.S. Government Printing Office.

years. Although they cannot be cured, chronic diseases can be treated to prevent premature death and maintain quality of life.[1]

Rethinking the Biomedical Model

A third trend that helped shaped the new field of health psychology was the need to go beyond the biomedical model to a more comprehensive model of health and disease. One shortcoming of traditional medicine is that it has difficulty explaining why the same set of physical risk factors sometimes triggers disease, and sometimes does not. Why, for example, does Frank—a middle-aged, overweight, cigarette-smoking, sedentary male with a family history of heart disease—suffer a fatal heart attack, while Malcolm—who has virtually the same risk factors—remains free of heart disease? Biomedicine's difficulty in predicting new cases of heart disease ultimately led researchers to discover that psychological factors—such as how a person reacts to stress—combine with physical risk factors to determine an individual's health risk.

A closely related problem for the biomedical model is explaining why one form of treatment (such as the use of a certain medication) may cure a particular illness in one person but not in another. Health psychologists have learned that whether a particular drug or some other form of treatment is effective is substantially influenced by psychological and social factors.

One such factor is the healing power of the **placebo effect,** or the faith of the patient and the practitioner in the therapeutic value of a certain treatment. *Placebo* is a Latin word that translates into English as "I shall please." In medicine, a placebo is an inactive substance or treatment presented in such a way that patients expect the substance or treatment to actually work. All treatments depend more or less on this faith, and that is why a particular treatment may be

placebo effect the power of a person's belief in the efficacy of a treatment to actually influence the treatment's effectiveness

[1]Note that the leading causes of death in the 1990s were not new diseases; they were present in earlier times, but fewer people died from them or they were called something else.

able to cure a particular disease by mobilizing the patient's own healing powers (Relman, 1998). Any medical procedure, from drugs to surgery, can have a placebo effect or, for that matter, a *nocebo* effect, in which a person attaches a negative rather than a positive expectation to a treatment. The doctor–patient relationship itself is a good example. Research studies have found, for example, that the amount of daily insulin required to stabilize diabetic patients fluctuates depending on the patient's rapport with his or her doctor.

Because of the credibility of modern science, treatments based on the most recent technologies (ultrasound, transcutaneous nerve stimulation) are especially susceptible to a placebo effect (Brody, 2000b). Placebo therapy has proved to be effective in a wide range of illnesses, including allergies, asthma, cancer, depression, diabetes, epilepsy, insomnia, migraines, multiple sclerosis, ulcers, and warts. We'll examine the placebo effect more fully in Chapter 14.

Rising Health Care Costs

A final factor that helped shape health psychology is the rapid rise in health care costs. In 1980, the annual cost of health care in the United States was $156 *billion,* or about $1000 per person. Today, health care costs consume more than 13 percent of the U.S. gross domestic product ($1.5 *trillion* dollars), or more than $3900 for every man, woman, and child (Figure 1.3).

These figures have helped focus attention on the cost-effectiveness of health promotion and maintenance. Health psychology's emphasis on modifying

Figure 1.3

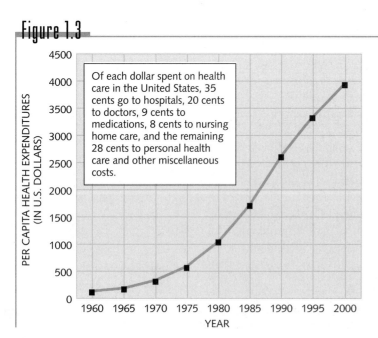

Of each dollar spent on health care in the United States, 35 cents go to hospitals, 20 cents to doctors, 9 cents to medications, 8 cents to nursing home care, and the remaining 28 cents to personal health care and other miscellaneous costs.

Per Capita Health Expenditures in the United States, 1960 to 2000

In 1980, the annual cost of health care in the United States was $156 billion. By 1995, this figure had increased to more than $989 billion. In 2000, health care costs consumed 13.4 percent of the U.S. gross domestic product. Although the U.S. health system spends a higher portion of its gross domestic product on health care than any other country, it ranks only thirty-seventh out of 191 World Health Organization member countries according to its overall performance.

Source: *Health, United States, 2000,* by U.S. Department of Health and Human Services, 2000, Washington, DC: U.S. Government Printing Office, p. 321.

people's risky health-related behaviors before they cause illness has the potential to reduce health care costs dramatically (Kaplan, 2000). For example, there are approximately 1 million new cases of cancer each year and nearly 500,000 cancer-related deaths. Many forms of cancer are preventable by reducing or eliminating smoking or by increasing the use of diagnostic tests that screen for cancer.

Perspectives in Health Psychology

You have seen how social and historical trends created the need for a new, broader model of health and illness. In fact, health psychologists have developed several models, or perspectives, to guide their work. As you read, remember that each perspective provides a different way of looking at the same thing. Together, they form a complete picture of health and illness.

Life-Course Perspective

In all stages of life, people face challenges to their health and overall well-being. From the moment of conception until the day we die, each of us is shaped by a unique collection of genetic, biological, and sociocultural factors. The **life-course perspective** in health psychology focuses on important age-related aspects of health and illness (Jackson, 1996). This perspective would consider, for example, how a pregnant woman's use of psychoactive drugs would affect her child's lifelong development. Her child might be born early and suffer from *low birth weight* (less than 2500 grams [$5\frac{1}{2}$ pounds]). One of the most common, and most preventable, problems of prenatal development, low birth weight has consequences that cast a shadow over the individual's physical and cognitive development for many years. Among these consequences are slowed motor, social, and language development; increased risk of cerebral palsy; and long-term learning difficulties (Liaw & Brooks-Gunn, 1993).

This perspective also examines the leading causes of death in terms of the age groups they affect. The chronic diseases that are the leading causes of death in the overall population are more likely to affect middle-aged and elderly adults. Young people are much more likely to die from accidents or unintentional injuries.

Yet another concern of this perspective is the way in which specific *birth cohort* experiences influence health. A **birth cohort** is a group of people who, because they were born within a few years of one another, experience similar historical and social conditions that affect their health and illnesses. People born in the late nineteenth or early twentieth centuries had to overcome enormous obstacles just to survive to the age of 50. Today, major shifts in public health policy have reshaped the future of existing cohorts of older adults in the United States. For example, in 1965, the U.S. Congress passed The Older

life-course perspective theoretical perspective that focuses on age-related aspects of health and illness

birth cohort a group of people who, because they were born at about the same time, experience similar historical and social conditions

■ **sociocultural perspective**
theoretical perspective that
focuses on how social and
cultural factors contribute to
health and disease

■ **gender perspective** theoretical perspective that focuses
on gender-specific health
problems and gender barriers
to health care

Americans Act, which provides every older person, regardless of income, with a variety of health benefits—from subsidized meals to counseling and other services provided by over 20,000 community agencies. As a result, older Americans have more opportunities today to remain in better health than their counterpart cohorts who reached late adulthood earlier in our nation's history.

Sociocultural Perspective

How social and cultural factors contribute to health and disease is the focus of the **sociocultural perspective.** When psychologists use the term *culture,* they refer to the enduring behaviors, values, and customs that a group of people have developed over the years and transmitted from one generation to the next. Within a culture, there may be one, two, or more *ethnic groups,* large groups of people who tend to have similar values and experiences because they share certain characteristics.

In multiethnic cultures such as those of the United States and most large nations today, wide disparities exist in the life expectancy and health status of ethnic minority groups and the majority population. Some of these differences undoubtedly reflect variation in *socioeconomic status (SES),* a measure of several variables, including income, education, and occupation. For example, the highest rates of chronic disease occur among people who are at the lowest SES levels (Flack et al., 1995).

Sociocultural variation is also apparent in health-related beliefs and behaviors. For example, traditional Native American health care practices are holistic and do not distinguish separate models for mental and physical illnesses (Johnson et al., 1995). As another example, Christian Scientists traditionally reject the use of medicine in their belief that sick people can be cured only through prayer. And Judaic law prescribes that God gives health, and it is the responsibility of each individual to protect it.

In general, health psychologists working from this perspective have found wide discrepancies not only among ethnic groups but also within these groups. Latinos, for example, are far from homogenous. The three major nationality groups—Mexican-Americans, Puerto Ricans, and Cubans—differ in education, income, overall health, and risk of disease and death (Bagley, Angel, Dilworth-Anderson, Liu, & Schinke, 1995).

Gender Perspective

The **gender perspective** in health psychology focuses on the study of gender-specific health problems and gender barriers to health care. Men and women differ in their risk of a variety of disorders. Throughout childhood, for example, boys outnumber girls in a range of behavioral and psychological disorders,

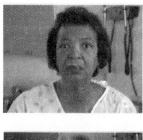 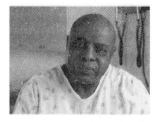 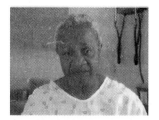 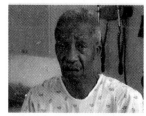
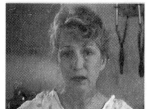 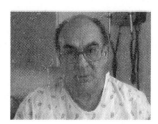 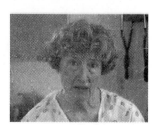 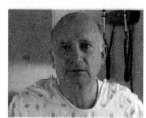

Sociocultural Bias in Diagnosis

Physicians were told that these supposed "heart patients" were identical in occupation, symptoms, and every other respect except age, race, and gender. Although catheterization was the appropriate treatment for the described symptoms, the physicians were much more likely to recommend it for the younger, white, male patients than for the older, female, or black patients.

Source: "The Effect of Race and Sex on Physician's Recommendations for Cardiac Catheterization," by K. A. Schulman, J. Berlin, W. Harless, J. F. Kerner, S. Sistrunk, B. J. Gersh, R. Dubé, C. K. Taleghani, J. E. Burke, S. Williams, J. M. Eisenberg, and J. Escarce, 1999, *New England Journal of Medicine, 340*, pp. 618–625.

including sleep and eating problems, hyperactivity, autism, and antisocial behavior. Conversely, from age 8 through adulthood, girls and women outnumber boys and men in the diagnosis of depression, anxiety, and eating disorders (Ussher, 1997). In addition, women tend to respond more actively than men to illness symptoms and to seek treatment earlier.

The medical profession has a long history of treating men and women differently. For example, research studies have shown that women treated for heart disease are given more prescriptions, are more likely to be put through unnecessary diagnostic procedures, and are not likely to receive the same quality of medical care as men (Ayanian & Epstein, 1991). In one study, 700 physicians were asked to prescribe treatment for eight heart patients with identical symptoms (Schulman et al., 1999). In fact, the "patients" were actors who differed only in gender, race, and reported age (55 or 70). Although diagnosis is a judgment call, most cardiac specialists would agree that diagnostic catheterization is the appropriate treatment for the symptoms described by each hypothetical patient. However, the actual recommendations revealed a small, but nevertheless significant, antifemale and antiblack bias. For the younger, white, and male patients, catheterization was recommended 90, 91, and 91 percent of the time, respectively; for the older, female, and black patients, 86, 85, and 85 percent of the time, respectively.

Problems such as these, and the underrepresentation of women as participants in medical research trials, have led to the criticism of gender bias in health research and care. In response, the National Institutes of Health (NIH) has issued detailed guidelines on the inclusion of women and minority groups in medical research (Burd, 1994). In addition, the NIH recently launched the Women's Health Initiative, a 15-year study of 160,000 postmenopausal women focusing on the determinants, and prevention, of disability and death in older

■ **biopsychosocial (mind–body) perspective** the viewpoint that health and other behaviors are determined by the interaction of biological mechanisms, psychological processes, and social influences

women. Among the targets of investigation in this sweeping study are osteoporosis, breast cancer, and coronary heart disease.

By now, it's probably clear to you that these perspectives overlap, that they all view health and illness as the product of interacting factors. They differ only in the factors they emphasize. Although these perspectives answer different questions about health, they complement, rather than contradict, one another. Together, they help explain human health and illness. In a sense, the sociocultural, life-course, and gender perspectives are subsumed under the biopsychosocial perspective because that model, whether directly or indirectly, deals with all the issues covered by the other perspectives. For that reason, our focus in this text will be on the biopsychosocial perspective, to which we now turn.

Biopsychosocial (Mind–Body) Perspective

As history tells us, looking at one causative factor paints an incomplete picture of a person's health or illness. Health psychologists therefore work from a **biopsychosocial (mind–body) perspective.** As depicted in Figure 1.4, this perspective recognizes that *bio*logical, *psycho*logical, and *social* forces act together to determine an individual's health and vulnerability to disease; that is, health and disease must be explained in terms of multiple contexts.

The Biological Context

All behaviors, including states of health and illness, occur in a biological context. Every thought, mood, and urge is a biological event made possible because of the characteristic anatomical structure and biological function of a person's body. Health psychology draws attention to those aspects of our bodies that influence health and disease: our genetic makeup and our nervous, immune, and endocrine systems (see Chapter 3).

Genes provide the blueprint for our biology and predispose our behaviors—healthy and unhealthy, normal and abnormal. For example, the tendency to abuse alcohol has long been known to run in some families (see

Figure 1.4

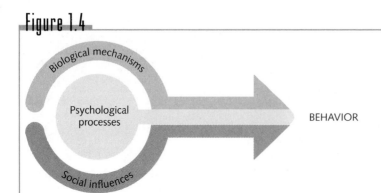

BEHAVIOR

The Biopsychosocial Model
According to the biopsychosocial perspective, all health behaviors are best explained in terms of three contexts: biological processes, psychological processes, and social influences.

Source: *Psychology: A Biopsychosocial Approach,* by C. Peterson, 1997, New York: Addison-Wesley Longman.

Chapter 8). One reason is that alcohol dependency is at least partly genetic, although it does not seem to be linked to a single, specific gene. Instead, some people may inherit a greater sensitivity to alcohol's physical effects, experiencing intoxication as pleasurable and the aftermath of a hangover as minor. Such people may be more likely to drink, especially in certain psychological and social contexts.

A key element of the biological context is our species' evolutionary history. Our characteristic human traits and behaviors exist as they do because they helped our distant ancestors to survive long enough to reproduce and send their genes into the future. For example, natural selection has favored the tendency of people to become hungry in the presence of a mouth-watering aroma (see Chapter 7). This sensitivity to food-related cues makes evolutionary sense in that eating is necessary for survival—particularly in the distant past when food supplies were unpredictable and it was advantageous to have a healthy appetite when food was available.

At the same time, biology and behavior constantly interact. For example, some individuals are more vulnerable to stress-related illnesses because they angrily react to daily hassles and other environmental "triggers" (see Chapter 4). Among men, increased amounts of the hormone testosterone are positively correlated with this type of aggressive reaction. This relationship, however, is reciprocal: Angry outbursts can also lead to elevated testosterone levels. One of the tasks of health psychology is to explain how (and why) this mutual influence between biology and behavior occurs.

The Psychological Context

The central message of health psychology is, of course, that health and illness are subject to psychological influences. For example, a key factor in how well a person copes with a stressful life experience is how the event is appraised or interpreted (see Chapter 5). Events that are appraised as overwhelming, pervasive, and beyond our control take a much greater toll on us physically and psychologically than do events that are appraised as minor challenges that are temporary and surmountable. Indeed, some evidence suggests that, whether a stressful event is actually experienced or merely imagined, the body's stress response is nearly the same. Health psychologists think that some people may be chronically depressed and more susceptible to certain health problems because they replay stressful events over and over again in their minds, which may be functionally equivalent to repeatedly encountering the actual event. Throughout this book we will examine the ways in which thinking, perception, motivation, emotion, learning, attention, memory, and other topics of central importance to psychology are implicated in health.

Psychological factors also play an important role in the treatment of chronic conditions. Consider the treatment of cancer—once a disease that automatically led to death. Although death is no longer automatic, treatments such as chemotherapy force patients to endure the sometimes miserable reactions, including severe nausea and vomiting, to the powerful drugs administered. The side effects can be so debilitating that some patients actually refuse to continue the potentially life-saving regimen. The effectiveness of medication is powerfully influenced by a patient's attitude toward treatment. A patient who believes a drug will only cause misery may experience considerable tension, which can actually worsen his or her physical reaction to the treatment. This reaction can set up a vicious cycle in which escalating anxiety before treatment is followed by progressively worse physical reactions as the treatment regimen proceeds. Psychological interventions can help patients learn to manage their tension, thereby lessening their negative reactions to treatment. Patients who are more relaxed are usually better able, and more motivated, to follow their doctors' instructions.

Psychological interventions can also assist patients in managing the everyday stresses of life, which seem to exert a cumulative effect on the immune system. Negative life events such as bereavement, divorce, job loss, or relocation have been linked to decreased immune functioning and increased susceptibility to illness. By teaching patients more effective ways of managing unavoidable stress, health psychologists may help patients' immune systems combat disease.

The Social Context

In placing health behavior in its social context, health psychologists are concerned with the ways in which we think about, influence, and relate to one another and to our environments. Your gender, for example, entails a particular socially prescribed role that gives you your sense of being a woman or a man. In addition, you are a member of a particular family, community, and nation; you also have a certain racial, cultural, and ethnic identity and live within a specific socioeconomic class. Each of these elements of your unique social context influences your beliefs and behaviors—including those related to health.

Consider the social context in which a chronic disease such as cancer occurs. A spouse, significant other, or close friend provides an important source of social support for many cancer patients. Women and men who feel socially connected to a network of caring friends are less likely to die of all types of cancer than their socially isolated counterparts (see Chapter 10). Feeling supported by others may serve as a buffer that mitigates the output of stress hormones and keeps the body's immune defenses strong during traumatic situations. It may also promote better health habits, regular checkups, and early screening of worrisome symptoms—all of which may improve a cancer victim's odds of survival.

Despite the significance of such social influences, remember that it would be a mistake to focus exclusively on this, or any one context, in isolation. Health behavior is not an automatic consequence of a given social context. For example, although, as a group, cancer patients who are married tend to survive longer than unmarried persons, marriages that are unhappy and destructive offer no benefit in this regard and may even be linked to poorer health outcomes.

Biopsychosocial "Systems"

As these examples indicate, the biopsychosocial perspective emphasizes the mutual influences among the biological, psychological, and social contexts of health. It is also based on a **systems theory** of behavior. According to this theory, health—indeed, all of nature—is best understood as a hierarchy of systems in which each system is simultaneously composed of smaller subsystems and part of larger, more encompassing systems. Thus, each of us is a system—a body made up of interacting systems such as the endocrine system, the cardiovascular system, the nervous system, and the immune system. Each of these biological systems is, in turn, composed of smaller subsystems consisting of tissues, nerve fibers, fluids, cells, and genetic material. Moving in the other direction, we are part of many larger systems, including our families, our neighborhoods, our societies, and our culture.

Applied to health, the systems approach emphasizes a crucial point: A system at any given level is affected by and affects systems at other levels. For example, a weakened immune system affects specific organs in a person's body, which in turn affect the person's overall biological health, which in turn might affect the person's relationships with his or her family and friends. Conceptualizing health and disease according to a systems approach allows us to understand the whole person more fully.

Applying the Biopsychosocial Model

To get a better feeling for the usefulness of biopsychosocial explanations of healthy behaviors, consider the example of *major depressive disorder,* which is diagnosed when signs of depression (including lethargy, feelings of worthlessness, and loss of interest in family and friends) last 2 weeks or longer without any notable cause.

Like most psychological disorders, depression is best explained in terms of several mechanisms (see Figure 1.5 on page 34). Research studies of families, identical and fraternal twins, and adopted children clearly demonstrate that people who have a biological relative who was diagnosed with depression before age 30 are much more likely to be diagnosed with depression than are people without a relative who suffers from depression (Pauls, Morton, & Egeland, 1992). In addition to genetics, other factors in the biological context of this disorder include low levels of certain brain neurotransmitters, especially norepinephrine and serotonin (see Chapter 3). Antidepressant medications (such as Prozac and Paxil), electroconvulsive shock therapy, and repetitive physical exercise (for example, running, swimming, and biking) are effective treatments largely because they increase the availability of these brain chemicals (Jacobs, 1994).

On the psychological side, there is considerable research evidence that negative thinking, including *self-defeating attitudes,* contributes to depression.

systems theory the viewpoint that nature is best understood as a hierarchy of systems, in which each system is simultaneously composed of smaller subsystems and larger, interrelated systems

Figure 1.5

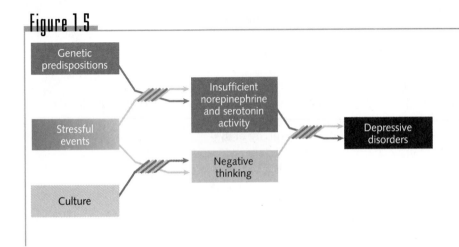

A Biopsychosocial Model of Depression
Depression is best understood as occurring in three contexts: biological (genetic predispositions and neurotransmitter imbalances), psychological (negative thinking and self-defeating beliefs), and social (stressful events, conditioned helplessness, and an individualistic culture that encourages self-blame for personal failure).

Source: *Psychology: A Biopsychosocial Approach,* by C. Peterson, 1997, New York: Addison-Wesley Longman.

Depressed people tend to think about themselves, their world, and the future in grim ways (see Chapter 5). When unavoidable or uncontrollable painful events occur, people who are vulnerable to depression tend to explain the events as due to causes that are internal ("It's all my fault"), global ("It's going to affect everything I do"), and stable ("I'll never get over this"). In *cognitive therapy,* psychologists work with depressed clients to challenge and redirect these negative beliefs.

On the social side, depression is often brought on by stressful experiences—losing a job or a loved one, getting divorced, anything that challenges a person's sense of identity and self-esteem (Kendler, Neale, Kessler, Heath, & Eaves, 1993). Martin Seligman (1991) has proposed that self-defeating beliefs and depression may be socially conditioned in people who learn that they cannot influence important events in their lives. Just as laboratory animals who receive unavoidable electric shocks become passive and withdrawn, so too do people who experience uncontrollable painful events.

As is true of other psychological disorders, culture exerts an important influence on a person's vulnerability to depression. Major depressive disorder is much more common among young Westerners—perhaps because of the rise of individualism, which encourages the self-focused individual to accept personal responsibility for all problems. In contrast, in more close-knit, cooperative non-Western cultures such as Japan, depression is much rarer—perhaps because problems are less likely to be tied to self-blame for personal failure (Seligman, 1995). Moreover, there is a birth cohort effect on depression: Young North American adults are three times as likely to report suffering depression today as were their grandparents *at any time during their lives* (Statistics, Canada, 1999).

Frequently Asked Questions about Health Psychology

W e have seen how views regarding the nature of illness and health have changed over the course of history, examined trends that helped shape the new field of health psychology, and discussed the various theoretical perspectives from which health psychologists work. But you may still have questions about the profession of health psychology. Here are answers to some of the most frequently asked questions.

What Do Health Psychologists Do?

Like all psychologists, health psychologists may serve as *teachers, research scientists,* and/or *clinicians.* Their role as teachers is obvious: They train the next generation of students in health-related fields. As research scientists, they identify the psychological processes that contribute to health and illness, investigate issues concerning why people do not engage in healthful practices, and evaluate the effectiveness of specific therapeutic interventions.

Health psychologists are on the cutting edge of research testing the biopsychosocial model in numerous areas, including HIV/AIDS, compliance with medical treatment regimens, and the effects of psychological, cultural, and social variables on immune functioning and various disease processes (for example, cancer, hypertension, diabetes, chronic pain). Because the biopsychosocial model was first developed to explain health problems, until recently the majority of this research has focused on diseases and health-compromising behaviors. However, a new movement in psychology, called *positive psychology,* is encouraging psychologists to devote more research attention to optimal, healthy human functioning (Seligman & Csikszentmihalyi, 2000). The scope of this research—covering topics as diverse as happiness, psychological hardiness, and the traits of people who live to a ripe old age—shows clearly that the biopsychosocial model guides much of it.

Applied health psychologists, who generally focus on health-promoting interventions, are licensed for independent practice in areas such as clinical and counseling psychology. As clinicians, they use the full range of diagnostic assessment and therapeutic techniques in psychology to promote health and assist the physically ill. Assessment approaches frequently include measures of cognitive functioning, psychophysiological assessment, demographic surveys, and lifestyle or personality assessment. Interventions may include stress management, relaxation therapies, biofeedback, education about the role of psychological processes in disease, and cognitive-behavioral interventions.

Both individual and group interventions are commonly used. Furthermore, interventions can be either direct or indirect. *Direct intervention* would involve, for example, designing and implementing a program of relaxation training to help a patient cope with chronic pain. An *indirect intervention* would be consulting with a patient's physician to determine whether the patient's psychological traits are influencing his or her medical treatment.

Interventions are not limited to those who are already suffering from a health problem. Healthy or at-risk individuals may be taught preventive healthy behaviors. Often health psychology interventions of this type focus on buffering the negative impact of stress by promoting enhanced coping mechanisms or improved use of social support networks.

As the Human Genome Project moves toward pinpointing the precise role of every human gene, society will confront an explosion of information, which promises wondrous advances in disease diagnosis, treatment, and prevention while raising challenging ethical and legal questions. Health psychologists are expected to play essential roles in providing the research and clinical support needed to grapple with this information. For example, in the research arena, health psychologists are likely to be called on to explore issues such as the age at which children should be permitted to give informed consent for medical treatment, the impact on the developing person of knowing that one is genetically vulnerable to a later chronic disease, and the impact of individual DNA profiles on interpersonal relationships.

Where Do Health Psychologists Work?

Traditionally, most psychologists accepted teaching or research positions at universities and four-year colleges. Because of declining college enrollments, however, faculty positions in many of psychology's subfields have not kept pace with the increasing numbers of interested applicants. Employment opportunities for health psychologists with applied or research skills, however, have been very good throughout the developed world, particularly in hospital settings (DeAngelis, 1995). In fact, the number of psychologists working in health-related fields more than doubled during the 1980s (Enright, Resnick, DeLeon, Sciara, & Tanney, 1990). This trend continues today, in response to society's increased emphasis on health promotion and meeting the needs of particular groups, such as the elderly (Kaplan, 2000).

Besides colleges, universities, and hospitals, health psychologists work in a variety of venues, including health maintenance organizations (HMOs), medical schools, pain and rehabilitation clinics, and in private practice (see Figure 1.6). An increasing number of health psychologists can be found in the workplace, where they advise employers and workers on a variety of health-related issues. They also help establish on-the-job interventions to help employees lose weight, quit smoking, and learn more adaptive ways of managing stress.

How Do I Become a Health Psychologist?

Preparing for a career in health psychology usually requires an advanced degree in any of a number of different educational programs. Some students enroll in medical or nursing school and eventually become nurses or doctors. Others train for one of the allied health professions such as nutrition, physical therapy, social work, occupational therapy, or public health. An increasing number of interested undergraduates continue on to graduate school in psychology and acquire the research, teaching, and intervention skills described earlier. Those who ultimately hope to provide direct services to patients typically take their training in clinical or counseling psychology programs.

Many students who wish to pursue a career in health psychology obtain general psychology training at the undergraduate level and then receive specialty training at the doctoral, postdoctoral, and internship levels. At the undergraduate level, health psychology courses currently are offered at about one-third of all colleges and universities. Because of health psychology's biopsychosocial orientation, students are also encouraged to take courses in anatomy and physiology, abnormal and social psychology, learning processes and behavior therapies, community psychology, and public health.

Most health psychologists eventually obtain a doctoral degree (Ph.D.) in psychology. To earn a doctorate in psychology, students complete a four- to six-year program, at the end of which they conduct an original research project. In 2000, there were 65 identified doctoral training programs in health psychology.

Graduate training in health psychology is generally based on a curriculum that covers the three basic domains of the biopsychosocial model. Training in the biological domain includes courses in neuropsychology, anatomy, physiology, and psychopharmacology. Training in the psychological domain includes courses in each of the major subfields (biological, developmental, personality, etc.) and theoretical perspectives (social-cultural, cognitive, behavior, neuroscience, etc.). And training in the social domain focuses on the study of group processes and the ways in which the various groups (family, ethnic, etc.) influence their members' health.

As we begin the new century, medicine is benefiting from a dazzling array of new techniques of diagnosis and treatment. In less than one hundred years, physicians have progressed from using leeches in bloodletting to the wonders of nuclear medicine, magnetic resonance imaging, and genetic engineering. Only 30 years ago, when President Nixon declared America's war on cancer, precious little was known about the basic cellular biology of diseases such as cancer. Oncologists had only the basic weapons of radiation, chemotherapy, and surgery at their disposal. Revolutionary new discoveries during the last

Figure 1.6

Where Do Health Psychologists Work?
Besides colleges, universities, and hospitals, health psychologists work in a variety of venues, including health maintenance organizations (HMOs), medical schools, pain and rehabilitation clinics, and in independent practice. An increasing number of health psychologists can be found in the workplace, where they advise employers and workers on a variety of health-related issues.

Source: *1993 Doctorate Employment Survey*, by M. Wicherski and J. Kohout, 1995, Washington, DC: American Psychological Association.

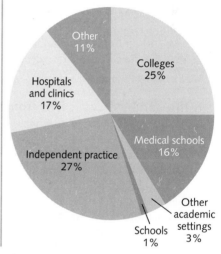

years of the 1990s have spawned many promising new treatments, including gene therapy, artificial antibodies, and the use of biological agents that choke off tumors by halting capillary growth (Brownlee & Shute, 1998). One can only wonder what new discoveries lie ahead.

Summing Up

Health and Health Psychology

1. Health is a state of complete physical, mental, and social well-being. Health psychology is concerned with the psychological aspects of health over the entire life span. Its specific goals are to promote health, prevent and treat illness, investigate the role of behavioral and social factors in disease, and evaluate and improve the formulation of health policy and the delivery of health care to all people.

2. The definition of health confirms that it is a positive, multidimensional state that involves three domains: physical health, psychological health, and social health. The three domains are not independent; they all influence one another.

Health and Illness: Lessons from the Past

3. In the earliest known cultures, illness was believed to result from mystical forces and evil spirits that invaded the body. Hippocrates' humoral theory was the first rational theory of disease. According to this theory, health of body and mind resulted from equilibrium among four bodily fluids called humors. Galen expanded the humoral theory of disease by developing an elaborate system of pharmacology that physicians followed for almost fifteen hundred years.

4. Under the influence of the medieval church, medicine advanced very little during the Middle Ages. Scientific studies of the body (especially dissection) were forbidden, and ideas about health and disease took on religious overtones. Illness was viewed as God's punishment for evildoing, and treatment frequently involved physical torture.

5. French philosopher René Descartes advanced his theory of mind–body dualism—the belief that the mind and body are autonomous processes, each subject to different laws of causality. Descartes' influence ushered in a new age of medical research based on the scientific study of the body.

6. Advances in measurement and microscopy led to several new models of disease. Based on his findings from hundreds of human autopsies, Morgagni advanced the idea that the causes of many diseases reside in problems in the internal organs and in the muscular and skeletal systems of the body (anatomical theory). The cellular theory of disease suggested that disease occurs when body cells malfunction or die. Louis Pasteur discovered that bacteria often cause cells to malfunction, giving rise to the germ theory of disease.

7. The dominant view in modern medicine is the biomedical model, which assumes that disease is the result of a virus, bacterium, or some other pathogen invading the body. Because it makes no provision for psychological, social, or behavioral factors in illness, the model embraces both reductionism and mind–body dualism.

8. In his treatment of patients suffering from biologically impossible ailments such as "glove anesthesia," Sigmund Freud introduced the idea that specific diseases could be caused by unconscious conflicts. Freud's views were expanded into the field of psychosomatic medicine, which is concerned with the treatment and diagnosis of disorders caused by faulty processes within the mind. However, psychosomatic medicine fell out of favor because it was grounded in psychoanalytic theory; arbitrary in regarding some diseases as physical and others as psychological; based on the sometimes faulty case study method; and predicated on the outmoded idea that a single problem is sufficient to trigger disease.

9. An outgrowth of the behaviorist movement in American psychology, behavioral medicine explores the role of classical and operant conditioning in health and disease. Unlike health psychology, which is a discipline-specific subspecialty of psychology, behavioral medicine draws its membership from many diverse academic fields.

Trends That Shaped Health Psychology

10. Several trends have led to the growth of health psychology:

   a. Average life expectancy increased by more than 20 years during the twentieth century.

b. The leading causes of death are now preventable "lifestyle diseases" rooted in health-compromising behaviors such as cigarette smoking, poor nutrition, and sedentary living. Each of these behaviors, to varying degrees, is controlled by psychological and social factors.

c. There has been a shift away from the biomedical model, first because it has difficulty explaining why the same set of risk factors sometimes triggers disease and sometimes does not. It also fails to explain why a particular treatment does or doesn't work with all people (for example, why the placebo effect works in some cases). Finally, the model fails to take into account the importance of the doctor–patient relationship in the efficacy of treatment.

d. Health promotion and disease prevention are the most cost-effective approaches to health care. Health psychology's emphasis on modifying the risky health behaviors of people before they become ill has the potential to reduce dramatically the burden of health care costs.

Perspectives in Health Psychology

11. Health psychologists approach the study of health and illness from four major overlapping perspectives. The life-course perspective in health psychology focuses attention on how aspects of health and illness vary with age, as well as how birth cohort experiences (such as shifts in public health policy) influence health. The sociocultural perspective calls attention to how social and cultural factors, such as ethnic variations in dietary practice and beliefs about the causes of illness, affect health. The gender perspective calls attention to male–female differences in the risk of specific diseases and conditions, as well as in various health-enhancing and health-compromising behaviors. The biopsychosocial perspective in effect combines these perspectives, recognizing that biological, psychological, and social forces act together to determine an individual's health and vulnerability to disease.

Frequently asked Questions about Health Psychology

12. Health psychologists are engaged in three primary activities: teaching, research, and clinical intervention. Health psychologists work in a variety of settings, including hospitals, universities and medical schools, health maintenance organizations, rehabilitation clinics, private practice, and, increasingly, in the workplace. Preparing for a career in health psychology usually requires a doctoral degree. Some students enter health psychology from the fields of medicine, nursing, or one of the allied health professions. An increasing number enroll in graduate programs in health psychology.

Key Terms and Concepts

health psychology, p. 4
health, p. 6
humoral theory, p. 12
epidemic, p. 14
mind–body dualism, p. 15
anatomical theory, p. 15

cellular theory, p. 16
germ theory, p. 16
biomedical model, p. 17
pathogen, p. 17
psychosomatic medicine, p. 18
case study, p. 18

behavioral medicine, p. 19
etiology, p. 21
average life expectancy, p. 22
placebo effect, p. 25
life-course perspective, p. 27
birth cohort, p. 27

sociocultural perspective, p. 28
gender perspective, p. 28
biopsychosocial (mind–body) perspective, p. 30
systems theory, p. 33

Health Psychology on the World Wide Web

The World Wide Web is full of resources related to health psychology. At the end of each chapter, a list of Web sites is provided to assist you in your study of health psychology. Some of the sites were chosen for another reason: to direct those of you with specific personal or family health questions in your search for authoritative sources of information and support.

Web Address	Description
http://web1.ea.pvt.k12.pa.us/medant/	Read essays on the history of medicine in ancient Rome and Greece and follow links to numerous resources on the history of medicine.
http://www.health-psych.org http://freud.apa.org/divisions/div38/	Division 38 (Health Psychology) of the American Psychological Association (APA) is a good place to start your search for the answer to any question related to psychology and health.
http://socbehmed.org/sbm/sbm.htm	The Society of Behavioral Medicine is an interdisciplinary resource on health and illness.
http://www.cdc.gov	The Centers for Disease Control and Prevention (CDC) site provides public information on infectious diseases.
http://www.chid.nih.gov	The CHID (Combined Health Information Database) is a bibliographic database produced by the National Institutes of Health and is a small, no-nonsense search engine that indexes articles on nearly any health topic.
http://www.noah.-health.org	Maintained by the City University of New York, this outstanding bilingual site (all information is available in English and Spanish) offers frequent updates and links to health newsletters.
http://is.dal.ca/~hlthpsyc/hlthhome.htm	The health psychology section of the Canadian Psychological Association provides information about and links to numerous health psychology topics.

Critical Thinking Exercise

Health Psychology on the Internet

Now that you have completed Chapter 1, take your learning a step further by testing your critical thinking skills on this psychological reasoning exercise. For an introduction to these exercises, turn to the Preface before you begin working.

Each chapter of this text concludes with a list of Internet sites. Some provide information on the latest relevant research. Others will help you answer questions about personal health concerns as well as list support services. If you have access to the Internet, you can easily find information about:

- Scientific research studies published in leading health journals such as the *Journal of the American Medical Association (JAMA), Health Psychology,* and *Behavioral Medicine.*

- Ongoing projects of federal and international health agencies, including the National Institutes of Health (NIH), the National Cancer Institute, and the World Health Organization (WHO).

- National health organizations such as the National Women's Resource Center, the American Heart Association, and the American Diabetes Association.

- Public and private health care providers, including hospitals, clinics, and support services in your part of the country.

- Health news in the popular media, such as *Consumer Reports, USA Today,* and the various network news agencies.

- Consumer-oriented material from organizations such as the Mayo Clinic.

- Electronic medical encyclopedias that allow you to look up health-related terms as well as provide information about specific medications, treatments, and conditions.

- Health forums and chat groups that bring together people with shared health interests.

- "Ask the expert" Web sites in which a team of health professionals answers users' questions.

Once you are connected to the Internet, a *Web browser* such as *Internet Explorer* or *Netscape Navigator* will give you two ways to navigate the Internet. The most direct method is to type in the address of a known Internet or World Wide Web site, such as those provided at the end of each chapter. The second is to conduct an online search using one of the *search engines* offered by your service provider.[2] Once at the search engine's main menu, you can type in the topic of interest. Say you are interested in looking up information related to AIDS and high-risk behaviors. If you enter the term "AIDS," your search engine will retrieve every Web site indexed to AIDS, probably thousands. By entering "AIDS and high-risk behaviors," however, you will narrow the search to only those Web sites that contain information related to both terms. The amount of information on the Internet is now so voluminous that narrowing your search is almost always a good idea.

Another approach is to consult a reputable commercial or noncommercial health site directly. Most have a news section, a library with reference books, frequently asked questions (FAQs), health articles, and an "ask the expert" section. Among the most notable biggies are webmd.com, mayohealth.org, medscape.com, mediconsult.com, and drkoop.com. Among the most reliable sites for research on health issues are Web pages maintained by major foundations such as the American Cancer Society (www.cancer.org), American Heart Association (www.americanheart.org), American Diabetes Association (www.diabetes.org), and Arthritis National Research Foundation (www.curearthritis.org).

The Internet is a great resource—but one that must be used with care. Because anyone can post information on the Internet, it is especially important that you think critically about what you find. Included among these skills is careful observation, asking questions, seeing connections among ideas, and analyzing information and the evidence on which it is based. Here are some tips.

■ *Don't believe everything you find on the Internet.* Be especially wary of information that is posted on Web sites by companies that are trying to sell health-related products. Be a skeptic and assume that their claims are merely advertising.

■ *Evaluate the source of information.* The most reliable sources are scientific journals, medical schools, universities, government agencies such as the National Institutes of Health (NIH), and major health organizations such as WHO, the American Medical Association (AMA), and the American Heart Association (AHA). These sites are reliable because the information they provide is subject to the rules and procedures of the scientific method. This means that postings generally have been carefully evaluated by several reputable research authorities.

■ *Make sure posted information is backed by a credible reference.* Scientists are not persuaded by opinion; they back up their arguments with references to empirical research studies. If a Web site claims that a particular medication, diet, or product reduces the incidence of a particular disease or condition, it should provide a citation from the scientific literature, including the name of the journal or periodical in which the study was published; the names of the authors; and the year, volume, and page numbers of the article. If this information is not provided, there's no way you can verify the accuracy of the information and you should be very skeptical. In some cases, universities, federal health agencies, and other scientific organizations will provide health-related information for the general public without citing the complete reference to the study on which the information is based. The organization's credibility as an authoritative source, however, would obviously permit you to consider such information reliable. Moreover, even when such organizations do not provide complete references, they almost always provide a hyperlink to the original source, or tell you how to request a complete citation.

Exercise: Find at least two Web sites that present conflicting information for a particular health treatment—say, for example, using Saint-John's-wort to improve memory or acupuncture to relieve pain. Then answer the following questions. (Hint: Two sites you might consult as a starting point are www.herbs.org, which boasts a library of 150,000 articles, and www.seanet.com/~vettf/Primer.htm, from the National Council on Reliable Health Information.)

1. What health treatment did you choose to research? Why?
2. What Web sites did you visit? How did you find them?
3. What agencies or groups maintain the Web sites? Are they credible authorities? How do you know?
4. What health claims are made for the product or treatment on each Web site? What evidence is presented to back up these claims? Is the evidence trustworthy?
5. Suppose a friend or relative asks you whether they should try the product or treatment. How should you respond?

---

[2]Some of the more powerful search engines are the ones provided by Yahoo, Infoseek, Microsoft Network, Excite, and Alta Vista, all of which have elaborate health categories with search engines, links, chats, and message boards. Use the category of "health" to locate information on almost any aspect of health, disease, and medicine.

2

Research in Health Psychology

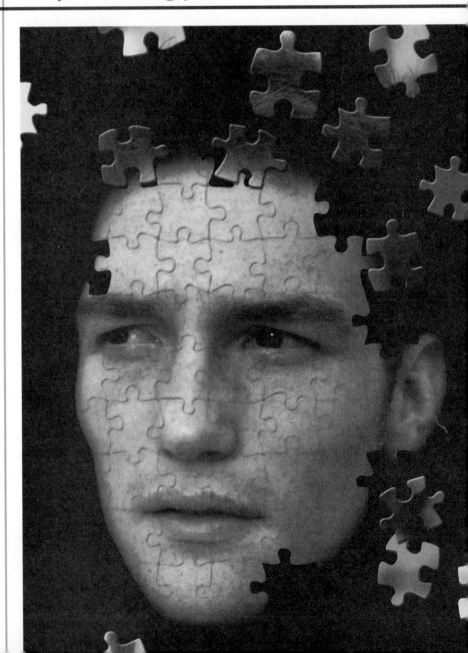

lorence Griffith Joyner, the 38-year-old three-time Olympic gold medalist who revolutionized women's sprinting, died at home on September 21, 1998. Known affectionately as "FloJo," Griffith Joyner not only ran faster than any woman before her, but she also displayed a spectacular flamboyance in the way she ran, dressing in one-legged spandex body suits and sporting 6-inch fingernails. As news of her sudden death spread, the collective reaction was disbelief. How could one of the world's greatest athletes die suddenly at such a young age?

Just 14 years earlier the world had similarly been shocked by the sudden death of another high-profile athlete—running guru Jim Fixx, who helped launch the running boom of the 1970s.

The deaths of these two apparently fit athletes prompted a predictable round of speculation about causes. Little was known of FloJo's medical history at the time of her death, so rumors spread quickly. Because she had shattered previous world records by such a huge margin and retired soon after the Seoul Olympics, some suspected that performance-enhancing steroids or human-growth hormones had damaged her heart. But FloJo passed every drug test she ever took, and toxicology tests showed only that she had recently taken Tylenol and the antihistamine Benadryl. There was no evidence of alcohol, recreational drugs, or performance-enhancing drugs in her body.

After several weeks of public speculation, the coroner finally concluded that FloJo died of suffocation after suffering a seizure while she slept. The seizure was apparently caused by a congenital abnormality of blood vessels in her brain. According to authorities, FloJo had been sleeping face down when the seizure apparently caused her to turn her head into her pillow, restricting the flow of oxygen into her lungs and causing her to become asphyxiated.

Fixx's sudden death while running was, regrettably, taken by many as proof that exercise offered no protection against cardiovascular disease. As with FloJo, however, this quick explanation was simply wrong. For most of his life, Fixx was overweight and consumed a high-fat, high-cholesterol diet. In addition, he had been a chain smoker, smoking three to four packs of cigarettes a day; and a workaholic, working 16 or more hours a day and getting only a few hours of sleep a night. Finally, Fixx was at high risk of heart disease because his father had died from a heart attack at the young age of 43 years. Fixx also had ignored warning symptoms. His fiancée has said that he had complained of chest tightness during exercise and had planned to travel to Vermont to see whether the fresh air there would alleviate his symptoms, which he believed to be due to allergy. The change of air did not help, and Fixx died while running on his first day in Vermont.

Fixx's autopsy showed severe coronary artery disease with near-total blockage of one coronary artery and 80 percent blockage of another. There was also evidence of a recent heart attack. On the day Fixx died, more than 1,000 other Americans succumbed to heart attacks. Had all the facts been available, people would have concluded that, at least with regard to his running, Fixx's death was an anomaly. We would have been provided with overwhelming evidence that heart attacks occur most commonly in males who have high blood pressure, smoke heavily, have high cholesterol levels, and maintain a sedentary lifestyle—a very different conclusion from that which sensationalized the one vivid case of America's "running guru." In fact, many experts believe that Fixx's regular exercise actually allowed him to outlive his father by 9 years.

Most of us read or listen to the news and take the reports at face value. Medical researchers and health psychologists must investigate again and again, comparing situations and symptoms and ensuring that all relevant factors have been considered. To avoid the trap of easy untested expla-nations for the causes of diseases or seemingly unexpected physiological events, researchers must abandon the infor-mal, unsystematic approach to explanation that we use in our everyday thinking and adopt an approach that has proved its ability to find reliable explanations. This ap-proach, called the scientific method, *and how it is applied to answer questions about health psychology are the central topics of this chapter.*

Critical Thinking: The Basis for Research

Health psychology touches on some of the most intriguing, personal, and practical issues of life. Does my family history place me at risk of developing breast cancer? Which of my lifestyle choices are healthy and which are unhealthy? Why can't I quit smoking? The answers to these and countless other vital health questions are by no means obvious. However, every day we seem to be bombarded with new "definitive" answers to these questions. For example, in the 1980s, researchers reported that caffeine leads to higher risk of heart disease and pancreatic cancer. In the early 1990s, they reversed themselves and asserted that limited amounts of caffeine were safe, even during pregnancy. In 1996, they alarmed all mothers-to-be with reports that pregnant women who drink three or more cups of coffee or tea daily were at increased risk of spontaneous abortion, while caffeine drinkers who were trying to conceive were twice as likely as noncaffeine drinkers to delay conception by a year or more. Less than two years later, the "experts" concluded that women who drink more than half a cup of caffeinated tea every day might actually *increase* their fertility. Most recently, researchers announced that the caffeine in coffee might offer protection against Parkinson's disease by reducing the destruction of nerve cells in the brain (Hughes et al., 2000). So, is coffee drinking safe? Which conclusion are you to believe?

At the heart of all scientific inquiry is a skeptical attitude that encourages us to evaluate evidence and scrutinize conclusions. The central feature of this attitude, which is also called *critical thinking,* is a questioning approach to all information. Whether listening to the evening news report, reading a journal article, or pondering a friend's attempt to persuade them to change their minds on a specific issue, critical thinkers ask questions. How did she arrive at that conclusion? What evidence forms the basis for this person's conclusions? Is there an ulterior motive? Can the results of a particular study be explained in another way? Until you know the answers to these and other questions, you should be cautious—indeed, downright skeptical—of all persuasive arguments, including health reports that appear in newspapers and magazines and on television. Learning which questions to ask will make you a much better informed consumer of health information.

The Dangers of "Unscientific" Thinking

In our quest for greater understanding of healthy behavior, we draw on the available information to formulate *cause-and-effect relationships* about our own and other people's behavior. This information derives from our personal experiences as well as from our beliefs and attitudes. Like the quick-reacting reporters who tried to make sense of the deaths of FloJo and James Fixx, in many instances we make a snap judgment, with little attention to its accuracy. Or, we base our explanations on hearsay, conjecture, anecdotal evidence, or unverified sources of information.

As scientists, psychologists have little confidence in the rationality of everyday thought processes and such *commonsense explanations*. These explanations fail because they are based on faulty reasoning. We make observations, and then *often incorrectly* infer the causes for the observed behavior. For example, seeing a lean, statuesque gymnast or dancer, we admire the person's obviously healthy eating and exercise habits, wishing we too could possess such willpower and well-being. When we later learn that the individual is actually anorexic or suffering from a stress fracture related to both poor diet and excessive and exercise-induced skeletal trauma, we are shocked.

One type of faulty reasoning is humorously illustrated in *Motel of the Mysteries,* a tongue-in-cheek book about Howard Carson, a twenty-fifth-century scientist studying the remnants of twentieth-century civilization, which was destroyed when an accidental reduction in postal rates caused all of North America to be buried under tons of third- and fourth-class brochures, fliers, and other junk mail. As Carson unearths a roadside motel, he begins the painstaking attempt to reconstruct twentieth-century life from the artifacts he finds there. Carefully brushing away centuries of earth from a toilet bowl (with a miraculously intact plastic toilet seat), the awestruck scientist leaps to a startling conclusion regarding the purpose of what he believed to be the "Sacred Urn" and "Sacred Collar":

> This most holy of relics was discovered in the Inner Chamber. It was carved from a single piece of porcelain and then highly polished. The Urn was the focal point of the burial ceremony. The ranking celebrant, kneeling before the Urn, would chant into it while water from the sacred spring flowed in to mix with sheets of Sacred Parchment.

Feeling an almost spiritual need to be connected to the ancient ritual of her ancestors, Carson's companion Harriet insisted that she be allowed to wear the Sacred Collar (you'll figure it out), matching headband, magnificent *plasticus* ear ornaments, and exquisite silver chain and pendant (see Figure 2.1).

All cultures develop incorrect beliefs about human behavior. Some people falsely believe that couples who adopt a child are later more likely to give birth to a child of their own and that more babies are born when the moon is full. Be on guard for examples of unscientific psychology in your own thinking.

Figure 2.1

Scientist Wears Sacred Collar and Headband Used in Twentieth-Century American Ritual
This fictional anthropologist's expectations of finding sacred relics from an archaeological excavation of a motel blinded her into thinking the plumbing fixtures must be sacred relics.

Source: *Motel of the Mysteries* (p. 37), by D. Macaulay, 1979, Boston: Houghton Mifflin. Copyright © 1979 by David Macaulay. Reprinted by permission.

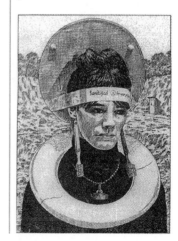

■ **belief bias** a form of faulty reasoning in which our expectations prevent us from seeing alternative explanations for our observations

■ **epidemiology** the scientific study of the frequency, distribution, and causes of a particular disease or other health outcome in a population

Although this example is far-fetched, real-life examples of faulty reasoning abound in all fields of science. In the early twentieth century, for example, thousands of Americans died from *pellagra,* a disease marked by dermatitis (skin sores), gastrointestinal disorders, and memory loss. Because the homes of many pellagra sufferers had unsanitary means of sewage removal, many health experts believed the disease was carried by a microorganism and transmitted through direct contact with infected human excrement. Although hygienic plumbing was certainly a laudable goal, when it came to pinpointing the cause of pellagra, the "experts" fell into one of the faulty reasoning traps that also led Carson astray—failing to consider alternative explanations for their observations. This type of leaping to unwarranted (untested) conclusions is an example of **belief bias,** which explains why two people can look at the same situation (or data) and draw radically different conclusions.

Fortunately, Surgeon General Joseph Goldberger's keener powers of observation allowed him to see that many pellagra victims were also malnourished. To pinpoint the cause of the disease, Goldberger conducted a simple, if distasteful empirical test: He mixed small amounts of the feces and urine from two pellagra patients with a few pinches of flour, rolled the mixture into little dough balls, which he, his wife, and several assistants ate! When none came down with the disease, Goldberger then fed a group of Mississippi prisoners a diet deficient in niacin and protein (a deficiency that he suspected caused the disease), while another was fed the normal, balanced prison diet. Confirming his hypothesis, within months the former group developed symptoms of pellagra, while the latter remained disease free (Stanovich & West, 1998). As this example illustrates, seeking information that confirms preexisting beliefs causes researchers to overlook alternative explanations of observed phenomenon.

Health Psychology Methods

Health psychologists use various research methods in their search to learn how psychological factors affect health. The method used depends in large measure on what questions the researcher is seeking to answer. To answer questions regarding how people cope with AIDS or cancer, for example, a psychologist might observe or ask questions of a large sample of victims of these deadly diseases. On the other hand, researchers investigating whether lifestyle factors contribute to the onset of these diseases might conduct laboratory studies under controlled conditions.

There are three major categories of research methods in psychology—descriptive, observational, and experimental (Table 2.1). Health psychologists also borrow methods from the field of **epidemiology,** which seeks to determine the frequency, distribution, and causes of a particular disease or other health

Table 2.1

Comparing Research Methods

Research Method	Research Setting	Data-Collection Method	Strengths	Weaknesses
Descriptive studies	Field	Case studies, surveys and interviews, naturalistic observation	In-depth information about one person; often leads to new hypotheses	No direct control over variables; subject to bias of observer; single cases may be misleading
Observational studies	Field or laboratory	Surveys, interviews, or observations that reveal a statistical correlation, which allows prediction	Detects naturally occurring relationships among variables	No direct control over variables; cannot determine causality; correlation may mask an underlying extraneous variable
Experimental studies	Usually laboratory	Statistical comparison of experimental and control groups	High degree of control over independent and dependent variables; random assignment eliminates preexisting differences among groups	Artificiality of laboratory may limit the generalizability of results; certain variables cannot be investigated for practical or ethical reasons
Epidemiological studies	Usually conducted in the field	Statistical comparisons between groups exposed to different risk factors	Useful in determining disease etiology, easy to replicate, good generalizability	Some variables must be controlled by selection rather than by direct manipulation; time-consuming; expensive
Meta-analysis	No new data are collected	Statistical combination of the results of many studies	Helps make sense of conflicting reports, replicable	Potential bias due to selection of studies included

outcome in a population. This section describes the research methods employed by psychologists and the tools they use to gather, summarize, and explain their data. The next section will explore the research methods of epidemiologists.

Descriptive Studies

In some cases a researcher wishes only to observe the behavior of an individual or group of people in specific circumstances without investigating a specific variable. This type of observation is frequently the first step in the research loop. In such a study, called a **descriptive study,** the researcher observes and records the participant's behavior, often forming hunches that are later subjected to more systematic study.

■ **descriptive study** research method in which researchers observe and record participants' behaviors, often forming hypotheses that are later tested more systematically; includes case studies, interviews and surveys, and observational studies

■ **case study** a descriptive study in which one person is studied in depth in the hope of revealing general principles

In most cases, descriptive studies are performed in the field, that is, in a real-world setting. Think about how a health psychologist might set about answering the following questions: What are the psychological and physiological health outcomes for victims of a grave national crisis, such as the "ethnic cleansing" of Albanians in Kosovo, who were driven from their homes during the 1999 war with Serbia? How can hospital staff reduce the anxiety of family members waiting to hear whether a loved one who is undergoing surgery will be okay? Does aggressive freeway driving occur more often among certain types of people? Clearly, the answers to each of these interesting questions will not be found in a university research laboratory. Instead, researchers look for answers about the behavior of an individual or a group of people as it occurs in the home, at work, or wherever people spend their time.

Several types of descriptive studies are commonly used: case studies, interviews and surveys, and observational studies.

Case Studies

As we noted in Chapter 1, among the oldest and best-known descriptive methods is the **case study,** in which psychologists study one or more individuals extensively over a considerable period of time in order to uncover principles that are true of people in general. The major advantage of the case study is that it permits a researcher to gather a much more complete analysis of the individual than ordinarily can be obtained in studies involving larger groups.

One of the most celebrated recent case studies involved Senator (and former astronaut) John Glenn of Ohio and his 1999 participation in shuttle mission STS-95. Millions of aging baby boomers watched the liftoff of the shuttle *Discovery* and eagerly followed the progress of the 9-day mission. In an "experiment of one" Glenn was subjected to a barrage of medical tests designed to study the normal effects of aging as reflected in the effects of space flight on an older person. The senator wore one monitor during the flight to measure his heart rhythms and blood pressure and another monitor to gauge his brain waves and eye movements while he was sleeping. He also provided blood and urine samples to determine how quickly his bones and muscles were deteriorating in zero gravity. Among the findings of this study were several intriguing parallels between the effects of space flight and those of aging: Both astronauts and the elderly suffer from loss of muscle and bone mass, sleep disturbances, and impairment of balance. As they analyze Glenn's data, scientists continue to look at characteristics of space flight that might help them understand why the elderly suffer these symptoms.

Although case studies are useful in suggesting hypotheses for further study, they do have one serious disadvantage: Any given person

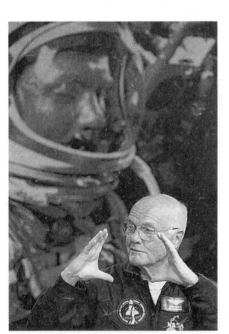

Astronaut-Senator-Septuagenarian John Glenn
In one of the most celebrated recent case studies, Glenn wore a variety of physiological monitors during his 1999 space shuttle mission to reveal possible similarities between the effects of aging and space flight on the body. In the background is a photograph of Glenn in 1962.

AP/Wide World Photos

may be atypical, limiting the "generalizability" of the results. John Glenn is hardly the typical septuagenarian; any findings regarding his body's responses to zero gravity must be subjected to rigorous study involving many typical older people.

In fact, case studies are not only limited in scope but can also be highly misleading. This is especially true given the human tendency to leap quickly from especially memorable (although unrepresentative) case studies to broad conclusions. For example, although researchers had long contended that "runners live longer," many people were quick to discount this view when they heard of jogging guru Jim Fixx's death ("Jim Fixx was a runner, wasn't he? He didn't live as long as my grandfather, who never exercised and was a lifelong cigar smoker."). As this example illustrates, personal experience and especially vivid case studies can often overshadow much stronger scientific evidence.

The point to remember: Individual case studies can provide fruitful leads and direct researchers to other research designs to uncover general truths. They can also be highly misleading.

Interviews and Surveys

Interviews and **surveys** examine individual attitudes and beliefs, but in larger numbers and in much less depth than the case study. In these *self-report measures,* research participants are asked to rate or describe some aspect of their own behavior, attitudes, or beliefs—from what they think of a new reputedly health-enhancing product to their opinion of the results of political elections and the state of the economy.

In an interview, researchers ask a sample of people a series of questions and record their answers to discover typical attitudes or behaviors. Clinical health psychologists also use the interview as they attempt to develop a supportive working relationship with a patient. It permits them to gather self-report and observational data from the patient and his or her family, significant others, and employers. The formality and style of an interview depend on what is being assessed, the personal preference of the researcher, and setting and time constraints. For example, interviews conducted prior to a patient's surgery are often unstructured in order to encourage the interviewer (in this example, a health care practitioner) to remain open to exploring areas of patient concern that may not have been anticipated.

Like interviews, surveys attempt to uncover typical attitudes or behaviors of a large sample of people. Unlike the interview, the survey may not involve a face-to-face confrontation. Surveys are mailed out, printed in magazines, conducted over the phone, or available through the Internet. The most extensive example of survey research is the U.S. Census, which is conducted every 10 years. Other familiar examples are Gallup polls, which tap opinions on a variety of subjects ranging from politics to television-viewing preferences. Surveys are among the most widely used research tools in health psychology because

■ **survey** a questionnaire used to ascertain the self-reported attitudes or behaviors of a group of people

■ **observational study** a nonexperimental research method in which a researcher observes and records the behavior of a research participant

■ **correlation coefficient** a statistical measure of the strength and direction of the relationship between two variables, and thus of how well one predicts the other

they are easy to administer, require only a small investment of time from participants, and quickly generate a great deal of data. In addition, they are invaluable because so many health-related behaviors—such as whether a person smokes, wears seatbelts, exercises, and eats a nutritious diet—stem from personal beliefs about the causes of health and disease.

Surveys are also frequently used by clinical health psychologists for diagnostic assessment as a first step in developing intervention programs. For example, chronic-pain patients may be asked to complete a questionnaire related to their problem that sheds light on previous treatments and the impact of their condition on their daily functioning. Reviewing this information with the patient not only steers the intervention away from treatments that have previously proved to be ineffective but is also a means of developing a supportive working relationship between the patient and the psychologist.

Observational Studies

In **observational studies,** the researcher records the relevant data regarding participants' behavior. Depending on the variable of interest, researchers may measure psychophysiological variables in response to a particular situation or event, or they may observe behavior in a laboratory or in a natural setting. The measurement of psychophysiological variables provides direct information about biological events such as heart rate or the consequences of biological events such as skin temperature. For example, a researcher interested in the physiological effects of everyday hassles on the body might have participants wear a heart rate monitor while commuting to and from school or work during rush hour traffic.

Observational studies may be unstructured or highly structured. Structured observations involve tasks such as role-playing as well as laboratory tests such as observing an individual's response to a very cold stimulus. In unstructured observations, referred to as *naturalistic observation,* the researcher attempts to be as unobtrusive as possible in observing and recording the subjects' behaviors. For example, a health psychologist might observe family members visiting a parent in a nursing home in an effort to gain insights into how various individuals cope with the acute stress of watching a beloved parent unable to fend for himself or herself. These observations may be audiotaped or videotaped and then quantified through rating methods or frequency scores.

Correlation

When descriptive studies suggest that one variable tends to accompany another, researchers say there is a *correlation* between them. To determine whether there is a correlation, or a tendency of two variables to accompany one another, researchers calculate a **correlation coefficient,** a statistical measure of the relationship between the two variables.

Correlation coefficients are calculated by a formula that yields a number, or *r value*, ranging from −1.00 to +1.00. The sign (+ or −) of the coefficient indicates the direction of the correlation (positive or negative). A positive correlation is one in which one variable increases in direct proportion to increases in another variable. In contrast, when two variables are negatively correlated, as one goes up, the other tends to go down. Notice that a correlation's being negative says nothing about the strength or weakness of the relationship between the variables; a negative correlation simply means the variables are inversely related. The researcher's ability to predict is no less with a negative correlation than it is with a positive correlation.

The absolute value of the correlation coefficient (from 0 to 1.00, regardless of whether the number is positive or negative) indicates the strength of the correlation, which determines how accurately a researcher can predict one variable from a known value of another. Correlation coefficients that are closer to 1.00 (either negative or positive) indicate stronger correlations than do coefficients that are closer to 0. However, coefficients that are relatively small may signify a reliable relationship between two variables if they are based on a very large number of observations. In most cases, however, such small correlations indicate that it is impossible to predict scores on one variable from knowledge of scores on the other variable.

Suppose, for example, that you are interested in the relationship between the percentage of body fat and systolic blood pressure. Perhaps you are testing your theory that a lean build lowers a person's risk of cardiovascular disease by reducing hypertension, a documented risk factor. To test your theory with an experiment would obviously be impossible. You would have to manipulate the body fat variable and then record blood pressure. Although measuring blood pressure is certainly possible, manipulating body fat is clearly not (or at best it is unethical). So, instead, you calculate a correlation coefficient. Richard Cooper, Charles Rotimi, and Ryk Ward (1999) did just that, measuring body mass index, or BMI (a measure of a person's weight-to-height ratio) and prevalence of hypertension in a large sample of participants of African descent from several countries. Figure 2.2 on page 52 displays a **scatterplot** of the results of their study. Each point on the graph represents two numbers for a sample of subjects from one country: average BMI and prevalence of hypertension.

A scatterplot (also called a scatter diagram) gives a good visual indication of two aspects of the relationship between two variables. The *strength* of the relationship is revealed by how closely together the points are clustered along an imaginary line. In a *perfect correlation,* the points in a scatterplot align themselves in a perfectly straight line. The second aspect of the relationship, *direction,* is what we mean when we say that a correlation is "positive" or "negative" (also called *inverse*). In a positive correlation the points in the scatterplot sweep upward, from the lower left to the upper right. In a negative, or inverse, correlation, the points sweep downward, from upper left to lower right. Notice

■ **scatterplot** a graphed cluster of data points, each of which represents the values of two variables in a descriptive study

Figure 2.2

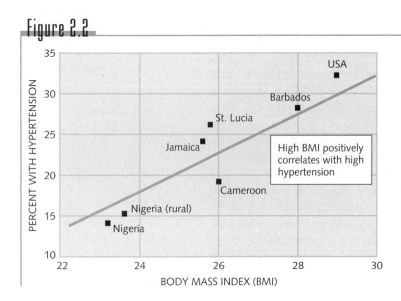

The Relationship between Body Mass Index and Hypertension in People of African Descent

Body mass index, or BMI, measures a person's weight-to-height ratio; BMIs over 25 are generally considered a sign of being overweight. In a study comparing key locations in the westward African migration, researchers found that as BMI increased, so did the prevalence of hypertension. The scatterplot reveals a strong positive correlation between BMI and hypertension. The solid line confirms this, showing an upward slope and fairly tight clustering of the data points.

Source: Based on data in "The Puzzle of Hypertension in African-Americans," by R. S. Cooper, C. N. Rotimi, and R. Ward, February 1999, *Scientific American*, p. 59.

in Figure 2.2 that the relationship appears to be both fairly strong (the points fall roughly along a straight line) and positive (the points sweep upward from lower left to upper right).

It is tempting to look at the Cooper study as a true experiment and draw cause-and-effect conclusions from the results. However, even when two variables are correlated, one does not necessarily cause the other. Maybe blood pressure is elevated in people with a high percentage of body fat because they tend to exercise less than people with a leaner build. In other words, correlations do not rule out the possible contributions of other hidden variables. Obviously, though, there can be no causation unless there is first correlation. In health psychology, correlations identify relationships that later may be subjected to closer study with experimental studies.

Another limitation of correlation is that even when the value of the correlation coefficient is large, it does not mean that it fully explains the health-related trait under consideration. Let's return to our example of body fat and blood pressure. The data depicted in Figure 2.2 represent a correlation coefficient of approximately r = +0.67, a fairly strong positive correlation. Assume for the moment that a high percentage of body fat *does* cause blood pressure to rise. But is every case of high blood pressure accompanied by a high percentage of body fat? We certainly would not expect body fat to be the *only* risk factor for high blood pressure. So, we would calculate an *explained variance*, a statistical measure of the percentage of variation in one variable that is accounted for, or explained, by another. This statistic is computed as the square of the correlation coefficient. Thus, in our example, the correlation coefficient of r = +0.67 tells us that body mass index explains roughly 45 percent of the variability in hypertension observed in our sample ($0.67 \times 0.67 = 0.45$). This means that about 55 percent of the variability in hypertension remains unexplained and must be the result of other variables.

Experimental Studies

Although descriptive studies and correlations are useful, neither can indicate the causes of the behaviors we observe. To pinpoint causal relationships, researchers conduct experiments. Considered the pinnacle of the research methods, experiments are commonly used in health psychology to investigate the effects of health-related behaviors (such as exercise, diet, and so on) on an illness (such as heart disease).

In contrast to descriptive studies, experiments test hypotheses by systematically manipulating (varying) one or more **independent variables** (the "causes") while looking for changes in one or more **dependent variables** (the "effects") and *controlling* (holding constant) all other variables. By controlling all variables except the independent variable, the researcher ensures that any change in the dependent variable is *caused* by the independent variable rather than by another extraneous variable.

Experiments often involve testing the effects of several different *levels* of the independent variable on different groups. For example, in an experiment testing the level at which noise (an independent variable) begins to cause stress (the dependent variable), participants in three different groups might be asked to complete a checklist of behavioral and psychological symptoms of stress (an operational definition of the dependent variable) while listening to 10-, 25-, or 50-decibel noise over headphones (different levels of the independent variable *noise*).

Typically, the researcher randomly assigns a sample of participants to two or more study groups and administers the condition or treatment of interest (the independent variable) to one group, the *experimental group,* and a different or no treatment to the other group, the *control group.* **Random assignment** is crucial because assigning research participants to groups by chance ensures that the members of all of the research groups are similar in every important aspect except in their exposure to the independent variable. For instance, random assignment would help prevent a large number of participants who were hypersensitive to noise from ending up in one group, thereby potentially masking the true effects of the independent variable.

Health psychology is somewhat unique among the subfields of psychology in that it studies a variety of variables as cause and effect. As possible "causes," health psychologists examine internal states (such as optimism and feelings of self-efficacy), overt behaviors (such as exercise and cigarette smoking), and external stimuli (such as a stressful job or a therapeutic program to promote

■ **independent variable** the factor in an experiment that an experimenter manipulates; the variable whose effect is being studied

■ **dependent variable** the behavior or mental process in an experiment that may change in response to manipulations of the independent variable

■ **random assignment** assigning research participants to groups by chance, thus minimizing preexisting differences among the groups

relaxation). As possible "effects," they investigate overt behaviors (such as coping reactions to stressful employment), biological traits (such as blood pressure or cholesterol levels), and psychological states (such as anxiety levels). Although correctly identifying the independent variable and the dependent variable is sometimes difficult, it is helpful to think of each person as a complex system that is influenced by information from the environment as well as feedback from his or her own behavior. Considered in this way, the "causes" may be stimuli that stem from external events as well as from internal biological and psychological states. Similarly, the "effects" may be overt behaviors as well as internal biological or psychological states.

Consider the following experimental study in health psychology. As we will explain more fully in Chapter 7, people often suppress their emotions, particularly negative emotions, as a way of regulating their mood and reducing stress. But is emotional suppression healthy? In a study designed to examine the short-term impact of thought suppression on the body's immune system, Keith Petrie, Roger Booth, and James Pennebaker (1998) randomly assigned 65 first-year medical-school students from the University of Auckland to one of four groups: emotional writing with and without thought suppression (the two experimental groups) and nonemotional writing with and without thought suppression (the two control groups).

As you can see in Figure 2.3, the immune systems of students in the control and experimental (emotional) writing groups who did not have to suppress their thoughts showed little effect, as measured by white blood cell count. In

Figure 2.3

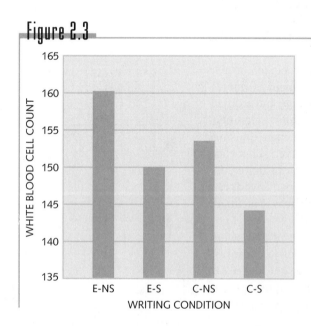

Results of the Thought Suppression Study

Participants in the control and experimental writing groups who did not have to suppress their thoughts after writing (C-NS and E-NS) had a higher total white blood cell count than did their counterparts who were instructed not to think about their writing topics (C-S and E-S).

Source: "The Immunological Effects of Thought Suppression," by K. J. Petrie, R. J. Booth, and J. W. Pennebaker, 1998, *Journal of Personality and Social Psychology, 75*(5), pp. 1264–1272.

contrast, thought suppression resulted in a significant decrease in the level of white blood cells, suggesting that the act of thought suppression produced a measurable effect on the immune system, whether the suppressed thoughts were emotional or unemotional.

Ex Post Facto Designs

When health psychologists cannot manipulate the variable of interest, they have other options: ex post facto designs, animal research, or qualitative research. An **ex post facto design** is similar to an experiment in that it involves two or more comparison groups. Unlike an experiment, an ex post facto design uses groups that differ from the outset on the variable under study (the *subject variable*). In addition, because the subjects in the *comparison* group are not equivalent to those in the experimental group at the start of the study, it is not a true experiment, and no cause-and-effect conclusions can be drawn. (Notice that we refer to a comparison group rather than a control group; this is because the group naturally differs from the experimental group and no variable is being controlled for.)

To illustrate an ex post facto design, suppose researchers wish to investigate—as they often do—the effect of a sedentary lifestyle on the development of cardiovascular disease; for ethical reasons, they cannot use humans in a standard experiment, so they must turn either to animals or to an ex post facto design. The subject variable is a sedentary lifestyle, the group consists of people who by their own admission get little or no exercise, and the comparison group would be people who exercise regularly. The health psychologist would accumulate data on the participants' base levels of daily physical activity over a defined period of time, then identify separate "active" and "sedentary" groups. These comparison groups would be followed for a period of years, with the researcher regularly reassessing the groups' activity levels and cardiovascular health.

Other subject variables used in ex post facto designs are age, gender, ethnicity, and socioeconomic status. In addition, researchers clearly cannot manipulate variables to produce extreme environmental stress, physical abuse, or natural disasters. In such cases, the researcher must wait for such events to occur and then study the variables of interest. Furthermore, like correlations, ex post facto designs do not allow researchers to determine cause and effect.

Life-Span Studies

In Chapter 1, we discussed the benefits of the life-span perspective in health psychology. Obviously, health psychologists working from the life-span perspective are concerned with the ways in which people change or remain the

ex post facto design a study in which the comparison groups differ on the variable of interest at the outset of the study

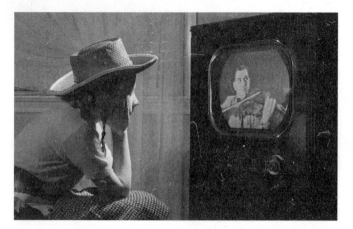

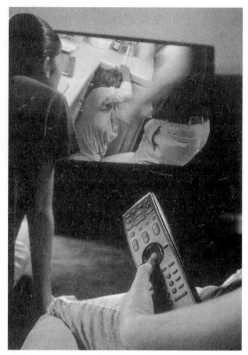

Cohort Differences

Researchers conduct longitudinal studies in order to rule out cohort effects. People born in the 1950s clearly have had different experiences from those born in the 1990s. Having been raised during one of the most peaceful periods of the twentieth century, the perspective and attitude of 1950s children are likely to be very different from those of children being raised today, where real as well as imagined violence is an everyday occurrence. In the 1950s, television was primarily a source of entertainment; today, it gives children a front-row view of domestic violence or even of wars taking place thousands of miles away. *(left)* © Bettmann/Corbis; *(right)* Ron Chapple, FPG International

■ **cross-sectional study** a study comparing representative groups of people of various ages on a particular dependent variable

■ **cohort differences** differences between comparison groups due to the impact of members having been born and raised at different moments in history

same over time. To answer questions about the process of change, researchers use two basic research techniques, *cross-sectional* and *longitudinal studies.*

In a **cross-sectional study,** the researcher compares representative groups of people of various ages to determine the possible effects of age on a particular dependent variable. Suppose we are interested in determining whether different age groups are more (or less) likely to eat a well-balanced, low-fat diet. An important consideration in cross-sectional research is that the various age groups be similar in other ways that might conceivably affect the characteristic being investigated (for example, in their ethnicity and socioeconomic status). To the extent that the groups are similar, any differences that exist among them can be attributed to age-related processes.

Matching different age groups for all subject variables other than age is difficult to do. Despite their best efforts, researchers using a cross-sectional design are well aware that the outcomes of such studies often produce **cohort differences** that reflect the impact of participants having been born and raised at a particular moment in history. A *cohort* is a group of people who share at least one demographic characteristic, such as age or socioeconomic status, in common. A cohort is similar to a generation, but the number of years separating two cohorts often is less than the number of years separating two adjacent generations.

How can a researcher rule out possible cohort effects and be sure that age, rather than some other variable, is the reason for differences in the characteristics of the different age groups? One way is to conduct a **longitudinal study,** in which a single group of individuals is observed over a long span of time. This allows information about a person at one age to be compared to the same information about the person at another age, revealing how this person changed over time.

Suppose you are interested in studying age-related changes in how people cope with stress. If you choose a cross-sectional approach, you might interview a sample of, say, 25 adults at each of five ages—for example 20, 30, 40, 50, and 60 years—and gather information about the ways in which they handle job stress, family quarrels, financial problems, and so forth. On the other hand, if you choose a longitudinal study to explore the same span of years, you (or, more likely, the researchers who will continue your study 40 years from now) would interview a group of 20-year-olds today and again when they are 30, 40, 50, and 60 years of age. The longitudinal study thus eliminates confounding factors such as differences in the types of stress encountered.

As this example makes clear, longitudinal studies are the "design of choice" from the life-span perspective. However, they have several drawbacks (Cairns & Cairns, 1994). For one thing, such studies are by definition very time-consuming and expensive to conduct. More important, over the span of years of longitudinal studies, it is common for some participants to drop out because they move away, die, or simply fail to show up for the next scheduled interview or observation. When the number of dropouts is large, the results of the study may become skewed. Another potential problem is that people who remain in longitudinal studies may change in the characteristic of interest but for reasons that have little to do with their advancing age. For example, our study of age-related coping responses to stress may show that older people cope more adaptively by not allowing everyday hassles to get to them. But suppose a large number of the participants dropped out of the study midway (or perhaps died of stress-related illnesses!) and those who remained tended to be those employed in low-stress occupations. Can the researcher conclude that age has produced the results?

Although both cross-sectional and longitudinal studies allow researchers to examine change over time, each method has flaws. For this reason, the two methods are sometimes combined to produce a **cross-sequential study** (also called a time-sequential design [Schaie, 1996]). In such a design, different age groups are tested initially (a cross-sectional study) and then retested later at various ages (a longitudinal study). Using a cross-sequential design to study age-related coping with stress, we would begin by selecting and testing subjects in each of the five age groups. We would then follow these subjects

longitudinal study a study in which a single group of people is observed over a long span of time

cross-sequential study a life-span research design that combines longitudinal and cross-sectional methods by studying groups of people of different ages over time

■ **heritability** the amount of variation in a trait among individuals that can be attributed to genes

■ **monozygotic (MZ) twins** genetically identical twins who develop from a single fertilized egg that splits in two

■ **dizygotic (DZ) twins** fraternal twins who develop from separate fertilized eggs

longitudinally, adding younger subjects along the way. That is, 10 years from now, our youngest cohort would be 30. To fill out the comparison groups we would select a new cohort of 20-year-old subjects. The cross-sequential design thus allows researchers to combine the advantages of cross-sectional and longitudinal studies in teasing apart the impact of age from cohort effects on health-related behaviors and traits.

Behavior Genetics Research Techniques

A fundamental question in life-span research is to what extent is our health—including our health behaviors and attitudes—shaped by our heredity (our nature) and by our life history (our nurture)? In an effort to answer questions about nature-nurture interactions, health psychologists and behavioral geneticists often estimate the **heritability** of a trait, that is, the amount of variation in a trait among a group of individuals that can be attributed to genes. In doing so, they employ two principal methods: twin studies and adoption studies.

Twin studies compare monozygotic twins with dizygotic twins. In both cases, the twins are raised in similar environments. However, **monozygotic (MZ) twins** develop from a single fertilized egg that splits in two and are genetically identical; **dizygotic (DZ) twins** develop from separate eggs and are genetically no more similar than nontwin siblings (they share half their genes). Because monozygotic twins are genetically identical, any observed difference between them must be attributable to environmental factors. In contrast, any observed differences between dizygotic twins can be attributed to a combination of environmental and genetic factors. Thus, differences between monozygotic and dizygotic twins raised in the same environment suggest a genetic influence. For example, a person whose identical twin has Alzheimer's disease has a 60 percent chance of also developing the disease. When a person's fraternal twin has the disease, the risk drops to 30 percent (Plomin, 1997). Such a difference suggests that genes play a considerable role in predisposing Alzheimer's disease.

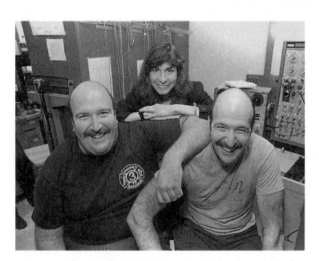

Monozygotic Twins

Because monozygotic twins develop from a single fertilized egg and are therefore genetically identical, any observed difference between them must be attributable to environmental factors. Gerald Levey and Mark Newman, shown here being questioned about physical and psychological similarities, were separated at birth and were not reunited until age 31. Although they were raised in different homes, they exhibited many similar characteristics—for example, both had chosen the same vocation, firefighting.

AP/Wide World Photos

However, we must be very careful in interpreting twin studies. A strong argument can be made that identical twins also share a more nearly identical environment than fraternal twins do. They are of the same sex, often are dressed alike, and are frequently confused with each other. To overcome this argument, researchers prefer to compare the characteristics of identical twins raised together with those of identical twins raised apart. Unfortunately, because of the time, expense, and the relatively infrequent occurrence of such arrangements, only a small number of such studies have been reported.

Adoption studies provide a way for researchers to eliminate the problem of similar environments. When a child is placed for adoption, two groups of relatives are created: genetic relatives (biological parents, brothers, and sisters) and environmental relatives (adoptive parents and siblings). Determining whether an adopted child more closely resembles his or her biological or adoptive parents with regard to a specific characteristic or behavior can be helpful in determining the effect of genetic inheritance in a different environment.

The strongest evidence of a genetic influence comes from the convergence of evidence from family studies, twin studies, and adoption studies. For example, if behavior geneticists discover that hypertension runs in families at a rate that is higher than would be expected by chance, that monozygotic twins are significantly more similar than dizygotic twins in their susceptibility to the disorder, and that adopted children resemble their biological parents more than their adopted parents in their susceptibility to hypertension, then a considerable genetic influence is suggested.

As you'll see, health psychologists are increasingly concerned with behavior genetics because family history is emerging as an important risk factor for a variety of chronic illnesses. At the same time, however, researchers are discovering that some genes may actually help *protect* our health, such as in the case of the lucky 1 to 5 percent of people of European descent who inherit a gene that appears to block the HIV-1 virus from infecting body cells.

Validating the Research

In any scientific investigation, there is always the possibility that researchers' procedures, expectations, and biases will influence their findings. This section discusses this potential problem and describes the steps researchers take to ensure that their results are as valid as possible. The specific steps a researcher takes will, of course, depend on the research method used.

Eliminating Expectancy Effects

When scientists have specific expectations about the results of their research, those expectations can actually influence the outcome. This is known as an **observer-expectancy effect.** Study participants, too, can influence the results of a study by behaving as they think they are expected to behave. This type of bias is called a **participant-expectancy effect.**

observer-expectancy effect
the outcome of an investigation is influenced by the researcher's expectations

participant-expectancy effect
the behavior of study participants is affected by their expectations, which influences the outcome of the study

■ **research bias** the outcome of an experiment is influenced by some extraneous factor other than the independent variable

■ **double-blind study** a technique designed to prevent observer- and participant-expectancy effects in which neither the researcher nor the subjects know the true purpose of the study or which subject is in which condition

In a classic study of participant expectancy (Roethlisberger & Dickson, 1939), researchers tried to increase worker productivity at an electric plant by shortening or lengthening coffee breaks, changing lighting conditions, and providing or taking away bonuses. Remarkably, no matter how conditions changed, productivity increased, indicating that the workers were simply responding to the knowledge that they were being studied.

Expectancy effects are a classic example of **research bias,** which occurs whenever the outcomes of a study are influenced by some nonrandom, or extraneous, factor other than the independent variable. Thus, research bias can occur in any of the research methods just discussed, as you will see.

Expectancy effects are especially likely to occur in survey research because obtaining valid, unbiased data from an interview or a questionnaire is not easy. In fact, surveys are more vulnerable to bias than most other research methods. For example, observer-expectancy effects can be obtained simply by altering the wording of a question. These *wording effects* occur when even a subtle change in the way in which a question is phrased affects respondents' answers. For instance, in a national survey, fully two-thirds of those surveyed responded that they felt there was too much sex and violence in the media and agreed that there should be "more restrictions on what is shown on television" (Lacayo, 1995). However, when essentially the same idea was reworded, less than one-third (27 percent) of them approved of "government censorship" of TV sex and violence.

A participant-expectancy effect can occur in survey research when respondents who do not have firm opinions on the topic in question make up answers just to satisfy the researcher. Or they give answers that they think the researcher expects or that they believe will make them appear "normal" or "good." For example, consider how you would respond to a probing questionnaire or face-to-face interview about your sexual behavior. Isn't it likely that you might not be entirely forthcoming in responding to certain embarrassing questions?

Despite these potential pitfalls, well-designed health surveys can be extremely valuable in allowing health psychologists to quickly and efficiently collect a large amount of data from a large group of people. There is a lesson here. Before accepting conclusions based on survey results, think critically: Could wording effects or subject-expectancy have biased the answers?

Similarly, expectancy effects can affect observational studies. Although researchers strive to be as unobtrusive as possible so that the participants will behave candidly, it is easier said than done. Particularly in a laboratory setting, participants may not act normally, instead behaving as they think a "normal" person would act or as they believe the researcher expects, or hopes, them to act.

Experimental studies provide the best tools for reducing research bias. To reduce the possibility of observer-expectancy effects, the person who actually collects data from subjects is often "blind," that is, unaware of either the purpose of the research or of which subjects are in which condition. This is a *single-blind study*. To further ensure that observer- or subject-expectancy effects do not contaminate the study, a **double-blind study** may be conducted. In such a case, neither the researcher nor the participants know the true purpose of the study or which participant is in which condition.

Avoiding Biased Samples

Researchers take great care to ensure that the participants they select constitute an unbiased **representative sample** that accurately reflects all the members of the group (the *population*) of individuals under investigation. The easiest way to select a large representative sample is to make it a random sample or a stratified sample.

In a *random sample,* each member of the entire population is equally likely to be questioned. Suppose, for instance, that a health psychologist wants to know the average age at which cigarette smokers took their first puff. Because she cannot survey every smoker in the population, she selects every tenth name on an alphabetical list of smokers. From her sample's self-reported age of first smoking, she calculates an average from which she makes an inference to smokers in general. And herein lies a possible pitfall: Survey respondents may not be representative of the population from which they are drawn. Virtually every type of study—from surveys to experiments—is subject to this type of *sampling error,* that is, to selecting participants who do not represent the population of interest.

To avoid sampling error, researchers generally select a *sample size* large enough that a few atypical cases will not distort the sample's depiction of the population as a whole. Suppose, however, that our health psychologist's sample consisted of only five smokers, one of whom did not begin smoking until age 40. In such a small group, even if the other four participants all began smoking before age 16, the one extreme score would skew the average substantially. With a larger sample, of, say, 100 smokers, one atypical case would not seriously distort the results.

However, small samples are sometimes unavoidable, even desirable. For example, if you wanted to measure students' opinions on risky sexual behavior at your college or university, you would want to make sure that all groups with a vested interest were equally represented, including women and men, first-year students, second-year students, members of various ethnic minorities, and students majoring in various subject areas. For this reason, selecting students to best represent the entire student body is best done by making them a **stratified sample.** In this method, particular subgroups (or "strata") within a population are identified, and then a representative sample is drawn from each subgroup.

Ensuring that a sample is representative is often a difficult task. For this reason, some researchers are a bit lax, particularly when conducting survey research. The lesson: Before accepting conclusions based on survey results, think critically. Is the sample on which the results are based representative of the entire population? How was the sample selected?

Avoiding Bias in Measurement

Ever since the nineteenth century when Sir Francis Galton attempted to equate intelligence with the size of people's heads, psychologists have led the way in

representative sample an unbiased subset of research subjects that accurately reflects the population of individuals under investigation

stratified sample a representative sample in which particular subgroups (or "strata") within a population are equally represented

standardization the process of establishing group norms on a psychometric test that serve as a source of comparison for evaluating an individual's performance

reliability a measure of the degree to which a psychometric test yields dependably consistent results

developing valid, reliable measures of human traits, behaviors, and abilities. In fact, one of psychology's most important contributions to epidemiology and behavioral medicine is its ongoing refinement of *psychometrics*—the science of measurement.

In general, two kinds of psychometric tests are used in clinical health psychology: broadband and narrow-focus measures (Belar & Deardorff, 1996). *Broadband measures* assess general measures of personality, whereas *narrowband measures* assess general psychological constructs, experiences, or symptoms. Health psychologists also use health-specific tests to diagnose particular health-related problems. Several psychometric tests will be described as relevant in different chapters.

For a psychometric assessment or some other measure to be useful and widely accepted, it must pass three tests: standardization, reliability, and validity.

Standardization

To say that a test has been **standardized** means that it was constructed with specific rules so that it is administered in exactly the same way every time (Anastasi, 1997). A standardized test includes scripted instructions that are to be read verbatim, precise timing of test segments, lists of allowed materials, and so forth. To standardize a test, researchers first give it to a large representative sample of people, called a *standardization group.* Doing so establishes group means, percentiles, standard deviations, and other scores against which individual scores can be compared. Knowing your raw score on a particular test would tell you next to nothing without a means of comparing it with other people's scores. Standardization thus establishes population averages, or *norms,* for tests that permit the researcher and the test-taker to interpret performance.

The reason for standardization is that any variation in scores on a test—say, the scores of a person prior to a health treatment and again following a health treatment or the scores of one group of subjects as compared to those of another—can be attributed to variations in the variable of interest (the treatment or subject variable differentiating the groups) and not to bias from variations in the test conditions. For example, after surveying a sample of smokers about the age at which they began smoking, our health psychologist might administer a standardized personality test to her sample to determine whether their traits match those of the standardization group.

Reliability

Comparing your score to those of the standardization group won't mean much unless the test is reliable. The **reliability** of a psychometric test is the extent to which it yields dependably consistent results. To ensure that a test is reliable, researchers have several techniques at their disposal. First, they may retest participants using parallel forms of the same test. If the two sets of scores correlate, the test is said to have *alternate form reliability.* Second, researchers may compare the test group's scores on one half of the test with their scores on the other half (*split-half reliability*). Third, researchers may compare scores on two or more separate administrations of the test to the same group (*test-retest reliability*). Finally, for tests that require the researcher to assess a person's behavior, he or she could compare the ratings of two or more judges observing the same behavior or phenomenon (*inter-rater reliability*).

Except for inter-rater reliability, reliability is customarily expressed as a correlation, indicating the degree to which the two sets of scores agree. High reliability correlation coefficients (such as +0.8 or +0.9) indicate that test-takers' scores were nearly the same on two separate administrations of the test, on alternate forms of the test, or on the two halves of one test. Inter-rater reliability is typically expressed in terms of the percentage of agreement among the observers' ratings. High percentages (such as 80 percent or 90 percent) indicate that the test's rating criteria elicit very similar judgments when different individuals administer the test.

Validity

Even if a test is reliable and produces consistent results, it may not have **validity.** There are three basic types of validity: content, predictive, and construct. *Content validity* is the degree to which the test actually measures what it is supposed to measure. If you used foot size to measure people's musical aptitude, chances are your data would have high reliability (consistency) but very low content validity. The issue of content validity is especially important in health research because many conventional psychological tests were developed for use with physically healthy people and thus may possess low content validity for medical problems.

Psychologists evaluate the content validity of a test in terms of how well it agrees with some independent *criterion.* Selection of a valid criterion is often difficult in health psychology. For example, what would be an appropriate criterion for assessing whether an obese patient is precisely following a prescribed weight-loss program consisting of dietary modification, moderate exercise, and certain medications? Weighing the person each day has the advantage of being a direct, objective measure and most likely would be included in the criterion. However, body weight may not be appropriate as the *only* criterion because the person may be able to lose weight by means other than those prescribed (for example, through crash dieting, excessive exercise, or sweat sessions in a sauna).

Tests are also evaluated in terms of how well they predict a future behavior or condition. In health psychology, *predictive validity* expresses how well

validity a measure of the degree to which a test actually measures what it is supposed to measure (content validity), predicts a future behavior or condition (predictive validity), or measures a particular construct that cannot be directly observed (construct validity)

a psychometric test predicts which participants in a sample will develop a particular disease or remain disease-free. For example, a variety of scales have been used to measure hypertension, cholesterol level, and other cardiovascular disease risk factors and to predict future morbidity or mortality among a sample of subjects (see Chapter 8). When initially healthy people who score high on such a test eventually have higher rates of heart disease or fatal heart attacks than those with low scores, the test is said to have predictive validity.

Construct validity refers to the extent to which a test measures some health-related concept—for example, perceived stress, Type A behavior, or defensive coping. Concepts such as these are constructs because they cannot be directly observed; instead, they must be inferred from other measures of behavior (such as a score on a test and other behaviors known to be linked to a particular disease). Health psychologists establish construct validity by checking a test against other measures with a known track record. For example, a researcher may use a known physiological index of anxiety (such as an increase in blood pressure or lowered skin resistance) obtained in a laboratory setting to evaluate the construct validity of a test of perceived stress.

Ruling Out Chance as a Factor

In a typical study, researchers test the hypothesis that the health outcomes or performance of two groups of subjects differ because of differential exposure to a specific independent variable. Even when a research study reveals that such a difference does in fact exist, it is still possible that the difference occurred purely by chance. For instance, in any group of people, some will tend to perceive greater personal control over the events in their lives than others do. If a researcher divides this group into separate experimental and control groups, it is quite possible that, by chance alone, more of one type ends up in one group than in the other. Suppose the researcher now compares the two groups on their perseverance in following a prescribed medical regimen that differs only in the type of verbal instructions given to the participants. If, at the end of the study, one group has followed the regimen more closely than the other, it could well be that the chance assignment of subjects, rather than the independent variable (the type of instructions), accounts for the results. To determine whether research results are simply due to chance, researchers apply a test of *statistical significance*. When group averages are based on many observations (sample size), when they are consistent within each group (sample variability), and when the difference between groups is large, researchers conclude the difference is *statistically significant*. In general, for a difference to be statistically significant, the odds that it has occurred by chance must be less than 1 in 20, or .05 (5 percent).

Epidemiological Research

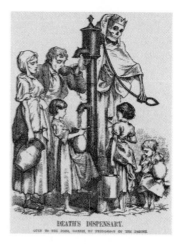

DEATH'S DISPENSARY.
OPEN TO THE POOR, GRATIS, BY PERMISSION OF THE PARISH.

The Pump Handle—Symbol of Effective Epidemiology
Since John Snow's pioneering efforts to eradicate cholera in nineteenth-century London, the pump handle has remained a symbol of effective epidemiology. Today, the John Snow Pub, located near the site of the once troublesome pump, boasts of having the original handle. This cartoon was published in 1866 in the London periodical *Fun* with the caption "Death's Dispensary, Open to the Poor, Gratis, By Permission of the Parish."

The Granger Collection, New York

When researchers consider the role of psychological and behavioral factors in health, among the first questions to be asked are: Who contracts which diseases, and what factors determine whether a person gets a particular disease? Such questions are addressed by the field of epidemiology.

Although health record-keeping can be traced back to ancient Greece and Rome (see Chapter 1), epidemiology was not formalized as a modern science until the nineteenth century, when epidemic outbreaks of cholera, smallpox, and other infectious diseases created grave public health threats. In many instances, these diseases were conquered largely as a result of the work of epidemiologists whose painstaking research gradually pinpointed their causes.

The modern era of epidemiology began with the work of John Snow, an English epidemiologist and founding member of the London Epidemiological Society (Frerichs, 2000). During the 1848 outbreak of cholera in London, Snow laboriously recorded each death throughout the city, eventually noticing that death rates were nearly ten times higher in one particular southern district of the city than elsewhere. Digging deeper, Snow discovered that in some instances, residents on one side of a residential street were stricken with the disease far more often than were their neighbors on the opposite side of the street. Like a good detective solving a mystery, Snow kept looking for clues until he found something different in the backgrounds of the high-risk groups. Polluted drinking water turned out to be the culprit. Although two separate water companies supplied most of the residents of south London, their boundaries were laid out in patchwork fashion so that residents living on the same street often received their water from different sources. Those unfortunate enough to be customers of one company were supplied with water from a highly polluted area of the Thames River; customers of the second company also received their water from the Thames but from a much cleaner area. By comparing the death rates with the distribution of customers of polluted and nonpolluted water, Snow inferred that the cholera came from an as-yet unidentified "poison" in the polluted water.

One incident during this epidemic became legendary. In the neighborhood at the intersection of Cambridge Street and Broad Street, the incidence of cholera cases was so great that the number of deaths reached over 500 in 10 days. After investigating the site, Snow concluded that the cause was centered on the Broad Street pump. After the doubtful but panicky town officials ordered the pump handle removed, the number of new cases of cholera dropped dramatically. Although the bacterium responsible for transmitting cholera would not be discovered for another 30 years, Snow devised an obvious intervention that broke the citywide epidemic: He simply forced the city to shut down the polluted water main.

- **morbidity** disease; as a measure of health, the number of cases of a specific illness, injury, or disability in a given group of people at a given time

- **mortality** death; as a measure of health, the number of deaths due to a specific cause in a given group of people at a given time

- **incidence** the number of new cases of a disease or condition that occur in a specific population within a defined time interval

- **prevalence** the total number of diagnosed cases of a disease or condition that exist at a given time

Since Snow's time, epidemiologists have described in detail the distribution of many different infectious diseases. In addition, they have identified many of the *risk factors* linked to both favorable and unfavorable health outcomes. In a typical study, epidemiologists measure the occurrence of a particular health outcome in a population, then attempt to discover why it is distributed as it is by relating it to the specific characteristics of people and the environments in which they live. For example, some forms of cancer are more prevalent in certain parts of the country than in others. By investigating these geographical areas, epidemiologists have been able to link certain cancers with the toxic chemicals found in these environments.

In discussing epidemiological findings, researchers employ several terms. The rate of **morbidity** refers to the number of cases of a specific illness, injury, or disability in a given group of people at a given time. The rate of **mortality** refers to the number of deaths due to a specific cause (such as heart disease) in a given group at a given time. Morbidity and mortality are outcome measures that are usually reported in terms of *incidence* or *prevalence*. **Incidence** refers to the number of new cases of a disease, infection, or disability that occur in a specific population within a defined time interval. An example is the number of cases of whooping cough during the previous year. **Prevalence** is defined as the *total* number of diagnosed cases of a disease or condition that exist at a given time. It includes both previously reported cases and new cases at a given moment in time. To express incidence and prevalence as percentages of the population being studied, epidemiologists use the following equations.

$$\text{Prevalence rate per 1,000} = \frac{\text{Number of cases of a disease present in the population at any given time}}{\text{Number of persons in the population at a specified time}} \times 1,000$$

$$\text{Incidence rate per 1,000} = \frac{\text{Number of new cases of a disease during a specified period of time}}{\text{Number of persons exposed to risk during that period of time}} \times 1,000$$

Thus, if an epidemiologist wished to know how many people overall have hypertension, she would examine prevalence rates. If, however, she sought to determine the frequency with which hypertension is diagnosed, she would look at incidence rates. Incidence and prevalence are obviously closely related.

To clarify the distinction between incidence and prevalence, consider Figure 2.4, which compares the incidence and prevalence of heart disease and AIDS between 1982 and 1994. As a result of greater public awareness of this epidemic disease, due in no small measure to epidemiological research, the incidence and prevalence of AIDS have decreased.

Although incidence and prevalence provide important information, scientists have recently developed measures that more accurately reflect the impact

Figure 2.4

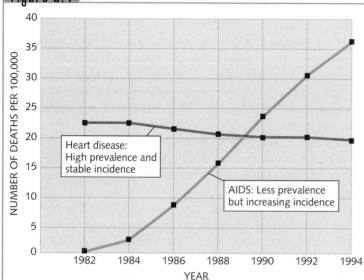

U.S. Death Rates for AIDS and Heart Disease in People Aged 25 to 44 Years
Between 1982 and 1988, AIDS was less prevalent than heart disease because it claimed fewer lives. However, the rapidly increasing incidence rate of AIDS meant that between 1990 and 1994, in this age group AIDS caused more deaths than heart disease did. Heart disease, on the other hand, has a high prevalence but a stable, or gradually decreasing, incidence.

Sources: *National Vital Statistics Reports*, July 2000, 48(11), p. 26; *National Vital Statistics Reports*, November 1998, 47(9), p. 26.

of diseases not only in shortening life but also in undermining the quality of life. Thus scientists now estimate the number of **disability-adjusted life years (DALYs)** lost in nonfatal conditions. DALYs indicate how many healthy years of life are lost to an illness, premature death, or disability. To calculate total DALYs for a given condition, the researcher estimates years of life lost and years lived with a disability of known severity and duration, then adds those numbers together to determine the total years of healthy life lost. For instance, if a 60-year-old is disabled with Parkinson's disease, then each year might be judged to provide only half the expected quality of life; if that person dies 20 years later, 10 DALYs would be considered lost. The estimated percentage of all DALYs lost to all diseases and disabilities in a population represents the **burden of disease** for that particular condition. Thus, the burden of disease takes the average number of years of life lost for each disease, factors in an estimate of how much a disabling (but not immediately fatal) disease reduces the quality of life, and expresses that total (in years) as a percentage of the number of years lost by the entire population due to all diseases.

Objectives

Epidemiologists use several research methods to obtain data on the incidence, prevalence, and *etiology* (origins) of disease. Like research methods in psychology, epidemiological research follows the logical progression from description to explanation to predication and control in the service of three fundamental

- **disability-adjusted life years (DALYs)** a measure of a population's health that indicates how many years of full vitality are lost to a particular disease or disability

- **burden of disease** a measure of a population's health that indicates the percentage of all DALYs lost due to all causes accounted for by a particular disease or disability

objectives (Frerichs, 2000): to pinpoint the etiology of a particular disease in order to generate hypotheses; to evaluate the hypotheses; and to test the effectiveness of specific preventive health interventions.

To determine the origins of a disease, epidemiologists first attempt to describe the overall health status of a population by counting current cases of an illness (prevalence) or measuring the rate at which new cases appear (incidence). They then analyze this information in order to generate hypotheses about differences between subgroups of the population that are responsible for the disease, just as Snow found differences between people who received their water from polluted sources and those who received it from unpolluted sources. A more recent example comes from efforts of epidemiologists to discern the etiology of hypertension in African-Americans (see Diversity and Healthy Living).

Once epidemiologists have identified the origins of a disease or health condition and generated hypotheses about its causes, they evaluate those hypotheses. For example, some doctors have noted that women who smoke are more likely than men who smoke to develop lung cancer. Could hormonal differences, or some other factor linked to gender, allow the cellular damage that cigarette smoking causes to occur more rapidly in women than in men? Only a large-scale epidemiological study can answer this type of question, and, indeed, epidemiological studies have reported this very finding (Prescott et al., 1998).

A closely related goal of epidemiological research is to test new hypotheses by attempting to predict the incidence and prevalence of diseases. If the predictions are borne out by the epidemiological data, researchers gain confidence that their understanding of the etiology of the disease is increasing.

The final goal of epidemiological research is to determine whether the intervention programs created as a result of research on the incidence and prevalence of a disease are effective. For example, AIDS intervention programs such as needle-exchange and safer-sex initiatives must be tested in a large group of high-risk subjects to determine their effectiveness in reducing the incidence of new cases of AIDS in targeted groups (see Chapter 11).

Research Methods

To achieve their purposes, epidemiologists use a variety of research methods, including *retrospective studies, prospective studies,* and *experimental studies.* Like research methods in psychology, each epidemiological method has its strengths and its weaknesses.

Retrospective and Prospective Studies

Like the cross-sectional studies described earlier, **retrospective studies** compare a group of persons who have a certain disease or condition with a group

■ **retrospective study** a "backward-looking" study in which a group of people who have a certain disease or condition are compared with a group of people who are free of the disease or condition, with the purpose of identifying background risk factors that may have contributed to the disease or condition

of people who do not; those with the condition of interest are considered "cases" and those without are "controls." The major distinction between cross-sectional and retrospective studies is that the former compare characteristics that are present in the cases and controls at the time of the study, while the latter attempt to determine whether the characteristics were present in the cases in the past, usually by a review of records.

Retrospective studies, looking backward in time, attempt to reconstruct the characteristics or conditions that led to the current health status of people who have a particular disease or condition. For example, retrospective research played an important role in identifying the risk factors that lead to AIDS. Initially, researchers observed a sharp increase in the incidence of a rare and deadly form of cancer called Kaposi's sarcoma among gay men and intravenous drug users. By taking extensive medical histories of the men who developed this cancer, epidemiologists were able to pinpoint unprotected anal sex as a common background factor among the first men to die from this deadly form of cancer. This was possible even though the AIDS virus, HIV, was not isolated for some years to come (see Chapter 11).

In contrast, **prospective studies** look forward in time to determine how a group of individuals changes or how a relationship between two or more variables changes over time. Identical to longitudinal research in life-span developmental psychology, a prospective epidemiological study begins by identifying a group of healthy participants and testing and retesting them over a period of time to determine whether a given condition, such as sedentary living or a high-fat diet, is related to a later health outcome, such as cancer or cardiovascular disease. Health psychologists frequently conduct prospective studies to pinpoint the risk factors that relate to various health conditions.

For example, there is some evidence that smoking may contribute to breast cancer, a cause of great concern considering the recent rise in smoking rates among women (see Chapter 8). In one prospective study that followed healthy women over a 6-year period, researchers found that women who smoked were 1.26 times more likely to die of breast cancer than were women who had never smoked. Among those who smoked two or more packs a day, the relative risk rose to 1.74, whereas those who smoked half a pack or less had a relative risk of only 1.19. In addition, women who started smoking before age 16 were 60 percent more likely to die from breast cancer than those who started after age 20 (Calle, Miracle-McMahill, Thun, & Heath, 1994).

Experimental Studies

Although both retrospective and prospective studies are helpful in identifying the various risk factors for illnesses, like the descriptive and observational methods in psychology, neither study can demonstrate causation in health outcomes. One exception is an *experimental prospective study*. Although most prospective studies are observational in nature, sometimes—when researchers

■ **prospective study** a longitudinal study that begins with a healthy group of subjects and follows the development of a particular disease in that sample

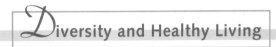

Diversity and Healthy Living

Hypertension in African-Americans: An Epidemiological "Whodunit"

Although almost 25 percent of all Americans experience rising blood pressure with age, for African-Americans the situation is much more serious: 35 percent suffer from hypertension that contributes to heart disease, stroke, and kidney failure. This disease accounts for 20 percent of the deaths among blacks in the United States—twice the number for whites.

In their never-ending effort to understand and control disease, epidemiologists have recently questioned the popular explanation that the disparity between blacks and whites is due to an "intrinsic genetic susceptibility." Scientists often invoke evolutionary theory to explain why a certain ethnic or racial group is at greater risk for a particular health outcome. The argument goes as follows: As a result of natural selection, some members of the group in question (and their genes) survived while others did not. If the survivors primarily mate with members of the same population, their genes are not mixed with those of other groups, and the resulting genetic traits begin to appear with increasing frequency among group members.

Some researchers have suggested that the voyages in slave ships caused exactly the kind of environmental pressure that would select for a predisposition to high blood pressure. During the voyages many died, often from "salt-wasting conditions" such as diarrhea, dehydration, and infection. Thus, the ability to retain salt might have had a survival value for Africans transported to America against their will. Today, of course, salt retention is *not* adaptive, linked as it is to hypertension.

Until recently, researchers have found it very difficult to abandon such conventional hypotheses about race. However, some now suggest that this type of easy explanation may mask underlying factors that may more directly contribute to hypertension, that is, that hypertension can arise through complex interactions among external factors (such as diet and the stress of economic problems), internal factors (such as the biological systems that regulate blood pressure), and genetic factors.

In 1991, Richard Cooper and his colleagues began a research project that concentrated on the African diaspora, the forced migration of West Africans between the sixteenth and nineteenth centuries caused by the slave trade. Knowing that the incidence and prevalence of hypertension in rural West Africa is among the lowest of any place in the world, the researchers attacked the problem on several fronts. First, they compared the prevalence of hypertension in West Africa with that in people of African descent in other parts of the world. The researchers found that people of African descent in other parts of the world, especially in the United States and the United Kingdom, have much higher incidences of hypertension. This suggests that something about the way of life of European and American blacks—rather than genes—was altering their susceptibility to high blood pressure.

To pinpoint an explanation, the researchers conducted widespread testing of people of African descent in Nigeria, Cameroon, Zimbabwe, St. Lucia, Barbados, Jamaica, and the United States. In addition to monitoring blood pressure, the researchers focused on high-salt diet, obesity, activity level, and other common risk factors for hypertension. After several years of investigation, the researchers concentrated on Africans in Nigeria, Jamaica, and Chicago as representative of three key points in the westward movement of Africans from their native lands. The findings were startling: Only 7 percent of those in rural Nigeria had high blood pressure, compared to 26 percent of black Jamaicans and 33 percent of black Americans. In addition, several risk factors for high blood pressure became increasingly prevalent as testing moved westward across the Atlantic. As we saw earlier (see Figure 2.2, page 52), body mass index, a measure of weight relative to height, rose steadily from Africa to Jamaica to the United States, along with hypertension. Being overweight and the associated lack of exercise and poor diet explained nearly 50 percent of the increased risk for hypertension that African-Americans face, as compared with Nigerians.

The researchers' data question the assumption that rising blood pressure is an unavoidable hazard of modern life for people of all skin colors. The human cardiovascular system evolved in a rural African setting in which obesity was uncommon, salt intake was moderate, the diet was low in fat, and high levels of physical activity were common. Because the life of subsistence farmers in Nigeria has not changed much, their blood pressure hardly rises with age and cardiovascular disease is virtually unknown. This group functions as an epidemiological control group against which researchers can test hypotheses about what causes elevated blood pressure in those of African descent.

For instance, blood pressure is higher in the nearby city of Ibadan, Nigeria, than in neighboring rural areas, despite only small differences in the overall level of obesity and salt intake. The researchers suspect that other variables, such as psychological and social stress and lack of physical activity, may help account for the increase. In North America and Europe, those of African descent face a unique kind of stress—racial discrimination. The effect of racism on blood pressure is, of course, difficult to establish, but it is worth noting that the average blood pressure of blacks in certain parts of the Caribbean, including Cuba and rural Puerto Rico, is nearly the same as that of other racial groups. Could it be that the relationships among races in these societies impose fewer insults on the cardiovascular system than those in the continental United States do?

Researchers are now also considering physiological factors related to kidney and liver functioning. They have found that many hypertensive people of African descent have elevated levels of *angiotensinogen II,* a hormone that increases blood pressure by causing blood vessels to constrict excessively, thereby increasing the risk for hypertension. Further, they have discovered that the average level of angiotensinogen for each sample studied increased significantly from Nigeria to Jamaica to the United States, paralleling increases in the rate of hypertension.

As a final piece to the puzzle, the researchers have found that some people carry variations of the gene that produces angiotensinogen. One form of this gene, known as 235T, is linked with higher levels of angiotensinogen and hypertension among people of European descent. Does this mean that hypertension among those who inherit this gene is entirely genetic in origin? Surprisingly, the researchers found that the 235T gene is twice as common among African-Americans as it is among European Americans, but blacks with this form of the gene are not at increased risk for hypertension compared with blacks who do not carry the gene (see Figure 2.5). This unexpected finding reveals how nurture may interact with nature to alter physiology and produce hypertension. But it also highlights the pitfalls of making sweeping generalizations. No single gene or environmental factor can explain why hypertension occurs and why it is so common in African-Americans. An individual with a given mix of genes may be susceptible to high blood pressure but only in a certain setting. To understand hypertension in African-Americans, scientists need to reevaluate the meaning of ethnic and racial divisions of the species.

Figure 2.5

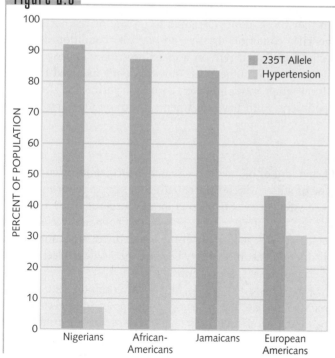

Incidence of the 235T Gene and Hypertension among Different Ethnic Groups
Epidemiologists expected that people who carried the 235T gene would have a higher incidence of hypertension. Surprisingly, 235T is common in certain groups (such as Nigerians), in whom hypertension is exceedingly rare. These findings suggest that both nature and nurture play a role in the development of high blood pressure.

Source: Redrawn from data in "The Puzzle of Hypertension in African-Americans," by R. S. Cooper, C. N. Rotimi, and R. Ward, February 1999, *Scientific American,* p. 62.

randomized clinical trial a true experiment testing the effects of one independent variable on individuals (single-subject design) or on groups of individuals (community field trials).

are able to select equivalent groups and manipulate independent variables—they can approximate a true experiment. Obviously, however, people who volunteer for prospective studies cannot always be placed randomly into experimental and control conditions, even if there are valid scientific reasons for doing so. For these and other practical and ethical considerations, experimental prospective studies are rare. To pinpoint cause and effect, health psychologists generally rely on "true" experiments.

There are three types of experimental studies in epidemiology: natural experiments, laboratory experiments, and clinical trials. In a natural experiment, a researcher attempts to study an independent variable under natural conditions that approximate a controlled study. Similar to the ex post facto design in psychological research, natural experiments are most common in health psychology when researchers compare two similar groups; one group is exposed (with their permission) to a health hazard (such as nicotine, occupational noise, or risky sexual behavior) and the other is not.

In a laboratory experiment, the researcher directly manipulates one independent variable rather than comparing groups of individuals who self-select their own exposure to a particular independent variable. Like experiments in psychology, epidemiological laboratory experiments use random assignment to ensure that the experimental and control groups are similar in every important way except the level of the independent variable to which they are exposed. Unfortunately, random assignment is not always possible. People cannot be randomly assigned to personality categories, such as introverts and extraverts. Nor can they be randomly assigned to disease or risk-factor categories, such as the HIV condition or the "no-seatbelt" condition. For this reason, health psychologists often rely on a *quasi-experimental design* (*quasi* means "resembling"), in which subjects are not randomly assigned to treatment conditions. In all other ways, however, a quasi-experimental design resembles a true experiment. Both have treatments, outcome measures, and so forth.

Clinical Trials

The so-called gold standard of biomedical research is the **randomized clinical trial.** From this type of study, which is essentially identical to the true experiment, researchers can safely draw conclusions about cause-and-effect relationships. Clinical trials test the effects of one or more independent variables on individuals (single-subject design) or on groups of individuals (community field trials). This distinction becomes blurry because the single-subject design, although it focuses on individuals, uses groups.

Although many variations are possible, the most common clinical trial involves measurement of a baseline (starting point) level of the condition followed by a measure of the effectiveness of the treatment. For example, in testing the effectiveness of an analgesic drug on migraine headaches, the researcher first records a baseline measure of the subject's pretrial level of headache pain, perhaps by having the subject regularly self-report using a pain scale. Once the baseline establishes a pretreatment reference value in the dependent variable (the subject's pain), treatment (the drug), which is the independent variable, is administered and the dependent measure is once again assessed. If the treatment data show improvement over the baseline data, the researcher concludes that the treatment is likely to be effective in the future. To be sure that the treatment itself, rather than some extraneous factor (such as the mere passage of time), produced the improvement, the researcher removes the medication, watches for the baseline condition to return, and then observes whether the symptoms reappear. If they do, the researcher can be even more confident in accepting the hypothesis that the drug produces a significant (clinical) improvement.

Clinical trials can also involve groups of individuals. In the most common type of design involving groups, pretreatment baseline measures of the dependent variable are taken, and the subjects are then randomly assigned to either an experimental group that receives the treatment of interest, such as a new headache medication, or a control group that receives a placebo (see Chapter 1). Also known as a *between-groups design* (because the effects of the independent variable on the dependent variable are compared between two or more groups), differences in the groups can be attributed to differences in the treatment—that is, the independent variable, assuming outside variables have been properly controlled.

Alternatively, clinical trials may involve repeated observations of a single group of subjects. An example of this *within-subjects design* would be a group of subjects pretested for headache pain, then treated with an analgesic and retested. In this procedure, each participant's self-report during treatment is compared with his or her own self-report during the baseline phase, making, as it were, each subject his or her own control.

In the final procedure, a *community field trial,* researchers compare people in one community to those in another. For example, children in one school might receive extensive educational information on the benefits of always wearing a helmet when bicycling, skateboarding, or using inline skates. A control group of children from another school would not receive the educational campaign.

Meta-Analysis

Traditionally, when a researcher began investigating a phenomenon, such as the relationship between cigarette smoking and breast cancer, the first step was a thorough review of the relevant research literature. Although the *literature review* has a long and noble history in the annals of science, such reviews are qualitative in nature and therefore subject to bias in how they are interpreted. No matter how skilled the person reviewing the literature may be, the way various results are interpreted essentially remains a subjective process, in which the reviewer's own biases, beliefs, overconfidence, and so forth may influence the outcome.

■ **meta-analysis** a quantitative technique that combines the results of many studies examining the same effect or phenomenon

To assist epidemiologists (and health psychologists) in sifting through the sometimes dozens of research studies that pertain to a particular hypothesis, statisticians have developed an observational procedure called **meta-analysis,** a quantitative technique that combines the results of studies examining the same effect or phenomenon. Just as an experiment examines the consistency in the responses of individual participants, a meta-analysis determines the overall consistency of individual studies that address the same topics. A meta-analysis does not replace individual studies; rather, it provides a systematic procedure for summarizing existing evidence about focused research hypotheses that already appears in the health psychology literature.

Meta-analysis has a number of advantages. First, by pooling the results of many studies, meta-analysis often reveals significant results simply because combined studies have more participants. Second, demonstrating that a finding holds up across different studies conducted by different researchers at different times and places and with different participants gives researchers much greater confidence in its validity. Finally, like good experiments, meta-analysis is subject to replication. That is, other researchers are able to repeat the series of statistical steps and should reach the same conclusions.

Some epidemiologists have criticized meta-analyses of nonexperimental studies, arguing that under certain circumstances, they may magnify spurious findings (Shapiro, 1994). Another possible pitfall is that the researcher still must decide which studies to include, how to group studies when operational definitions of variables differ, and other important factors (Friedman & Booth-Kewley, 1987).

Inferring Causality

No matter which research method they use, epidemiologists can infer a cause-and-effect relationship between a particular risk factor and a particular disease or other adverse health outcome only if certain basic conditions are met (Beaglehole, Bonita, & Kjellstrom, 1993). *The research evidence must be consistent.* As is true of all research findings, before we accept epidemiological conclusions, studies that report an association between a risk factor and a health outcome must have been replicated. When evidence is not entirely consistent (as is often the case in health research), a convincing majority of the evidence must support the alleged association. If not, causality cannot be inferred.

■ *The alleged cause must have been in place before the disease actually appeared.* Although obvious, the importance of this criterion cannot be overstated. For example, if a woman starts smoking after her breast cancer is diagnosed, smoking obviously could not have caused the disease. You would be surprised at how often this seemingly obvious criterion is overlooked.

- *The cause-and-effect relationships must make sense.* This means that the explanation must be consistent with known physiological findings. In the case of the relationship between smoking and breast cancer, for example, a wealth of other evidence suggests several plausible biological links between smoking and other forms of cancer, including that the chemicals in tobacco smoke increase cellular damage caused by free radicals in the body.

- *There must be a systematic, dose-response relationship between a possible risk factor and a health outcome. Dose-response relationships* are systematic associations between a particular independent variable, such as cigarette smoking, and a particular dependent variable, such as breast cancer. Such relationships pinpoint the relative risk associated with specific *levels* of an independent variable. Thus, the morbidity rate of breast cancer is highest among women who smoke heavily, somewhat less for women who smoke moderately, less still for light smokers, and lowest among women who do not smoke.

- *The strength of the association between the alleged cause and the health outcome (relative risk) must suggest causality.* **Relative risk** is statistically defined as the ratio of the incidence or prevalence of a health condition in a group exposed to a particular risk factor to the incidence or prevalence of that condition in a group not exposed to the risk factor. Any relative risk value above 1.0 indicates that the exposed group has a greater relative risk than the unexposed group. For example, a relative risk of 2.0 indicates that the exposed group is twice as likely to develop a health outcome than an unexposed group. Conversely, a relative risk of 0.50 means that the incidence or prevalence rate of the condition in the exposed group is only half that of those in the unexposed group.

- *The incidence or prevalence of the disease or other adverse health outcome must drop when the alleged causal factor is removed.* Although dose-response and relative-risk relationships are necessary to infer causality, they are not sufficient. Before we can infer that smoking causes breast cancer, we must have evidence that women who quit smoking have a reduced risk of this disease. Recent research has, in fact, shown this very thing to be true, thus meeting our fifth criterion (Manjer et al., 2000). When all conditions are met, epidemiologists are able to infer that a causal relationship has been established, even when a true experiment cannot be conducted.

relative risk a statistical indicator of the likelihood of a causal relationship between a particular health risk factor and a health outcome; computed as the ratio of the incidence (or prevalence) of a health condition in a group exposed to the risk factor to its incidence (or prevalence) in a group not exposed to the risk factor

Animal and Qualitative Research

Experimentation involving health outcomes is somewhat unique because of the ethical considerations of such studies. Humans who might be randomly assigned to the control group, for example, cannot be prevented from exercising, nor could those in the experimental group be forced to do so.

In addition, for both practical and ethical reasons, not all variables of interest in health psychology can be manipulated in human subjects. For this reason, researchers sometimes turn to nonhuman subjects to investigate the effects of variables such as diet and exercise on health outcomes.

Although the majority of research studies we have examined to this point have used humans, the use of animals for research and testing in health psychology is fairly common. As in other areas of research, notably medicine and pharmacology, animal studies are often used in health psychology as an initial step in exploring hypotheses, which are then carried over to research with humans.

One important research area that frequently involves animals seeks to answer questions about the genetic basis of high-risk behaviors. For example, when Neil Grunberg, Jerry Singer, and I (Straub, Singer, & Grunberg, 1986) sought to determine the extent to which genes influenced aggressiveness and *atherosclerosis* (narrowing of the coronary arteries)—two possible risk factors in promoting cardiovascular disease—we chose Mongolian gerbils as our laboratory subjects. Gerbils were selected for two reasons. First, they have cardiovascular systems that are excellent models of the human cardiovascular system. Second, gerbils have a very short gestation period (28 days, on average), allowing us to breed the animals selectively over several generations in a relatively brief period of time.

At the start of the study we used several standard behavioral tests to identify the most naturally aggressive and least naturally aggressive male and female gerbils out of a sample of 24 (half female and half male). Afterward, males and females of each type were paired as mates and allowed to reproduce. When their offspring reached maturity, they received the same battery of behavioral tests as their parents had, were classified according to their aggressiveness, were paired with mates of similar temperament, and so forth. We continued this regimen of testing and selective breeding for several generations, allowing the animals to live out their lives normally, with no further interference. As individual animals died, an animal pathologist conducted an autopsy on each gerbil, identifying the cause of death and measuring the extent of atherosclerosis in each subject's coronary arteries. After four generations, gerbils in the most aggressive group were found to have significantly greater narrowing of their coronary arteries than animals in the least aggressive group. This study demonstrated that heredity might play a role in the development of both aggressiveness and coronary disease in animals. In addition, the study suggested that similar results might be found in humans, if one is willing to generalize from gerbils to humans.

Over the past several decades, researchers have used animals to investigate numerous health topics ranging from the genetic basis of disease, obesity, and addiction to the physiological impact of stress, secondhand smoke, and other cancer-causing agents. In many cases, animal research is the only practical way to answer an important question. For example, selective breeding studies such as the one described above enable researchers to study genetic influences on a trait over several generations in a period of only a few years. The same study with humans, if it could be done, would require 100 or more years.

Animal studies have been important in moving health psychology forward on a theoretical level, playing key roles in the development of the biopsychosocial model and the emerging field of psychoneuroimmunology. For example, the discovery that the immune system was subject to basic laws of learning occurred in a study with laboratory rodents (Ader, Felten, & Cohen, 2001). This hallmark research alerted psychologists to previously unanticipated connections among the immune system, the brain, and the endocrine system.

Despite these apparent advantages, the use of animals in research remains a sensitive and controversial topic for both ethical and scientific reasons. Some ask whether it is justifiable to use animals to advance our understanding of our own species, even when doing so may alleviate suffering among people, lead to cures for disease, and prolong life. Some animal rights activists argue that animal researchers use distorted logic by justifying the scientific validity of animal models of human health conditions because of our similarities, while rationalizing the moral validity of animal research by calling attention to our differences (Ulrich, 1991). Other critics suggest that animal research not only is wasteful but can also be downright misleading (Barnard & Kaufman, 1997).

In a striking example of the sometimes inadequate reliability of animal models, scientists in the 1960s concluded from numerous animal studies that inhaled tobacco smoke did not cause lung cancer. Although they did find that tar from smoke painted on animals' skin caused tumors to develop, these results were considered irrelevant to cigarette smoking. For years, tobacco industry lobbyists pointed to these studies to deny that tobacco use caused cancer. Human epidemiological studies later provided conclusive evidence of the tobacco–cancer link. As it turns out, cancer research is especially sensitive to physiological differences between humans and animals. Mice, rats, and many other animals used in medical research produce proportionately much greater levels of vitamin C and other antioxidants than do humans. In addition, certain carcinogens—including tobacco's benzo(a)pyrene—appear to have a special affinity for human genes.

In the place of animal studies, some critics point to better epidemiological methods, such as clinical intervention trials, along with new imaging tools for examining neuroanatomy and physiology noninvasively. The emerging science of *molecular epidemiology,* which relates genetic, metabolic, and biochemical factors to epidemiological data on disease incidence and prevalence, also promises to improve researchers' ability to pinpoint the causes of human disease. Even with these techniques, however, animal studies remain a valuable research tool for both health psychologists and epidemiologists.

In this chapter, we have introduced a variety of research methods for studying biological, psychological, and social factors. It is natural to ask, Which one is best? Some researchers might quickly answer that the laboratory experiment is most desirable because only in such studies are the variables of interest directly manipulated while all other variables are controlled. But we have also seen that some questions of vital interest to health psychologists (as well as patients in need of more effective health interventions) do not lend themselves to experimentation for ethical and/or practical reasons. Moreover, experiments are often criticized for being artificial and having little relevance to behavior in the real world.

Increasingly, researchers are combining experimental and nonexperimental methods in order to make their investigations more comprehensive (Murray & Chamberlain, 1999). For example, suppose a researcher was interested in determining whether an educational campaign about safer sex behaviors would induce college students to modify their behavior. Conceivably, the researcher might design an experiment in which a randomly assigned group of students who received educational materials related to this issue (the independent variable) was compared to a control group that received unrelated material in terms of their stated intentions to practice safe sex. However, the researcher would surely want to know whether the educational campaign was equally effective with women, men, members of various ethnic minorities, and so forth. After reading this chapter, it should be obvious that subject variables such as these cannot be manipulated experimentally. Together, however, experimental and nonexperimental methods complement one another and, most important, give health psychologists a large tool kit with which to study their subject.

This chapter has presented you with the basic tools of the health psychology trade—critical thinking that guards against faulty everyday reasoning, and research methods that guide researchers in their quest for valid and reliable answers to health-related questions. Armed with this background, you are now ready to begin to ask those questions.

Summing Up

Critical Thinking: The Basis for Research

1. Our everyday thinking is prone to bias for a variety of reasons, including reaching snap conclusions.

Health Psychology Methods

2. Descriptive studies, which observe and record the behavior of participants, include case studies, interviews and surveys, and observational studies.

3. Observational studies take research a step further by determining whether lawful relationships exist among the variables of a study. The strength and direction of a relationship between two sets of scores are revealed visually by scatterplots and statistically by the correlation coefficient. Correlation does not imply causality.

4. In an experiment, a researcher manipulates one or more independent variables while looking for changes in one

or more dependent variables. Experiments typically compare an experimental group, which receives a treatment of interest, with a control group, which does not.

5. When health psychologists study variables that cannot be manipulated, they use an ex post facto design. In this design subjects are selected on the basis of age, gender, ethnicity, or some other subject variable; assigned to groups; and then followed.

6. In a cross-sectional study, researchers compare representative groups of people of various ages to determine the possible effects of age on a particular dependent variable. Cross-sectional studies may also reflect cohort differences stemming from cohort members having been raised at a particular moment in history.

7. In a longitudinal study, a single group of individuals is followed over a long span of time. To correct the problem of subjects dropping out over the lengthy span of years such studies require, researchers have developed a cross-sectional study, in which different age groups are tested initially and then retested later at various ages.

8. Behavior genetics uses methods such as twin and adoption studies to pinpoint the heritability of specific characteristics and disorders. Monozygotic twins develop from a single fertilized egg that splits in two. Dizygotic twins develop from separate eggs. Differences between monozygotic and dizygotic twins raised in the same environment suggest a genetic influence.

Validating the Research

9. Researchers take several steps to ensure that their findings are valid. To reduce the possibility of observer- and subject-expectancy effects, researchers avoid bias in the wording of survey questions and use double-blind controls.

10. To avoid biased samples, researchers select large, representative samples or, in some cases, stratified samples to ensure that key subgroups are represented. To prevent ambiguity in how variables are defined, researchers provide an operational definition of each variable. Doing so also allows other researchers to replicate their studies.

11. To avoid bias in measurement, psychologists use psychometric tests, which must have group norms and be administered the same way each time (standardization). They must also yield dependably consistent results (reliability) and measure what they claim to measure (content validity), predict what they claim to predict (predic-

tive validity), and measure a construct that cannot be observed (construct validity).

12. To rule out chance as a factor in research findings, researchers apply a test of statistical significance. Such a test takes into account several factors, especially sample size, sample variability, and the measured difference between groups being compared.

Epidemiological Research

13. Epidemiological research studies measure the distribution of health outcomes, seek to discover the etiology (causes) of those outcomes, and test the effectiveness of specific preventive health interventions. Among the commonly used epidemiological statistics are morbidity, mortality, incidence, prevalence, disability-adjusted life years (DALYs), and burden of disease.

14. Epidemiologists use several basic research designs. In a retrospective study, comparisons are made between a group of people who have a certain disease or condition and a group that does not. In contrast, prospective studies look forward in time to determine how a group of people changes or how a relationship between two or more variables changes over time. There are also several types of experiments in epidemiology, including laboratory experiments, natural experiments, and randomized clinical trials.

15. Meta-analysis analyzes the data from already published studies, statistically combining the size of the difference between the experimental and control groups to enable researchers to evaluate the consistency of findings.

16. In order to infer causality in epidemiological research, research evidence must be consistent and logically sensible and exhibit a dose-response relationship. In addition, the alleged cause must have been in place before the health outcome in question was observed and must result in a reduced prevalence of the condition when removed.

Animal and Qualitative Research

17. When it is unethical to use humans for experimentation, animals serve as valuable research subjects. Animals have provided important insights into such health topics as the genetic basis of disease, obesity, and addiction and the physiological impact of stress and secondhand smoke. Many health psychologists now combine experimental and nonexperimental studies for more accurate results.

Key Terms and Concepts

Health Psychology on the World Wide Web

http://psych.hanover.edu/APS/exponent.html — The American Psychological Society's guide to research on the Internet. Visiting this site will not only introduce you to the wide range of research questions studied by psychologists but will also give you an idea of what it's like to be a research participant.

http://www.criticalthinking.org — The Web site of the Critical Thinking Community; includes a collection of articles and chat room discussions focused on the background and theory of critical thinking.

http://www.stat.uiuc.edu/~stat100/cuwu — Champaign-Urbana Web University; a hands-on Web site with activities to enhance your understanding of basic statistical principles, including correlation coefficients.

http://www.apa.org/science/animal2.html — APA Web page discussing animal research in psychology and how it continues to be essential for answering some fundamental questions.

Critical Thinking Exercise

Exercise and Mood

Now that you have completed Chapter 2, take your learning a step further by testing your critical thinking skills on this scientific reasoning exercise.

Lauren, who teaches aerobics at a local health club, believes that regular aerobic exercise improves people's mood and overall sense of well-being. She announces her hunch to one of her classes of longtime aerobics enthusiasts, many of whom respond enthusiastically to her request for volunteers to participate in a one-month test of her hypothesis. Ten volunteers from the class are assigned to the experimental group and instructed to complete a mood questionnaire each day after their weekly aerobics class. For the control group, Lauren recruits volunteers from a group of people waiting to go in to see a movie at the theater next to the health club. After describing the purpose of her study, Lauren asks for volunteers, promising them five free movie passes for their participation. She then arranges for the 10 control subjects to return to the theater one day each week for the next month, during which time they watch a documentary film that lasts exactly the same amount of time as the aerobics class. After each film the control subjects also complete the mood questionnaire. After the one-month period, Lauren is delighted to find that the average mood rating of the subjects in the exercise group is substantially higher than that of the participants in the control group.

1. What type of research study is this? In your answer, be sure to include the method, research setting, and data-collection method.

2. What is Lauren's hypothesis?

3. What is the independent variable? How is it operationally defined?

4. What is the dependent variable? How is it operationally defined?

5. List three variables that are controlled in this study.

6. List several variables that are not controlled and explain how they might have affected Lauren's findings.

7. Was this study a valid test of Lauren's hypothesis? Explain your reasoning.

3

Biological Foundations of Health and Illness

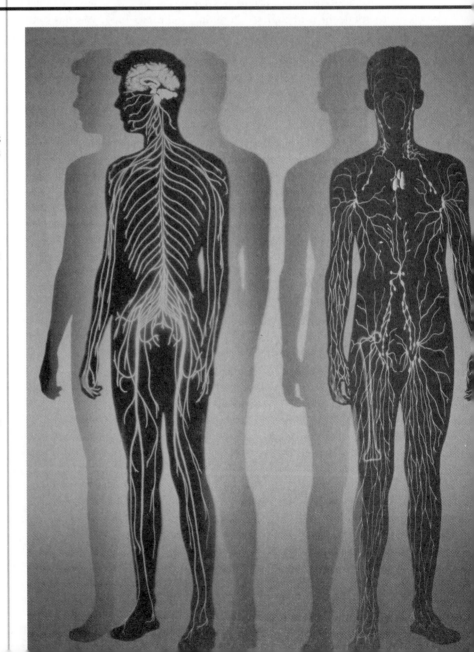

*L*akeesha's story begins in the spring of 1975, with a difficult, slow birth that required the use of excessive anesthetics and forceps to pull her roughly into the world. Together, these medical procedures choked off the supply of oxygen to her young brain. Although she survived, Lakeesha's complicated delivery, coupled with her low birth weight and her mother's heavy use of alcohol during her pregnancy, meant that her problems were just beginning. Lakeesha was born with mild spastic cerebral palsy (CP), a movement disorder that results from damage to the brain's motor centers.

Once thought to be solely caused by medical procedures, cerebral palsy is now thought to have multiple causes, including genetic vulnerability, prenatal exposure to toxins (such as alcohol), low birth weight (less than 35 ounces), or a birthing process that includes anoxia (a temporary lack of oxygen that can cause brain damage). Although CP's most obvious symptom is a person's inability to move body parts the way he or she normally would, other symptoms may occur. These include seizures, mental retardation, and hearing and vision problems.

As the months and years went by, it became apparent that these biological factors were to cast a lifelong shadow over Lakeesha's health, affecting not only her continuing physical development but her psychological and social development as well. Among the first problems her parents and pediatrician noticed were mild mental retardation, visual and hearing impairment, slight deformities in her teeth and joints, and scoliosis (curvature of the spine). Later, when other children were learning to speak, Lakeesha was having speech difficulties caused by her muscular problems.

Like many physically challenged kids, Lakeesha found that everything was harder. From the beginning, she seemed to need extra self-confidence and persistence to master tasks that were routine for other children. During early childhood, when she desperately wanted to be like everyone else, Lakeesha too often found that she couldn't do the same things, look the same way, or keep up with other children. Realizing that her handicap was permanent caused Lakeesha to become depressed and angry.

Lakeesha's condition also challenged the members of her family. Like many parents of disabled children, after learning that their child had CP, Lakeesha's mom and dad experienced grief, guilt, and disappointment. They found that it took more time and effort to raise their daughter than it had to raise her older sister. To make matters more difficult, other people often were hurtful in their comments and behavior toward Lakeesha.

Fortunately, interventions were available for Lakeesha and her family in each of the three domains—biological, psychological, and social. Although cerebral palsy cannot be cured at this time, many victims of CP can enjoy near-normal lives if their neurological problems are properly managed. Dental treatments and orthopedic surgery on Lakeesha's heel cords, hamstrings, adductor muscles, and hips corrected most of her facial and posture problems. Speech and behavior therapy helped Lakeesha improve her muscular control, balance, and speech.

By age 8, Lakeesha's development had progressed far enough that she was able to attend a "normal" elementary school for the first time. In some areas her skills were poor (writing with a pencil was extremely difficult, for example, and continuing vision problems hampered Lakeesha's efforts to learn to read). In other areas, however, her skills were *average, or even advanced (she was one of the first in her class, for example, to understand multiplication and division).*

Throughout her childhood, Lakeesha's emotional and psychological needs remained strong, but they were met. Her anger, low self-esteem, and perception of herself as damaged, or different, were corrected with therapy. Similarly, joining a support group and working with a cognitive-behavior therapist helped her parents recognize and cope with their feelings.

Today, at 25 years of age, Lakeesha is living independently, working part-time in an electronics store, and attending classes at the local community college. She maintains a close, warm relationship with her parents (who live nearby) and has a small but close-knit circle of friends. Most important, she feels good about herself and has confidence in her ability to overcome life's obstacles. Compared to what she's already managed to conquer, the road ahead seems easy.

Lakeesha's story illustrates the biopsychosocial perspective. Biological, psychological, and social factors all contributed to Lakeesha's health problems, and all of these were addressed as part of her triumphant survival. Recall also from Chapter 1 that the biopsychosocial perspective advocates a systems approach, the idea that the human body is a system made up of many interconnected subsystems and externally related to several larger systems such as society and culture.

The story also makes clear one of health psychology's most fundamental themes: The mind and body are inextricably intertwined. Whether they are focusing on promoting health or treating disease, health psychologists are concerned with the various ways our behaviors, thoughts, and feelings affect the functioning of the body.

Although not all of health psychology is directly concerned with biological activity, health and illness are ultimately biological events. An understanding of the body's physical systems is therefore necessary to appreciate how good health habits help prevent disease, while poor habits do the opposite.

This chapter lays the groundwork for our investigation into health psychology by reviewing the basic biological processes that affect health. These processes are regulated by the nervous system, the endocrine system, the cardiovascular system, the respiratory system, the digestive system, the immune system, and the reproductive system. For each system, we describe its basic structure and healthy functioning. In later chapters we describe the major diseases and disorders to which that system is vulnerable.

The chapter ends with a discussion of the mechanisms of heredity and the techniques used by behavior geneticists to evaluate genetic and environmental contributions to health, disease, and various traits.

Because the material in this chapter is fundamental to an understanding of the specific aspects of health and illness discussed in later chapters, you will probably want to refer back to it frequently.

The Nervous System

Major control over the operation of our body's systems belongs to the nervous system, made up of the brain, the spinal cord, and all the peripheral nerves that receive and send messages throughout the body. Without the nervous system, our muscles would not expand or contract, our heart would not beat, our pancreas would not know to release insulin. Let's begin our discussion of the body's nervous system with its building blocks, the neurons.

Neurons

Neurons, or nerve cells, are specialized to send and receive signals. There are three types of neurons: *sensory neurons,* which carry information coming from the environment; *interneurons,* which transmit signals from one neuron to another; and *motor neurons,* which transmit instructions to the muscles and glands of the body. These three types of cells are connected in a variety of neural circuits, ranging from the simplest reflex to the complicated interactions that form the basis of thinking and problem solving.

Although they come in a variety of shapes and sizes, all neurons share a basic structure, including a *cell body,* which contains the nucleus and metabolic mechanism of the cell; branching *dendrites* that receive stimulation from other cells; and an *axon* that conducts its signal (the neural impulse) to other cells (Figure 3.1, page 86). Unlike the shorter dendrites, which are specialized to receive input from adjacent neurons, axons may be up to several feet in length. Many axons are covered by a *myelin sheath,* a layer of fatty tissue that insulates the axon and increases the speed of neural impulses.

Synaptic Transmission

The tips of axons branch into swellings called *axon terminals,* which lie next to the dendrites of adjacent neurons. The junction between the axon and an adjoining dendrite is called a **synapse,** and the space between two neurons is the synaptic gap or cleft. When a neural impulse reaches the axon terminal, chemical messengers called **neurotransmitters** cross the synaptic cleft and bind to receptor sites on the receiving neuron's dendrite—rather like a key fits into a lock. In binding to the receptor sites, neurotransmitters unlock tiny channels that allow electrically charged atoms to flow into the receiving neuron, thereby altering its readiness to generate a neural impulse. If the postsynaptic cell is a muscle cell, the neurotransmitter causes the cell to contract. If the postsynaptic cell is another neuron, the neurotransmitter alters the cell's readiness to fire.

Each neuron has synapses with hundreds or even thousands of other neurons. Some of these are *excitatory synapses.* Neurotransmitters at these sites

neuron a nerve cell, including the cell body, dendrites, and axon (which is sometimes insulated by a myelin sheath). There are three types: sensory neurons, interneurons, and motor neurons

synapse the junction between one neuron's axon and the dendrites of an adjoining neuron, across which a nerve impulse may be transmitted

neurotransmitters chemical messengers released by a neuron at synapses that diffuse across the synaptic cleft and alter the electrical state of a receiving neuron

Figure 3.1

The Neuron

(a) A neuron may receive messages from other neurons on any of the dendrites or the cell body, and then transmit each message down the long axon to other neurons. Nerve impulses travel in one direction only, down the axon of a neuron to its axon terminal. When a nerve impulse reaches the axon terminal, chemical messengers called neurotransmitters cross the synapse and bind to receptor sites on the receiving neuron's dendrite or cell body—rather like a key fits into a lock. (b) Scanning electron micrograph of three neurons in the human brain. Secchi-Lecague/Roussel-Uclaf/CNRI/Science Photo Library/Photo Researchers

(b)

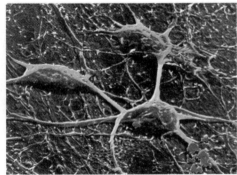

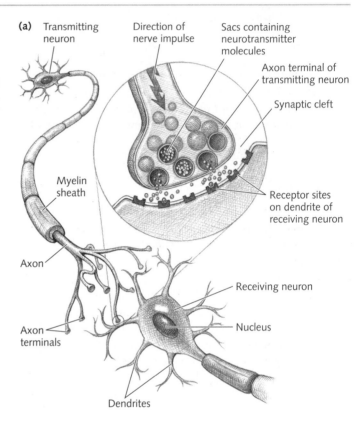

(a)

Transmitting neuron

Direction of nerve impulse

Sacs containing neurotransmitter molecules

Axon terminal of transmitting neuron

Synaptic cleft

Myelin sheath

Receptor sites on dendrite of receiving neuron

Axon

Receiving neuron

Axon terminals

Nucleus

Dendrites

increase the neuron's readiness to fire. At *inhibitory synapses,* neurotransmitters decrease the neuron's readiness to fire. If the total excitatory signals minus the total inhibitory signals exceed a minimum intensity, or **threshold,** the neuron generates a neural impulse. Increasing the imbalance between excitatory and inhibitory signals, however, will not increase the intensity of a neural impulse, which is an *all-or-none response.* (Neurons are like guns in that they either fire or they don't. Squeezing the trigger harder will not affect the speed or intensity of the gun [or axon's] response.)

Although each neural impulse is an all-or-nothing event, the effect a given neuron has is not. The more intense a stimulus, the faster the frequency at which neural impulses are initiated in the axon. This frequency varies from zero when the neuron is at rest to up to several hundred neural impulses each second.

 threshold the minimum change in electrical activity required to trigger an action potential in a neuron

Divisions of the Nervous System

The human nervous system contains billions of neurons and trillions of synapses, most of which are in the brain. These neurons form two major divisions: the **central nervous system (CNS),** which consists of the brain and the spinal cord, and the **peripheral nervous system (PNS),** which contains the remaining nerves of the body.

The PNS is further divided into two divisions: the *somatic nervous system,* which includes the nerves that carry messages from the eyes, ears, and other sense organs to the CNS, and from the CNS to the muscles and glands; and the *autonomic nervous system,* the nerves that link the CNS with the heart, the intestines, and other internal organs. Because the skeletal muscles that the somatic nerves activate are under voluntary control, the somatic nervous system is often referred to as the voluntary nervous system. In contrast, the autonomic, or involuntary, nervous system controls the organs over which we customarily have no control.

The autonomic nervous system is itself composed of two divisions (Figure 3.2, page 88). The *sympathetic nervous system* consists of groupings of neuron cell bodies called *ganglia* that run along the spinal cord and connect to the body's internal organs. The sympathetic division prepares the body for "fight or flight," a response generated when a person experiences stress or perceives a threat (see Chapter 4). It does so by increasing the heart rate and breathing rate, decreasing digestive activity (this is why eating while under stress can lead to a stomachache), increasing blood flow to the skeletal muscles, and releasing energizing sugars and fats from storage deposits. Because all the sympathetic ganglia are closely linked, they tend to act as a single system, or "in sympathy" with one another.

Unlike the ganglia of the sympathetic division, the ganglia of the *parasympathetic nervous system* are not closely linked and therefore tend to act more independently. Furthermore, this system has opposite effects; in helping the body to recover after arousal, it decreases heart rate, increases digestive activity, and conserves energy.

The Brain

In all likelihood the most complex and highly organized structure in the universe, the human brain weighs about 1,400 grams (3 pounds), is thought to consist of perhaps 100 billion (100,000,000,000) individual neurons, and has the consistency of a soft cheese.

The anatomical organization of the human brain is difficult to learn because it seems to make little sense. As new brain structures developed over the course of evolution, older structures remained but often assumed new

central nervous system the brain and spinal cord

peripheral nervous system all the neurons outside the central nervous system; consists of both the somatic nervous system and the autonomic nervous system, which includes the sympathetic and parasympathetic nervous systems

Figure 3.2

The Autonomic Nervous System

The autonomic nervous system is subdivided into the sympathetic and parasympathetic nervous systems. The sympathetic division prepares the body for action, accelerating heartbeat, stimulating the secretion of adrenaline, and triggering other elements of the "fight-or-flight" response. The parasympathetic division calms the body by slowing heartbeat, stimulating digestion, and triggering other restorative activities of the body.

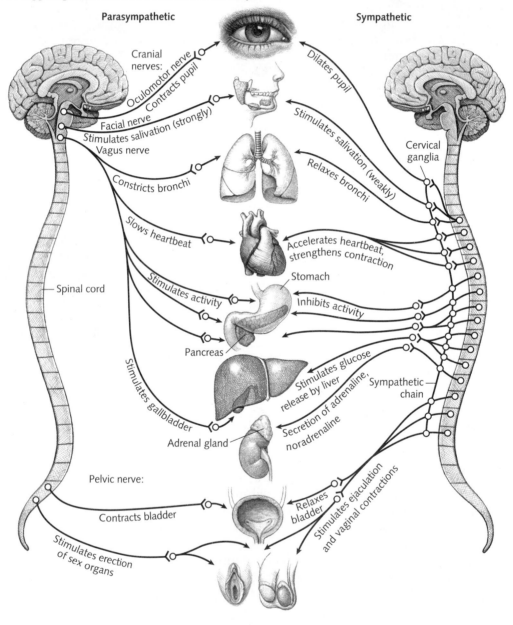

Parasympathetic | Sympathetic

Cranial nerves:
Oculomotor nerve
Contracts pupil
Dilates pupil
Facial nerve
Stimulates salivation (strongly)
Stimulates salivation (weakly)
Vagus nerve
Cervical ganglia
Constricts bronchi
Relaxes bronchi
Slows heartbeat
Accelerates heartbeat, strengthens contraction
Spinal cord
Stimulates activity
Stomach
Inhibits activity
Pancreas
Stimulates gallbladder
Stimulates glucose release by liver
Sympathetic chain
Secretion of adrenaline, noradrenaline
Adrenal gland
Pelvic nerve:
Contracts bladder
Relaxes bladder
Stimulates ejaculation and vaginal contractions
Stimulates erection of sex organs

roles. The structure of the brain makes sense only when viewed in the context of evolution, organized in layers that emanate outward from a central core.

Figure 3.3 is a diagram of the three principal regions of the brain: the brainstem, the cerebellum, and the cerebrum. Refer to it frequently as you read the following sections.

Lower-Level Structures

Located at the point where the spinal cord swells as it enters the skull, the **brainstem** is the first region of the vertebrate brain that evolved. Remarkably similar from fish to humans, the brainstem contains the medulla, the pons, and the reticular formation. Together, they control basic and involuntary life-support functions via the autonomic nervous system. (This is why a blow to the head at the base of the skull is so dangerous.) The brainstem is also the point at which most nerves passing between the spinal cord and the brain cross over, so that the left side of the brain sends and receives messages from the right side of the body, and vice versa.

The **medulla** controls several vital reflexes, including breathing, heart rate, salivation, coughing, and sneezing. It also receives sensory information about blood pressure and then, based on this input, varies the constriction or dilation of blood vessels to maintain an optimal state. Damage to the medulla is often fatal. An overdose of an opiate drug such as morphine or heroin may disrupt (or even suppress) breathing because of the drug's effects on the medulla.

As the spinal cord's sensory input travels up through the brain, branch fibers stimulate the **reticular formation,** a brainstem circuit that governs arousal and sleep. The reticular formation is also responsible for alerting the brain during moments of danger and prioritizing all incoming information. When this region is damaged, a person may lapse into a coma and never awaken.

Above the brainstem is the **thalamus.** Consisting of two egg-shaped groups of nuclei, the thalamus sorts sensory information received from the brainstem and routes it to the higher brain regions that deal with vision, hearing, taste, and touch.

Figure 3.3

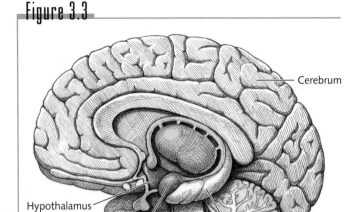

Hypothalamus
Pituitary gland
Amygdala
Brainstem
Cerebrum
Cerebellum
Hippocampus

The Brain

This cross section of the human brain shows its three principal regions: the brainstem, which controls heartbeat and respiration; the cerebellum, which regulates muscular coordination; and the cerebrum, which is the center for information processing. Surrounding the central core of the brain is the limbic system, which includes the amygdala, hippocampus, and hypothalamus. The limbic system plays an important role in emotions, especially those related to sexual arousal, aggression, and pain.

- **brainstem** the oldest and most central region of the brain; includes the medulla, pons, and reticular formation
- **medulla** the brainstem region that controls heartbeat and breathing
- **reticular formation** a network of neurons running through the brainstem involved with alertness and arousal
- **thalamus** the brain's sensory switchboard. Located on top of the brainstem, it routes messages to the cerebral cortex

■ **cerebellum** located at the rear of the brain, this brain structure coordinates voluntary movement and balance

■ **limbic system** a network of neurons surrounding the central core of the brain; associated with emotions such as fear and aggression; includes the hypothalamus, amygdala, and hippocampus

■ **amygdala** two clusters of neurons in the limbic system that are linked to emotion, especially aggression

■ **hippocampus** a structure in the brain's limbic system linked to memory

■ **hypothalamus** lying just below the thalamus, the region of the brain that influences hunger, thirst, body temperature, and sexual behavior; helps govern the endocrine system via the pituitary gland

Lying at the back of the brain, the **cerebellum,** or "little brain," is shaped like the larger brain. Its main function is to maintain body balance and coordinate voluntary muscle movement. Damage to the cerebellum produces a loss of muscle tone, tremors, and abnormal posture. In addition, specialized parts of the cerebellum contribute to memory, language, and cognition. Learning-disabled children, for example, often have damaged cerebellums.

The Limbic System

Surrounding the central core of the brain is the **limbic system,** which includes the amygdala, hippocampus, hypothalamus, and the septal area. The limbic system is believed to play an important role in emotions, especially those related to sexual arousal, aggression, and pain.

In 1939, neurosurgeons Heinrich Kluver and Paul Bucy surgically lesioned (destroyed) the **amygdala** of an especially aggressive rhesus monkey's brain. The operation transformed the violent creature into a docile pussycat. Other researchers have discovered that electrical stimulation of the amygdala will reliably trigger rage or fear responses in a variety of animals.*

Another limbic circuit involves areas within the **hippocampus,** which are thought to be involved in learning and memory. When the hippocampus is injured, people typically develop a form of amnesia in which they are unable to form new memories but retain their memory for previously learned skills. In a famous case, a talented composer and conductor, Clive Wearing, suffered damage to his hippocampus; he now lives from one moment to the next, always feeling as though he has just awakened.

Lying just below (hypo) the thalamus, the **hypothalamus** interconnects with numerous regions of the brain. Neuroscientists have pinpointed hypothalamic nuclei that influence hunger and regulate thirst, body temperature, and sexual behavior. One intriguing function of the hypothalamus is its role in the brain's reward system, a discovery made in 1954 by neuroscientists James Olds and Peter Milner. The researchers were attempting to implant electrodes in the brainstems of laboratory rats when they accidentally stimulated an area in the hypothalamus. Much to the researchers' surprise, the rats kept returning to the precise location in their cages where they had previously been stimulated by the errant electrode. Recognizing that the animals were behaving as if they were seeking more stimulation, Olds and Milner continued on to conduct a series of experiments that validated their discovery of the brain's reward circuitry. Indeed, rats have been known to "self-stimulate" their hypothalamic reward centers as many as 7,000 times per hour. As you will see in Chapter 8, some researchers believe that certain addictions—perhaps to food, alcohol, and other drugs—may stem from a genetic *reward deficiency*

---

*Given that amygdala lesions transform violent animals into docile ones, might the same procedure work with violent humans? Although this type of psychosurgery has been attempted in a few cases involving patients with severe brain abnormalities, the results have been mixed.

syndrome in which the brain's reward circuitry malfunctions and leads to powerful cravings.

The Cerebral Cortex

The *cerebrum,* which represents about 80 percent of the brain's total weight, forms two hemispheres (left and right) that are primarily filled with synaptic connections linking the surface of the brain to its other regions. The thin surface layer of the cerebrum, called the **cerebral cortex,** is what makes human beings what they are. Within this 3-millimeter-thick sheet of some 30 billion nerve cells are found neural centers that give rise to our sensory capacities, skilled motor responses, language abilities, and aptitude for reasoning.

The cortex in each hemisphere can be divided into four principal regions, or lobes; each lobe carries out many functions, and in some cases several lobes work together to perform a function (Figure 3.4, page 92). The *occipital lobe,* located at the back of the cortex, receives visual information from the retina of each eye. The *parietal lobe,* in the center of the cortex, receives information from the skin and body. Auditory information from the ear projects to the *temporal lobes.* The *frontal lobes,* lying just behind the forehead, are involved in reasoning, planning, and controlling body movement.

In the parietal lobe, on the edge of the frontal lobe, is the **sensory cortex,** which processes body sensations such as touch. The **motor cortex,** at the back of the frontal lobes, lies just in front of the sensory cortex. In 1870, German physicians Gustav Fritsch and Eduard Hitzig discovered that electrical stimulation of this arch of neurons triggered movement in the limbs of laboratory animals.

Little more than half a century later, neurosurgeon Wilder Penfield mapped the motor cortex in conscious patients during surgery to remove brain tumors. In addition to mapping the cortex according to the body parts it controlled, Penfield made the remarkable discovery that the amount of motor cortex devoted to a specific body part is proportional to the degree of control we have over that body part. The muscles of the face and fingers, for example, have much more representation in the cortex than does the thigh. Penfield also mapped the sensory cortex and found that the amount of cortical representation was proportional to the sensitivity of that body part.

The basic functional organization of the primary sensory and motor areas of the cerebral cortex is virtually identical in all mammals, from the rat to the human (Thompson, 2000). However, this accounts for only about one-fourth of the total area of the human cerebral cortex. Researchers are just beginning to understand the functions of the remaining areas, which are called **association cortex.** These areas are responsible for higher mental functions such as thinking and speaking. Interestingly, although humans do not have the largest brains (porpoises, whales, and elephants have much larger brains), as one ascends the evolutionary scale it is obvious that more intelligent animals have much greater amounts of "uncommitted" association areas.

cerebral cortex the thin layer of cells that covers the cerebrum; the seat of conscious sensation and information processing

sensory cortex lying at the front of the parietal lobes, the region of the cerebral cortex that processes body sensations such as touch

motor cortex lying at the rear of the frontal lobes, the region of the cerebral cortex that controls voluntary movements

association cortex areas of the cerebral cortex not directly involved in sensory or motor functions; rather, they integrate multisensory information and higher mental functions such as thinking and speaking

Figure 3.4

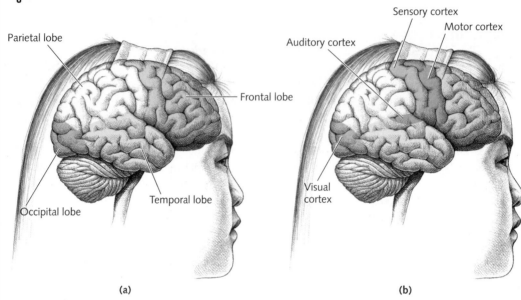

(a)

(b)

The Cerebral Cortex
(a) The four lobes, or regions, of the cerebral cortex; each lobe performs various functions, sometimes separately and more often in conjunction with another region.
(b) Within these regions are the neural centers that give rise to our sensory capacities, skilled motor responses, language ability, and reasoning ability.

*R*eality *Check*

Reacting to Health Problems

This chapter covers the body's major systems. The diseases and disorders that occur when a system malfunctions will be described in greater detail in later chapters. Before reading about these problems and the ways in which they can be dealt with, you might want to see how you generally react to illness or injury; as you read later sections, you will have a more personal sense of the importance of the biopsychosocial perspective.

COPING WITH HEALTH: INJURIES AND PROBLEMS SCALE

The following are ways of reacting to health problems, such as illness, sicknesses, or injuries. We are interested in your last illness, sickness, or injury. Please number from 1 (not at all) to 5 (very much) for each of the following items. Indicate how much you engaged in these types of activities when you encountered this health problem.

1 = not at all   2 = a little   3 = occasionally
          4 = fairly often   5 = very often

___ 1. Think about better times.

___ 2. Stay in bed.

___ 3. Find out more information.

___ 4. Wonder "why me?"

___ 5. Be with others.

___ 6. Rest when tired.

___ 7. Seek treatment quickly.

___ 8. Feel angry.

___ 9. Daydream.

___ 10. Sleep.

___ 11. Focus on getting better.

___ 12. Become frustrated.

___ 13. Enjoy attention from people.

___ 14. Conserve energy.

___ 15. Learn more.

___ 16. Think about things I can't do.

___ 17. Plan for the future.

___ 18. Stay warm.

___ 19. Comply with advice.

___ 20. Fantasize about being healthy.

___ 21. Listen to music.

___ 22. Make surroundings quiet.

___ 23. Follow doctor's advice.

___ 24. Wish it hadn't happened.

___ 25. Invite company.

___ 26. Stay quiet.

___ 27. Take medications on time.

___ 28. Think about being vulnerable.

___ 29. Have nice things around.

___ 30. Get comfortable.

___ 31. Find out about treatments.

___ 32. Worry about my health.

Scoring: People cope with adverse health conditions in a variety of ways. This test consists of four subscales, each of which is associated with a different style of coping with injury or illness. Each subscale consists of 8 test items. To obtain your score for each subscale, add the numbers you wrote next to the 8 items according to the following information.

Items 2, 6, 10, 14, 18, 22, 26, and 30 measure *palliative coping*—a self-help strategy that aims to reduce the unpleasant-ness of the condition. Among a group of college men and women, mean scores of 22.72 and 24.79, respectively, were obtained on this subscale.

Items 3, 7, 11, 15, 19, 23, 27, and 31 measure *instrumental coping*—a task-oriented strategy closely associated with problem-focused coping, which we'll discuss fully in Chapter 5. A person who copes with an injury or disease instrumentally might actively seek more information, such as by consulting a doctor, researching symptoms, or checking family history for signs of genetic vulnerability for the condition. Mean scores of 28.72 and 29.54 were obtained for college-age men and women, respectively.

Items 1, 5, 9, 13, 17, 21, 25, and 29 measure *distraction coping*—a strategy of avoidance in which the person tries hard not to think about his or her plight by seeking out the company of others, keeping busy, and keeping the mind focused on pleasant thoughts. College-age women and men averaged scores of 22.0 and 20.16, respectively.

Items 4, 8, 12, 16, 20, 24, 28, and 32 assess *emotional preoccupation coping*—in which a person simply can't get his or her mind off the problem. Like cows chewing their cud, people who frequently engage in this type of rumination play their condition over and over again in their mind. As we'll see in Chapter 5, health psychologists have found that emotional preoccupation with health conditions is often associated with greater distress and poorer recovery from the injury or illness. Mean scores of 28.76 and 29.41 were obtained among groups of college-age men and women, respectively.

How did you score on each of the four subscales? Were your scores close to the average of other college women or men? Did you score substantially higher (or lower) on one or more scales than other students? Keep these scores in mind as you continue your exploration of health psychology. One of the major themes of the biopsychosocial model is that how you think about events and conditions strongly influences the impact these events and conditions have on your health.

Source: "Coping with Health Problems: Developing a Reliable and Valid Multidimensional Measure," by N. S. Endler, J. D. A. Parker, and L. J. Summerfeldt, 1998, *Psychological Assessment, 10,* pp. 195–205.

The Endocrine System

Closely connected with the nervous system in regulating many bodily functions is the second of the body's communication systems, the endocrine system (see Figure 3.5, page 94). The two systems are very different, however. Whereas the nervous system communicates through neurotransmitters, the endocrine system communicates through chemical

Figure 3.5

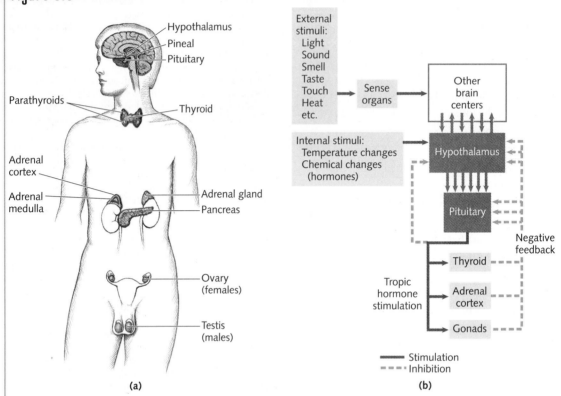

(a)

(b)

━━━ Stimulation
- - - - Inhibition

The Endocrine Glands and Feedback Control
(a) Under the direction of the brain's hypothalamus, the pituitary releases hormones that, in turn, regulate the secretions of the thyroid, the adrenal glands, and the reproductive organs. (b) The production of many hormones is regulated by a complex negative feedback system. As the levels of hormones produced in target glands rise in the blood, the hypothalamus and pituitary decrease their production of hormones, and the secretion of hormones by the target glands also slows.

hormones chemical messengers, released into the bloodstream by endocrine glands, that have an effect on distant organs

messengers called **hormones.** And, unlike the much speedier nervous system, which is chiefly responsible for fast-acting, short-duration responses, the endocrine system primarily governs slow-acting responses of longer duration.

Endocrine glands secrete hormones directly into the bloodstream, where they travel to various organs and bind to receptor sites. When binding is achieved, the organ is stimulated or inhibited depending on the type of receptor and hormone. In this section, we'll describe the activity of four important endocrine glands—the pituitary, adrenal, and thyroid glands, and the pancreas.

The Pituitary and the Adrenal Glands

The **pituitary gland** secretes a number of hormones that influence other glands. These include hormones that influence growth, sexual development, reproduction, kidney functioning, and aging.

Although the pituitary gland is often referred to as the *master gland* of the endocrine system, the brain's hypothalamus more properly deserves this title because it directly (and rigidly) controls pituitary functioning. Together, the hypothalamus and pituitary act as a master control system. For example, during a stressful moment, the hypothalamus secretes the hormone *corticotrophin-releasing hormone (CRH)*, which travels in the bloodstream to the anterior pituitary, where it stimulates the pituitary to secrete *adrenocorticotropic hormone (ACTH)*. ACTH binds to receptor cells on the adrenal cortex, causing this gland to release cortisol into the bloodstream. The increased level of cortisol in the blood acts back on the hypothalamus and pituitary gland to inhibit the release of additional CRH and ACTH. This example of *feedback control* is similar to the mechanism by which a household thermostat regulates temperature by turning on and turning off a furnace or air conditioner as needed.

Located atop the kidneys, the **adrenal glands** secrete several important hormones that play a crucial role in the body's response to stress and emergencies. In a moment of danger, for example, *epinephrine* and *norepinephrine* are released from the innermost region of the gland (the adrenal medulla) into the bloodstream, where they travel to receptor sites on the heart. These hormones increase heart rate, blood pressure, and blood sugar, providing the body with a quick surge of energy. A third hormone, *cortisol*, is secreted from the outermost region (the adrenal cortex). Cortisol is a steroid that helps to reduce swelling and inflammation following an injury to the body.

The Thyroid Gland and the Pancreas

Located in the front of the neck, the *thyroid gland* is shaped like a butterfly, with the two wings representing the left and right thyroid lobes that wrap around the windpipe. The thyroid gland produces the hormone thyroxin, which helps regulate the body's growth and metabolism (energy utilization). Located just behind the thyroid are four parathyroid glands. The hormones secreted by these glands regulate the level of calcium in the body.

Another endocrine gland, the *pancreas,* produces glucagon and insulin, two hormones that act in opposition to regulate the level of the sugar glucose in the blood. Glucagon raises the concentration of glucose in the blood, while insulin controls the conversion of sugar and carbohydrates into energy by promoting the uptake of glucose by the body's cells (see Chapter 7).

- **pituitary gland** the master endocrine gland controlled by the hypothalamus; releases a variety of hormones that act on other glands throughout the body
- **adrenal glands** lying above the kidneys, the pair of endocrine glands that secrete epinephrine, norepinephrine, and cortisol, hormones that arouse the body during moments of stress

■ **arteries** blood vessels that carry blood away from the heart to other organs and tissues. A small artery is called an arteriole

■ **veins** blood vessels that carry blood back to the heart from the capillaries

The Cardiovascular System

In the fourth week after conception, a primitive beating heart and blood vessels form, making the cardiovascular system the first organ system to become active. About the size of a clenched fist and weighing only about 11 ounces, the heart pumps 5 or more quarts of blood a minute through your circulatory system. Over the course of your life, your heart will beat more than 2.5 *billion* times.

The cardiovascular system—consisting of the heart, blood vessels, and blood—serves as the body's transportation system; through the pumping action of the heart, the blood vessels carry blood rich in nutrients and oxygen to our cells and tissues and remove waste products through the lungs, liver, and kidneys. We begin our journey through the cardiovascular system with the basic terminology you'll need to understand how this transportation system works.

Blood and Circulation

Human blood is a living tissue; it contains three types of cells that perform different functions. Red blood cells, or *erythrocytes,* carry oxygen from the lungs to the cells of the body. Formed in the bone marrow, red blood cells contain *hemoglobin,* the iron-rich substance that gives blood its reddish tint. Hemoglobin is the means by which the blood is able to pick up oxygen in the lungs while releasing the carbon dioxide it has picked up from the cells. Blood also carries nutrients from the digestive system to cells and transports cellular waste to the kidneys for excretion in urine.

The white blood cells (*leukocytes*) carried by the blood are part of the immune system, and the *platelets* are small cell fragments that stick together (coagulate) when necessary to form clots along the walls of damaged blood vessels. Without leukocytes we would have no defenses against infection. Without platelets we would bleed to death from wounds, even from a small cut from a razor blade.

Blood is transported throughout the body by the *circulatory system,* which consists of several types of blood vessels. **Arteries** carry blood from the heart to the other organs and tissues. The arteries branch into increasingly narrower blood vessels called *arterioles,* which eventually connect with *capillaries.* The smallest of the blood vessels, capillaries carry blood directly to the individual cells. **Veins** return blood from the capillaries to the heart.

The vessels of the circulatory system move blood throughout the body by dilating and contracting as needed. When arteries narrow (constrict), resistance to blood flow increases. Blood pressure is a measure of the force necessary to overcome this resistance. This force is highest during *systole,* when the heart contracts in order to force the blood out. During *diastole,* the heart relaxes as blood flows into the heart, and blood pressure drops. Thus, diastolic blood pressure is lower than systolic blood pressure.

A blood pressure level of 120/80 ("120 over 80") mm Hg (millimeters of mercury) is considered normal. Systolic BP above 140 mm Hg and/or diastolic BP above 90 mm HG indicates the presence of hypertension.

The Heart

Musicians, artists, and writers all romanticize the heart. In fact, the heart is nothing more than a muscular pump—although an extremely effective one. Just as a gasoline pump pulls the gas from underground tanks through a hose to your car, the heart pumps blood through your lungs and other organs and into all the cells of the body.

In birds and mammals, the heart is separated into four parts, or chambers: the right and left *atria* in the upper section of the heart and the right and left *ventricles* in the lower section of the heart. These chambers work in coordinated fashion to bring blood into the heart and then to pump it throughout the body (Figure 3.6). Blood returning from the body enters the *right atrium* through two large veins. After expanding to receive the blood, the right atrium contracts, forcing the "used" blood into the *right ventricle.* Depleted of oxygen, this "used" blood is sent into the pulmonary artery (*pulmonary* refers to lungs), then through the capillaries of the lungs, where it picks up oxygen for

Figure 3.6

The Cardiovascular System
The heart is separated into four parts, or chambers, the right and left atria in the upper section of the heart and the right and left ventricles in the lower section of the heart.

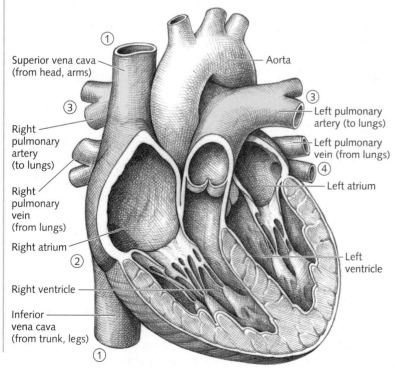

Superior vena cava (from head, arms)

Aorta

Right pulmonary artery (to lungs)

Left pulmonary artery (to lungs)

Left pulmonary vein (from lungs)

Right pulmonary vein (from lungs)

Left atrium

Right atrium

Left ventricle

Right ventricle

Inferior vena cava (from trunk, legs)

① Oxygen-depleted blood returns to the heart from the body through the superior and the inferior vena cava. . . .

② This blood is pumped from the right atrium into the right ventricle. . . .

③ And from there through capillaries of the lungs, where it picks up fresh oxygen and disposes of carbon dioxide. . . .

④ The freshly oxygenated blood is pumped through the pulmonary vein into the left atrium and from there into the left ventricle, from which it flows into the arterial system.

later distribution to cells and disposes of waste carbon dioxide (CO_2) (which will be exhaled). The now oxygen-rich blood flows into the pulmonary vein to the superior and inferior vena cavas, and pumping action of cardiac muscles forces that blood into the left atrium and then into the left ventricle. The left ventricle propels the oxygen-rich blood into the aorta, from which it flows into the arterial system carrying nutrients to all parts of the body. If you listen to your heartbeat, the "lubb-dup, lubb-dup" sound represents the closing of the valves between the atria and ventricles ("lubb"), followed by the closing of the valves between the ventricles and the arteries ("dup"). When one of the heart's valves is damaged, as occurs following rheumatic fever, blood leaks back through the valve and produces the "ph—f—f—t" sound of a "heart murmur."

The Respiratory System

Respiration has two meanings. At the level of the individual cell, it refers to energy-producing chemical reactions that require oxygen. At the level of the whole organism, it refers to the process of taking in oxygen from the environment and ridding the body of carbon dioxide.

The Lungs

The most important organ in the respiratory system is, of course, the lung (see Figure 3.7). After air enters the body through the mouth or nose it passes to the lungs through the *pharynx* and *trachea*, from which it travels through the **bronchi** that branch into smaller tubes, called *bronchioles*. Each bronchiole ends in a cluster of small bubble-like sacs, called *alveoli*. The membranous wall of each alveolus is thin enough to permit the exchange of gases, allowing oxygen to be exchanged for carbon dioxide. Alveoli are surrounded by millions of capillaries so that gases can be transferred efficiently from the bloodstream.

How do the muscles that control lung expansion "know" when it's time to breathe? Sensors in capillaries monitor the chemical composition of the blood. As the level of carbon dioxide rises, this information is relayed to the brain's medulla, which signals the muscles of the diaphragm to contract and cause you to inhale. Sensing that the level of carbon dioxide is low, the medulla signals the muscles to slow the rate of breathing until the carbon dioxide level returns to normal.

The respiratory system also has protective mechanisms that eliminate airborne dust particles and other foreign matter from the body. The two reflex mechanisms are sneezing when the nasal passages are irritated and coughing when the larger airways of the throat are irritated. In addition, the air passages in the nose, mouth, and trachea are lined with tiny hairs called **cilia** that trap germs. Moving in wavelike fashion, the cilia force the mucus that coats them gradually up toward the mouth, where it is either expelled in a cough or swallowed.

bronchi the pair of respiratory tubes that branch into progressively smaller passageways, the bronchioles, culminating in the air sacs within the right and left lungs (alveoli)

cilia the tiny hairs that line the air passageways in the nose, mouth, and trachea; moving in wavelike fashion, the cilia trap germs and force them out of the respiratory system

Figure 3.7

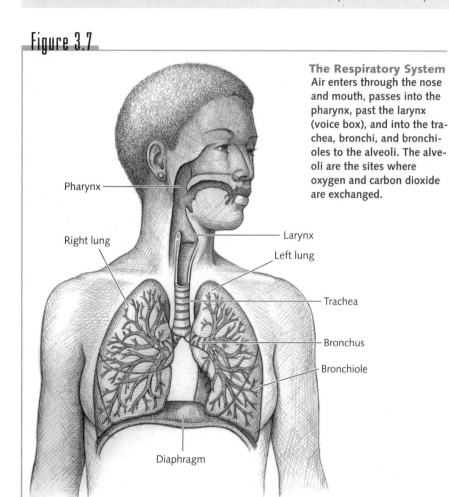

The Respiratory System
Air enters through the nose and mouth, passes into the pharynx, past the larynx (voice box), and into the trachea, bronchi, and bronchioles to the alveoli. The alveoli are the sites where oxygen and carbon dioxide are exchanged.

Pharynx

Right lung

Larynx

Left lung

Trachea

Bronchus

Bronchiole

Diaphragm

The Diversity and Healthy Living box, pages 100–101, discusses asthma as an example of what can happen when a system malfunctions and of how health psychology contributes to the care and well-being of sufferers.

The Digestive System

Digestion is the breaking down of food into molecules that can be absorbed by the blood and distributed to individual cells as nutrients for energy, growth, and tissue repair. The heart of the digestive system, or the **gastrointestinal system,** is the *digestive tract*—a long convoluted tube that extends from the mouth to the anus (Figure 3.8, page 102). The digestive system also includes the salivary glands, the pancreas, the liver, and the gallbladder.

■ **gastrointestinal system** the body's system for digesting food; includes the digestive tract, salivary glands, pancreas, liver, and gallbladder

Diversity and Healthy Living

Asthma

Asthma is a chronic noninfectious lung disease characterized by hypersensitivity and responsiveness of the trachea (windpipe) and bronchi (main airway) to some type of trigger that causes narrowing of the airways. Ninety percent of childhood cases of asthma are allergic reactions triggered by animal dander, pollens, dust, or mold. In the nonallergic form of asthma, which is more likely to affect adults, the trigger may be as simple as a common cold. Cold air, viral infections, secondhand smoke, and household chemicals can also trigger an asthma attack. According to the National Institute of Allergy and Infectious Diseases (NIAID), there are an estimated 6 million chemicals in the environment and 2,800 of these have allergenic, or contact-sensitizing, properties. Many people with asthma find that strong emotions, stress, or anxiety can make symptoms of asthma worse, especially during a severe attack. Sometimes asthma symptoms appear for no apparent reason.

When an asthma attack occurs, the muscles surrounding the bronchi in the lungs constrict, obstructing the flow of air. In addition, the bronchi become inflamed and filled with mucus, further reducing the supply of oxygen. The major symptoms of an asthma attack include wheezing, a whistling sound that may occur throughout the chest or in a local area where the airway has become blocked; coughing as the body attempts to rid itself of any foreign substance (mucus) or irritant (smoke); and shortness of breath caused by fast, shallow breathing as the body attempts to take in sufficient oxygen through narrowed airways.

Although asthma can develop at any age, it usually begins in childhood—it is now the most common chronic childhood disease in the United States—and affects more boys than girls. Elderly adults and members of minority groups are particularly susceptible to asthma. In the United States, the prevalence of asthma is greater for African-Americans (6.1 percent) than for Caucasians (5.0 percent); among Hispanics, prevalence ranges from a low of 2.7 percent among Mexican-American children living in the Southwest to 11.2 percent for Puerto Rican children living in New York City. Taken overall, both hospitalization and mortality rates among blacks are nearly three times those among whites.

Asthma was rare in 1900, but now it has grown into an epidemic: There are more than 15 million people with asthma in the United States and 10 times that many around the world (World Health Organization, 2000). The prevalence of asthma is highest in Western countries, particularly English-speaking ones; the disease is rare in parts of rural South America and Africa. Each year in the United States about 500,000 asthma-related hospitalizations occur and 5,000 people die, mostly older adults. Worldwide, there are more than 180,000 asthma deaths each year.

Although having one parent with asthma—or, worse still, two parents with asthma—increases a child's risk, geographical variations in the prevalence of asthma are probably due to environmental and lifestyle factors rather than genetic ones. Precisely what elements are involved is not entirely clear. Among the candidates is the tendency of children to spend more time indoors than did those in earlier generations, thus increasing their exposure to household allergens, including dust mites, animal dander, and indoor pests such as cockroaches. According to one theory, the immune systems of Western children, unlike those in developing countries, are weaker because they are not conditioned to live with parasites, and so the children become more vulnerable to asthma and other allergic diseases such as hay fever.

How Food Is Digested

Digestion begins in the mouth, where chewing and the chemical action of salivary enzymes begin to break food down. Most mammals have teeth that assist in the tearing and grinding of food. As food is chewed, it is moistened by saliva so that it can be swallowed more easily. Saliva contains a digestive enzyme called *amylase* that causes starches to begin to decompose.

Once food is swallowed, it passes into the *esophagus*, a muscular tube about 9.3 inches (25 centimeters) long in the typical adult. The muscles of the esoph-

Asthma has been increasing at an alarming rate in the United States, more than doubling since 1980 and contributing to at least 25 percent of missed school days (NIAID, 2001). To find out why, ongoing research is focusing on each domain of health: biological, psychological, and social. For instance, in the first search of the entire human genome in African-Americans, European Americans, and Hispanics with asthma, researchers from the National Heart, Lung, and Blood Institute analyzed data on 380 children and adults with asthma (117 African-Americans, 48 Hispanics, and 215 Caucasians). Preliminary results indicate strong **genetic linkage** among genes at 11 chromosomal sites associated with asthma-promoting traits such as bronchial hyperresponsivity and allergic sensitivity. Genetic linkage is a statistical measure of the proximity of two or more genes on a chromosome; the stronger (closer together) the linkage between the genes, the lower the probability that they will be separated during DNA repair or replication, and hence the greater the probability that they will be inherited together. Of the 11 chromosomal regions identified, all but one was unique to only one racial or ethnic group, suggesting that gene–environment interactions in promoting asthma vary with race or ethnicity.

Other research studies have focused on nongenetic risk factors for asthma, such as whether a child's mother smoked during her pregnancy, poverty, and living in an inner city. In the largest study of its kind ever conducted, researchers at the National Institute of Allergy and Infectious Diseases recently completed a 5-year study of more than 1,500 children, ages 4 to 11, living in inner cities. About 75 percent of the children were African-Americans and 20 percent were Hispanic. In a powerful validation of the biopsychosocial model, the researchers found that a wide variety of factors, rather than a single cause, were responsible for the recent increase in asthma morbidity. Among these factors were environmental toxins, such as indoor allergens and passive smoke; psychological problems of both the children and their caretakers; and problems with access to medical care. On the latter point, asthma was most severe among children whose families reported significant barriers to access to medical care. In view of the findings, researchers developed a broad-based intervention centered on the use of an asthma counselor who instituted educational, behavioral, and environmental interventions tailored to the specific needs of individual children and their families. Over the course of the 5-year study, these interventions resulted in significant reductions in symptoms and the need for medical treatment.

Although asthma cannot be cured, it can be managed with asthma medications, with muscle relaxation techniques that improve breathing, and by reducing exposure to allergens. On this last subject, modifying the asthmatic's environment can be a real pain and a real expense, but it does work. Depending on the severity of the case, environmental interventions can take one, or all, of the following steps:

- removing stuffed animals and books
- sealing mattresses and pillows in high-quality dust-proof enclosures
- removing all carpeting, draperies, and curtains
- removing upholstered furniture
- purchasing high-efficiency particle arresting (HEPA) air filters
- finding new homes for cats and dogs
- converting forced air heating systems to dust-free systems such as radiant (hot-water) ones
- frequent damp mopping (rather than vacuuming) of flooring

agus contract rhythmically, propelling the food downward in an involuntary reflexive motion called *peristalsis*. This reflex is so efficient that you are able to swallow food and water even while standing on your head.

In the stomach, the food is mixed with a variety of gastric juices, including hydrochloric acid and *pepsin*, an enzyme that breaks down proteins. At this point, the food has been converted into a semiliquid mass. The secretion of gastric juices (including saliva) is controlled by the autonomic nervous system. Food in the mouth, or even the sight, smell, or thought of food, is sufficient to trigger the flow of gastric juices. Conversely, fear inhibits digestive activity.

- **genetic linkage** a statistical measure of the proximity of two or more genes on a chromosome; the stronger (closer together) the linkage between the genes, the greater the probability that they will be inherited together

Figure 3.8

The Digestive System
The heart of the digestive system is the digestive tract—a long convoluted tube that extends from the mouth to the anus. The digestive system also includes the salivary glands, the pancreas, the liver, and the gallbladder.

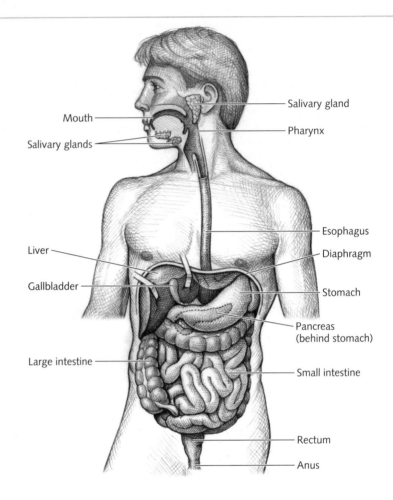

Mouth
Salivary glands
Salivary gland
Pharynx
Liver
Esophagus
Diaphragm
Gallbladder
Stomach
Pancreas (behind stomach)
Large intestine
Small intestine
Rectum
Anus

When you are in danger or under stress, your mouth becomes very dry and food sits like an uncomfortable, undigested lump in your stomach.

Stomachs vary in capacity. Depending on their success in hunting, carnivores such as hyenas may eat only once every few days. Fortunately, their large-capacity stomachs can hold the equivalent of 30 to 35 percent of their own body weight. In contrast, mammals that eat more frequent, smaller meals typically have much smaller stomachs. The capacity of the average college student's stomach is roughly 2 to 4 liters of food—about 2 to 3 percent of the average person's body weight—roughly equal to a burger, fries, and a Coke.

About 4 hours after eating, the stomach empties its contents into the small and large intestines. Digestive fluids from the pancreas, liver, and gallbladder are secreted into the small intestine through a series of ducts. These fluids contain enzymes that break down proteins, fats, and carbohydrates. For example, the liver produces a salty substance called *bile* that emulsifies fats almost as effectively as dishwashing liquid, and the pancreas produces the hormone insulin, which assists in transporting glucose from the intestine into body cells.

The breakdown of food that began in the mouth and stomach is completed in the small intestine. The inner lining of the small intestine is composed of gathered circular folds, which greatly increase its surface area. In fact, fully extended, the small intestine would be almost 20 feet (approximately 6 meters) in length, giving a total surface area of 3,229 square feet (300 square meters)—roughly the size of a basketball court. This vast area is lined with tiny fingerlike projections of mucus, called *villi*, through which water and nutrient molecules pass into the bloodstream. Once in the bloodstream, nutrients travel to individual cells.

Food particles that have not been absorbed into the bloodstream then pass into the large intestine, or *colon,* where absorption, mainly of water, continues. In the course of digestion, a large volume of water—approximately 7 liters each day—is absorbed. When this process is disrupted, as occurs in diarrhea and other gastric disorders, dehydration becomes a danger. Indeed, dehydration is the reason diarrhea remains the leading cause of infant death in many developing countries.

Completing the process of digestion, food particles that were not absorbed earlier are converted into feces by colon bacteria such as *Escherichia coli.* Fecal matter is primarily composed of water, bacteria, cellulose fibers, and other indigestible substances.

The Immune System

At this moment, countless numbers of microorganisms surround you. Most are not dangerous. Indeed, many, such those that assist in digestion and the decomposition of waste matter, play an important role in health. However, **antigens**—bacteria, viruses, fungi, parasites, and any foreign microorganism—are dangerous to your health, even deadly. Defending your health against these invaders is the job of the immune system.

You may be exposed to antigens through direct bodily contact (handshaking, kissing, or sexual intercourse) or through food, water, insects, and airborne microbes. Antigens may penetrate body tissue through several routes, including the skin, the digestive tract, the respiratory tract, or the genitourinary system. Their impact depends on the number and virulence of the microorganisms and the strength of the body's defenses.

antigen a foreign substance that stimulates an immune response

Figure 3.9

The Immune System
Positioned throughout the body, the organs of the immune system are home to lymphocytes, white blood cells that are the basis of the body's immune defense against foreign agents or antigens. Other components of the system are the bone marrow, where lymphocytes are produced, the thymus, spleen, and the tonsils.

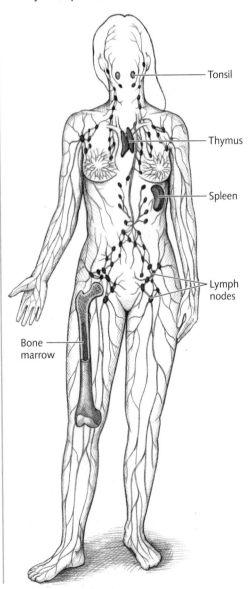

Tonsil

Thymus

Spleen

Lymph nodes

Bone marrow

Structure of the Immune System

Unlike most other systems, the immune system is spread throughout the body in the form of a network of capillaries, lymph nodes (glands), and ducts that comprise the *lymphatic system,* along with the bone marrow, thymus, and tonsils (see Figure 3.9). Lymphatic capillaries carry *lymph,* a colorless bodily fluid formed by water, proteins, microbes, and other foreign substances that are drained from the spaces between body cells. Lymph takes its name from the billions of white blood cells it circulates called **lymphocytes.** These cells, which are produced in the bone marrow, patrol the entire body, searching for bacteria, viruses, cancerous cells, and other antigens.

The lymph nodes contain filters that capture infectious substances and debris; as lymph passes through the lymph nodes, the lymphocytes destroy the foreign particles collected there. During an immune response, the lymphocytes expand, which produces swelling and inflammation. You may have noticed how your lymph nodes swell when you are fighting an infection.

Two structures play a role in the activity of lymphocytes: the thymus and the tonsils. The thymus, which also functions as part of the endocrine system, secretes the hormone *thymosin,* which plays a crucial role in controlling the maturation and development of lymphocytes. Interestingly, the thymus is largest during infancy and childhood and slowly shrinks (atrophies) throughout adulthood, which may partially explain why immune responses are generally more efficient during childhood and aging is associated with reduced immune efficiency (see Chapter 15). Finally, the tonsils are masses of lymphatic tissue that seem to function as a holding station for lymphocytes as well as a garbage can for worn-out blood cells.

The Immune Response

The body's immune reactions can be divided into two broad categories: *nonspecific immunity* and *specific immunity.* Nonspecific immune defenses defend against any antigen, including one never before encountered. Specific immune defenses occur only when a particular antigen has been encountered before, creating a kind of immunological *memory* for the intruder.

Nonspecific Immune Responses
The body's first line of defense against most antigens consists of the several layers of tightly knit cells that make up the skin.

Chemicals found in perspiration, such as the oily *sebum* secreted by glands beneath the skin, prevent most bacteria and fungi from growing on the skin.

The nose, eyes, and respiratory tract—although they lack the tough, protective barrier of the skin—also provide a first line of defense. The mucus membranes of the nose and respiratory tract are armed with hairlike cilia, which, as noted earlier, catch dust, microbes, and other foreign matter. A powerful enzyme in tears and saliva destroys the cell walls of many bacteria. Similarly, gastric acids are able to destroy most antigens that enter the digestive system.

When an antigen penetrates the skin cells, it encounters a second line of defense, called *phagocytosis,* in which two specialized lymphocytes called phagocytes and macrophages attack the foreign particles. *Phagocytes* are large scavenger cells that prowl the blood and tissues of the body for antigens. Phagocytes destroy antigens by engulfing and digesting them. *Macrophages* ("big eaters") are phagocytes found at the site of an infection, as well as in the lymph nodes, spleen, and lungs. These specialized white blood cell "sentries" pass into body tissues, where they hunt antigens and worn-out cells. A single phagocyte can digest 5 to 25 bacteria before dying itself from an accumulation of toxic wastes.

Suppose, for instance, that your skin was punctured by a splinter. Neighboring cells in the area of the wound immediately release several chemicals, particularly *histamine,* which increases blood flow to the area. Circulating phagocytes and macrophages, attracted by these chemicals, rush to the site of the wound, where they begin to engulf the inevitable bacteria and foreign particles that enter the body through the wound. At the same time, blood clots form, sealing off the wound site, and additional histamine is released, creating a hot environment unfavorable to bacteria.

As a consequence of this sequence of nonspecific immune reactions, collectively referred to as the *inflammatory response,* the injured area becomes swollen, red, and tender to the touch. In addition, some lymphocytes release proteins that produce *systemic effects* (that is, effects throughout the entire body), one of which is fever. In addition to its role in destroying invading microorganisms, inflammation helps restore bodily tissues that have been damaged. Figure 3.10, page 106, illustrates this process of inflammation.

In addition to the phagocytes and macrophages, the immune system's nonspecific defenses include smaller lymphocytes called *natural killer,* or NK, cells, which patrol the body for diseased cells that have gone awry. Researchers are just now learning how NK cells distinguish normal body cells, or what is *self,* from virus-infected and cancerous cells that are *non-self.* NK cells destroy their targets by injecting them with lethal chemicals. They also secrete various forms

■ **lymphocytes** white blood cells produced in the bone marrow that fight antigens

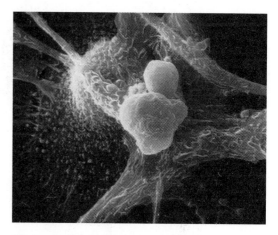

**The Immune System in Action:
A Macrophage Attacks**
Macrophages ("big eaters") are specialized white blood cell "sentries" that pass into body tissues, where they hunt antigens and worn-out cells. A single macrophage can digest 5 to 25 bacteria before dying itself from an accumulation of toxic wastes.
Microworks/Phototake

Figure 3.10

The Inflammatory Response

When an infection or, as in this case, an injury breaches the body's first line of defense, histamine and other chemicals are released at the site of the wound. These chemicals increase blood flow to the area, attract white blood cells, and cause a clot to form, sealing off the wound site. Some of the white blood cells engulf foreign particles, while others release a protein that produces fever.

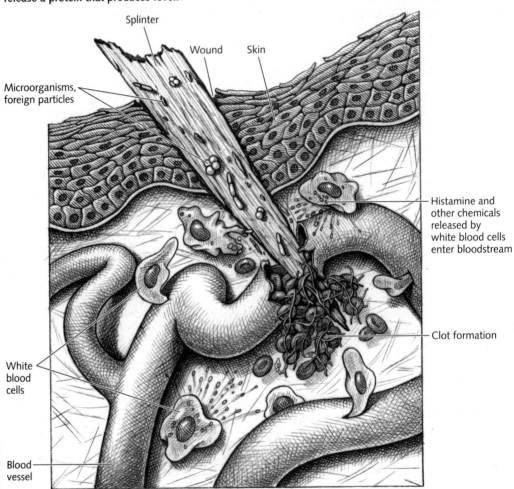

Splinter

Wound   Skin

Microorganisms, foreign particles

Histamine and other chemicals released by white blood cells enter bloodstream

Clot formation

White blood cells

Blood vessel

of *interferon,* an antimicrobial protein that inhibits the spread of viral infections to healthy cells. Interferons, which differ from species to species, work by preventing viruses from replicating. The subject of intensive biomedical research, interferons have the potential for treating influenza, the common cold, and other diseases.

Specific Immune Responses

Some antigens either elude the body's nonspecific defenses or are too powerful to be handled by phagocytes, macrophages, and NK cells alone. In such cases, the immune system calls upon its strongest line of defense: specific immune responses. These reactions occur when a particular antigen has been encountered before. Some specific immunities are acquired when a nursing mother passes a specific immunity to her child through breast milk. Others develop when a person successfully weathers a disease such as measles, or is *immunized*. As a child, you probably were vaccinated against mumps, chickenpox, whooping cough, polio, and other diseases, making your body artificially resistant to these diseases should you ever be exposed to them. Your body's ability to develop "memory" for specific antigens is the basis of acquired immunity. When a child is vaccinated, a dead or nonvirulent form of a specific virus is injected, allowing the body to create a memory for it.

Specific immune responses involve two special lymphocytes, called *B cells* and *T cells*, which recognize and attack specific invading antigens. B cells attack foreign substances by producing specific antibodies, or *immunoglobulins*, proteins that chemically suppress the toxic effects of antigens, primarily viruses and bacteria. A particular antibody molecule fits into receptors on an invading antigen as precisely as a key fits a lock. When a B cell is activated by a particular antigen, it divides into two types: a plasma cell capable of making 3,000 to 30,000 antibody molecules per second and an antibody-producing memory cell (Figure 3.11, page 108). The rapid response of memory cells, called the *primary response,* is the basis of immunity to many infectious diseases, including polio, measles, smallpox, and mumps.

Unlike the plasma cell, which lives only a few days, memory cells may last a lifetime, producing a stronger, faster antibody reaction should the particular antigen be encountered a second time. When a memory cell encounters the same antigen during a subsequent infection, the *secondary immune response* is triggered.

For many years, scientists believed that circulating antibodies produced by B cells were the sole basis of immunity. They now know that the immune system has a second line of defense, called *cell-mediated immunity,* in which T cells directly attack and kill antigens without the aid of antibodies.

There are three major varieties of T cells: *cytotoxic cells, helper cells,* and *suppressor cells*. Cytotoxic T cells, known as "killer cells," are equipped with receptors that match one specific antigen. When that antigen is encountered, the killer cell receptor locks onto it and injects it with a lethal toxin. Current estimates are that each person is born with enough killer T cells to recognize at least 1 million different kinds of antigens.

Helper T cells and suppressor T cells are the principal mechanisms for regulating the immune system's overall response to infection. They do so by secreting chemical messengers called *lymphokines,* which stimulate or inhibit activity in other immune cells. Helper cells are sentries that travel through the bloodstream hunting antigens. When they find them, they secrete chemical messengers that alert B cells, phagocytes, macrophages, and cytotoxic T cells to

Although 95 percent of kindergarteners in the United States are immunized (a law in most states), only 40 to 60 percent of preschoolers are—a lower rate than in many developing countries. One in five of these is a child without health insurance.

Figure 3.11

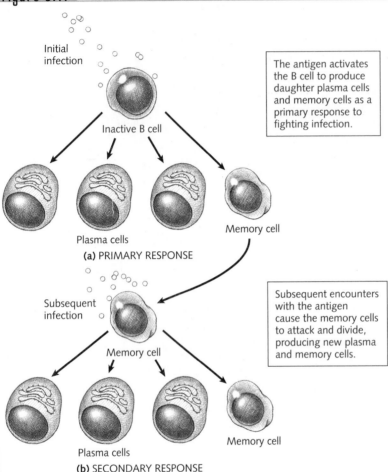

Initial infection

Inactive B cell

The antigen activates the B cell to produce daughter plasma cells and memory cells as a primary response to fighting infection.

Plasma cells

Memory cell

(a) PRIMARY RESPONSE

Subsequent infection

Memory cell

Subsequent encounters with the antigen cause the memory cells to attack and divide, producing new plasma and memory cells.

Plasma cells

Memory cell

(b) SECONDARY RESPONSE

Primary and Secondary Responses of the Immune System
(a) When a B cell is activated by an antigen, it divides into plasma cells, which manufacture antibodies, and memory cells. (b) When memory cells encounter the same antigen during a subsequent infection, the secondary immune response occurs. Memory cells release antibodies that attack the antigen and also divide, producing a new generation of plasma cells and memory cells.

attack. Suppressor T cells serve a counterregulatory function. By producing chemicals that suppress immune responding, these cells ensure that an overzealous immune response doesn't damage healthy cells. Suppressor cells also alert T cells and B cells when an invader has been successfully vanquished.

The Reproductive System and Behavior Genetics

The human reproductive system is, of course, where life and health begin. The separate development of the female and male reproductive systems begins during prenatal development, when a hormonal signal from the hypothalamus stimulates the pituitary gland to produce the *gonadotropic hormones,* which direct the development of the *gonads,* or sex glands—the ovaries in females and the testes in males. One of these hormones in particular, *GnRH (gonad releasing hormone),* directs the ovaries and testes to dramatically increase the production of sex hormones, especially *estrogen* in girls and *testosterone* in boys.

The Female Reproductive System

On either side of the female's uterus are two almond-shaped *ovaries,* which produce the female sex hormones estrogen and progesterone. The outer layer of each ovary contains the *oocytes,* from which the *ova* (eggs) develop. The oocytes begin to form during the third month of prenatal development. At birth, an infant girl's two ovaries contain some 2 million oocytes—all that she will ever have. Of these, about 400,000 survive into puberty, and some 300 to 400 reach maturity, generally one at a time, approximately every 28 days from the onset of puberty until menopause, which typically occurs at about age 50. Each ovum is contained in the ovary within a *follicle,* or capsule.

The menstrual cycle is divided into four phases, each of which is timed and controlled by the hypothalamus in a complex feedback system (see Figure 3.12, page 110). During the first phase, the *proliferative phase,* which lasts 9 or 10 days, estrogen and progesterone are quite low. Sensing these low levels, the hypothalamus instructs the pituitary to release *follicle-stimulating hormone (FSH)* and *lutenizing hormone (LH).* When FSH reaches the ovaries, it stimulates some follicles to mature and begin producing estrogen, which causes the inner layer of the uterus, called the *endometrium,* to thicken, or "proliferate," in preparation for a possible pregnancy.

During the second phase, the *ovulatory phase,* peak estrogen levels cause one or the other of the ovaries to discharge a mature ovum near the fallopian tubes, or *oviducts,* from where it begins its passage to the uterus. When the hypothalamus detects the elevated levels of estrogen, it instructs the pituitary to release additional FSH and LH. Surging levels of LH trigger ovulation within 12 to 24 hours.

The third phase of the cycle, called the *secretory,* or *luteal,* phase, begins just after ovulation and continues to the beginning of the next menstrual phase. Under the continued production of LH, the cells of the emptied follicle enlarge, becoming the *corpus luteum* ("yellow body"). LH also triggers the corpus luteum to begin producing large amounts of estrogen and progesterone. As the hormone levels increase, estrogen and progesterone inhibit further production of GnRH by the hypothalamus and thus of LH and FSH by the pituitary.

If the released ovum is not fertilized by a sperm, it remains in the uterus for approximately 14 days, after which the corpus luteum is reabsorbed, hormone levels drop, and the corpus luteum is flushed from the body along with the endometrium during the final phase of the cycle, the *menstrual phase.*

Figure 3.12

The Menstrual Cycle

Timed and controlled by the hypothalamus, the menstrual cycle has proliferative, ovulatory, secretory (luteal), and menstrual phases. This illustration shows three categories of biological changes: (a) changes in blood levels of hormones, (b) follicular changes, and (c) changes in the development of the uterine lining.

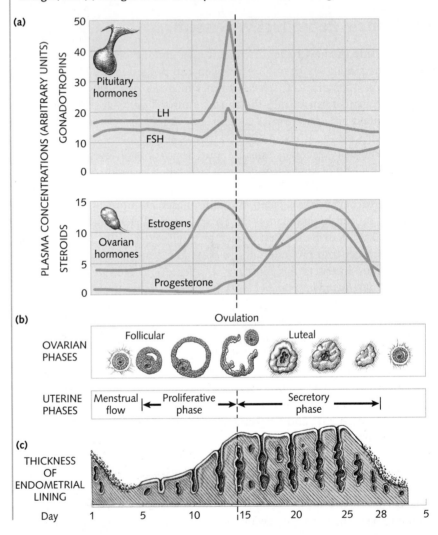

The Male Reproductive System

From puberty until old age, the testes of human males produce an average of several hundred million sperm each day. The testes form during the embryonic phases of prenatal development and are subdivided into some 250 individual compartments, each of which is packed with coiled *seminiferous* ("seed-bearing") *tubules.* It is in these tubules that sperm cells are formed over a period of 8 to 9 weeks. Taken together, the two testes contain a total of approximately 500 meters of tubules.

In contrast to the female's cyclical changes in hormone levels, males maintain fairly constant blood hormone levels. However, the same pituitary hormones that regulate the ovaries—LH and FSH—regulate the testes. FSH stimulates the actual production of sperm, while LH stimulates the testes to secrete testosterone.

As in the female, in the male the hypothalamus monitors blood levels of sex hormones by way of a tight *feedback loop.* Low testosterone levels cause the hypothalamus to secrete a releasing hormone that signals the pituitary to release LH, which in turn causes the testes to secrete testosterone. When testosterone levels rise to an adequate level, the hypothalamus orders the pituitary to cease further production of LH.

Fertilization and the Mechanisms of Heredity

At the moment of conception, a *sperm cell* from the male finds its way upward from the uterus into the fallopian tubes, where it fertilizes an ovum from the female. After fertilization, the resulting single-celled organism, called a **zygote,** travels down the fallopian tube, where the first cellular divisions take place. About 36 hours after fertilization, the zygote divides in half; at 60 hours, the two cells divide again to form four cells. These four cells soon become eight, then sixteen, and so on.

By five days after fertilization, the developing organism consists of approximately 120 cells and embeds itself in the uterine wall in a process known as *implantation.* Implantation triggers the hormonal changes that halt the woman's usual menstrual cycle and enables the connective web of the placenta to develop and nourish the organism over the next 9 months or so.

The zygote contains all the inherited information from both parents that will determine the unborn child's characteristics. Each ovum and each sperm contain 23 *chromosomes,* the long, threadlike structures that carry our inheritance. At conception, the 23 chromosomes from the egg and the 23 from the sperm unite, bequeathing to the newly formed zygote a full complement of 46 chromosomes. As the cells of the developing person divide, this genetic material is replicated time and again so that the nucleus of every cell in the person's body contains the same instructions written at the moment of conception.

The twenty-third pair of chromosomes determines the zygote's sex. The mother always contributes an **X chromosome;** the father can contribute either an X or a **Y chromosome.** If the father's sperm also contains an X chromosome, the child will be a girl; a Y chromosome will produce a boy. Y chromosomes contain a single gene that triggers the testes to begin producing testosterone, which in turn initiates the sexual differentiation in appearance and neural differentiation during the fourth and fifth months of prenatal development.

■ **zygote** a fertilized egg cell

■ **X chromosome** the sex chromosome found in males and females. Females have two X chromosomes; males have one

■ **Y chromosome** the sex chromosome found only in males; contains a gene that triggers the testes to begin producing testosterone

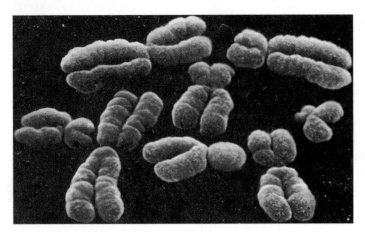

Human Chromosomes
At conception, the 23 chromosomes from the egg and sperm unite, bequeathing to the newly formed zygote a full complement of 46 chromosomes. As the cells of the developing zygote divide, this genetic material is replicated time and again so that the nucleus of every cell in a person's body contains the same instructions written at the moment of conception. Biophoto Associates/ Science Source/Photo Researchers

Each chromosome is composed of strings of *genes*—the basic units of heredity that determine our growth and characteristics. Genes are discrete particles of deoxyribonucleic acid, or *DNA* for short. Each cell in the body contains 50,000 to 80,000 genes that determine everything from the length of your toenails to whether you have a tendency toward schizophrenia, a major psychological disorder.

Before the last decade, scientists knew relatively little about the specific effects of specific genes. Today, with the Human Genome Project, they have been able to map—locate and determine the role of—many of those genes. Remarkably, the first stage of this massive project was finished little more than 100 years after Mendel's work, which marked the beginning of the science of genetics.

Genes and Environment

Most human characteristics are not determined by genes alone, but rather by a combination of factors. In other words, most human characteristics are both *multifactorial*—that is, influenced by many different factors, including environmental factors—and *polygenic*—that is, influenced by many different genes.

The sum total of genes that a person inherits is that person's **genotype.** The observable physical and nonphysical traits that are actually expressed constitute the person's **phenotype.** This distinction is important because each of us inherits many genes in our genotype that are not expressed in our phenotype. In genetic terminology, we are *carriers* of these unexpressed bits of DNA; although we may not manifest them in our own phenotype, they may be passed on to our offspring, who will then have them in their genotype and may or may not express them in their phenotype. For any given trait, a person's phenotype is determined by two patterns of genetic interaction: gene–gene and gene–environment.

Gene–Gene Interactions One common pattern of gene–gene interaction is called *additive* because the resulting phenotype simply reflects the sum of the contributions of individual genes. Genes that determine height and skin color, for example, usually interact additively. For other traits, genes interact in a *nonadditive* fashion. With these traits, the resulting phenotype depends on the influence of one gene more than on the other. A familiar example of nonadditive interaction is the *dominant-recessive pattern.* Some traits occur in the presence of a single dominant gene, with its paired recessive gene making little or no contribution. Many physical characteristics, including eye color, follow the dominant-recessive pattern.

Gene–Environment Interaction Worldwide, genes also interact with a person's environment in determining phenotype. When behavior geneticists refer to envi-

■ **genotype** the sum total of all the genes present in an individual

■ **phenotype** a person's observable characteristics; determined by the interaction of the individual's genotype with the environment

ronment, they are referring to everything that can influence a person's genetic makeup from the beginning of prenatal development until the moment of death. Environmental influences include the direct effects of nutrition, climate, and medical care, as well as indirect effects brought on by the particular economic, cultural, and historical context in which the individual develops.

Health psychologists now recognize that most or all health behaviors are influenced by genetic predispositions and physiological states. As the mind–body perspective reminds us, however, health behaviors are also influenced by personality and thinking style and by social and cultural circumstances. In subsequent chapters you'll see how physical systems combine and interact with psychological and sociocultural factors to determine health behaviors, as well as overall states of wellness or illness.

Summing Up

The Nervous System

1. A neuron is a specialized cell that receives signals through its dendrites and cell body and transmits electrical signals down its axon. An above-threshold stimulus causes a neural impulse to flow down the axon to the axon terminal and release chemical neurotransmitters across the synapse.

2. The central nervous system consists of the brain and the spinal cord. The remaining neurons comprise the peripheral nervous system, which itself has two main divisions: the somatic nervous system, which controls voluntary movements, and the autonomic nervous system, which controls the involuntary muscles and endocrine glands through the sympathetic and parasympathetic nervous systems.

3. As the oldest and most central region of the brain, the brainstem, including the reticular formation, thalamus, and cerebellum, controls basic life-support functions via the autonomic nervous system. The limbic system includes the amygdala, which plays an important role in aggression and other emotions; the hippocampus, which is involved in learning and memory; and the hypothalamus, which influences hunger, thirst, body temperature, and sexual behavior.

4. The cerebral cortex is the thin layer of cells that covers the cerebrum. The cortex is the seat of consciousness and includes areas specialized for speaking and decision making (frontal lobe), vision (occipital lobe), hearing (temporal lobe), and touch (parietal lobe). The association cortex includes areas that are not directly involved in sensory or motor functions. These areas integrate information and are involved in higher mental functions such as thinking and speaking.

The Endocrine System

5. Operating under the control of the hypothalamus, the pituitary gland secretes hormones that influence growth, sexual development, reproduction, kidney functioning, and aging. Other glands augment the nervous system in regulating the functioning of heart rate and blood pressure (adrenal medulla), reducing inflammation (adrenal cortex), regulating growth and metabolism (thyroid), and regulating blood glucose levels (pancreas).

The Cardiovascular System

6. The heart is separated into four chambers. Oxygen-depleted blood returning from the body is pumped from the right atrium into the right ventricle, and from there through the capillaries of the lungs, where it picks up fresh oxygen and disposes of carbon dioxide. The freshly oxygenated blood is pumped through the pulmonary vein into the left atrium of the heart, and from there into the left ventricle, from which it flows into the arterial system.

The Respiratory System

7. After air enters the body through the mouth or nose, it travels to the lungs via bronchial tubes that branch into the smaller bronchioles and air sacs of the lungs

(alveoli). The thin walls of the alveoli permit the exchange of oxygen and carbon dioxide.

The Digestive System

8. Digestion begins in the mouth, where chewing and salivary enzymes begin to break food down. Once food is swallowed, the rhythmic movements of the esophageal muscles propel food downward to the stomach, where it is mixed with a variety of gastric enzymes under the control of the autonomic nervous system. Digestive fluids from the pancreas, liver, and gallbladder are secreted into the small and large intestines, where—several hours after eating—the breakdown of food is completed.

The Immune System

9. The body's first line of defense against health-threatening pathogens includes the protective barrier provided by the skin, the mucus membranes of the nose and respiratory tract, and gastric enzymes of the digestive system. A pathogen that penetrates these defenses encounters an army of white blood cells (lymphocytes) that filter out infectious substances and debris with the passage of fluids through the lymphatic system. Other nonspecific immune defenses include the action of the antigen-engulfing phagocytes, macrophages, and NK cells. NK cells also secrete antimicrobial proteins called interferon and play a role in the body's inflammatory response.

10. Specific immune reactions occur when B cells and T cells attack specific antigens. B cells accomplish this when memory cells produce specific antibodies that kill antigens previously encountered. In cell-mediated immunity, T cells directly attack and kill antigens by injecting them with lethal toxins. Immune functioning improves throughout childhood and early adolescence and begins to decline as people approach old age.

The Reproductive System and Behavior Genetics

11. The reproductive system, under the control of the hypothalamus and the endocrine system, directs the development of the primary and secondary sex characteristics. Timed and controlled by the hypothalamus, the menstrual cycle has proliferative, ovulatory, secretory (luteal), and menstrual phases. These phases involve three categories of biological changes: changes in blood levels of hormones, follicular changes, and changes in the development of the uterine lining. In contrast to females, males maintain fairly constant blood hormone levels. As in the female, the hypothalamus monitors these levels.

12. The sum total of all the genes a person inherits is the person's genotype. How those genes are expressed in the person's traits is the phenotype. Human development begins when a sperm cell fertilizes an ovum, resulting in a single-celled zygote that contains the inherited information from the 23 chromosomes inherited from each parent. The twenty-third pair of chromosomes determines the zygote's sex. Genes are segments of DNA that provide the genetic blueprint for our physical and behavioral development. For any given trait, patterns of gene–gene and gene–environment interaction determine the observable phenotype. Two common patterns of gene–gene interaction are additive and dominant-recessive.

Key Terms and Concepts

neuron, p. 85
synapse, p. 85
neurotransmitters, p. 85
threshold, p. 86
central nervous system (CNS), p. 87
peripheral nervous system (PNS), p. 87
brainstem, p. 89
medulla, p. 89
reticular formation, p. 89
thalamus, p. 89
cerebellum, p. 90
limbic system, p. 90

amygdala, p. 90
hippocampus, p. 90
hypothalamus, p. 90
cerebral cortex, p. 91
sensory cortex, p. 91
motor cortex, p. 91
association cortex, p. 91
hormones, p. 94
pituitary gland, p. 95
adrenal glands, p. 95
arteries, p. 96
veins, p. 96

bronchi, p. 98
cilia, p. 98
gastrointestinal system, p. 99
genetic linkage, p. 101
antigen, p. 103
lymphocytes, p. 104
zygote, p. 111
X chromosome, p. 111
Y chromosome, p. 111
genotype, p. 112
phenotype, p. 112

Health Psychology on the World Wide Web

Web Address	Description
http://www.nhgri.nih.gov/	National Human Genome Research Institute—the latest human genetics news.
http://www.amhrt.org/	American Heart Association.
http://sln.fi.eud/biosci/heart.html	The Heart: An Online Exploration—a multimedia tour of the cardiovascular system.
http://www.niaid.nih.gov/default.htm	National Institute of Allergy and Infectious Diseases—links to research aimed at developing better ways to diagnose, treat, and prevent infectious, immune, and allergic diseases.

Critical Thinking Exercise

Genetic Screening

Now that you have completed Chapter 3, take your learning a step further by testing your critical thinking skills on this scientific reasoning exercise.

As we move closer to the day when genetic screening and engineering become commonplace, many scientists are raising concerns about the social, ethical, and political implications of this genetic revolution. Who should decide what constitutes a genetic "defect"? Should genetic screening be required? Who would decide who must be screened?

Another worry concerns safeguarding the privacy of the individual. In nations that do not have universal health insurance, critics fear that insurance companies might require genetic screening before writing a policy, using this information either to deny coverage or to charge exorbitant premiums to those individuals who carry defective genes that might lead to chronic illness.

Another fear is that some may want to use genetic screening and gene therapy to "improve" individuals with traits that are not lethal but simply less desirable. Should a parent, for example, be permitted to use genetic engineering to make a short child taller or a hyperactive child quieter?

To help bring your own thoughts on these controversial issues into sharper focus, answer the following questions.

1. Would you want to know that you carried a gene for a disease that can't be treated? How would you feel about knowing you carried a gene that *might* cause a disease to develop years later?

2. Should parents know if an unborn child might develop an incurable disease? What impact would such knowledge have on each domain of the child's health?

3. Should genetic screening be required of every couple? For some couples? Who should decide who must be screened?

4. What are some of the negative effects of genetic technology on the individual? On the family? On society?

2

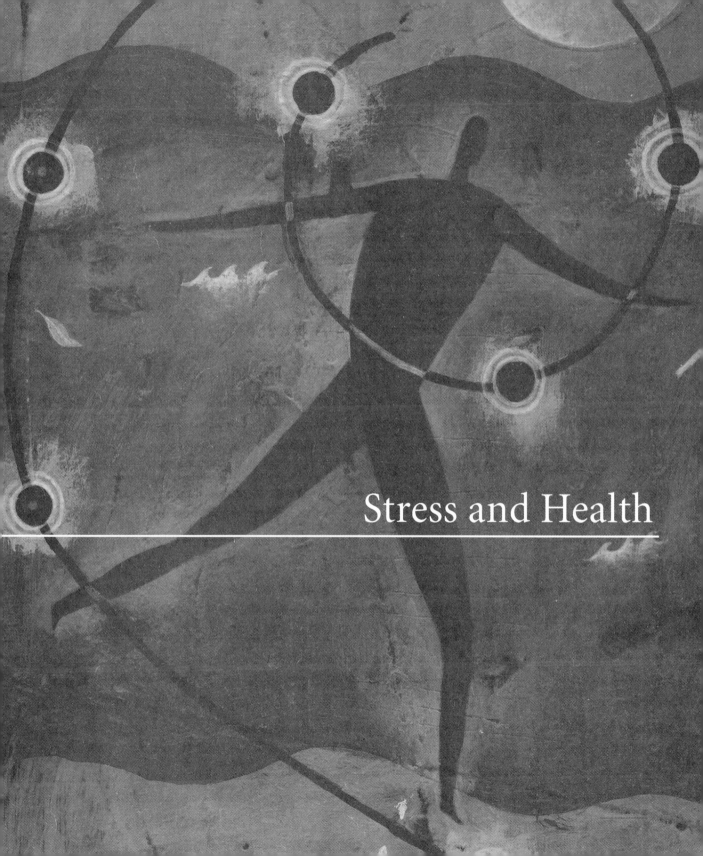

Stress and Health

4

Stress

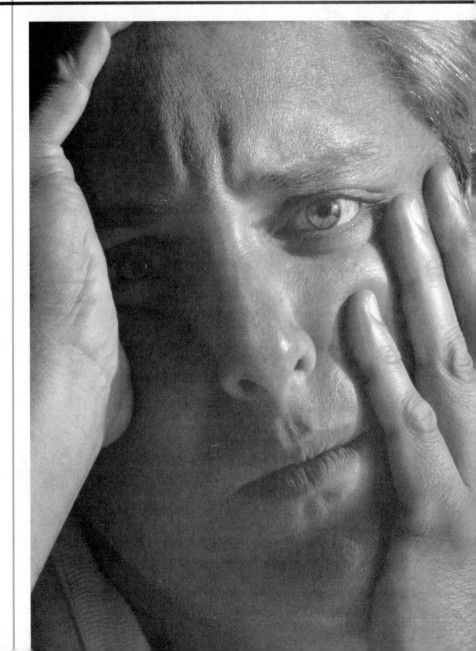

*J*avier, don't forget that you have to work tonight," the restaurant manager called out as Javier was rushing to leave for his afternoon psychology class. It was the day of the final exam and Javier was already running late. To make matters worse, he still had to stop by the campus bookstore to purchase the special answer booklet Professor Roosevelt required for her essay exams. (He could still remember the look of horror on his friend Sandy's face when her midterm was returned marked down one full grade because she had used the "wrong" answer booklet.)

A college sophomore, Javier had to work full-time to support himself while carrying a heavy load of courses at the college. Working in the restaurant paid well, and his elderly boss was nice, but he just didn't seem to realize that Javier was first and foremost a student, not a candidate for a fast-track/fast-food career.

Exhausted, Javier turned the key of the 10-year-old "beater" car he'd managed to buy from his meager savings. "Please don't fail me now," he pleaded as the car's engine coughed to life. Always tired when exam week rolled around, Javier worked a rotating shift schedule that invariably forced him to forgo sleep in order to study.

As he drove to the campus, Javier's mind momentarily shifted to other worries. His parents had been pressuring him for months to declare a college major. ("Will I ever be able to decide on a career," Javier wondered, "or will I remain a student forever, sampling classes in an endless variety of subjects?") They were also anxious for Javier and Ally, his girlfriend of 5 years, to make plans for their future. "Aren't you two ever going to set the wedding date?" they had complained during their most recent phone call. On top of all this, Javier just could not seem to shake the cold that had plagued him since midterms.

Javier breathed a sigh of relief as he pulled into the students' parking lot. There was one parking space open in the normally full lot. With only 10 minutes to go until the start of class, he realized that if he sprinted to the bookstore, he just might be able to buy the answer booklet and make it to class after all.

As the tests were being passed out, Javier began to breathe faster and his heart began to pound. What was it they had talked about in class last week? Oh yeah, the "fight-or-flight" response. That's what he was feeling now.

Grabbing his calculator and answer booklet from his backpack ("The statistics portion of the exam is going to be a real bear"), Javier took a deep breath and willed himself to relax.

As he began to work on the first question, the display on Javier's calculator slowly began to fade and then disappeared. "Oh no! The batteries can't be dead now. What am I going to do?"

Javier felt like his world was spinning out of control.

Javier's situation is not uncommon. Each of us experiences stress in our every-day lives. Stress can come from many directions, including school, family and friends, interactions with strangers, and the job. Fortunately, in most cases stress is a brief experience—as when you are forced to juggle the ever-changing demands of school, job, family, and friends. On other occasions stress may persist for a long time—as when a person loses a loved one or is forced to retire or is laid off. The idea that persistent, or chronic, stress influences a person's vulnerability to disease is, in fact, a major theme in health psychology.

Stress has been a central concept in medicine and health since antiquity. The idea that the body "gears up" to meet environmental demands has appeared many times. For example, Hippocrates (460–377 B.C.) made a clear distinction between the specific symptoms of discomfort caused by a disease *(pathos)* and the general discomfort, or stress, caused as the body struggles to resist the disease *(ponos)*.

Most of what we know today about stress has come to light in the past 50 years, as researchers formally attempted to examine stress in both humans and animals. This chapter looks at what stress is, how it is measured, where it comes from, and its impact on the body; Chapter 5 deals with the ways we cope with stress. To begin, we will look at how researchers define stress.

What Is Stress?

You probably had no trouble feeling empathy for Javier's plight because you've been in similar situations. How do you feel when you are "under a lot of stress"? If you are like most people, you probably feel tense, irritable, and unable to concentrate easily on things that you normally do automatically.

Stimulus or Response?

Despite the pervasiveness of such experiences, psychologists have not had an easy time coming up with an acceptable definition of stress. The word *stress* is sometimes used to describe a threatening situation or *stimulus* ("Javier's stressful work schedule really did him in before the exam"), and at other times to describe a *response* to a situation ("When Javier realized his calculator batteries were dead, he really stressed out").

Perhaps the simplest approach to stress is to view it as a stimulus, that is, as a property of the events and situations we face. We see this when a friend says that his class schedule this semester is unusually "stressful" or when a relative wants to switch careers in order to escape his "high-stress job."

The stimulus concept of stress can be traced to seventeenth-century engineering analyses of loads (the amount of force applied to an object) and strain (the resulting damage to the object). Researchers who follow this approach have analyzed the load created by a variety of sources of stress, including noise, crowding, natural disasters, and major life events such as the loss of a loved one.

A second approach considers stress to be a person's response to a threatening event or situation. Just before giving an important oral presentation in a class, for example, you may feel "stressed out." Your response includes both psychological and physiological components. The psychological component includes emotions (such as anxiety or fear), behaviors (such as nervous laughter or smoking), and thoughts (such as pessimistic self-talk). The physiological component includes the various symptoms of bodily arousal: dry mouth, butterflies in the stomach, and perspiration. We'll examine the physiology of the stress response later in the chapter.

So, is stress a stimulus or is it a response? Well, it is both—but also something more. Health psychologists distinguish the stimulus properties of stress from its response properties. Following this distinction, **stressors** are demanding stimulus events or situations that trigger coping adjustments in a person. In the example at the beginning of the chapter, the stressors that Javier experienced included the exam, the dead calculator batteries, and his pressing workload. **Strain** refers to the physical and emotional *responses* that accompany the person's perception of the stressors. Javier's pounding heart, shallow breathing, and feeling that the "world was spinning out of control" are examples of strain. **Stress** is thus most completely defined as a *process* by which a person both perceives and responds to events that are judged to be challenging or threatening.

- **stressor** any event or situation that triggers coping adjustments

- **strain** the physical and emotional wear and tear reaction of a person attempting to cope with a stressor

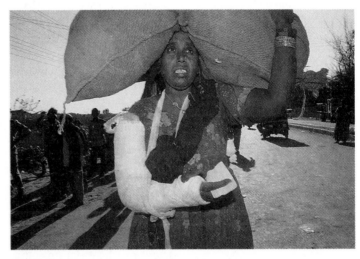

Stress Is . . .

Floods, tornadoes, and other catastrophic events provide real-world examples of stress as both a stimulus and a response. The catastrophic event that triggers coping behavior is the stressor (the stimulus), and the person attempting to flee the event or trying to compensate for the destruction it causes illustrates the response. This Indian woman, her arm broken in a February 2001 earthquake that killed 14,200 people and left an estimated 600,000 homeless, carries wheat from a Red Cross campsite in Bhuj, India. John McConnico/AP/Wide World Photos

- **stress** the process by which we perceive and respond to events, called stressors, that are perceived as harmful, threatening, or challenging

- **transactional model** Lazarus' theory that the experience of stress depends as much on the individual's cognitive appraisal of a potential stressor's impact as it does on the event or situation itself

Stress as a Transaction

The most influential model describing stress as a process is the **transactional model** (also called the *relational model*), proposed by Richard Lazarus and his colleagues (Lazarus, 1993; Lazarus & Launier, 1978). The fundamental idea behind this model is that we cannot fully understand stress by examining environmental events (stimuli) and people (responses) as separate entities; rather,

■ **primary appraisal** a person's initial determination of an event's meaning, whether irrelevant, benign-positive, or threatening

■ **secondary appraisal** a person's determination of whether his or her own resources and abilities are sufficient to meet the demands of an event that is appraised as potentially threatening or challenging

■ **cognitive reappraisal** the process by which potentially stressful events are constantly reevaluated

we need to consider them together as a transaction, in which each person must continually adjust to daily challenges.

According to the transactional model, the *process* of stress is triggered whenever stressors exceed the personal and social resources a given person is able to mobilize in order to cope (Steptoe, 1997). If a person's coping resources are strong enough, there is no stress, even when—to another person—the situation is seemingly unbearable. On the other hand, if a person's coping resources are weak or ineffective, stress occurs, even when—to another person—the demands of a situation can easily be met.

When the demands of an event or situation do create stress, our response is not static but, rather, involves continuous interactions and adjustments—called *transactions*—between the environment and our attempts to cope. Each of us is an active agent who can dramatically alter the impact of a potential stressor through our own personal resources.

Lazarus believes that the transactions between a person and his or her environment are driven by the individual's *cognitive appraisal* of potential stressors. Cognitive appraisal involves assessing (1) whether a situation or event threatens a person's well-being, (2) whether there are sufficient personal resources available for coping with the demand, and (3) whether the person's strategy for dealing with the situation or event is working.

When a person confronts a potentially stressful event, such as hearing the blaring sound of a car horn, he or she engages in a **primary appraisal** to determine the event's meaning. The primary appraisal is equivalent to asking the question, "Is this situation going to mean trouble for me?" The outcome of the primary appraisal is that the event is interpreted in one of three ways: as *irrelevant*; as *benign-positive*; or as challenging, harmful, or *threatening* (Figure 4.1).

Once an event has been appraised as a challenge or threat, **secondary appraisal** answers the question, "What can I do to cope with this situation?" At this point, the person assesses his or her coping abilities to determine whether they will be adequate to meet the challenge, potential harm-loss, or threat. If these resources are deemed adequate, little or no stress occurs. When a threat or challenge is high and coping resources are low, stress is likely to occur.

Finally, the transactional model emphasizes the ongoing nature of the appraisal process as new information becomes available. Through **cognitive reappraisal** the person constantly updates his or her perception of success or failure in meeting a challenge or threat. New information may allow the person to turn a previously stressful appraisal into a benign-positive one, as when a student gains confidence in her ability to do well on a long-feared exam after successfully answering the first few questions.

Cognitive reappraisal does not always result in less stress, however; sometimes it increases stress. An event originally appraised as benign or irrelevant can quickly take on a threatening character if a coping response fails or if the person

Figure 4.1

The Transactional Model of Stress
The impact of a potential stressor, such as the startling sound of a honking horn, depends on a three-step process of cognitive appraisal. During primary appraisal, events perceived as neutral or benign pose no threat as a source of stress. Events perceived as challenging, harmful, or threatening are subjected to a secondary appraisal, in which the individual determines whether his or her coping resources are sufficient to meet the challenge posed by the stressor. Finally, in the reappraisal process, feedback from new information or ongoing coping efforts is used to check on the accuracy of both primary and secondary appraisals.

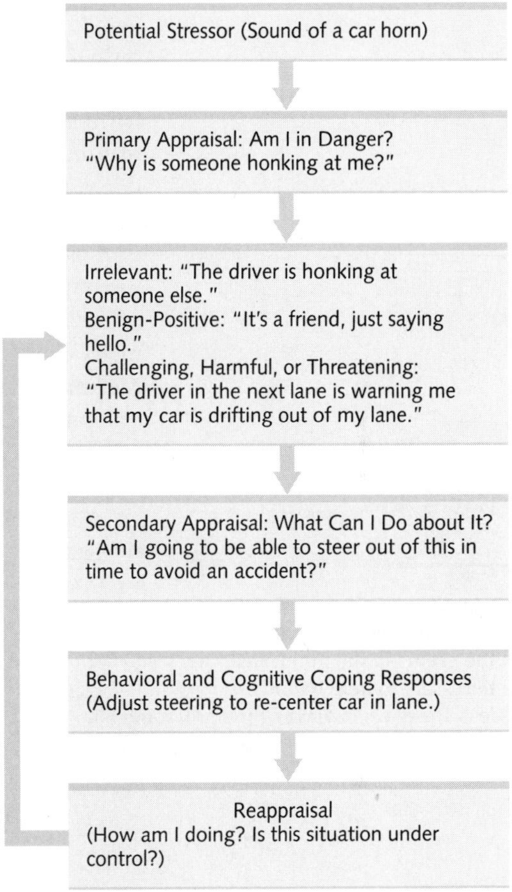

Potential Stressor (Sound of a car horn)

↓

Primary Appraisal: Am I in Danger?
"Why is someone honking at me?"

↓

Irrelevant: "The driver is honking at someone else."
Benign-Positive: "It's a friend, just saying hello."
Challenging, Harmful, or Threatening: "The driver in the next lane is warning me that my car is drifting out of my lane."

↓

Secondary Appraisal: What Can I Do about It? "Am I going to be able to steer out of this in time to avoid an accident?"

↓

Behavioral and Cognitive Coping Responses (Adjust steering to re-center car in lane.)

↓

Reappraisal
(How am I doing? Is this situation under control?)

begins to see the event differently. For example, a job interview that seems to be going very well may become very stressful when the interviewer casually mentions the large number of well-qualified individuals who have applied for the position.

Let's look at an example of cognitive appraisal and reappraisal. As I was jogging through my neighborhood one day last winter, a car approached from the opposite direction, slowed, and then stopped alongside me. The icy road offered only a narrow shoulder, and when the driver honked her horn I became angry at her unwillingness to share the road. As I was about to shake my fist at her, the driver smiled and waved—not at me, but at a neighbor just stepping out his front door to collect his newspaper. Chiding myself for a short fuse, I quickly reappraised the event as irrelevant and experienced no stress. My neighbor, on the other hand, heard the car horn, immediately recognized his neighbor, and appraised the situation as benign-positive—a desirable event that does not cause stress.

Types of Cognitive Appraisal

According to Lazarus and as shown in Figure 4.1, appraising an event as stressful means seeing it as a potential challenge, a source of harm, or as a threat to one's future well-being. A *challenge* is perceived when a situation is demanding but ultimately can be overcome, and the person can profit from the situation. For example, hearing a honk and noticing that your car has drifted over into the next lane is a potentially stressful situation. Realizing that you have time to make the necessary steering adjustments to avoid an accident allows you to appraise the event as a surmountable challenge. As another example, a person who is fired from her job undoubtedly experiences some level of stress, but she may also see this as a surmountable problem (and, perhaps, an opportunity to improve her life by starting a better career).

Appraisals of harm-loss or threat refer to less positive outcomes. *Harm-loss* is the assessment that some form of damage has already occurred as a result of a situation, such as an illness, an injury, or the lost income and lowered self-esteem that may follow from being laid off from work. An event may be appraised as a *threat* when the person anticipates that a situation may bring about loss or harm at some point *in the future*. For example, hearing the honk of a horn and realizing that the car behind you is going to crash into your car would most certainly involve an appraisal of threat (quickly followed, in all likelihood, by a cognitive reappraisal of harm-loss stemming from a damaged automobile or injury).

A classic series of studies conducted by Lazarus and his colleagues illustrates the importance of cognitive appraisal in the experience of stress. In one study college students watched a gruesome film depicting shop accidents such as a metal worker being impaled by a plank driven through his abdomen (Koriat, Melkman, Averill, & Lazarus, 1972). Before viewing the film, the students were randomly assigned to one of three experimental conditions. One group was told that the events in the film had been staged, that no one was actually hurt during filming, and that the film was designed to improve worker safety. A second group was told that the events were real but that the film would help to improve worker safety. A third group of students (the control group) was not given any explanation whatsoever.

What were the results? On the basis of the students' autonomic arousal (their heart rate and blood pressure) and their self-reported level of anxiety, the researchers found that both sets of explanations were effective in reducing arousal during the film. As shown in Figure 4.2, the gruesome film was perceived to be less stressful when viewers were told the events in the film were staged (Group 1) or were necessary to help improve worker safety (Group 2). Groups 1 and 2 experienced considerably less stress than the group that was not given an explanation, presumably because the instructions permitted the students to appraise the film in a less threatening manner. Thus, this study demonstrates that stress was not a property of the film itself but depended on the viewer's appraisal of it.

Implications of the Transactional Model

Lazarus' transactional model has three important implications. First, situations or events are not inherently stressful or unstressful; any given situation or event may be appraised (and experienced) as stressful by one person but not by another. Second, cognitive appraisals are extremely susceptible to changes in mood, health, and moti-

Figure 4.2

The Impact of Cognitive Appraisal on the Perception of Stress
Compared with students in the control group who were not given an explanation, students who were told the events in the film were either staged or real but necessary to help improve worker safety experienced less stress when viewing the gruesome film.

Source: Based on data from "The Self-Control of Emotional Reactions to a Stressful Film," by A. Koriat, R. Melkman, J. R. Averill, and R. Lazarus, 1972, *Journal of Personality, 40*(4), pp. 601–619.

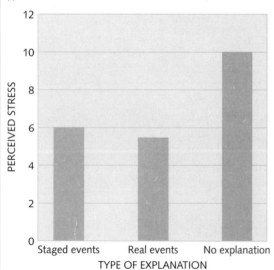

vational state. You may interpret the same event or situation in very different ways on separate occasions. Being forced to wait in traffic may be a minor annoyance on most days; on the day when you are late for an exam it may seem an insurmountable obstacle. Third, some evidence suggests that the body's stress response is nearly the same, whether a situation is actually experienced or merely imagined. This means that even recalled or imagined appraisals of a situation may elicit a stress response. Clinical psychologists think that some people may be chronically depressed because they replay stressful events over and over again in their minds, a situation that may be functionally equivalent to actually encountering the stressful event repeatedly.

Measuring Stress

Health psychologists measure stress either through self-report instruments or through physiological and behavioral assessments. Self-report instruments include checklists, life events scales, and everyday hassles inventories (see Reality Check, pages 126–127). Physiological and behavioral measures of stress, the subject of this section, include examining the body's physiological changes as stressors are encountered and adjusted to, and measuring how a person's performance on a familiar task changes in response to a stressor.

Physiological Measures

Stress affects nearly every system in the body. The simplest way to assess the physiological arousal that stress triggers is to measure changes in a person's heart rate, blood pressure, rate of breathing, or **galvanic skin response (GSR).** GSR is a measure of the skin's resistance to electricity. Experiencing stress, a person may begin to perspire, causing a measurable increase in the skin's ability to conduct an imperceptible electric current. These measurements are often made jointly using a **polygraph,** a machine that records several arousal responses that accompany stress and other emotions, including heart rate, blood pressure, respiration rate, and skin resistance.

In a typical study, participants are asked to sit quietly for 20 to 30 minutes in order to stabilize their blood pressure, heart rate, and so on; these physiological functions are then measured to give a comparison, or baseline, score for relaxation. Participants are then exposed to a demanding task or stressful situation, such as working a difficult puzzle or viewing a stressful film, while the experimenter carefully watches the polygraph for signs of increased bodily arousal.

■ **galvanic skin response (GSR)** a measure of the skin's resistance to electricity. Experiencing stress, a person may begin to perspire, causing a measurable increase in the electrical conductivity of the skin

■ **polygraph** often called a *lie detector,* a machine that measures several of the physiological responses that accompany stress and other emotional states

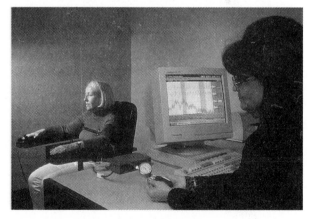

Measuring Stress—the Polygraph
A polygraph (lie detector) recording of a subject during a baseline measure of relaxation. The physiological measures depicted include GSR (galvanic skin response), heart rate, and blood pressure. Index Stock Imagery

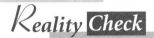

Is There Too Much Stress in Your Life?

This questionnaire is concerned with your thoughts about various aspects of a potentially stressful situation such as an upcoming examination, losing a job or scholarship, contracting AIDS or some other chronic disease, or living through some sort of natural disaster. There are no right or wrong answers. Pick one such event and respond to the following questions according to how you view the situation right NOW.

THE STRESS APPRAISAL MEASURE (SAM)

Please answer ALL questions. Answer each question by writing the appropriate number on the line, according to the following scale.

1 = not at all	2 = slightly	3 = moderately
	4 = considerably	5 = extremely

___ 1. Is this a totally hopeless situation?

___ 2. Does this situation create tension in me?

___ 3. Is the outcome of this situation uncontrollable by anyone?

___ 4. Is there someone or some agency I can turn to for help if I need it?

___ 5. Does this situation make me feel anxious?

___ 6. Does this situation have important consequences for me?

___ 7. Is this going to have a positive impact on me?

___ 8. How eager am I to tackle this problem?

___ 9. How much will I be affected by the outcome of this situation?

___ 10. To what extent can I become a stronger person because of this problem?

___ 11. Will the outcome of this situation be negative?

___ 12. Do I have the ability to do well in this situation?

___ 13. Does this situation have serious implications for me?

___ 14. Do I have what it takes to do well in this situation?

___ 15. Is there help available to me for dealing with this problem?

___ 16. Does this situation tax or exceed my coping resources?

___ 17. Are there sufficient resources available to help me in dealing with this situation?

___ 18. Is it beyond anyone's power to do anything about this situation?

___ 19. To what extent am I excited thinking about the outcome of this situation?

___ 20. How threatening is this situation?

___ 21. Is the problem unresolvable by anyone?

___ 22. Will I be able to overcome the problem?

___ 23. Is there anyone who can help me to manage this problem?

___ 24. To what extent do I perceive this situation as stressful?

___ 25. Do I have the skills necessary to achieve a successful outcome to this situation?

___ 26. To what extent does this event require coping efforts on my part?

___ 27. Does this situation have long-term consequences for me?

___ 28. Is this going to have a negative impact on me?

Scoring The SAM, which was designed to measure your primary appraisal of a future event, contains three dimensions: threat (the potential for harm/loss), challenge (the anticipation of gain or growth from the experience), and centrality (the perceived importance of the event for well-being). It also contains three secondary appraisal measures that reflect your appraisal of available coping resources: controllable-by-self, controllable-by-others, and uncontrollable-by-anyone. Finally, the SAM includes a general perceived stressfulness subscale. To score your appraisals, calculate the mean for each subscale by adding together your responses for the items on each subscale and dividing this sum by 4.

Threat: Items 5, 11, 20, 28

Challenge: Items 7, 8, 10, 19

Centrality: Items 6, 9, 13, 27

Control-self: Items 12, 14, 22, 25

Control-others: Items 4, 15, 17, 23

Uncontrollable: Items 1, 3, 18, 21

Stressfulness: Items 2, 16, 24, 26

To interpret your scores, compare your mean on each subscale with those found in a large comparison group of col-

	Exam	Unemployment	AIDS	Natural Disaster
Threat	2.6	2.6	3.2	2.8
Challenge	3.0	3.5	2.5	2.3
Centrality	3.6	3.7	3.5	3.6
Control-Self	3.9	3.8	3.1	3.2
Control-Others	3.7	3.4	3.3	3.3
Uncontrollable	1.6	2.2	2.8	2.9
Stressfulness	3.4	3.0	3.0	3.1

lege students (see table). Based on information discussed in the chapter, how realistic (and adaptive) is your appraisal process? Do you, for instance, appraise an upcoming examination as a controllable challenge that is important but that will not have a central impact on your sense of well-being?

Source: "The Stress Appraisal Measure (SAM): A Multidimensional Approach to Cognitive Appraisal," by E. Peacock and P. Wong, 1990. *Stress Medicine, 6*, pp. 227–236.

Although physiological measures are useful for charting the body's physical response to stress, they have several drawbacks. First, measuring arousal requires expensive and extremely sensitive instruments that are not easily moved beyond the confines of a laboratory setting. A second difficulty concerns the interpretation and reliability of results. Because physiological responses are much the same from one emotion to another, polygraphs can't distinguish among guilt, stress, and anxiety—all appear as physiological arousal. Finally, the measuring procedures may themselves prove stressful for some people.

Performance Measures

Most people are aware that they perform differently when they are under stress. Some may "rise to the occasion" when they are overloaded with work, while others may crumble under the pressure and perform below their capability. Assessing performance, then, provides one method of measuring stress.

Performance tests typically compare how well a person accomplishes a task under normal conditions with how well he or she does in the presence of an acute stressor. Typical stressors include crowding, loud noise, and electric shock. If the participant's performance deteriorates after exposure to a stressor, the researcher assumes that the poor performance is due to stress.

In one early study, David Glass and Jerome Singer (1972) demonstrated that persistent environmental noise reduced the speed and accuracy of people's performance on simple cognitive tasks. The researchers put students to work on a variety of paper-and-pencil tasks while exposing them to random bursts of noise over a 25-minute period. At the end of the noisy period the students were given additional cognitive tasks to perform, including proofreading an article for accuracy and working difficult puzzles. Compared to students who had earlier worked in a quiet control group, those who had earlier been exposed to the random noise consistently performed more poorly on these subsequent tasks.

Research has also shown that people tend to develop a form of "tunnel vision," in which they narrow their focus and become less socially aware when stressed—a tendency that can be especially disruptive to the performance of groups or teams. In a recent study, James Driskell, Eduardo Salas, and Joan Johnston (1999) asked naval cadets to participate in a computer simulation of a naval warfare decision-making task. Using radar, the cadets had to determine whether the ships surrounding them were friendly or hostile and "target" the unfriendly ones. The cadets completed the task either individually or on interdependent teams. Members of interdependent teams were required to cooperate with one another to complete the task. Some teams performed the exercise under high stress as they were subjected to constant chatter over earphones, frequent interruptions to remind them of time constraints, and numerous threats from hostile ships. The results showed that the interdependent teams completed the task more efficiently than individuals did, showing higher levels of team perspective. But under stress the team perspective broke down for the interdependent teams and performance deteriorated to no better than that of individuals.

Given the interdependent nature of many jobs and situations, it is worth considering the practical implications of this research. As external demands (and stress) increase, teamwork behaviors, such as attending to others, may be neglected as the attention of individual group members shifts to cues involved in performing their own immediate tasks. When effective teamwork is critical, it may be necessary to structure tasks to make them less demanding so that attention can be maintained on teamwork.

"Good" Stress and Improved Performance Most people think that stress always has a negative impact on well-being, but researchers have found that some types or amounts of stress actually *improve* performance on some tasks. For instance, when I compete against other runners in a road race, the stress generally brings out a faster performance compared to when I cover the same distance running by myself. Similarly, musicians, actors, and actresses generally give stronger performances in front of an audience than they do during rehearsal. Canadian scientist Hans Selye proposed the terms *distress* for unpleasant, damaging stress, and *eustress* for beneficial, or good, stress.

The Optimum Level of Arousal In Selye's view, the most important aspect of a stressor is its impact on the body. To meet stressful demands, whether good or bad, the body becomes aroused and expends energy. It is this arousal and energy expenditure that constitutes stress.

Following this line of reasoning, for each person there is an *optimum level of arousal* at which he or she performs and feels best on a given task (Hebb, 1955). The stress of worrying about whether you will pass an exam may motivate you to study, or the stress of performing in front of an audience may help a musician or athlete perform at a peak level.

Let's examine this theory more carefully. Although there are individual differences in the optimum level of arousal, too little or too much arousal impairs *anyone's* functioning. Figure 4.3 illustrates this **optimum level of arousal hypothesis** (also called the *inverted-U hypothesis*). At low arousal (low stress levels) performance is below par; an athlete would say that he or she is not "psyched up" (Weinberg & Gould, 1995). As arousal/stress increases, so too does performance—up to an optimal point at which the person's performance is at its peak. Further increases in arousal, however, are accompanied by a decline in performance; an athlete might say that he or she "choked" under too much arousal. So, this hypothesis is represented by an inverted "U" graph that reflects high performance at the optimum level of arousal and low performance when arousal level is either very low or very high.

We now turn our attention to how stress affects the body. For it is there that we will see why health psychologists and medical epidemiologists consider stress to be a key risk factor in many chronic illnesses.

Figure 4.3

The Optimum Level of Arousal Hypothesis
At low arousal levels, performance on many tasks (such as a gymnast's execution of a difficult routine) is below par. As arousal/stress levels increase, so too does performance—up to an optimal point where peak performance occurs. Further increases in arousal are accompanied by a decline in performance.

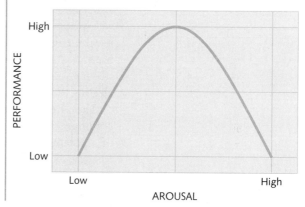

The Physiology of Stress

One of the first to use the term *stress* was the medical researcher Walter Cannon (1932). Cannon observed that extremes of temperature, lack of oxygen, and emotion-arousing incidents all had a similar arousing effect on the body. He called this effect *stress* and he believed that it was a common cause of medical problems.

In one of Cannon's studies, cats were frightened by the sound of a barking dog. Cannon discovered that large amounts of the hormone epinephrine could later be detected in the cats' blood. Cannon called this response to stressful events the body's *fight-or-flight reaction*. An outpouring of epinephrine, along with cortisol and other hormones, helps prepare an organism to defend itself against a threat either by attacking or by running away.

This emergency response system seems highly functional and adaptive. It undoubtedly was essential to our ancestors' survival in a time when human beings faced numerous physical threats, such as possible attacks by wild animals. In response, our ancestors had to either fight or run away. Although today, in our modern, highly developed societies, our stresses are apt to be psychological rather than physical, our body's reaction has not changed: The body still reacts to today's stresses as thought it were facing a standoff with a wild animal. Let's now look at what's going on inside the body when you feel stress.

optimum level of arousal hypothesis the idea that there is an optimal level of arousal, or behavioral activation, at which behavior and mental processes are most efficient

- **anabolism** the constructive form of metabolism in a plant or animal by which food is converted into living tissue

- **catabolism** the destructive form of metabolism in which living tissue is broken down for energy

Research conducted in the mid-1990s demonstrated that the bacterium *Helicobacter pylori*—not stress—is the major cause of most ulcers. Nevertheless, 60 percent of Americans continue to believe stress causes ulcers. Even some physicians continue to recommend that their patients with ulcers take antacids rather than the recommended antibiotics.

The Role of the Brain and Nervous System

The body's overall reaction to stress is regulated by the central nervous system. Recall from Chapter 3 that the nervous system consists of two parts, the *central nervous system* (the brain and the spinal cord) and the *peripheral nervous system*. The peripheral nervous system is also divided into two major branches: the *autonomic nervous system* (ANS) and the *somatic nervous system*. Finally, the ANS is further divided into two branches: the *sympathetic nervous system* (SNS) and the *parasympathetic nervous system* (PNS).

When a potential stressor is first perceived by your sense organs, sensory neurons in the somatic nervous system transmit nerve impulses to lower-level brain regions announcing the impending threat. Running like a rope through the middle of the brainstem, the *reticular formation* plays a central role in alerting the brain to an impending threat or challenge.

The reticular formation coordinates two neural pathways of brain–body communication. Through the first, it routes information about the existence of a potential stressor, such as the perception of a dangerous situation on the freeway, to the *thalamus,* which sorts this sensory information and relays it to the *hypothalamus,* the *limbic system,* and to higher brain regions in the cerebral cortex that interpret the meaning of the potential stressor. Through the second pathway, the reticular formation carries neural instructions back from the higher brain regions to the various target organs, muscles, and glands controlled by the sympathetic nervous system; as a result of these instructions, the body is mobilized for defensive action.

Arousal of the SNS also causes a change in the body's overall metabolic state. Most of the time the cells of the body are occupied with activities that build the body (**anabolism**). When the brain perceives an impending threat or challenge, however, anabolic metabolism is converted into its opposite, **catabolism,** which breaks down tissues to provide energy. Interestingly, the long-term consequences of stress, when taken together, look very much like aging (see Chapter 14). Hypertension, wasted muscles, ulcers, fatigue, and increased risk of chronic disease are common signs of both aging and chronic stress.

Under instructions from the SNS, the adrenal glands release hormones that cause the fight-or-flight response in which heart rate increases, the pupils dilate, stress hormones are secreted, and digestion slows. In addition, SNS activation increases blood flow to the muscles and causes stored energy to be converted to a form that is directly usable by the muscles.

The region of the brain that most directly controls the stress response is the hypothalamus. Nearly every region of the brain interacts in some way with the hypothalamus. For this reason, the hypothalamus reacts to a variety of stimuli, from actual threats to memories of stressful moments to imagined stressors.

Within the hypothalamus the region most directly concerned with stress is the *periventricular nucleus (PVH).* Roughly half a square millimeter in area and containing 10,000 neurons, the PVH contains *endocrine neurons* that secrete *releasing hormones* (also called *releasing factors*) that coordinate the activity of the endocrine system. The endocrine system's hormones play a key role in how we respond to stress.

The Role of the Endocrine System

As we saw in Chapter 3, the endocrine system is the body's relatively slow-acting communication system consisting of a network of glands that secrete hormones directly into the bloodstream. Under stress, the hypothalamus orders the pituitary gland to secrete *adrenocorticotrophic hormone (ACTH)*, which is taken up by receptors in the *adrenal glands,* a pair of small endocrine glands lying just above the kidneys (see Figure 4.4, page 132).

Each of these remarkable structures consists of two nearly independent glands: a central region called the *adrenal medulla* and an outer covering called the *adrenal cortex.* When so ordered by the hypothalamus via the pituitary gland, the adrenal medulla secretes *epinephrine* (also called adrenaline) and *norepinephrine* (also called noradrenaline) into the blood. These hormones help trigger the familiar fight-or-flight responses that are noticeable almost immediately: The heart pounds, the mouth becomes dry, and sweat pours from the palms of the hands and armpits. These endocrine reactions last much longer than those generated directly by the SNS. Taken together, the interaction of the SNS and adrenal medulla is called the **sympathoadreno-medullary (SAM) system.**

The endocrine system is involved in stress in a second, equally important way. This system involves the hypothalamus, the pituitary gland, and the adrenal cortex, or what has been called the **hypothalamic-pituitary-adrenocortical (HPAC) system.** While the SAM system is the body's initial, rapid-acting response to stress, the HPAC system is a delayed response that functions to restore the body to its baseline state, a process known as **homeostasis.** The HPAC system is activated by messages relayed from the central nervous system to the hypothalamus, which in turn secretes *corticotrophin releasing hormone (CRH).* CRH stimulates the production of *adrenocorticotrophic hormone (ACTH)* by the pituitary gland, which then activates the adrenal cortex to secrete **corticosteroids,** steroid hormones that combat inflammation, promote healing, and help mobilize the body's energy resources.

Fortunately, the endocrine system has a mechanism that can halt the body's stress response before it damages the body. It involves *cortisol,* a hormone secreted by the adrenal glands. Cortisol has a potent effect on all the body's tissues, increasing the level of glucose in the blood, stimulating the breakdown of proteins into amino acids, and inhibiting the uptake of glucose by the body tissues but not by the brain. In a finely tuned feedback mechanism, the released cortisol acts back on the hypothalamus and the

■ **sympathoadreno-medullary (SAM) system** the body's initial, rapid-acting response to stress, involving the release of epinephrine and norepinephrine from the adrenal medulla under the direction of the sympathetic nervous system

■ **hypothalamic-pituitary-adrenocortical (HPAC) system** the body's delayed response to stress, involving the secretion of corticosteroid hormones from the adrenal cortex

■ **homeostasis** the tendency to maintain a balanced or constant internal state; the regulation of any aspect of body chemistry, such as the level of glucose in the blood, around a particular set point

■ **corticosteroids** hormones produced by the adrenal cortex that fight inflammation, promote healing, and trigger the release of stored energy

Figure 4.4

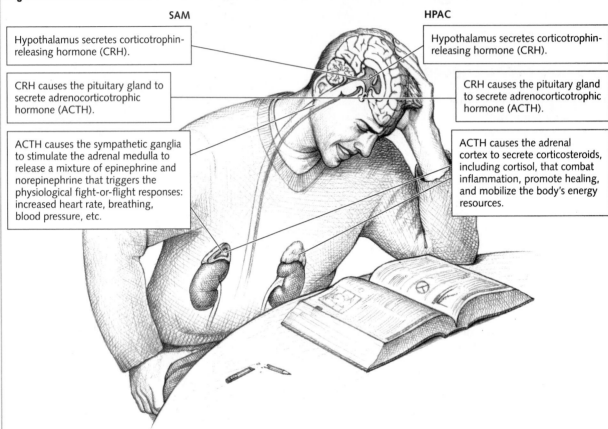

SAM

Hypothalamus secretes corticotrophin-releasing hormone (CRH).

CRH causes the pituitary gland to secrete adrenocorticotrophic hormone (ACTH).

ACTH causes the sympathetic ganglia to stimulate the adrenal medulla to release a mixture of epinephrine and norepinephrine that triggers the physiological fight-or-flight responses: increased heart rate, breathing, blood pressure, etc.

HPAC

Hypothalamus secretes corticotrophin-releasing hormone (CRH).

CRH causes the pituitary gland to secrete adrenocorticotrophic hormone (ACTH).

ACTH causes the adrenal cortex to secrete corticosteroids, including cortisol, that combat inflammation, promote healing, and mobilize the body's energy resources.

The Body's Response to Stress
During a moment of stress, the hypothalamus secretes releasing factors that coordinate the endocrine responses of the pituitary and adrenal glands. As part of the sympathoadreno-medullary system (SAM), the adrenal medulla releases the stress hormones epinephrine and norepinephrine as the body's initial, rapid-acting response to stress. Epinephrine and norepinephrine increase heart rate, breathing, and blood pressure; slow digestion; and dilate the pupils. A second, delayed response involves the hypothalamic-pituitary-adrenocortical (HPAC) system, which triggers secretion of corticosteroids from the adrenal cortex. These steroid hormones fight inflammation, promote healing, and trigger the release of stored reserves of energy.

pituitary to suppress the further release of CRH and ACTH. As the amount of ACTH in the blood decreases, the adrenal cortex shuts down its production of cortisol.

The rate of cortisol secretion is remarkably sensitive to psychological factors (Thompson, 2000). For some people, even a seemingly ordinary event such as boarding an airplane can trigger a large increase in cortisol, which means, of course, that CRH has already been released from the hypothalamus and ACTH from the pituitary.

All of these endocrine system actions help the organism deal with stress. Faced with a threat, the brain needs energy in the form of glucose, which cortisol helps provide. But too much cortisol can have negative consequences, leading to hypertension, a decrease in the body's ability to fight infection, and perhaps to psychological problems as well. Interestingly, hypersecretions of cortisol have been observed in patients suffering from major depression (Gold, Goodwin, & Chrousous, 1988).

Sources of Stress

Everyone experiences stress. How and why we experience stress may change as we journey through life, but none of us escapes. Each of us experiences the events of life in a unique way. What you find stressful your roommate may not. Similarly, some of the leisure activities that you find relaxing are probably too stressful to be enjoyable to your parents. Research has focused on several sources of stress: major life events, daily hassles, environmental stress, job-related stress, and sociocultural factors. In all cases, you will notice that it is not the event alone but the person's appraisal of the event that results in stress, as pointed out in the transactional model of stress.

Major Life Events

What impact do major life events, such as changing jobs, having a child, or losing a loved one, have on the quality of our health? In the late 1950s psychiatrists Thomas Holmes and Richard Rahe of the University of Washington substantially advanced our understanding of how the events of our lives affect our health. They interviewed more than 5,000 people to identify which events forced people to make the most changes in their lives. Then they assigned each event a value in *life change units (LCUs)* to reflect the amount of change that was necessary. For example, a divorce disrupts many more aspects of one's life than does taking a vacation and thus it would be assigned a larger number of LCUs. The events Holmes and Rahe investigated covered a wide range, even including occasions that called for celebration, such as marriage or a promotion. They then ranked these events and devised the *Social Readjustment Rating Scale (SRRS),* which attempts to quantify the impact of life changes on health. (Table 4.1 on page 134 is the College Undergraduate Stress Scale, a variation of the original SRRS directed specifically at college students.)

Holmes and Rahe theorized that the total number of LCUs a person had accumulated during the previous year could predict the likelihood that he or she would become sick over the next several months. In one study (Rahe, Mahan,

Stress may also take a toll on the unborn. Women who reported high levels of stress on a life events scale were more likely to experience a spontaneous abortion (miscarriage) at 11 weeks or later (Boyles et al., 2000). (See Chapter 15.)

Table 4.1

The College Undergraduate Stress Scale

Copy the "stress" rating number into the last column for any item that has happened to you in the last year, then add the numbers.

Event	Stress Ratings	Your Items	Event	Stress Ratings	Your Items
Being raped	100		Lack of sleep	69	
Finding out that you are HIV-positive	100		Change in housing situation (hassles, moves)	69	
Being accused of rape	98		Competing or performing in public	69	
Death of a close friend	97				
Death of a close family member	96		Getting in a physical fight	66	
Contracting a sexually trans- mitted disease (other than AIDS)	94		Difficulties with a roommate	66	
			Job changes (applying, new job, work hassles)	65	
Concerns about being pregnant	91		Declaring a major or concerns about future plans	65	
Finals week	90				
Concerns about your partner being pregnant	90		A class you hate	62	
Oversleeping for an exam	89		Drinking or use of drugs	61	
Flunking a class	89		Confrontations with professors	60	
Having a boyfriend or girlfriend cheat on you	85		Starting a new semester	58	
			Going on a first date	57	
Ending a steady dating relationship	85		Registration	55	
Serious illness in a close friend or family member	85		Maintaining a steady dating relationship	55	
Financial difficulties	84		Commuting to campus or work, or both	54	
Writing a major term paper	83		Peer pressures	53	
Being caught cheating on a test	83		Being away from home for the first time	53	
Drunk driving	82				
Sense of overload in school or work	82		Getting sick	52	
			Concerns about your appearance	52	
Two exams in one day	80		Getting straight A's	51	
Cheating on your boyfriend or girlfriend	77		A difficult class that you love	48	
			Making new friends; getting along with friends	47	
Getting married	76				
Negative consequences of drink- ing or drug use	75		Fraternity or sorority rush	47	
			Falling asleep in class	40	
Depression or crisis in your best friend	73		Attending an athletic event (e.g., football game)	20	
Difficulties with parents	73				
Talking in front of a class	72		Total		

Note: Of 12,000 U.S. college students who completed this scale, scores ranged from 182 to 2,571, with a mean score of 1,247. Women reported significantly higher scores than men, perhaps because most of the students used in pretesting items were women. This being the case, items that are stressful for women may be overrepresented in the scale.
Source: "A Life Stress Instrument for Classroom Use," by M. J. Renner and R. S. Mackin, 1998, *Teaching of Psychology, 25,* p. 47.

& Arthur, 1970), researchers obtained SRRS scores on naval crewmen who were about to depart on a 6-month cruise. Over the course of the voyage, the researchers found a positive correlation between life change units and illness rates. Those sailors who reported the highest LCUs were more likely to fall ill than those who reported the lowest LCUs. The message: When life brings many changes at once, the stress that results may make us more vulnerable to health problems.

Although the research of Holmes and Rahe was groundbreaking and influential, the value of the scale for predicting stress and illness has been criticized for several reasons (Monroe & Simons, 1991):

- Many of the items on the SRRS are vague and open to subjective interpretation. "Change in living conditions" or "revision of personal habits," for example, can mean almost anything.

- Assigning specific point values to events fails to take into consideration individual differences in the way events are appraised (and therefore experienced). A divorce, for example, may mean welcome freedom for one person but a crushing loss to another.

- The SRRS lumps all events together—whether positive, negative, chance, or willfully chosen. Many studies have found that unexpected or uncontrollable negative events, such as the premature death of a family member, are much more stressful than are events that are positive, expected, or under one's control, such as changing to a different line of work or taking a vacation (Bandura, Cioffi, Taylor, & Brouillard, 1988; Gump & Matthews, 2000).

- Reactions to life events are also influenced by one's mood. Being in a pessimistic mood, for instance, substantially increases the likelihood of reporting symptoms of illness (Brett, Brief, Burke, George, & Webster, 1990).

- There is wide variation in how readily people admit to feeling stressed. Some people are more ready than others to report stress in their lives (Brett et al., 1990).

- The SRRS does not differentiate between resolved and unresolved stressful events. There is evidence that stressors that have been successfully resolved have substantially weaker adverse effects on the person's health than events that linger unresolved (Turner & Asvison, 1992).

Despite its apparent flaws, the SRRS represents the first systematic effort to establish a link between stress and illness. And newer research studies *have* found a general link between multiple life changes and a wide range of negative health outcomes. In further defense of the SRRS, one measure of a good theory is that it generates research that leads to new understanding, even if it also leads to its own demise. If nothing else, the tremendous number of studies conducted using the SRRS have revealed that there is no simple, direct

Research has found that college students who were perfectionists were more likely than other students to react to stressful life events with symptoms of depression (Flett, Hewitt, Blankstein, & Mosher, 1995).

connection between life stress and illness: Subjected to the same stressors, one person will get sick while another will not. Stress and its health consequences arise not from events per se but rather from how we appraise them.

Daily Hassles

Major life changes occur infrequently; everyday hassles obviously happen all the time and thus may be the most significant sources of stress (Lazarus, 1990; Ruffin, 1993). These minor annoyances range from missing a commuter train to work, not having the required answer booklet for an exam, or losing a wallet to arguing with a professor or living with an aggravating roommate.

Richard Lazarus—who, you'll recall, developed the transactional model of stress—believes that the impact on health of such hassles depends on their frequency, duration, and intensity. In addition, how a person reacts to minor hassles is influenced by his or her personality, the individual's style of coping, and how the rest of the day has gone.

The counterpart to daily hassles is daily *uplifts:* mood-lifting experiences such as receiving an approving nod from the boss, hearing your favorite song at just the right moment, or even getting a good night's sleep. Just as hassles may cause physical and emotional stress that may result in illness, uplifts may serve as buffers against the effects of stress.

Lazarus and his colleagues have devised a scale to measure people's experiences with day-to-day annoyances and uplifts (Kanner, Coyne, Schaefer, & Lazarus, 1981). The *Hassles and Uplifts Scale* consists of 117 events that range from small pleasures to major problems. In one study, middle-aged adults completed the scale over a 9-month period while the researchers simultaneously tracked their psychological symptoms, such as anxiety and depression (Kanner et al., 1981). Along with these measures, the participants recorded the occurrence of any potentially stressful major life events, such as those included in the SRRS. Table 4.2 shows the 10 most frequent hassles and uplifts as reported by this sample of adults, together with the percentage of time each event was checked.

How well did a person's hassles and uplifts predict his or her overall psychological well-being? Hassles proved to be a better predictor of health problems than both major life events and the frequency of daily uplifts. This finding has been confirmed many times. Everyday hassles or mundane irritants and stressors negatively affect physical and mental health to a degree that exceeds the adverse consequences of major life events (Burks & Martin, 1985; Eckenrode, 1984; Weinberger, Hiner, & Tierney, 1987).

Despite the promise of early research indicating the link between daily hassles and stress, critics have argued that some of the items listed as hassles may actually be *symptoms of stress* rather than stressors. Items relating to appearance, for example, may tap lowered self-esteem that *results from* rather than contributes to stress (Dohrenwend & Shrout, 1985). In addition, some items

Table 4.2

Common Hassles and Uplifts

Hassles	Percentage of Times Checked Over 9 Months	Uplifts	Percentage of Times Checked Over 9 Months
1. Concern about weight	52.4	1. Relating well with your spouse or lover	76.3
2. Health of family member	48.1	2. Relating well with friends	74.4
3. Rising prices of common goods	43.7	3. Completing a task	73.3
4. Home maintenance	42.8	4. Feeling healthy	72.7
5. Too many things to do	38.6	5. Getting enough sleep	69.7
6. Misplacing or losing things	38.1	6. Eating out	68.4
7. Yardwork or outside home maintenance	38.1	7. Meeting responsibilities	68.1
8. Property, investment, or taxes	37.6	8. Visiting, phoning, or writing someone	67.7
9. Crime	37.1	9. Spending time with family	66.7
10. Physical appearance	35.9	10. Home pleasing to you	65.5

Source: Adapted from "Comparison of Two Modes of Stress Management: Daily Hassles and Uplifts versus Major Life Events," by A. D. Kanner, C. Coyne, C. Schaefer, and R. S. Lazarus, 1981, *Journal of Behavioral Medicine, 4,* p. 14.

refer to alcohol and drug use, sexual difficulties, physical illness, and personal fears—all possible consequences of stress.

In addition, other researchers have suggested that individuals who are high in anxiety to begin with will find daily hassles more stressful (Kohn, Lafreniere, & Gurevich, 1991). Paul Kohn and his colleagues found that having an anxious personality triggered stress as often as did daily hassles. This suggests that an overly anxious person may overreact to daily hassles in a way that magnifies their impact. Those who are predisposed not to overreact may be less vulnerable to the physical and psychological impact of daily hassles.

Daily hassles also have been demonstrated to interact with long-term *background stressors,* such as job dissatisfaction (Frankenhaeuser & Gardell, 1976), commuting (Singer, Lundberg, & Frankenhaeuser, 1978), and crowded living conditions (Harburg et al., 1973). A dramatic illustration of this interaction is the skyrocketing rates of divorce, murder, suicide, and stress-related diseases that occurred in Russia during the 4 years that immediately followed the breakup of the former Soviet Union (Holden, 1996). It is suspected that persistent social and economic background stress during this difficult period caused many people to overreact to everyday stressors that they would normally have shrugged off. Remarkably, during this same period of time, life expectancy for Russian men fell from about 64 years to 59 years.

Environmental Stress

Crowded subways, noisy street corners, and pollution are daily facts of life for many of us. Unless we are able to escape by moving to a remote part of the world, these largely uncontrollable potential stressors are likely to affect us for many years. Over time, do these environmental stressors take a toll on our health and well-being? Let's see.

Noise

As a student living in New York City, I lived for 2 years in an unair-conditioned fifth-floor apartment that looked out on an elevated subway train track less than 100 feet from my window. With the window open in summer, a train rumbling by literally shook the building, and I was forced to shout to be heard by a friend sitting in the same room. Still, the rent-controlled apartment was all I could afford, and I inadvertently became a case study of the physical and psychological impact of chronic noise.

Using both field studies and laboratory studies, health psychologists have uncovered a number of negative health consequences of long-term living in noisy environments. In one study, children around airports in Munich, Germany, compared to a control group, were found to have higher systolic and diastolic blood pressure levels and elevated levels of cortisol and other stress hormones (Evans, Hygge, & Bullinger, 1995).

Animal studies also confirm the damaging effects of chronic noise. The blood pressure of rhesus monkeys exposed to loud noise for 9 months was elevated by one-third, and it persisted more than 1 month after the cessation of noise. Thus chronic exposure to high intensity noise may increase the risk of cardiovascular problems (Hygge, 1997).

Researchers have also focused on the impact of chronic noise on academic performance. In the Evans study cited earlier, the motivation, long-term memory, and reading and word skills of the children living near noisy airports were impaired. Similarly, Sheldon Cohen, David Glass, and Jerome Singer (1973) found that children who lived in noisy apartments had greater difficulty detecting subtle differences in sounds and had more reading problems than did children who lived in quieter apartments. The longer the children had lived in their present apartment, the greater the discrepancy. Another study found that children attending school in classrooms facing noisy railroad tracks had lower reading scores than did children attending classes in rooms on the quieter side of the building (Bronzaft & McCarthy, 1975).

Just as I did in my noisy apartment, most people attempt to cope with chronic noise by tuning out extraneous sounds and focusing their attention only on relevant cues (such as the voice of a person to whom you are talking). Because they are young, however, children are less likely than adults to be able to differentiate appropriate and inappropriate cues. This may explain why chronic noise is more disruptive to children. Children may have more difficulty with verbal skills because they are more likely to "tune out" verbal elements (along with other noise) in their environment. To test this idea, health psychologists have also investigated the impact of noise on health in the more controlled setting of the laboratory. In such studies, researchers have demonstrated that fairly high levels of noise (80 to 90 decibels in random bursts) disrupt our ability to attend to even simple cognitive tasks, as well as our short-term memory (Hygge, 1997).

Noise alone doesn't necessarily cause stress. The individual's cognitive appraisal plays an important role, as demonstrated by a study that asked people who lived on a busy street about their overall health, sleep, anxiety level, and attitude toward their noisy environment (Nivision & Endresen, 1993). Although noise levels were not significantly correlated with poor health, loss of sleep, or increased anxiety, the residents' subjective attitudes toward noise were strongly linked to the number of their health complaints.

A key factor in how a person appraises noise is the potential he or she has for controlling the noise level. In one study, David Glass and Jerome Singer (1972) demonstrated that college students who were given the possibility of controlling a loud, distracting noise reported less stress than students who had no opportunity to control the noise. This may explain why "self-administered" noise—such as that experienced at rock concerts—is generally appraised as benign, even enjoyable.

Crowding

In a classic study of the effects of crowding on the behavior of animals, John Calhoun (1970) provided ideal living conditions to a group of rats, allowing them to eat, drink, and reproduce freely. When living space was plentiful, the rats behaved normally, forming stable social groups, mating successfully, and rearing their offspring to healthy maturity.

As the population increased, however, the formerly good "citizenship" of rats began to deteriorate. Frequent fights broke out, as male rats began to stake out and attempt to defend a more crowded territory. In addition, infant mortality increased sharply, the sexual receptivity of females declined, and some rats became cannibalistic.

What about crowding among humans? In yet another example of the importance of cognitive appraisal in the process of stress, some researchers say that we need to make a distinction between crowding and **population density,** which refers to the number of people living in given area. Crowding is a *psychological* state in which people *believe* they do not have enough space to function as they wish.

Density is necessary to produce crowding, but crowding is not an inevitable consequence of density. Being in a crush of people during a New Year's Eve celebration, for example, may not be perceived as crowding, despite the extreme population density. Conversely, the presence of one other family of campers in a wilderness campground may represent an intolerable crowd to a vacationer seeking solitude.

Crowding has been linked to increased aggression, withdrawal from interpersonal relations, and increased crime rates (Sundstrom, 1978). Crowding

population density a measure of crowding based on the total number of people living in an area of limited size also increases unwanted social interactions, a condition that often triggers social withdrawal as a means of coping. In studies of prison inmates, for example, rates of psychiatric commitments and death were higher in years when the prison population was higher. Inmates who live under dense conditions also have higher blood pressure and stress hormone levels (Freedman, 1975).

Other studies have demonstrated that the design of residential space can have far-ranging effects on physical health and subjective well-being. Studies of student housing, for example, reveal that suite-type clusters of dormitory rooms are preferred over the more traditional arrangement of rooms branching off of long corridors. Residents of corridor rooms feel more crowded, report lower feelings of control, are more competitive, and react more negatively to minor annoyances.

Natural Disasters

Imagine how you would react to learning that a toxic substance contaminates your neighborhood's water supply or that plans have been approved for the construction of a nuclear plant near your home. Although pollution is not a recent phenomenon, modern technology has increased the potential for serious accidents in the handling of dangerous substances. Health psychologists increasingly are turning their attention to the physiological and psychological effects of such disasters.

On March 28, 1979, the worst commercial nuclear accident in the history of the United States happened at Three Mile Island, a nuclear power plant in Middletown, Pennsylvania. A pump in the reactor cooling system failed, causing an increase in pressure and temperature. For 2 hours, a stuck valve allowed contaminated, radioactive water that had cooled the reactor's core to evaporate into the atmosphere. Shortly after the incident, Andrew Baum and his colleagues began one of the first systematic health psychology studies of toxic pollution. For more than a year after the accident, residents faced a chronically high level of stress, fearing that they had been exposed to radiation (Baum & Fleming, 1993). This fear manifested itself in excessively high blood pressure as well as elevated levels of cortisol, epinephrine, and norepinephrine.

Responses to the Three Mile Island incident were not unique. Researchers have uncovered a number of similar responses in situations involving both human error and natural phenomena. For example:

- Hypertension, heart disease, and other stress-related ailments tripled in the Republic of Belarus during the stressful aftermath of the world's worst nuclear accident—the Chernobyl nuclear disaster in April 1986 (Nuclear Energy Agency, 1995).

- A meta-analysis of over 50 studies of the community impact of floods, fires, and hurricanes revealed that, after the disaster, rates of psychological disorders, especially depression and anxiety, rose by 17 percent (Rubonis & Bickman, 1991).

- During the 12-month period following the 1988 crash of the 747 jumbo jet at Lockerbie, Scotland, residents experienced a 38 percent increase in acute illnesses (Paton, 1992).

- Refugees who uproot their families in order to flee disasters in their homeland report significantly increased rates of psychological disorders (Williams & Berry, 1991).

Thankfully, most of us will never experience nuclear plant meltdowns, airline crashes, and other disastrous events. Nevertheless, environmental stress is a fact of life. Noise and crowding may cause us to feel anxious and irritable and leave us more vulnerable to physical disorders. For some of us, these reactions, and the stressors that trigger them, come to a point of sharp focus in the workplace.

Job-Related Stress

In recent years an extensive amount of research has been devoted to examining the causes and consequences of job-related stress. These studies are important for two reasons. First, almost all people at some time experience stress related to their work. Second, work-related stress may be one of the most preventable health hazards and thereby provides a number of possibilities for intervention.

For most of us, job stress is brief in duration and does not pose a serious threat to our health. For some people, however, job stress may be chronic, continuing for years. As the following job-stress findings reveal, more workers today than in the past report high levels of stress (Miller, Smith, Turner, Guijarro, & Hallet, 1997).

- The Occupational Safety and Health Administration has declared stress a hazard of the workplace. Among federal government workers, for instance, compensation claims for "emotional illness" increased more than 400 percent between 1981 and 1990.

- In terms of absenteeism, reduced productivity, and workers' compensation benefits, stress costs American industry more than $300 billion annually, or $7500 per worker per year.

- 75 to 90 percent of all physician office visits are for stress-related ailments and complaints. Stress is linked to the six leading causes of death—heart disease, cancer, lung ailments, accidents, cirrhosis of the liver, and suicide.

- People who handle money on the job, those who work at night, and/or those who work in the inner city are most likely to report stress from fears of being killed on the job. For women, homicide is the leading cause of death in the workplace; for men, it is the third leading cause of death.

Let's take a look at some other factors that can make certain jobs more stressful than others.

Work Overload

One source of occupational stress is *work overload*. People who feel they have to work too long and too hard at too many tasks feel more stressed (Caplan & Jones, 1975). They also have poorer health habits (Sorensen, 1985), experience more accidents (Quick & Quick, 1984), and suffer more health problems than do other workers (Repetti, 1993).

It is important to note, however, that the total number of hours a person works is not a reliable indicator of stress (Herzog, House, & Morgan, 1991). Work overload has a subjective, as well as an objective, component. One worker may feel a crushing weight from a schedule that another handles easily. This fact is, of course, consistent with a major theme of this chapter: Stress is in the eye of the beholder.

Role Overload

Work stress sometimes occurs when people attempt to balance several different jobs at the same time and experience *role overload*. The problems associated with juggling multiple roles simultaneously have been particularly great for women. In one study exploring role overload among employed mothers, participants rated their activities and completed mood questionnaires several times a day for an 8-day period. The results were very clear: Role overload associated with juggling heavy work and home responsibilities reduced the enjoyment of *all tasks* and worsened mood (Williams, Suls, Alliger, Learner, & Wan, 1991).

Overall, though, research on the question of whether having a job as well as a home and family enhances or threatens a woman's health is sparse and contradictory (Bonebright, Clay, & Ankenmann, 2000). Studies have supported two competing hypotheses. One, the *scarcity hypothesis*, maintains that because they have only so much time and energy, women with competing demands suffer from role overload and conflict. The other, the *enhancement hypothesis*, argues that the benefits of meaningful work in enhancing a worker's self-esteem outweigh the costs.

To study this issue further, Ulf Lundberg of the University of Stockholm developed a "total workload scale" to quantify the number of competing demands in women's lives (Lundberg, Mardberg, & Frankenhaeuser, 1994). Using this scale, Lundberg found that age and occupational level don't make much difference in women's total workload. The presence of children, however, makes a huge difference. In families without children, men and women each average 60 hours of work a week. In a family with three or more children, women average 90 hours a week in paid and unpaid work, while men still aver-

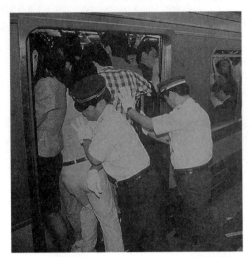

Job-Related Stress
Japan is notorious for its long work hours and lack of vacation time. Workers begin their stress-filled day with an equally stress-filled subway ride to their jobs. The number of people crowding into the subway became so dangerous that the system had to hire people to manage the overloads.

Work has become such a deeply entrenched ethic in Japanese culture that they have created a term, *karoshi,* to describe death that results from work overload. Under Japanese law, bereaved family members may be entitled to special financial compensation if they are able to prove that the cause of their family member's death was *karoshi.* Paul Chesley/Stone

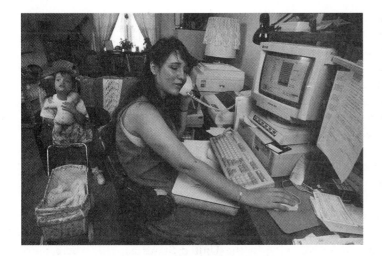

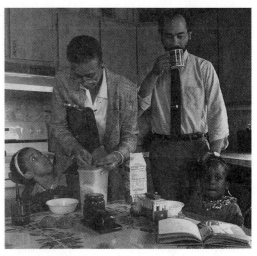

Role Overload

The task of managing multiple roles affects both men and women, but the increase in employment of women has triggered more research on role overload and job-related stress in women. Some research findings regarding the stress of role overload have been contradictory; however, the overall conclusion seems to be that what matters most is the quality of a working mother's experiences in her various roles. Fortunately, the computer and enhanced telecommunications have enabled women to select their work sites. Some, such as the woman who must care for a daughter with Down syndrome (*left*), are better able to balance their responsibilities while working at home; others, whose children are school-age, are comfortable working outside the home (*right*). *(left)* © Rob Crandall / The Image Works; *(right)* © Judy Gelles / Stock Boston

age only 60. "Women's stress is determined by the interaction of conditions at home and work," notes Lundberg, "whereas men's stress is determined more by situations at work."

In another study of psychological and physiological responses related to work and family, Lundberg and Marianne Frankenhaeuser (1999) investigated female and male managers in high-ranking positions. While both women and men experienced their jobs as challenging and stimulating, women were more stressed by their greater unpaid workload and by a greater responsibility for duties related to home and family. Physiologically, women had higher norepinephrine levels than men did, both during and after work, which reflected their greater workload. Women with children at home had significantly higher norepinephrine levels after work than did the other participants.

Although findings such as Lundberg's seem to support the scarcity hypothesis, other researchers have found that employed women are generally healthier than unemployed women (LaCroix & Haynes, 1987). Moreover, for many working mothers, employment is an important source of self-esteem and life satisfaction. Indeed, researchers have found that those adults—both men and women—who *balance* vocational, marital, and parental roles generally are healthier and happier than adults who function in only one or two of these roles (Hochschild, 1997; Milkie & Peltola, 1999).

From research studies such as these, researchers have concluded that what matters most is not the number of roles a woman occupies, but the quality of her experience in those roles (Baruch & Barnett, 1986). Having control over one's work (Rosenfield, 1992), a good income, adequate child care, and a

burnout a job-related state of physical and psychological exhaustion

supportive family combine to help reduce the likelihood that multiple role demands will be stressful.

Many researchers believe that the gender differences in job stress will eventually disappear as cultural values shift. These values are reflected in many ways, including degree of equal employment opportunity and the social support made available to working families. A study comparing female managers in Sweden and the former West Germany, for example, reveals a striking difference: In Sweden, the majority of the women managers had at least two children; in Germany, most had no children. Why the difference? Researchers suspect it is because Sweden offers high-quality child care to any family that requests it. Reading signals from their society, German women apparently feel that they must forsake family for work, whereas Swedish women are apt to take it as their right to combine both roles (Bonebright, et al., 2000).

Cultural values are changing in the United States as well, where most married mothers are in the labor force, including 77 percent of those whose youngest child is still in school and 61 percent who have children under age 3 (U.S. Bureau of the Census, 1999). Of these women, 96 percent have husbands who are also in the labor force, most of whom share domestic chores with their wives. Moreover, recent studies report that in the happiest and least-stressed couples, both spouses contribute to the household income and to the unpaid work of maintaining a household (Moen & Yu, 1999). More specifically, neither spouse works either very long hours (more than 60 per week) or very short hours outside the home. As a result of this shift to a new cultural ideal of "coparenting," many children are now being raised with gender-free expectations about their future roles and those of their future spouses (Cabrera, Tamis-LeMonda, Bradley, Hofferth, & Lamb, 2000).

Burnout

Burnout has been defined as a job-related state of physical and psychological exhaustion that can occur among individuals who work with other people in some capacity (Maslach, 1986). More specifically, burnout is a multidimensional syndrome characterized by *emotional exhaustion, depersonalization,* and *reduced personal accomplishment.* Emotional exhaustion refers to feelings of being drained of emotional resources, with a corresponding loss of energy and feelings of fatigue. Depersonalization refers to a loss of idealism in the workplace, triggering negative attitudes toward the recipients of the employee's service or care. Reduced personal accomplishment refers to a loss of feelings of work-related competence and achievement. Burnout is most common among employees whose long-term involvement in work environments that are highly frustrating and emotionally demanding gradually leads to a loss of purpose and ambition.

Jobs that involve responsibility for other people, rather than responsibility for products, appear to cause high levels of burnout (Sears, Urizar, & Evans, 2000). Health care workers seem to be especially susceptible to this type of job stress. One study demonstrated that one-third of nurses report stress-related symptoms that are severe enough to be considered a warning sign of increased risk of psychiatric problems (Tyler & Cushway, 1992). Nursing has one of the highest rates of suicide among professional groups (Gillespie & Gillespie, 1986). Oncology (cancer treatment) nurses who provide care to chemotherapy patients report feeling stressed most often when dealing with the death of patients or when interacting with physicians and when observing suffering (Florio, Donnelly, & Zevon, 1998). Interestingly, when doctors are asked what causes stress in their work, they report work overload as the main cause (Firth-Cozens, 1997). But when asked to write about stressful days over the past month, they are more likely to remember heart-wrenching individual patients, followed by difficult relationships with other doctors and the fear of making medical mistakes (Firth-Cozens & Morrison, 1989).

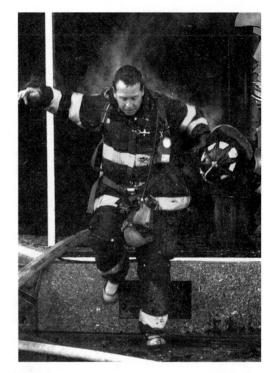

Burnout
Firefighters have stressful jobs, partly because of their responsibility for others' lives, which makes them highly susceptible to burnout. © Jim Mahoney/The Image Works

Burnout levels in dentists, paramedics, air traffic controllers, and firefighters are also unusually high (Firth-Cozens, 1997). And burnout is equally common among workaholics and others facing overwhelming workloads who become so consumed by their work that they neglect social relationships and leisure activities.

Although burnout customarily develops over a period of years, its warning signs may appear early on. These signs include

- Feelings of mental and physical exhaustion
- Loss of meaning in one's work and life in general
- Difficulty concentrating
- An increase in stress-related ailments, such as headaches, backaches, and depression
- Shortness of temper

It is important to note that burnout is not an inevitable consequence of employment in certain professions. As the biopsychosocial model reminds us, susceptibility to most health conditions—favorable or unfavorable—is the product of overlapping factors in every domain of health. For instance, nurses who maintain a hopeful, optimistic view of life are much less likely to experience burnout than their more pessimistic counterparts on chronic care wards, thereby highlighting the protective function of certain personality styles (Sherwin, Elliott, Rybarczyk, & Frank, 1992).

Lack of Control over Work

Workers feel more stress when they have little or no control over the procedures, pace, and other aspects of their jobs (Steptoe, Fieldman, & Evans, 1993). The relationship between lack of control and illness was clearly revealed in Marianne Frankenhaeuser's (1975) classic study of Scandinavian sawmill workers. Compared with workers who had more say over aspects of their jobs, those working at dull, repetitive, low-control jobs had significantly higher levels of stress hormones, higher blood pressure, more headaches, and more gastrointestinal disorders, including ulcers.

Other studies have consistently confirmed the relationship between perceived control and work-related stress. A study of British civil servants, for example, found that workers in lower-grade, low-control occupations had poorer health, even after adjustments were made for smoking, diet, and exercise (Hewison & Dowswell, 1994).

Secretaries, waitresses, factory workers, and middle managers are among those with the most stressful occupations marked by repetitive tasks and having little control over events. Common to these jobs are complaints of too many demands with too little authority to influence work practices. The sense of powerlessness that results often creates crushing stress (Miller & Smith, 1998).

Other Sources of Job-Related Stress

Several other aspects of jobs increase stress among workers, including these:

- *Role ambiguity or conflict* Role ambiguity occurs when workers are unsure of their jobs or the standards used to evaluate their performance. Role conflict occurs when a worker receives mixed messages about these issues from different supervisors or coworkers.

- *Shiftwork* Shiftwork involves continuous staffing of a workplace by groups of employees who work at different times. Shiftworkers face disruption to their family and domestic lives, as well as to their *biological rhythms.* Most human functions have a rhythm with peaks and valleys that occur over a regular 24- to 25-hour cycle. Shiftwork desynchronizes these rhythms and may lead to a number of health complaints, including headaches, loss of appetite, fatigue, sleep disturbances, gastrointestinal problems, and heart disease (Taylor, 1997; Waterhouse, 1993).

- *Job loss* Downsizing, layoffs, mergers, and bankruptcies cost thousands of workers their jobs each year. The loss of a job can have a serious impact on a worker's well-being, putting unemployed workers at risk for physical illness, anxiety, depression, and even suicide (Vinokur, Schul, Vuori, & Price, 2000). Job insecurity and the threat of unemployment have been linked to higher levels of several health-compromising risk factors. One study reported higher blood pressure and serum cholesterol levels among Michigan autoworkers who faced the closing of their factory (Kasl, 1997). Other studies have reported increased smoking, alcohol consumption, use of prescription drugs, body weight, and hospital admissions among laid-off workers (Hammarstrom, 1994).

- *Gender harassment* To find out what makes certain jobs especially stressful for women, researchers at the University of North Carolina and the National Institute for Occupational Safety and Health conducted a survey of 213 female construction workers and 392 female factory workers around the United States (Goldenhar, Swanson, Hurrell, Ruder, & Deddens, 1998). The team of researchers explored several sources of job stress, including harassment by male coworkers. A startling 41 percent of the women reported mistreatment because they were women. Over one-third reported that coworkers had made unwanted sexual references or suggestions to them. And 10 percent said that they had been threatened physically while on the job.

- *Inadequate career advancement* People who feel that they have been promoted too slowly or that they are not getting the recognition they deserve on the job experience more stress and have higher rates of illness (Catalano, Rook, & Dooley, 1986; Cottington, Matthews, Talbott, & Kuller, 1986).

- *Retirement* Closely related to the issue of job loss is the issue of retirement. Although many workers enter this season of life with great enthusiasm, some quickly become disenchanted. Jobs not only provide economic support but also impose time structure on the day, provide for regular contacts with other people, give workers a sense of status and identity, and promote an active lifestyle (Jahoda, 1979). For many workers, these losses make retirement almost unbearable. Many retirees also find living on their retirement income an additional hardship.

    Retirement often poses different challenges for women. After raising their children and beginning a career at a later age, women may find themselves pressured to retire prematurely by already retired spouses. And once they retire, women may find that they do not have the same leisure opportunities their male counterparts do. After just hitting their stride in their careers, they may leave their jobs only to face years of caregiving for ailing parents and spouses (Yee et al., 1996).

Although job-related stress is difficult to avoid, there are ways to buffer its negative impact. Better ways of responding include knowing what to expect from certain aspects of work (and coworkers), expressing your feelings to increase your perception of control, keeping things in perspective, and avoiding self-defeating thoughts and overreactions. We'll take up the topic of coping with stress much more fully in Chapter 5. Now, however, we turn our attention to the unique stress experienced by ethnic minorities, immigrants, those who are poor, and women (see Diversity and Healthy Living, pages 148–149).

Diversity and Healthy Living

Sociocultural Factors in Stress

Many researchers have argued that sociocultural factors may have a greater impact on health than discrete events of everyday life. Several studies have shown that being African-American, poor, an immigrant, or female can be a source of chronic life stress (Greenwood et al., 1996).

African-Americans, for example, report significantly more stresses in their everyday lives than do nonminority individuals (Young & Zane, 1995). Much of this, of course, stems from the racism and subtle oppression that marginalized people feel because their needs often seem peripheral to the concerns of most Americans.

Poverty People with the lowest *socioeconomic status (SES)* are more likely to suffer ill effects from stress for at least two reasons. First, they invariably experience a greater number of sources of stress, such as overcrowded housing, neighborhood crime, and single parenthood. Second, they are least likely to have the financial resources to help themselves cope with stress (Adler & Matthews, 1994).

Homelessness is one problem faced by many poor people. Between 50,000 and 100,000 U.S. children are homeless each night (Jencks, 1994). These children have more fears, more fights, fewer friends, more chronic illnesses, and more changes of school than their peers and are about 14 months behind them academically. Homeless families as a unit also lack a supportive social network to assist them in coping with life. Finally, many homeless families are headed by single mothers striving to cope with the after-effects of an abusive relationship.

Immigrant Stress Immigrants are pressured to become **acculturated**—that is, to adopt the cultural values and behaviors of the dominant group in a country. In a diverse, multicultural country such as the United States, acculturation is an issue of increasing concern to health psychologists. In 2000, 28.4 million foreign-born people lived in the United States, representing 10.4 percent of the total population. Among these, 51.0 percent were born in Latin America, 25.5 percent in Asia, 15.3 percent in Europe, and the remaining 8.1 percent in other regions of the world (U.S. Bureau of the Census, 2000). How do the stresses of acculturation affect health?

There are two major views of acculturation stress (Griffith, 1983). The *melting pot model* maintains that immigrants who quickly strive to become more like the people who make up the dominant culture experience less acculturation stress. According to this theory, immigrants would minimize their adjustment stress by learning and speaking English and taking up the customs of mainstream American society.

According to the *bicultural theory*, immigrants experience less stress when they maintain their traditional values and customs while also adapting to the mainstream culture. According to this perspective, a flexible combination of ethnic identity and efforts to adapt to the mainstream culture promote well-being.

Although some health problems have been linked with a *failure* to become acculturated, the opposite is more often true. Adapting to a new culture is nearly always stressful, especially when one is a member of a marginalized minority group. Consider:

- Highly acculturated Mexican-Americans who were born in the United States have higher rates of depression and substance abuse than those born in Mexico (Hartung, 1987).

- Highly acculturated Hispanic-American women are more likely to be heavy drinkers than are low-acculturated Hispanic-American women (Caetano,

■ **acculturation** the process in which a member of one ethnic or racial group adopts the values, customs, and behaviors of another

Models of Stress and Illness

Stress is a fact of life. But when it overtaxes our coping resources, stress can damage our health. No single topic in health psychology has generated more research than how stress can sometimes promote illness. Links between stress and illness have been established for many disorders, including

1987). Less rigid American gender roles and a loosening of traditional Latin American constraints on drinking among women may explain this finding.

- Highly acculturated Hispanic-American high school girls are more susceptible than less acculturated girls to eating disorders such as anorexia. Acculturation may make Hispanic-American girls more vulnerable to stereotypes of female attractiveness in mainstream U.S. culture (Pumariega, 1986).

Stress for acculturating persons is usually lower when migration is voluntary rather than forced (that is, for immigrants versus refugees); when there is a functioning social support group (when there is an ethnic community willing to assist during the settlement process); when there is tolerance for diversity within the mainstream culture; and when income, education level, and other background factors help ease the transition from one country to another (Berry, 1997). On this final point, the data are not very encouraging. Consider:

- In 1999, 16.8 percent of foreign-born U.S. residents were living below the poverty level, compared with 11.2 percent of U.S.-born residents (U.S. Bureau of the Census, 2000).
- Immigrants are less likely to have graduated from high school than native-born residents (67.0 percent and 86.6 percent, respectively). In 1999, more than one-fifth of the foreign born had less than a ninth grade education (22.2 percent) compared with about one-twentieth of native-born residents (4.7 percent). Interestingly, the proportions with a college bachelor's degree (or higher) were not significantly different for foreign-born and native-born residents (25.8 and 25.6 percent, respectively).

Gender Do men or women experience more life stress? In one large-scale study (Silverman, Eichler, & Williams, 1987), 23 percent of the women and 18 percent of the men reported experiencing significant stress during a 2-week period. Based on these figures, nearly 20 million women and 14 million men regularly feel "a lot" of stress. More recent studies have corroborated this gender difference (Greenglass & Noguchi, 1996).

Marianne Frankenhaeuser (1991) notes that many women today face a particularly heavy daily workload because they have to handle not only an outside job but also most of the chores at home. As people grow older, this gender discrepancy increases even more. Women age 65 and older are twice as likely as men to report a lot of stress in their lives. Furthermore, significantly more women (49 percent) than men (38 percent) believe that stress has had "a lot" or "some" effect on their health.

In addition to causing stress themselves, sociocultural factors may increase an individual's vulnerability to the ill effects of discrete stressors. It is important to recognize, however, that there is no simple correspondence between a given stressor and health. The extent to which situations are stressful is largely determined by how the individual understands, interprets, and feels about a situation. However, longitudinal studies clearly demonstrate that the impact of a given stressor on a person depends on the total number of stressors he or she is experiencing and on the degree to which these affect the overall patterns of everyday life. One classic study reported that children coping with only one major stressor such as poverty were *no more likely* to develop serious psychological problems than children living without this particular stressor. As the number of serious stressors children had to cope with increased, however, the percentage of children diagnosed with serious psychological health problems also increased (Rutter, 1979).

cancer, heart disease, and hypertension. In this section we'll examine several theoretical models of how stress affects physical health.

The General Adaptation Syndrome

Surely the most significant contribution to our understanding of stress and illness came from the research of Canadian scientist Hans Selye. Selye's research

Figure 4.5

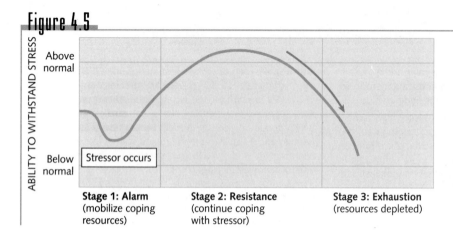

Stage 1: Alarm (mobilize coping resources)

Stage 2: Resistance (continue coping with stressor)

Stage 3: Exhaustion (resources depleted)

The General Adaptation Syndrome
Under stress, the body enters an alarm phase during which resistance to stress is temporarily suppressed. From this it rebounds to a phase of increased resistance to stress. The body's resistance can last only so long. In the face of prolonged stress, the stage of exhaustion may be reached. During this final stage, people become more vulnerable to a variety of health problems.

on stress began almost accidentally. In searching for a new sex hormone, Selye injected laboratory rats with extracts of ovary tissue. Inexplicably, these injections produced three unexpected effects: enlargement of the adrenal glands, bleeding ulcers, and shrinkage of the thymus gland (which produces the disease-fighting lymphocytes). Realizing the importance of this unexpected outcome, Selye followed up with an elegant series of experiments, finding that extracts of other tissues caused the same three physiological responses, as did exposure to x-rays, extreme heat or cold, and prolonged bouts of exercise.

From these observations, Selye devised his concept of stress as a "nonspecific response of the body to any demand" (1974, p. 27). The body's reaction to stress was so predictable that Selye called it the **general adaptation syndrome (GAS).**

As Figure 4.5 shows, the GAS consists of three stages. Stage 1, the *alarm reaction,* is essentially the same as the *fight-or-flight* response. Adrenal activity and cardiovascular and respiratory functions increase rapidly. This fast-acting arousal is the result of hormones secreted by the endocrine system: The pituitary gland releases ACTH, which stimulates the adrenal medulla to release epinephrine and norepinephrine and the adrenal cortex to secret cortisol into the bloodstream. The strength of the alarm reaction depends on the degree to which the event is perceived as a threat.

When a stressful situation persists, the body's reaction progresses to Stage 2, the *resistance stage.* In this stage, physiological arousal remains high (but not as high as during the alarm reaction) as the body tries to adapt to the emergency by replenishing adrenal hormones. At the same time, there is a decrease in the individual's ability to cope with everyday events and hassles. One manifestation of this deficit is that people often become irritable, impatient, and increasingly vulnerable to health problems.

If the stressful situation persists, and resistance is no longer possible, the body enters the final stage of the GAS—the *stage of exhaustion.* At this point the body's energy reserves are depleted. If stress persists, disease and physical

general adaptation syndrome (GAS) Selye's term for the body's reaction to stress, which consists of three stages: alarm, resistance, and exhaustion

deterioration or even death may occur. For example, one result of exhaustion is increased susceptibility to what Selye referred to as *diseases of adaptation.* Among these are allergic reactions, hypertension, and common colds, as well as more serious illnesses caused by immune deficiencies.

Numerous studies have reinforced Selye's basic point: Prolonged stress exacts a toll on the body. People who have endured the prolonged stress of combat, child abuse, or a chronic disease may suffer enlarged adrenal glands, bleeding ulcers, damage to the brain's hippocampus, and abnormalities in several other cerebral areas. The hippocampus, which plays a crucial role in the formation and storage of new memories, is highly activated during the fight-or-flight response. In one recent study, laboratory rats were chronically stressed by being tightly held in wire mesh restrainers for 6 hours a day for 21 days (Conrad, Magarinos, LeDoux, & McEwen, 1999). Compared to unrestrained control rats, the restrained rats suffered significant atrophying of neurons in the hippocampi of their brains. As shown in Figure 4.6, both the number and length of branch points on the dendrites of these neurons were reduced—deficits that could have far-reaching neural and cognitive implications.

Atrophy of the human hippocampus is associated with recurrent clinical depression, post-traumatic stress disorder—which we will discuss shortly— and mild cognitive impairment in normal aging (Lupien et al., 1998). Although some memory loss occurs with age, stress may play an even more important role than simple aging. In one study older people with low stress hormone levels tested as well as younger people on cognitive tests; those with higher stress levels tested between 20 and 50 percent lower (McEwen & Magarinos, 1997). If stress is chronic or extremely severe, memory loss due to hippocampal damage may become permanent. For instance, in one study, severely stressed Vietnam veterans and women who suffered from sexual abuse displayed up to 8 percent shrinkage in the hippocampus (Sapolsky, 1996). Severe stress may even break down the blood-brain barrier—the physiological mechanism that helps protect the brain from toxins, bacteria, and other potentially harmful substances that may be carried in blood.

Selye's belief that all stressors produce the same physiological reactions has been revised in the face of more recent evidence. Newer research demonstrates that stress responses are more specific; that is, they are patterned according to the situations encountered and individual coping behaviors (Steptoe, 1997). In one of the earliest demonstrations of physiological specificity, John Mason (1975) found different patterns of epinephrine, norepinephrine, and corticosteroid secretion when stressors differed in their predictability. Some stressors led to increases in epinephrine, norepinephrine, and cortisol, whereas others increased only one or two of these stress hormones.

In another classic study of the role of appraisal in stress responses, Mason (1975) compared the adrenal responses of two groups of dying patients to a mild physical stressor (heat application). One group consisted of patients who

Figure 4.6

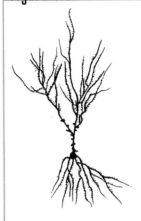

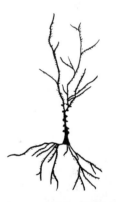

Stress-Induced Atrophy of Hippocampal Neurons
Neuronal tracings from laboratory rats subjected to 21 days of restraint stress. Both neurons are oriented with the dendrites on top. Compared with the neuron from an unstressed control rat (top), the neuron from a chronically stressed rat shows reduced dendritic branching and decreased total dendritic length (bottom).

Source: "Repeated Restrain Stress Facilitates Fear Conditioning Independently of Causing Hippocampal CA3 Dendritic Atrophy," by C. D. Conrad, A. M. Magarinos, J. E. LeDoux, and B. S. McEwen, 1999, *Behavioral Neuroscience, 13,* pp. 902–913.

diathesis-stress model the model that proposes that two interacting factors determine an individual's susceptibility to stress and illness: predisposing factors in the person (such as genetic vulnerability) and precipitating factors from the environment (such as traumatic experiences)

remained in a coma until the moment of death; the other was made up of patients who remained conscious until the moment of death. Post-mortem examination revealed that the conscious groups showed symptoms of stress in response to the heat applications, such as enlarged adrenal glands, whereas the coma patients displayed no such symptoms. Results such as these have demonstrated that stress requires the conscious appraisal of potential harm.

The Diathesis-Stress Model

Evidence that the stress response is more specific and varies with how a particular stressor is perceived has led researchers to propose several other models that highlight the interaction of biological and psychosocial factors in health and illness (Fowles, 1992; Levi, 1974). The **diathesis-stress model** proposes that two continuously interacting factors jointly determine an individual's susceptibility to stress and illness: *predisposing factors* that establish a person's vulnerability to illness and *precipitating factors* from the environment.

Some individuals are more vulnerable to illness because they react more strongly to specific environmental triggers (Gatchel, 1993). This reactive predisposition (diathesis) is customarily believed to be genetic in origin, but some theorists have suggested that acquired behavioral or personality traits (such as being overly aggressive or prone to anger) may also make some persons more susceptible to stress-related illnesses (Zubin & Spring, 1977). Table 4.3 lists the physical, psychological, and social effects of stress on health and well-being.

Consider an example that may hit close to home. Every student experiences test anxiety to varying degrees. Most of us, however, learn to cope with the stress of exam-taking by studying and keeping things in perspective. In some rare instances, however, test anxiety can spiral out of control, causing a student to react to exams with a large increase in heart rate and blood pressure. After years of stressful exams, this abnormally intense cardiovascular reactivity (diathesis) may make the student more vulnerable to cardiovascular disorders than a student with better coping resources.

A recent study reported that cardiac reactivity to stress does indeed bear a strong relationship to risk of heart attack and stroke (Kamarck & Lichtenstein, 1998). The researchers studied the responses of 901 Finnish men on a simple test of memory that was designed to elicit a mild state of mental stress. The men under age 55 who displayed the strongest blood-pressure reaction during the test also had the most severe blockages in their carotid arteries. The researchers speculate that like cholesterol, over time blood pressure reactions to stress may injure coronary vessels and promote coronary disease.

The diathesis-stress model highlights the fact that different people have different vulnerabilities, resulting in many possible health consequences due to stress combined with diathesis. As an extreme case in point, consider post-traumatic stress disorder (PTSD).

Table 4.3

Stress-Related Health Problems

Physical Problems		
stiff or tense muscles	vomiting	weight loss or gain
grinding teeth	tiredness	sweating
tension headaches	shakiness	upset stomach
choking feeling	muscle tremors	nausea
skin rashes	hypertension	allergic reactions
painful menstruation	rapid or irregular heart beat	

Psychological Problems		
anxious thoughts	anger	depression
memory difficulties	fatigue	anger
resentment	inability to relax	poor concentration

Behavioral Problems		
fidgeting	crying	avoidance of tasks
sleep problems	clenched fists	substance abuse
changes in eating	short temper	withdrawal from relationships

Note: These conditions are not inevitable consequences of stress, nor does the presence of several symptoms necessarily indicate that stress is the cause.

Post-Traumatic Stress Disorder (PTSD)

Historically, a diagnosis of **post-traumatic stress disorder (PTSD)** was reserved for cases in which a person had experienced an overwhelming event so fearful as to be considered *outside the range of normal human experience*. More recently, PTSD has been expanded to include "exposure to an extreme traumatic stressor involving direct personal experience of an event that involves actual or threatened death or serious injury" (APA, 1994, p. 424).

Although the traumatic event most often studied is military combat, researchers now also focus on physical attack, diagnosis of a life-threatening illness, or a catastrophic environmental event such as an earthquake or flood (Steinglass & Gerrity, 1990). Car accidents are the most frequent cause of trauma in men, and sexual assault is the most frequent source of trauma among women (Blanchard & Hickling, 1997). It has been estimated that up to 45 percent of the some 3 million people each year who are involved in serious automobile accidents later suffer from PTSD. PTSD has also been known to stem from witnessing (or learning about) the death or injury of a relative or friend. Children who live in violent neighborhoods or in one of the world's war zones may also show symptoms of PTSD (Garbarino, 1991).

post-traumatic stress disorder (PTSD) a psychological disorder triggered by exposure to an extreme traumatic stressor, such as combat or a natural disaster. Symptoms of PTSD include haunting memories and nightmares of the traumatic event, extreme mental distress, and unwanted flashbacks

Symptoms of PTSD include haunting memories and nightmares of the traumatic event, sleep disturbances, excessive guilt, and impaired memory, as well as extreme mental and physical distress. Victims may also suffer unwanted flashbacks in which feelings and memories associated with the original event are reexperienced. Other complaints include muscle pains, sensitivity to chemicals and sunlight, and gastrointestinal problems.

In a recent study, psychologists Todd Buckley, Edward Blanchard, and Edward Hickling (1998) assessed 158 automobile accident survivors for PTSD and other psychological disorders. The 5-year study found that nearly 40 percent of the accident survivors developed PTSD within 1 year of their accident. The main symptoms were unwanted reexperiencing of the event and an increase in general feelings of anxiety. In addition, over 15 percent developed a driving phobia sufficiently intense to cause them to completely stop or dramatically reduce their driving. And at least 90 percent of the crash survivors avoided the site of their accident and did not drive in weather and road conditions similar to those on the day of their traumatic experience.

Despite its increased prominence in the media, PTSD is actually a new name for a collection of symptoms that have been observed for centuries. During the industrial revolution, for example, shock reactions stemming from railroad accidents were fairly common. During World War I, combat stress cases were referred to as *shell shock*. Physicians of that time sought biomedical explanations for stress. They generally believed that the concussive change in air pressure caused by exploding artillery shells somehow damaged neural tissue and caused the resulting psychological disturbances. By the end of World War I, however, the number of cases of shell shock among noncombatants was large enough to force physicians to concede that the disorder might be psychological in origin. The observations of field physicians and psychologists during World War II and the Korean War served to reinforce the conclusion that traumatic stress could indeed inflict serious psychological damage.

PTSD was made an independent diagnostic category during the Vietnam War. Although it is impossible to determine whether PTSD was more common among Vietnam veterans than among veterans of earlier wars, it has been suggested that clinicians were more aware of stress-related disorders and therefore more likely to diagnose them from ambiguous symptoms (Baum & Spencer, 1997). This increasing awareness of traumatic stress has also been characteristic of the most recent conflicts in the Persian Gulf and the Middle East, as well as following cataclysmic events such as the eruption of Mount Saint Helens and the bombing of the federal office building in Oklahoma City.

Those suffering from PTSD show increased cortisol, epinephrine, norepinephrine, testosterone, and thyroxin activity that lasts over an extended period of time (Mason, Kosten, Southwick, & Giller, 1990). A review of studies for the National Center for PTSD found that PTSD sufferers consistently respond to combat-related scenes and audiotapes with elevated heart rate, blood pressure, skin conductivity, and muscle tension (Gottlieb, 1996).

One of the most striking aspects of PTSD is the frequent simultaneous occurrence (comorbidity) of other psychological disorders. Approximately 84 percent of combat veterans with PTSD are also diagnosed with substance abuse problems, 68 percent with major depressive disorder, 53 percent with panic disorder, 53 percent with generalized anxiety disorder, and 26 percent with personality disorder (Keane & Wolfe, 1990). In fact, PTSD patients are twice as likely to meet the diagnostic critera for another major psychological disorder as non-PTSD patients (Helzer et al., 1987).

Most combat-stress veterans, however, do not suffer from PTSD and are living successful lives. The prevalence of PTSD in the general population is estimated at only about 1 percent (Helzer et al., 1987), compared to 20 percent of wounded Vietnam veterans and 35 percent of women who have been the victims of a life-threatening crime (Resnick, Kilpatrick, Best, & Kramer, 1992). The rarity of the disorder has led some skeptics to argue that PTSD is a fad diagnosis (Young & Kane, 1995).

Several ongoing studies are expected to shed light on the origins, treatment, and prevention of PTSD (Gottlieb, 1996; Macklin et al., 1998). The largest study, which so far has evaluated more than 10,000 veterans of the Gulf War, was started by the U.S. Department of Defense in 1994. Of these veterans, 37 percent have thus far been diagnosed with a psychiatric condition, the most common being depression (11 percent), PTSD (5 percent), adjustment disorder (4 percent), and mild anxiety (2 percent). Among the early findings of the studies are these:

- Individuals who develop the symptoms of PTSD are also more vulnerable to emotional disorders.

- People who feel a lack of social support are more likely to develop symptoms of PTSD, as are soldiers who score lower on *personal hardiness,* a measure of how people cope with stress and adversity.

- Soldiers who develop PTSD tend to display more avoidance, wishful thinking, and self-blame than other soldiers. In remembering their childhood, they also believe their families were less cohesive and communicative than others were.

- Female soldiers who reported experiencing harassment or sexual assault report higher-than-average symptoms of PTSD.

- People with lower intelligence are more likely to develop PTSD after a traumatic experience. Researchers who studied Vietnam combat veterans found that those with PTSD symptoms had lower pre- and post-combat scores on standardized intelligence tests, as well as fewer years of total education. The researchers are careful to point out that PTSD does not lower intelligence scores, and that PTSD is caused by a traumatic event, not lower intelligence. Still, they maintain that there is a reasonable explanation for their controversial results: Individuals who have more cognitive resources may be better equipped to cope with combat stress.

As results of these studies surface, researchers are hopeful that they will be able to pinpoint the origins of PTSD. Doing so will go a long way in helping health psychologists develop effective intervention strategies for the treatment and prevention of PTSD.

Psychoneuroimmunology

One day in 1974, in a laboratory at the University of Rochester School of Medicine, psychologist Robert Ader made an accidental discovery that would forever change the face of medicine. Ader had been conducting a classic Pavlovian learning experiment, attempting to condition laboratory rats to avoid saccharin-flavored drinking water (see Chapter 1). The design of the study was simple (Figure 4.7). After the rats were given a drink of the artificially sweetened water (a neutral stimulus), they received an injection of the drug cyclophosphamide (unconditioned stimulus), which made them sick (unconditioned response)—sick enough so that a single pairing of the two stimuli should have been sufficient to establish a *conditioned aversion* to the water.

But Ader soon discovered a problem. Over the course of several weeks of training and testing, a number of the rats became sick and died. Puzzled by this development, Ader discovered that the number of virus- and infection-fighting T lymphocytes (see Chapter 3) was significantly reduced in the bodies of the unfortunate experimental animals. The nausea-inducing drug apparently had a more serious impact on the rats—it suppressed their immune responses.

What was most remarkable in Ader's experiment was that during the study, these same rats had later been given saccharin-flavored water alone, without the cyclophosphamide; the animals' immune systems responded as if the drug was actually circulating in their bloodstream. Classical conditioning had cre-

Figure 4.7

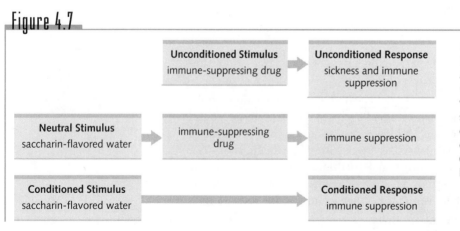

Conditioning the Immune Response
After Robert Ader and Nicholas Cohen paired saccharin-flavored water with an immune-suppressing drug, the taste of the sweetened water alone elicited a conditioned response (immune suppression) in laboratory rats.

ated a learned association between the taste of the water as a conditioned stimulus and the suppression of T cells as a conditioned response. Over time, conditioned responding made the animals increasingly susceptible to disease as their immune reserves were weakened with each drink of sweetened water.

Before Ader's study, most biomedical researchers believed that the mind and body were, for the most part, independent systems that had no influence on one another. So entrenched was this belief that Ader himself had difficulty accepting the results of his own research.

Good science demands replication of findings, so Ader teamed up with immunologist Nicholas Cohen to see if his initial findings were a fluke. They were not. In a subsequent series of experiments, Ader and Cohen demonstrated that the immune system could be conditioned, just as Ivan Pavlov had demonstrated that the salivary response could be conditioned in hungry dogs.

Ader and Cohen's research gave rise to a new model of stress and illness (and, in fact, an entire new field of biomedical research) known as **psychoneuroimmunology (PNI).** The name of this field describes a great deal about its focus: *psycho* for psychological processes, *neuro* for the neuroendocrine system (the nervous and hormonal systems), and *immunology* for the immune system (Ader & Cohen, 1985; Bachen, Cohen, & Marsland, 1997). PNI identifies three areas of functioning that at one time were believed to be relatively independent.

Since Ader and Cohen's watershed studies, the evidence for coordinated interactions among the brain, the neuroendocrine system, and the immune system has quickly mounted. Much of this research has focused on the three-way link among stress, immune system activity, and disease. Various research studies have demonstrated that exposing laboratory animals to electric shock, loud noise, or separation from the mother, for example, all adversely affect immune functioning. In one study, researchers injected stressed rats with malignant tumor cells and monitored the resulting change in natural killer cell activity and tumor development (Ben-Eliyahu, Yirmiya, Liebeskind, Taylor, & Gale, 1991). Immune activity was weakest and tumors developed most rapidly in rats stressed within 1 hour of being injected with the malignant cells. When the stress manipulation was delayed 24 hours, the tumor cells metastasized no more rapidly than those injected into a control group of unstressed animals.

Research with human participants has yielded similar findings. Adverse changes in immune functioning (immunosuppression) have been demonstrated following a divorce, bereavement, unemployment, and stressful bouts of exercise; during exam periods; and when experiencing occupational stress. Among these changes are reduced numbers of natural killer cells, T cells, and total lymphocytes (Kiecolt-Glaser, Malarkey, Cacioppo, & Glaser, 1994). And there seems to be a "dose-response" relationship between stress and immunosuppression. College students with the highest levels of overall life stress or the tendency to overreact to stressful events, for instance, show the greatest deficit

psychneuroimmunology (PNI) the field of research that emphasizes the interaction of psychological, neural, and immunological processes in stress and illness

in their immune response during exam weeks (Kiecolt-Glaser et al., 1984; Workman & La Via, 1987).

Research studies also demonstrate the importance of social relationships to healthy immune functioning (Cohen & Herbert, 1996). Loneliness, for example, appears to adversely affect immune functioning, as does relationship stress (Glaser, Kiecolt-Glaser, Speicher, & Holliday, 1985). Immunosuppression has been linked to interpersonal conflict among married couples (Kiecolt-Glaser et al., 1997), women recently separated from their husbands (Kiecolt-Glaser et al., 1987), and men whose wives have recently died (Schleifer, Keller, Camerino, Thorton, & Stein, 1983). More recent studies have demonstrated that impaired immunity associated with the loss of a loved one occurs primarily among those people who become depressed in response to their bereavement (Zisook et al., 1994).

The caregiving role, in which one person provides the bulk of care for a relative with a chronic illness, can also be stressful and adversely affect immune functioning. A recent study demonstrated that family members who provide care for a relative with Alzheimer's disease reported more depression and lower life satisfaction than those in the control group (matched family members with no caregiving responsibilities). The same study reported that the caregivers also had lower percentages of T cells and other measures of immunosuppression (Kiecolt-Glaser, Glaser, Gravenstein, Malarkey, & Sheridan, 1996).

There is mounting evidence that stress is also linked to lowered immune resistance to viral infections (Solomon, Segerstrom, Grohr, Kemeny, & Fahey, 1997). For example, among a group of 276 students inoculated with common cold viruses, those who reported the most severe acute chronic stressors (1 month or longer) were most likely to develop colds (Cohen et al., 1998). Other studies demonstrate that both children and adults, when subjected to chronic stress, suffer more bouts of flu, herpes virus infections (cold sores and genital lesions), chicken pox, mononucleosis, and Epstein-Barr virus (Cohen & Herbert, 1996).

Pathways from Stress to Disease

Exactly how stress influences the immune system and promotes disease is the subject of a great deal of ongoing research. Two hypotheses have been suggested. According to the *direct effect hypothesis,* immunosuppression is part of the body's natural response to stress. Alternatively, the *indirect effect hypothesis* maintains that immunosuppression is an aftereffect of the stress response (Baum, Davidson, Singer, & Street, 1987).

Consider the example of the rate at which wounds heal. As discussed in Chapter 3, wound healing progresses through several overlapping stages. In the initial inflammatory stage, vasoconstriction and blood coagulation are followed by platelet activation and the release of growth factors. Growth factors stimulate the migration of phagocytes to the wound site, triggering a subsequent phase of healing that involves the recruitment and replication of cells necessary for tissue regeneration and capillary regrowth. This process may continue for weeks or months.

Research studies with both humans and animals demonstrate that stress delays the healing of wounds. One recent study reported that in mice subjected to the stress of being held in a restraining harness, a standardized punch biopsy wound healed an average of 27 percent more slowly than in unstressed mice (Kiecolt-Glaser, Page, Marucha, MacCallum, & Glaser, 1998). Among humans, dental students who received standardized wounds 3 days before a major test healed an average of 40 percent more slowly than those whose wounds were received during summer vacation (Marucha, Kiecolt-Glaser, & Favagehi, 1998).

The Indirect Effect Hypothesis According to the indirect effect hypothesis, stress-induced delays in healing may occur because stress alters immune processes *indirectly* by encouraging maladaptive behaviors that disrupt immune functioning (Kiecolt-Glaser et al., 1998). Among the behavioral risk factors that could delay wound healing through their effects on the immune system are smoking, alcohol and drug abuse, fragmented sleep, and poor nutrition, each of which has been associated with increased stress (Steptoe, Wardle, Pollard, & Canaan, 1996). Smoking, for instance, slows healing by weakening the normal proliferation of macrophages at wound sites and by reducing the flow of blood through vasoconstriction (Silverstein, 1992). In addition to healing more slowly, smokers are more likely to develop infections following surgical procedures, perhaps because nicotine and other toxins in cigarette smoke suppress both primary and secondary immune responses by reducing the activities of white blood cells (see Chapter 3).

As another example of how stress indirectly alters immune processes, consider that deep sleep is associated with the secretion of growth hormone (GH), a hormone that facilitates wound healing by activating macrophages to kill bacteria at the wound site (see Chapter 3). Loss of sleep, or fragmented sleep, results in reduced GH secretion and delayed healing (Leproult, Copinschi, Buxton, & Van Cauter, 1997).

The Direct Effect Hypothesis Another possibility is that stress may *directly* affect immune efficiency through the activation of neuroendocrine mechanisms that cause the release of cortisol, epinephrine, and other hormones and neurotransmitters that may reduce the body's defenses against infection and disease (Bachen et al., 1997). As we discussed earlier in this chapter, activation of the HPAC and SAM systems are two possible direct routes. T cells and B cells have receptors for corticosteroid "stress" hormones (which produce immunosuppression), and lymphocytes have catecholamine (epinephrine and norepinephrine) receptors. Stress activates these systems; the hormones released attach to the receptors of T cells, B cells, and lymphocytes, suppressing the immune response.

Evidence in support of a direct stress effect has also been reported. For example, in the study described earlier involving restraint stress in mice, the researchers also tested the hypothesis that the slower rate of wound healing reflected activation of the HPAC system (Kiecolt-Glaser et al., 1998). This was done in two ways: by assessing serum corticosteroid levels and by blocking the activity of naturally circulating stress hormones in restraint-stressed animals with a chemical that binds to corticosteroid receptor sites. In both cases, the results supported the hypothesis: Corticosteroid levels in the stressed mice were six times higher than in the unstressed mice. When their corticosteroid receptors were blocked, the stressed mice healed as well as control animals.

The Brain and Stress

There is also mounting evidence that the brain itself might directly affect the immune response. The brain closely monitors the activity of the immune system. Damage to the hypothalamus, for example, can either enhance or suppress the body's response to allergens. Moreover, when antigens induce an immune response, cells in the hypothalamus become more active. This may occur when T cells that have been activated by antigens release *lymphokines*. These chemicals, which attract macrophages and stimulate phagocytosis at wound and infection sites, are similar in structure to neurotransmitters. In other words, the lymphokines are like sheep in wolves' clothing: They look enough like neurotransmitters to bind to receptor sites on brain cells and trigger nerve impulses. Lymphocytes also have receptors for beta-endorphin, a chemical released from the pituitary gland in response to stress that can produce immunosuppression (Jemmott & Locke, 1984). The apparent interchangeability between neurotransmitters and lymphokines suggests that the immune system's lymphocytes may, in effect, act as circulating "language translators," converting information from their direct contact with pathogens into the language of the central nervous system so that the brain can monitor and regulate the immune response.

To sum up, PNI research studies reveal that the immune system does not work in isolation. Rather, it functions as part of a coordinated system involving the brain and the hormone-secreting endocrine system. The brain regulates the production of stress hormones, which in turn influence the body's immune defenses. We have only sketched the outline of the PNI model here. This model will be examined more fully in later chapters in conjunction with our exploration of the causes of cancer, AIDS, and other chronic diseases.

In concluding this chapter, it is worth remembering that although stress is inescapable, it does offer mixed blessings. Some stress arouses and motivates us and, in the process, often brings out our best qualities and stimulates personal growth. A life with no stress whatsoever would be boring and would leave us unfulfilled. The price we pay, of course, is the toll that stress may take on our physical health. Too much stress can overtax our coping abilities and leave us vulnerable to stress-related health problems. Fortunately, there are many things we can do to keep stress at a manageable level. It is to this topic that we turn our attention in the next chapter.

Summing Up

What Is Stress?

1. Stress has been a central concept in medicine and health for centuries. Early research on stress focused on the physiological processes involved. Modern research on stress began with Walter Cannon's description of the fight-or-flight reaction.

2. Stress has been defined as both a stimulus and a response. Researchers distinguish among stimulus events that are stressful (stressors), the physical and emotional responses of a person to a stressor (strain), and the overall process by which a person perceives and responds to threatening or challenging events (stress).

3. According to the transactional model, a key factor in stress is cognitive appraisal. In primary appraisal, the person assesses whether an event is benign-positive, irrelevant, or a potential threat or challenge. In secondary appraisal, the person assesses the coping resources available for meeting the challenge. Through reappraisal the person constantly updates his or her perception of success or failure in meeting a challenge or threat.

4. Stress has been measured in several ways, including self-report measures such as life events scales, physiological reactivity to an acute stressor through such devices as a polygraph, and in terms of changes in performance during persistent stress.

The Physiology of Stress

5. The body's response to stress involves the brain and nervous system, the endocrine glands and hormones, and the immune system. During a moment of stress, the hypothalamus secretes releasing factors that coordinate the endocrine response of the pituitary and adrenal glands. The sympathoadreno-medullary (SAM) system is the primary or first response to stress. Activation of the SAM system leads to increased blood flow to the muscles, increased energy, and higher mental alertness.

6. The hypothalamic-pituitary-adrenocortical (HPAC) system is a slower-reacting response to stress that is activated by messages from the CNS. HPAC activation functions to restore homeostasis to the body. Excessive cortisol production from the adrenal glands, however, may impair immune efficiency.

Sources of Stress

7. Among the sources of stress that have been investigated are major life events, daily hassles, environmental stress, and job-related stress. Major life events and daily hassles have been studied in relation to the prevalence of illness. Daily hassles may interact with anxiety and background stressors to influence a person's vulnerability to illness. Research exploring environmental stress has focused on noise, crowding, pollution, and cataclysmic events.

8. Among the factors that make work stressful are work overload, burnout, role conflict or ambiguity, inadequate career advancement, and lack of control over work. Events perceived as predictable and controllable are generally less stressful than those perceived as unpredictable and uncontrollable.

Models of Stress and Illness

9. Hans Selye outlined the general adaptation syndrome (GAS) to describe the effects of chronic stress. This syndrome consists of an alarm reaction, a stage of resistance, and a stage of exhaustion. Persistent stress may increase a person's susceptibility to a disease of adaptation.

10. The diathesis-stress model suggests that some persons are more vulnerable to stress-related illnesses because of predisposing factors such as genetic weakness. A good example of how this works is seen in post-traumatic stress disorder.

11. Psychoneuroimmunology is a multidisciplinary field that focuses on the interactions among behavior, the nervous system, the endocrine system, and the immune system. According to the direct effect hypothesis, immunosuppression is part of the body's natural response to stress.

12. The indirect effect hypothesis maintains that immunosuppression is an aftereffect of the stress response. Animal and human research studies demonstrate that the brain regulates the production of stress hormones, which in turn influence the body's immune defenses.

Key Terms and Concepts

stressor, p. 121
strain, p. 121
stress, p. 121
transactional model, p. 121
primary appraisal, p. 122
secondary appraisal, p. 122
cognitive reappraisal, p. 122
galvanic skin response (GSR), p. 125
polygraph, p.125
optimum level of arousal hypothesis, p. 129

anabolism, p. 130
catabolism, p. 130
sympathoadreno-medullary (SAM) system, p. 131
hypothalamic-pituitary-adrenocortical (HPAC) system, p. 131
homeostasis, p. 131
corticosteroids, p. 131
population density, p. 139

burnout, p. 144
acculturation, p. 148
general adaptation syndrome (GAS), p. 150
diathesis-stress model, p. 152
post-traumatic stress disorder (PTSD), p. 153
psychoneuroimmunology (PNI), p. 157

Health Psychology on the World Wide Web

Web Address	Description
http://helping.apa.org	The American Psychological Association's comprehensive Internet *Help Center,* providing access to resources to help people cope with modern stressors.
http://www.stress.org/	The American Institute of Stress, a nonprofit clearinghouse for information on all stress-related subjects. Hans Selye, Norman Cousins, and Linus Pauling were among the founding members.
http://www.stressfree.com	A wealth of resources for coping with job-related stress.
http://www.dartmouth.edu/dms/ptsd/	Web site of the National Center for Post-Traumatic Stress Disorder.

Critical Thinking Exercise

Post-Traumatic Stress Disorder

Persistent stress often leads to impaired performance and stress-related health problems, sometimes lingering even after the stressor has been terminated. As described in the chapter, post-traumatic stress disorder (PTSD) is one of the most dramatic examples of the aftereffects of stess. As a class assignment, you have been asked to prepare a brief presentation on PTSD that focuses on different theoretical views of the disorder and the controversy surrounding its increased prevalence. Answer the following questions to organize your presentation.

1. How would a researcher working from the biopsychosocial perspective explain PTSD? What are some of the

specific biological, psychological, and social factors in the disorder?

2. How would a researcher working within the diathesis-stress model explain PTSD? What are some of the specific predisposing and precipitating factors in PTSD?

3. How would a researcher working within the field of psychoneuroimmunology explain PTSD? What are some possible mind–body pathways to the disorder?

4. What evidence supports those who claim that PTSD is a genuine condition that is triggered by a traumatic event?

5. What evidence supports skeptics who claim that PTSD is at least partly a cultural or social phenomenon?

5

Coping with Stress

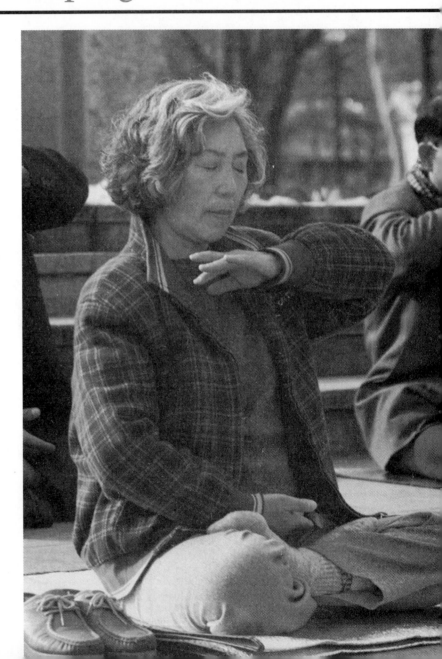

S pring break!" shouted Raheema, as she and her two sorority sisters stepped out of the airport into the blessedly warm Florida sunshine. The frozen winter semester at their Michigan college seemed to go on forever, but now they had a whole week to cut loose, soak up some rays, and recharge before midterms. Brittany and Latrice laughed as their roommate, eager to get the adventure under way, snatched the keys of their rental car from the agent's hand before he'd finished giving them directions to the parking lot. For 2 years now, ever since they'd arrived in Ann Arbor as scared freshmen, the three had been inseparable.

"To the beach!" Raheema commanded.

The traffic was light, so Raheema found it easy to drive and still put in her "two cents" as she and her passengers argued about where to go and what to do first. As the conversation grew more animated, she took her eyes off the road for just an instant, glancing back to express her displeasure with Brittany, who had suggested they stop for groceries and sun block before heading to the hotel and beach. Latrice's scream told Raheema that she'd made a terrible mistake.

The light had turned green, but as the women's compact convertible entered the intersection a large sport utility vehicle plowed into their driver's side door, killing Raheema instantly. The driver of the SUV, who was legally drunk, later admitted that the light had turned yellow before he entered the intersection. "It was very close," he stammered. "I thought they saw me coming through."

Miraculously, Brittany and Latrice's injuries were relatively minor and they were hospitalized for only a few days. Back at school a few weeks later, however, their bodies were healed but their hearts and minds were not. Brittany seemed unable to overcome her grief, shock, and feeling that she was at least partly responsible for her friend's death. "If only I hadn't disagreed with Raheema when she wanted to head straight to the beach," she ruminated. "She'd still be alive." As the days passed, neither Latrice nor anyone else could dissuade Brittany from believing that it was she, and not the drunken SUV driver who ran the stoplight, who was to blame for the tragic accident.

After taking some time off at home to mend her head and heart, Latrice was ready to get back to her studies. She missed Raheema dearly, and still cried every now and then over her senseless death, but she was putting her life back together. The loving support of her mother and father had helped a lot, and she'd talked things over with a psychologist at the college's counseling center, who was helping her work through her grief. And to honor her friend's memory, she'd enrolled in the fitness class the two of them had been pledging to join for more than a year.

Brittany, however, seemed to be in a downward psychological and physical spiral, alternating between states of denial and self-blame. She hadn't gone back to class since the accident, or home for that matter. "My parents wouldn't understand," she said. "Nobody could." To cope with her grief, she tried hard to keep from thinking about the accident. She slept a lot, and when she was awake she was glued to the television, usually with a beer in her hand. When her friends suggested that she talk to a counselor or join a grief support group, Brittany shook her head and said it was hopeless. Asked what she planned to do, she simply said, "My tuition, room, and board are paid up through the end of the school year. I'll worry about it then."

■ **coping** the cognitive, behavioral, and emotional ways in which people manage stressful situations

As you saw in Chapter 4, appraising a situation or event as stressful does not automatically lead to an adverse physiological and psychological response. In fact, how people deal with stressful events is at least as important as the stressors themselves in determining health or illness.

In this chapter we examine the factors that affect how people deal with stress, including differences in coping styles, personality traits, mood or outlook on life, perception of control, and amount of social support. Through our journey into the psychology of responding to stress, we will see ample evidence supporting the connection between mind and body and the biopsychosocial model. We will see that at every turn, biological, psychological, and social forces interact in determining our response to stress. The chapter concludes with a discussion of stress management techniques that can help minimize the ill effects of stress. Among these are exercise, relaxation, biofeedback, and hypnosis. Quite often, clinical health psychologists use such techniques to assist people in developing their ability to manage stress.

Responding to Stress

When we talk about how people respond to stress, we generally use the word *cope*. **Coping** refers to the cognitive, behavioral, and emotional ways that people manage stressful situations (Moss-Morris & Petrie, 1997). Implicit in this definition is the understanding that coping includes *any attempt* to preserve mental and physical health—even if it has limited value.

Coping is a dynamic process, not a one-time reaction; that is, it is a series of responses involving the interaction of a person and his or her environment. For example, when you break up with a girl- or boyfriend, you experience a number of physical and emotional reactions, perhaps an overall sadness and an inability to sleep or eat, maybe even nausea. These reactions may in part be triggered by environmental influences and later may be affected by those same influences (for example, friends' sympathetic comments may constantly remind you of your situation, as can revisiting places where the two of you spent some happy times). Together, these responses form the person's style of coping with stress.

Coping Strategies

Coping strategies—the ways people deal with stressful situations—are intended to moderate, or buffer, the effects of stressors on physical and emotional well-being (Ingledew, Hardy, & Cooper, 1997). Not all coping strategies are equally effective, however. Some strategies provide temporary relief in the short run, but tend to be maladaptive in the long run. For example, although psychological defenses (such as choosing not to think about a problem) allow people to distance themselves from the stressful situation by denying its existence, they do not eliminate the source of stress. Similarly, alcohol or other drugs push the stress into the background but do nothing to get rid of it. As another example, an overworked, frustrated executive may displace his or her pent-up aggression onto lower-level employees, who are less threatening than the demanding boss who caused the problem in the first place. These behaviors are maladaptive because they do not confront the stressor directly and are likely to make the situation worse.

In some cases, it doesn't matter which coping strategy the person uses; the stressor cannot be eliminated nor can its recurrence be prevented. Instead, the strategies may simply help a person tolerate or accept a situation (Moos & Schaefer, 1987). Facing the unrelenting stress of living in a war-torn country, for example, residents can only hope to survive until the danger passes.

Several attempts have been made to classify people's coping strategies. In this chapter we present the approach developed by Richard Lazarus (1984), which seems to be most useful in describing the varied responses to stress. With this approach, coping strategies are classified as either emotion focused or problem focused.

Emotion-Focused Coping

In **emotion-focused coping,** people use behavioral and cognitive strategies to manage their emotional reactions to stress. Behavioral strategies include seeking out others who offer social support, using alcohol or other psychoactive drugs, or keeping themselves busy to distract attention from the problem. Cognitive strategies involve changing how a stressor is appraised or denying unpleasant information.

People tend to rely on emotion-focused coping when they believe little or nothing can be done to alter the stressful situation or when they believe that their coping resources or skills are insufficient to meet the demands of the stressful situation (such as the loss of a loved one).

There are three types of emotion-focused coping: escape-avoidance, distancing, and positive reappraisal. With *escape-avoidance,* an individual physically or psychologically separates himself or herself from a stressor. Fearing failure in college, a student may stop attending classes or fantasize about miraculous solutions to his or

■ **emotion-focused coping**
coping strategy in which the person tries to control his or her emotional response to a stressor

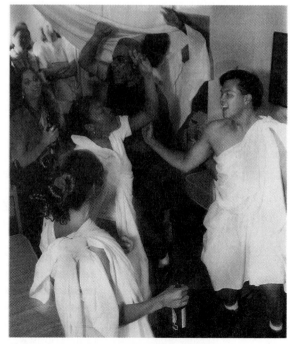

Coping with Stress, the Unhealthy Way
People do not always choose healthy ways of coping with stress. This is particularly true of teenagers and young adults, who have a sense of invincibility. © Greg Mancuso/ Stock Boston

■ **problem-focused coping**
coping strategy for dealing
directly with a stressor, in
which the person either
reduces the stressor's
demands or increases his or
her resources for meeting its
demands

■ **proactive coping** a type of
problem-focused coping in
which people attempt to
anticipate or detect potential
stressors and act in advance
to prevent them or to mute
their impact

■ **combative coping** a reactive
problem-focused coping
strategy in which a person
reacts to, or attempts to
escape from, a stressor that
cannot be avoided

her dilemma. Another student might begin sleeping excessively or abusing alcohol.

Distancing involves psychologically detaching oneself from a stressor. Learning that she is suffering from dangerously high blood pressure, for example, an obese woman might choose not to think about her health or might make light of her weight problem.

Positive reappraisal requires reinterpreting a situation in order to turn a negative into a positive. For example, an athlete may redouble her commitment to training after finishing poorly in a swim meet by reappraising the disappointing result as a challenge to her level of fitness.

Problem-Focused Coping

In **problem-focused coping,** people deal directly with the stressful situation either by reducing its demands or by increasing their capacity to deal with the stressor. They tend to rely on problem-focused coping strategies when they believe their resources and situations are changeable (Lazarus & Folkman, 1984). For example, people who are caring for terminally ill patients are likely to rely on problem-focused strategies during the caretaking period prior to their loved one's death. After the person's death, however, they are likely to see the situation as beyond their control and so lean toward emotion-focused coping (Moskowitz, Folkman, Collette, & Vittinghoff, 1996).

There are two types of problem-focused coping: proactive coping and combative coping. In **proactive coping** (also called *preventive coping*), people attempt to anticipate or detect potential stressors and act in advance to prevent them or to mute their impact (Aspinwall & Taylor, 1997). They do this by applying any of several mechanisms—for example, by using their problem-solving skills, by developing a stronger network of social support, by improving their financial assets, or by boosting their self-esteem—all of which require long-term efforts. For instance, a student who tackles a seemingly overwhelming course load by breaking her assignments into a series of smaller, manageable tasks is using one of these strategies, as is a recovering alcoholic who joins a support group to share experiences.

In **combative coping,** a person reacts to, or attempts to escape from, a stressor that cannot be avoided. Because the stressor is unavoidable, the person may have to rely on outside help to cope with the situation. As you'll learn later in the chapter, certain relaxation techniques and biofeedback have been helpful in this regard. Thus, a person who suffers from hypertension because of a stressful job may adopt a more nutritious diet and start a program of aerobic exercise to reduce body weight and control the hypertension. Alternatively, the person may resort to some form of meditation to calm the inner turmoil.

An important distinction between proactive and combative coping is in the amount of time and effort the two techniques require. Proactive coping skills often involve a long-term effort because the person may have to modify long-held attitudes, cognitive styles, and behaviors. On the other hand, many combative coping skills such as relaxation techniques and biofeedback often can be learned quickly.

What determines whether a person uses emotion-focused or problem-focused coping strategies? An important factor is the nature of the stressful event or circumstance. School- or work-related challenges lend themselves naturally to problem-focused coping strategies, such as seeking assistance from friends or using problem-solving skills to tackle the stressor directly. Any situation in which constructive action is possible favors problem-focused coping strategies. In contrast, some health problems, the loss of loved ones, and other situations that simply have to be accepted are more likely to trigger emotion-focused coping.

Think of your own style of coping with stressful situations. Which of these strategies have you employed? When? Did they help?

Evaluating the Emotion-Focused/Problem-Focused Model

Despite the prominence of the emotion-focused/problem-focused model of coping strategies, some researchers have argued that describing coping in either-or terms is misleading because the two strategies are often used together (Ingledew et al., 1997). Consider the college freshman who experiences stress at the start of the school year when adding up all of her course assignments. Although her initial reaction might be frustration with her professors, even anger at the seemingly insurmountable task facing her, she quickly calms down and realizes this won't help the situation. So she takes out her daily planner and begins mapping out a schedule that will allow her to meet the demands of each course. This example illustrates emotion-focused coping in controlling her initial angry impulse and problem-focused coping in developing a plan for the semester.

Differences in Coping Strategies

Each of us has our own way of coping with stress. In order to help us better understand those differences, researchers have attempted to categorize ways of coping by gender, ethnicity, and socioeconomic status.

Gender

Do men and women differ in how they react to and cope with stress? As is often the case in psychological research, there is no simple answer.

Men and women exhibit a number of different physiological reactions to stress. For example, women tend to have higher heart rates and sympathetic nervous system (SNS) tone at rest and greater stress-induced increases in heart rate and overall SNS tone. Men tend to exhibit stronger blood pressure and hormone reactivity during and immediately after stress (Baum & Grunberg, 1991). In addition, whereas men display greater increases in the hormones adrenaline and noradrenaline in response to stress, women exhibit a stronger cortisol response (Gallucci, Baum, & Laue, 1993). These neurochemical differences may in part reflect the tendency of men to be more aggressive or hostile than women. And, as we'll see in later chapters, these physiological differences may also help explain gender differences in sudden coronary death, arteriosclerosis, and other chronic diseases.

Other research studies have demonstrated that men exhibit larger increases in low-density lipoprotein cholesterol (LDL) and blood pressure during stressful laboratory tasks (Stoney, Matthews, McDonald, & Johnson, 1988). Chronic LDL cholesterol increases have been linked with atherosclerosis and coronary artery disease—another possible reason for the greater incidence of heart disease in men than in women. There is, however, no reason to suspect that transient changes in LDL in response to an acute stressor have serious implications for long-term health, especially when diet, exercise, body weight, and other factors are taken into consideration.

In explaining gender differences in emotional reactivity to stress, researchers report that women are consistently better than men at reading emotional cues. When students are shown a brief, soundless film clip of an upset person's face, women are significantly more accurate than men at detecting which emotion is being displayed. This sensitivity to body language helps in part to explain women's greater emotional responsiveness in stressful situations (Grossman & Wood, 1993). It also may explain why both men and women are more likely to seek emotional understanding and support from women than from men when attempting to cope with problems.

Another commonly cited gender difference in emotional reaction to stress is that men are more likely to use problem-focused coping strategies in dealing with stress, whereas women are more likely to rely on emotion-focused strategies (Endler & Parker, 1990; Zuckerman, 1989). However, several researchers have suggested that gender differences in coping styles may have less to do with being female or male than with the scope of coping resources available (see Diversity and Healthy Living, pages 172–173). When women and men of similar socioeconomic status are compared, gender differences in coping strategies often disappear (Greenglass & Noguchi, 1996).

Ethnicity and Socioeconomic Status

Stressful experiences are likely to be common occurrences for many ethnic minority families, who tend to be overrepresented among groups of low socioeconomic status (SES) (Taylor, Roberts, & Jacobson, 1997). Indeed, one-third of African-American families and nearly one-half of African-American children live below the poverty line (U.S. Bureau of the Census, 2000). Impoverished families experience more pollution, substandard and overcrowded housing, crime, and dangerous traffic than do more affluent families (Myers, Kagawa-Singer, Kumanika, Lex, & Markides, 1995). They also suffer poor nutrition, limited education, low-paying work, and a lack of health insurance and access to health care (Johnson et al., 1995). Moreover, children from low-SES homes are more likely to experience divorce, frequent school transfers, and harsh and punitive parenting, events that have been linked with a variety of behavioral and emotional difficulties (Taylor et al., 1997). Unemployment is also common among many minorities and low-SES groups. For African-American workers, for example, the unemployment rate is approximately twice that of European Americans.

The research has consistently found that people of low socioeconomic status rely less on problem-focused coping than do people with more education and higher incomes (Billings & Moos, 1981). Why? A possible answer is that because of the social experiences noted above, disadvantaged people have developed a feeling of hopelessness that causes them to believe they have little or no control over events in their lives. So, with repeated exposure to stress and no way to break the cycle, their only recourse is to try to control their emotional responses to stress—since they've learned that they can't control the situation itself.

Research by Judith Stein and Adeline Nyamathi (1999) demonstrates not only that impoverished people have more difficulty coping with stress but also that women in this situation have more problems than men do. The researchers examined a sample of 486 impoverished men and women of African-American, Latino, and European descent who were recruited to participate in a community-based AIDS prevention program. Compared with their male counterparts, the impoverished women reported greater stress and higher levels of depression, and they were more likely to resort to *avoidant coping* strategies. These strategies fell into three categories: *passive behaviors,* such as avoiding people and not thinking about their problems; *antisocial behaviors,* such as escapist drug use, risky sexual behaviors, and taking their problems out on others; and *fantasizing,* such as wishing their problems would go away or hoping for a miraculous intervention. The researchers suggest that the subordinate positions of impoverished women make them even more vulnerable than men to developing feelings of hopelessness in the face of grinding stress. This finding points to the need for gender-specific interventions in helping people cope with chronic stress.

One of the best-documented effects of low SES on coping behavior has to do with the effect of environmental stress on parents' relations to their children. One study of African-American mothers living in one- and two-parent households found that family disruption and work-related stress were powerfully linked to decreases in the mother's self-esteem (Ballie, 1986). Mothers who developed negative views of themselves seemed less able to engage in problem-focused coping that would benefit their children. In this way, environmental stress is linked to parental distress, which is linked to harsh parenting and additional problems for children.

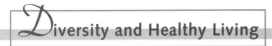

Diversity and Healthy Living

Understanding Gender Differences in Coping Styles

Think back to a moment of significant stress in your family when you were growing up, perhaps a life-threatening illness or loss of a job, an encounter with a tornado or hurricane, a serious traffic accident, or some other crisis. Were there differences in how the men and women around you coped with the stressful situation?

Two competing hypotheses have been offered to explain differences in how women and men cope with stress: socialization and role-constraint. The *socialization hypothesis* suggests that because of traditional stereotypes women and men are brought up to cope with stress in very different ways. Traditionally, men are encouraged to take action and remain stoically independent, whereas women are socialized to seek social support from others and to express their emotions freely. As a result, men tend to cope with stress in a *problem-focused* mode, while most women cope in an *emotion-focused* mode.

Although many research studies have reported evidence consistent with the socialization hypothesis (Brems & Johnson, 1989; Carver, Scheier, & Weintraub, 1989), others have failed to find gender differences in emotion- or problem-focused coping (Stern, Norman, & Komm, 1993). In some studies, the predicted results have actually been reversed, with men reporting greater use of certain emotion-focused strategies (such as denial), and women greater use of problem-focused strategies (Rosario, Shinn, Morch, & Huckabee, 1988).

Mixed results such as these were the impetus for the *role-constraint hypothesis,* which contends that when stressors are the same for men and women, gender is irrelevant in predicting coping reactions (Ptacek, Smith, & Zanas, 1992). According to this view, women and men have different social roles, which, in turn, make them more likely to experience different types of stressors. Any differences in coping are therefore due to differences in the types of stressors encountered.

In a fascinating test of the two hypotheses, Hasida Ben-Zur and Moshe Zeidner of the University of Haifa, Israel (1996), compared the coping reactions of Israeli women and men during a stressful national crisis with their reactions during a period of more typical daily stress. During the 10-day Gulf War in 1991, 39 Iraqi missiles were launched at the cities of Haifa and Tel Aviv, causing one death, 290 injuries, and untold damage to homes, buildings, and shops. For Israelis, the Gulf War was a grave national event, which exposed all citizens to a similar environmental stressor.

The researchers surveyed men and women regarding their coping behavior during the Gulf War and again 3 months after the crisis had ended. The participants in both surveys completed the *COPE Inventory*—a personality test consisting of 15 separate subscales that measure various aspects of problem-focused and emotion-focused coping, including denial, disengagement, humor, religion, venting of emotions, and seeking social support. Each participant indicated the extent to which he or she relied on each of the coping strategies, using a scale that ranged from 0 (not at all) to 3 (a great extent).

When the study was concluded, several of the subscales showed an interaction between gender and type of stress (see Figure 5.1, which plots the problem-focused and emotion-focused coping scores separately for men and women during war stress and under everyday stress). During the war, for example, women scored higher than men on the active and planning subscales (problem-focused coping), whereas during the postwar period they scored lower than men on these subscales. Men scored lower than women on seeking emotional social support during the stress of the war than during the postwar period, but reported more acceptance and types of avoidance behavior, including denial, behavioral disengagement, alcohol/drug use, and humor during the war than they did under everyday stress.

Women also reported using a wider range of coping strategies, scoring higher on 12 out of the 15 subscales during the war period and on 10 out of the 15 subscales during the postwar period. Differences between men and women were small after the war, both in total reported coping and in type of coping strategy, with men reporting slightly more emotion-focused strategies in daily life.

Thus, the data are not entirely consistent with either hypothesis. According to the socialization hypothesis, women

Figure 5.1

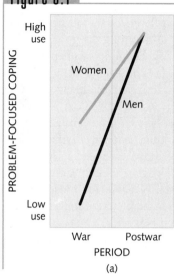

(a)

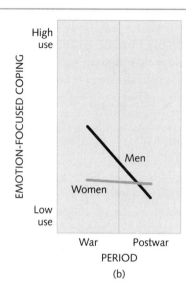

(b)

Gender Differences in Coping Strategies
(a) During a national crisis, women were more likely than men to report problem-focused coping, while men were more likely to report emotion-focused coping. (b) The differences between women and men were smaller after the war, with women reporting slightly more emotion-focused coping strategies in dealing with everyday stressors.

Source: Adapted from "Gender Differences in Coping Reactions under Community Crisis and Daily Routine Conditions," by H. Ben-Zur and M. Zeidner, 1996, *Journal of Personality and Individual Differences*, *20*(3), pp. 331–340.

should have exhibited more emotion-focused coping and men more problem-focused coping in dealing with everyday events, but especially during periods of war stress. According to the role-constraint hypothesis, men and women should have exhibited similar reactions during the war because it constituted a similar stressor for both sexes, but not necessarily after the war, when men and women presumably encountered different stressors.

Researchers have suggested possible reasons for the inconsistency between the data and both hypotheses. The socialization hypothesis is not entirely correct because it was based on traditional gender stereotypes that are disappearing in many modern cultures. Women today are expected to have a career of their own, and thus are more likely to be socialized toward greater assertiveness, independence, and active coping.

The role-constraint hypothesis also missed the mark, possibly because although the threat was the same for everyone, men and women may have perceived it differently. For example, many of the coping options that could help protect individuals were related to creating a safe home environment. Under threat of being bombed by missile warheads with poisonous chemical compounds, families had to stay indoors in a sealed environment, stock up on food, and so forth. Although traditional gender roles are undoubtedly merging, the specific demands of the war situation may have encouraged women to take charge. In contrast, Israeli men, whose defense response more often involves active military service, may have perceived fewer tasks to accomplish. This may explain their relatively higher level of emotion-focused coping.

Think back again to your family crisis. Is either hypothesis consistent with the men and women you saw coping? What about you? Is your coping style more the product of socialization or role-constraint? Do these hypotheses make sense for women and men of your generation?

Other dysfunctional attempts to cope with stress have been found to play a role in the morbidity and mortality of people who have low socioeconomic status. Hector Myers and his colleagues (1995) reviewed evidence on five high-risk behaviors: cigarette smoking, poor diet, obesity, sedentary lifestyle, and alcohol consumption among African-Americans, Asian/Pacific Islanders, Latinos, and Native Americans. Substantial differences in the prevalence of these health-compromising behaviors were found among the groups. Obesity, for example, was found to be a prevalent risk factor in women within all groups, but especially among African-Americans and Pacific Islanders. An excessive intake of dietary fat and an inadequate intake of dietary fiber were found to be particularly prevalent among African-Americans. It is important to note that Myers' study included only members of ethnic minorities; as a general rule, high-risk behaviors such as smoking, sedentary living, and poor diet are more prevalent in all low-SES groups, regardless of ethnicity.

The researchers are quick to point out, however, that there is a limited amount of basic health behavior information available for most groups of people of color. Moreover, the research that is available often makes it difficult to separate cultural influences from other factors, such as socioeconomic differences. That is, most studies simply compare an undifferentiated sample of members of one ethnic group with those of other ethnic groups. Researchers working from the biopsychosocial perspective emphasize that studying a variable such as ethnicity or SES in isolation will at best yield an incomplete understanding of how that variable relates to health. At worst, it may lead researchers to reach erroneous conclusions. Additional studies on socioeconomic, age, gender, and other subgroups within each ethnic group are vital to help researchers avoid these pitfalls.

Factors Affecting the Ability to Cope

Most of us resist the idea that we should work on our psychological makeup in order to improve our health. We do this even though we all know that certain life stresses (such as final exams) tend to give us headaches, queasy stomachs, and other ailments, whereas exhilarating or uplifting experiences (such as a ski weekend or a new intimate relationship) make us feel on top of the world.

Why this reluctance to relate psychological factors to health and illness? The main reason is that we are used to thinking of the body (and health) as separate from the mind. As you'll recall from Chapter 1, this dualistic thinking—which characterizes the traditional biomedical model of health—was unable to explain psychologically based physical symptoms, leading researchers to develop the biopsychosocial model of health. In this section we explore several psychosocial factors that affect how well people cope with potential stressors and, by extension, how this affects their health. Keep in mind that no one factor by itself determines your well-being. Health is always a result of biopsychosocial factors interacting in various ways.

Hardiness

Do you know people who approach life with enthusiasm, who always seem to be taking on more challenges, who remain healthy in the face of adversity? This zest for life keeps these people from becoming overwhelmed. Psychologists Salvatore Maddi and Suzanne Kobasa (1991) have identified three stress-buffering traits—*commitment, challenges,* and *control*—that have a substantial effect on how people react to threatening events. Together, these traits form a personality style called **hardiness.**

According to Kobasa and Maddi, hardy people tend to view the everyday demands of life as challenges rather than as threats. They are also committed to their families, jobs, communities, or other groups or activities that give their lives a sense of meaning. And, most important, they have a sense of control over their lives, of having access to needed information, and of being capable of making good decisions regarding the demands of life.

In this view, hardy people are healthier because they are less likely to become aroused by stressful situations. As a result, they avoid stress-related physical and psychological processes that lead to illness. Is there evidence to support such contentions? In a 1982 study, Kobasa collected personality data from 670 middle- and upper-level managers and attempted to relate these to stress and illness experienced during the next 2 years (Kobasa, Maddi, & Kahn, 1982). As Figure 5.2 (page 176) shows, managers who experienced high levels of stress also reported more illness; however, those in this group who were high in hardiness experienced significantly lower levels of illness than did those low in hardiness.

Overall, hardiness has been found to be an effective indicator of adaptation or adjustment to numerous health problems, including cancer, chronic obstructive pulmonary disease, cardiovascular disease, diabetes, epilepsy, HIV infection, hypertension, kidney transplant, and stroke (see Pollock, 1986, for a review). Hardiness has also been linked to lower levels of anxiety, active coping styles, decreased caregiver burden, reduced vulnerability to depression in older people living in a long-term care facility, better adaptation of professional women to the stress of multiple roles, greater spiritual well-being in elderly people, and fewer negative health outcomes during periods of extended stress (Drory, Florian, & Kravetz, 1991; Florian, Mikulincer, & Taubman, 1995).

Psychological hardiness has also been studied on the battlefield. Victor Florian and his colleagues at Bar-Ilan University collected data on hardiness,

hardiness a cluster of stress-buffering traits consisting of commitment, challenges, and control

Figure 5.2

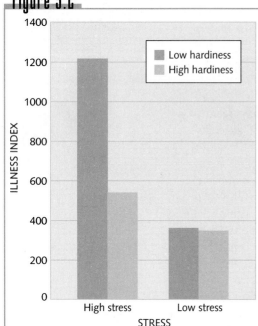

Stress, Hardiness, and Illness
High levels of stress clearly are more likely than low levels to cause illness. However, hardiness can buffer the effects of stress. Hardy managers who reported high levels of stress experienced significantly lower levels of illness than did those low in hardiness. The measure of stress was an adaptation of the familiar *Social Readjustment Rating Scale,* which subjectively quantifies the stressfulness of numerous events (see Chapter 4). Note that the illness index is a composite measure of the frequency and severity of 126 commonly recognized physical and mental symptoms and diseases.

Source: Based on data from "Hardiness and Health: A Prospective Study," by S. C. Kobasa, S. R. Maddi, and S. Kahn, 1982, *Journal of Personality and Social Psychology, 42*(1), pp. 168–177. Copyright 1982 by the American Psychological Association. Adapted with permission.

mental health, and coping style from Israeli military recruits just before and just after a stressful 4-month tour of combat duty (Florian et al., 1995). The results revealed that two traits of hardiness—commitment and a sense of control—were especially accurate in predicting mental health. Recruits who reported greater commitment to their mission reported fewer negative symptoms than did the others. In addition, they relied less on emotion-focused strategies, which would be less useful in coping with stress in these situations. A sense of control improved mental health by increasing the soldiers' tendency to reappraise stressful events in more positive terms and promoting their use of problem-solving and support-seeking coping strategies.

Evaluating the Hardiness Hypothesis

Despite the large number of studies in support of the idea that psychologically healthy people are buffered against stress, the concept of hardiness has received its share of criticism. Some researchers have suggested that the hardiness-health relationship is more applicable to men than women. For instance, Lori Schmied and Kathleen Lawler (1986) examined hardiness, stress, and illness in a group of women secretaries. Although a strong association between overall stress and illness was found, there were no differences in hardiness among women who reported high levels of both stress and illness and those who reported high stress but low levels of illness. Other critics have questioned the use of subjective self-report measures of stress and illness, as well as Kobasa and Maddi's fundamental idea that hardiness consists of certain specific core constructs. On this latter point, Lois Benishek (1996) has used *factor analysis*—a statistical procedure that identifies clusters of items on self-report tests that measure a common trait (such as hardiness)—to show that hardiness actually comprises one to four factors, rather than the three proposed by Kobasa and Maddi. The number of factors seems to depend on the measures used and the population studied. Another methodological critique is that hardiness research generally has ignored individual differences in the perceived severity of a given stressor in favor of merely tallying its frequency (Benishek & Lopez, 1997). As you learned in Chapter 4, how stress is *appraised* is a crucial factor in its impact on the individual.

Recent studies have also reported mixed support for hardiness as a buffer against certain stress-related health problems. Take the case of job-related stress—burnout, in particular. Recall that health care workers are especially prone to the physical and mental exhaustion of burnout, and at least two studies have found that nurses working in cancer and AIDS wards who scored high in hardiness were less likely to later develop symptoms of burnout than were their low-scoring counterparts (Constantini, Solano, DiNapoli, & Bosco, 1997; Duquette, Kerouac, Sandhu, Ducharme, & Saulnier, 1995). Another study, however, found that hardiness did not reduce symptoms of burnout among nurses when other factors such as age, temperament, and coping resources were ruled out (Rowe, 1997).

Are hardy people healthier because they have greater personal resources, such as income, education, social support, coping skills, even younger age (to go along with a "youthful outlook" on life)? To determine whether the health benefits of hardiness are actually the result of other protective factors, Kobasa interviewed stressed executives who after scoring high on the Social Readjustment Rating Scale (see Chapter 4) had remained in good health or become sick. Those who remained healthy were not younger, wealthier, or better educated than their sicker counterparts. However, they experienced more commitment in their lives, felt more in control, and had a greater appetite for challenge (Kobasa et al., 1982). In another study, hardiness was shown to have a stronger protective effect against illness than exercise or social support (Kobasa, Maddi, Puccetti, & Zola, 1985). These and other studies in which hardiness and health-enhancing behaviors were measured separately indicate that hardiness is an independent trait not caused by other variables.

On balance, the results of research studies on hardiness do seem to demonstrate that some people handle stress more effectively because they view themselves as choosing to live challenging lives. They also appraise potentially stressful events more favorably, seeing them as enriching their lives rather than as intensifying pressure. When confronted with stressful situations, they are more likely to reappraise negative conditions as positive ones (Williams,

■ **resilience** the quality of some children to bounce or spring back from environmental stressors that might otherwise disrupt their development

Wiebe, & Smith, 1992). This reappraisal allows them to feel in control of, rather than controlled by, stressors they encounter. Equally important, hardy people strive to solve their problems with active coping strategies—such as problem-focused coping and seeking social support—rather than trying to avoid them (Williams et al., 1992). Finally, hardy people, who are high in commitment, have a sense of purpose in life that allows them to find meaning in potentially stressful events and makes them more likely to adopt active coping strategies.

Resilience

Closely related to hardiness is the concept of **resilience,** a term that has been applied to children who show a remarkable ability to develop into competent, well-adjusted people despite having been raised in extremely disadvantaged environments (Garmezy, 1983). Variously defined as the ability to develop coping strategies despite adverse conditions, to bounce back when bad things happen, and to flourish in the face of stress, resilience allows these remarkable children to shrug off potential stressors.

Psychiatrist Steven Wolin (1993) describes the case of Jacqueline, who at 2 years of age was placed by her birth parents in a foster home. Eighteen months later, Jacqueline's foster father murdered his wife and Jacqueline was moved to another foster family. After 2 relatively stable years, Jacqueline's birth mother appeared without explanation, taking her daughter to live with her for the next 4 years. During those years, Jacqueline's mother had a string of dysfunctional relationships with men who moved in and out of the house, some of whom physically abused Jacqueline. At age 10, Jacqueline was once again displaced, this time to an orphanage, where she stayed until she was 17. Although many theories of psychosocial development would predict that Jacqueline would develop into an antisocial, problem-ridden woman, this did not happen. Throughout her childhood, she excelled in school, was a leader among her peers, and remained optimistic about her future. Now an adult, she has a stable marriage and finds great joy in being "the parent to my children that I never had."

Where does such resilience come from? Research points to two groups of factors. One group relates to individual traits, the other to social support. Resilient children have well-developed social, academic, or creative skills; easy temperaments; high self-esteem; self-discipline; and strong feelings of personal control (Werner, 1997). These elements of *social cognition* seem to foster healthy relationships with others that help such children adjust to otherwise adverse conditions. They also help these children to deflect many of the problems they may face at home (Ackerman, Kogos, Youngstrom, Schoff, & Izard, 1999).

Studies of resilient children also point to the importance of at least one consistently supportive person in the life of a child at risk (Garmezy, 1993). This person can be an aunt or uncle, older sister or brother, grandparent, family friend, or teacher. Often a model of resilience, this person plays a significant role in convincing at-risk children that they can and will beat the odds.

Although early studies of resilience implied that there was something remarkable about these children, recent research suggests that resilience is a more common phenomenon that arises from the ordinary resources of children, their relationships, and their communities (Masten, 2001). Echoing the theme of the positive psychology movement (see Chapter 1), the resilience research now focuses on understanding how these adaptive processes develop, how they operate under adverse conditions, and how they can be protected (or restored).

Stamina

Another concept related to hardiness is **stamina,** a term used to describe successful coping among the elderly. Elizabeth Colerick (1985) collected data on 70- to 80-year-old women and men to determine how people deal with the difficult life events that often occur during old age. Using questionnaires and interviews, Colerick differentiated two groups: a high stamina group and a low stamina group. People in the high stamina group—characterized by a "triumphant, positive outlook during periods of adversity"—were found to cope more effectively with everyday stresses than those in the low stamina group. Said one, "I realize that setbacks are a part of the game. I've had 'em, I have them now, and I've got plenty more ahead of me. Seeing this—the big picture—puts it all into perspective, no matter how bad things get" (page 999).

This ability to reframe potentially stressful events, to shift focus from a cup that is half empty to one that is half full, is a major cognitive component of hardiness—and a clear example of emotion-focused coping. People with high stamina remain healthier and more involved in community service and make regular efforts at personal growth (such as continuing education and travel) throughout their lives.

Explanatory Style

Hardiness describes how you respond to stress. **Explanatory style**—your general propensity to attribute outcomes always to positive causes or to negative causes, such as personality, luck, or another person's actions—determines your response. People who look on the bright side of life—who see a light at the end of the tunnel—have a positive explanatory style. People who see only the dark side—who expect failure because they believe that the conditions that lead to failure are all around them or even within them—have a negative explanatory style. The research literature views these two explanatory styles as extremes along a single continuum of optimism, although in common usage people with negative explanatory styles are referred to as pessimists. Are you at either extreme? Which one? See the Reality Check on page 180 which will help you to identify your usual explanatory style.

- **stamina** the quality of some elderly adults to remain positive and upbeat in the face of adversity

- **explanatory style** a person's general propensity to attribute outcomes always to positive causes or always to negative causes, such as personality, luck, or another person's actions

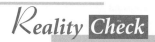

Your Outlook on Life

Your outlook on life, which is reflected in your explanatory style, influences your ability to cope effectively with stress. Michael Scheier and Charles Carver (1985) have developed the Life Orientation Test to measure individual differences in pessimism and optimism.

LIFE ORIENTATION TEST

Answer "true" or "false" to each of the following items.

T F   1. In uncertain times, I usually expect the best.
T F   2. It's easy for me to relax.
T F   3. If something can go wrong for me, it will.
T F   4. I always look on the bright side of things.
T F   5. I'm always optimistic about my future.
T F   6. I enjoy my friends a lot.
T F   7. It's important for me to keep busy.
T F   8. I hardly ever expect things to go my way.
T F   9. Things never work out the way I want them to.
T F 10. I don't get upset too easily.
T F 11. I'm a believer in the idea that "every cloud has a silver lining."
T F 12. I rarely count on good things happening to me.

Scoring: To score yourself, drop filler items 2, 6, 7, and 10. Items 1, 4, 5, and 11 are worded in the optimistic direction. Give yourself 1 point for each "true" answer; subtract 1 point for each "false" answer. Items 3, 8, 9, and 12 are worded in the pessimistic direction. Give yourself 1 point for each "false" answer; subtract a point from your total for each "true" answer. Total your score and see how optimistic you are. The higher your total (out of a possible maximum of 8), the greater your optimism.

If your score on the Life Orientation Test was very low, you probably have a pessimistic viewpoint. And such pessimism can leave you more vulnerable to the physical and emotional effects of stress, which in turn increase stress. This negative stress cycle in which stress activates health-compromising systems and these systems increase stress is illustrated in Figure 5.3.

Pessimists' self-defeating interpretation of stressful life events is often the result of automatic thoughts, beliefs, and attitudes. For example, if you get caught in a traffic jam, you might think: "Why me?" "Why now?" "I'm not going to be able to handle this" or "This is going to be a rotten day!" These responses often appear before you've taken a moment to ratio-

Figure 5.3

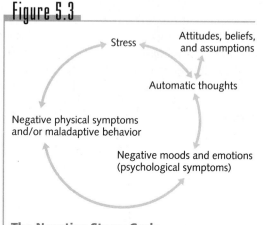

The Negative Stress Cycle
Stressful events interpreted through a pessimistic, self-defeating style create a negative mood that leads to stress-related physical symptoms and fuels additional stress. Fortunately, this vicious cycle can be interrupted at any point.

nally evaluate your situation. Here are examples of the major types of defeatist thinking: Do you recognize any?

- Magnification: exaggerating situations in extreme ways—for example, interpreting a pounding heart as a heart attack.

- All-or-none thinking: evaluating situations in extreme ways—for example, concluding that a D on one exam makes you a total failure.

- Personalization: assuming responsibility for a negative situation when there is no basis for doing so—for example, feeling inadequate and somehow responsible for a friend's depression.

- Jumping to conclusions: interpreting situations in the worst possible light, whether or not such a view is justified by the facts—for example, interpreting a friend's lack of response to an e-mail as not wanting to talk to you.

- Overgeneralization: viewing a single bad situation as part of a continual pattern—for example, assuming that you'll never get a date at all after you were turned down by one person.

When you become aware of your thought processes, you can modify them through various techniques. Once you can do this, you can utilize the following four-step approach for reducing stress developed by Herbert Benson and Eileen Stuart (1996).

Stop Whenever you encounter a stressful situation, STOP, before your thinking jumps to the worst possible conclusion about what will happen. Doing so will interrupt the negative stress cycle before it gets under way.

Breathe Breathing deeply will release physical tension and help trigger relaxation. Deep breathing will also further divert your attention from the stressor.

Reflect When you break the automatic tendency to magnify every stressful event, you can focus your energy on the cause of the problem at hand. This process of reflection will help you identify the source of the stress, appraise/reappraise the situation, and understand why you are reacting as you are. Ask yourself these questions: "What's going on here? Why am I feeling stressed? Are things really as bad as they seem? Is there another way to look at this situation? Can I handle this?"

Choose After you have stopped your automatic thinking and taken a deep breath to promote relaxation, then, reflecting on the cause of your stress, you can choose the best strategy for dealing with the problem at hand. The following skills provide a variety of coping strategies:

■ *Think Twice, Act Once.* This doesn't mean procrastinate. Sometimes, temporarily putting off a problem until it can be dealt with more effectively is the best strategy. Listing the pros and cons of possible solutions to a problem can help you take a new perspective. It can also reduce stress by demonstrating that you do have some options.

■ *Reappraise.* Reappraisal, or reframing, is the ability to interpret an event from a different perspective. The classic example is how you "see" a glass that is filled to its middle: Is it half empty or half full? In thinking about her failure to get a part in the school play, a student who had originally been very stressed by "failure" reframed the experience with the old saying: "I'm not a failure if I don't succeed; I'm a success because I tried."

■ *Don't Ruminate.* Some people dwell too long on a problem before taking action, playing it over and over again (ruminating) in their minds for fear of taking the wrong step. Rather than becoming paralyzed into a state of inaction, sometimes the best thing to do is to act immediately (and directly) to solve a problem. Worried about a festering situation with a friend, for example, a student may simply decide to confront the problem head-on. The friend is likely to appreciate her honest concern for their relationship, which makes a good starting point for working out the problem.

■ *Seek Social Support.* Seeking others for support should always be considered an option in coping with a stressful event or situation. Friends, relatives, coworkers, and professionals can be sources of instrumental and emotional support during times of stress.

Stress is a fact of life, but it is a fact you can learn to manage in ways that do not compromise your physical or psychological well-being. Each time you encounter a stressful situation, *make a conscious effort* to apply the four-step model:

Stop → Breathe → Reflect → Choose

Why are some people more prone to one style or the other? The difference lies in part with individual attribution styles—whom or what we blame for our failures. Martin Seligman and his colleagues (1995) believe that negativity and "epidemic hopelessness" are largely responsible for the prevalence of depression among Western people. When failure and rejection are (inevitably) encountered in life, maintains Seligman, the self-focused Westerner is more likely to assume personal responsibility. In non-Western cultures, where individualism is subordinate to cooperation and a sense of community, depression is less common, perhaps because it is less likely to be linked with self-blame for failure.

Pessimism

A recipe for severe depression is preexisting pessimism encountering failure.
—Martin Seligman (1995)

Those with a negative explanatory style tend to explain failures in terms that are global ("Everything is awful"), stable ("It's always going to be this way"), and internal ("It's my fault, as usual"). Anger, hostility, suppressed emotions, anxiety, depression, and pessimism are all associated with a negative explanatory style and are believed to lead to harmful health-related behaviors (smoking and alcohol and drug abuse, for example) and disease (Scheier & Bridges, 1995).

Pessimism has also been related to earlier mortality. In a study of personality data obtained from general medical patients at the Mayo Clinic between 1962 and 1965, Toshihiko Maruta and his colleagues examined the patients' scores on the Optimism-Pessimism (PSM) scale of the Minnesota Multiphasic Personality Inventory (MMPI). Over the ensuing years, patients who were more pessimistic (had higher PSM scores) had significantly higher (19 percent) mortality (Maruta, Colligan, Malinchoc, & Offord, 2000). Reviewing the growing literature on pessimism and early mortality, Martin Seligman (Seligman & Csikszentmihalyi, 2000) has identified four mechanisms by which pessimism might shorten life: (1) Pessimists experience more unpleasant events, which have been linked to shorter lives; (2) believing that "nothing I do matters," pessimists are less likely to comply with medical regimens and take fewer preventive actions (such as exercising) than optimists; (3) pessimists are more likely to be diagnosed with major depressive disorder, which itself is associated with mortality; and (4) pessimists have weaker immune systems than optimists. Despite this bleak prognosis, Seligman is quick to note that pessimism is identifiable early in life and can be changed.

Optimism

People with an upbeat, optimistic explanatory style, on the other hand, tend to enjoy good health (Peterson & Bossio, 1991). They lead healthier, longer lives than do their gloom-and-doom counterparts. They also have shorter hospital stays, faster recovery from coronary artery bypass surgery, and greater longevity when battling AIDS (Scheier, Matthews, Owens, & Magovern, 1989). Optimists also respond to stress with smaller increases in blood pressure and are much less likely to die from heart attacks (Everson, Goldberg, Kaplan, & Cohen, 1996). Among college students, optimists—those who agree with statements such as, "In uncertain times, I usually expect the best" and "I always look on the bright side of things"—report less fatigue and fewer aches, pains, and minor illnesses (Scheier & Carver, 1985).

Why is optimism beneficial to health? According to the *broaden-and-build theory*, positive emotions increase people's physical, cognitive, and social resources, which in turn helps them cope more effectively with stressful experiences and live healthier lives (Frederickson, 2001). For example, by shortening the duration of negative emotional arousal, positive emotions may stave off stress-related cardiovascular activation, elevated blood pressure, and other disease-promoting processes. As another example, among children, the positive emotions experienced during play help build social skills, which in turn foster lasting social bonds and attachments (Aron, Norman, Aron, McKenna, & Heyman, 2000). In support of this theory, a recent study found that people who consistently experienced positive emotions with their families as children, and again as adults with their own families, were half as likely to display high levels of cumulative wear and tear on their bodies (Ryff, Singer, Wing, & Love, 2001). Another study of older Hispanic-Americans reported that those who generally reported positive emotions were half as likely as those who were more pessimistic and cynical to become disabled or to have died during the two-year duration of the study (Ostir, Markides, Black, & Goodwin, 2000).

Optimism may also help sustain immune functioning under stress. A recent study demonstrated exactly that: Persistent stress—in this case, caused by the pressure of first-semester law school—took a less negative toll on immune activity in students who were optimistic about their academic success, compared to students who were pessimistic (Segerstrom, Taylor, Kemeny, & Fahey, 1998). As Figure 5.4 shows, the number of CD4 cells in the optimists' bloodstream rose by 13 percent, compared with a 3 percent drop in the number of cells in the pessimists. Similarly, NK cell activity rose by 42 percent in the high-scoring optimists but only by 9 percent in pessimists. (As we saw in Chapter 3, CD4 cells and NK cell activity are immune system factors that help fight infection.)

This is not an isolated finding. For example, other studies have reported that people with AIDS who believe their illness is controllable also display increased T cell counts over time and live longer. In contrast, HIV-positive men who are pessimistic about their fate display a decrease in T cell counts and faster onset of AIDS symptoms over the same period of time (Segerstrom, Taylor, Kemeny, Reed, & Visscher, 1996).

One interesting unanswered question raised by the law-student study is, Why does optimism enhance immune function under stress? Segerstrom and Taylor believe that their optimistic students had healthier attitudes and better health habits than did the pessimists. Optimists, for example, were more likely to appraise their course work as a challenge (and therefore perceive less stress), to exercise more, and to avoid smoking, alcohol abuse, and other health-compromising behaviors. These health-enhancing behaviors thus contributed to stronger immune systems and better functioning under stress.

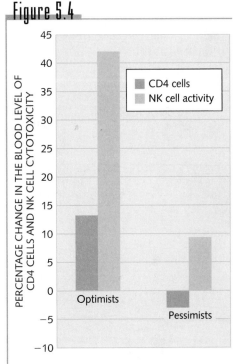

Figure 5.4

Optimism and Immune Function

Two months after beginning law school, optimistic law students showed a 13 percent increase in the blood level (estimated total number) of CD4 cells in the bloodstream, as compared with a 3 percent drop in the number of cells in the bloodstream of pessimists. Similarly, natural killer cell cytotoxicity (a measure of cell activity level) rose by 42 percent in the optimists but only by 9 percent in pessimists.

Source: Based on data from "Optimism Is Associated with Mood, Coping and Immune Change in Response to Stress," by S. C. Segerstrom, S. E. Taylor, M. E. Kemeny, and J. Fahey, 1998, *Journal of Personality and Social Psychology, 74*(6), pp. 1646–1655. Copyright 1998 by the American Psychological Association. Adapted with permission.

■ **rumination** repetitive focusing on the causes, meanings, and consequences of stressful experiences

■ **personal control** the belief that we make our own decisions and determine what we do or what others do to us

This and other studies reveal not only the differences in how optimists and pessimists physically react to stress but also differences in how they cope with stress. Whereas optimists are more likely to try to alter stressful situations or to take direct problem-focused action against a stressor (Scheier, Weintraub, & Carver, 1986), pessimists are more likely to **ruminate,** that is, to obsess and be overwhelmed by persistent thoughts about stressors (Nolen-Hoeksema, Parker, & Larson, 1994); this has been linked to a negative explanatory style, self-criticism, a history of past depression and excessive dependency on others (Spasojevic & Alloy, 2001).

Interestingly, those who tend to ruminate about stressful events feel they have less social support from others and are more likely to suffer from depression than those who are more optimistic (Nolen-Hoeksema & Davis, 1999). Optimists also perceive they have more control over stressors, which in turn leads to more effective coping responses, including seeking treatment when illness strikes (Lin & Peterson, 1990; Scheier & Bridges, 1995). In contrast, pessimists are more likely to be depressed and sad and to perceive the world as being uncontrollable (Keltner, Ellsworth, & Edwards, 1993).

Personal Control

Consider the following scenario. After a routine physical examination, your doctor tells you that your blood pressure is too high. Because you do not have any other symptoms or a family history of hypertension or coronary heart disease, she suspects that your lifestyle is to blame. She warns you that you'd best gain control over whatever health-compromising behaviors are elevating your blood pressure now.

How do you respond to your doctor's warning? Ideally, you consider how you might alter your diet, activity level, stress level, and other aspects of your daily routine because you believe you can exert a significant degree of control over your blood pressure. Conversely, if you believe that you cannot influence your health or that there is nothing you can do to make your situation better, you do nothing.

Personal control is the belief that we make our own decisions and determine what we do or what others do to us (Rodin, 1986). As children, we gradually develop a sense of control over our surroundings. Albert Bandura and other researchers have called this sense of control *self-efficacy* (Bandura, 1977). More precisely, self-efficacy refers to people's beliefs in their capabilities to organize and execute the courses of action required to deal with potentially stressful situations (Bandura, 1997).

Personal Control and Coping Strategies

People with a strong sense of personal control are more likely to engage in adaptive problem-focused coping. In one study, health care workers facing layoffs completed questionnaires assessing their levels of stress, personal resources, coping styles, and illness at the beginning of the study and again one year later (Ingledew et al., 1997). The results revealed that increases in perceived level of stress were generally accompanied by increases in emotion-focused coping, but to a lesser degree in those who perceived strong personal control over their lives—for those workers, feelings of control and self-efficacy led to more problem-focused coping.

A classic example of the health benefits of perceived control was reported by Ellen Langer and Judith Rodin (1976) in a study that manipulated the amount of responsibility allowed elderly residents on two floors of a nursing home. Residents on one floor were permitted to assume more responsibility and control over their daily lives—for example, they were allowed to arrange the furniture in their rooms as they wished, given houseplants to care for, and encouraged to select their own recreational activities. In comparison, residents on the neighboring floor—while similar in age, gender, prior socioeconomic status, and physical and psychological health—had most of these decisions made for them. For example, they were assigned to various recreational activities, and their houseplants were to be fed and watered by the nursing home staff. The results of the study were striking. After only 3 weeks, residents who had control over their lives were happier, more active and alert, and reported a higher overall level of well-being than their counterparts who had little control. Most striking was that while 93 percent of the residents who were given responsibility showed some psychological and physical improvement, 71 percent of the no-responsibility residents actually became *less* active, less alert, and more physically debilitated.

Remarkably, $1\frac{1}{2}$ years later the residents in the responsibility group continued to be healthier. They were more active, more sociable, happier, and had half the rate of mortality of their no-control counterparts. As researcher Ellen Langer (1983) noted, "Perceived control is basic to human functioning . . . for the young and old alike." Most striking was the difference in the mortality rates of the two groups 18 months after the study began: 15 percent of the experimental group had died, compared with 30 percent of the control group.

Those who feel a strong sense of psychological control are more likely to exercise direct control over health-related behaviors. Niall Pender and colleagues (1990) studied a sample of 589 employees enrolled in six employer-sponsored health-promotion programs. Employees who believed that they exerted greater control over their health were far more likely to stick with wellness programs than were employees who felt less responsible for their well-being. In a similar vein, patients in medical and clinical settings who are well informed prior to stressful procedures experience less stress. Results such as these indicate that the opportunity to control aversive events plays a crucial role in determining a person's response to a stressful situation.

Personal Control and Biological Effects

While our sense of control or self-efficacy affects the behavioral responses that influence our health, it also plays a role in how the biological processes

■ **regulatory control** the various ways in which people modulate their thinking, emotions, and behavior over time and across changing circumstances

activated by stressors will or will not alter our health. Recall from Chapter 4 that stressful situations activate several biological events. The degree to which our bodies' systems are activated depends on our sense of control. For example, in response to stress, the autonomic nervous system (ANS) increases heart rate, slows digestion, dilates arteries, and cools us with perspiration. People with a strong sense of self-efficacy can experience stressors with minimal arousal by the ANS and thus not risk damage to their health.

Our sense of control over a stressor also affects the release of cortico-steroids—the endocrine hormones released by the adrenal cortex that mobilize the body's fight-or-flight response. When a stressor is uncontrollable or inescapable—or when we perceive we have no control over it—our body releases more corticosteroids than when the stressor can be avoided or terminated (Swenson & Vogel, 1983).

The perception of control affects yet another endocrine response during stressful moments. When we believe we have no control over a stressor, pain-relieving beta-endorphins are released by the brain and various immune cells throughout the body. In one laboratory study, college students subjected to mild inescapable electric shocks experienced endorphin-based pain relief; those subjected to escapable shocks experienced no such relief (Jackson, Maier, & Coon, 1979).

Last but not least, the perception of control has an impact on the immune system. A weak sense of control tends to impair the functioning of the immune system sufficiently to increase a person's susceptibility to bacterial and viral infection and accelerates the rate of progression of disease (Schneiderman, McCabe, & Baum, 1992). In contrast, stress that is aroused while a person is gaining a sense of mastery over a threatening situation can actually enhance immune functioning (Bandura, 1992).

Regulatory Control

Have you ever been so angry with a rude driver that you felt like exploding, yet you didn't? Or perhaps you've been at a religious service when you found something hysterically funny but needed to stifle your laughter? In such situations, you strive to control which emotions are experienced and which are expressed. **Regulatory control,** which refers to the capacity of people to modulate their thoughts, emotions, and behaviors, is an everyday occurrence. In fact, nine out of ten college students report making an effort to control their emotions at least once a day (Gross, 1998).

Controlling your responses and emotions has broad implications for many aspects of your health. On the positive side, self-regulation is associated with success in dieting (Herman & Polivy, 1980), quitting smoking (Russell, 1971), and maintaining good interpersonal relationships (Kelly & Conley, 1987). In addition, children who have good self-control are calmer, more resistant to frustration, better able to delay gratification (an important factor in later resisting substance abuse), and less aggressive (Muraven, Tice, & Baumeister, 1998). Conversely, undercontrolled people are more likely to become aggressive (Baumeister, 1997), experience depression (Wenzlaff, Wegner, & Roper, 1988), and dwell obsessively on self-defeating thoughts (Martin & Tesser, 1989).

Exercising too much self-control, however, may adversely affect health, especially if control over negative emotions that are allowed to fester inside is too tight. This idea is not a new one, having been a cornerstone of the psychosomatic movement of the 1930s (see Chapter 1). People who chronically inhibit their sadness or anger, for example, were once believed to be more susceptible to respiratory disorders such as asthma and cardiovascular disorders such as hypertension (Alexander, 1939). Although many of the alleged associations between tight control of specific emotions and illnesses have not withstood the scrutiny of contemporary research, some have, such as that between chronic hostility and cardiovascular disease (Steptoe, Fieldman, & Evans, 1993).

Individual differences in regulatory control are related to individual differences in how people cope with stressful events and experiences. People with good self-control are less likely to resort to maladaptive coping responses such as angry venting of emotions and avoidant coping (Aronoff, Stollak, & Woike, 1994). Similarly, children with good regulatory control are reported by their mothers to be likely to use constructive, problem-focused coping responses and unlikely to use avoidant or aggressive coping responses in stressful situations (Fabes, Eisenberg, Karbon, Troyer, & Switzer, 1994).

Vagal Tone and Regulatory Control Because of the relationship between self-control and physical arousal, researchers are exploring the use of heart rate and other physiological markers to identify individual differences in how people cope with stress (Fabes & Eisenberg, 1997; Gross, 1998). One such marker is *vagal tone,* which, broadly defined, is a measure of the changes in heart rate that occur during social and emotional responses.

How does it work? Most changes in heart rate, such as those that occur in response to challenging physical and emotional demands, are controlled by the vagus cranial nerve (Porges, Doussard-Roosevelt, & Maiti, 1994). When a healthy person inhales, the vagus nerve becomes less active, increasing heart rate; when he or she exhales, vagal activity increases and heart rate decreases. In response to stress, for example, the autonomic nervous system speeds heart rate (to meet the metabolic demands of the body's emergency response system) by decreasing vagal action on the heart.

Vagal tone is thus a measure of the relationship between the rhythmic increases and decreases in heart rate associated with breathing in and breathing out. High vagal tone, measured as greater variability in heart rate as a person

Figure 5.5

Vagal Tone and Coping with Stress
(a) Students with high vagal tone were less likely than students with lower vagal tone to experience high levels of negative emotional arousal in response to everyday hassles and stress. (b) They were also more likely to rely on constructive coping measures.

Source: "Regulatory Control and Adults' Stress-Related Responses to Daily Life Events," by R. A. Fabes and N. Eisenberg, 1997, *Journal of Personality and Social Psychology, 73*(5), pp. 1107–1117. Copyright 1997 by the American Psychological Association. Adapted with permission.

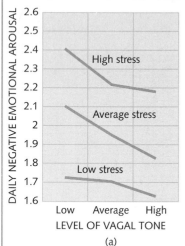

(a)

> High vagal tone is inversely related to negative emotional arousal and positively related to constructive coping.

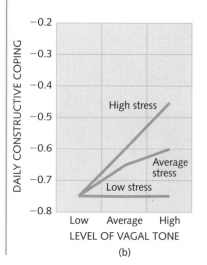

(b)

breathes in and out, reflects greater regulatory control by the vagus nerve. In contrast, low vagal tone (measured as a more stable heart rate pattern) reflects weaker regulatory control.

Many researchers believe that these differences in regulatory control influence how effectively people cope with stress. When a person is faced with stress, high vagal tone (regulatory control) dampens the intensity of any negative emotions that are aroused and leads to more adaptive coping responses.

Richard Fabes and Nancy Eisenberg (1997) have investigated the relationship among vagal tone, daily stress, and coping responses in college students. Vagal tone was computed from the students' electrocardiograph responses during a brief meditation film depicting dolphins swimming to a soundtrack of calm music. Daily stress levels were monitored with a diary kept by the students over a 2-week period. For each entry, the student would describe the most stressful experience over the past 24 hours, then rate the degree to which they felt or responded to the stress (on a scale from 0 = not at all to 3 = a lot). Students also rated the degree to which they used each of 13 different coping responses (using the same 4-point scale). The coping responses included both constructive strategies (active coping, seeking social support, positive reinterpretation, emotion-focused coping) and maladaptive strategies (psychological and physical distancing, venting of emotion, alcohol/drug use).

As Figure 5.5 shows, students with high vagal tone were less likely than students with lower vagal tone to experience high levels of negative emotional arousal in response to everyday hassles and stress. They were also more likely to rely on constructive coping measures.

The lesson to be learned: Regulatory control, when too tight or too loose, may adversely affect physical health. Just how this happens is currently a subject of intense research, but many experts believe that faulty self-control leads to abnormal physiological responses that, over time, take a toll on health (Gross, 1998; Krantz & Manuck, 1984). Emotional suppression, for example, has been shown to activate the sympathetic division of the autonomic nervous system, functioning much like a stressor in triggering the fight-or-flight response (Gross & Levenson, 1997).

Repressive Coping Sometimes we are not aware that we are controlling our emotions. In laboratory studies of stress some individuals will report feeling relaxed while performing challenging tasks, but physiologically and behaviorally, they show signs of significant stress, such as slower reaction times, increased muscle tension, and rapid heart rate. This extreme form of regulatory control—in which there is a discrepancy between verbal and physiological measures of stress—is called **repressive coping** (Weinberger, Schwartz, & Davidson, 1979). Using this emotion-focused coping style, *repressors* attempt to inhibit their emotional responses so they can view themselves as emotionally imperturbable. Newton and Contrada (1992) found that repressors displayed the greatest discrepancy between self-report and physiological measures of anxiety when their behavior was being observed. This suggests that repression is most likely to occur in a social context.

Is repression healthy? Accumulating evidence suggests not. Recent studies have found that disclosure of stressful experiences is not only healthy but can also enhance health (Cameron & Nicholls, 1998). Researchers have demonstrated that keeping a daily journal of thoughts and feelings can reduce health clinic visits, improve immune functioning, decrease absenteeism, and even improve grade-point averages among college students (Pennebaker & Francis, 1996; Petrie, Booth, & Davison, 1995).

Learned Helplessness

What happens when you have no control over a stressful event or situation? To find out, Martin Seligman strapped dogs into harnesses and delivered repeated, unavoidable electric shocks (Seligman & Maier, 1967). Then, he removed the harnesses and put the dogs in a different test situation, one in which they could escape the punishing shocks. Remarkably, the dogs did nothing but passively cower in the corner of the test apparatus. Seligman called the resigned, passive behavior **learned helplessness.**

Additional studies by Seligman and others have demonstrated that humans, when faced with repeated uncontrollable stress, may also learn that they cannot affect what happens to them. In concentration camps, prisons, even in factories and nursing homes, people who repeatedly fail at a goal often stop trying. Even more important, they often also are unresponsive in other environments where success is more likely. For example, college students were faced with uncontrollable stress in the form of repeated bursts of noise (Krantz, Glass, & Snyder, 1974). Later, when they could control the noise, they made only the feeblest attempts to do so.

Elderly people living in long-term care or nursing home facilities, as well as those suffering from chronic illnesses, are particularly vulnerable to learned helplessness. Unwittingly, the well-intentioned staff of many nursing homes (as well as those who provide care in a home setting) encourage passive, helpless behavior in the elderly and chronically ill by denying them the responsibility for

repressive coping an emotion-focused coping style in which people attempt to inhibit their emotional responses, especially in social situations, so they can view themselves as imperturbable

learned helplessness the passive, hopeless resignation of a person or animal in the face of persistent uncontrollable stress

■ **social support**
companionship from others
that conveys emotional
concern, material assistance,
or honest feedback about a
situation

even the most fundamental aspects of their care (recall the Langer and Rodin study described earlier).

Seligman believes that learned helplessness is rooted in the belief that some stressors are *noncontingent*—that is, the person can do something or nothing; it doesn't matter because the results will be the same. When a person comes to believe that the outcomes of his or her behavior are not contingent on that behavior, there are significant motivational, emotional, and behavioral consequences. People who feel helpless either do not engage in health-enhancing behaviors or they abandon those behaviors before they have time to exert a positive effect on health. Because of the link between helplessness and depression, and the link between depression and health-compromising behaviors such as substance abuse, there is even reason to believe that feelings of helplessness can be life threatening (Wallston, Wallston, Smith, & Dobbins, 1997).

Social Support

So far, we have focused on a person's *internal* resources for dealing with stress. These resources—psychological hardiness, optimism, and personal control—certainly play important roles in our response to stress. Another important factor—an external factor—is the degree of social support we receive. Social ties and relationships with other people powerfully influence us, in both positive and negative ways.

Social support is companionship from others that conveys emotional concern, material assistance, or honest feedback about a situation. In stressful situations, people who perceive a high level of social support may experience less stress and may cope more effectively.

A study of residents near the site of the Three Mile Island nuclear accident in 1978 revealed that people who perceived a high level of social support felt less stress than those with fewer sources of social support. They also reported significantly fewer stress-related physical symptoms such as headaches, nausea, and shortness of breath (Fleming, Baum, Gisriel, & Gatchel, 1982).

While you may not live by a nuclear power plant, at one time or another you will experience some kind of illness. At such times, social support becomes important to your wellness in several respects:

1. *Faster recovery and fewer medical complications:* Social support has been associated with better adjustment to and/or faster recovery from coronary artery surgery, rheumatoid arthritis, childhood leukemia, and stroke (Magni, Silvestro, Tamiello, Zanesco, & Carl, 1988). In addition, women with strong social ties have fewer complications during childbirth (Collins, Dunkel-Schetter, Lobel, & Scrimshaw, 1993), and both women and men with high levels of social support are less likely to suffer heart attacks (Holahan, Holahan, Moos, & Brennan, 1997).

2. *Lower mortality rates:* Peter Williams and colleagues (1992) studied coronary artery disease patients. Over a 9-year period, patients with low social support (defined as being unmarried and without a confidant) had a 50 percent survival rate as compared with 82 percent for those with the most social support. The beneficial effect of social support was independent of initial health and socioeconomic status. Similarly, another study showed that cancer patients with the fewest contacts each day were 2.2 times more likely to die of cancer over a 17-year period than were those with greater social support (Spiegel, 1996).

3. *Less distress in the face of terminal illness:* AIDS patients who perceive a strong network of social support seem to experience less depression and hopelessness than do patients lacking social support (Varni, Setoguchi, Rappaport, & Talbot, 1992).

4. *Vulnerability to illness and mortality:* Having a number of close social relationships is also associated with a lower risk of dying at any age. The classic example of this relationship comes from a survey of 7,000 adults in Alameda County, California, conducted by epidemiologists Lisa Berkman and Leonard Syme (1994). The researchers found that having a large number of social contacts enabled women to live an average of 2.8 years longer and men an average of 2.3 years longer. These benefits to longevity remained, even when health habits such as smoking, alcohol use, physical activity, obesity, and differences in socioeconomic status and health status at the beginning of the study were taken into account.

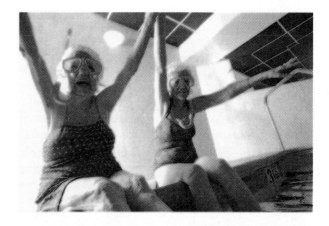

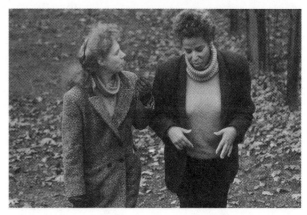

Friends Can Prevent or Eliminate Stress
Throughout our lives, friends are an important stress-busting resource. The important point is our perception of social support. If we perceive a high level, we are better able to cope with stress. Research has also found that social support is associated with faster recovery and fewer medical complications after surgery, lower mortality rates, and less distress in the face of a terminal illness. © Photex/Corbis; © Mark Antman/The Image Works

In a prospective study of mortality rates in Sweden, Kristina Orth-Gomer and her colleagues (1993) collected data on 50-year-old men, including the results of a standard physical examination, several measures of perceived social support, and the number of stressful life events during the preceding 12 months. A 7-year follow-up revealed that social support was inversely related to mortality: Participants with *high* levels of support had the *lowest* mortality rates. Moreover, the impact of low levels of social support on mortality was comparable in magnitude to that of cigarette smoking.

■ **buffering hypothesis** theory that social support produces its stress-busting effects indirectly, by helping the individual cope more effectively

■ **direct effect hypothesis** theory that social support produces its beneficial effects during both stressful and nonstressful times by enhancing the body's physical responses to challenging situations

How Social Support Makes a Difference

Clearly, the support of others can benefit our health, but how? The most common view is that social relationships act as a buffer against the effects of stress. According to the **buffering hypothesis,** social support mitigates stress indirectly, by providing resources "on the spot" to help the individual cope more effectively (Cohen & McKay, 1984; Cohen & Wills, 1985). For instance, people who perceive strong social support are less likely to ruminate in an effort to cope with stressful experiences. In general, rumination tends to be counterproductive; instead, it leads to more negative interpretations of events, triggers recall of unpleasant memories, interferes with problem solving, and reduces the ruminator's interest in participating in enjoyable activities (Lyubomirsky, Caldwell, & Nolen-Hoeksema, 1998; Lyubomirsky & Nolen-Hoeksema, 1995; Spasojevic & Alloy, 2001).

Another theory maintains that a sense of connection with other people may convey direct physical benefits not only during moments of stress but during nonstressful times as well. According to the **direct effect hypothesis,** social support produces its beneficial effects by enhancing the body's physical responses to challenging situations (Pilisuk, Boylan, & Acredolo, 1987). For example, in times of stress, the presence of others who are perceived as supportive may dampen sympathetic nervous system arousal, perhaps by reducing the release of *corticotropin-releasing hormone* from the hypothalamus.

Support for the hypothesis comes from a standard classical conditioning procedure devised by Stanford University psychologist Seymour Levine. He exposed a group of squirrel monkeys to a series of trials in which a flash of light (the conditioned stimulus) was paired with a mild electric shock (the unconditioned stimulus). As conditioning proceeded, the animals' stress reactions included a sharp rise in blood levels of the stress hormone cortisol. If a monkey was conditioned in the presence of another monkey, however, the increase in cortisol level was 50 percent less than when the monkey was alone.

In another study, researchers investigated the relationships among self-reported stress levels, the availability of social support, and circulating levels of prostate-specific antigen (PSA) in men participating in a screening program for prostate cancer (Stone, Mezzacappa, Donatone, & Gonder, 1999). Men with the highest levels of self-reported stress also had significantly higher levels of PSA—a biological marker of prostate malignancy—than their less-stressed counterparts. Although stress was positively associated with PSA levels, there was an *inverse* correlation between PSA levels and the participants' perceived level of social support, as demonstrated by their scores on the 6-item *Satisfaction with Social Contacts (SSC)* scale (see Figure 5.6). The SSC includes items such as, "How has the number of people that you feel close to changed in the past 6 months?" and "How satisfied are you with the amount of social contact you have?" Those low in social support had significantly higher PSA levels than their more socially connected counterparts.

This issue of how social support benefits health continues to be hotly debated. It may be that social support makes potentially stressful events more benign by diffusing or minimizing their initial impact. For example, having a supportive friend may make it less likely that you will interpret a low exam grade as evidence of low intelligence. Or perhaps the belief that other people care about you increases your self-esteem and gives you a more positive outlook on life. The result: greater resistance to disease and a greater chance of adopting health-enhancing habits.

Measuring the Effects of Social Support

How can researchers tell that observed effects are actually due to social support? Two major approaches have been used. In one approach, a *social integration score* is computed by adding the number of social relationships in which a person participates. This approach tallies such variables as whether a person is married, has relatives living nearby, knows his or her neighbors, belongs to a school or community organization, or is a member of a religious group (Wills, 1998).

Another approach is to measure the extent to which a person *perceives* support to be available from his or her current social network. Among the types of support measured are

- *emotional support*—the availability of friends in whom one can confide feelings and problems.

- *instrumental support*—the availability of tangible assistance in the form of finances, home repairs, child care, and transportation.

- *informational support*—the availability of advice and practical information.

- *social companionship*—the availability of persons to share recreational activities.

When researchers calculate a social integration score, they find evidence of direct physical effects of social support. When they look at the more subjective measure of *perceived* social support (such as the extent to which a patient feels that others are available to provide help), they find buffering effects.

Who Receives Social Support—and Who Benefits?

Why are some people more likely than others to receive social support? The answer is predictable: People with better social skills—who relate well to others and who are caring and giving—create stronger social networks and thus receive more social support. Some evidence comes from a study of college freshmen (Cohen, Sherrod, & Clark, 1986). Researchers categorized incoming students according to their social competence, social anxiety, and

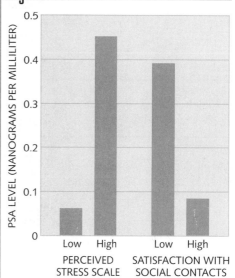

Figure 5.6

Stress, Social Support, and Prostate-Specific Antigen (PSA)
Level of prostate-specific antigen (PSA) was positively associated with stress and inversely related to the satisfaction with social contacts. Participants who perceived low levels of stress and high satisfaction with social contacts had significantly lower levels of PSA, a biological marker of prostate malignancy.

Source: "Psychosocial Stress and Social Support Are Associated with Prostate-Specific Antigen Levels in Men: Results from a Community Screening Program," by A. A. Stone, E. S. Mezzacappa, B. A. Donatone, and M. Gonder, 1999, *Health Psychology, 18*(5) p. 485.

self-disclosure skills. Over the course of the study, they discovered that students with greater social skills were the most likely to form strong social networks. These findings lend support to the idea that it may not be the availability of social support as an external resource but rather preexisting personality traits that determine the ability to structure a network of social support.

Cathleen Connell and Anthony D'Augelli (1990) have developed an explanation of how this works. According to their model, having the personality traits of affiliation (seeking others' company), succorance (receiving help), and nurturance (giving help) increases a person's social skills, their perceived social support, and the size of their social network. In support of Connell and D'Augelli's model, John Hardy and Timothy Smith (1988) found evidence that angry or hostile people tend to receive less social support than agreeable people do. Hostile people also report a greater number of daily hassles and more negative life events than those who are more approachable. Results such as these suggest an obvious health intervention: To help people increase their social support, help them learn to be friendlier and less hostile.

Social skills aside, other factors also play a role in the amount of social support you receive—and the health benefits you derive from that support. Consider the following statements:

- Women profit more from social support than men do.
- Married people live longer than single, divorced, or widowed people.
- People with close social networks are healthier and live longer.

Although the popular wisdom would say that all three statements are true, the research evidence is not clear-cut. Let's examine each one.

Some researchers believe that women profit more than men from social support, perhaps because women tend to have closer, more emotionally intimate relationships (Argyle, 1992). In fact, research has shown that *both* men and women prefer to have women as confidants (Sapadin, 1988). Relationships of this type may convey a greater health advantage than the cooler, less trusting relationships that men tend to form.

Studies have also reported a gender difference in the impact of a spouse's death. Knud Helsing and his colleagues (1981) found that widowed men died at a much higher rate than married men but that widowed women were in no more danger of death than married women. The researchers also found that widowed men who remarried lived longer than those who remained single, but once again, widowed women who remarried experienced no such advantage. Furthermore, men are more likely than women to become lonely and depressed when a spouse dies. This places them at increased risk of alcohol abuse, poor eating habits, other health-compromising behaviors, and even suicide. Such negativity may stress the immune and cardiovascular systems.

Attempting to make sense of these gender differences in the social support–health relationship, Ralf Schwarzer and Anja Leppin (1992) reasoned that the loss of a spouse places both men and women at increased risk of dying during the period of bereavement. However, because women tend to be younger than their spouses, they are less likely to die soon after their partners' passing. In addition, because women generally have a larger network of social support than do men, they are more likely to receive support when their spouses die.

So, statement 1 is mostly true. What about statement 2? Most people believe that marriage conveys protective health benefits by providing social support and that married adults live longer than those who are divorced or who never married (House, Robbins, & Metzner, 1982). Recent studies, however, have found that adults who have not married by midlife are at no greater risk of dying before 80 years of age than are married adults, particularly if they have at least one person in whom they can confide their feelings (Tucker, Friedman, Wingard, & Schwartz, 1996).

While marriage may not significantly affect longevity (as suggested by statement 2), social networks do promote longer, healthier lives, as suggested by statement 3. George Kaplan and colleagues (1988) found that unmarried Finnish men who were socially isolated were 1.5 to 2.0 times more likely to die from cardiovascular disease than those who had many social connections. Another study discovered that men and women aged 65 and older who perceived the greatest social support had the lowest levels of depression (Oxman, Berkman, Kasl, Freeman, & Barrett, 1992).

While older people often enjoy relationships with young people, they cherish their long-term friendships (Rawlins, 1995). By late adulthood, many members of a social network have been together for decades. This helps explain why older people's overall satisfaction with life is more strongly related to the quantity and quality of their contact with friends than with the quantity or quality of their contact with younger members of their own family (Ulbrich & Bradshjer, 1993). For men, such friends are equally like to be male or female; for unmarried women, the friend is nearly always female (Akiyama, Elliott, & Antonucci, 1996).

It would seem, then, that the secret to a long healthy life is to construct a large social network. But can a person be too socially connected? Can some social connections adversely affect our health?

When Social Support Is Not Helpful

Sometimes social support does not reduce stress and benefit health. In fact, it may produce opposite results. There are several reasons for this surprising fact. First, although support may be offered, a person may not *perceive* it as beneficial (Wilcox, Kasl, & Berkman, 1994). This may occur because the person does not want the assistance, thinks the assistance offered is inadequate, or is too distracted to notice that help has been offered. For example, in the first hours of coping with the loss of a loved one, a person may want only to be alone with his or her grief.

Second, the type of support offered may not be what is needed at the moment. For example, a single mother who is struggling to complete her college degree may feel stress during exam weeks. Although what she may need most is *instrumental social support,* such as assistance with child care, all that may be offered is *emotional support,* such as encouragement to study hard. Instrumental social support is especially valuable for controllable stressors, whereas emotional support is more helpful for uncontrollable stressors, such as a cataclysmic event or the loss of a loved one. In one study of young widows, for example, the stress of losing a spouse was best buffered by emotional support (particularly from their parents). Conversely, among working women with young infants the only effective buffer was instrumental support from their spouse (Lieberman, 1982). The role of social support in promoting health, then, is quite specific.

Third, too much social support may actually increase a person's stress. Perhaps you know someone who is a member of too many organizations or is overwhelmed by intrusive social and family relationships. During periods of stress, this person may feel under siege in the face of all the advice and "support" that is offered (Shumaker & Hill, 1991). The critical factor appears to be having at least one close friend to confide in and share problems with. Having five, six, or even a dozen more may convey no more—perhaps less—benefit than having one or two (Langner & Michael, 1960).

Fourth, the relationship itself may exert a negative influence on the person and make him or her more vulnerable to stress-related health problems. Arguments with friends and relatives, for example, can be especially stressful.

And finally, under some circumstances, social relationships can impair a person's health (Burg & Seeman, 1994). For example, peer group influence is especially strong during adolescence, so an adolescent may engage in health-compromising behaviors—smoking cigarettes, eating too many unhealthy foods, driving recklessly, or avoiding exercise—just to be part of the group.

Stress Management

Each of us has coping skills that we have acquired over the years. These include strategies that have worked in the past, techniques we have read about, and behaviors we have observed in other people. In most situations, these skills are probably adequate to keep us from experiencing undue stress. Sometimes, however, the demands of a situation may exceed our coping resources.

Stress management describes a variety of psychological methods designed to reduce the impact of potentially stressful experiences (Steptoe, 1997). Originally introduced in clinical settings to help patients adapt to chronic illnesses and stressful medical procedures, these techniques are now used widely. For example, occupational groups (especially health care providers, emergency services personnel, students, and teachers) and people in disadvantaged personal circumstances, such as family caregivers, single parents, the unemployed, and victims of assault or abuse, all benefit from stress-management techniques.

There are many techniques available to help people manage stress more effectively. In this section we consider exercise, relaxation, biofeedback, hypnosis, and some of the more effective cognitive therapies.

Exercise

A sedentary lifestyle has been linked to such disorders as cardiovascular disease, obesity, osteoporosis, and back problems. It is also associated with a reduced ability to cope with stress, increased risk of depression, lower work productivity, and greater absenteeism (Long & van Stavel, 1995).

In contrast, many studies demonstrate that regularly taking part in sustained moderate-level exercise can have significant health-protective benefits (Owen & Vita, 1997). The most commonly advocated type of exercise is *aerobic exercise,* such as walking, cycling, or running, which elevates the heart rate through sustained activity. *Anaerobic exercise,* such as weight lifting, on the other hand, is quick or of very high intensity and elevates the heart rate in brief bursts. Both types of exercise offer significant, but different, health benefits.

How, exactly, does exercise help us cope with stress? Two kinds of explanations have been offered: physiological and psychological.

Physiological Effects of Exercise

According to the physiological view, stress results from abnormal biochemical processes in the central nervous system. A number of researchers therefore consider regular physical activity to be *the most effective* strategy for minimizing the impact of stressful events on physiological health (Thayer, Newman, & McClain, 1994).

Exercise has a profound affect on physiology. It enhances blood flow to the brain, stimulates the autonomic nervous system, and triggers the release of a variety of hormones. For these reasons, exercise may trigger a neurophysiological "high" that produces an antidepressant effect in some people, an antianxiety effect in others, and, at the very least, an enhanced sense of well-being in most (Sacks, 1990).

In one study, researchers gave groups of runners and sedentary control subjects lists of anagrams to unscramble without telling them that the scrambled

■ **stress management** the various psychological methods designed to reduce the impact of potentially stressful experiences

People who take regular vacations are less likely to die prematurely, especially from heart disease. Bring along your pager or cell phone, however, and you won't reap the full stress-busting effects of time off—you'll be on guard for potential stress (Gump & Matthews, 2000).

"words" actually were unsolvable (Brown, 1991). After their inevitable failure at the rigged task, the subjects were informed that their sorry performance was "well below average." Not surprisingly, both groups of subjects displayed increased muscle tension, blood pressure, and self-reported anxiety in the face of the frustrating task, but the runners showed significantly smaller increases. However, it remains unclear whether the runners showed a lower stress response because they found it easier to shrug off the mild stressor or because their higher level of fitness made their cardiovascular systems stronger.

Other evidence that exercise can moderate the effects of stress and help protect against disease (especially stress-linked disorders):

- Physically fit college students report fewer stress-related health problems than less active students (Roth & Holmes, 1985).

- Regular exercise may offer protection against cancer. Examining men who regularly walk, cycle, swim, run, and play tennis, researchers have found an inverse relationship between level of physical activity and deaths from lung cancer and digestive tract cancer (Wannamethee, Shaper, & Macfarlane, 1993).

- Exercise can dampen the effect of laboratory stress—caused by trying to solve anagrams and math problems, for example—on cardiac reactivity in hypertensive subjects (Perkins, Dubbert, Martin, Faulstich, & Harris, 1986).

- Adolescents who exercise regularly are less vulnerable to the harmful effects of stressful life events (Brown, 1991; Brown & Siegel, 1988). One team of researchers measured stressful life events, amount of daily exercise, and symptoms of illness in adolescent girls between 12 and 16 years old. The analysis revealed that life stress predicted illness only in those subjects who were physically inactive. Among the physically fit girls, life stress had little relationship to illness.

- Exercise reduces blood pressure, resting heart rate, and cardiovascular reactivity, all of which tend to increase in stressful situations (Dimsdale, Alper, & Schneiderman, 1986). Gary Jennings and his colleagues (1986) collected data on 19- to 27-year-old sedentary individuals who had not exercised regularly during the preceding year. The results revealed that participants who exercised regularly reduced their resting heart rate and their blood pressure.

Psychological Effects of Exercise

According to the psychological view, like other activities such as going to a movie, reading a book, or relaxing, exercise relieves stress simply by offering a change of pace. In support of this view, some studies have found that subjects who rested in a recliner or ate lunch with friends in a pub experienced the same reduction in anxiety level as did people who exercised (Bahrke & Morgan, 1978).

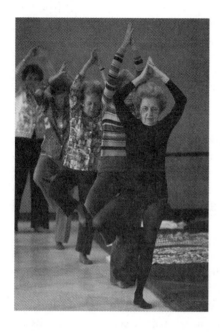 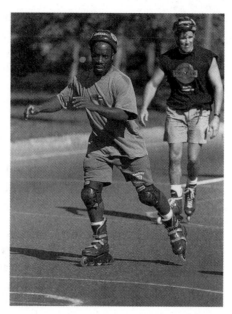

Exercise Protects against Stress and Illness
Regular exercise, whether for a half or several hours, has a profound effect on physiology, enhancing blood flow to the brain, stimulating the autonomic nervous system, and triggering the release of various hormones. All these physiological effects tend to protect the individual against illness, especially stress-related health problems. And you are never too old to exercise; just choose something appropriate to your ability—senior citizens practice yoga, while younger people prefer the challenge of in-line skating. © Ted Spiegel/Corbis; © Michael A. Dwyer/Stock Boston

Exercise may produce additional psychological benefits because it helps people to feel better about their appearance. Nancy Norvell and Dale Belles (1993) assigned one-half of a group of law enforcement officers to a weight-training program and one-half to a nonexercising control group. Over the four months of the study, participants in the weight-training group reported significantly lower levels of anxiety. The researchers concluded that improved body appearance as well as the time out from stressful work accounted for the results of their study.

Exercise and Depression Depression, perhaps the most common of psychological disorders, may be particularly responsive to exercise. A growing body of research suggests that physically active people have lower rates of anxiety and depression than sedentary people (Statistics Canada, 1999). Consider a classic study in which Lisa McCann and David Holmes (1984) randomly assigned one-third of a group of mildly depressed female college students to an aerobic exercise program, another third to a program of relaxation exercises, and the final third to a no-treatment condition (the control group). Ten weeks later, the subjects in the exercise group reported the largest decrease in depression.

Norepinephrine and serotonin, two neurotransmitters that increase arousal and boost mood, are low in depressed people. Aerobic exercise such as running may counteract depression in part by increasing the serotonin activity in the brain and thus replacing depression's state of low arousal. In this manner, running does naturally what antidepressant drugs such as Prozac, Zoloft, and Paxil do (Jacobs, 1994).

Aerobic exercise can also be an effective adjunct to counseling or other forms of psychotherapy in decreasing anxiety, improving self-esteem, and reducing depression (Hinkle, 1992). In one study, depressed subjects were randomly assigned to a running therapy group, a traditional group psychotherapy program, or a relaxation-training group. Those in the running therapy group received no other form of treatment (they were even forbidden to discuss their depression during the study). During the clinical trial, running therapy patients ran with a group leader in small groups for 1 hour three to four times a week. After 12 weeks, all the subjects reported lower levels of depression. However, 3 months later, only the running and relaxation groups continued to show improvement in their psychological well-being. Patients who had received traditional psychotherapy actually showed some regression toward higher levels of depression.

Interestingly, the type of exercise seems in part to determine its benefits. In one study, researchers induced a depression-like state of reduced activity level and impaired sex drive in rats by administering the drug clomipramine (Dunn, Reigle, Youngstedt, Armstrong, & Dishman, 1996). They then allowed one group of the drugged rats 24-hour voluntary access to an activity wheel for 12 weeks. A second group of drugged animals was forced to run on a treadmill for 1 hour each day, 6 days a week, for 12 weeks. A third group was given the antidepressant drug imipramine for the last 6 days of the 12-week experiment. A fourth, control group received no treatment whatsoever—no medication and no exercise—for the duration of the experiment. The rats that received imipramine showed increased brain concentrations of both norepinephrine and serotonin—classic signs that the antidepressant drug was counteracting the drug-induced state of depression. The two exercise groups also showed increases in both neurotransmitters. But only the rats in the voluntary exercise group also displayed increased behavioral and sexual activity, the *behavioral* measures the researchers used to rate depression.

Other studies with human subjects have found that significant reductions in tension, anxiety, and stress are more likely to occur following exercise in which the subjects exercised at 60 to 80 percent of their *VO2 max*—a measure of the maximum rate at which oxygen can be utilized by a person's body (Farrell, Gates, Maksud, & Morgan, 1982). This finding is intriguing, since athletes, personal trainers, and exercise physiologists know that in order to receive aerobic benefit from exercise, it is necessary for the participant to exercise at this intensity; otherwise, little, if any, cardiorespiratory benefits are derived.

Research studies such as these imply that simply "prescribing" exercise may not guarantee improved psychological health. Although the forced-exercise treadmill rats in the study described earlier exercised more than the voluntary-exercise activity-wheel rats, the wheel runners displayed the greatest behavioral benefits, indicating that fitness may only be part of the reason that exercise improves mental health in people. The ultimate benefits of exercise are probably the result of a combination of biological, psychological, and social factors. And although *any* physical activity is better than none, to derive the greatest benefit—both physically and psychologically—you probably need to exert yourself somewhat.

Relaxation Therapies

Perhaps the simplest psychological interventions are the relaxation training therapies. These include progressive muscle training, the relaxation response (meditation), and autogenic training (Lehrer, Carr, Sargunaraj, & Woolfolk, 1994).

Although relaxation techniques have been used since antiquity, modern use is usually traced to Edmond Jacobson (1938), whose **progressive muscle relaxation** technique forms the cornerstone for many modern relaxation procedures. In progressive relaxation, individuals are instructed first to tense a particular muscle (such as the forehead) and to hold this tension for about 10 seconds. They are then instructed to slowly release the tension, focusing on the soothing feeling as the tension drains away. Finally, they are told to first tense, then relax other major muscle groups, including the mouth, eyes, neck, arms, shoulders, thighs, stomach, calves, feet, and toes. After practicing the relaxation technique for several weeks, the individuals are urged to identify the particular spots in their bodies that tense up during moments of stress, such as the jaw or fists. As they become more aware of these reactions, they can learn to relax these muscles at will.

In another training technique, the **relaxation response,** subjects assume a meditative state (as described below) in which metabolism slows and blood pressure lowers. Cardiologist Herbert Benson became intrigued with the possibility that meditation might be an antidote to stress when he found that experienced meditators could lower their heart rate, blood lactate level (a byproduct of physical exercise that creates the "burn" of muscular exertion), blood pressure, and oxygen consumption (Benson, 1996). Benson identified four requirements for achieving the relaxation response:

- A quiet place in which distractions and external stimulation are minimized.
- A comfortable position such as sitting in an easy chair.
- A mental device such as focusing your attention on a single thought or word and repeating it over and over.
- A passive attitude.

■ **progressive muscle relaxation** a form of relaxation training that reduces muscle tension through a series of tensing and relaxing exercises involving the body's major muscle groups

■ **relaxation response** a meditative state of relaxation in which metabolism slows and blood pressure lowers

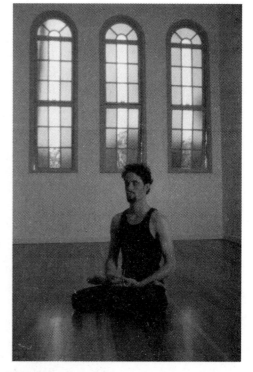

Meditation
Many people find meditation to be an effective technique for managing stress. According to research by Herbert Benson, experienced meditators can lower their heart rate, blood lactate level, blood pressure, and oxygen consumption, and so reduce or even eliminate the effects of stress. However, other studies have not shown that meditation reliably achieves these results.
© Bruce Burkhardt/Corbis

■ **autogenic training** a relaxation-promoting form of self-hypnosis involving a series of exercises that induce feelings of heaviness and warmth in the body's limbs

■ **biofeedback** a system that provides audible or visible feedback information regarding involuntary physiological states

Another relaxation technique is **autogenic training (AT).** This technique, developed in the 1930s by the German physician Johannes H. Schulz, has been used extensively in Europe but less in North America. A form of self-hypnosis, AT consists of a series of exercises in six hierarchical stages that induce feelings of heaviness and warmth in the body's limbs.

The person uses verbal triggers such as, "My left arm feels heavy," "My left arm is warm and relaxed," "My heartbeat is slow and steady," "My breathing is deep, even, and relaxed," and "My forehead is cool" to create the desired feelings in parts of the body, and eventually to relax those parts. Autogenic training usually takes several months of daily, 30- to 60-minute practice sessions to master (Weinberg & Gould, 1995).

There is now considerable evidence that progressive muscle relaxation training and autogenic training can help patients cope with a variety of stress-related problems, including hypertension, tension headaches, depression, lower back pain, adjustment to chemotherapy, and anxiety (Carlson & Hoyle, 1993; Hermann, Kim, & Blanchard, 1995; Lehrer, Carr, Sargunaraj, & Woolfolk, 1994). Underlying the effectiveness of these techniques is their ability to reduce heart rate, muscle tension, and blood pressure, as well as self-reported tension and anxiety (English & Baker, 1983). Moreover, these techniques have generally been found to be more effective than placebos in reducing pain and alleviating stress.

To date, there have been few studies evaluating the effectiveness of the relaxation response or other forms of meditation in helping people cope with stress. Those studies have, however, reported that meditative relaxation is effective in helping people cope with work site stress (Murphy, 1996) and anxiety (Miller, Fletcher, & Kabat-Zinn, 1995). Still, although popular belief holds that during meditation people experience unique physiological states of profound rest, several quasi-experimental studies have shown that meditation is not reliably linked with differences in heart rate, brain wave activity, body metabolism, breathing rate, or blood pressure (Holmes, 1984; Lichstein, 1988).

Biofeedback

Biofeedback is a technique for converting certain supposedly involuntary physiological responses—such as skin temperature, muscle activity, heart rate, and blood pressure—into electrical signals and providing visual or auditory feedback about them. It is based on the principle that we learn to perform a specific response when we receive information (feedback) about the consequences of that response and then make appropriate adjustments (Gatchel, 1997).

Using an electronic monitoring device that detects and amplifies internal responses, biofeedback training begins by helping the person gain awareness of the maladaptive response. Next, the person focuses attention on a tone, light, or some other signal that identifies desirable changes in the internal response. By attempting to control this biofeedback signal, the patient learns to control his or her physiological state. Finally, the individual learns to transfer control from the laboratory setting to everyday life.

David Shapiro and colleagues (1969) were the first to show that humans could control their blood pressure via biofeedback. The amount their participants could lower their systolic blood pressure during a single session was small, however, typically averaging only 5 mm Hg. Today, with more sophisticated equipment and better training, many people are able to achieve even greater success using biofeedback to lower their blood pressure.

The most common biofeedback technique in clinical use is *electromyography (EMG) feedback*. EMG biofeedback detects skeletal muscle activity by measuring muscle tension via the electrical discharge of muscle fibers. Electrodes are attached to the skin over the muscles to be monitored. The biofeedback machine responds with an auditory signal that reflects the electrical activity (tension) of the muscle being measured. EMG biofeedback to decrease muscle tension has been used to treat facial tics, spasmodic movements, and other muscular disorders. It has also been used to treat headaches and lower back pain.

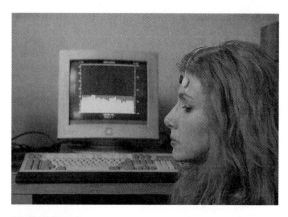

Biofeedback
Biofeedback has been firmly established as a viable means of treating a variety of anxiety and stress-related disorders in some people. Using computerized imaging, the person affects physiological functions using visual/sound feedback. Although biofeedback does seem to enable control of internal functions, evidence to date suggests that it conveys no advantage over other, less expensive relaxation techniques. © Leonard Lessin/Peter Arnold, Inc.

Another common technique, *thermal biofeedback,* is based on the principle that skin temperature tends to vary in relation to a person's perceived level of stress. The rationale for this technique is that high stress, which often causes blood vessels in the skin to constrict, may be linked with cooler surface skin temperatures. Accordingly, by placing a temperature-sensitive instrument on the skin's surface (most often the fingertips), people sometimes are able to raise their skin temperature by monitoring an auditory or visual feedback signal (Sedlacek & Taub, 1996). Thermal biofeedback is often used to help people cope with stress and pain, such as that associated with *Raynaud's disease,* a cardiovascular disorder in which the fingers and toes suffer from a cold, numb aching due to severely reduced circulation. Thermal biofeedback is also frequently used with migraine and tension headache patients (Compas, Haaga, Keefe, Leitenberg, & Williams, 1998).

How Effective Is Biofeedback?

Biofeedback has proved to be somewhat beneficial in treating stress-related health problems in some people. For example, one early study reported that patients suffering from chronic tension headaches who were given biofeedback regarding muscle tension in their foreheads later reported fewer headaches than control subjects (Budzynski, Stoyva, Adler, & Mullaney, 1973). Most impressive of all was that the subjects continued to report fewer headaches 3 months following the intervention.

Some researchers have suggested that biofeedback may be more effective with children than with adults, perhaps because children tend to be more enthusiastic about gadgetry, less skeptical about trying out new procedures, and more likely than adults to keep up their training at home (Andrasik & Attanasio, 1985). In fact, many children approach a biofeedback session much like a game, an attitude that in itself helps them to relax and achieve positive results.

Despite some promising results, several important questions remain as to how medically effective biofeedback actually is. To date, there have been relatively few well-controlled clinical outcome trials using large numbers of patients who have confirmed medical conditions (Gatchel, 1997). Two limitations have emerged in clinical evaluations of biofeedback (Steptoe, 1997). First, people often cannot generalize the training they receive in clinical settings to everyday situations. Second, research has not successfully confirmed that biofeedback itself enables people to control their internal, involuntary responses. Even when biofeedback is effective, it is not clear why, which raises the possibility that relaxation, suggestion, an enhanced sense of control, or even a placebo effect may be operating (Gatchel, 1997; Turk, Meichenbaum, & Berman, 1979).

Similar mixed findings have been obtained from the few available studies on the use of biofeedback in treating other maladies, such as lower back pain and hypertension. For instance, although biofeedback alone may be no more effective than a drug placebo in treating lower back pain (Bush, Ditto, & Feuerstein, 1985), when biofeedback is combined with cognitive-behavioral therapy, it may convey some advantages (Flor & Birbaumer, 1993). And although psychologists have reported some success in using biofeedback to treat patients with mild hypertension (Nakao et al., 1997; Paran, Amir, & Yaniv, 1996), the effect apparently is short-lived, disappearing after only a few months (McGrady, 1994).

Equally troubling for advocates of biofeedback therapy is the finding that patients with lower back pain or migraine and tension headaches typically report less pain over time, *even without any form of treatment* (Bush et al., 1985). Although this finding seriously undermines the credibility of those who claim that biofeedback is causally linked with improved health, it partially explains why testimonials regarding biofeedback's effectiveness abound. Because people with moderate pain are likely to improve anyway, any form of treatment that they tried in the interim may, as a result of coincidence, seem effective. We'll explore this issue further in Chapter 14, when we take up the topic of alternative medicine.

After reviewing a number of studies, Paul Lehrer and colleagues (1994) concluded that although biofeedback can help reduce autonomic arousal, it conveys no advantage over other behavioral techniques (such as simple relaxation training), which are easier and less expensive to use. In short, the positive effects of biofeedback are more general than its pioneers had originally believed and may be the result of enhanced relaxation, a placebo effect, the passage of time, or suggestion, rather than direct control of the physical underpinnings of stress.

Although results from biofeedback studies are mixed, and it remains unclear how control occurs, the method has been firmly established as a viable means of treating anxiety and stress-related disorders in *some* people. So what is the bottom line for those seeking relief from stress and pain? To date, research studies suggest that biofeedback alone is probably not a wise choice for treating migraine or tension headaches, lower back pain, or high blood pressure.

Hypnosis

Hypnosis is a psychological state that results from a social interaction in which one person (the hypnotist) suggests to another (the hypnotized person) that certain thoughts, feelings, perceptions, or behaviors will occur. To some extent, nearly everyone is suggestible—and can be hypnotized—although there are vast individual differences in this trait. For example, the most hypnotizable people tend to be those who can engage freely in fantasy (Kihlstrom, 1985). Also, suggestibility seems to change with age. It is greatest in children between the ages of 7 and 14, then declines during adolescence and remains stable throughout adulthood (Place, 1984).

Hypnosis has been used for a variety of purposes, from overcoming fear of exams or public speaking to treating self-maladaptive behaviors such as overeating to helping people with chronic diseases such as stabilizing blood sugar levels in diabetics. The benefits include reduction of anxiety and fear, increased comfort during difficult medical procedures, and more stable autonomic processes such as blood pressure (Olness, 1993). For example, a clinician may use a *posthypnotic suggestion*—suggesting a behavior to be carried out after the hypnosis session has ended—such as, "Each and every time you put a cigarette to your lips, you will immediately experience a terrible taste in your mouth."

Posthypnotic suggestions have also been shown to help treat asthma and stress-related disorders of the skin and headaches, but when applied to problems in self-control such as cigarette smoking, the most suggestible people show no greater benefit than do those who are less suggestible. A major review of outcome studies of hypnosis drew a distinction between "self-initiated"

■ **hypnosis** a social interaction in which one person (the hypnotist) suggests to another that certain thoughts, feelings, perceptions, or behaviors will occur

dissociation a division in consciousness that presumably allows some thoughts and behaviors to occur simultaneously with others

problems such as overeating, smoking, and alcoholism and "nonvoluntary" problems such as warts, asthma, and clinical pain. The researchers concluded that the effects of hypnosis for self-initiated problems are largely nonspecific and placebo based (Wadden & Anderton, 1982). This finding suggests that the benefits of the treatment are not due to hypnosis per se (Bowers & LeBaron, 1986).

Is Hypnosis Effective?

Those who study hypnosis are frequently frustrated by its persistent myths—for example, that hypnosis can improve recall of forgotten events. In fact, hypnosis is often unpredictable and as likely to contaminate memory with false recollections as it is to trigger real ones (Barnier & McConkey, 1992). Controlled research studies of the therapeutic effects of hypnosis have shown that its benefits often are no greater than other techniques that merely promote relaxation. For example, Spanos (1991) found that hypnosis can accelerate the disappearance of warts but no more effectively than when the same suggestions were given to subjects who are awake but relaxed. Hypnosis can be effective in stress management, but it does not appear to be any more effective than other techniques that merely promote relaxation.

On the other hand, hypnosis does appear to be more powerful than a placebo in helping people cope with pain and other stress-related problems (Jacobs, Kurtz, & Strube, 1995). However, this effectiveness varies with the hypnotic suggestibility of the patient. For people who are low in hypnotizability, hypnotic suggestions of analgesia are no more effective than drug placebos (Miller, Barabasz, & Barabasz, 1991). For people who are easily hypnotized, hypnotherapy can be an effective intervention for migraine and tension headaches (ter-Kuile et al., 1994), the anxiety of cancer treatment (Genuis, 1995), and the pain and stress of childbirth (Mairs, 1995).

Some authorities, such as Ernest Hilgard (1992) and Joseph Barber (1996), believe that hypnosis is an altered state of consciousness in which there is a division or **dissociation** in the person's consciousness. This split in consciousness presumably allows some thoughts and behaviors to occur simultaneously with others. According to this theory, hypnosis is an effective therapy for stress-related conditions such as pain because it separates the *sensation* of pain (of which the subject is still aware) from its *emotional* suffering.

In one study, Hilgard (1965) found that for a small percentage of highly suggestible subjects, hypnosis could completely eliminate the pain of placing one's arm in a bowl of icy water. In pain elimination, however, it is not hypnosis alone but the suggestion that no pain (analgesia) will be felt that is crucial. People hypnotized without a suggestion of analgesia reported almost as much pain as did unhypnotized control subjects (Miller, Barabasz, & Barabasz, 1991). In laboratory pain studies, hypnosis with a suggestion of analgesia is also superior to nonhypnotic suggestions of analgesia (Jacobs, Kurtz, & Strube,

1995) or acupuncture (Moret, Forster, Laverriere, & Lambert, 1991). For people who are not *highly suggestible,* then, hypnotic analgesia is no more effective than a placebo medication (Orne, 1980). But highly suggestible people do experience substantially greater hypnotic analgesia than with a placebo. This intriguing finding suggests that for highly suggestible people the hypnotic state is not merely a placebo effect.

Skeptics note that these and other behaviors induced through hypnosis can also be induced without it, suggesting that hypnotic phenomena merely reflect a state of heightened deep concentration or relaxation (Spanos & Coe, 1992) or that hypnosis is merely a form of highly focused attention, as when an injured athlete, caught up in the heat of competition, ignores excruciating pain until after the game is over. It also seems that the hypnotic state can be triggered while a person reads a book, listens to music, or even watches television (Olness, 1993).

Other skeptics, such as Theodore Barber (1977), view hypnosis as a social phenomenon in which imaginative people are merely acting out the role of "good hypnotic subjects." Advocates of this **social influence theory** maintain that hypnosis is not a unique physiological state and that hypnotic phenomena are merely an extension of everyday behavior (Spanos, 1994, 1996).

Cognitive Therapies

Cognitive therapy is based on the view that our way of thinking about the environment, rather than the environment itself, determines our stress level. If thinking can be changed, stress can be reduced. There are a variety of interventions that use cognitive strategies, including distraction, calming self-statements, and cognitive restructuring. In distraction procedures, people learn to direct their attention away from unpleasant or stressful events. Use of pleasant imagery (also called visualization), counting aloud, and focusing attention on relaxing stimuli (such as a favorite drawing, photograph, or song) are examples of distraction.

Individuals can also be taught to silently or softly make calming, relaxing, and reassuring self-talk statements that emphasize the temporary nature of a stressor ("Let it go, that rude driver won't get to me"), are aimed at reducing autonomic arousal ("Stay calm now, breathe deeply and count to 10"), or are directed at preserving a sense of personal control ("I can handle this").

Cognitive restructuring is a generic term that describes a variety of psychological interventions directed at replacing maladaptive, self-defeating thoughts with healthier adaptive ones. These interventions are aimed at breaking the vicious cycle of negative thinking (the negative stress cycle described earlier in this chapter), which distorts perception of everyday events and prevents adaptive coping behaviors (Belar & Deardorff, 1996). Typical forms of treatment involve teaching clients to reinterpret their thoughts in a

social influence theory the idea that hypnosis is a social phenomenon in which a highly suggestible person merely acts out a role

cognitive therapy the category of treatments that teach people healthier ways of thinking

■ **rational-emotive therapy** a confrontational form of cognitive therapy, developed by Albert Ellis, which challenges people's irrational ideas and attitudes

less negative way and to raise their awareness of distorted and maladaptive thinking.

This reciprocal relationship between maladaptive thinking and behavior is well documented. For example, focusing on a negative experience at work can affect your mood and lead to a tension headache. Having a tension headache can alter your mood, which can, in turn, affect your thoughts.

Rational-Emotive Therapy

One of the first and most effective forms of cognitive restructuring, **rational-emotive therapy (RET),** was developed by Albert Ellis (1962). RET is based on the premise that stress appraisal processes, such as we examined in Chapter 4, become dysfunctional when people engage in irrational thinking. There are many examples of irrational thinking, including *catastrophizing,* which occurs when an unpleasant event that might be perceived as a minor inconvenience is psychologically blown out of proportion into a global disaster from which the individual may never recover. Other examples are the tendency to expect negative events at every turn ("I just know something awful is about to happen to me"), to underestimate one's ability to cope with stressful events ("I can't live if she dumps me"), and to tie one's sense of self-worth to performance on a particular task ("I am worthless if I don't get an 'A' in this class"). Other examples of this type of maladaptive thinking can be found in the Reality Check presented earlier in this chapter.

A considerable amount of research has demonstrated that a tendency to engage in this type of irrational thinking is hazardous to health. For instance, Christopher Peterson and his colleagues analyzed the relationship between explanatory style and mortality among participants in the Terman Life Cycle Study, a longitudinal study of men and women born around 1910 and followed from the 1920s to the present. The participants completed a variety of open-ended questionnaires in 1936 and 1940, including ones that tapped their explanatory style. Catastrophizing (attributing unpleasant events to global causes) strongly predicted mortality, especially among men, and especially deaths due to accidental causes and violence (Peterson, Seligman, Yurko, Martin, & Friedman, 1998).

Once irrational beliefs and thought processes are identified, the rational-emotive therapist can attack them and challenge the person to restructure them into more rational, adaptive thought patterns such as, "If I do poorly on this test, it's not the end of the world. I'll just have to study harder next time," or "My grade in this class doesn't reflect my worth as a person," or "Just because she dumped me, it doesn't mean that I'm unlovable."

Thus, Ellis believes people can learn to deal rationally with their problems, use logic to analyze their belief systems, and minimize the impact of unpleasant situations. Escaping a stressor may not always be possible, but learning to manage the situation—especially one's emotional response—is possible.

Stress Inoculation Training

In a different approach to stress, **stress inoculation training** begins by teaching people to confront stressful events with a variety of coping strategies that can be used before the events become overwhelming. In this way, individuals are able to "inoculate" themselves against the potentially harmful effects of stress (Meichenbaum, 1985). Many stress inoculation programs offer an array of techniques, so that the person can choose those skills that work best for him or her.

Stress inoculation training is a three-stage process, with the therapist using a weakened dose of a stressor in an attempt to build immunity against the full-blown stressor.

■ Stage 1: *Reconceptualization.* Patients reconceptualize the source of their stress. Consider the example of a person agonizing over an upcoming medical procedure, such as a prostate exam. During the first stage of stress inoculation training, the individual would learn that his discomfort is at least partially the result of psychological factors, such as dwelling on how much the procedure is going to hurt. Once the individual has been convinced that some of his pain is psychological in nature, he is then more likely to accept that cognitive-behavior therapy can offer some relief.

■ Stage 2: *Skills acquisition.* The patient is taught relaxation and controlled breathing skills. The logic is inescapable: Being relaxed is incompatible with being tense and physically aroused. Therefore, learning to relax at will is a valuable tool in managing pain. Other techniques that may be taught include the use of pleasant mental imagery, dissociation, or humor.

■ Stage 3: *Follow-through.* The patient learns to use coping skills in everyday life. At this time, patients are also encouraged to increase their physical activity and to take medication on the basis of a timed daily schedule (rather than whenever they feel pain). Other family members are taught ways of reinforcing healthy behaviors in their loved one.

By itself, stress inoculation training has proved to be effective in helping people cope with a variety of stress-related problems, including hypertension (Amigo, Buceta, Becona, & Bueno, 1991), test anxiety (Schneider & Nevid, 1993), anger, anxiety, and depression (Wilcox & Dowrick, 1992). In combination with other techniques, such as progressive muscle relaxation, cognitive restructuring, and biofeedback, stress inoculation has proved to be an effective stress management technique.

Although our everyday coping skills are sufficient to prevent us from experiencing undue stress in most situations, stressful events may become overwhelming. The good news is that the level of stress we experience depends as much on us as it does on the situation. Engaging in regular aerobic exercise and drills that promote relaxation can help buffer the toxic effects of stress and improve our physiological and psychological well-being. So relax, look at life with a positive attitude, and don't let stress get to you.

■ **stress inoculation training** a form of cognitive therapy that helps people to confront stressful events with a variety of coping strategies that can be used before the event becomes overwhelming

Summing Up

Responding to Stress

1. Coping refers to the various ways—sometimes healthy, sometimes unhealthy—in which people attempt to prevent, eliminate, weaken, or simply tolerate stress. Emotion-focused coping refers to efforts to control your emotional response to a stressor, either by distancing yourself from it or by changing how you appraise it. Problem-focused coping refers to efforts to deal directly with a stressor by applying problem-solving skills to anticipate and prevent potential stressors (proactive coping) or by directly confronting the source of stress (combative coping).

2. Compared to women, men react to stress with larger increases in blood pressure, low-density lipoprotein cholesterol, and certain stress hormones. In general, women report more symptoms of stress and are more emotionally responsive to stressful situations. When women and men of similar SES are compared, gender differences in coping styles disappear.

3. People of higher SES are more likely than those of lower SES to use problem-focused coping strategies in dealing with stress. Low SES is often accompanied by a stressful lifestyle that limits a person's options in coping with stress. Many ethnic group differences in morbidity and mortality are due to differences in behavioral risk profiles (smoking, alcohol consumption, obesity, diet, and sedentary lifestyle).

Factors Affecting the Ability to Cope

4. Hardy people may be healthier because they are less likely to become overwhelmed by stressful situations. Along with hardiness, resilience (in children) and stamina (in older adults) are positively correlated with physical and mental health.

5. People whose explanatory style is negative tend to explain failures in terms that are global, stable, and internal. This, in turn, may increase their sensitivity to challenging events and promote self-blame, pessimism, and depression. In contrast, optimists may be healthier and more resistant to stress. Optimism also is related to greater perceived control and self-efficacy, which in turn are related to more effective coping responses.

6. The opportunity to control aversive events plays a crucial role in determining a person's response to a stressful situation. Biologically, exposure to stressors without the perception of control activates the autonomic system. The perception of control buffers stress-related arousal, leads to the release of pain-relieving beta-endorphins, and enhances immune activity.

7. Repeated exposure to noncontingent stressors such as shock may lead to the resigned, passive behavior of learned helplessness. Studies of elderly persons and nursing home residents show that helplessness can also lead to depression, a shortened life span, and a variety of health-compromising behaviors.

8. Physiological responses such as vagal tone may serve as accurate markers of individual differences in regulatory control during moments of stress. People with high vagal tone may be less likely to experience negative emotional arousal in response to stress. They are also more likely to rely on constructive coping measures than are people who exercise less regulatory control. Repressive coping is an emotion-focused coping style in which the person attempts to inhibit his or her emotional responses.

9. People who perceive a high level of social support may cope with stress more effectively than people who feel alienated. Along with companionship, social ties can provide emotional support, instrumental support, and informational support. Social support produces its beneficial effects indirectly, by helping people cope more effectively (buffering hypothesis), or directly, by enhancing the body's responses to challenging events (direct-effect hypothesis).

10. People with better social skills—who relate well to others and who are caring and giving—create stronger social networks and thus receive more social support. Some researchers believe that women profit more than men from social support, perhaps because women tend to have closer, more emotionally intimate relationships than men do. Social support does not always reduce

stress and benefit health. Sometimes support is perceived as intrusive; other times the type of support offered is not what is needed.

Stress Management

11. Regular physical activity can improve a person's psychological and physiological ability to cope with stress. Exercise produces an antidepressant/antianxiety effect in many people, enhances the efficacy of the immune system, and lowers blood pressure and cardiovascular reactivity. Relaxation techniques such as progressive muscle relaxation, the relaxation response (meditation), and autogenic training can help people cope with a variety of stress-related problems, including hypertension, headaches, chronic pain, and anxiety.

12. Biofeedback is a technique for converting certain supposedly involuntary physiological responses—such as skin temperature, muscle activity, heart rate, and blood pressure—into electrical signals and providing visual or auditory feedback about them. Although results from studies of biofeedback effectiveness are mixed, and it remains unclear how "control" over autonomic processes is developed, the method has been firmly established as a viable means of treating anxiety and stress-related disorders.

13. Although hypnosis remains a controversial treatment, most psychologists now agree that hypnosis is a state of heightened suggestibility to which people are subject in varying degrees, and that hypnosis is effective in helping suggestible people cope with pain. Although some researchers believe that hypnosis is an altered state involving dissociation between levels of consciousness, most psychologists admit that hypnosis is, at least in part, a by-product of everyday social phenomena.

14. Cognitive therapies are aimed at breaking the cycle of irrational thought patterns that distort people's perception of everyday events and prevent them from adopting appropriate coping behaviors. Rational-emotive therapy is a confrontational form of therapy that challenges people's irrational beliefs. Stress inoculation training is a form of cognitive-behavioral therapy that helps people to confront stressful events with coping strategies that can be put in place before stressors become overwhelming.

Key Terms and Concepts

coping, p. 166
emotion-focused coping, p. 167
problem-focused coping, p. 168
proactive coping, p. 168
combative coping, p. 168
hardiness, p. 175
resilience, p. 178
stamina, p. 179
explanatory style, p. 179
rumination, p. 184

personal control, p. 184
regulatory control, p. 186
repressive coping, p. 189
learned helplessness, p. 189
social support, p. 190
buffering hypothesis, p. 192
direct effect hypothesis, p. 192
stress management, p. 197
progressive muscle
    relaxation, p. 201

relaxation response, p. 201
autogenic training (AT), p. 202
biofeedback, p. 202
hypnosis, p. 205
dissociation, p. 206
social influence theory, p. 207
cognitive therapy, p. 207
rational-emotive therapy (RET), p. 208
stress inoculation training, p. 209

Health Psychology on the World Wide Web

Web Address	Description
http://helping.apa.org	The American Psychological Association's Internet *Help Center,* providing access to resources to help people cope with modern stressors.
http://www.stressfree.com	A wealth of resources for coping with job-related stress.

Critical Thinking Exercise

Humor and Health

There ain't much fun in medicine, but there's a heck of a lot of medicine in fun.

— *Josh Billings, Humorist*

Everyone likes a good joke. A sense of humor can help people through difficult situations and can make setbacks seem less serious. In one of the best-known personal accounts of coping with chronic disease, Norman Cousins (1979) described how a daily dose of viewing comedy films helped relieve his pain, thus crediting laughter with helping him to regain his health. Cousins referred to the healing processes of laughter as *internal jogging.*

Although personal accounts such as Cousins' are captivating, they provide only anecdotal evidence of the health-enhancing effects of humor. But is there really something to this bit of folk wisdom? Is there scientific evidence that laughter is an effective stress buster?

To date, only a few studies have systematically investigated humor and stress. In one study, Rod Martin and Herbert Lefcourt (1983) divided college students into two groups: those who scored high on a measure of sense of humor and those who scored low on the same measure. The researchers found that students who had a good sense of humor had better self-concepts and higher self-esteem than the others. They also seemed better able to shrug off setbacks and cope more effectively with everyday stressors. In a similar study, Arthur Nezu and his colleagues (Nezu, Nezu, & Blissett, 1988) found that humor helped students deal with depression.

Two theories have been offered to explain how humor buffers stress. The first is that humor gives you a time out from ongoing stress and buys time for appraising/reappraising the situation, evaluating your options, and altering your otherwise automatic stress response. The second theory is that a sense of humor enhances immune functioning. Among people who report high levels of daily stress, those who use humor to cope have higher levels of immunoglobulin A, a protein-based antibody synthesized by the B cells of the immune system. One study demonstrated that immunoglobulin A increased in subjects after they had watched a comedy film, but did not increase in subjects who watched an instructional film.

On the other hand, some recent evidence suggests that cheerfulness and a sense of humor may not always be beneficial to health. Howard Friedman and colleagues, for example, have found that humor may help people cope effectively in the short run, but that in the long run, humor may actually be maladaptive (Friedman et al., 1993; Friedman et al., 1995a; Friedman et al., 1995b).

Friedman's data come from Lewis Terman's famous research with gifted children. Beginning in 1921, Terman studied more than 1,500 California schoolchildren, 8 to 12 years old, with IQ scores above 135. Over the next six decades, Terman carefully followed this group of gifted people, collecting data on their physical development, emotional well-being, and academic success. After Terman's death in 1956, other researchers continued to study the sample, as well as their children and their grandchildren. Contrary to the popular myth that gifted children are often socially and emotionally maladjusted, these people were found to be unusually healthy, well adjusted, and academically successful.

With this wealth of longitudinal data in hand, Friedman set out to determine whether psychosocial traits of the study participants *as children* could be used to predict their longevity. Terman and his colleagues had collected enough data to permit Friedman to test six psychosocial dimensions: sociability, self-esteem, conscientiousness, sense of humor, physical energy, and emotional stability.

Of all these factors, only two correlated with longevity: conscientiousness and humor. Adults who scored high in conscientiousness *as children* did live longer. In fact, childhood conscientiousness predicted how long a child would live just about as well as variables such as diet, exercise, cholesterol level, and blood pressure. Friedman speculates that conscientious people are more likely to take better care of themselves and to engage in fewer risky or health-compromising behaviors throughout their lives.

Surprisingly, Friedman found that children who scored high on the humor dimension tended to have shorter lives than those who scored lower on this dimension. Friedman speculates that while a sense of humor often is helpful in coping with short-term stressors, excessive humor may also lead to an unrealistic belief that things will always turn out for the best and may cause some people to underestimate the dangers of health-compromising behaviors such as cigarette smoking, sedentary living, or a poor diet.

The safest conclusion thus seems to be that laughter can help people feel better and buffer some of the psychological effects of stress. Whether the physical effects of humor in promoting health are significant remains to be demonstrated.

1. Suppose a health psychologist wished to test her hunch that humor relieves stress. How would she set about doing this? What factors should she consider in designing her study?

2. Why don't health psychologists consider anecdotal accounts such as Norman Cousins' as valid evidence for testing research hypotheses? What *would* constitute valid evidence?

3. Suppose a friend asks for your opinion regarding whether or not having a sense of humor helps buffer the effects of stress. What should your response be?

3

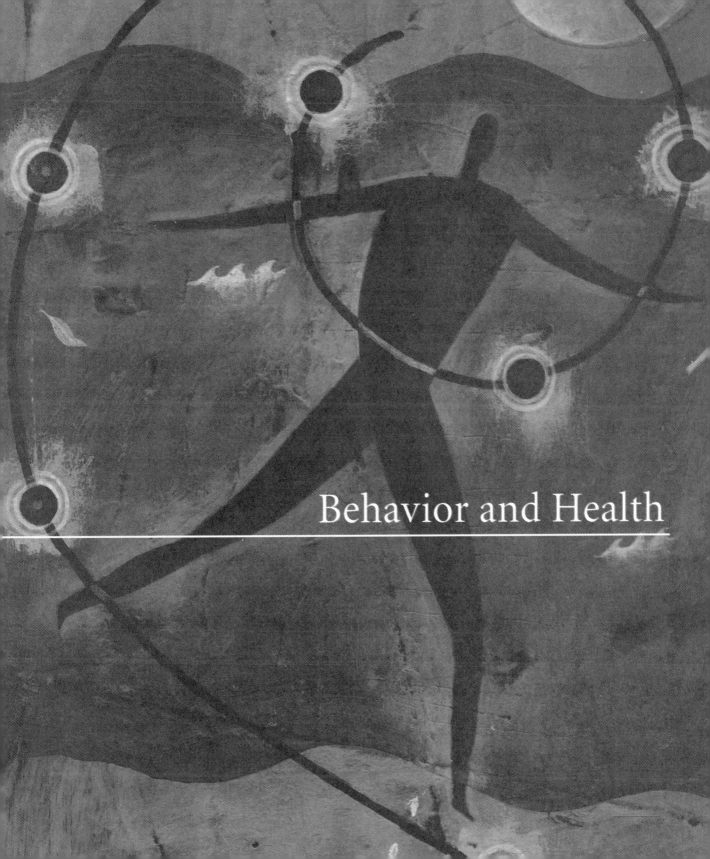

Behavior and Health

6

Staying Healthy

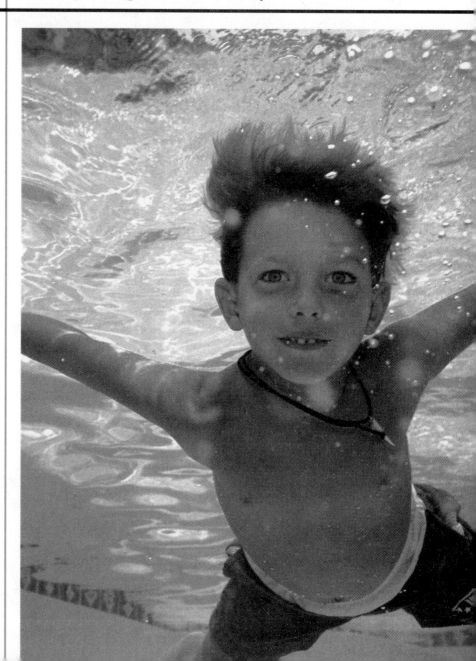

Anthony, a 20-year-old college sophomore, is very casual about his health. Although he can knowledgeably discuss the hazards of cigarette smoking, poor nutrition, and unsafe sex, Anthony engages in all these health-compromising behaviors.

Most days, Anthony's breakfast consists of a cup of coffee, a doughnut, and a cigarette grabbed in a mad dash to get to class on time. Lunch and dinner are almost always a burger and fries from the local drive-through. Anthony hasn't settled down with a girlfriend yet but he's had a number of intimate partners and, despite knowing better, sometimes fails to use a condom. Still, he doesn't worry about contracting HIV or that he will develop a sexually transmitted disease.

Anthony's parents are worried about their son. Over semester break, Anthony seems terribly run down and irritable and has obviously gained a lot of weight. To make matters worse, he seems to be behaving recklessly. For example, although he's on an urban campus and not driving so much, he behaves like a future Nascar driver. He doesn't even wear his seatbelt anymore. Anthony tells his parents that accidents are inevitable and that people who don't wear seatbelts are no more likely to be seriously injured than are those who wear them.

His more health-conscious friends think Anthony acts as though he is going to be 20 years old forever and nothing bad can ever happen to him. Anthony isn't intentionally trying to make others worry. Sure, his life is fast-paced, but he feels there is plenty of time to make improvements once the pressures of school are behind him. He knows he should quit smoking but is afraid that he'll become even more overweight if he does. Similarly, he knows he should practice safe sex, but he doesn't know how to bring it up at the right time and he's worried about what his friends would think.

Do you know someone who, like Anthony, seems to have a complete disregard for his (or her) health? Someone who seems more concerned about his appearance and acceptance by friends than about his lifelong well-being? How does a person form such attitudes about health? Researchers have found that unhealthy habits such as Anthony's tend to be related, just as healthy behaviors also tend to go together. Excessive drinking, drug use, violence, and unprotected sexual activity often co-occur to form a single behavioral syndrome (Fisher & Feldman, 1998; Jessor, 1992). People who engage in these behaviors are also less likely to eat nutritiously, wear seatbelts, or practice other health-enhancing behaviors (Hawkins, 1992).

Are such foolhardy behaviors the result of ignorance? On the contrary, researchers have found that most people are well aware of the risks of such behaviors. They know, for example, which kinds of sexual behaviors are safe and which are not (Gerrard & Luus, 1995). When asked whether they intend to engage in high-risk behaviors, they frequently say "no" and then do so anyway (Zabin, 1993).

Although people take risks at any age, adolescents tend to take risks more frequently because their behaviors are sometimes not well thought out. This may explain why more than 80 percent of adolescent pregnancies are unplanned (Brown & Eisenberg, 1995). Another reason is peer influence: Adolescents seldom engage in smoking, reckless driving, excess drinking, and other risky behaviors by themselves. When they do consider whether to take risks, the social consequences of their actions play a large role in their decisions (Gibbons, Gerrard, Blanton, & Russell, 1998). Like Anthony, many young adults engage in risky behaviors because the *immediate* social rewards for doing so outstrip the health benefits that are only reaped years later.

Fortunately, not all students are as reckless with their health as Anthony is. In fact, over the past 25 years the "wellness" movement has gained considerable momentum. Several factors have combined to engender the movement. One is the increasing tendency of people to assume more responsibility for their own health and welfare. Another is the exponential rise in health care costs, which has encouraged researchers to seek more effective ways of promoting health (and containing costs) in addition to developing new treatments for disease.

This chapter begins an exploration of factors that promote health and prevent illness. We first consider how our individual lifestyles influence our health, then turn to some of the barriers that prevent wellness. Next, we examine several prominent theoretical models of health-related attitudes and behaviors. The chapter concludes with a discussion of various approaches to changing people's health-related attitudes and habits.

Health and Behavior

Remember from Chapter 1 that at the turn of the twentieth century the leading causes of mortality were infectious diseases such as pneumonia, influenza, and tuberculosis. Our ancestors succumbed to these illnesses because antibiotics were unavailable to eradicate infection, and public health standards were so poor that disease spread rapidly. In developed countries today, illnesses such as these are rarely fatal. Indeed, whereas in 1900 about 12 percent of all deaths in the United States were caused by pneumonia and influenza, by the end of the twentieth century this figure had decreased to less than 3 percent, and most of these victims were elderly or already seriously ill.

Today, chronic diseases have replaced infectious diseases as the primary causes of mortality in developed countries. Heart and blood vessel diseases account for 50 percent of all deaths in the United States. Cancer is the second leading cause of mortality in this country; experts estimate that one of every three Americans will be diagnosed with cancer at some point during his or her life, and one of every four will die of cancer (McGuire, 1999). These diseases are strongly influenced by behavioral and environmental factors such as cigarette smoking, lack of exercise, excessive eating, and a hostile temperament. Indeed, by some estimates, more than two-thirds of cancer cases are linked either to smoking cigarettes or eating unwisely (Doll & Peto, 1981; Visser & Herbert, 1999). For this reason, the focus has shifted from strictly physiological causes of disease to physiological and/or psychological causes.

Another reason lifestyle behaviors have come under closer scrutiny is that promoting health is considerably less costly than treating disease. Annual health care costs in the United States currently total over $1 trillion. Seventy percent of this amount stems from the treatment of preventable conditions (Scott, 1999). Smoking is an excellent example, because it is so costly to individual smokers and to all of society. Annually, over 400,000 preventable deaths in the United States are attributed to smoking (Prochaska, 1996a). Globally, the problem is even more catastrophic. Worldwide, some 3 million deaths a year are estimated to be attributable to smoking. Of all people currently alive in the world today, approximately 500 million will die from smoking—a cumulative "cost" of 5 billion years of life due to tobacco use (Peto et al., 1996).

Behavioral Immunogens and Pathogens

It is difficult to imagine an activity or behavior that does not influence health in some way—directly or indirectly, immediately or over the long term, for better or worse. Excessive use of alcohol is an example of a health-related behavior that has a direct negative impact on physical health. Other behaviors

■ **behavioral pathogen** a health-compromising behavior or habit

■ **behavioral immunogen** a health-enhancing behavior or habit

influence health indirectly, through their association with behaviors that have a direct impact on health. Hostility, for example, may increase the risk of heart disease because it is linked with cigarette smoking and other coronary-prone risky behaviors such as unhealthy eating and sleeping habits and poor stress management (Scherwitz & Rugulies, 1992).

Some behaviors affect health immediately—for example, being involved in an automobile accident while not wearing a seatbelt. Others, such as eating a high-fat diet, have a long-term effect. And some behaviors, such as exercising or cigarette smoking, have both an immediate and a long-term effect on health.

Some health-related behaviors could have both a positive and a negative impact on health. For example, exercise and dieting can lead to a beneficial loss of weight; if carried to the extreme, though, they can trigger a "yo-yo" pattern of weight loss and gain that might be hazardous to your health (Lowe, 1993).

Lifestyle behaviors or habits that damage health are called **behavioral pathogens** (Matarazzo, 1984). Among the more common behavioral pathogens are smoking, excessive eating, substance abuse, dangerous driving practices, and risky sexual behavior. Other pathogens compromise health in less obvious ways. For example, anger contributes to coronary heart disease in two ways: in the way a person expresses it and through the health-compromising behaviors that angry people tend to exhibit.

Behaviors or habits that have a protective effect on health are called **behavioral immunogens** (Matarazzo, 1984). Exercising regularly, using sunscreen, eating a low-fat diet, practicing safe sex, and wearing seatbelts—all these behaviors help "immunize" you against disease and injury. Less obvious examples of immunogens include pleasurable hobbies, meditation, laughter, regular vacations, and even owning a pet. These activities help many people manage stress and retain an upbeat outlook on life.

Health-related behaviors interact and often are interrelated. A person who smokes, for example, often also drinks alcohol and excessive amounts of coffee (Carmody, 1985). Moreover, the combined effect of these pathogenic behaviors on health is stronger than if the person engaged in only one such behavior. Similarly, exercising, eating healthy foods, and drinking lots of water usually come together but in a positive way. Sometimes, a person may engage in both pathogenic behaviors and immunogenic behaviors—for example, drinking alcohol and exercising. In such cases, one may offset the effects of the other. Finally, a behavioral immunogen may replace a behavioral pathogen. For example, many ex-smokers find that regular aerobic exercise provides a healthy (and effective) substitute for nicotine.

What is the potential impact of adopting a healthier lifestyle? By one estimate, the incidence of seven of the ten leading causes of mortality (heart disease, cancer, stroke, automobile accident, diabetes, arteriosclerosis, and cirrhosis) could be substantially re- duced if more people would modify just five behaviors: cigarette smoking, alcohol consumption, diet, exercise, and stress management (U.S. Department of Health and Human Services, 1991).

In one classic epidemiological study begun in 1965, Lester Breslow and Norman Breslow (1993) began to track the health and lifestyle habits of the residents of Alameda County, California. Over the many years of this landmark study, the salutary effects of seven healthy habits—sleeping 7 to 8 hours daily, never smoking, being at or near a healthy body weight, moderate use of alcohol, regular physical exercise, eating breakfast, and avoiding between-meal snacking—have proved striking (Figure 6.1).

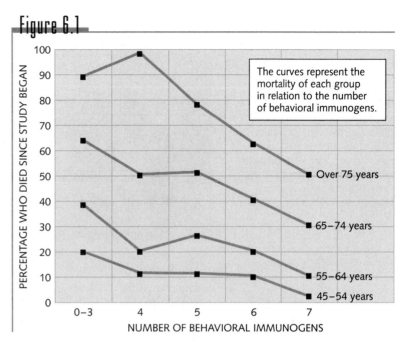

Figure 6.1

The curves represent the mortality of each group in relation to the number of behavioral immunogens.

Behavioral Immunogens and Death Rate

Nine-and-a-half years into the famous Alameda Health Study, the mortality of men who regularly practiced all seven health habits (sleeping 7 to 8 hours daily, never smoking, being at or near a healthy body weight, moderate use of alcohol, regular physical exercise, eating breakfast, and avoiding between-meal snacking) was 28 percent of the mortality of those who had practiced three or fewer healthy behaviors.

Source: "Health Practices and Disability: Some Evidence from Alameda County," by L. Breslow and N. Breslow, 1993, *Preventive Medicine, 22*, pp. 86–95.

Longevity and the Span of Healthy Life

Another way to confirm or deny whether a behavioral immunogen has health-protecting effects is to study the characteristics of people who live long lives. First, however, you need to understand some basic terms regarding mortality.

Average life expectancy is defined as the age at which 50 percent of a group of people born in a given year are still alive. In the United States, for example, the life expectancy for children born in 1900 was 47 years; in 1999, the average life expectancy at birth was 79.7 years for women and 73.8 years for men (World Health Organization, 2000). Based on mortality rates in 1998, women are expected to outlive men by an average of 5.9 years, and white Americans are expected to outlive black Americans by an average of 6.0 years. White females have the highest average life expectancy at birth (79.9 years), followed by black females (74.7 years), white males (74.3 years), and black males (67.2 years). Between 1996 and 1997, black males enjoyed the single largest increase in average life expectancy (1.1 years). Although an increasing suicide rate has shortened the average life expectancy of Japanese men in recent years, in 1999 the average life expectancies of Japanese men (77.6) and women (84.3) remained the highest in the world.

■ **average life expectancy** the number of years the average child born in a given year is likely to live

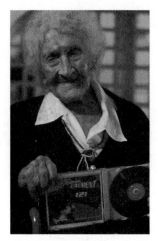

Jeanne Calment, the World's Oldest Person
The longest-living person with a birth certificate was Jeanne Calment of Arles, France. Calment, who was born on February 21, 1875—about 10 years after Abraham Lincoln was assassinated—entered the Guinness Book of Records in 1993 as the oldest living person whose birth date could be authenticated. Calment died quietly at her home in 1997 at age 122. © Pascal Parrot / Corbis Sygma

■ **life span** the oldest age that members of a particular species live under ideal circumstances. In humans, this age is estimated to be between 110 and 113 years

Life span refers to the maximum age reached by the last surviving member of a group of people born in a given year. The life span of a baby born this year is estimated to be between 110 and 113 years. Although our potential life span is the same today as it was at the turn of the twentieth century, the number of centenarians (people who reach 100 years of age) has increased dramatically. In 1900, only 1 in 400 people in the United States had reached the age of 100. By the 1990s, this figure had risen to 1 in 87; at the beginning of the twenty-first century estimates indicate that more than 52,000 Americans will pass this milestone (Warshofsky, 1999). This increase results in large part from lifestyle changes that enable people to improve their health (see Reality Check).

Three areas of the world—in Abkhasia, Georgia; in Peru; and in Pakistan—are renowned for the longevity of their people. Abkhasia, a remote mountainous region in the former Soviet Union, is a place of almost mythical longevity. Some of the "supercentenarians" living there, most of whom are illiterate farmers, have reportedly reached 120 or 130 years of age (Chopra, 1993). Although accurate birth records aren't available to confirm many of these claims, Abkhasia appears to have a higher-than-average proportion of long-lived adults.

What enables this longevity? Although heredity undoubtedly plays a large role, a number of lifestyle factors have also emerged as common traits of long-lived people (Pitskhelauri, 1982). These include

■ a moderate diet that discourages overeating and is low in meat and saturated fat and high in fresh vegetables and fruit.

■ regular exercise and relaxation. Most of the long-lived walk extensively (for both pleasure and out of necessity), take a daily nap, and spend time each day socializing with friends and family members.

■ an active work life that extends well into old age. Many centenarians help with child-care and household tasks.

■ little or no use of alcohol and nicotine.

Reality Check

Calculating Your Life Expectancy

Compared to others of your age and gender, is your lifestyle likely to lengthen (or shorten) your life? This table will give you an approximate idea of how your life expectancy varies from the norm. Use the table at right to find the average life expectancy of your age group. Then consult the table opposite, adding or subtracting years based on the risk factors listed.

Age	Female	Male	Weighting Risk Factors
20–59	80	73	use table as shown
60–69	81	76	reduce loss or gain by 20%
70–79	82	78	reduce loss or gain by 50%
80+	add 5 yrs. to current age		reduce loss or gain by 75%

Health	+3 Years	+2 Years	+1 Year		−1 Year	−2 Years	−3 Years	Tally
Blood Pressure	Between 90/65 and 120/81	Less than 90/65 without heart disease	Between 121/82 and 129/85	130/86	Between 131/87 and 140/90	Between 141/91 and 150/95	More than 151/96	
Diabetes	—	—	—	None	Type II (adult onset)	—	Type I (juvenile onset)	
Total Cholesterol	—	—	Less than 160	161–200	201–240	241–280	More than 280	
HDL cholesterol	—	—	More than 55	45–54	40–44	Less than 40	—	
Compared with others my age, my health is	—	—	Excellent	Very good or fair	—	Poor	Extremely poor	
Lifestyle	**+3 Years**	**+2 Years**	**+1 Year**		**−1 Year**	**−2 Years**	**−3 Years**	**Tally**
Cigarette smoking	None	Ex-smoker, no cigarettes for more than 5 yrs.	Ex-smoker, no cigarettes for 3–5 yrs.	Ex-smoker, no cigarettes for 1–3 yrs.	Ex-smoker, no cigarettes for 5 mons.–1 yr.	Smoker, 0–20 per day	Smoker, more than 20 per day	
Secondhand-smoke exposure	—	—	—	None	0–1 hour per day	1–3 hours per day	More than 3 hours per day	
Exercise average	More than 60 min. per day of exercise (e.g., walking) for more than 3 yrs.	More than 30 min. per day for more than 3 yrs.	More than 20 min. per day for more than 3 yrs.	More than 10 min. per day for more than 3 yrs.	More than 5 min. per day for more than 3 years	Less than 5 min per day	None	
Saturated fat in diet	—	Less than 20%	20%–30%	31%–40%	—	More than 40%	—	
Fruits and Vegetables	—	—	5 servings per day	—	None	—	—	
Family	**+3 Years**	**+2 Years**	**+1 Year**		**−1 Year**	**−2 Years**	**−3 Years**	**Tally**
Marital status	—	Happily married man	Happily married woman	Single woman, widowed man	Divorced man, widowed woman	Divorced woman	Single man	
Disruptive events in the past year*	—	—	—	—	One	Two	Three	
Social groups, friends seen more than once/month	—	Three	Two	One	—	None	—	
Parents' age of death	—	—	Both lived past 75	One lived past 75	—	—	Neither lived past 75	

* Deaths of family members, job changes, moves, lawsuits, financial insecurity, etc.

Source: *Real Age: Are You as Young as You Can Be?* by M. F. Roizen, 1999, New York: Cliff Street Books.

Estimated Life Expectancy:	Total

As the table indicates, an individual's life expectancy is determined by many factors, including overall health, lifestyle, and family history. By how many years did your predicted life expectancy change (for better or worse) as a result of the above factors?

■ **disability-adjusted life expectancy (DALE)** the number of years of life that a person can expect to spend free from disease or disability

■ **well year** a year of life that is free of any serious health-related problem

■ **primary prevention** health-enhancing efforts to prevent disease or injury from occurring

■ **secondary prevention** actions taken to identify and treat an illness or disability early in its course

Clearly then, how we react to our environment biologically, psychologically, and socially has a lot to do with how long we live. Together, these factors in large measure determine whether we come close to reaching our species' life span or die prematurely.

Although longevity is a universal goal, many older adults today are focusing instead on making sure that they not only live for a long time but that these are healthy years. They are changing their lifestyles to increase their **disability-adjusted life expectancy (DALE)** and number of **well years,** that is, the number of years a person is not sick or sidelined by health-related problems. Many health psychologists believe that the concept of well years may be the best measure of the effectiveness of health-promotion interventions in older adults (Kaplan & Bush, 1982).

DALE, which is also called *health expectancy,* is a measure of the probability of health and the number of well years in the life span. In effect, it is average life expectancy minus the disability-adjusted life years (see Chapter 2) for all diseases and disabilities for a person of a given age and gender. DALE is estimated from three kinds of information: the fraction of the population surviving to each age, the prevalence of each type of disability at each age, and the overall weight assigned to each type of disability, defined in terms of its impact on the individual (World Health Organization, 2000). Throughout the world an average of about 7 well years are lost to disability—a loss that is somewhat less for richer, low-mortality regions and somewhat higher for poorer, high-mortality ones (see Table 6.1). Disability has a greater impact in poor countries in part because some disabilities—injury, blindness, paralysis, and tropical diseases such as malaria—strike children and young adults more often in these countries than in more affluent ones.

Preventing Injury and Disease

The relationship between lifestyle and health has triggered a massive research effort aimed at preventing injury and disease. We usually think of prevention solely in terms of efforts to modify one's risk *before* disease strikes. In fact, researchers have differentiated three types of prevention that are undertaken before, during, and after a disease strikes.

Primary prevention refers to health-promoting actions that are taken to prevent a disease or injury from occurring. Examples of primary prevention include wearing seatbelts, practicing good nutrition, exercising, avoiding smoking, and going regularly for health screening tests. Behavioral immunogens are examples of primary prevention.

Secondary prevention involves actions taken to identify and treat an illness early in its course. In the case of a person who has high blood pressure, for example, secondary prevention would include regular examinations to monitor symptoms, the use of blood pressure medication, and dietary changes.

Table 6.1

Average Life Expectancy and Disability-Adjusted Life Expectancy for Representative World Regions*

WHO Region	Men		Women	
	Average Life Expectancy	Disability-Adjusted Life Expectancy	Average Life Expectancy	Disability-Adjusted Life Expectancy
AFRICAN REGION				
Chad	47.3	38.6	50.1	40.2
Sierra Leone	33.2	25.8	35.4	26.0
THE AMERICAS				
United States	73.8	67.5	79.7	72.6
Ecuador	67.4	59.9	70.3	62.1
EASTERN MEDITERRANEAN				
Saudia Arabia	71.0	65.1	72.6	64.0
Egypt	64.2	58.6	65.9	58.3
EUROPE				
France	74.9	69.3	83.6	76.9
Latvia	63.6	57.1	74.6	67.2
SOUTHEAST ASIA				
Thailand	66.0	58.4	70.4	62.1
India	59.6	52.8	61.2	53.5
WESTERN PACIFIC				
Japan	77.6	71.9	84.3	77.2
Malaysia	67.6	61.3	69.9	61.6

*For each of the World Health Organization's regions, data regarding disability-adjusted life expectancy and the average life expectancy of men and women are presented for two representative countries: first, the country with the lowest mortality rates in that region, and then the country with the highest mortality rates. Of the 191 member countries in the World Health Organization, Japan ranks first in average life expectancy and DALE, and Sierra Leone ranks last. Note also that while women have greater average life expectancy and DALE than men in most regions of the world, in some regions (such as Africa) DALE is nearly equal in women and men and in some regions DALE is greater in men than in women (Eastern Mediterranean, for example).

Source: *The World Health Report: Health Systems: Improving Performance* (2000, June). Geneva: World Health Organization, Annex Table 2, pp. 156–163; Annex Table 5, pp. 176–182.

■ **tertiary prevention** actions taken to contain damage once a disease or disability has progressed beyond its early stages

Tertiary prevention involves actions taken to contain or retard damage once a disease has progressed beyond its early stages. An example of tertiary prevention is the use of radiation therapy or chemotherapy to destroy a cancerous tumor. Tertiary prevention also strives to rehabilitate people to the fullest extent possible.

Although less cost-effective and less beneficial than primary or secondary prevention, tertiary prevention is by far the most common form of health care.

Tertiary care is much easier to accomplish because the appropriate target groups (those who are ill or injured) are readily identifiable. In addition, patients under tertiary care typically have the greatest motivation to comply with treatment and to engage in other health-enhancing behaviors.

Health psychologists have contributed to disease prevention in several ways. They encourage doctors and other health care professionals to take the time to give advice to their patients. As effective as this personalized attention would seem to be, many doctors find it hard to follow through with preventive measures. One reason for their difficulty is that medical schools have traditionally placed little emphasis on preventive measures. Another is a lack of time, given the number of people they have to see during a single day.

Health psychologists also promote health by encouraging legislative action and by conducting educational campaigns in the media. These efforts are focused at many levels, from the individual to the community to society as a whole. Table 6.2 illustrates a comprehensive program of primary, secondary, and tertiary disease

Table 6.2

Levels and Timing of Prevention

Level	Primary	Secondary	Tertiary
Individual	Self-instruction guide on HIV prevention for uninfected lower-risk people	Screening and early intervention for HIV	Designing an immune-healthy diet for an HIV+ person
Group	Parents gather to gain skills to communicate better with teens about risky behaviors	Needle exchange program for low SES, high-risk IV-drug users	Rehabilitation program for groups of AIDS patients
Work site	Work site educational campaign focusing on how HIV is transmitted	Work site safer sex incentive program (e.g., free condoms, confidential screening)	Extending leave benefits so employees can care for HIV+ relatives
Community	Focused media campaign to promote safer sex behaviors	Establishing support networks for HIV+ people	Providing better access to recreational facilities for those with AIDS
Society	Enforcing felony laws for knowingly infecting another person with HIV	Enacting antidiscrimination policies for HIV+ people	Mandating the availability of HIV medications for uninsured AIDS patients

Source: Adapted from "A Framework for Health Promotion and Disease Prevention Programs," by R. A. Winett, 1995, *American Psychologist, 50*(5), 341–350.

prevention based on the three major national health goals established by the U.S. Department of Health, Education, and Welfare as part of its *Healthy People 2000 Campaign*. As discussed in Chapter 1, these goals are to increase the span of healthy life, to decrease the disparities in health between different segments of the population, and to provide universal access to preventive services.

The Rocky Road to Wellness

Despite its acknowledged importance, preventive health care accounts for only a small percentage of the total health dollars spent in the United States (and in the world). Sadly, in developing countries some of the deadliest diseases are the cheapest to prevent. Worldwide, it is estimated that 1,500 people, mostly children and young adults, die each hour from tuberculosis, malaria, measles, diarrhea, pneumonia, flu, and other infectious diseases, many of which could be prevented for less than the cost of a few bottles of aspirin (Neergaard, 1999).

In more affluent, developed countries, many infectious diseases have been brought under control with effective primary and secondary prevention measures. However, far too many people in these countries continue to jeopardize their health by eating fattening foods, smoking, and practicing many other risky behaviors. Why isn't everyone striving to prevent chronic illness and promote optimal health?

Many of the world's deadliest diseases are cheap to prevent. For instance:

- Drugs that treat AIDS may be too expensive for many developing countries, but just $14 for a year's supply of condoms could prevent infection in the first place.
- An insecticide-soaked bednet to protect people from malaria-carrying mosquitoes costs $10.
- One dose of measles vaccine costs 26 cents.
- Five days of antibiotics for pneumonia costs 27 cents.

—Neergaard, 1999

Barriers to Health Promotion

As we explained in Chapter 1, the biopsychosocial (or mind–body) perspective applies a *systems approach* to health psychology—viewing health and other behaviors as being determined by the interaction of biological mechanisms, psychological processes, and social influences. In order to understand the barriers to health promotion, therefore, we must consider the behavior not only of the individual but also of family members, health care professionals, and the community.

Individual Barriers

People are sometimes their own worst enemies in the battle for health. In their teens and twenties when people are developing their health-related habits, they are usually quite healthy. Smoking cigarettes, eating a high-fat diet, and avoiding exercise at this time seem often to have no effect on health. So, young people have little immediate incentive for practicing good health behavior and correcting poor health habits.

■ **gradient of reinforcement**
the principle that immediate
rewards and punishments are
much more effective than
delayed ones

This **gradient of reinforcement**—the principle that immediate rewards and punishments are more effective than delayed ones—operates throughout life. Many health-enhancing behaviors such as engaging in vigorous exercise and pursuing a low-fat diet are either less pleasurable or more effortful than their less healthy alternatives. If engaging in a behavior (such as eating when you are depressed) causes immediate relief or gratification, or if failing to engage in this behavior provides immediate discomfort, the behavior is difficult to eliminate.

High-risk sexual behaviors that may result in HIV infection and AIDS are a tragic example of the gradient of reinforcement. Within 3 to 6 weeks after first exposure, some HIV-positive persons develop a sore throat, fever, and a rash that often looks like measles. This early form of the HIV illness usually disappears and is often so mild that it is not even remembered. Months or years may pass without any overt symptoms. During this time, of course, HIV is being actively produced and weakening the immune system. The precise length of time before AIDS develops for any individual is not known. Some researchers believe the *incubation period*—the time between exposure to the virus and when the first symptoms of AIDS appear—may be as long as 20 years. Once full-blown AIDS appears, death (if not prevented by new treatments) usually follows within the next 2 years. The point is, of course, that at the height of passion, the far-removed *potential* negative consequences of risky behavior too often are overshadowed by the immediate pleasures of the moment.

Family Barriers

Health habits are typically acquired from parents and others who model health-compromising behaviors. Parents who smoke, for example, are significantly more likely to have children who smoke (Chassin, Presson, Sherman, & McGrew, 1987; Schulenberg, Bachman, O'Malley, & Johnston, 1994). Similarly, obese parents are more likely to have obese children, and the children of problem drinkers are themselves at increased risk of abusing alcohol (Grilo & Pogue-Geile, 1991; Mirin & Weiss, 1989; Schuckit & Smith, 1996).

Although there may be a genetic basis to these behaviors, children also may acquire their expectancies about risky health-related behaviors by observing the behaviors of family members and the consequences. A study conducted by Elizabeth D'Amico and Kim Fromme (1997) of the University of Texas, Austin, convincingly demonstrated the impact of older siblings on the behavior and attitudes of their younger adolescent siblings. Their results suggest that vicarious learning from an older sibling is one mechanism through which adolescents form expectancies about risky health-related behaviors. A number of other family variables have been linked with risky health-related behaviors among adolescents. These include parental conflict and inconsistencies, absence of parental supervision, absence of the father, diffuse family relationships, coercive parent–child relationships, and parental drug and alcohol use (Metzler, Noell, Biglan, & Ary, 1994).

Health System Barriers

Because medicine tends to focus on treating conditions that have already developed, early warning signs of disease and contributing risk factors often go undetected in health care. People who are not experiencing symptoms of illness see little reason to seek advice regarding potential risk factors, and doctors are oriented toward correcting conditions rather than preventing future problems. Even when doctors press their patients for information regarding health-related habits, many patients misrepresent or even distort their condition or symptoms.

Although health care has begun to change—physicians today are receiving much more training in health promotion—economic forces often undermine the efforts of health care workers to promote preventive measures. Some health insurance plans, for example, still do not cover preventive medical services such as cholesterol screening. And more than 43 million Americans, 16 percent of the population, do not have insurance and therefore are unlikely to undergo preventive screening. Over the next 10 years, the number of uninsured Americans is projected to grow to between 52 and 54 million (Kaiser Foundation, 2000).

Who are the uninsured, and why aren't they covered? More than 8 out of every 10 uninsured are from working families and only 27 percent come from families with income below the federal poverty level (about $16,450 for a family of four in 1998).

As for other characteristics of the uninsured, single adults are at high risk because they can obtain health benefits solely through their own employment, are more likely to have low incomes, and usually do not qualify for government-supported programs like Medicaid. Some ethnic groups are at much higher risk of being uninsured. As Figure 6.2 shows, over one-third of Hispanic-Americans and one-quarter of both African-Americans and Native Americans have no health insurance (Kaiser Foundation, 2000).

As for why people lack health coverage, about 10 percent say they are not covered because they don't feel they need health insurance. More than two-thirds of the uninsured cite the high cost of insurance as the main reason. The costs of health insurance have skyrocketed over the past two decades, causing employers to pass a greater share of the costs on to their employees. In 1999, workers paid more than three times as much for health benefits as in 1977 (Kaiser Foundation, 2000).

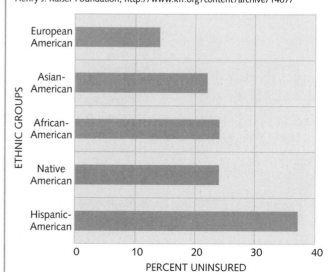

Figure 6.2

Ethnic Groups That Are More Likely to Be Uninsured
Over a third of Hispanic-Americans are uninsured, and nearly one-quarter of African-Americans and Native Americans have no health coverage. **Source:** *Uninsured in America: A Chart Book,* May 2000. Henry J. Kaiser Foundation, http://www.kff.org/content/archive/1407/

Not having insurance can have a devastating impact on a person's health and financial security. Medical bills can quickly wipe out a family's savings, and fear of high bills is a barrier that prevents many of the uninsured from seeking health care. Uninsured adults are four times as likely as those who are insured to report delaying or forgoing needed health services. For example, only 16 percent of uninsured women have recommended mammograms each year, compared to 42 percent of insured women (Kaiser Foundation, 2000). Is it any wonder that uninsured women are 40 percent more likely to be diagnosed with late stage breast cancer and 40 to 50 percent more likely to die from breast cancer than insured women?

To make matters worse, health insurance companies are using managed care to reduce behavioral health care benefits substantially more than other benefits. Overall, behavioral health care as a percentage of total health care benefits—with its emphasis on primary prevention—fell from its already low 6.2 percent in 1988 ($154.08 per covered individual) to 3.1 percent in 1997 ($69.61 per person). In comparison, the value of other benefits dropped only 7 percent, from $2,326.86 per covered individual in 1988 to $2,155.60 in 1997 (Kaiser Foundation, 2000).

Community Barriers

The community can be a powerful force for promoting or discouraging healthy living. People are more likely to adopt health-enhancing behaviors when these behaviors are promoted by community organizations, such as schools, governmental agencies, and the health care system. In recent years, society has made significant progress in changing attitudes toward exercise and proper nutrition. People also are much better informed about the importance of reducing their risk factors for cancer, cardiovascular disease, and other serious chronic conditions. However, there are still powerful social pressures that lead people to engage in health-compromising behaviors.

Consider alcohol use. National surveys indicate that alcohol use is more prevalent among American college students than among their peers who do not attend college (Quigley & Marlatt, 1996). Other surveys reveal that binge drinking among college students is associated with several social risk factors, including living in certain "party" residence halls (Larimer, 1992). For some students, the excitement of being together in a largely unsupervised environment can trigger such risky behaviors (Lightfoot, 1997).

Fortunately, most peer-inspired risk taking is a short-lived experiment that is outgrown before irreversible, long-term consequences are felt. Although drinking rates increase significantly in the transition from high school to the college freshman year (Baer, Kivlahan, Fromme, & Marlatt, 1994), heavy drinking declines as students grow older and assume increased responsibilities (Donovan, Jessor, & Costa, 1988).

Medical Compliance

Surprisingly, even when people seek health care, many simply ignore (or fail to closely follow) the treatment that is prescribed for them. Every health care professional can tell stories about this phenomenon: the patient who cheats on a special diet; the coronary case who, without consulting her doctor, stops taking her hypertension medication; or the accident victim who misuses a prescribed painkiller.

Compliance (also called *adherence*) is broadly defined as closely following the advice of a health care professional (Ley, 1997). This includes advice pertaining to medications, lifestyle changes (for example, losing weight or quitting smoking), as well as recommendations about preventive measures such as avoiding fatty foods or starting an exercise program. Compliance is both an attitude and a behavior. As an attitude it entails a willingness to follow health advice; as a behavior it is related to the actual carrying out of specific recommendations. Noncompliance would include refusal to adhere to instructions or the lack of sustained effort in following a treatment regimen.

The potential costs associated with noncompliance are enormous. By one estimate noncompliance causes 10 to 20 percent of patients to require an otherwise unnecessary refill of prescription medications, 5 to 10 percent to require further visits to their doctor, and another 5 to 10 percent to need additional days off from work (U.S. Department of Health and Human Services, 1997).

Researchers measure compliance in two ways. *Direct measures* include pill counts and urine and blood screening for the presence of a specific medication or microorganism. *Indirect measures,* which are easier to conduct and more frequently used, involve asking the health care practitioner or patient to estimate compliance. The subjective character of the indirect method, however, leaves the data open to various forms of bias, including overestimates by patients regarding the extent to which they comply with prescribed treatment. This problem is particularly acute in the elderly, who might also be suffering from memory problems. In one case, an 82-year-old woman swore she was taking a blood pressure pill every day, but a check of the pill bottle showed that no pills were missing since the last count.

How Widespread Is Noncompliance?

Philip Ley (1988) reviewed nine studies comparing patients' self-reports of compliance with more direct methods. Although 75 percent of patients stated that they had followed their treatment regimens, the more direct methods indicated the actual percentage to be closer to 46 percent.

In a later study (1997), Ley found that clinicians were even worse in estimating their patient's compliance. Their estimates had an average correlation of only +0.21 with direct measures of compliance. Although this weak correlation is due in part to the clinician's reliance on the patient's self-report, it is

> **compliance** a patient's willingness to follow a prescribed regimen of treatment and success in actually doing so

also a function of the physician's failure to ask his or her patients whether they complied fully with the treatment regimen.

Estimating the prevalence of noncompliance is difficult because noncompliance takes so many different forms. For example, a patient may not show up for a scheduled appointment or may fail to complete the course of an antibiotic. A person may "cheat a little" in adhering to a special diet, completing rehabilitative strength exercises, or following some other treatment regimen. In other words, there are many degrees of both compliance and noncompliance.

In broad terms, the average rate of compliance to medical advice is estimated to be only about 60 percent—only three out of every five patients follow their treatment regimens closely (DiMatteo, 1994). Here are some specifics:

- Only 20 to 40 percent of participants in treatment programs for smoking, alcohol, and drug abuse continue to comply with treatment after one year.

- In the treatment of obesity, between 10 and 13 percent of participants stop attending program meetings after 2 to 3 months, and from 42 to 48 percent after 3 to 4 months.

- Half of all appointments scheduled by health care providers are missed (except when children are the patients). However, if patients schedule their own appointments, compliance rates increase to 75 percent.

- Only 50 percent of patients comply fully with physician-directed dietary restrictions. Up to 80 percent of patients drop out of programs that prescribe other lifestyle changes (for example, fitness programs).

What Factors Predict Compliance?

Are some people more likely than others to comply with treatment? Is compliance more likely for certain kinds of treatment than for others? In their search for answers to these questions, biomedical researchers have examined three broad categories of variables: *patient variables, doctor–patient communication,* and *treatment regimen variables.*

Patient Variables Although a substantial amount of compliance research has focused on age, gender, ethnicity, education, and income, it is now generally understood that sociodemographic factors are not very accurate predictors of patient compliance (Symister & Friend, 1996). In general, this is because people themselves are surprisingly inconsistent in their individual compliance behaviors. A patient who follows a medication regimen, for example, may not necessarily adhere to a dietary regimen (Eitel, Hatchett, Friend, & Griffin, 1995). In short, there seem to be very few who are strictly "compliers" or "noncompliers."

Gender is a poor predictor because there is little difference in the overall adherence rates of women and men. For example, women and men are equally likely to stick with (or drop out of) exercise programs (Emery, Hauck, & Blumenthal, 1992; Lynch et al., 1992). Some differences do exist, however. For example, women are more likely than men to comply with dietary regimens (Laforge, Greene, & Prochaska, 1994).

The relationship between age and compliance is complex. Among adults, adherence to treatment regimens for heart disease, hypertension, and diabetes tends to increase as people get older (Sherbourne, Hays, Ordway, DiMatteo, & Kravitz, 1992). For colorectal cancer screening, however, William Thomas and colleagues (1995) found that 70-year-olds were the most compliant, whereas those younger than 55 or older than 80 were least compliant.

At the patient level, what does affect compliance? Having the support of family and friends (Doherty, Schrott, Metcalf, & Iasiello-Vailas, 1983), being in a good mood, and having optimistic expectations are all important factors (Leedham, 1995). Conversely, being depressed reduces compliance (Carney, Freedland, Eisen, Rich, & Jaffe, 1995).

Doctor–Patient Communication Robin DiMatteo (1993) conducted a 2-year study of patient compliance with medication, exercise, and dietary restrictions prescribed by 186 doctors who were treating patients for heart disease, diabetes, and high blood pressure. Among the factors that correlated with patient compliance were the doctor's level of job satisfaction, the number of patients seen per week, the doctor's communication style (for example, his or her willingness to answer a patient's questions), and the patient's satisfaction with his or her physician.

At the heart of the doctor–patient relationship is the nature and quality of communication. Patients too often emerge from consultations with insufficient information or even a misunderstanding of their problems. Particularly during difficult consultations, patients often are under considerable stress and find it difficult to take in everything the doctor says. To improve the situation, communication-skills training is now regarded as an integral component of the medical school curriculum (Weinman, 1997). This seems appropriate.

Doctors who are good communicators, who are less businesslike, and who meet their patients' expectations regarding the information they are entitled to receive tend to have patients who are more likely to adhere to treatment recommendations (Thompson, Dahlquist, Koenning, & Bartholomew, 1995). Physicians' nonverbal skills are also linked with patient satisfaction and compliance. We will explore the subject of communication and patient behavior more fully in Chapter 12.

Treatment Regimen Variables Patients are more likely to follow recommendations that they believe in and that they are capable of carrying out (DiMatteo, 1994). Even when a treatment is deemed useful, whether the patient is actually able to carry out the regimen depends on how difficult the regimen is to follow and the support available to the patient. Researchers have generally found that the more complex a treatment regimen, the lower the likelihood of complete compliance.

Health care providers can take several steps to improve compliance in their patients, including the following (Jeffery et al., 1993):

The simpler the treatment regimen, the greater the compliance. One study found that as the number of prescribed pills per day increased from one to four, the rate of compliance decreased from nearly 90 percent to less than 40 percent (Cramer, Mattson, Prevey, Scheyer, & Ouellette, 1989). This is significant, since more than 44 percent of Americans take prescription drugs daily and 8.8 percent take five or more (American Society of Health-System Pharmacists in *USA Today*, 2001).

- Keep the treatment regimen as simple and short in duration as possible.
- Tailor the treatment to fit the patient's lifestyle. Anything that makes a treatment regimen easier to follow, such as daily reminders about taking medicine, individually packaged meals for those on a restricted diet, or breaking down a complicated or long-term regimen into smaller segments, tends to increase adherence to treatment.
- Simplify instructions with clear language to ensure that the patient understands the amount, timing, and duration of treatment.
- Make sure that the individual understands enough of the treatment rationale to gain confidence in the treatment schedule.
- Involve family members, friends, and other people in the patient's treatment.
- Provide feedback about progress.

Interpreting and Understanding Illness

Despite the current emphasis on health and illness prevention, the average person remains largely ignorant about illness. Even those who are well educated often have erroneous beliefs about their health, partly because when people encounter new information, they tend to reconstruct it in order to integrate it into their existing beliefs. When people receive new information that seems to contradict long-held beliefs, they usually find it easier to modify or discount this information than to change their existing knowledge structure.

Leventhal's Four-Component Theory

Psychologist Howard Leventhal and his colleagues have investigated four components in how people conceptualize illness. The first component, *identifying the disease,* refers to how people label the disease when they first notice symptoms. Labels provide a cognitive framework within which symptoms are interpreted. In one study, the researchers gave people either false information that their blood pressure was high or correct information indicating normal blood pressure (Baumann, Cameron, Zimmerman, & Leventhal, 1989). Those whose blood pressure was labeled "high" (whether or not it actually was) were more likely to report symptoms commonly associated with hypertension than those told that their blood pressure was normal.

The second component is the *time line.* Researchers have found that people's understanding of the duration of illness is often inaccurate. People with chronic hypertension, for example, tend to view their condition as temporary; with treatment, the symptoms are expected to be cured (Meyer, Leventhal, & Gutmann, 1985).

The *perceived consequences* of disease are the third component in Leventhal's model. How a person views the consequences of a particular diagnosis may have an enormous impact on his or her response. For example, finding a lump in a testicle may cause one man to immediately schedule an appointment with a doctor so that treatment can be started immediately. Another may delay in making an appointment, not because he fails to recognize the lump as a possible symptom of cancer but because he fears that a cure is impossible.

The final component in Leventhal's model is *determining the cause* of the disease. The need to attribute symptoms to a cause is strong (Benyamini, Leventhal, & Leventhal, 1997). For instance, Shelley Taylor, Rosemary Lichtman, and Joanne Wood (1984) interviewed women diagnosed with breast cancer and found that 95 percent of them had formed an attribution about the cause of their cancer—for example, that it was due to their use of estrogen supplements. Other researchers have found that the need to make causal attributions increases with the severity of the diagnosis and the longer the time since diagnosis (Turnquist, Harvey, & Anderson, 1988).

Attributing a particular illness to a particular cause has important implications. Researchers have found that people are less likely to seek professional treatment for symptoms that are not perceived to be the result of natural or emotional causes. This is significant because people who are diagnosed with a chronic disease often accept explanations of their symptoms that are not based on empirical medical evidence. For instance, when symptoms are mild and slow to develop, they may be interpreted as "normal" signs of aging rather than disease. As another example, symptoms whose onset coincides with recent stressful life events such as exams, family quarrels, and so forth may be attributed to stress rather than illness (Cameron, Leventhal, & Leventhal, 1995). Both attributions may delay someone from seeking health care.

Researchers have also discovered that attributions for illness may be unrelated to an individual's level of knowledge or experience. In one remarkable study, a group of college biology majors gave explanations of illness that were no more accurate than control students who had not taken a single course in biology (Bibace & Walsh, 1979). Biology and non-biology students alike frequently attributed colds to lack of sleep, inclement weather, or failure to dress warmly. Such explanations differ very little from those offered by a third group of "experts"—7-year-old children. Other researchers have found that some college students attribute the development of illnesses such as AIDS to sin and God's will (Landrine & Klonoff, 1994).

The Optimistic Bias

Just as our attributions about the causes of disease are often faulty, so are our estimates of how likely we are to succumb to disease. In one study, Neil Weinstein (1982) asked college students to complete a health questionnaire estimating their risk of developing a variety of health problems. The students were asked to estimate on a 7-point scale ranging from "much above average" to "much below average" their risk, for example, of becoming a drug addict or alcoholic; developing coronary disease, ulcers, lung cancer, or diabetes; and becoming seriously obese.

■ **optimistic bias** the tendency of some people to believe that they are less likely to become ill than other adults of their own age and gender

■ **invincibility fable** the irrational belief, common in adolescents, that one is immune to the dangers of engaging in risky behaviors

The results of Weinstein's study revealed that the students believed that they were *much less likely* than their peers to develop all of the above health problems except one: ulcers. These results were not a fluke. Later research studies in which similar questions were posed to 18- to 65-year-old adults around the country reveal that most people also have an **optimistic bias**—that is, they believe that they are less likely to become ill than other adults of their own age and gender (Peterson, 2000; Weinstein & Klein, 1996).

Other research has shown that in the face of actual environmental threats, this optimistic bias often disappears. Shortly after the Chernobyl nuclear explosion in Ukraine, for example, a group of students exposed to radioactive fallout were asked to speculate about their future health. Although they believed that they were less likely than other students (in the same community) to develop heart disease or become disabled through injury, they felt that their risk of developing cancer and radiation-induced illness over the next several years was unusually high. Similarly, residents of communities hit by severe tornadoes are less optimistic about their vulnerability to future natural disasters than residents of communities that have been spared in recent years (Weinstein, Lyon, Rothman, & Cuite, 2000).

So, is it more advantageous to be unrealistically optimistic or pessimistic about your health? The answer is not a simple one. On the one hand, as we saw in Chapter 5, optimism conveys health advantages. On the other hand, research has demonstrated that people who feel somewhat vulnerable to specific health problems are more likely to practice preventive health behaviors (Becker, Kaback, Rosenstock, & Ruth, 1975).

Changing Attitudes about Illness over the Life Span

Developmental psychologists have long recognized that every age has its own special way of viewing the world. Childhood concepts of disease often include magical notions about causality. Only at a later age do children begin to understand the concept of contagion and the mechanisms by which infectious diseases are transmitted. Still later, as their concept of self-efficacy continues to mature, they begin to realize that they can take steps to control their health (Burbach & Peterson, 1986).

During adolescence, thinking is typically distorted by a self-view in which teenagers regard themselves as more significant than they actually are. This *adolescent egocentrism* manifests itself in many ways. One that potentially influences health is the **invincibility fable,** in which some young people believe that they will never be seriously harmed by dangerous actions. As a result of this false sense of security, they are more likely to engage in risky behaviors such as cigarette smoking, substance abuse, unsafe sexual behavior, and dangerous driving.

During late adulthood, *ageist* stereotypes, which are widely held among health care professionals and even by some older adults, can be significant barriers to achieving and maintaining good health. Chief among these are the views that old age is a period of inevitable decline, that elderly people are generally unable or unwilling to change their lifestyles and behaviors, that their compliance with treatment regimens and preventive interventions is poor, and that the benefits gained from lifestyle and behavioral interventions at this stage of life are minimal. This is unfortunate, since most people aged 65 years or older suffer from at least one chronic health condition and many suffer from two or more—and in many cases these conditions can be cured or at least controlled.

Ageist stereotypes may also prevent older adults from seeking (or receiving) optimal preventive health care. For instance, cancer screening programs often are not directed at people over age 65, despite the increased prevalence in this age group (Black, Sefcik, & Kapoor, 1990). Ageist stereotypes can also be a barrier to older adults' motivation to adopt healthier lifestyles aimed at increasing their overall health expectancy. Fortunately, research studies indicate that many elderly people remain optimistic about their health status—a good thing, since self-assessed health is the strongest predictor of life satisfaction during old age (Hart, 1997). We'll take up the topic of life-span issues in health psychology more fully in Chapter 15.

Theories of Health Behavior

Health psychologists have developed a number of theories to explain why people do or do not engage in certain healthy behaviors. In this section, we discuss several of the most influential ones, which are broadly divided into two categories: *non-stage theories* and *stage theories.*

The non-stage theories focus on predicting how people make decisions regarding a particular behavior (Weinstein, Rothman, & Sutton, 1998). Most are based on the idea that people are rational and engage in a process of weighing the pros and cons of engaging in a particular behavior that could affect their health. In contrast, stage theories assume that the decision to adopt a particular health behavior is a dynamic process that involves more than one decision and usually requires several steps or stages (Prochaska & DiClemente, 1984).

Non-Stage Theories

A friend was diagnosed with breast cancer. On her doctor's recommendation, she immediately decided to undergo a lumpectomy (surgical removal of the tumor), followed by radiation therapy and chemotherapy. Her doctor further suggested (strongly) that she take the drug tamoxifen to reduce the likelihood of her developing tumors in the future. However, because the medication produced several uncomfortable side effects, she decided to forgo this part of the treatment.

Non-stage theories of health behavior attempt to identify variables that influence health-related behaviors and combine them into a formula that

■ **health belief model (HBM)** non-stage theory that identifies three beliefs that influence decision making regarding health behavior: perceived susceptibility to a health threat, perceived severity of the disease or condition, and perceived benefits of and barriers to the behavior

predicts the probability that a particular individual will act in a certain way in a given situation. In the example above, these theories would look for the variables that influenced my friend's decision to switch from health-enhancing behaviors to potentially health-compromising behaviors.

The Health Belief Model

According to the **health belief model (HBM),** decisions regarding health behavior are based on three interacting factors that influence a person's perceptions about an illness or disease (Strecher & Rosenstock, 1997). As depicted in Figure 6.3, the factors are these:

■ *Perceived susceptibility* to a health threat. Some people worry constantly about their vulnerability to health threats such as HIV; others believe they are not in danger. The greater the perceived susceptibility, the stronger the motivation to engage in health-promoting behaviors. As you'll recall from the opening vignette, Anthony, like many adolescents, has a false sense of "invulnerability" that gives him little motivation to change his risky behaviors.

■ *Perceived severity* of the disease or condition. Among the factors considered are whether pain, disability, or death may result, as well as whether the disease will have an impact on family, friends, and coworkers. Although Anthony's parents worried about their son's irritability, weight gain, and symptoms of exhaustion, Anthony did not believe that these symptoms were a cause for concern. Moreover, Anthony was able to convince himself that he had plenty of time to change when things settled down in his life.

Figure 6.3

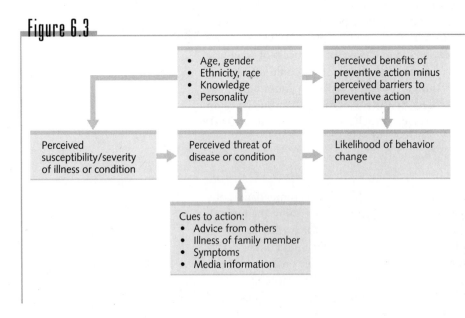

The Health Belief Model
This non-stage theory emphasizes three beliefs that influence decision making regarding health behavior: perceived susceptibility to a health threat, perceived severity, and perceived benefits and barriers. If a person believes that an available course of action will reduce his or her susceptibility to or the severity of the condition, then he or she will engage in that health behavior.

Source: "The Health Belief Model," by V. J. Strecher and I. W. Rosenstock, 1997. In A. Baum, S. Newman, J. Weinman, R. West, & C. McManus (Eds.), *Cambridge Handbook of Psychology, Health, and Medicine* (p. 115). Cambridge, UK: Cambridge University Press.

- *Perceived benefits and barriers of treatment.* In evaluating the pros and cons of a particular health behavior, a person decides whether its perceived benefits—such as enabling him or her to avoid a potentially fatal disease—exceed its barriers—such as causing unpleasant side effects or triggering a negative reaction from peers. Anthony's reluctance to quit smoking for fear of becoming obese (and unattractive) as well as his failure to consistently practice safe sex are classic examples of succumbing to perceived social pressures.

- *Cues to action.* The HBM also recognizes that advice from friends, media health campaigns, and sociodemographic factors such as age, socioeconomic status, and gender will influence the likelihood that the person will act.

In summary, the health belief model is a commonsense theory proposing that people will take action to ward off or control illness-inducing conditions if they regard themselves as susceptible to the condition; if they believe the condition has serious personal consequences; if they believe a course of action available to them will reduce either their susceptibility to or the severity of the condition; and if they believe that the costs of taking the action are outweighed by the benefits of doing so (Strecher & Rosenstock, 1997).

How effective is the health belief model in predicting health behaviors? Research has been extensive, but the results paint a mixed picture. On the one hand, the HBM has been shown to predict preventive dental care (Ronis, 1992), safer sex behaviors (Zimmerman & Olson, 1994) and other AIDS risk-related behaviors (Aspinwall, Kemeny, Taylor, Schneider, & Dudley, 1991), breast self-examination (Champion, 1994), and use of mammography services (Champion, 1994). However, some studies have found that health beliefs only modestly predict health behaviors, and that other factors, such as perceived barriers to being able to practice a health behavior, are more important determinants (Janz & Becker, 1994). For instance, in a major prospective study, Ruth Hyman and her colleagues (Hyman, Baker, Ephraim, Moadel, & Philip, 1994) found that perceived susceptibility to breast cancer did *not* predict their participants' use of mammography services, although both perceived benefits and barriers (such as having an accessible clinic and a physician who recommended a mammogram) did. The same study also found that a woman's ethnicity was the best predictor of all, with African-American women being significantly more likely to obtain regular mammograms than European Americans. In response to mixed results such as these, some researchers have expanded the HBM to include concepts from other theories, to which we now turn.

The Theory of Reasoned Action

Like the health belief model, the **theory of reasoned action (TRA)** specifies the relationships among beliefs, attitudes, intentions, and behavior (Ajzen & Fishbein, 1980). As depicted in Figure 6.4 (page 240), the theory assumes that a person's intention to perform a certain health behavior is shaped by two factors.

■ **theory of reasoned action (TRA)** the theory that decision making regarding healthy behavior is shaped by a person's attitude toward the behavior and his or her motivation to comply with the views of others regarding the behavior in question

■ **subjective norm** an individual's interpretation of the views of other people regarding a particular health-related behavior

The first is a person's *attitude toward the behavior,* which is determined by his or her belief that engaging in the behavior will lead to certain outcomes. For example, a person's judgment that reducing the amount of saturated fat in his or her diet is a good thing to do may be based on his or her belief that reducing fat will lead to weight loss and greater personal attractiveness. Similarly, Anthony rationalized his inconsistent use of a seatbelt by arguing that accidents are unavoidable and that people who don't wear seatbelts are no more likely to be injured than those who wear them.

The second determinant of intention to act is the **subjective norm,** which reflects the individual's motivation to comply with the views of other people regarding the behavior in question. Shifting to a low-fat diet, for example, may or may not be deemed appropriate, depending on whether the individual wants to bring his or her eating behavior in line with those of friends and relatives. People will have strong intentions to act when their attitude toward the behavior is positive and they believe that others also think the behavior is appropriate.

How well does the theory of reasoned action predict health behaviors? With regard to specific health-promoting behaviors, researchers have found the theory to be moderately accurate in predicting use of mammograms (Montano, Thompson, Taylor, & Mahloch, 1997), performing regular breast self-examinations (Lierman, Kasprzyk, & Benoliel, 1991), attending child-

Figure 6.4

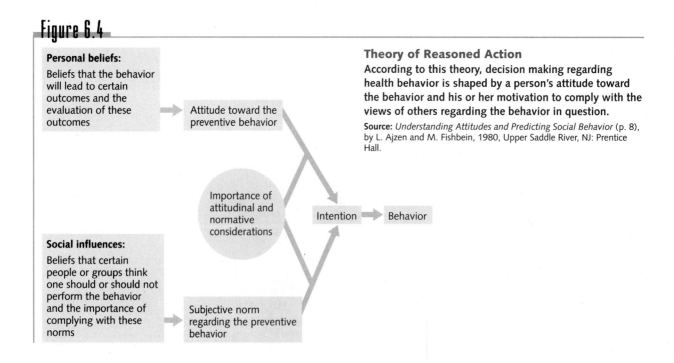

Personal beliefs:

Beliefs that the behavior will lead to certain outcomes and the evaluation of these outcomes

Attitude toward the preventive behavior

Importance of attitudinal and normative considerations

Intention → Behavior

Social influences:

Beliefs that certain people or groups think one should or should not perform the behavior and the importance of complying with these norms

Subjective norm regarding the preventive behavior

Theory of Reasoned Action
According to this theory, decision making regarding health behavior is shaped by a person's attitude toward the behavior and his or her motivation to comply with the views of others regarding the behavior in question.

Source: *Understanding Attitudes and Predicting Social Behavior* (p. 8), by L. Ajzen and M. Fishbein, 1980, Upper Saddle River, NJ: Prentice Hall.

birth health-information classes (Michie, Marteau, & Kidd, 1992), and trying to quit smoking (Sutton, 1989). More generally, a meta-analysis of 87 studies that applied the theory of reasoned action to a diverse range of topics (not all of which were health related) reported a moderately strong mean correlation of +0.53 for the intention–behavior relationship and a somewhat stronger mean correlation of +0.66 for predicting intention from attitude and the subjective norm (Sheppard, Hartwick, & Warshaw, 1988). Stated differently, it is estimated that the theory of reasoned action typically explains about 25 percent of individual differences in a given health behavior from intention alone and slightly less than 50 percent of individual variation in intentions (Sutton, 1997). Although significant, and at least as accurate as the health belief model in predicting health behaviors, these effects indicate that the theory of reasoned action is incomplete as an explanation of intention and behavior.

■ **theory of planned behavior (TPB)** a theory that predicts health behavior on the basis of three factors: personal attitude toward the behavior, the subjective norm regarding the behavior, and perceived degree of control over the behavior

The Theory of Planned Behavior

An extension of the theory of reasoned action, the **theory of planned behavior (TPB)** emphasizes the importance of perceived control in attitude formation and behavior change (Ajzen, 1991; Doll & Ajzen, 1992; Millstein, 1996). The more resources and opportunities to affect a behavior change people believe they have, the greater their beliefs that they can, in fact, change their behavior. As depicted in Figure 6.5, the TPB predicts behavior on the basis of three factors: personal attitude toward the behavior, the subjective norm regarding the behavior, and perceived degree of control over the behavior.

Although the theory of planned behavior has not generated nearly as much empirical research as the health belief model or the theory of reasoned action, researchers have found that whether it predicts behavior more accurately than the other theories depends on the perceived controllability of the behavior in

Figure 6.5

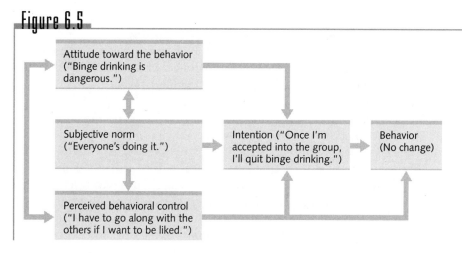

Theory of Planned Behavior This theory predicts that a person's decision to engage in a particular health behavior is based on three factors: personal attitude toward the behavior, the subjective norm regarding the behavior, and perceived degree of control over the behavior.

Source: "The Theory of Planned Behavior," by S. Sutton, 1997. In A. Baum, S. Newman, J. Weinman, R. West, & C. McManus (Eds.), *Cambridge Handbook of Psychology, Health, and Medicine* (p. 178). Cambridge, UK: Cambridge University Press.

behavioral intention (BI) in theories of health behavior, the rational decision to engage in a health-related behavior or to refrain from engaging in the behavior

prototype/willingness theory (P/W) a decision-making theory that assumes that health behavior is a function of a person's motivation to engage in that behavior (behavioral willingness) and the social image associated with that behavior (social prototype)

behavioral willingness (BW) in theories of health behavior, the reactive, unplanned motivation involved in the decision to engage in risky behavior

question (Madden, Ellen, & Ajzen, 1992). For highly controllable behaviors such as scheduling a medical appointment, differences between the two models in predicting behavior are insignificant. However, for behaviors that are deemed more difficult—such as modifying one's temperamental style in order to be less hostile toward others—the TPB is more accurate.

Susan Millstein (1996) compared the TRA and TPB in predicting physicians' intentions and their subsequent behaviors in discussing HIV transmission with their adolescent patients. Only those physicians who were confident that they could change their patients' tendency to engage in risky sexual behavior followed through with this important health intervention.

A central tenet of the theories discussed so far is that health behaviors involve planning. This being the case, the best way to predict whether the behavior will occur is to measure a person's **behavioral intention (BI)**—that is, his or her decision to engage in a health-related behavior or to refrain from engaging in the behavior. Indeed, the models are most accurate in predicting *intentional* behaviors that are goal-oriented and fit within a rational framework (Gibbons et al., 1998). In some cases, the TRA and TPB have successfully predicted health-compromising behaviors such as excess drinking (Schlegel, D'Avernas, Zanna, & DeCourville, 1992), smoking (Godin, Valois, Lepage, & Desharnais, 1992), and reckless driving (Parker, Manstead, Stradling, & Reason, 1992); in other cases, such as substance abuse (Morojele & Stephenson, 1994) and drunk driving (Stacy, Bentler, & Flay, 1994), they have been less successful. The next theory, the prototype/willingness theory, recognizes that many health behaviors are not based on rational decision making and so is more successful at predicting such behaviors.

The Prototype/Willingness Theory

The **prototype/willingness theory (P/W)** is based on the assumption that for many people, especially adolescents and young adults, health behaviors are often reactions to social situations. Behavioral pathogens are prime examples of socially oriented behaviors. For example, young people may attend a party where others are smoking marijuana or drinking excessively or agree to the demands of an overzealous girlfriend or boyfriend who wants to have sex. As Frederick Gibbons (1998) has noted, in such settings, "What are you willing to do?" probably describes a young person's predicament (and predicts his or her subsequent behavior) more accurately than "What do you plan to do?"

Although the prototype/willingness theory shares many assumptions with the other theories discussed so far, it adds two new constructs: behavioral willingness and social prototypes. **Behavioral willingness (BW)** refers to a person's motivation at a given moment to engage in risky behavior. Like *behavioral intention*—the focus of other non-stage theories—behavioral willingness is a function of subjective norms. The perception that significant others, especially peers, engage in and approve of the behavior in question is associated with greater behavioral willingness. Also like behavioral intention, greater behavioral willingness is linked to the individual's own positive attitudes toward the behavior. Finally, previously engaging in the behavior is associated with greater intention and willingness to engage in the behavior again.

Behavioral willingness differs from behavioral intention in that it is reactive rather than deliberative (Gibbons, Gerrard, Blanton, & Russell, 1998). Risky, health-compromising behaviors are often spontaneous social events, in which people follow the group's lead rather than make a personal decision to engage in the behavior. People (especially young people) rarely engage in these behaviors by themselves. For this reason, risky behaviors often have clear social images that influence a person's momentary willingness to engage in those behaviors.

Research in social cognition suggests that when people consider joining a particular group (such as people who engage in risky sexual behavior) they will often compare themselves with the **social prototype** associated with that group. A *prototype* is a mental image or best example that incorporates all the features we associate with a particular category (Rosch, 1978). The closer our self-concept matches a social prototype, the greater our interest in joining the group. By engaging in risky behaviors with their friends, for instance, adolescents acquire the image of the prototype in the eyes of their peers.

Frederick Gibbons and Meg Gerrard (1995) conducted a longitudinal study of 679 college students at the start of the students' freshman year. The students' social prototypes associated with four risky behaviors (smoking, drinking, reckless driving, and unprotected sex) were assessed, as was the frequency with which the students engaged in each of the risky behaviors. These same measures were repeated 6 or 7 months later.

The results revealed a strong reciprocal relationship between social prototypes and risky behaviors. Students who more frequently engaged in risky behaviors at the start of the study had more favorable prototypes of those behaviors than did participants who engaged in those behaviors less frequently. Students who reduced their risky behavior over the course of the study adjusted their social prototypes by *lowering* their evaluations of people who tended to engage in risky behaviors. Students who reported an increase in risky behaviors over the course of the study *raised* their evaluations of the prototypical risk taker. Each student's tendency toward social comparison moderated the impact of social prototypes on his or her risky behavior. This study

■ **social prototype** the predominant social image an individual associates with a particular group of people

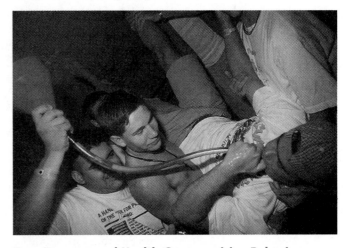

Peer Pressure and Health-Compromising Behavior
For many young adults, health behaviors are often reactions to social situations rather than rationally planned decisions. They drink because their friends drink, not because they have made a conscious decision that they enjoy alcohol. © Bruce Lee Smith / Liaison Agency

emphatically suggests that young people who are strongly inclined to compare their behaviors with significant others (high social comparison) tend to be most strongly affected by social prototypes.

Putting the Non-Stage Theories to the Test

Non-stage theories assume that people evaluate the perceived pros and cons of their actions and behave according to the outcome of this evaluation. These theories were the first health models subjected to extensive research, which generally has been supportive of the basic assumptions of the models (Strecher & Rosenstock, 1997).

- People's self-reported attitudes and intentions predict a variety of health-promoting actions, including weight loss (Schifter & Ajzen, 1985), exercise (Godin, Valois, & Lepage, 1993), reducing dietary fat (Sparks & Shepherd, 1992), condom use (Fisher, Fisher, & Rye, 1995), smoking behavior (Fishbein, 1982), breast and testicular self-examination (Lierman, Kasprzyk, & Benoliel, 1991), mammography utilization (Brubaker & Wickersham, 1990), cancer screening (Conner & Sparks, 1996), and willingness to donate blood (Bagozzi, 1981).

- People are more likely to have regular dental checkups, practice safe sex, and engage in other health-protective behaviors if they feel susceptible to the various health problems that might stem from failure to do so (Abraham & Sheeran, 1994).

- Educational interventions aimed at changing health beliefs do increase health-protective behaviors. For example, women who receive educational messages aimed at enhancing their knowledge of the benefits of mammography are nearly four times more likely to seek mammography than women in a control group (Champion, 1994).

- Cues to action such as postcard reminders of scheduled dental and medical appointments increase people's likelihood of engaging in preventive health measures (Agars & McMurray, 1993).

- A substantial amount of recent research supports the concept of behavioral willingness in health-related behaviors. Surveys conducted with sexually active teens, for example, demonstrate that sexual activity often is reactive rather than planned (Ingham, Woodcock, & Stenner, 1991). The same is apparently true of driving while drinking (Gerrard, Gibbons, Benthin, & Hessling, 1996).

- Support for the idea of reasoning by prototypes comes from evidence that the more favorable an adolescent's image of smokers, the more likely he or she is to smoke (Chassin et al., 1987). Adolescent images of the typical drinker have also been shown to predict changes in drinking behavior among adolescents and college students (Blanton, Gibbons, Gerrard, Congder, & Smith, 1997). In addition, adolescents who have a favorable image of the typical unwed teenage parent report a greater willingness to engage in unprotected sex (Gibbons & Gerrard, 1995).

Shortcomings of the Non-Stage Theories

One difficulty with the non-stage theories is that people do not always do what they intend (or claim they intend) to do. People's attitudes predict some health-related behaviors, such as drinking, but not others, such as driving and drinking (Stacy, Bentler, & Flay, 1994).

Another shortcoming is that the predictive power of the non-stage theories is greater for some groups (such as those with above-average income and education) than for others. And as we have seen, in some studies, ethnicity or socioeconomic status has proved to be a better predictor of health-screening behaviors than attitudes and perceived benefits or barriers.

The theories also ignore a person's past experiences with a specific health-related behavior. One study pitted the theory of reasoned action and the theory of planned behavior against a modified version of the theory of reasoned action that included a specific past health behavior, use of alcohol (O'Callaghan, Chang, Callan, & Baglioni, 1997). Although *intention* to drink accurately predicted drinking behavior, *past drinking behavior* along with the perception of what peers valued (subjective norms) most accurately predicted *intention*. Thus, the modified theory that included past behavior achieved the greatest overall accuracy in predicting alcohol use among young adults.

Attempts to explain the influence of past experiences on current health behavior suggest that these experiences may increase the degree of control people perceive over the behavior in question. When people believe that they can control their behavior, they are more likely to attempt to do so. For example, people who believe that they can be successful in losing weight are more likely to attempt to do so than those who do not (Schifter & Ajzen, 1985).

Stage Theories

An overweight uncle of mine continued to smoke and eat a high-fat diet despite his doctor's recommendation to modify these health-compromising behaviors. When pressed to explain why he wasn't changing his poor health habits, he replied that he was well aware of the risks and believed that he should improve his lifestyle—but he wasn't "ready." A few months later, after a nearly fatal heart attack, he declared that he was ready to quit smoking. And he did so. Unfortunately, he also "quit" 6 months later, and again this past winter. He struggled to reach his goal until the very end of his life. Does my uncle remind you of anyone you know?

Non-stage theories of health behavior attempt to identify variables that influence health-related behaviors and combine them into a formula that predicts the probability that a particular individual will act in a certain way in a given situation. For example, the theory of planned behavior might predict that my uncle

transtheoretical model (TTM) a widely used stage theory that contends that people pass through five stages in altering health-related behavior: precontemplation, contemplation, preparation, action, and maintenance

precaution adoption process model (PAPM) a stage model theory based on the assumption that people pass through seven discrete stages on their way to adopting precautionary health behaviors

continued to smoke because he had a positive attitude about smoking, because it was the accepted thing to do among his friends, and because it gave him control over his life. Stage theories, on the other hand, maintain that behavior often changes systematically through qualitatively distinct stages of development.

Stage theories are a familiar concept in psychology. Rather than resembling stages of cognitive or physical development, however, stages of health behavior do not follow a steady, linear process. Like my uncle, people who are struggling to lose weight, quit smoking, or become aerobically fit often take one step forward and two steps back before reaching their final goal. Although there may be a direct, linear path to the goal, multiple paths often exist. Stage theories recognize these possible variations and argue that attempting to use a single equation to model health-related behaviors distorts and oversimplifies the processes (Weinstein, Rothman, & Sutton, 1998).

The Transtheoretical Model

The **transtheoretical model (TTM)** is the most widely used stage theory in health psychology. Initially developed to explain smoking behavior, the model has been applied to a variety of health-related behaviors, including exercise, mammography, and safe sex (Prochaska, Redding, Harlow, Rossi, & Velicer, 1994; Sutton, 1997).

The TTM contends that people progress through five stages in altering health-related behaviors. The stages are defined in terms of past behavior and intentions for future action.

Stage 1: Precontemplation. During this stage, people are not seriously thinking about changing their behavior. They may even refuse to acknowledge that their behavior needs changing.

Stage 2: Contemplation. During this stage, people acknowledge the existence of a problem (such as smoking) and are seriously considering changing their behavior (quitting smoking) in the near future (typically within 6 months).

Stage 3: Preparation. This stage includes both thoughts and action. In preparing to quit smoking, for example, a person obtains a prescription for a nicotine patch, joins a support group, enlists family support, and makes other specific plans.

Stage 4: Action. During this stage, people have actually changed their behavior and are trying to sustain their efforts.

Stage 5: Maintenance. People in this stage continue to be successful in their efforts to reach their final goal. Although this stage can last indefinitely, its length is often set arbitrarily at 6 months.

The TTM recognizes that people move back and forth through the stages in a nonlinear fashion. Like my uncle, many recently reformed ex-smokers relapse from *maintenance* to *preparation*, cycling through stages 2 to 5 one or more times until they have completed their behavioral change.

The TTM also acknowledges that different behavioral, cognitive, and social processes may come to the forefront as people struggle to reach their ultimate health goal. These include consciousness raising (for example, seeking more information about a health-compromising behavior), counterconditioning (substituting alternative behaviors for the target behavior), and reinforcement management (rewarding oneself or being rewarded by others for success).

The Precaution Adoption Process Model (PAPM)

Neil Weinstein and his colleagues have refined the transtheoretical model to explain why some people find it easier than others to move through stages of health promotion (Weinstein & Sandman, 1992; Weinstein et al., 1998). The **precaution adoption process model (PAPM)** is based on the assumption that people pass through seven discrete stages on the way to adopting precautionary health behaviors (see Figure 6.6).

To understand these stages, consider the issue of binge drinking among college students. In stage 1, a new student is unaware of the importance of the issue to his or her health. In stage 2, the student becomes aware of the issue (perhaps by reading a magazine article or by observing the drinking behavior of other students) but does not feel that it concerns him or her (you may recognize this as an example of the optimistic bias). In stage 3, the student becomes engaged by the issue (perhaps in response to social pressures to drink more often) and feels that he or she needs to make a personal decision regarding drinking. The decision may be not to take any precautionary steps—not to change his or her drinking behavior—at least for the moment (stage 4) or to adopt the precaution by setting a personal limit to drinking or stopping the behavior completely (stage 5). If the student opts to maintain his or her drinking behavior, obviously the process ends at stage 4. If the student chooses to change the behavior, he or she enters stage 6, initiating the behavior change. Stage 7 entails successful maintenance of the new habit (or absence of the old habit) over some period of time.

Although similar to the transtheoretical model, the PAPM has several unique features. First, it distinguishes between people who are unaware of a health issue and those who are aware of the issue but have not considered its personal significance (stages 1 and 2). Second, it

Figure 6.6

Stage 7 (Maintenance)
"I haven't consumed more than 3 drinks on one occasion in over a year. I'll never go back to my old binge drinking lifestyle."

Stage 6 (Implementation)
"I've begun to avoid parties where binge drinking is likely to occur, in order to change my drinking habits."

Stage 5 (Intention to change)
"I'm going to let my friends know that I've decided to avoid binge drinking."

Stage 4 (No change)
"Binge drinking may be hazardous to my health, but I have to go along with my friends, at least for now."

Stage 3 (Engagement)
"I really need to make a decision about binge drinking since it's happening at so many of the parties I attend."

Stage 2 (Optimistic bias)
"I've heard that binge drinking may be dangerous, but I don't think anything can happen to me."

Stage 1 (Ignorance)
"I really don't know anything about the health aspects of binge drinking."

The Precaution Adoption Process Model
The precaution adoption process model (PAPM) is based on the assumption that when people consider new behaviors aimed at protecting their health, they pass through seven discrete stages. This theory takes into account several factors that are not considered in other theories—for example, whether the person has considered the issue and then how that affects his or her decision to act.

differentiates between people who have decided not to act (stage 4) and those who are not acting because they have not considered the issue (stages 1 and 2). Finally, as noted earlier, it identifies several of the factors that determine why some people find it harder than others to move from one stage to the next. Perceptions of personal vulnerability to the health threat, for example, are believed to be important in determining whether a person decides to take precautionary action (move from stage 3 to stage 5). Situational obstacles are thought to play a large role in moving from an intention to act (stage 5) to the action itself (stage 6).

Putting the Stage Theories to the Test

The approach used most often to test stage theories is to compare the health attitudes of people whose behaviors place them in different stages. In general, the research has supported the validity of these theories. For example, Hans De Vries and Esther Backbier (1994) compared pregnant women whose smoking behavior placed them in the categories of precontemplators, contemplators, or actors. As the transtheoretical model predicted, contemplators and actors professed stronger beliefs regarding the hazards of smoking than did precontemplators, whereas actors were more likely to believe they could quit smoking than either precontemplators or contemplators.

The stage theories have been applied successfully to a variety of health-related behaviors: home radon testing (Weinstein & Sandman, 1992), osteoporosis prevention (Blalock et al., 1996), vaccination against hepatitis B (Hammer, 1997), smoking (DiClemente, 1991), breast cancer testing (Rakowski, Fulton, & Feldman, 1993), safe sex behaviors (Bowen & Trotter, 1995), HIV prevention (Prochaska et al., 1994), and diet (Glanz, Patterson, Kristal, & DiClemente, 1994).

Other research has shown that these theories have a very practical advantage: They promote the development of more effective health interventions by providing a "recipe" for ideal behavior change (Sutton, 1996). This enables clinical health psychologists and other practitioners to match an intervention to the specific needs of a person who is "stuck" at a particular stage (Perz, DiClemente, & Carbornari, 1996).

Let's take an example. Attempting to convince an obese person who is in the precontemplation stage to lose weight is likely to fail because people in this stage do not believe that they have a health problem. The most effective intervention at this time would be to encourage the person to *consider* changing his or her behavior, perhaps by providing information about the health hazards of obesity. On the other hand, a person in the preparation or action stage doesn't need additional persuasion to change his or her behavior. What he or she may need, however, are specific tips about how to enact an effective plan of action.

Updating Our Understanding of Health Behavior Theories

Research on the theories we've discussed reveals that they all predict health-related behavior moderately well. For example, they all identify variables that generally are more accurate than demographic factors in predicting health-related behaviors. Why, then, do health-related behaviors remain difficult to predict? Why aren't models of health behavior more precise? Several reasons have been suggested.

- The theories say little or nothing about how intentions are translated into actions.

- The theories are unrealistically complex. Many people consider only one or two aspects of a health threat before making a decision about preventive measures.

- Health habits are only modestly related. Knowing one health habit does not necessarily enable you to predict another. The person who exercises faithfully is not necessarily the person who wears a seatbelt. A teammate of mine on a competitive track team occasionally chews tobacco.

- Health habits are unstable over time. A person may stop smoking for a year but take it up again during a period of stress. Why? Different health habits are controlled by different factors, and these may shift over the course of a lifetime. Smoking may be related to stress, whereas exercise may depend on ease of access to sports facilities.

- It is unrealistic to expect that one theory will be sufficiently comprehensive to predict health-seeking behaviors for all disorders. The same underlying factors do not determine all health-related behaviors.

- For many people (especially the very young, the very old, and the very ill), health care decisions are made by another person, such as a parent or a caregiver.

- Although most theories recognize the existence of some type of barrier to seeking health care, the number of possible barriers is almost unlimited.

- For many people, the barriers to preventive measures are beyond the life experiences of the researchers. For example, barriers to health care for affluent European Americans are typically quite different from those of poor Hispanic-Americans or African-Americans (Cochran & Mays, 1990).

- No allowance is made in the theories for barriers such as racism and poverty.

■ **cognitive dissonance** the psychological tension we experience when our behavior conflicts with our beliefs or attitudes regarding that behavior

Health Attitudes and Behavior: A Reciprocal Relationship

Most theories of health-related behavior maintain that beliefs about health and illness—such as one's perceived vulnerability to a certain disease—guide decisions to engage in preventive behaviors (Harrison, Mullen, & Green, 1992). Recent evidence suggests that the relationship is bidirectional: Health-related behaviors also affect health beliefs.

The idea that behavior influences attitudes is not new. More than 40 years ago social psychologist Leon Festinger (1957) outlined his theory of **cognitive dissonance,** which is based on three central ideas. First, people prefer consistency in their beliefs and behaviors. For example, the belief "smoking causes cancer" is consistent with the behavior of not smoking. Second, when a person's beliefs and behaviors are inconsistent (such as when a person who believes smoking is harmful smokes), the result is an unpleasant state, similar to having a guilty conscience, called *dissonance.* Third, when people experience dissonance, they always take steps to reduce it, just as they do when experiencing other aversive states such as hunger, thirst, or being uncomfortably cold. Festinger argued that people reduce the psychological tension associated with their hypocritical behavior by either changing their behavior or changing their attitude. In our example, a smoker could quit smoking, decide that the smoking–cancer link isn't well established, or decide that the pleasures of smoking outweigh its costs.

Meg Gerrard and her colleagues at Iowa State University (1996) examined the reciprocal relationship between health beliefs and three risky adolescent behaviors: reckless driving, drinking, and smoking. Gerrard found that adolescents' perceptions of vulnerability increased as their participation in those behaviors increased. This indicates that adolescents do understand the relationship between risky behavior and vulnerability. Instead of denying the potential hazards associated with their risky behavior, the participants in Gerrard's study manipulated their thinking in order to allow them to deal with the inherent contradiction between their behavior and their knowledge of the danger. First, the teenagers overestimated the prevalence of risky behaviors among their peers, apparently reasoning that "If everyone is doing it, it can't be too dangerous." Second, they downplayed the influence of their health and safety concerns on their behavior. That is, they put such issues out of their mind. As the researchers note, in doing so the adolescents engaged in what appears to be a "Scarlett O'Hara strategy" in which they said to themselves, "I won't think about this now. I'll think about it tomorrow."

Gerrard's study has important implications for our understanding of the origins of risky health-related behaviors. Adolescents whose initial experimentation leads them to enjoy a specific risky behavior will begin to associate with others who engage in that behavior, which leads them to believe that the behavior is more prevalent than it actually is. Faulty reasoning such as this can have dramatic health consequences. Deborah Prentice and Dale Miller (1993) have demonstrated that college students who mistakenly believe that others share their accepting attitudes about excessive drinking are motivated to conform to their misperception that binge drinking is both common and expected.

Recent neuroimaging research suggests a potential physiological factor in the faulty reasoning that allows some adolescents to engage in impulsive, high-risk behaviors. Using *functional magnetic resonance imaging,* Abigail Baird and her colleagues (1999) compared the brain activity of a group of youths, ages 10 to 18, with that of a group of adults, ages 23 to 32, all of whom were shown a photograph of a person displaying extreme fear. Teenagers looking at the photograph, especially the youngest ones, displayed sharply increased activity in the amygdala, which plays an important role in the regulation of emotions (see Chapter 3). In contrast, the older adolescents and adults showed the greatest brain activity in their frontal lobes—the brain region involved in planning, insight, and rational thinking. Based on these findings, the researchers suggest that the frontal lobe may begin maturing only at age 17 or so, perhaps making it more difficult for young adolescents to think rationally about many issues, including the long-term hazards of high-risk behaviors.

The results of these studies suggest an obvious health intervention for adolescents. Given that most teens at least experiment with a variety of risky behaviors at an early age, it is important to examine cognitive shifts that promote the progression from experimentation to acceptable behavior. John Graham, Gary Marks, and William Hansen (1991) believe that health education programs should include efforts to correct teens' misperceptions about the prevalence of risky behaviors among their peers. In addition, educational interventions should encourage young adolescents to develop their frontal lobes by teaching them to think rationally about risky health behaviors.

Changing Health-Related Beliefs and Behaviors

Theories derive their greatest value from their application to real-world problems. In health psychology, a good theory enables psychologists to develop interventions that will help promote better health. Health campaigns have been divided into three categories: work site wellness programs, health education campaigns, and behavioral interventions.

Work Site Wellness Programs

The workplace is an ideal site for promoting health for several reasons. First, workers find such programs convenient to attend. Some employers even permit their employees to participate in prevention programs during the workday. In addition, the workplace offers the greatest opportunity for continuing contact, follow-through, and feedback. Finally, coworkers are available to provide social support and help motivate people during difficult moments.

Work site programs began to emerge at a rapid pace with the advent of the wellness movement during the 1980s. In the United States today, more than 80 percent of organizations with 50 or more workers offer some sort of health-promoting program (Scott, 1999). Work site wellness programs offer a variety of activities, including weight management, nutrition counseling, smoking cessation, preventive health screenings, educational seminars, stress management, low back care, fitness centers, immunization programs, and prenatal programs. In one effective low-cost program, a company simply replaced junk-food vending machines in dining areas with machines that dispense more nutritious foods and posted the nutritional value of such foods (Anderson, Cacioppo, & Roberts, 1995).

At the heart of the wellness movement was the realization that preventing disease is easier, cheaper, and far more desirable than curing disease. Worldwide, health care costs have risen from about 3 percent of world gross domestic product (GDP) in 1948 to 7.9 percent today. The United States currently spends 13.7 percent of its GDP on health care (World Health Organization, 2000). As noted earlier, an ever-increasing proportion of these costs has been passed along to employers who pay their employees' health insurance premiums. According to a 1999 William B. Mercer study, 97 percent of corporate health benefits costs are spent on treating preventable conditions such as cardiovascular disease, lower back problems, hypertension, stroke, bladder cancer, and alcohol abuse. Employers have realized that work site programs that are even modestly successful in improving employees' health can result in substantial savings.

Are such programs effective? A number of careful studies reveal that they are. The cost of the programs is more than offset by reductions in work-related injuries, absenteeism, and worker turnover. For instance, Union Pacific Railroad employees in a wellness group lowered their risk of high blood pressure (45 percent) and high cholesterol (34 percent), moved out of the at-risk range for obesity (30 percent), and quit smoking (21 percent), yielding a net savings to the company of $1.26 million (Scott, 1999).

Research studies have revealed that, to be successful, work site programs should

- be voluntary.
- include health screenings, which have the greatest impact on a work site's health costs.
- relate to health behaviors of interest to employees.
- ensure confidentiality of health information.
- be convenient and have company support.

- offer additional incentives, such as health insurance rebates, monetary bonuses, or other prizes for success.

Health Education Campaigns

There is probably a greater emphasis on health promotion today than at any other time in history. Substantial effort is devoted to shaping the public's views on health issues through educational campaigns in advertisements; on public transportation; in magazines and newspapers; and on television, radio, and Web sites. The importance of these campaigns is revealed in research controversies over how information should be presented (for example, should HIV-prevention campaigns emphasize safer sex or abstinence?).

Health education refers to any planned intervention involving communication that promotes the learning of healthier behavior (Kok, 1997). The most widely used model in health education and health promotion is the *precede/proceed model* (Green & Kreuter, 1990). According to the model, planning for health education begins by identifying specific health problems in a targeted group or community. Next, lifestyle and environment elements that contribute to the targeted health problem (as well as those that protect against it) are identified. Then, background factors that predispose, enable, and reinforce these lifestyle and environmental factors are analyzed to determine the possible usefulness of health education and other interventions. During the final, implementation phase, health education programs are designed, initiated, and evaluated.

Let's examine how the precede/proceed model would apply to a health education campaign for lung cancer. First, health psychologists would identify the target group for the intervention. Next, they would investigate environmental factors that might affect the target group because the disease might result from unhealthy working or living conditions in which people are exposed to hazardous pollutants. In addition, health psychologists would consider psychological and social factors. They would begin by determining who smokes. When did they start smoking? Why? Researchers have found that smoking typically begins during adolescence, largely in response to social pressures (Flay, 1985). These pressures include the imitation of family members, peers, and such role models as well-known actors and athletes. Many adolescents find it very difficult to resist social pressure. Being accepted by one's peers is an extremely important source of reinforcement. There are also strong enabling factors: Cigarettes are generally very easy to obtain and sanctions against smoking are minimal.

Having determined which factors contributed to the health problem, health psychologists would design a health education program to counteract those factors. For example, if social pressure was found to be a major factor, they might design a health education program that focused on improving the ability of teens to resist social pressure. Such programs might involve role models urging teens not to smoke, adopting antismoking policies in public buildings,

health education any planned intervention involving communication that promotes the learning of healthier behavior

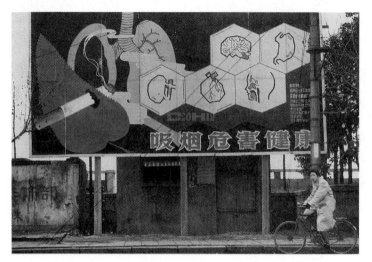

Antismoking Campaign in China
Although the number of smokers in the United States has decreased recently, the reverse seems to be occurring in other countries, such as China. Billboards such as this one can be understood by everyone, no matter what their native language. © David Wells / The Image Works

imposing stricter sanctions against the sale of cigarettes, and/or levying higher taxes on cigarettes.

How effective are health education campaigns? Researchers have found that education campaigns that merely inform people of the hazards of health-compromising behaviors are typically ineffective in motivating people to change long-held health habits (Green & McAlister, 1984). For example, antismoking messages and other drug education programs by themselves often have little effect—or a negative effect. In one study, teenagers who had participated in a school-sponsored drug education program were actually *more likely* to use alcohol, marijuana, and LSD than a control group of students who had not participated in the course (Stuart, 1974). Simply finding out that one's lifestyle is not as healthy as it could be is often is insufficient to provoke change because many people believe they are exempt or invulnerable to the negative consequences of their risky behavior.

Generally speaking, multifaceted community campaigns that present information on several fronts work better than "single-shot" campaigns. For example, antismoking campaigns that combine school intervention programs with communitywide mass media messages have proved to be more effective in reducing smoking among fourth- to sixth-grade students than campaigns consisting only of school intervention.

Community programs are on the rise because a large body of research evidence indicates that rates of morbidity and mortality are linked to social conditions such as poverty, unstable living conditions, community disorganization, poor education, social isolation, and unemployment (Adler & Matthews, 1994; Williams & Lund, 1992). The goal of community-based intervention is to create a social infrastructure that supports the efforts of each community member to improve the quality of his or her life (Heller, King, Arroyo, & Polk, 1997).

Community programs have several important advantages. First, they can promote changes that are difficult for individuals to accomplish, such as creating bike paths and other public exercise facilities or banning smoking in public offices. Second, unlike interventions that concentrate on high-risk individuals, community programs reach out to a broader cross section of the public, potentially reaching those in the lower- to moderate-risk categories earlier in the process of disease (Altman, 1995). Third, community programs combine information with the social support of friends, neighbors, and family members.

One of the earliest community campaigns was initiated in 1972 for residents of a rural county in Finland with a very high incidence of coronary heart disease (Kottke, Puska, Salonen, Tuomilehto, & Nissinen, 1984). Organized by the government, the program's goal was to reduce smoking, cholesterol, and blood pressure levels through informational campaigns. The initial 5-year follow-up study demonstrated a 17.4 percent reduction in these coronary risk factors among men and an 11.5 percent reduction among women. In addition, coronary disability payments had declined by approximately 10 percent, much more than enough to pay for the entire community program. A 10-year follow-up showed a 22 percent decrease in mortality from coronary heart disease.

Not all community interventions are successful, however. Campaigns are expensive to run and require massive organization efforts to reach all the residents (Susser, 1995). In addition, community campaigns must continue for several years before noticeable effects occur.

Message Framing

An important factor in the effectiveness of health education is how information is worded, or *framed*. Health messages generally are framed in terms of the benefits associated with a particular preventive action or the costs of failing to take preventive action (Rothman & Salovey, 1997).

Gain-Framed Messages versus Loss-Framed Messages

Gain-framed messages focus on the positive outcome from adopting a health-promoting behavior ("If you get a mammogram, you are likely to find out that you are healthy") or on avoiding an undesirable outcome ("If you get a mammogram, you decrease the risk of an undetected, potentially life-threatening tumor"). **Loss-framed messages** emphasize the negative outcome from failing to take preventive action ("If you don't utilize mammography, you increase the risk of an undetected, potentially life-threatening tumor"). Loss-framed messages may also emphasize missing a desirable outcome ("If you don't get a mammogram, you will not know whether you are healthy").

Which are more effective in promoting behavior change, gain-framed or loss-framed messages? Researchers have discovered that it depends on the type of behavior in question. For **detection behaviors**—behaviors aimed at identifying symptoms of illness such as health screening—loss framing has a strong advantage. In one study, undergraduate women received videotaped messages or informational pamphlets about breast self-examination and mammography; the messages were either gain- or loss-framed. A follow-up revealed that participants who received loss-framed messages were more likely than those who received gain-framed messages to obtain mammograms within one year (Banks et al., 1995; Meyerowitz, Wilson, & Chaiken, 1991). Loss-framed messages have also proved effective in promoting skin cancer screening (Block & Keller, 1995) and HIV testing (Kalichman & Coley, 1995).

gain-framed message a health message that focuses on attaining positive outcomes, or avoiding undesirable ones, by adopting a health-promoting behavior

loss-framed message a health message that focuses on a negative outcome from failing to perform a health-promoting behavior

detection behaviors behaviors designed to identify symptoms of sickness, such as health screening

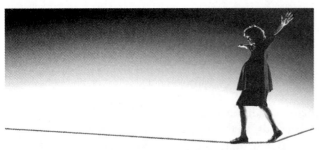

Don't Put Your Baby's Health On The Line.

Get Prenatal Care Early • Call 1-800-311-2229 • Confidential

Take Care of Yourself So You Can Take Care of Your Baby.

Message Wording Makes a Difference
Educational campaigns may use gain-framed or loss-framed messages, as shown here. However, research has found that the message's effectiveness depends on the behavior to be changed. Loss-framed messages ("Don't put your baby's health on the line") work best for detection behaviors. Gain-framed messages are most appropriate for prevention behaviors. For example, a gain-framed message regarding prenatal care would probably say, "Take care of yourself while you are pregnant and you'll have a healthy child." Courtesy of The Advertising Council / Healthy Start

Loss-framed messages are more effective than gain-framed messages because they highlight the immediate consequences of engaging in detection behavior. The reasoning goes as follows: First, detection behaviors such as breast and testicular self-examinations, mammography, and HIV screening are performed to see if people are sick, not to see if they are healthy, and so they entail an element of risk (Rothman & Salovey, 1997). Second, because behaviors are frequently evaluated in terms of their short-term consequences (Herrnstein, 1990), decisions to engage in risky behaviors have little immediate reinforcement. Detection behaviors provide long-term rather than immediate benefits. Third, their benefits are indirect at best. A detection behavior detects the illness; long-term benefits (reinforcement) depend on subsequent treatment (Rothman & Salovey, 1997.) To the extent that performing illness-detecting actions is perceived to involve risk, loss-framed messages should be more effective because they highlight an immediate consequence for engaging in such behaviors.

In contrast to detection behaviors, **prevention behaviors**—behaviors designed to stave off illness, such as using sunscreen—provide a relatively certain, desirable outcome (maintaining healthy skin and averting skin cancer). Given that loss-framed messages facilitate preferences for risky options, they might actually undermine prevention behaviors such as sunscreen use. Conversely, gain-framed information might promote prevention-oriented health behaviors. Indeed, gain-framed messages have led to stronger intentions to exercise (Robberson & Rogers, 1988), use infant car seats (Christophersen & Gyulay, 1981), use sunscreen (Rothman, Salovey, Antone, & Keough, 1993), and engage in other skin cancer prevention behaviors (Block & Keller, 1995).

Loss-Framed Fear Appeals

In a ninth-grade health class I remember watching a brutally graphic film showing the rotting sores of victims of "venereal disease." Despite the good intentions of the film in promoting personal hygiene, the implicit message of the film seemed to be *NEVER, EVER, HAVE SEX.*

Are fear-arousing messages effective in promoting attitude and behavior change? To find out, Irving Janis and Seymour Feshbach (1953) compared the effectiveness of messages that aroused various levels of fear in promoting

■ **prevention behaviors** behaviors designed to stave off sickness, such as wearing sun block

changes in dental hygiene. Janis and Feshbach discovered that messages that aroused moderate levels of fear were more effective than more extreme messages in getting junior high school students to change their dental hygiene habits. In accounting for their results, the researchers suggested that individuals and circumstances differ in the optimal level of fear for triggering a change in attitude or behavior. When this level is exceeded, people may resort to denial or avoidance coping measures.

A key factor in determining the effectiveness of threatening health messages is the recipient's perceived *self-efficacy*. Before they can be persuaded, people must believe that they have the ability to follow through on recommendations. In one study, Carol Self and Ronald Rogers (1990) presented highly threatening messages regarding the dangers of sedentary living with or without information indicating that the subjects could perform the health-enhancing behavior (such as exercise) and succeed in enhancing their health. What did they find? Threat appeals worked only if participants were convinced that they could cope with the health threat; attempts to frighten participants without reassuring them were ineffective.

Scare tactics that arouse tremendous fear, such as photographs of grossly decayed or diseased gums, tend to upset people. As a result, such messages may backfire and actually *decrease* a person's likelihood of changing his or her beliefs and hence his or her behavior (Beck & Frankel, 1981). Such messages increase the person's anxiety to such a level that the only coping avenue they perceive open to them is a refusal to face the danger.

Behavioral Interventions

Behavioral interventions in health promotion are based on principles of learning. With this strategy, the health psychologist identifies the target behavior to be modified (for example, high blood pressure), measuring the current status of the behavior (including the context in which it occurs and its antecedent cues) and examining its consequences. The antecedents and consequences are manipulated in an effort to modify the behavior's rate of occurrence. The key to this process is removing reinforcement for health-compromising behaviors and providing reinforcers for healthy behaviors. This approach has proved useful for increasing a variety of healthy behaviors, including practicing good dental hygiene and controlling obesity.

Traditional behavior therapy derives from two forms of learning (see Chapter 1): classical conditioning (also called Pavlovian conditioning or respondent conditioning) and operant conditioning. One form of behavior modification that derives from classical conditioning is **aversion therapy,** which involves following an undesired behavior (such as eating foods high in cholesterol) with a negative consequence (such as nausea). The effectiveness (as well as the

aversion therapy a type of behavior therapy in which the person learns to associate a negative consequence with an undesired behavior

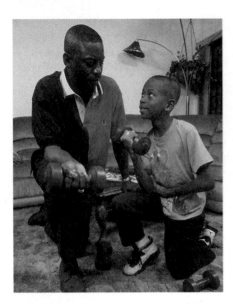

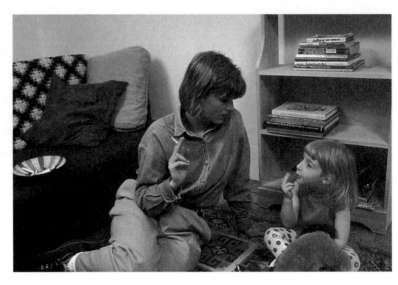

Behavior Learned by Imitation

According to Bandura's social learning theory, a major form of learning involves the imitation of significant, usually authoritative people we respect. As young children, we tend to imitate the behavior of our parents, then extend our modeling to teachers and others we admire. However, modeling is not restricted to "good" behaviors; people also model smoking, drinking, hitting, or some other negative behavior.
© Jeffrey Dunn/Stock, Boson Inc./PictureQuest; © Will Hart/PhotoEdit/PictureQuest

■ **token economy** an operant conditioning procedure in which desired behavior is rewarded with tokens that can be exchanged for various types of reward

■ **modeling** learning by observing (and imitating) a role model

ethics) of aversive conditioning have been the subject of heated debate, but a number of research studies demonstrate its effectiveness in dealing with smoking, overeating, and the paraphilias (nontraditional sexual behaviors).

Two notable and widely used types of behavioral techniques are *token economies* and *modeling*. In a **token economy,** small tokens (such as marbles) are awarded for desirable behavior (and sometimes taken away for undesirable behavior) and can later be exchanged for favored rewards such as money or special privileges. In an institutional setting, the token economy creates the orderliness of a market economy, in which certain behaviors are assigned specific values within the parameters of a monetary system (Davison, 1997).

Modeling involves learning a desired behavior by observing and imitating a role model. It is widely used as an efficient way to teach complex patterns of behavior. Because of the many social influences that cause teens to begin smoking, preventive interventions have often been based on peer modeling procedures. One of the best known is the 3-year Houston Project (Evans et al., 1981), which was based on Albert Bandura's social learning theory. The premise behind this study was that adolescents acquire expectations about smoking by observing others—for example, seeing popular artists and musicians smoke and then receiving positive reinforcement (social approval), adolescents are more likely to smoke themselves.

The Houston Project developed a program of persuasive intervention aimed at inoculating adolescents against the social influences that caused them to smoke. It included films and posters of highly admired role models to educate students about effective techniques for resisting social pressures to smoke. Other messages presented information about the negative physical consequences of smoking. Since the 1980s, efforts such as these have generally reported good success rates, reducing smoking onset rates by 50 percent or so in typical samples of subjects.

Behavioral methods have also proved effective in increasing mammography use (Lerman & Rimer, 1995) and participation in DNA testing for cancer risk (Glanz et al., 1994). They have shown success in promoting dietary changes (Brownell & Wadden, 1992), changes in smoking behavior (Lichtenstein & Glasgow, 1992), increases in physical exercise (Dubbert, 1992), and HIV risk reduction (Jemmott & Jemmott, 2000).

Although behavior therapies have proved useful for increasing a number of health behaviors, the effectiveness depends on several factors, including the types of reinforcement used; the age, gender, ethnicity, and sociocultural background of the person; and the person's level of motivation. For example, in changing smoking behavior, strength of motivation is important, but age, over a certain level, does not seem to be a factor.

In this chapter we have explored a number of factors that promote health and prevent illness, as well as factors that are potential barriers to wellness. More important than any single factor is getting people to realize their vulnerability to behavior-related health problems. Only then will they make an effort to modify their health-compromising behaviors. An especially important health-related behavior—eating wisely—is the subject of the next chapter.

Summing Up

Health and Behavior

1. Most behaviors affect health in some way: for better (behavioral immunogens) or worse (behavioral pathogens), directly or indirectly, immediately or over the long term.

2. Although the estimated human life span has not changed since the turn of the twentieth century, average life expectancy and the number of well years have increased dramatically. This increase has been attributed to people's efforts to modify their lifestyles in ways that will increase their DALE and well years.

3. Researchers distinguish three categories of injury and disease prevention. Primary prevention refers to actions to prevent a disease or injury from occurring. Secondary prevention involves actions to treat an illness early in its course. Tertiary prevention involves actions taken to contain damage once a disease has progressed beyond its early stages. Most medical care is tertiary in nature.

The Rocky Road to Wellness

4. There are a number of barriers to health promotion. At the individual level behavioral immunogens and pathogens are subject to a gradient of reinforcement in which the immediate reinforcement for pleasurable health-compromising behaviors such as smoking outstrips the long-term rewards of many health-promoting behaviors. At the family level, the health habits and attitudes of family members exert powerful influences on the individual. Within the health system, prevention remains a relatively minor focus in traditional medicine, and many people cannot afford health coverage. At the community level, people are more likely to adopt health-enhancing behaviors when these behaviors are promoted by community organizations, such as schools, governmental agencies, and the health care system.

5. It is estimated that only three out of every five patients comply fully with their medical treatment regimens.

Many factors are related to compliance, including the patient's satisfaction with his or her physician, the quality of doctor–patient communication, the complexity of the treatment, and patient confidence in a treatment regimen.

6. Leventhal investigated four components in how people conceptualize illness: identifying the disease, understanding the time line, perceiving consequences, and determining the causes. Researchers have also found reasoning about illness varies with age and is often faulty. For example, most people have an optimistic bias and believe they are not likely to become ill.

Theories of Health Behavior

7. Non-stage theories assume that people make a single, rational decision regarding a particular health-related behavior. The health belief model and the theory of reasoned action assume that personal belief about health and illness, attitudes toward certain health behaviors, and social influences are important factors in determining health behavior. The theory of planned behavior emphasizes the importance of believing that one can control his or her health (self-efficacy) in promoting actual change in health behaviors.

8. The prototype/willingness theory, also a non-stage theory, is based on the assumption that many health behaviors are unplanned reactions to social situations. This being the case, behavioral willingness and social prototypes associated with certain health behaviors may be more important in determining whether a person engages in risky behavior than are deliberate behavioral intentions.

9. Stage theories assume that health behavior is usually not a steady, linear process. The transtheoretical model outlines five stages through which people progress in altering health-related behaviors. The precaution adoption progress model outlines seven stages of behavior change and identifies several factors that determine why some people find it difficult to move from one stage to the next. Stage theories may promote the development of more effective interventions by enabling practitioners to match an intervention to the needs of a person at a particular stage.

10. Several reasons have been suggested for why health behavior theories don't always predict health-related behaviors. For one, different habits are often controlled by different factors, and these may change. In addition, the theories may not place enough importance on interpersonal processes, public policy, and various barriers such as racism or poverty.

Changing Health-Related Beliefs and Behaviors

11. Health campaigns have been divided into three categories: work site wellness programs, health education campaigns, and behavioral interventions. Today, most organizations with 50 or more workers offer some form of work site wellness program. The cost of such programs has proved to be more than offset by reductions in work-related injuries, absenteeism, and worker turnover.

12. Carefully planned health education campaigns that present information on several fronts and are community based often can promote changes that are difficult for individuals to accomplish. Community programs reach out to a broader cross section of the public.

13. Message framing is a critical factor in the effectiveness of health education. Research on messages that promote detection behaviors has shown strong support for the advantage of loss-framed messages. Gain-framed messages tend to be more effective in promoting prevention behaviors. Fear-arousing messages tend to be more effective with adults than with young children. Such messages may backfire, however, and actually decrease a person's likelihood of changing his or her behaviors.

14. Behavioral interventions such as aversion therapy, modeling, and token economies have proved useful for promoting a number of health behaviors.

Key Terms and Concepts

behavioral pathogen, p. 220
behavioral immunogen, p. 220
average life expectancy, p. 221

life span, p. 222
disability-adjusted life expectancy (DALE), p. 224

well year, p. 224
primary prevention, p. 224
secondary prevention, p. 224

Health Psychology on the World Wide Web

Web Address	Description
www.awhp.org	Web site of the Association for Worksite Health Promotion.
http://www.behavior.net/	An on-line gathering place for those interested in the applied social and behavioral sciences.
www.healthpsych.com	An educational forum pertaining to all facets of health psychology, including risk management, wellness programs, and cognitive-behavioral interventions in medical settings.

Critical Thinking Exercise

Risky Health-Related Behaviors

In the chapter opening, you were introduced to Anthony, a 20-year-old college sophomore, who is very casual about his health. Although he is aware of the hazards, he engages in health-compromising behaviors.

Researchers have found that unhealthy habits such as Anthony's tend to be related, just as healthy behaviors also tend to go together. Although people take risks at any age, young adults like Anthony seem to be especially prone to risk taking. Using the biopsychosocial model to guide your thinking, prepare answers to the following questions as you diagnose the roots of Anthony's risky health-related behaviors.

1. What are some of the biological influences on the tendency of young adults to take health-related risks?

2. What are some of the psychological influences on the tendency of young adults to take health-related risks?

3. What are some of the social influences on the tendency of young adults to take health-related risks?

4. Which of the models of health behavior discussed in the chapter makes the most sense in accounting for a risk taker such as Anthony? Explain your reasoning.

5. Suppose you were asked by your college or university to design a health campaign to reduce risky health-related behaviors among students. Based on the research discussed in the chapter, what types of interventions are likely to be effective? What types of interventions are likely to be ineffective?

7

Nutrition, Obesity, and Eating Disorders

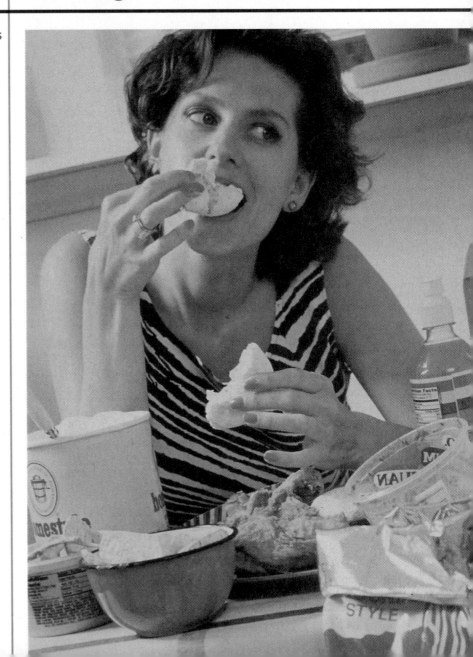

Jodi is 26 years old and weighs 78 pounds. She was once a sleek and muscular 800-meter track champion and an academic All-American. Before that she was valedictorian of her high school graduating class and voted "most likely to succeed." Today she is hospitalized with serious coronary complications resulting from her 12-year battle with disordered eating. But even now, Jodi sees herself not as emaciated and malnourished but as bloated and obese.

Growing up in an upper-middle-class home, Jodi had two loving parents and a terrific older sister. Yet ever since she was a child, she felt pressure to live up to her family's high expectations. She found it particularly difficult to follow in the footsteps of her talented and popular sister. By the time she entered college, Jodi felt that she had to be perfect at everything.

Unfortunately, her major imperfection was that she did not look like the swimsuit models and actresses many of her friends admired. Jodi had a short, powerful build that was well suited for running fast. Even though she was the top runner on her high school and college teams, her coaches and trainers believed that she could run faster if she would only shed a few pounds.

Jodi tried her best to lose weight, but her body simply wouldn't cooperate for very long. She tried several diet plans but felt so tired and hungry that she was unable to concentrate on her schoolwork and never stayed on a diet for very long. Her weight bounced up and down like a yo-yo.

Then one day Jodi found the answer to her weight problem: She would eat whatever and whenever she wanted and then either make herself throw up or take a large dose of laxatives. She also redoubled her training efforts, increasing her daily running mileage and adding cross-training workouts of lap swimming or spinning on a bicycle trainer. She still felt tired, but at least she was gaining some control over her weight.

Because she maintained a fairly stable weight, Jodi was able to hide her bingeing and purging throughout high school and college; when she was living on her own, however, she started eating less and less and her weight loss soon became obvious. One holiday, while visiting her family, she fainted while playing basketball with her father. When he picked her up, he realized that she weighed little more than a child.

Jodi's parents insisted that she see a doctor, who quickly placed her into a treatment program in which she was force-fed for a week. Although Jodi's weight has increased, the years of disordered eating have taken a severe toll on her body, and her prospects for regaining her health are not promising.

■ **obesity** excessive accumulation of body fat

Throughout most of history, a full figure was considered a sign of prosperity and health. How ironic, then, that today **obesity** (having excess body fat) threatens the health of more than half the citizens of the richest nation in the world (see Figure 7.1). Although 61 percent of the adult population in the United States are overweight or obese—easily qualifying the condition for epidemic status—obesity is even more prevalent elsewhere, such as in Western Samoa and several other Pacific islands (Gibbs, 1996).

More people are treated for obesity in this country than for all other health conditions combined. A staggering $30 billion is spent each year on commercial weight-loss programs alone (Gura, 1997). Add to this the $15 billion spent in treating the many chronic diseases caused by it, including diabetes, heart disease, gallstones, and hypertension, and the $23 billion in indirect costs for missed days of work and you begin to understand the scope of the problem—a problem that sends approximately 300,000 women and men to early graves each year.

Still, each year dozens of new weight "solutions" appear, from liquid diets to appetite-suppressing "aroma sticks," most of which fail (in controlled clinical trials) to reduce the weight of even a handful of obese participants for any length of time.

Although losing weight has clear benefits for obese people, they are not the only ones concerned about weight. We are bombarded with media images of movie stars, sports figures, and other celebrities that shape our standards of attractiveness. The current emphasis on thinness strongly influences how we feel about our bodies. Most American women, for example, feel that they weigh somewhat more than men prefer, and much more than the ideal body weight for women. This negative body image has been reported in girls as young as 10 years of age. Although men are generally more satisfied with their bodies, most believe that the ideal masculine physique is more muscular than their own.

Figure 7.1

Prevalence of Overweight and Obese Americans
Data from the National Health and Nutrition Examination Survey (NHANES) reveal that 25 years ago, 47 percent of Americans were classified as overweight or obese; today, 61 percent of U.S. adults between the ages of 20 and 74 years are overweight or obese. Americans are fatter today than their parents and grandparents ever were, and they are getting fatter every year.

Source: Centers for Disease Control and Prevention, National Center for Health Statistics, National Health and Nutrition Examination Surveys (http://www.cdc.gov/nchs/products/pubs/pubd/hestats/obese/obse99t2.htm).

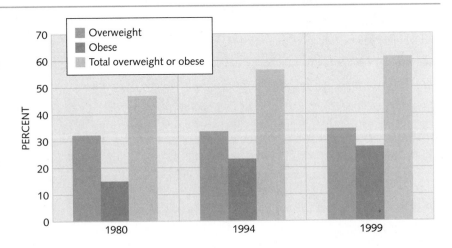

The goal of health psychology is to help people attain and maintain a *healthy weight*, not necessarily the cultural ideal. To this end, psychologists have joined forces with molecular biologists, genetic engineers, nutritionists, and other health professionals in the search for answers to some of eating behavior's most puzzling questions. Why is obesity becoming more prevalent, not just in the United States but also in developed countries throughout the world? Why is it relatively simple to lose a little weight but nearly impossible to keep it off? How is it that some people can eat whatever they want without gaining weight, while others remain overweight despite constant dieting? Why do some of the best and brightest teenagers literally starve themselves to death in order to reduce their body fat from 3.5 percent to 3 percent?

We begin our exploration of eating behavior and weight regulation by examining the components of food and their role in maintaining health.

- **calorie** a measure of food energy equivalent to the amount of energy needed to raise the temperature of 1 gram of water 1 degree Celsius

- **kilocalorie** a measure of food energy equal to 1,000 calories

Nutrition: Eating the Right Foods

How many times have you heard it? You are what you eat. In 1948, a healthy American breakfast consisted of a plate of fried eggs, a rasher of bacon, and several pieces of buttered toast. People spooned sugar and fatty cream from the top of milk bottles into their coffee. Given this nutritional nightmare researchers descended on the town of Framingham, Massachusetts, to find out why 1 in 4 men age 55 or older developed heart disease. Doctors didn't know what was killing their patients, often listing acute indigestion as the cause of death.

After 50 years and over 1,000 scholarly research papers, the Framingham Heart Study has shown that poor nutrition is a leading risk factor in the development of heart disease (Dawber, 1980). A healthy diet that focuses on fruits and vegetables while limiting the consumption of total fat and saturated fat provides the body with the nutrients it needs to protect and repair itself.

The Components of a Healthy Diet

The average adult male requires approximately 2,300 to 3,100 calories per day to maintain body weight; the average woman needs approximately 1,600 to 2,400 calories. A **calorie** is the amount of heat necessary to raise the temperature of 1 gram of water 1 degree Celsius (1°C). No matter what their source, all calories supply the same amount of energy. Because the calorie refers to such a small amount in comparison to the energy requirements of humans and other animals, physiologists commonly use the **kilocalorie** (kcal) as a unit of reference (1 kcal = 1,000 calories). Nutritionists also use the kcal as the standard unit for measuring dietary energy; they refer to it as the *Calorie*, which is always capitalized to differentiate it from 1 calorie.

To calculate the number of calories in a certain food, multiply the number of grams of fat, protein, and carbohydrates in the food by the number of calories each food group provides (9, 4, and 4, respectively). Then add the total.

■ **marasmus** a growth-inhibiting disease of infancy caused by severe protein-calorie malnutrition

■ **kwashiorkor** a childhood disease resulting from protein-calorie deficiency

In addition to daily caloric energy, our bodies require forty-six *nutrients* (essential substances found in food) to remain healthy. A major source of nutrition is water, which helps transport nutrients throughout the bloodstream, removes wastes, and regulates the body's temperature. Besides water, the remaining nutrients are grouped into five categories: proteins, fats, carbohydrates, minerals, and vitamins. Each of these nutrient groups offers unique contributions to bodily function and health, and in the case of proteins, fats, and carbohydrates, the caloric energy our bodies need to meet the demands of daily living.

■ *Proteins* (including meat, fish, soybean products, and other vegetables such as legumes) are the building blocks of muscle, bone, hair, blood, antibodies, hormones, and virtually all other body tissues. Proteins are composed of twenty-two different organic molecules called *amino acids.* The body is able to manufacture thirteen of these amino acids from other fats and carbohydrates; the remaining nine, called *essential amino acids,* must be obtained directly through the foods we eat.

The typical diet in developed nations includes plenty of protein to meet the daily needs of the average person. Although protein deficiencies are rare in the United States and other developed countries, they are fairly common in developing countries around the world. For example, children in the first year of life may suffer severe protein-calorie malnutrition, which causes **marasmus,** a condition in which growth stops, the body wastes away, and death follows swiftly. Toddlers with protein deficiencies can develop **kwashiorkor,** a disease in which the child's stomach, face, and legs swell with water, often making the starving child appear well fed. The primary cause of these disorders in developing countries is an early switch from breast- to bottle-feeding. Although powdered infant formulas provide a balanced, nutritious diet, their value is undermined by the dirty water and unhygienic conditions under which they are often prepared; the result may be diarrhea followed by dehydration and malnutrition from lack of protein.

■ *Carbohydrates* constitute the major source of energy in our diet. They are also stored as a form of muscle fuel called *glycogen.* Carbohydrates are grouped into two categories: *complex carbohydrates* and *simple carbohydrates.* Complex carbohydrates are found in breads and cereals, cruciferous vegetables (broccoli, cauliflower, and cabbage), dark green leafy vegetables, legumes, pasta, root vegetables (potatoes and yams), citrus fruits, and yellow fruits and vegetables (melon, squash, and carrots). Because of their power-packed energy calories, these foods are the favorite pre-event meals of athletes who practice *carbo-loading* before important competitions.

Another type of complex carbohydrate, *dietary fiber,* includes pectin, cellulose, and the structural parts of plants that the body can't digest. Most of the dietary fiber that we consume passes undigested through the body, along the way helping to reduce blood cholesterol levels, regulate bowel

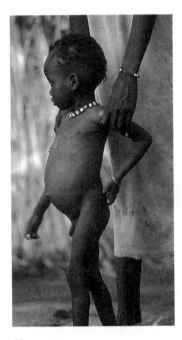

Marasmus
This young victim of the famine in southern Sudan (Pachalla) suffers from marasmus, which is caused by severe protein-calorie malnutrition. With this condition, growth stops and the body begins to waste away, and death follows shortly. © Alexis Duclos/Liaison Agency

function, and protect against heart disease and certain cancers. Despite the popular misconception that carbohydrates are fattening, complex carbohydrates are low in fat and calories. Nutritionists recommend that about half your daily calories should consist of complex carbohydrates.

Simple carbohydrates include *lactose,* which is the sugar found in dairy products; *maltose,* which is found in cereals and legumes; *glucose,* which is found in animal products; and *fructose,* or fruit sugar. Although simple carbohydrates are a rich source of quick energy, they have little nutritional value. In addition, a diet that is high in simple carbohydrates is often deficient in other important nutrients.

- *Fats,* or *lipids,* are the densest sources of food energy: 1 gram provides 9 calories, compared with 4 calories for each gram of carbohydrate or protein. The message is clear: You will consume twice as many calories from fats as you will from the same amount of carbohydrates or proteins. The body also converts fat into cholesterol, so consumption of high levels of fat increases the risk of certain diseases, such as colon cancer and heart disease.

  Fats are present in various amounts in a wide range of foods, including vegetable oils, cookies and cakes, dairy foods, and fatty cuts of meat. They are composed of three types of *fatty acids: saturated, monounsaturated,* and *polyunsaturated.* The greater the percentage of saturated fat in one's diet, the greater the impact on the body's cholesterol level.

- *Vitamins* are organic compounds that regulate a variety of vital functions, including *metabolism*—the process by which food energy is converted into body energy. Vitamins, which are found in small amounts in many foods, including eggs, vegetables, fruits, vegetable oils, and dairy products, also produce hormones and break down waste products.

  There are thirteen known vitamins, which are classified as either *fat-soluble* or *water-soluble.* Fat-soluble vitamins—A, D, E, and K—are carried in the fats we eat and are stored in the body's fatty tissue. Water-soluble vitamins, such as the B vitamins and vitamin C, travel in the bloodstream. The body stores only a small supply of water-soluble vitamins. The excess amounts are excreted in the urine.

- *Minerals* are inorganic elements, such as calcium, phosphorus, sodium, magnesium, iron, zinc, and selenium, which are found in many foods, including seafood, meats, grains, green leafy vegetables, and dairy products. Along with vitamins, minerals play an important role in many different physiological processes. Calcium is essential for strong muscle contraction, bone formation, and nerve transmission. Phosphorus plays a crucial role in building bones and cell division. Sodium is an *electrolyte* (a nutrient that conducts electricity) that is involved in the conduction of neural impulses through the nervous system. Magnesium is essential for efficient nerve functioning and bone mineralization. Iron is crucial for the production of

A Balanced Diet

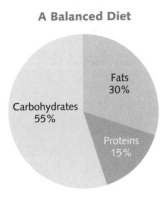

hemoglobin, the reddish pigment in red blood cells that transports oxygen. Zinc is involved in healing and growth, DNA synthesis, and healthy immune functioning. Selenium plays a role in the destruction of metabolic waste products called *free radicals,* which are unstable molecules that damage cells. Free radicals have been implicated in aging, cancer, and more than 50 other age-related diseases (Harman, 1993).

Nutritionists recommend a balanced diet in which 50 to 60 percent of our daily calories come from carbohydrates, 15 percent from protein, and no more than 30 percent from fat. However, their advice is frequently ignored (Mayo Clinic, 2001). Jane Wardle (1995) surveyed the dietary habits of 16,000 students (and their parents), including their efforts to avoid animal fat, salt, sugar, and food additives; to emphasize fiber and fruit in their nutrition; and to never skip breakfast. The disappointing results revealed only modest compliance; surprisingly, the students reported significantly *fewer* healthy habits than did their parents. Those who valued health highly, believed in the importance of diet in determining health, and felt responsible for determining their health most often practiced healthy dietary practices. This was true across all dietary practices—in both men and women—offering convincing support for cognitive models of health behaviors such as the theory of reasoned action (see Chapter 6).

The results of this survey may not surprise students, who often rely on fast foods to satisfy their appetites within the time constraints of a busy lifestyle. Consider breakfast—a meal that can be a mixture of the most and least nutritious foods. Nutritionists have observed an unhealthy trend in fast-food breakfasts: "dessert for breakfast" (Nutrition Action Newsletter, 2001). Health- and calorie-conscious students who would never consider having ice cream after a meal might be surprised to learn that an almond croissant or cinnamon scone from a popular coffee chain contains 630 calories, five teaspoons of sugar, and 16 to 18 grams of saturated fat—the equivalent of more than two ice cream bars.

Diet and Disease

Early dietary habits may set a lifelong pattern. And this pattern may lead to problems in later life. In fact, the foods we eat are implicated in five of the ten leading causes of death: heart disease, cancer, stroke, diabetes, and atherosclerosis (World Health Organization, 1990).

Excess dietary fat has been widely acknowledged as a major behavioral pathogen (Willett, 1994). Once inside the body, dietary fat becomes body fat very efficiently. The body expends only 3 calories to turn 100 calories of fat into body fat. In contrast, the body burns about 25 calories to turn the same amount of carbohydrates into body fat. To make matters worse, we crave fat, perhaps a legacy from our prehistoric ancestors, who lived in a time when regular meals and survival were both uncertain. As a result of this craving, about 40 to 45 percent of the total calories in the average Western diet come from fat.

Coronary Heart Disease

Consumption of fat, which becomes dietary cholesterol in the body, is a contributing factor in many adverse health conditions, including coronary heart disease. Cholesterol is a waxy substance essential for strong cell walls, myelination of nerve cells, and the production of hormones. However, the cholesterol we take in from the fats in our foods is nonessential because the liver manufactures all the cholesterol that the body needs. Dietary cholesterol—which comes from animal fats and oils, not from vegetables or plant products—circulates in the blood and so is called *serum cholesterol* (serum is the liquid part of the blood).

Serum cholesterol is found in several forms of proteins called *lipoproteins*. There are three types of lipoproteins, distinguished by their density. *Low-density lipoprotein (LDL)* and *very low-density lipoprotein (VLDL)* have been linked to the development of heart disease, whereas *high-density lipoprotein (HDL)* may offer some protection against heart disease. Cholesterol carried by LDL and VLDL is therefore often called "bad cholesterol," while HDL is referred to as "good cholesterol" because it helps clear away cholesterol deposits from cell walls and carries them to the liver, where they are broken down and then removed from the body.

Serum cholesterol level is expressed in milligrams (mg) of cholesterol per deciliter (dl) of serum. Therefore, a serum cholesterol level of 300 means 300 mg of cholesterol per deciliter of blood. The National Cholesterol Education Program (NCEP) therefore recommends keeping serum cholesterol below 200 mg/dl, LDL and VLDL levels below 100 mg/dl, and HDL levels above 40 mg/dl. They also call for everyone, beginning in their twenties, to obtain a complete serum cholesterol profile (total cholesterol, LDL cholesterol, HDL cholesterol, and triglycerides) every 5 years (NCEP, 2001).

A long-term prospective study of white males found that their serum cholesterol levels at age 22 accurately predicted their cardiovascular health decades later (Klag et al., 1993). At the beginning of the study, the participants were separated into three groups based on their average serum cholesterol level. Those in the high-risk group at age 22 (serum cholesterol between 209 mg and 315 mg) were 70 percent more likely to develop heart disease than were those in the low-risk group (cholesterol levels between 118 mg and 172 mg.)

Although cholesterol levels tend to increase with age, lowering blood cholesterol may not be important for people over the age of 70. Data from the Framingham study demonstrate a positive relationship between serum cholesterol level and death from coronary disease only up to age 60 (see Chapter 9). In older adults, serum cholesterol may provide some protection from heart disease, particularly among women (Kronmal, Cain, Ye, & Omenn,

1993). The Framingham study thus revealed an important point: The best predictor of heart disease is not total level of serum cholesterol; instead, the culprit is the amount of "bad cholesterol" (LDL and VLDL) in the body.

Even people with lower levels of total serum cholesterol are at increased risk of developing atherosclerosis if their HDL levels are very low. HDL levels below 35 mg/dl are considered unhealthy. Smoking, physical inactivity, and a high dietary intake of cholesterol and saturated fats are linked with increased levels of LDLs and decreased levels of HDLs. Certain types of polyunsaturated and monounsaturated fats, vitamin E, and a low-fat, high-fiber diet may protect against heart disease by elevating HDL levels.

Serum cholesterol level is determined partly by heredity. Some people seem to be able to consume a diet rich in fat without elevating serum cholesterol; others may have high cholesterol levels even though their diet is low in saturated fat. For most people, however, diet and lifestyle play a major role in the amount of serum cholesterol circulating in their bodies.

Cancer

Diet is implicated in one-third of all cancer deaths in the United States (Lichtenstein et al., 1998). The major dietary culprit in cancer is saturated fat, especially that found in animal products. Saturated fat has been linked to several cancers, including breast cancer, prostate cancer, and colorectal cancer (Toribara & Sleisenger, 1995).

Fortunately, there is also evidence that certain foods may protect us against cancer. Vegetables and fruits are rich in *beta-carotene,* which the body processes into vitamin A—a nutrient that helps ensure healthy immune system functioning. Along with beta-carotene, small amounts of the mineral selenium, found in fish, whole grains, and certain vegetables, may help prevent some forms of cancer (Glauert, Beaty, Clark, Greenwell, & Chow, 1990). A diet rich in vitamins C and E may also help prevent cancer by protecting body cells from the damaging effects of free radicals. Such a diet may also protect against carcinogenic *nitrosamines,* which are produced in the stomach when you eat foods laced with nitrates, nitrites, and other preservatives.

Weight Determination: Eating the Right Amount of Food

Naturally, it's not only what you eat but also how much you eat in relation to your body's caloric needs that determine your weight and your health. Before we discuss obesity—its causes and treatment—you first need to understand the basic mechanisms by which the body determines the type and amount of calories needed.

Basal Metabolic Rate and Caloric Intake

Body weight remains stable when the calories your body absorbs from the food you eat equal the calories it expends for basic metabolic functions plus physical activity. How many calories does your body need? This figure, called the **basal metabolic rate (BMR),** is the minimum number of calories your body needs to maintain bodily functions while at rest. Although BMR is not easily determined—because it depends on a number of variables, including your age, gender, current weight, and activity level—a rough estimate of your daily calorie needs *to maintain your current weight* can be calculated by multiplying your body weight (in pounds) by 13 (Mayo Clinic, 1996).

Individual differences in BMR help explain why it is possible for two people of the same age, height, and apparent activity level to weigh the same, even though one of them has a voracious appetite while the other merely picks at food. Several factors determine your BMR. First, heredity influences BMR: Some people have a naturally higher metabolic rate than others, even when they're asleep. Other people need fewer calories for the same amount and level of physical activity. Second, younger people and those who are active generally have a higher BMR than do older adults and those who are sedentary. Third, fat tissue has a lower metabolic rate (burns fewer calories) than muscle does. Thus, once you add fat to your body, you require less food to maintain your weight than you did in order to gain the weight in the first place. Finally, because men have more muscle, their bodies burn 10 to 20 percent more calories at rest than women's bodies do.

The Set-Point Hypothesis

Many people believe that their body weights fluctuate erratically, but in fact their bodies actually balance energy intake and expenditure quite closely. A typical adult consumes roughly 900,000 to 1 million calories a year. Subtract from this figure the energy costs of BMR and you'll discover that less than 1 percent of the calories you eat are stored as fat, a remarkable degree of precision in energy balance (Gibbs, 1996).

Evidence of such precision supports the **set-point hypothesis,** the idea that each of us has a body weight "thermostat" that continuously adjusts our metabolism and eating to maintain our weight within a genetically predetermined range, or set point (Keesey & Corbett, 1983). Early evidence for the set-point hypothesis came from experimental studies of voluntary starvation and overeating. During World War II, Ancel Keys studied 36 men who volunteered to participate in a study on semistarvation as an alternative to military service (Keys, Brozek, Henschel, Mickelsen, & Taylor, 1950). For the first 3 months of the study, the participants ate normally. Then, for 6 months, they received half their normal caloric intake, with the goal of reducing their body weight by 25 percent. Initially, the men lost weight rapidly. As time passed, however, the pace of weight loss slowed, forcing the men to consume even fewer calories in

■ **basal metabolic rate (BMR)** the minimum number of calories the body needs to maintain bodily functions while at rest

■ **set-point hypothesis** the theory that each person's body weight is genetically set within a given range, or set point, that the body works hard to maintain

order to meet their weight-loss goal. An even more dramatic result of this study was its findings regarding the psychological effects of semistarvation. The subjects did nothing but think and talk about food; they even spent time collecting recipes.

Why is it so difficult to bring your weight down? As a study by George Bray (1969) showed, with continued dieting, the body defends its precious fat reserves by decreasing its metabolic rate. When obese dieters reduced their daily intake from 3,500 to 450 calories for 24 days, their bodies quickly started burning fewer calories until their BMRs had dropped by 15 percent. The result: Although their body weight initially dropped 6 percent, with a lower BMR, they found it difficult to lose more weight. These findings will surely strike a chord with dieters who suffer the frustrating experience of losing a few pounds relatively quickly but then find it harder to lose additional weight as their dieting (and reduced metabolism) continues.

If starvation has this effect on metabolism, what effect does overeating have? To find out, researchers persuaded a group of volunteers to overeat until their weights increased by 10 percent (Leibel, Rosenbaum, & Hirsch, 1995). The results mirrored those of the semistarvation studies. After an initial period of rapid gain, further weight increases came slowly and with great difficulty, even though the participants had access to an abundance of delicious food and kept calorie-burning physical activity to a minimum. Like the men in the semistarvation study, the overfed volunteers found the experiment unpleasant. Food became repulsive and they had to force themselves to eat. Some even failed to reach their goal weight gain even though they more than doubled the number of calories consumed each day. At the end of the experiment, however, most lost weight quickly.

These studies clearly indicate that people find it extremely difficult to alter their weight substantially and that even if they are able to do so, the weight differential is difficult to maintain. The body defends its set point by adjusting its basal metabolic rate as necessary.

Why is the body so good at maintaining its set point? An interesting theory traces this ability back to our ancestors. In the course of evolution, the capacity to store excess calories as fat was an important survival mechanism, especially for species that were able to eat only infrequently. Animals that hibernate and those that must endure periods of nutritional scarcity—as did the human species throughout much of our history—store internal energy reserves when food is plentiful and live off these reserves when food is in short supply. Natural selection favored those human ancestors who developed "thrifty genes," which increased their ability to store fat from each feast in order to sustain them until the next meal. If you hunted and gathered your food, excess fat came in handy when food was scarce. All you needed to do was tap the energy stored in your fat cells. Although those of us who live in well-stocked developed countries no longer need to store so much fat, many of us continue to do so.

The Biological Basis of Hunger and Satiety

Our basal metabolic rate determines how many calories we need to maintain bodily functioning, but what sets off the initial hunger pangs we all feel? No single question has generated more research in health psychology than this: Precisely what triggers hunger and its opposite—*satiety?* Although it once seemed obvious that hunger and satiety occur in the stomach, this simplistic notion was soon dismissed in the face of evidence that hunger persists in humans and laboratory animals that have had their stomachs removed (Tsang, 1938).

Turning their attention to other possible signals, researchers discovered that feelings of hunger rise and fall with levels of glucose and insulin in the body. As you'll recall from Chapter 3, the pancreas produces the hormone insulin and assists the body in converting glucose into fat. When glucose levels fall, insulin increases and we feel hunger. Conversely, when glucose rises, hunger and insulin levels decrease. In terms of hunger, as time passes since the last meal, the level of glucose drops in the blood. Low blood glucose triggers a release of stored fat from body cells. As fat is depleted, the hypothalamus arouses hunger, motivating us to replenish our fat and glucose stores by eating. Other gastrointestinal hormones have been implicated in the regulation of hunger, including *cholecystokinin (CCK),* which suppresses appetite even when injected into starving animals (Thompson, 2000).

Increased feelings of hunger have also been linked to an increase in the number of fat cells in the body. The typical adult has about 30 billion fat cells, or **adipocytes.** Adipocytes are collapsible storage tanks that can be plump and full of *lipids* or empty and shrunken. In a thin person, the adipocytes remain relatively empty; in an obese person, however, they may swell to three times their normal size. When adipocytes reach their volume, they divide—a condition called *fat-cell hyperplasia.* Once the number of fat cells increases in a person's body, as a result of genetic predisposition or overeating, they never decrease. People who are not obese have 25 to 30 billion fat cells. Those who are severely obese may have 200 billion or more.

Another signal for hunger and satiety seems to be a neurotransmitter in the brain. Researchers happened upon this fact when analyzing the effects of appetite-suppressing (*anorexigenic*) diet drugs. Like many psychoactive drugs, a number of these anorexigenic drugs produce their effects by altering the activity of synaptic neurotransmitters. The reasoning is straightforward: If these drugs reduce hunger by binding to neural receptor sites in the brain, then there must be a naturally occurring neurotransmitter that does the same thing. This substance has not yet been found, however.

■ **adipocytes** collapsible body cells that store fat

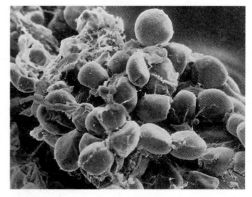

Adipocytes
Typically, we all have about 30 billion of these fat cells, or adipocytes. They are like little storage tanks. In a thin person, the fat cells are relatively empty; as the person gains weight, the cells begin to fill up. Each of the cells in this electron photomicrograph is filled by a single lipid droplet, mostly formed by triglycerides. Connective tissue fibers, in the upper left, provide support for the fat cells. © Professor P.
Motta / Department of Anatomy / University "La Sapienza," Rome / Science Photo Library / Photo Researchers

Not all ancient cultures valued a stout build. Obesity was stigmatized in medieval Japan because it was viewed as the karmic consequence of a moral failing in Buddhism. In some parts of Europe obesity was frowned upon as a sign of the Christian sin of gluttony.

Other researchers have tackled the problem by asking *where* the signals for hunger and satiety are processed in the brain. During the 1960s, researchers located appetite centers in two areas of the hypothalamus: a side region called the *lateral hypothalamus (LH)*, which seemed to trigger hunger, and a lower area in the middle called the *ventromedial hypothalamus (VMS)*, which seemed to trigger satiety. Animal experiments during the 1960s demonstrated that electrical stimulation of the LH causes an animal that has eaten to the point of fullness to begin eating again; when this area is lesioned, even an animal that has not eaten in days shows no signs of hunger. Conversely, when the VMH is stimulated, animals stop eating; when this area is destroyed, they overeat to the point of extreme obesity (Hoebel & Teitelbaum, 1966). Likewise, hypothalamic brain tumors have been linked to obesity in some human patients (Miller, Holicky, Ulrich, & Wieben, 1995).

Assuming that the LH and VMH integrate the various internal signals for hunger and satiety, *how* does the brain maintain the body's weight near the set point? One theory proposes that the hypothalamus regulates the number of fat cells directly. Until recently, fat cells were believed by most researchers to be a passive system of storage. Researchers now consider fat to be a type of endocrine tissue, complete with its own chemical hormones. In a relatively recent study, researchers at the Salk Institute discovered a new hormone, named $15d\text{-}PGJ_2$, that is produced inside fat cells and seems to trigger the formation of new ones, especially in children (Saez et al., 1998).

Obesity: Some Basic Facts

People are concerned about what and how much they eat because of the negative physiological and psychological effects of obesity. Being overweight carries a social stigma in many parts of the world today, indicating the importance that many societies place on physical appearance. Obese children are frequently teased and, as adults, are often perceived as ugly and sloppy (Harris, Walters, & Waschull, 1991) and as lacking in willpower (Friedman & Brownell, 1995).

Measuring Obesity

How do we define obesity? From the 1940s through the 1960s, tables prepared by the Metropolitan Life Insurance Company were used. Based on the mortality records of people of various heights and weights, the tables classified a person obese if he or she was 20 percent or more above ideal weight. Although widely used, weight tables don't account for differences in body composition, such as the amount of water, muscle, bone, or fat in a person's body. Nor will a conventional bathroom scale or "mirror test" account for these differences. Small shifts in scale weight usually reflect changes in body fluids, which, in turn, depend on the foods you eat, your activity level, and even the weather. For this reason, people may be mistakenly classified as overweight even though they actually have average or below-average body fat. Athletes, for example, often are statistically overweight because of a large frame or muscle development.

In recent years, the definition of obesity has been refined to mean the presence of excess body fat. A person with an acceptable weight and figure but too much body fat could be considered obese and his or her health could be at risk. Thus, you can be thin or fat at the same weight—it all depends on your individual fat-to-muscle content.

Given this more accurate definition of obesity, researchers were challenged to find new measurement techniques. Several methods have been used. A fairly common one involves measuring body fat by determining the size of skinfolds. Special calipers are used to pull and measure a pinch of skin that contains a double layer of skin plus the fat underneath. Skin pinches are taken at several defined parts of the body, such as the back of the upper arm and the abdomen, and then used to estimate the percentage of body fat.

Another method of assessing body fat is based on **bioelectrical impedance analysis** (BIA). In this method, a low-frequency electrical current is passed through the body. Because it is more difficult for electricity to flow through body fat than through moisture in muscle tissue, the amount of fat can be estimated from the body's electrical resistance to this imperceptible current.

The most accurate method of measuring the amount and percentage of body fat, **hydrostatic weighing,** is based on the principle that fat tends to float. The person is weighed underwater, then out of the water. The difference between the two weights enables the accurate calculation of the amount and percentage of body fat. When a person is in the water, the floating fat has no weight, so the amount by which the on-land weight is higher is assumed to be due to fat.

Because hydrostatic weighing requires a great deal of expensive, specialized equipment and is difficult to do on large numbers of people, another method, also relatively accurate, is frequently used. The most frequently used measure of obesity today is the **body mass index (BMI),** which is strongly correlated with percentage of body fat.

The BMI is computed by dividing your body weight (in kilograms) by the square of your height (in meters): BMI = weight in kg/height in m^2. Here's how to determine your BMI: multiply your weight in pounds (without shoes or clothes) by 700. Divide this product by your height in inches. Then divide it again by your height. Alternatively, you could use the BMI calculators at the NIH Web Site (www.nhlbisupport.com/bmi/) or the Calorie Control Council (www.caloriecontrol.org/bmi.html). For example, if you weigh 140 pounds

■ **bioelectrical impedance analysis** a method of determining the percentage of body fat by analyzing the electrical resistance as an imperceptible electric current is passed through the body

■ **hydrostatic weighing** a method of determining the percentage of body fat by comparing a person's weight underwater with his or her dry weight

■ **body mass index (BMI)** a measure of obesity calculated by dividing body weight by the square of a person's height

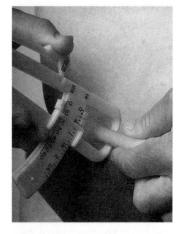

Measuring Obesity
Using special calipers, the researcher takes skin pinches at several specified parts of the body, such as the upper arm and the abdomen. The skin pinch consists of a double layer of skin plus the fat underneath. Together, these skin pinches are used to estimate the percentage of body fat. © Grantpix/Photo Researchers

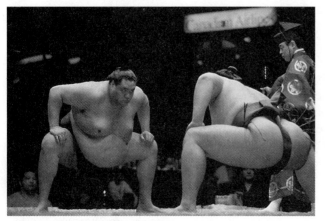

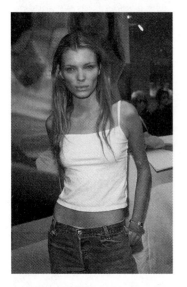

and are 5′6″, you would calculate your BMI as follows:

$$140 \times 700 = 98{,}000$$
$$98{,}000 \div 66 \text{ inches} = 1{,}485$$
$$1{,}485 \div 66 = 22.5$$
$$\text{BMI} = 22.5$$

To put these calculations into perspective, this person would have a normal BMI, while a person who is 5 feet, 8 inches tall and weighs 200 pounds *barely* exceeds the threshold of obesity. Researchers classify a person with a BMI between 25 and 30 as **overweight**—exceeding the desirable weight for a person of a given height, age, and body shape. A person with a BMI greater than 30 is labeled obese—not only exceeding the desirable weight but also possessing excessive body fat. A person with a BMI of 40 or greater—the clinical definition of *morbid obesity*—has reached the point where the excess body fat begins to interfere first with agility and then with day-to-day movement. As obesity increases, body weight begins to interfere with breathing and cause *hypoxemia* (decreased blood oxygen saturation). Morbid obesity is equivalent to 294 pounds for a 6-foot man or 247 pounds for a woman 5 feet 6 inches tall. The risk of death from all causes is much higher among women and men with the highest body mass indexes. Interestingly, the mortality risk associated with a high BMI is greater for European Americans than for African-Americans (Calle, Thun, Petrelli, Rodriguez, & Heath, 1999).

In defining obesity as excess body fat, researchers do not establish a set ideal amount for all people because the amount of body fat changes with age. During the first few years of life, you form new fat cells rapidly. Newborns have about 12 percent body fat; by 6 months of age, they have about 30 percent. But over the next 10 years, body fat decreases to about 18 percent in both sexes. At puberty, it increases dramatically in women and decreases slightly in men. By age 18, men have about 15 to 18 percent body fat and women have about 20 to 25.5 percent. Between 20 and 50 years of age, the body fat of men doubles while that of women increases by about 50 percent. In healthy adults, acceptable levels of body fat range from 25 to 30 percent in women and from 18 to 23 percent in men (Mayo Clinic, 1996) (see Byline Health on pages 278–279).

While the overall amount of body fat is important, the evidence indicates that *where* body fat is distributed may be even more significant. The excess upper body and abdominal fat (an apple-shaped body) associated with **male pattern obesity** has been linked to atherosclerosis, hypertension, and diabetes (Morris & Rimm, 1991), and—pound for pound—a greater overall health risk than fat that is concentrated on the hips and thighs (the

Two Weight Extremes
A Sumo wrestler clearly has a BMI above 30, which puts him well into the obese category. At the other end of the scale, sinewy model Esther Canadas checks in at 5′10″ and 101 pounds, for an unhealthy BMI of 14.4. © Steve Jay Crise/Corbis; © Evan Agostini/Liaison Agency

pear-shaped body of **female pattern obesity**). However, the health hazards of a high waist-to-hip ratio apply to both women and men (Sjostrom, 1992) and may even be a more accurate predictor of mortality from all causes than body mass index. To measure your waist-to-hip ratio:

1. Measure your waist at its slimmest point.
2. Measure your hips at the widest point.
3. Divide your waist measurement by your hip measurement:
   _____ (waist in inches) / (hips in inches) = _____

Thus, a woman with a waist of 29 inches and a hip measurement of 37 would have a ratio of 0.78, while a man with a 34-inch waist and a 40-inch hip measurement would have a ratio of 0.85. Both ratios fall within the healthy range. As a rule, the desirable waist-to-hip ratio is less than 0.8 for women and less than 0.95 for men.

One study of a large sample of Iowa women reported that the higher the waist-to-hip ratio, the higher the death rate (Folsom, Krahn, Naim, & Gold, 1993). This relationship remained significant even after BMI, smoking, education level, marital status, alcohol consumption, and use of estrogen were factored out. More recently, the Nurses' Health Study showed that women with a waist-to-hip ratio of 0.88 or greater were three times as likely to develop coronary heart disease as were women with a waist-to-hip ratio under 0.72 (Rexrode et al., 1998).

Hazards of Obesity

The National Institutes of Health (NIH) cite obesity as second only to cigarette smoking as a behavioral factor in mortality rates. Although being slightly overweight appears to pose no health risks (Ernsberger & Koletsky, 1999; Miller, 1999), obesity presents a major risk: As body fat accumulates, it crowds the space occupied by internal organs and contributes to many chronic health problems. Consider:

- The incidence of hypertension in people who are 50 percent or more overweight is three to five times that of normal-weight people.
- Obesity increases the body's demand for, and resistance to, insulin. For this reason, obesity is a leading cause of Type II diabetes.
- The liver manufactures more triglycerides (the most common form of dietary fat in the bloodstream) and cholesterol in those with excess body weight, in turn increasing the risk of arthritis, gout, and gallbladder disease.
- Complications following surgery, including infection, occur more often among the obese.

overweight body weight that exceeds the desirable weight for a person of a given height, age, and body shape

male pattern obesity the "apple-shaped" body of men who carry excess weight around their upper body and abdomens

female pattern obesity the "pear-shaped" body of women who carry excess weight on their thighs and hips

When It Comes to Food, Guys Have All the Luck
William Grimes

The subject of gender differences in food behaviors has fascinated researchers for decades. Do men and women eat and think about food differently, and if so, why?

In life's grand lottery, men have made out pretty well when it comes to food. Nature allows them to eat more of it every day, without gaining weight, than women can. Better yet, the social pressures that make food a love-hate object for women barely exist for the male of the species. A man with fat hips and a fat wallet is, in social terms, a slim man.

In short, men eat differently than women do, and think about food differently than women do for biological and social reasons. Neither is very well understood, but the differences are visible enough, and important enough, to interest researchers.

Adult males can consume about 2,500 calories a day and maintain equilibrium; that's about 700 calories more than women can consume. The body's ratio of fat to muscle tissue, which is more or less the same for both sexes up to adolescence, allows men to metabolize food faster, which means they can consume more food without gaining weight. Not surprisingly, women regard the calorie as a unit of fat. Most men see it as a unit of energy.

Add to this natural advantage the lack of a serious social penalty for being overweight, and you get an upbeat, extroverted approach to food, a sharp contrast to the complex, often tortured relationship experienced by women, who account for 90 percent of the cases of eating disorders.

Men may be coarser in their pleasures, however, gourmands rather than epicures. "Men tend to eat large quantities," said Dr. Thomas Wadden, the director of the Weight and Eating Disorders Program at the University of Pennsylvania Medical School. "There's almost a machismo about being able to pack it away, like downing a six-pack. Women are more discerning eaters, more attentive to taste and texture."

Women, of course, traditionally spend more of their lives preparing food. But there may also be a physical basis to greater taste sensitivity in women. Dr. Linda Bartoshuk, a professor at Yale University's School of Medicine who studies sensory processes and nutrition, has found that about 35 percent of women, and only 15 percent of men, are what she calls supertasters—that is, they have unusually dense clusters of taste buds that perceive a test chemical, known as PROP, as extremely bitter.

Supertasters are hypersensitive to bitterness, sweetness, and the texture of fat. At the other end of the scale are nontasters, who cannot detect the presence of PROP at all. "The winners of the booby prize are white males," Dr. Bartoshuk said. "Thirty-five percent of white men are nontasters versus 10 percent of women." Men also eat more quickly, and in larger bites, researchers have found. No surprise there. But the urge to eat large amounts seems to be counterbalanced, in men ages 20 to 35, by an internal gauge that accurately records how much food is being wolfed down.

- There is a strong correlation between obesity and cardiovascular diseases in both men and women, even after statistical adjustments are made for blood pressure, cholesterol, smoking, age, and diabetes.
- Obesity increases the risk of certain cancers.

Given the health hazards that obesity poses, it will come as no surprise that being significantly overweight can cut life short. A recent large-scale study of German women and men reported a relationship between the degree of obesity and mortality rates from all causes (Bender, Trautner, Spraul, & Berger 1998). A BMI score under 32 was unrelated to death rates from all causes combined, a BMI of 36 (moderate obesity) was linked to slightly increased mortality rates, and a BMI above 40—in both women and men—more than doubled the all-cause mortality rates. Similarly, a massive recent study following

"We've found interesting data showing that normal-weight men seem very tuned in to responding appropriately to the calories they are given," said Barbara Rolls, the director of the Laboratory for the Study of Human Ingestive Behavior at Pennsylvania State University. "If they are given a high-calorie dish, they will cut back their intake on the next course."

There is evidence that this internal monitoring system breaks down with age. In a 1994 study conducted by Susan Roberts, the director of the Energy Metabolism Laboratory at Tufts University in Boston, male subjects were put on diets that caused them to add or lose weight. The young men in the study quickly returned to their normal weight, but the men over 65 did not.

When men do put on weight, the health consequences are more likely to be more severe, since men tend to develop abdominal obesity, which is associated with diabetes and heart disease. Women tend to develop lower-body obesity.

Men, moreover, are more likely to resist seeing themselves as overweight and more likely to put off dealing with the problem. "They are less concerned about it until they have a health scare," Dr. Wadden said. "Then they get G.I. Joe, ready-to-go."

The military reference is not far off. "Men tend to come at healthy eating from a very physical mind-set, perhaps because the first instruction they get on the subject is from a coach," said Linda Gilbert, the president of Health Focus, a company that tracks consumer attitudes about health and nutrition. "They're performance oriented. They want to know, 'Will this food raise my energy level?' whereas women are more likely to choose food for a medical purpose."

Ms. Gilbert's surveys have found that men are less likely to say they enjoy eating healthful food; more likely to feel that if a package says "low-fat" or "no-fat" it will not taste good, and more likely to disbelieve the health claims on packages.

Women, when organizing a healthier diet, will maximize their choices within a narrow range of food groups to keep life interesting, but men will not, which may give them a jaundiced view of good-nutrition programs in general. And if weight control is an issue as well, they would rather meet the enemy on the playing field. "Men will exercise rather than diet," said Adam Drewnowski, the director of the Nutrition Sciences Program at the University of Washington. "Dieting is a last resort."

When the will to diet does break down, women and men tend to surrender to different cravings. Both sexes want fat, but women lust for fat and sugar, while men want fat and salt. "That means hot dogs, pizza and nachos," said Mr. Drewnowski. "For half the human race, that adds up to one fine, exquisitely balanced meal.

Source: New York Times.com, February 17, 1999.

Exercises

1. Are the gender differences in food behaviors discussed in this article consistent with your experiences as a woman or a man?

2. Which gender differences in food behaviors are likely the result of biological factors? Which differences are more likely the result of psychological and social factors?

3. How might a health psychologist working from an evolutionary perspective explain gender differences in food behaviors? (Hint: What possible advantage might male–female differences in taste sensitivity, fat storage, and body composition convey to the human species?)

more than 1 million Americans over a 14-year period reported that white men and women with the highest BMI (40 or higher) had two to six times the relative risk of death of their thinner counterparts with a BMI of 24 (Calle et al., 1999). For both women and men, however, being slightly overweight was less of a risk factor (see Figure 7.2, page 280).

Although generally speaking, thinner people live longer, Figure 7.2 also demonstrates that people who are extremely thin do not have the lowest death rates, indicating that the relationship between body weight and health hazards is probably U-shaped (Durazo-Arvizu, McGee, Cooper, Liao, & Luke, 1998). Just such a relationship was found in a recent study that followed a large sample of women over a 26-year period (Lindsted & Singh, 1997). Mortality rates were highest among the very thinnest and the very heaviest individuals.

Figure 7.2

Mortality Rates as a Function of Body Mass Index (BMI)
Generally speaking, thinner women and men live longer. At a BMI of 40, a woman's risk of dying is approximately 50 percent higher than that of a person with a BMI of 24; for men with a BMI over 40, the risk of death is about 2.5 times higher. However, very thin people do not have the lowest mortality rates, indicating that the relationship between weight and poor health is actually U-shaped, were the graph extended to BMIs below 18.

Source: "Body-Mass Index and Mortality in a Prospective Cohort of U.S. Adults," by E. E. Calle, M. J. Thun, J. M. Petrelli, C. Rodriguez, and C. W. Heath, 1999, *New England Journal of Medicine, 341*, pp. 1097–1105.

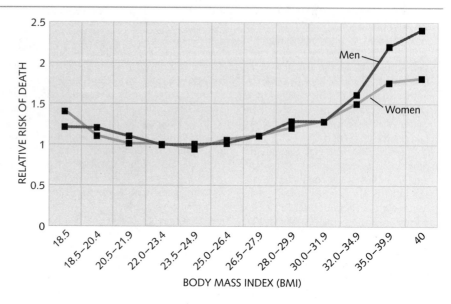

It should be noted that the hazardous consequences of a BMI between 25 and 30 remain controversial, with some experts suggesting that people who are short, elderly, African-, Latino, or Asian-American suffer no ill effects unless they become truly obese (Strawbridge, Wallhagen, & Shema, 2000). For instance, among African-American women and men, the lowest mortality rates occur among those with a BMI of 27; among European Americans, the lowest mortality rates occur among those with a BMI of 24 to 25 (Durazo-Arvizu et al., 1998).

Another factor that complicates the obesity-health relationship is age. Being overweight increases the risk of death from all causes among young and middle-aged adults (Oster, Thompson, Edelsberg, Bird, & Colditz, 1999; Stevens et al., 1998). After about age 65, however, *losing* weight is actually associated with increased risk of dying from all causes (Diehr et al., 1998). This is because losing weight in late adulthood generally means less muscle, thinner bones, and greater risk of accidents and chronic disease.

Even psychological well-being is affected by obesity, although how it is affected depends on gender. For instance, overweight women are more likely to be depressed, even suicidal, than their thinner counterparts (Carpenter, Hasin, Allison, & Faith, 2000). Interestingly, *underweight* men are more likely to be diagnosed with clinical depression than their heavier counterparts. Kenneth Carpenter and his colleagues (2000) have suggested that this puzzling gender difference may be a direct result of being underweight, or an indirect result, in that married men tend to be heavier and happier, and a disproportionate number of unmarried men are thin.

While being excessively under- or overweight is hazardous to health, equally hazardous is **weight cycling,** a pattern of repeated weight gain and loss. An ongoing study of Harvard alumni (see Chapter 2) has reported that men who maintained a stable weight had significantly lower death rates from all causes (including cardiovascular disease) than did alumni who had either gained or lost a significant amount of weight over the years (Lee & Paffenbarger, 1992). More recently, a study of middle-aged and older men showed that *extreme* weight loss increased risk of death from all causes, even when the weight loss was intentional (Yaari & Goldbourt, 1998).

■ **weight cycling** repeated weight gains and losses through repeated dieting

Factors That Contribute to Obesity

Derived from the root words from *ob*, or "over," and *edere*, "to eat," the literal definition of obesity implies that it is a single entity that results from a single cause. Although it is tempting to take the view that obesity is simply the result of overeating, research shows that this is an oversimplification. Those who are overweight often do *not* eat more than their thin friends do. Rather, obesity is a complex phenomenon involving biological, social, and psychological factors in both its causes and consequences.

Biological Factors

Research on the biological factors that contribute to obesity has focused on the roles of heredity, the brain, and hormones in regulating appetite.

Heredity

Genes contribute approximately 50 percent to the likelihood of obesity. This is because you inherit a tendency toward obesity from your biological parents. Approximately 60 percent of those who are clinically overweight had overweight biological parents.

Heredity influences different factors that contribute to obesity. For example, basal metabolic rate is determined by genes. People with a naturally lower BMR burn fewer calories than their thinner counterparts. Overall body shape, which influences your tendency to gain weight, is also genetically determined. Rounded *endomorphs,* who have the largest capacity for storing body fat, will probably never have the lean build of *ectomorphs* (who have the smallest fat-storage capacity) or the muscular body of the *mesomorph.* Genes also affect how the body absorbs nutrients. For example, our blood cholesterol levels are not equally responsive to changes in dietary cholesterol (Gylling & Miettinen, 1997). Some people, for example, are "nonresponders" whose

■ **ob gene** a gene that controls several physiological systems involved in obesity. Animals with a defective ob gene become hugely obese

■ **leptin** the weight-signaling hormone monitored by the hypothalamus as an index of body fat

serum cholesterol stays the same even when their intake of eggs and other cholesterol-rich foods is reduced (Brody, 1995).

The role of heredity in obesity is illustrated by a massive study in which researchers analyzed the weights of more than 3,500 adopted Danish children and their biological and adoptive parents (Meyer & Stunkard, 1994). The study found a strong relationship between the body weights of adoptees and their biological parents but little or no relationship between the weights of offspring and their adoptive parents. Additional evidence comes from the strong correlation (0.74) between the body weights and BMIs of identical twins, even when they are raised in separate households (Plomin, Defries, McClearn, & Rutter, 1997). The much lower correlation between the body weights and BMIs of fraternal twins (0.32) suggests that genes account for approximately two-thirds of individual differences in BMI (Maes, Neale, & Eaves, 1997). It is therefore not surprising that the body weights of adopted siblings (who share the same family diet but no genes) are not correlated at all.

Because most studies to date have used primarily European American samples to investigate the genetics of BMI, it is fair to ask whether these estimates of heritability apply equally to all races and ethnic groups. There are, in fact, slight ethnic differences in body composition—African-Americans, for example, generally have a greater bone mineral density and body protein content than do European Americans (Wagner & Heyward, 2000). Nevertheless, a recent examination of BMI among black and white schoolchildren from Philadelphia found no significant differences in estimates of heritability between the two groups (Katzmarzyk, Mahaney, Blangero, Quek, & Malina, 1999).

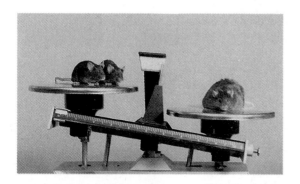

Fat Genes and Hormones
The mouse on the right inherited the defective ob gene for producing the fat-signaling hormone leptin. Together, the two mice on the left do not weigh as much; they do not have the defective ob gene. © John Sholtis, The Rockefeller University

Genetic Disorders, the Brain, and Hormones

Why do some people apparently have more potential to become fat than do others? Molecular biologists speculate that genetic disorders may interfere with the body's ability to regulate the number of fat cells, thereby causing people to gain weight. For example, researchers have discovered that laboratory mice with a defective **ob gene** cannot control their hunger and tend to become obese (Gura, 1997). The ob gene appears to regulate the production of **leptin,** a hormone produced by fat, which the hypothalamus monitors as an index of obesity. The amount of leptin is generally correlated with how much fat is stored in the body, with greater levels of leptin in people with higher BMIs and reduced levels in those with lower body fat. Because they have higher body fat content, women generally have higher leptin levels than men do. Leptin levels do, however, vary greatly from person to person. For example, the amount of leptin for some obese patients with BMIs above 40 is the same as that of patients with BMIs less than 20.

As body fat increases, increased levels of leptin signal the normal brain to suppress hunger. Animals with defective ob genes produce too little leptin and overeat. They become hugely obese and diabetic, and they have a substantially lower basal metabolic rate than their genetically normal counterparts (Zhang, Proenca, Maffei, & Barone, 1994). When given daily injections of leptin, they eat less, they become more active, and their body weights eventually return to normal (Halaas et al., 1995).

The discovery of the ob gene and leptin has renewed support for set-point theory. According to this line of reasoning, if the body's set point is something like a thermostat, leptin acts like the thermometer (Gibbs, 1996). As a person gains weight, he or she may produce more leptin. This shuts off appetite, increases energy expenditure, and triggers other mechanisms to restore body weight to the set point. Conversely, as a person loses weight (as in dieting), levels of leptin decrease, hunger increases, and metabolism falls until the person's weight returns to its targeted level.

However, other researchers are not yet sure whether a defective gene also accounts for obesity in humans. Some believe that the leptin receptors of obese people are simply less sensitive to leptin (Considine & Caro, 1996). Reduced sensitivity to leptin could explain why more leptin is found in obese people, who must produce the hormone at a greater rate to compensate for a faulty signaling process (Nakamura et al., 2000).

Leptin's signaling ability may also explain why most dieters regain lost weight. After dieting, less leptin is available to signal the brain, possibly increasing hunger and slowing metabolism. In normal mice, leptin levels dropped 40 percent after a 3-day fast and 80 percent after a 6-day fast (Nakamura et al., 2000). Interestingly, in genetically diabetic mice, leptin levels did not drop after 15 days of restricted food. After 28 days of dieting, however, leptin fell precipitously (Friedman & Brownell, 1995).

Destiny? Genetics versus Environmental Factors

Despite the mounting evidence for the role of biological factors in obesity, it is important to recognize that heredity alone does not destine a person to be fat. Obesity is a product of genetic vulnerability and environmental factors or maladaptive behaviors. What appears to be inherited is a *tendency* to be overweight; the amount a person becomes overweight is affected by diet *and* activity level. Regular activity and a moderate diet that is low in fat can limit genetic tendencies toward obesity (Brownell & Wadden, 1992).

Psychosocial Factors

Hunger and eating behavior are not controlled by physiological factors alone. Psychosocial factors also come into play. From an early age we are conditioned to associate eating with holidays, personal achievements, and most social occasions. And the giving of food is among the first symbols of love between a parent and child. Should we be surprised that people are conditioned to turn to food when they are upset, anxious, or under stress (Arnow et al., 1992)?

Neil Grunberg and I (Grunberg & Straub, 1992) asked groups of nonsmoking men and women seated in a comfortable living room to watch either a stressful film about eye surgery or a pleasant travelogue. Within the subjects' reach were bowls of salty peanuts, bland rice cakes, and sweet M & M candies. The bowls were weighed before and after each session to determine how much of each snack food the subjects ate. All the men and those women who reported little concern about dieting and body weight ate fewer sweets when watching a stressful film than did those who watched the nonstressful film. Only those women who reported being especially conscious of their weight and who had a history of frequent dieting consumed more sweets when stressed. Stress did not influence the participants' preferences for salty or bland foods.

Why should most people have less of an appetite for sweets when they are stressed? One possibility is that stress may indirectly increase a person's blood sugar level by lowering the level of insulin. The elevated blood sugar may reduce the desire (or taste) for additional sweets.

Culture, Socioeconomic Status, and Gender

Genes and other physiological factors also cannot explain why overweight and obesity are more prevalent today than in the past; why, to put it another way, the average woman's dress size has increased from size 12 in 1951 to size 16 today (Merriman, 1999). Twenty-five years ago, 47 percent of Americans were classified as overweight (BMI of 25 or over) or obese (BMI of 30 or more); today this figure has jumped to 61 percent of U.S. adults between the ages of 20 and 74 years (National Center for Health Statistics, 2000). Americans are fatter today than their parents and grandparents ever were, and they are getting fatter every year. Similar trends are apparent in Australia, Canada, Asia, Europe, and in Central and South America (WHO, 2000).

Within the United States, obesity is more prevalent among African-Americans, Hispanic-Americans, Native Americans, and other minority groups (National Center for Health Statistics, 2000). Socioeconomic factors may help to explain this relationship. Researchers have found an inverse relationship between obesity and socioeconomic status (SES), with people of lower SES more likely to be overweight than those who are more affluent. The fact that members of minority groups are disproportionately represented among lower-SES groups helps explain why they are more likely to be overweight (McMurtrie, 1994).

SES, as you will recall, is determined from a person's education level and income. Among all young people between 16 and 24 years of age, those who are overweight tend to have lower personal incomes and to have completed fewer years of education than their normal-weight counterparts (Gortmaker, Must, Perrin, & Sobol, 1993). However, the relationship among income, ethnicity, and weight also varies with gender. Figure 7.3 shows that there is a clear

Figure 7.3

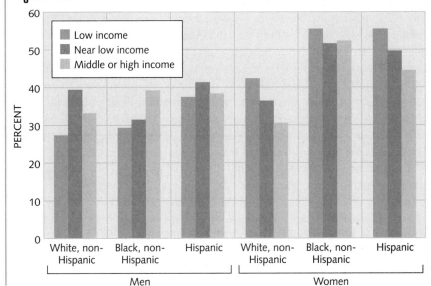

Prevalence of Overweight Adults by Income, Gender, and Ethnicity

Among women of all ethnicities, there is a clear income gradient in overweight prevalence, with overweight prevalence for poor women 1.4 times that of women with middle incomes and 1.6 times that for women with high incomes. In contrast, there is little evidence of an income-related gradient in the prevalence of overweight among men.

Source: Centers for Disease Control and Prevention, National Center for Health Statistics, National Health and Nutrition Examination Surveys (www.cdc.gov/nchs/nhanes.htm, 2000).

income gradient in overweight prevalence among women: Poor women are 1.4 times as likely to be overweight as women with middle incomes and 1.6 times as likely to be overweight as women with high incomes. For men of all races, however, there is little evidence of an income-related gradient in the prevalence of overweight.

Overweight and obesity are also inversely related to education level. Men and women of all races with a college degree are less likely to be overweight than men and women with fewer than 12 years of education. Among women, however, the relationship between education and overweight is becoming weaker. In addition, since the mid-1970s the prevalence of overweight and obesity among men and women has increased steadily at all education levels (National Center for Health Statistics, 2000).

Why are lower-SES people at increased risk for obesity? Compared with more affluent, better-educated people, those of lower SES have more limited access to health care services and less knowledge about the importance of a healthy diet and the hazards of obesity, and they tend to exercise less. It has also been suggested that the greater daily stress associated with poverty—resulting from prejudice, crowding, and crime, for example—may trigger increased eating as a defensive coping mechanism. Thus, it is not surprising that obesity is less prevalent among minority Americans who live in more affluent neighborhoods than among those living in lower-SES neighborhoods (Hazuda, Mitchell, Haffner, & Stern, 1991).

Ethnocultural differences in dietary customs and body image may also be a factor in some group differences in body weight (see Diversity and Healthy

■ **restraint theory** the theory that heightened sensitivity to norms for body weight triggers a pattern of eating that vacillates between strict dieting and binge eating

Living on pages 302–303). For example, there is some evidence that African-Americans are less concerned about adhering to a thin ideal for women than are European Americans (Biener & Heaton, 1995). Generally speaking, however, thinness tends to be more highly valued among women in developed countries, which in turn leads to an emphasis on dieting and avoiding a sedentary lifestyle—especially among those who are relatively affluent (Sobal & Stunkard, 1989). Interestingly, as immigrant groups become acculturated to American norms, which generally discourage being overweight, obesity tends to decline (Stunkard, 1979). In contrast, in most developing countries today—and especially those in which famine is a real danger—being overweight is considered a sign of affluence and elevated social status (Furnham & Baguma, 1994).

Acculturation of dietary customs can cut both ways, however. Japanese-American men, for example, are nearly three times as likely to be obese as their countrymen living in Japan. This is because, like most American males, the average Japanese-American male consumes far more fat in his diet than do his counterparts living in Japan (Curb & Marcus, 1991).

Food Cues, Restraint, and Hunger

One influential psychological theory proposed that obese and nonobese people respond to different food cues (Schachter, 1971). According to the *internality-externality hypothesis,* feelings of hunger and satiety in normal-weight people are closely tied to internal stimuli such as stomach fullness, whereas obese persons are more responsive to external cues such as the time of day or the taste, smell, or appearance of food. More recent studies, however, have failed to find consistent differences in the responsiveness of obese and normal-weight people to food-related cues. For example, Judith Rodin (1981) discovered that body weight did not predict externality or internality. Some obese people *do* respond to internal cues, whereas many normal-weight people (especially those who are dieting) do not.

To help explain the apparent contradictions in the varying behaviors of obese and nonobese people, Peter Herman and Janet Polivy (1975) developed the **restraint theory** of eating behavior. This theory contends that heightened sensitivity to body-weight norms results in a pattern of eating that vacillates between strict dieting (restrained eating) and overindulging (unrestrained eating). According to this theory, external sensitivity is a consequence of dietary restraint.

A series of studies by Herman and Polivy (1980) found that externality was tied to restrained eating rather than to body weight. In one study, obese and nonobese college students were divided into high- and low-restraint groups based on their answers to questions such as "How often are you dieting?" and "Do you give too much time and thought to food?" Ostensibly participating in a taste test, half the students in each group were asked to drink a large milkshake "preload" before rating several varieties of ice cream. In fact, the researchers were interested only in how much ice cream each student consumed. As expected, unrestrained eaters ate less ice cream following the milkshake preload than their counterparts in the no preload condition. Restrained eaters, who claimed to be dieting frequently and to think a lot about food, however, actually ate more after having just consumed a large milkshake.

In another study, restrained eaters who were told that they had just eaten a high-calorie pudding ate 61 percent more food in a subsequent tasting experiment than those who were told that they had just eaten a low-calorie diet pudding (Polivy, 1996). This paradoxical loss of control over eating when restraint is disrupted has been called **disinhibition,** or *counterregulation.* Restrained eaters who are "forced" off their normally strict diet overeat in the presence of external cues.

The overeating that results from disinhibition is often triggered by an event, emotion, or behavior. Several studies have reported an association between dietary restraint and emotional eating. Restrained eaters eat more than unrestrained eaters when they are depressed and when they are feeling stress (Polivy & Herman, 1987; Wardle & Beales, 1988).

Although the restraint theory has garnered considerable support in the last two decades, it has been criticized by some as being overly simplistic (Lowe, 1993). Skeptics doubt that a behavior as complex as eating can be fully explained by restraint or any other single factor. Researchers are now focusing on *all* the possible factors—biological, social, and psychological—that contribute to obesity and are attempting to determine any interaction among those factors. They are also focusing more on why some obese individuals suffer negative psychological consequences while others do not (Friedman & Brownell, 1995).

■ **disinhibition** overeating triggered by an event, emotion, or behavior that causes a restrained eater to abandon his or her restraint

Treatment of Obesity

Obesity is highly stigmatized. Beginning in nursery school, children show a dislike of fatness, rating drawings of fat children more negatively than those of children with physical disabilities (Richardson, 1971). And it continues into adulthood, with discrimination against the obese occurring in housing, college admissions, and employment (Pingitore, Dugoni, Tindale, & Spring, 1994). In one clever study, Regina Pingitore and her colleagues videotaped job interviews in which applicants either appeared to be of normal weight or wore makeup and padding that made them appear 30 pounds heavier. When made up to appear obese, the same applicants, using the same well-rehearsed presentation, received a significantly lower "employability rating" from a group of college students posing as potential employers. The discriminatory bias was especially pronounced when the applicant was a woman.

Because antifat prejudice is so strong and because fat people are generally held responsible for their condition, some psychologists maintain that weight discrimination is even greater than race and gender discrimination and that it affects every aspect of employment, including hiring, promotion, and salary (Dejong, 1980; Roehling & Winters, 2000).

This prejudice against obesity has led to the proliferation of different weight-reduction regimens, which will be described in the following sections.

Dieting

A stroll through any bookstore will give you a quick idea of the vast array of dieting strategies—everything from preplanned meals with strict calorie limits to single-food plans to hypnosis. It's easy to be cynical about the number of choices. Needless to say, if any of them were truly effective, there would not be a market for such variety. Clearly, the main beneficiaries of most of these books are their authors.

For most overweight adults, weight loss is a healthy goal. On the other hand, many people (especially women who are not overweight) are trying to shed pounds for reasons that have little or nothing to do with health. The increasing popularity of dieting has been attributed to the growing cultural pressure to be slim.

How Effective Are Diets?

Research shows that dieting alone usually does not work to take weight off and keep it off. The best way to lose weight and keep it off is to develop sound eating habits and to engage in regular physical exercise to raise the basal metabolic rate.

Even though most diets fail, dieting is on the rise. The value of the diet business in the United States is estimated to be over $50 billion (Wardle, 1997). National surveys suggest that at any given time about 20 percent of the population is on a diet, with more than 72 percent of women and 44 percent of men having dieted at some point in their adult lives (Serdula, Collins, Williamson, Anda, Pamuk, & Byers, 1993). In a 1999 Gallup poll, 52 percent of U.S. residents—up from 31 percent in 1951—said they would like to lose weight.

At all ages, women are twice as likely as men to be dieting, even though there is only a small gender difference in the prevalence of obesity (Serdula et al., 1999). Dieting is increasingly prevalent among adolescents, which is cause for concern because of the potential hazards to growth and development. About 65 percent of high school girls and 21 percent of high school boys are dieting at any given time (French, Story, Downes, Resnick, & Blum, 1995).

Why Diets Fail

One reason diets fail is that many people are not very good at calculating the number of calories their bodies need or the size of the food portions they are eating. Underestimating calorie consumption is a common problem in many failed diets. In one study, for example, obese dieters reported eating an average of 1,028 kcal per day but their actual intake was 2,081 kcal, more than twice as many calories as reported. To make matters worse, the self-reported daily activity level of the dieters was also substantially in error (Lichtman, Pisarska, Berman, & Prestone, 1992).

Diets also fail because people find it nearly impossible to comply with them for very long (Garner & Wolley, 1991). In effect, many dieters practice what has been called "yo-yo" dieting—achieving temporary success, then quitting the diet, regaining weight, and eventually going on a diet again. This itself is cause for concern, since weight cycling may be more hazardous to health than a high but stable weight (Wardle, 1997) (see also p. 281).

The most successful diets are clinical interventions that include some form of post-treatment following weight loss, such as social support, exercise programs, or continued contact with the therapist. One study found that 18 months after finishing a diet program, those who did not participate in a post-treatment phase regained 67 percent of their weight, compared with 17 percent of dieters who participated in a post-treatment program combining exercise and social support (Perri, 1998).

Diet Pills

During the 1950s and 1960s, diet pills (most often stimulants such as amphetamines) were widely prescribed. The treatment caught on because the drugs boosted metabolism, reduced appetite, and often resulted in quick weight loss. Like many psychoactive drugs, however, amphetamines lose their effectiveness at a given dose level, so the amount has to be steadily increased. The resulting physical dependence often proves to be a greater health hazard than being overweight.

A variety of other weight-loss drugs—both prescription and nonprescription—quickly followed the amphetamines. Prescription weight-loss drugs include those that slow stomach emptying; drugs that interfere with pancreatic enzymes; synthetic hormones that signal the body to burn fat rather than sugar; and drugs that curb appetite by mimicking serotonin, dopamine, and other brain neurotransmitters. Nonprescription drugs include the many over-the-counter appetite suppressants that line your pharmacist's shelves. Although most of these products temporarily reduce hunger, their benefits are generally small and temporary at best. Fewer than 5 percent of respondents in a 1993 *Consumer Reports* survey, for example, were satisfied with nonprescription diet pills.

Despite the abundance of pharmaceutical "remedies," there are no entirely acceptable, safe, and effective drugs to treat obesity. For example,

■ **gastroplasty** a radical treatment for obesity in which a portion of the stomach is removed or stapled shut

■ **liposuction** a radical form of cosmetic surgery in which fat tissue is suctioned from the body

phenylpropanolamine (PPA), a substance found in many nonprescription diet pills, has been linked to heart and kidney damage, hypertension, lung disease, and stroke (Abenhaim et al., 1996). In December 1994, Pam Ruff at the Merit-Care Medical Center noted two unusual cases involving leaky heart valves in young women. From their medical charts, she realized that both women had taken the popular combination of diet pills known as *fen-phen* (fenfluramine and phentermine), which have since been taken off the market. Over the next 2 years, Ruff collected 20 more files, most involving women in their thirties and forties, who developed heart valve problems while taking fen-phen. Fen-phen alters serotonin levels in the body, possibly damaging heart valve tissue (Cannistra, Davis, & Bauman, 1997). Normal heart valves permit blood to move in only one direction; when the valves are damaged, blood flows backward, forcing the heart to work harder, in some cases to the point of *congestive heart failure* (Connolly et al., 1997).

Surgery

For the very obese, pill-taking is inadequate for losing the needed amount of weight, so they must turn to a more radical treatment: surgery. **Gastroplasty** is a form of surgery in which a portion of the stomach is removed or stapled shut to reduce its volume. Although used infrequently in this country, gastroplasty has proven effective elsewhere in treating extreme cases of obesity. A study of 1,150 obese gastroplasty patients in Sweden, for example, reported an average decrease of 66 pounds over a 2-year period (Gibbs, 1996).

In another form of gastroplasty, *intestinal bypass,* a portion of the intestines is surgically removed, allowing the patient to eat normally but preventing food from being absorbed and thereby reducing the number of calories metabolized by the body. Other surgical treatments for obesity include the insertion of *gastric balloons* (which create a sensation of fullness when inflated) and wiring of the jaw to restrict eating to low-calorie liquid meals.

In addition to risking the complications that can accompany any type of major surgery, many gastroplasty patients suffer digestive complications such as nearly constant diarrhea, which can lead to vitamin and mineral deficiencies as well as increased risk of dehydration. And for some, gastroplasty is ineffective in promoting weight loss: It is merely an inconvenience that forces them to eat smaller, more frequent meals (Kral, 1992).

Another radical method of losing weight is **liposuction,** in which fat tissue is suctioned from the body. Although liposuction does not control obesity, it does allow a cosmetic recontouring of body shape. For this reason, the expensive (and uncomfortable) procedure has become the most common form of plastic surgery (Brownell & Rodin, 1994).

Behavioral Treatment

Behavior modification, particularly if it is practiced in conjunction with cognitive intervention techniques, has become a mainstay of many contemporary weight-loss programs. Although the jury is still out about the effectiveness of behavioral programs, at least they generally have few, if any, adverse side effects (Brownell & Wadden, 1992).

Behavior modification programs typically include the following components:

- *Stimulus control* procedures to identify and limit the number of cues that trigger eating (for example, confining eating to one particular place).

- *Self-control* techniques to slow the act of eating (for example, chewing each bite a set number of times, putting down silverware between bites).

- *Contingency contracts* in which therapist-delivered or self-controlled reinforcement is made dependent upon reaching weight-loss goals (for example, the client puts up a sum of money to be earned back as goals are attained).

- *Social support* of family members and friends, who are enlisted to provide additional reinforcement for success and compliance.

- *Careful self-monitoring* and recordkeeping to increase awareness of what foods are eaten and the circumstances under which eating occurs.

Self-monitoring is often sufficient, in and of itself, to promote weight loss. Raymond Baker and Daniel Kirschenbaum (1998) examined self-monitoring of eating behaviors during three holiday periods (Thanksgiving, Christmas/Hanukkah, and New Year's Eve). Compared to the controls who gained weight, those participants who were the most thorough in recordkeeping actually lost weight during the holiday weeks.

In recent years, advocates of behavioral treatments have shifted their emphasis from a focus on eating cues and techniques to a greater concern with the types of foods consumed, the need for exercise and coping skills to aid in overcoming high-risk relapse situations, responses to violating diet and/or binge eating, and primary prevention of obesity during childhood.

Despite the success of behavioral interventions in terms of initial weight loss in both adults and children, behavior therapies in isolation have tended to be relatively ineffective in sustaining long-term weight loss (Lewis, 1997). One study reported that 5 years after participating in a behavioral weight-loss program, participants were slightly heavier on average than they were before the program began (Stalonas, Perri, & Kerzner, 1984).

Greater success has been obtained when behavioral methods are combined with cognitive techniques recognizing that overweight people often start treatment with unrealistic expectations and self-defeating thoughts. *Cognitive behavior therapies (CBT)* focus on the reciprocal interdependence of feelings, thoughts, behavior, consequences, social context, and physiological processes (Meichenbaum, 1997). The underlying premise of these therapies is that eating habits and attitudes must be modified on a permanent basis for weight loss and the maintenance of that loss to occur.

As noted in Chapter 1, cognitive behavior programs use many different techniques to change dietary habits. Rather than attempting to force quick and dramatic weight losses, all of these techniques focus on the gradual loss of 1 to 2 pounds per week, using a combination of operant conditioning, self-control, and cognitive restructuring techniques, in which the person learns to control self-defeating thoughts about body weight and dieting.

The balance of evidence suggests that the most effective forms of cognitive behavior therapy for weight control are those that do not necessarily focus on weight loss but rather on encouraging clients' perceptions that they *can* gain control over their weight and improve their body image. In addition, CBT is aimed at modifying dieting emotions—in particular, emotional overeating and binge eating (Lewis, 1997).

Stepped Care

Today, health psychologists recognize that patients differ in which treatment will be most effective for them. Kelly Brownell and Thomas Wadden (1991) have proposed the *stepped-care* process for determining which intervention is most appropriate for a given person (see Figure 7.4). The first step is to classify the person on the basis of degree of obesity. A seriously obese person clearly may require more aggressive and intensive treatment than someone who is moderately obese. After considering relevant factors about the client, the safest, least intensive intervention is put into place. In step 2, based on information obtained about the patient, the psychologist structures an intervention that meets that person's needs. Only if this treatment is ineffective is a more intensive intervention warranted. Steps 3 through 5 are geared for the very obese, people who are 40 percent or more overweight.

Marlene Schwartz and Kelly Brownell (1995) asked 33 weight-loss experts from several fields (psychology, nutrition, internal medicine, surgery, and neuroendocrinology) to compare 11 popular weight-loss approaches, including self-directed dieting, *Weight Watchers,* behavioral programs, medication, and surgery (see also Reality Check on page 294). Among their findings:

- Self-directed dieting was recommended for those with mild to moderate obesity, except for people with a history of weight cycling.
- Commercial programs with group support, such as *Weight Watchers,* were recommended for an initial weight-loss attempt or for people who could not diet on their own.

- Very low-calorie diets and surgery were recommended only for those with a medical problem complicated by their obesity.

- Medical supervision was considered necessary for people with diabetes and others with medical conditions that are likely to change with dieting.

- Individual counseling and behavioral weight-loss programs were considered appropriate for those with eating disorders.

The idea of matching individuals to treatment is appealing because of the likelihood that people with different personality styles, levels of obesity, eating practices, and so on will respond differently to various treatments.

Figure 7.4

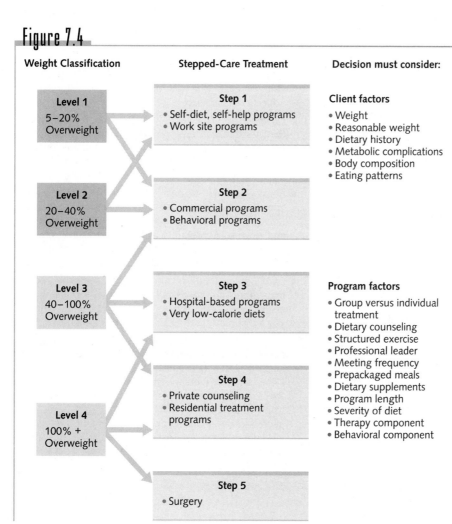

Weight Classification	Stepped-Care Treatment	Decision must consider:
Level 1 5–20% Overweight	**Step 1** • Self-diet, self-help programs • Work site programs	**Client factors** • Weight • Reasonable weight • Dietary history • Metabolic complications • Body composition • Eating patterns
Level 2 20–40% Overweight	**Step 2** • Commercial programs • Behavioral programs	
Level 3 40–100% Overweight	**Step 3** • Hospital-based programs • Very low-calorie diets	**Program factors** • Group versus individual treatment • Dietary counseling • Structured exercise • Professional leader • Meeting frequency • Prepackaged meals • Dietary supplements • Program length • Severity of diet • Therapy component • Behavioral component
	Step 4 • Private counseling • Residential treatment programs	
Level 4 100% + Overweight	**Step 5** • Surgery	

Stepped Care in the Treatment of Obesity

In general, people at levels 1 or 2 should be able to lose weight through steps 1 and 2. At level 3, treatment should begin with step 2 and extend through 4. Those at level 4 who have medical problems may need surgery to solve their weight-loss problems. However, before a health psychologist sets up a program, he or she considers all factors related to both the client and the program (as listed on the right).

Source: "The Heterogeneity of Obesity: Fitting Individuals to Treatments," by K. D. Brownell and T. A. Wadden, 1991, *Behavior Therapy, 22,* pp. 153–177.

Reality Check

How Much Should You Weigh?

People who choose to diet should establish reasonable weight-loss goals based on heredity, body shape, and diet history rather than on a table of ideal weights (Foster, 1997; Wadden, Steen, Wingate, & Foster, 1996). This decreased emphasis on ideal weights is underscored by the National Academy of Sciences, which considers successful weight loss to be a 5 percent reduction in body weight that is maintained for at least one year. Many health conditions improve significantly with a modest weight loss of 5 to 10 percent, even when patients remain considerably overweight (Blackburn, 1995). Moreover, modest changes in weight and behavior are more successfully maintained than are more dramatic ones (Wadden, Foster, & Letizia, 1994).

Unfortunately, many people set unrealistic weight-loss goals. Before beginning a 48-week treatment program, 60 obese women (BMI = 36.3) were asked to define their goal weight loss. On average, their weight-loss goal was a 32 percent reduction in body weight—quite different from the 5 to 10 percent recommendations of health experts. Naturally, then, although the average weight loss at the end of treatment was a healthy 16 kg, 47 percent of the participants were disappointed.

The best way to determine whether you need to lose weight is to evaluate how "healthy" your current weight is. Answer the following questions, listed in order of importance (Mayo Clinic, 2001):

- Do I have a health condition that would benefit if I lost weight? Examples of weight-sensitive health problems are high blood pressure, atherosclerosis, diabetes, high serum cholesterol, and arthritis.
- Am I genetically vulnerable to these problems as I get older? Determine whether your family history makes it more likely that you will develop a chronic disease related to weight.
- Is my weight outside the acceptable range? Follow the guidelines in the body of the text to determine whether your BMI and body fat percentage indicate that you have excess weight.
- Do I overeat, smoke cigarettes, have more than two alcoholic drinks a day, or live with uncontrolled stress?

When combined with these behaviors, obesity is even more hazardous to your health.

If you were able to answer "no" to all the above questions, you probably shouldn't worry about your weight. Conversely, if you answered "yes" to one or more, it might be wise to consider losing some weight.

Here are some healthful tips if you decide to lose weight:

- *Be clear on your motivation.* Lose weight because you want to, not to please someone else or to look like a supermodel.
- *Set a realistic goal.* Accept the reality that healthful weight loss is a slow process and set weekly or monthly goals that will allow you to monitor (and achieve) regular success.
- *Eat more healthful foods.* Appetite suppressants and the latest fad diets are generally ineffective. They may also harm your health. Complex carbohydrates boost metabolism and are not as easily converted to body fat as are dietary fats.
- *Boost your BMR.* Regular, 20-minute sessions of sustained aerobic exercise are the best way to lose body fat. Good choices are walking, bicycling, swimming, and running. Moderate weight/strength training will also increase metabolism, although not as effectively as sustained aerobic exercise.
- *Gain some stimulus control.* Keep tempting, no-preparation fast foods out of reach. Make eating a deliberate decision. Never shop for groceries when you are hungry.
- *Develop healthy eating habits.* Many overweight people starve themselves by skipping breakfast and lunch in order to eat one "normal" meal at dinner. Doing so slows metabolism and makes it much easier for calories to be stored as body fat. Other bad habits to guard against are eating when you are anxious or depressed (emotional eating), binge eating, and eating late at night, especially if you're sitting or lying down afterward.

Eating Disorders

For some dieters, especially young, overachieving women like Jodi—the young woman we met at the beginning of the chapter—obsession with weight control may turn into a serious eating disorder.

Derived from the Greek roots *an*, meaning "without," and *orexis*, meaning "a desire for," **anorexia nervosa** is an eating disorder characterized by refusal to maintain body weight above a BMI of 18, intense fear of weight gain, disturbance of body image, and amenorrhea (cessation of menstruation) for at least 3 months (APA, 1997). Because attainment of a given percentage of body fat is necessary for menstruation, post-pubescent women develop amenorrhea if they lose enough weight.

Anorexia can lead to starvation and many other serious medical complications:

- slowed thyroid function
- irregular breathing and heart rhythm
- low blood pressure
- dry and yellowed skin
- brittle bones
- anemia, light-headedness, and dehydration
- swollen joints and reduced muscle mass
- intolerance to cold temperatures

The other major eating disorder is **bulimia nervosa,** which derives from the Greek roots *bous*, meaning "ox" or "cow," and *limos*, meaning "hunger." Bulimia involves compulsive bingeing followed by purging through self-induced vomiting or large doses of laxatives. Some people purge regularly, others only after a binge. For example, they may consume as many as 5,000 to 10,000 calories at one time, eating until they are exhausted, in pain, or out of food. Bulimia patients also engage in compulsive exercise to try to control their weight. And, unlike those with anorexia, people with bulimia typically maintain a relatively normal weight (Hsu, 1990)—as Jodi initially did until she moved out on her own and began reducing her food intake.

Although as many as half of all college women report having binged and purged at some time (Fairburn & Wilson, 1993), most would not be considered bulimic. The criteria for a clinical diagnosis include at least two bulimic episodes a week for at least 3 months; lack of control over eating; behavior designed to avoid weight gain; and persistent, exaggerated concern about weight (APA, 1997).

■ **anorexia nervosa** an eating disorder characterized by self-starvation, a distorted body image, and, in females, amenorrhea

■ **bulimia nervosa** an eating disorder characterized by alternating cycles of binge eating and purging through such techniques as vomiting or laxative abuse

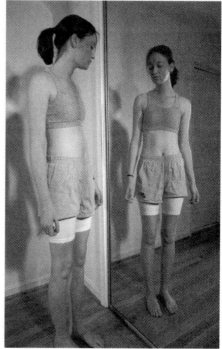

Anorexia
Young girls with anorexia look at themselves in the mirror and see—not the superthin person we see—but someone who is overweight and still needs to shed more pounds. If she continues to lose weight, this girl's systems will become overburdened with the job of trying to maintain a functioning system with minimal caloric intake. At the extreme, the heart may stop pumping.
© Richard T. Nowitz/Corbis

Unlike anorexia, which has a mortality rate of 2 to 15 percent, bulimia is rarely fatal. But it puts sufferers at risk for many serious health problems, including:

- laxative dependence.

- hypoglycemia (low blood sugar) and lethargy from eating an unbalanced diet (often one high in sweets but lacking in sufficient fatty acids).

- damaged teeth from purging since hydrochloric acid from the stomach erodes tooth enamel. (Dentists are often the first health care professionals to suspect bulimia.)

- bleeding and tearing of the esophagus from purging.

- anemia (a condition involving a lack of hemoglobin in the blood) and electrolyte imbalance caused by loss of sodium, potassium, magnesium, and other body minerals.

Bulimic episodes are reported by 40 to 50 percent of anorexic patients. It is possible for an individual to meet criteria for both disorders if they are both underweight and binge.

History and Demographics

Richard Morton reported the first documented case of anorexia nervosa in 1689. Over the next two centuries only a handful of additional cases were reported. In London, Sir William Gull studied several cases of self-starvation during the 1860s, concluding that the disorder was psychological in origin and later giving the disorder its name, which means "nervous loss of appetite." Bulimia nervosa has only been recognized as a distinct disorder in the past 20 years or so (Russell, 1979).

Anorexia and bulimia are unique among psychological disorders in having a strong gender bias (a 10 to 1 ratio of women to men) and in the substantial increase in these disorders during the twentieth century. Before the 1970s, eating disorders also were far more common among upper- and upper-middle-class women in Western cultures (Garfinkel & Garner, 1984). Since then disordered eating has been increasing among other populations, leading researchers to conclude that SES and ethnocultural identity are no longer reliable predictors (Dolan & Ford, 1991; Whitaker, 1989).

Today, approximately 0.5 to 1 percent of young adult and adolescent females are anorexic, and between 1 and 3 percent are clinically bulimic (APA, 1997). College women are at particular risk, as are young women between 15 and 19 who attend ballet or modeling academies. Athletes also are at increased risk of eating disorders, even those who participate in sports that do not emphasize appearance or an overly thin body. Men make up about 5 to 10 percent of all anorexia victims. Male athletes—especially swimmers, rowers, and wrestlers—are especially vulnerable (Weinberg & Gould, 1995).

Applying the Biopsychosocial (Mind–Body) Model

As with many issues discussed in this book, researchers have discovered that biological, psychological, social, and cultural factors may all be involved in disordered eating. Until the late 1930s, many doctors linked anorexia with a pituitary gland disorder, but this view soon lost favor. During the 1940s and 1950s, psychiatrists hypothesized that anorexia involved a denial of femininity and a fear of motherhood, but this view too was discarded in the face of mounting evidence that anorexia is a learned syndrome. Recent emphasis has been on describing the disorder in terms of multiple components, reflecting the emphases of the biopsychosocial (or mind–body) model.

Biological Factors

A number of researchers have reported that a young person's body image at the onset of puberty may foretell healthy or disordered eating behaviors (Graber, Brooks-Gunn, Paikoff, & Warren, 1994). Girls who perceive the timing of their development to be early tend to feel the least positive about their bodies, whereas girls who perceive their development to be on time feel the most attractive and have the most positive body images (Richards, Boxer, Petersen, & Albrecht, 1990). Early maturing girls may feel less comfortable with their bodies because, at a time when peer acceptance is crucial to self-esteem, their bodies are different from those of the majority of their peers. On-time development may present the least psychological challenge to adolescent girls.

Biochemical abnormalities at all levels of the hypothalamic-pituitary-adrenal axis are associated with both anorexia and bulimia. These include abnormal levels of norepinephrine and other neurotransmitters that may promote clinical depression (Fava, Copeland, Schweiger, & Herzog, 1989). There is also evidence that bulimia may be caused in part by disturbances in the brain's supply of *endorphins,* the opiatelike neurotransmitters linked to pain control and pleasure (Jonas & Gold, 1988). Researchers have found that *opiate antagonists,* which block the action of the endorphins, may be an effective treatment in reducing the frequency of binge-purge episodes. For example, the drug naltrexone, which is an opiate antagonist, flushes endorphins from brain receptor sites, rendering them useless.

Biochemical theories are inconclusive, however, because neurotransmitter levels often return to normal when disordered eating stops. It is possible that abnormal brain biochemistry, caused by an unrelated factor, could alter mood and lead to abnormal eating. If this is the case, and there is mounting evidence that it is, biological abnormalities may be consequences rather than causes of eating disorders (Wardle, 1997).

Might people inherit a predisposition to eating disorders? Studies of eating disorders within families and among twins reveal a possible genetic influence on anorexia and bulimia. Consider:

- When one twin has bulimia, the chances of the other twin's sharing the disorder are substantially greater if they are identical twins (a 75 percent concordance rate) rather than fraternal twins (a 27 percent rate) (Walters & Kendler, 1995).

- The chances that a young adult woman will be diagnosed with a clinical eating disorder are much greater if she has a female relative who is anorexic (Strober, Morrell, Burroughs, Salkin, & Jacobs, 1985).

- Individuals with eating disorders tend to have a family history of major depression, obsessive-compulsive disorder (OCD), and anxiety. Those with anorexia have a high rate of depression before the onset of disordered eating.

Psychological Factors

Other theorists argue that the roots of eating disorders can be found in certain psychological situations, such as the competitive, semiclosed social environments of some families, athletic teams, and college sororities (Lester & Petrie, 1998).

The families of anorexia patients tend to be high achieving, competitive, overprotective, and characterized by intense interactions and poor conflict resolution (Minuchin, Rosman, & Baker, 1978; Pate, Pumariega, Hester, & Garner, 1992). The families of bulimia patients have a higher-than-average incidence of alcoholism, drug addiction, obesity, and depression (Miller, McCluskey-Fawcett, & Irving, 1993). Researchers caution, however, against assuming that all children of parents addicted to alcohol are alike. Eating disorders are *not* a telltale sign of an alcohol abuser's home environment (Mintz, Kashubeck, & Tracy, 1995). Young women with anorexia and bulimia rate their relationships with their parents as disengaged, unfriendly, and even hostile (Wonderlich, Klein, & Council, 1996). They also feel less accepted by their parents, who are perceived as overly critical, neglectful, and poor communicators (Calam, Waller, Slade, & Newton, 1990).

Until recently, researchers have focused almost entirely on the role of the mother in her daughter's disordered eating, tracing its roots to the relationship between infant and primary caregiver (Bruch, 1982). Following this model, the mother of the girl with anorexia was described as overnurturing, overprotective, and demanding, whereas the mother of the girl with bulimia was seen as undernurturing, rejecting, and unaffectionate. Although research studies of this model are sorely limited, there *is* evidence that the mothers of daughters with an eating disorder tend to be more controlling and demanding (Humphrey, 1987) as well as critical of the weight and appearance of their daughters (Pike & Rodin, 1991).

More recent research has shown that both parents play important roles in influencing the development of healthy eating behaviors in their children. These studies also encourage a shift away from the once popular "blame mother" view of adolescent eating disorders. For example, Amy Swarr and Maryse Richards of Loyola University (1996) investigated family relationships and disordered eating in adolescent females. Positive relationships with *both* parents predicted healthier eating scores both concurrently and in the future. Girls who felt close to both mom and dad reported the fewest weight and eating concerns during the seventh, eighth, and ninth grades. Those who spent more time with both parents reported fewer eating problems 2 years later.

Sociocultural Factors

Sociocultural factors may explain why anorexia and bulimia occur more often in women than in men and more often in weight-conscious Western cultures, and why the prevalence of eating disorders has increased in recent years. According to the sociocultural view, dieting and disordered eating are women's understandable responses to women's social roles and to cultural ideals of beauty (Seid, 1994). Thus, binge eating, self-starvation, and thin standards of female beauty have characterized female cohorts who reached adolescence in periods when educational opportunities for women increased but did not characterize cohorts who reached adolescence when educational opportunities remained stable or decreased (Perlick & Silverstein, 1994).

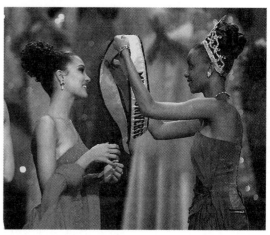

Thin Is Good, Skinny Is Better
Over the years, judges have selected increasingly thin women as Miss Universe, showing the current idealization of the "skinny" Western-style woman around the world. © AFP/Corbis

Interestingly, the "thin is beautiful" standard is absent in many developing countries. In Niger, West Africa, for instance, fat is the beauty ideal for women, who often compete to be crowned the heaviest (Onishi, 2001). Among the Calabari of southeastern Nigeria, brides are sent to "fattening farms" before their weddings, where they gorge themselves on food and take steroid drugs to gain bulk and other pills to increase their appetites. At the end of their stay, they are paraded in the village square where their fullness can be admired.

In recent years, Western cultures have increasingly emphasized the positive attributes of slender bodies, in particular for women. As Roberta Seid has noted, "Our culture has elevated the pursuit of a lean, fat-free body into a new religion. It has a creed: 'I eat right, watch my weight, and exercise.' Indeed, anorexia nervosa could be called the paradigm of our age, for our creed encourages us all to adopt the behavior and attitudes of the anorexic" (Seid, 1994). Nowhere is this "religion" more apparent than in how women's bodies are represented in the media.

Body Image and the Media

The ideal female weight—represented by actresses, supermodels, and Miss Americas—has progressively decreased to that of the thinnest 5 to 10 percent of American women. Consequently, over three-fourths of normal-weight women think they weigh too much and more than half are dieting at any given time (Mintz & Kashubeck, 1999).

A survey of 15,000 American women between the ages of 17 and 60 revealed an average weight-loss goal of 30 pounds, which, if attained, would have made most of them underweight (Williamson, Serdula, Anda, Levy, & Byers, 1992). Another survey of American dieters found that those who were most likely to diet were young, well-educated, employed, and least likely to need to diet. In fact, half these dieters had a BMI under 25 (Biener & Heaton, 1995). Most disturbing of all is that even very young girls are now preoccupied with body weight. One study reported that 80 percent of fourth-grade girls in the San Francisco Bay area were watching their weight (Kilbourne, 1994).

Society's current emphasis on thinness may be the clearest example of the power of advertising to influence cultural norms and individual behavior. Like clothing styles, body types go in and out of fashion and are promoted by advertising. The images constantly reinforce the latest ideal. The impact of the media in establishing role models is undeniable. In the United States, women of European ancestry are particularly vulnerable to these role models (Cash & Henry, 1995). With increasing Americanization and globalization, body image dissatisfaction is becoming more common among young women in Egypt, Russia, Japan, Brazil, and many other nations (Nasser, 1997).

The question of why advertisers became preoccupied with thinness is difficult to answer. In a controversial line of reasoning, O. Wayne Wooley (1994) has argued that the cultural shift to a thin body image ideal was triggered by the feminist movement and its attempts to counteract female pornography. A major goal of the feminist movement was to get more women into the workplace—and on an equal footing with men. In addition, the movement began at a time when pornographic images of women, which tended to emphasize the "fat" parts of a woman's body, began to reach a wider public audience than ever before. "If women were going to be able to go out into the workplace," argues Wooley, "they needed representations of their bodies that could compete with, and answer, the messages of pornography. They needed a new ideal body that they could carry in their minds . . . the counterimage had to be thinner."

Although advertisers will undoubtedly continue to play to the public's fears, Jean Kilbourne (1994) believes the situation is not hopeless. "We can learn a lot from the public policy advocates who have been battling the alcohol and nicotine industries with success," she notes. "As a result, norms for smoking have changed dramatically. This is a result of many things, including warning labels on the packs, advertising restrictions, product liability suits, and increased health information. We can change the norms about diet and thinness with many of the same measures."

On a more encouraging note, a recent study found that long-term exposure to ultrathin celebrities and magazine models does not automatically lead to excessive dieting and other unhealthy behaviors. Eric Stice and his colleagues (1998) randomly assigned 13- to 17-year-old girls either to a group that received a 15-month subscription to *Seventeen* magazine or to a control group that did not receive the magazine. Over the next 20 months, only those who initially expressed body dissatisfaction experienced significant increases in dieting, depression, and symptoms of bulimia.

The researchers suggest that previous studies probably found that brief exposure to ads showing lean, sinewy models resulted in sharply decreased satisfaction with personal appearance because the studies were nearly always conducted in a laboratory environment. Over a longer period of time in the more natural home environments of their participants (as in the study by Stice and his colleagues), the feedback of supportive parents, peers, and dating partners might overshadow the media's influence. The researchers caution, however, that their findings don't mean that media influences should be discounted, since teenagers with poor body images might be more likely to read fashion magazines to learn more about weight-loss techniques.

Putting It All Together

Eating disorders appear to be multifactorial disorders determined by the interaction of biological, psychological, social, and cultural factors. The changes in fat distribution in adolescent girls, particularly those who mature early, may provide the foundations for body image dissatisfaction. A social and family environment in which there is an emphasis on slimness may foster additional frustration with body weight. At the individual level, competitiveness and perfectionism combined with the stresses of adolescent peer pressure may promote the decision to diet. Once food restriction and weight loss occur, a range of metabolic and neuroendocrine responses takes place that may help perpetuate disordered eating. Once weight loss has occurred, many become more weight-phobic as they adapt to a new body shape in which any fat is regarded with horror.

The Psychology behind the Need to Lose Weight

In a society that stigmatizes obesity it makes sense that obese women are more dissatisfied with their bodies than lean women are (Sarwer, Wadden, & Foster, 1998). Gary Foster and his colleagues at the University of Pennsylvania assessed body image, as measured in 59 obese women before, during, and after 48 weeks of weight-loss treatment. Weight loss was associated with significant improvements in the participants' ratings of appearance and body satisfaction. Surprisingly, improvements in body image during treatment were not related to the total amount of weight lost. Those who lost an average of 12 kg at week 24 showed the same improvement in body image as those who lost 27 kg by this time. Other researchers have also found that small reductions in weight improve body image, and further weight loss confers no additional advantage.

It bears repeating that the increasing idealization of the thin-and-fit look in many developed countries is a clear example of a cohort effect that arose in

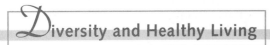

Diversity and Healthy Living

Eating Disorders and Ethnocultural Identity

Traditional American standards of attractiveness are oppressive for many women, but especially for those whose own body ideals do not stem from European American culture.

Cultures differ in the flexibility of the ideal body image. Colleen Rand and John Kuldau (1990) compared body image satisfaction in African-Americans and European Americans, finding a greater tolerance for diversity of body type and shape in the former group. Similar differences among college students have been reported. One study found that African-American college women had a less restricted definition of ideal body weight and were less likely to become depressed after binge eating (Gray, Ford, & Kelly, 1987).

Most eating disorder research has focused on white women, to the exclusion of other racial or ethnic groups. Maria Root (1990) identified stereotypes, racism, and ethnocentrism as reasons underlying this lack of attention. She suggested that many have adopted the stereotype of the individual with an eating disorder as a white, upper-class woman, despite evidence that African-American women do suffer from eating disorders (Abood & Chandler, 1997; Wilfley et al., 1996).

It has also been suggested that many experts believe that certain factors within minority cultures, such as an ap-preciation of a healthier (larger) body size and less emphasis on physical appearance, make minority women invulnerable to eating disorders. Although research has demonstrated that African-American women generally do have more positive attitudes toward their bodies, food, and weight than white women (Abood & Chandler, 1997), they certainly are *not* immune to developing hazardous patterns of eating.

Newer studies reveal that for women of color, eating disorders may be "a means of suppressing one's ethnocultural concept of beauty by replacing it with a Eurocentric one of thinness" (Harris & Kuba, 1997). According to this view, eating disorders among members of minority groups are a symptom of identity confusion. Although the *Diagnostic and Statistical Manual of Mental Disorders* (DSM-IV) includes ethnicity and culture in its review of anorexia nervosa and bulimia nervosa, it does not refer to compulsive eating. This is problematic, given that many women of color suffer from this eating disorder. In a recent study of women assessed for eating disorders, 84 percent of African-American women were diagnosed as bulimic (Harris & Kuba, 1997).

For the adolescent who is attempting to assimilate into a different culture, learned ways of behavior may conflict with the messages from the majority community and result in a crisis. Thus, if the Latin American culture accepts a

response to a unique combination of social and historical circumstances (see Diversity and Healthy Living). Many women strive to lose weight because they are needlessly dissatisfied with their bodies. It is a sad truth that at some point in her development, nearly every young woman in today's developed nations has a distorted body image and considers herself too fat (Mintz & Kashubeck, 1999).

This current fat aversion and body image dissatisfaction is so pervasive in the United States that it represents a "normative discontent" among women of all shapes and sizes (Striegel-Moore, Silberstein, & Rodin, 1993). Judy Rodin has argued that women too often are brought up to believe that their appearance is not solely their own business. How daughters look, for instance, is an open topic of conversation in many families, making them feel their bodies are fair game for public scrutiny. Sadly, to the degree that there is a gap between their *actual selves* and *ideal selves*, many come away feeling exposed and shamed. The increased prevalence of eating disorders during the last

How much blame for girls' plump body image should be placed on the unrealistic body dimensions of Barbie and other popular dolls? By one estimate, to achieve "Barbie doll proportions" a female of average height would have to gain 12 inches in height, lose 5 inches in her waistline, and gain 4 inches in her bustline!

robust figure but the European American culture values thinness, young Latina women may find themselves in conflict over the appropriate body image and eating behaviors. Similarly, Toshiaki Furukawa (1994) reported that Japanese exchange students developed maladaptive eating patterns (and experienced weight changes) during their time in the United States.

Ethnocultural identity develops as children learn about themselves in relation to the norms and expectations of others within their group. Most models of identity formation among people of color identify four or five distinct psychological states (Helms, 1995).

- *Precultural awakening.* Those in this stage often experience low self-esteem as they struggle to identify with a majority frame of reference. The roots of disordered eating can often be found in this struggle. For example, a young African-American woman may decide to stop eating certain foods because she is preoccupied with the size of her hips or thighs as she compares herself with European American actresses.

- *Dissonance stage.* In the next stage, the individual becomes aware of her internal conflict and vacillates between the desire to be thin and to accept her body as it is. She may develop bulimic symptoms that represent the push and pull of two different cultures.

- *Immersion-emersion.* The third stage is characterized by greater self-appreciation as the young person immerses herself in her culture of origin. Although it may appear that she has formed a healthy identity, she may exaggerate her ethnocultural stereotype, even rejecting any attempt to appear physically attractive. Anger and mood swings are a predominant emotional theme of this stage. Compulsive eating may reflect this stage of thinking.

- *Internalization stage.* The final stage is marked by improved self-esteem and an integration of positive attitudes toward self and culture, with less anger and a greater appreciation for differences in attractiveness across cultures.

One implication of these models is the need for preventive interventions that are sensitive to each individual's stage of identity development. When the patient is in the precultural awakening stage, an appropriate strategy is to increase the young person's awareness of her ethnocultural legacy as well as the prejudice inherent in majority cultures. Intervention during the dissonance stage should focus on the grief caused by the client's sense of loss of her culture. Development beyond this stage might be hastened by encouraging contact with others of similar ethnocultural identity.

half-century has coincided with this epidemic body image dissatisfaction (Feingold & Mazzella, 1996). Figure 7.5, page 304, illustrates one test of the *self-ideal discrepancy* that has been widely used in body image dissatisfaction research.

Treatment of Eating Disorders

A range of therapies has been used to treat anorexia and bulimia, from force-feeding to family therapy. Experts agree that treatment must address both the behavior and the attitudes that perpetuate disordered eating.

Restoring body weight is, of course, the first priority in treating anorexia. In extreme cases, inpatient treatment includes force-fed diets that gradually increase from about 1,500 to 3,500 calories per day. In many cases, a number of secondary biological and psychological disturbances are reduced once body weight is restored.

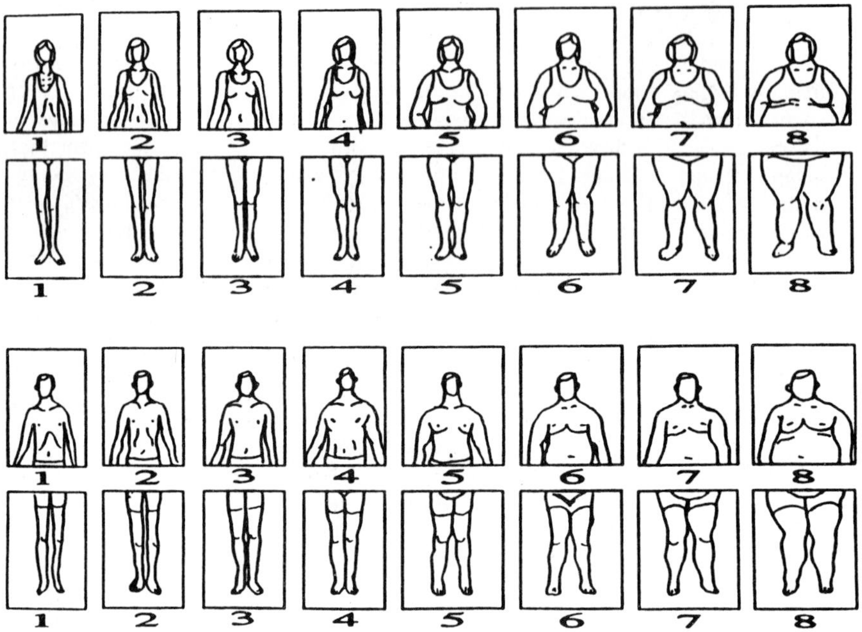

Figure 7.5

Self-Ideal Body Image Discrepancy

Working first with the top part (head to waist) of the drawings for your gender, choose the number below the figure that best illustrates (A) how you think you currently look (that is, the figure that best represents your actual size). Then choose the figure that illustrates (B) how you would like to look (your ideal figure). Each figure has a number associated with it, so you can calculate your body discrepancy score. The numerical difference between your views of how you think you look and how you would like to look (A − B) represents your self-ideal discrepancy. Repeat the same procedure for the figures from waist to feet. Finally, rate how ashamed you are of any body image discrepancy from 0 (not at all) to 5 (extremely). If you have a shame score of 3 or more, you should consider talking to a close friend or counselor about these feelings.

Source: *Body Traps* (pp. 76–77), by J. Rodin, Ph.D. 1992, New York: William Morrow. Reprinted by permission of HarperCollins Publishers, Inc.

■ **exposure-response prevention** a behavioral treatment of bulimia nervosa that attempts to prevent purging (and therefore, reinforcement) following binge eating

Many different drugs have been used in the treatment of binge eating. These include antidepressants, appetite suppressants, and opiate antagonists. Pharmacological treatments remain controversial, however, and have an especially high relapse rate. For this reason, most clinicians view such treatment as supplementary and consider psychotherapy as the treatment of choice for most patients. Antidepressants and other drugs are generally prescribed only when there is clear evidence of a coexisting affective- or impulse-control disorder, especially one that preceded the onset of the eating disorder (Fairburn & Wilson, 1993).

Behavioral Treatments

Behavioral treatments for eating disorders are based on the assumption that self-starvation is a learned habit maintained by some source of reinforcement. Following this reasoning, one form of treatment for bulimia, called **exposure-response prevention,** attempts to prevent purging after bingeing (Rosen & Leitenberg, 1982). This treatment is based on an anxiety model of bulimia nervosa, in which binge eating is believed to increase anxiety (over weight gain), which in turn is relieved by purging. When purging is prevented, a powerful source of negative reinforcement for bingeing (relief from anxiety) is removed. Over time, and in conjunction with interventions that promote more realistic thinking about food and body image, binge eating may disappear (extinction).

Other aspects of behavioral programs include relapse prevention training in which the patient learns to identify circumstances that trigger disordered eating and to develop strategies to avoid those situations or to cope more effectively. Relaxation training and stress-management skills are also taught.

Since the 1970s, cognitive behavior therapy has become the most widely used method of treating both anorexia and bulimia (Agras, 1993). (Recall that this therapy is also most effective in helping people to lose weight and keep it off.) The procedure is straightforward: First, therapists monitor food intake, binge-eating episodes, and stimulus triggers of those episodes. They then use this information to gradually mold the patient's eating into a pattern of three or more meals per day, introduce feared foods into the diet, and change faulty thinking and distorted attitudes about food intake, weight, and body image.

How Effective Are Treatments for Eating Disorders?

Anorexia remains one of the most difficult behavior disorders to treat because many victims see nothing wrong with their eating behavior and resist any attempt to change. Consequently, from 5 to 18 percent will eventually die from starvation, cardiac arrest, or suicide (Wardle, 1997).

Although there are relatively few controlled studies comparing the results of treatments for anorexia, most therapies result in some weight restoration in the short term but a high relapse rate (often in excess of 50 percent) and poor long-term outcome (Wardle, 1997). Longer-term follow-up studies show that the majority of anorexia patients persist in their preoccupation with food and weight and that many continue to show psychological signs of the disorder, have low weight, and exhibit social or mood disturbances (Sullivan, Bulik, Fear, & Pickering, 1998).

There have been more controlled clinical trials of the treatment of bulimia, which is more prevalent than anorexia. As with anorexia, longer-term evaluations have not produced entirely favorable results (Wardle, 1997). One study compared the effectiveness of behavior therapies and cognitive behavior therapies. The behavior therapy group received eight sessions of individualized treatment that focused on restructuring the patient's environment to gain greater control over environmental triggers for disordered eating. The group was also taught self-monitoring, contingency contracts, and relapse prevention strategies. The cognitive behavior therapy group received the behavioral training as well as treatment sessions designed to challenge irrational food attitudes, to promote coping skills, and to prevent relapse. A third, control group received training in self-monitoring. At the end of the treatment phase, all three groups experienced a significant decrease in binge-purge episodes. Six months later, only 15 percent of the control subjects and 38 percent of the behavior therapy group remained free of binge-purge episodes. In contrast, 69 percent of the cognitive behavior therapy group remained free of such episodes (Thackwray, Smith, Bodfish, & Meyers, 1993).

Cognitive behavior therapy has also proved to be fairly effective as a primary prevention for binge eating in high-risk women (Kaminski & McNamara, 1996). The researchers recruited college women with warning signs for eating disorders: low self-esteem, poor body image, perfectionism, and a history of repeated dieting. The students were randomly assigned to either a treatment group or a control group. The treatment group received training in cognitive strategies for increasing self-esteem, challenging self-defeating thinking, improving body image, and combating social pressures for thinness. After 7 weeks, students in the treatment group showed greater improvement in self-esteem and body image than did students in the control group. They also had reported significantly fewer disordered eating episodes.

Christopher Fairburn, a leading bulimia researcher, has suggested that the long-term success rate of all eating disorder interventions is a function of two participant variables: self-esteem and body image. Regardless of the type of treatment used, patients with lower self-esteem and persistent body-image distortions tend to be less successful in terms of their long-term recovery (Fairburn & Wilson, 1993).

Controlled studies of treatments for disordered eating show dropout rates ranging from 0 to 34 percent and long-term abstinence from disordered eating ranging from 20 to 76 percent. As Stewart Agras (1993) has noted, out of a treatment group of 100 binge eaters treated with cognitive behavior therapy (generally the most effective treatment), 16 will probably drop out of treatment and 40 will be abstinent by the end of treatment. A failure rate of 60 percent suggests that researchers have not yet found the ideal treatment for eating disorders.

Some programs fail because they try to do too many things at one time. Traci Mann and colleagues at Stanford University (Mann, Nolen-Hoeksema, Huang, & Burgard, 1997) evaluated an eating disorder intervention aimed at both primary and secondary prevention in a sample of female college freshman. (As described in Chapter 5, primary prevention is aimed at preventing new cases of eating disorders from arising and so is targeted at healthy, at-risk individuals. Secondary prevention is aimed at reducing the severity and duration of eating disorders by detecting and treating them early on and so is targeted at people in the early stages of bulimia and anorexia.) The intervention consisted of a 90-minute group discussion of issues in disordered eating. The discussion was led by two older students, one who had recovered from anorexia and the other a bulimia patient who, while still exhibiting some symptoms of disordered eating, was no longer clinically diagnosable. Students also filled out surveys at the beginning of the freshman year and again 4 weeks and 12 weeks after the intervention program. The surveys assessed disordered eating symptoms, including bingeing, purging, dieting, and loss of control over eating. The results were extremely disappointing: Students who attended the program actually reported slightly more symptoms of eating disorders than did students who did not attend.

Because of their very different aims, the ideal primary and secondary prevention strategies often oppose each other. As Mann suggests, to prevent disordered eating in healthy young women (primary prevention), the ideal strategy might be to stress the abnormal and hazardous nature of anorexic and bulimic behaviors. In contrast, to encourage those who already have problems to come forward for help (secondary prevention), it might be advisable to suggest the opposite—that eating disorders are common and easy to treat. The researchers therefore suggest that interventions for eating disorders may be more effective if they do not try to simultaneously achieve both primary and secondary prevention. Instead, efforts should be made to assess the needs of students and to evaluate which would benefit from a primary and which from a secondary intervention (Mann et al., 1997).

Despite the relatively dismal success rate of formal treatment programs and preventive interventions for eating disorders, there is evidence that some people with eating disorders respond to simple interventions, such as instruction in self-help techniques. Jacqueline Carter, Christopher Fairburn, and their colleagues (1998) found that pure self-help and guided self-help had a substantial and sustained impact on eating behavior, with almost half the participants ceasing to binge eat at the end of treatment and at treatment follow-ups 3 and 6 months later.

There is also good news in the finding that some victims of eating disorders may recover on their own with the passage of time. A recent longitudinal study followed a cohort of 509 women and 206 men who were teenagers in the late 1970s and early 1980s, a period when eating disorders were prevalent. The researchers surveyed the participants' eating attitudes and behaviors while in college and again 10 years later (Heatherton, Mahamedi, Striepe, & Field, 1997). The results showed that body dissatisfaction, chronic dieting, and eating disorder symptoms generally diminished among many of the women in the 10 years following college, with rates of apparent eating disorder dropping by more than half. However, a substantial number of the women, particularly those who were dissatisfied with their body weight or shape in college, continued to have eating problems 10 years after college. More than 1 in 5 of the women who met clinical criteria for an eating disorder in college also did so 10 years later.

These results suggest that some degree of disordered eating may be normative for college women and that diminution of these problems after graduation is also normative. However, body dissatisfaction and chronic dieting remain a problem for a substantial number of women. Changes in maturation and gender role status may partly explain why eating problems diminish after college.

It is also possible that these findings reflect a more general societal trend. Todd Heatherton, Patricia Nichols, and their colleagues (1995) compared the eating behavior of college students in 1982 and 1992. They found that eating disorder symptoms, dieting, and body dissatisfaction declined during that decade. Heatherton attributes the decline in eating disorders to greater public awareness. The increased media focus may have increased awareness of the potential consequences of fasting or bingeing and purging.

Along with greater awareness of disordered eating, today there is an increased emphasis on healthful eating and nutritious low-fat rather than low-calorie diets. Sociocultural messages about thinness have changed somewhat as well, again with greater emphasis on health and less on actual weight.

Summing Up

Nutrition: Eating the Right Foods

1. Besides water and daily caloric energy, the body requires 46 nutrients, which are grouped into five categories: proteins, fats, carbohydrates, vitamins, and minerals. Carbohydrates are the major source of energy in our diet; fats, or lipids, are the densest source of food energy; proteins are the building blocks of all body tissues. Chronic protein deficiencies in the diet—which are rare in this country but common in developing parts of the world—can lead to severe disorders such as marasmus and kwashiorkor.

2. Poor nutrition has been implicated in five of the ten leading causes of death: heart disease, cancer, stroke, diabetes, and atherosclerosis. There are three types of lipoproteins: Low-density lipoprotein (LDL) and very low-density lipoprotein (VLDL) have been linked to heart disease, whereas high-density lipoprotein (HDL) may protect against atherosclerotic plaques. Saturated fat has been implicated as a dietary factor in some forms of cancer.

Weight Determination: Eating the Right Amount of Food

3. Basal metabolic rate, or BMR, depends on a number of variables, including your age, gender, current weight, and activity level. Many people believe that their body weights fluctuate erratically, but in fact their bodies actually balance energy intake and expenditure quite closely. This supports the concept of a body weight set point. In an obese person, fat cells, or adipocytes, may swell to three times their normal size and then divide (fat-cell hyperplasia). Once the number of fat cells in a person's body increases, it never decreases.

4. Researchers have located appetite centers in two areas of the hypothalamus: a side region called the lateral hypothalamus (LH), which may trigger hunger, and a lower area in the middle called the ventromedial hypothalamus (VMS), which may trigger satiety. Approximately 59 percent of American adults are obese, and the number of obese children has increased dramatically during recent years.

Obesity: Some Basic Facts

5. Obesity is a risk factor for many diseases. In addition, the obese also have social problems because they are the objects of discrimination. Body fat can be estimated by skinfold measurement, electrical resistance of body tissue, and underwater weighing. The most frequently used measure of obesity today is the body mass index (BMI), which is strongly correlated with percentage of body fat. Distribution of fat is also important, with abdominal (male pattern) fat being less healthy than lower-body (female pattern) fat. Furthermore, weight cycling may be more hazardous to health than a high but stable weight.

Factors That Contribute to Obesity

6. Obesity is partly hereditary. Researchers have discovered that laboratory mice with a defective ob gene cannot control their hunger and tend to become obese. The ob gene appears to regulate the production of leptin, a hormone produced by fat, which the hypothalamus monitors as an index of obesity. The amount of leptin is generally correlated with how much fat is stored in the body.

7. Hunger and eating behavior are not controlled by physiological factors alone. Psychosocial factors, such as stress, socioeconomic status, and culture also come into play. For example, as immigrant groups become acculturated to American norms, which generally discourage being overweight, obesity tends to decline.

8. According to the internality-externality hypothesis, feelings of hunger and satiety in normal-weight people are closely tied to internal stimuli such as stomach fullness, whereas obese persons are more responsive to external cues such as the time of day or the taste, smell, or appearance of food. In contrast, the restraint theory of eating proposes that external sensitivity is the result of dietary restraint. Restrained eaters vacillate between strict dieting and overeating triggered by disinhibition.

Treatment of Obesity

9. At all ages, women are twice as likely as men to be dieting, even though there is only a small gender difference in the prevalence of obesity. Dieting is increasingly prevalent among adolescents, which is cause for concern because of the potential hazards to growth and development.

10. Despite the abundance of pharmaceutical "remedies," there are no entirely acceptable, safe, and effective drugs to treat obesity. Gastroplasty and liposuction are surgical procedures sometimes used with the very obese. Behavior modification may be the safest approach to weight loss.

11. Today, health psychologists recognize that patients differ in which treatment will be most effective for them. The stepped-care process can be used for determining which intervention is most appropriate for a given person.

Eating Disorders

12. Anorexia nervosa is an eating disorder characterized by refusal to maintain body weight above a BMI of 18, intense fear of weight gain, disturbance of body image, and amenorrhea for at least 3 months. Bulimia nervosa involves compulsive bingeing followed by purging through self-induced vomiting or large doses of laxatives. Women with low self-esteem are particularly likely to have a negative body image and to be vulnerable to eating disorders. The families of bulimia patients have a higher-than-usual incidence of alcoholism, obesity, and depression. Anorexia patients often come from families that are competitive, overachieving, and protective. Eating disorders may also be partly genetic and linked to abnormal levels of certain neurotransmitters.

13. Cultural factors may explain why anorexia and bulimia occur more often in women than in men and more often in weight-conscious Western cultures, and why the prevalence of eating disorders has increased in recent years. Eating disorders are more common among women in occupations that emphasize appearance (for example, dance).

14. A range of therapies has been used to treat anorexia and bulimia, from force-feeding to family therapy. Experts agree that treatment must address both the behavior and the attitudes that perpetuate disordered eating. One behavioral treatment for bulimia, called exposure-response prevention, is based on an anxiety model of bulimia nervosa, in which binge eating is believed to increase anxiety (over weight gain), which in turn is relieved by purging. The most widely used therapy for anorexia and bulimia, cognitive behavior therapy, attacks faulty thinking about food intake, weight, and body image and gradually molds the patient's eating into a healthier pattern.

Key Terms and Concepts

obesity, p. 264
calorie, p. 265
kilocalorie, p. 265
marasmus, p. 266
kwashiorkor, p. 266
basal metabolic rate (BMR), p. 271
set-point hypothesis, p. 271
adipocytes, p. 273

bioelectrical impedance analysis, p. 275
hydrostatic weighing, p. 275
body mass index (BMI), p. 275
overweight, p. 276
male pattern obesity, p. 276
female pattern obesity, p. 277
weight cycling, p. 281
ob gene, p. 282

leptin, p. 282
restraint theory, p. 286
disinhibition, p. 287
gastroplasty, p. 290
liposuction, p. 290
anorexia nervosa, p. 295
bulimia nervosa, p. 295
exposure-response prevention, p. 304

Health Psychology on the World Wide Web

Web Address	Description
www.nal.usda.gov/fnic	The U.S. Department of Agriculture's resource center for information on food and nutrition.
www. cspinet.org/nah/index.htm	The Nutrition Action Newsletter published by the Center for Science in the Public Interest. This Web site is a great resource for information on the nutritional content of food products, including fast-food meals.
www.fda.gov	The Food and Drug Administration's Web site, with a wealth of information related to food safety.
http://odp.od.nih.gov/ods/	The Office of Dietary Supplements, which tracks bona fide research on substances from kava to gingko.
www.something-fishy.com/ed-f.htm	Eating disorder Web site.
http://library.advanced.org/10991/bmr.html	An on-line source that will calculate your BMR.
www.medscape.com/23373.rhtml	Medscape's weight-management resource center, offering a collection of the latest medical news and information on obesity and approaches to weight loss and weight maintenance.
www.hungersite.com	The hunger site, including much information about the worldwide hunger crisis, as well as links to CARE, UNICEF, and other organizations devoted to wiping out hunger.

Critical Thinking Exercise

The "Weighting" Game

Now that you have completed Chapter 7, take your learning a step further by testing your critical thinking skills on this practical problem-solving exercise.

Tanya and Maysoun have been good friends since meeting as first-year students in their freshman dormitory. Although they are about the same height and age, their body weights are very different. Tanya, whose parents are both obese, has always had a BMI between 30 and 35. Although acquaintances assume that she is lazy, lacks willpower, and is a gluttonous eater, Tanya's close friends know that she is none of these. Maysoun's BMI has nearly always hovered around 20, as has that of both her mother and father.

As a project in their health psychology class, Tanya and Maysoun decided to make themselves the subjects of an experiment. For one month, the two friends ate the same total number of calories per day, spread across several small, healthy meals that were low in fat and included plenty of fruits, vegetables, and whole grains. They also added a 30-minute daily aerobics class to their daily routines. At the end of the month, Tanya and Maysoun weighed themselves for the first time since beginning the project. Although Tanya was delighted to find that she had lost some weight, Maysoun had lost more. When they presented their results to the class, several students suggested that Tanya had either "fudged" on her diet by underestimating her daily food intake or simply hadn't employed as much willpower as Maysoun had, and that was why Maysoun lost more weight.

1. What factors in Tanya's background might have contributed to her elevated BMI?

2. What factors in Maysoun's background might have contributed to her normal BMI?

3. Why did Maysoun lose more weight than Tanya, even though she consumed the same number of calories, ate the same types of food, and did the same amount of exercise?

8

Substance Abuse

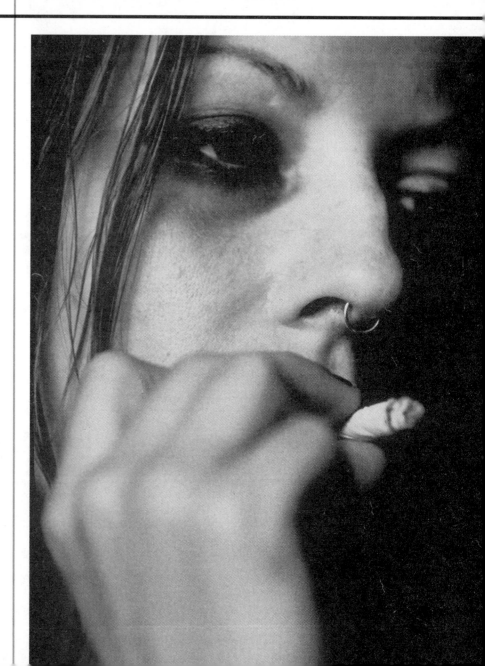

*J*ack was one of the first students I met when I entered Columbia University's graduate program in the fall of 1975. Like the rest of us, Jack was a highly motivated overachiever, eager to get on with the business of becoming a research psychologist.

But Jack was different, too. He seemed older and surer of himself and what it took to be successful. And he was smart. I admired his ability to "think on his feet" during a particularly stressful seminar taught in the Socratic style. Confident in his preparation for each class and a gifted speaker, Jack would not be intimidated when questioned by cranky full professors eager to reduce a young student to a quivering mass of jelly.

We all looked up to Jack, but we also worried about him. While the rest of us spent our nights studying in the library stacks, Jack had a part-time job as a New York cab driver. Although each of us received a teaching or research fellowship that covered tuition and provided a modest monthly stipend for living expenses, Jack apparently couldn't make it on this amount alone. Some of us suspected that he was sending money to some less fortunate relative who was unable to work. Or maybe he didn't want to admit, like the rest of us mere mortals, that the first year of graduate school required his full, undivided attention.

For a few months, Jack seemed unfazed by the double workload. I don't know when he slept or studied, but he seemed fully functional in class, and except for an occasional yawn during a particularly boring lecture, he performed about as well academically as any of us.

But the loss of sleep and mounting academic pressure eventually took its toll on Jack. Something had to give, and we first noticed it when our classmate stopped attending bull sessions, post-exam parties, and other social functions. Soon Jack began coming late to class—a cardinal sin in graduate school—then missing an occasional seminar, or—worst of all—showing up unprepared to discuss the day's reading assignment.

When Jack did make it to class, his appearance belied his lifestyle. He appeared haggard and worn out, with huge circles under his eyes. He looked to be 50 or 60 years of age rather than 22. Rumor had it that he was drinking heavily and using an assortment of pills—"uppers" and "downers" mostly—to medicate himself into a "functional state." When a group of us confronted Jack's roommate, he shrugged off our concern about Jack's drug use, saying, "Don't worry about Jack. He knows what he's doing. Those pills are all prescription drugs, and Jack never takes more than the prescribed dosage."

Well, you can guess what happened. A few weeks later, the department chairman interrupted our seminar in physiological psychology to inform us that Jack's body had been found early that morning. Jack had died of an apparent overdose of alcohol and barbiturate tranquilizers.

drug abuse the use of a drug to the extent that it impairs the user's biological, psychological, or social well-being

drug use the ingestion of a drug, regardless of the amount or effect of ingestion

Since antiquity, human beings have sought ways of altering mood, thought processes, and behavior. This chapter examines the different facets of substance, or (more commonly) drug, abuse—its causes, effects, and prevention. While the first section discusses drug use generally, the chapter focuses on the two most popular drugs: tobacco and alcohol. The good news is that scientists are closing in on these "everyday" drugs. New research findings point to a biopsychosocial common ground in the origins of addiction to many habit-forming substances, including tobacco and alcohol.

Substance Use and Abuse: Some Basic Facts

The spread of drug use is often described as a global pandemic, with similarities to epidemic diseases. The most widely used drug is tobacco. According to the World Health Organization (2000), globally one in three people aged 15 or older, or 1.1 billion people, smoke. Although tobacco use is decreasing in high-income countries, since the 1970s its use has climbed steadily in low- and middle-income countries. Note that **drug abuse** is the use of any chemical substance to the extent that it impairs the user's well-being *in any domain of health:* biological, psychological, or social. By this definition, legal drugs—such as prescription medicines—can also be abused. **Drug use,** on the other hand, is simply the ingestion of any drug, regardless of the amount taken or its effect.

Next to tobacco, alcohol is the most widely used and abused drug and is available in all but the most isolated areas of the world and in a few countries with strict religious prohibitions (World Health Organization, 2000). In the United States, approximately 10 million people abuse alcohol (Thompson, 2000). Although alcohol consumption has recently declined in many developed countries, its use has been increasing in developing countries. Moreover, alcohol problems are now occurring in many Asian and Western Pacific countries where they did not exist before.

Use of illegal drugs has also increased throughout the world in recent years. Based on estimates of the United Nations Drug Control Program, the annual global rate of illegal drug use is in the range of 3.3 to 4.1 percent of the world's population. Globally, marijuana (*cannabis*) is the most commonly used illicit drug, with an estimated 141 million users (2.5 percent of the world population, mostly in developed countries) (World Health Organization, 2000). Among students, marijuana use is followed by MDMA, or ecstasy (a synthetic *designer drug* that is increasingly used at dance clubs and "raves"), steroids, and heroin.

Despite years of efforts to focus public attention on drug abuse, drug experimentation and even abuse is increasing and has reached down to the grade-school level. Students surveyed in 2000 also showed that personal disapproval of drug use had decreased in the past 5 years (Monitoring the Future Study, 2000). In addition, smoking is on the rise among women, ethnic minorities, and lower socioeconomic groups.

The health hazards and costs of drug abuse are incalculable. The abuse of illegal drugs, alcohol, and tobacco is the cause of more deaths, illnesses, and disabilities than any other preventable health condition (Robert Wood Johnson Foundation, 2001). The National Institute on Alcohol Abuse and Alcoholism estimates that alcohol is implicated in 44 percent of the more than 40,000 annual traffic fatalities (NIAAA, 2001). Half of all murders in the United States involve alcohol or some other drug, and 80 percent of all suicide attempts follow the use of alcohol. And tobacco abuse, the number one preventable cause of death in the United States, claims more than 400,000 lives and costs $50 billion in direct medical expenses each year. According to one World Health Organization study, the global disease burden due to alcohol and tobacco, measured in years of life lost to disability, is greater than that due to poor sanitation or hypertension (World Health Organization, 2000).

Why, despite these enormous financial, health, and social costs, do people continue to use and abuse drugs? To answer this question, you first need to know how drugs move through and affect the body.

Mechanisms of Drug Action

As a first step, the drug must be ingested, or administered. Drugs are administered in one of six ways: orally, rectally, by injection, by inhalation, and by absorption through the skin or the mucous membranes. The manner in which a drug is administered can alter its physiological effects. Because they enter the bloodstream faster, drugs that are injected or inhaled usually have stronger and more immediate effects than those that are swallowed.

Within minutes after a drug is absorbed from its point of entry, it is distributed by the bloodstream to its site of action (receptors). How quickly a drug reaches its target receptors depends on the rate of blood flow to the target and how easily the drug passes through cell membranes and other protective barriers in the body. Blood flow to the brain is greater than to any other part of the body. Therefore, drugs that are able to pass through the network of cells that separate the blood and the brain — the **blood-brain barrier** (Figure 8.1, page 316) — quickly arrive in the central nervous system. The ease with which a drug passes through this barrier depends on its lipid (fat) solubility. Most recreational drugs as well as those that are widely abused are lipid soluble, which means they easily pass through the barrier to their target receptor sites in the brain.

Fat-soluble drugs that cross the blood-brain barrier are usually also able to permeate the *placental barrier* that separates the blood of a pregnant

■ **blood-brain barrier** the network of tightly packed capillary cells that separates the blood and the brain

Figure 8.1

The Blood-Brain Barrier
Unlike the porous blood capillaries in most other parts of the body, those in the brain are tightly packed, forming a fatty glial sheath that provides a protective environment for the brain. The glial sheath develops from the nearby astrocyte cells. In order to reach the brain, a drug must first be absorbed through the capillary wall and then through the fatty sheath.

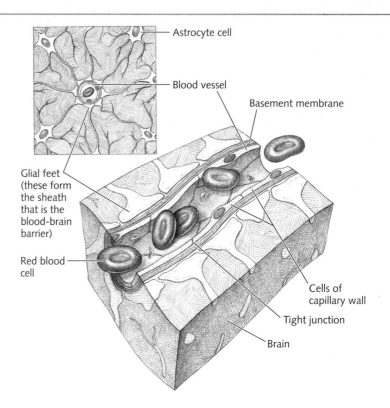

Astrocyte cell

Blood vessel

Basement membrane

Glial feet
(these form
the sheath
that is the
blood-brain
barrier)

Red blood
cell

Cells of
capillary wall

Tight junction

Brain

woman from that of her developing child. For this reason, any alcohol, nicotine, or other drugs as well as chemicals in cosmetics, foods, and elsewhere in the environment absorbed by the mother can affect her unborn child. Scientists now understand a great deal about **teratogens**—drugs, pollutants, and other substances that cross the placental barrier and damage the developing person. Alcohol, tobacco, heroin, and marijuana, for example, can stunt fetal growth and can permanently damage the developing brain. The extent of their effect, however, depends on when exposure occurs; exposure to particular teratogens causes the greatest damage during critical periods of development when specific organs and systems are developing most rapidly.

■ **teratogens** drugs, chemicals, and environmental agents that can damage the developing person during fetal development

Drugs and Synapses

Once in the brain, drugs affect behavior by influencing the activity of neurons at their synapses (see Chapter 3). Drugs can achieve their effects in one of three ways: by mimicking or enhancing the action of a naturally occurring neurotransmitter, by blocking its action, or by affecting its reuptake.

Drugs that produce neural actions that mimic or enhance those of a naturally occurring neurotransmitter are **agonists** (see Figure 8.2). Recall that synaptic receptors are cellular locks that wait for neurotransmitters with a particular shape to act like a key and trigger activity within the cell. For example, nicotine is an acetylcholine agonist, which means that it fits the lock meant for

■ **agonist** a drug that attaches to a receptor and produces neural actions that mimic or enhance those of a naturally occurring neurotransmitter

Agonists and Antagonists

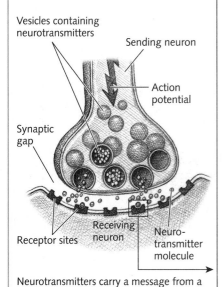

Vesicles containing neurotransmitters

Sending neuron

Action potential

Synaptic gap

Receiving neuron

Receptor sites

Neuro-transmitter molecule

Neurotransmitters carry a message from a sending neuron across a synapse to receptor sites on a receiving neuron.

This neurotransmitter molecule has a molecular structure that precisely fits the receptor site on the receiving neuron, much as a key fits a lock.

Neurotransmitter molecule

Receiving cell membrane

Receptor site on receiving neuron

(a)

This agonist molecule excites. It is similar enough in structure to the neuro-transmitter molecule that it mimics its effects on the receiving neuron. Morphine, for instance, mimics the action of endorphins by stimulating receptors in brain areas involved in mood and pain sensations.

Agonist mimics neurotransmitter

(b)

This antagonist molecule inhibits. It has a structure similar enough to the neurotransmitter to occupy its receptor site and block its action, but not similar enough to stimulate the receptor. Botulin poisoning paralyzes its victims by blocking ACh receptors involved in muscle movement.

Antagonist blocks neurotransmitter

(c)

■ **antagonist** a drug that blocks the action of a naturally occurring neurotransmitter or agonist

■ **drug addiction** a pattern of behavior characterized by physical as well as possible psychological dependence on a drug as well as the development of tolerance

■ **physical dependence** a state in which the use of a drug is required for a person to function normally

■ **withdrawal** the unpleasant physical and psychological symptoms that occur when a person abruptly ceases using certain drugs

acetylcholine and binds to postsynaptic receptors on the same neuron, thus enhancing activation of the receiving neuron and causing the tobacco user to feel more alert. Similarly, LSD is structurally similar to serotonin. Because of this resemblance, LSD is able to bind to serotonin receptors, function as an artificial agonist, and trigger alterations in perception, thinking, and emotion. Other agonists stimulate the release of neurotransmitters. Amphetamine, for example, stimulates the release of norepinephrine and dopamine from storage sites, which may elevate mood, induce euphoria, increase alertness, and reduce fatigue.

Drugs that produce their effects by blocking the action of neurotransmitters or agonist drugs are **antagonists.** Caffeine, for example, is an antagonist that blocks the effects of *adenosine,* a neurotransmitter that normally inhibits the release of other transmitters that excite (cause to fire) postsynaptic cells. Thus, the excitatory cells continue firing, resulting in the stimulation felt when caffeine is ingested.

Finally, drugs can alter neural transmission by enhancing or inhibiting the reuptake of neurotransmitters in the synapse, that is, the natural breakdown or reabsorption of the neurotransmitter by the presynaptic neuron. Cocaine, for example, produces its stimulating effects by blocking the reuptake of norepinephrine and dopamine. Because these neurotransmitters are not reabsorbed by the sending neuron, they remain in the synapse and continue to excite (or inhibit) the receiving neuron.

Addiction, Dependence, and Tolerance

Not everyone who starts using a drug becomes addicted. How can you tell whether a person is addicted? As used by health experts today, **drug addiction** describes a behavior pattern characterized by overwhelming involvement with the use of a drug, a preoccupation with its supply, and a high probability of relapse if the drug is discontinued (Grunberg, Brown, & Klein, 1997). Drug addiction also involves the development of physical and psychological dependence on a substance.

Physical dependence is a state in which the body has adjusted to the repeated use of a drug and requires its presence in order to maintain "normal" physiological functioning. In this context, *normal* refers to the absence of the withdrawal symptoms that will appear when use of a drug is discontinued. Drug **withdrawal** (also called *abstinence syndrome*) refers to the unpleasant physical and psychological symptoms that occur when a person abruptly ceases using a drug. The symptoms of withdrawal, which vary widely from drug to drug, are generally the direct opposite of a drug's primary effects. Amphetamines and other stimulants, for example, create a primary rush of euphoria. Amphetamine withdrawal triggers its opposing state of depression. Other symptoms include nausea and vomiting, sleep disturbances, anxiety, and even death.

The complementary effects of drug use and drug abstinence have led to a general theory of withdrawal—the *hypersensitivity theory*—which proposes that addiction is the result of efforts by the body and brain to counteract the effects of a drug in order to maintain an optimal internal state. Take nicotine as an example. Among its many physical effects, nicotine accelerates heart rate. To compensate and maintain a constant internal state, the brain and nervous system stimulate the vagus nerve, slowing the heart rate. Over time, regular use of nicotine and the associated increase in vagus nerve activity could, in effect, create a new, higher "set point" for vagus nerve activity. Should the person quit smoking, vagal tone would remain high, higher than usual in fact, since there is no nicotine in the system to increase the heart rate.

One sign of physical dependence is the development of **drug tolerance,** a state of progressively decreasing responsiveness to a frequently used drug. As a person's body adjusts to a drug, increased dosages are necessary to produce the effect formerly achieved by a smaller dose. Although all addictive drugs give rise to tolerance, not all drugs to which tolerance develops are addictive. For example, tolerance develops rapidly to LSD and a number of other drugs that do not appear to induce physical dependence.

There are at least two reasons that tolerance develops. With repeated use, some drugs are metabolized at a faster rate by the liver, so that more of the drug must be administered simply to maintain a constant level in the body. Second, brain receptors adapt to the continued presence of a particular drug either by increasing the number of receptor sites or by reducing their sensitivity to the drug. In either case, more of the drug is required to produce the same biochemical effect.

Psychological dependence, the other side of addiction, occurs particularly for drugs that relieve stress. Psychological dependence involves the compulsive use of a drug even in the absence of physical dependence. Some drugs, such as marijuana, can lead to psychological dependence, even though they do not appear to cause physical dependence. Most drugs, including alcohol, nicotine, and heroin, give rise to both physical and psychological dependence. For example, alcohol, which seems to produce biochemical changes in the brain (see page 329), also seems to improve mood and allow a person to forget his or her problems. For many former drug users, memories of the "highs" once experienced fade slowly and are constant triggers for relapse.

Psychoactive Drugs

Most of the drugs used for recreational purposes (and therefore most likely to be abused) are classified as **psychoactive drugs**—chemical substances that act on the brain to alter mood, behavior, and thought processes. Psychoactive drugs are grouped into three major categories: *stimulants, depressants,* and *hallucinogens.*

■ **drug tolerance** a state of progressively decreasing responsiveness to a frequently used drug

■ **psychological dependence** an emotional and cognitive compulsion to use a drug

■ **psychoactive drugs** drugs that affect mood, behavior, and thought processes by altering the functioning of neurons in the brain; they include stimulants, depressants, and hallucinogens

Stimulants

Stimulants, including nicotine, caffeine, cocaine, and the amphetamines, make people feel more alert and energetic by boosting activity in the central nervous system. At low doses, the stimulants reduce fatigue, elevate mood, and decrease appetite. In higher doses, however, the stimulants may cause irritability, insomnia, and anxiety. Because the effects of stimulants mimic the actions of adrenaline—one of the neurotransmitters that activate the fight-or-flight response of the sympathetic nervous system—stimulants are often referred to as *sympathomimetic agents.*

Like most psychoactive drugs, stimulants produce their behavioral and psychological effects by altering the action of neurotransmitters at synapses. The stimulants have a dramatic impact on several neurotransmitters, including acetylcholine, the catecholamines, dopamine, and, to a lesser extent, norepinephrine. Recall that nicotine is an acetylcholine agonist and that cocaine blocks the reuptake of dopamine and norepinephrine. Like nicotine, the amphetamines are agonists, stimulating the release of dopamine from presynaptic storage sites in nerve terminals. The alertness that follows this release derives from the resulting overstimulation of dopamine receptors in postsynaptic neurons.

Because of their powerful reward effects, stimulants are widely abused. Physical and psychological dependence develop rapidly along with tolerance that forces the addict to take progressively higher doses. Withdrawal symptoms associated with amphetamines include increased appetite, weight gain, fatigue, sleepiness, and, in some people, symptoms of paranoia.

Depressants

Central nervous system (CNS) depressants dampen activity in the brain and spinal cord. Also called *sedatives, tranquilizers,* and *hypnotics,* these drugs include the barbiturates, opiates, alcohol, general anesthetics, and antiepileptic drugs. Low doses reduce responsiveness to sensory stimulation, slow thought processes, and lower physical activity. Higher doses result in drowsiness, lethargy, and amnesia; they can also lead to death by shutting down vital physiological functions such as breathing.

One group of depressants, *barbiturates,* is used to block pain during surgery and to regulate high blood pressure. They are also popular street drugs because they produce a mild sense of euphoria that can last for hours. Up until about 1960, the barbiturates were also the most commonly prescribed drugs for treating anxiety and insomnia. However, because they are highly addictive and were implicated in thousands of suicides, accidental overdose deaths, and dependency, barbiturates are no longer prescribed for these complaints. To take their place, researchers developed synthetic tranquilizers, the benzodiazepines, which are much less toxic than the older sedative-hypnotics. *Librium* and *Valium,* for example, were synthesized in the 1960s and are now widely used to treat anxiety and insomnia.

Barbiturates are considered particularly dangerous because, taken in combination with another drug, their effects will increase the effects of that drug, a reaction known as **drug potentiation.** In combination with alcohol, for example, a barbiturate may suppress the brain's respiratory centers and cause death. Another example of this type of drug interaction involves the concurrent use of alcohol and marijuana. The driving ability of a person under the influence of both alcohol and marijuana will be profoundly impaired because of the interaction of the two drugs. Drug potentiation may have caused the death of Jack, whom we met at the opening of the chapter.

Another group of depressants, the *opiates,* such as morphine, heroin, and codeine, derive from the opium poppy. One of the most potent painkillers (analgesics), morphine has been used for more than a century as an analgesic. In one of medicine's greatest historical ironies, heroin was developed following the Civil War to be a *nonaddictive* alternative to morphine. So many war veterans returned from the battlefield addicted to morphine (the "soldiers' disease") that physicians sought to synthesize a nonaddictive analgesic. The truth, of course, is that heroin induces physical dependence even more rapidly than morphine. Indeed, there are approximately 1 million heroin addicts in the United States today (World Health Organization, 2000).

Opiates produce their effects by mimicking the body's natural opiates, the *endorphins.* As you'll recall, endorphins are neurotransmitters that help regulate our normal experience of pain and pleasure. When the brain is flooded with artificial opiates such as heroin, molecules of these synthetic drugs bind to the receptor sites for the endorphins, and the brain stops producing its own naturally occurring opiates. If the drug is discontinued, withdrawal symptoms soon occur, including rapid breathing, elevated blood pressure, severe muscle cramps, nausea and vomiting, panic, and intense cravings for the drug.

Hallucinogens
Also called psychedelic drugs, hallucinogens such as marijuana, LSD, and mescaline alter sensory perception and induce visual and auditory hallucinations as they separate the user from reality. These drugs also disrupt thought processes and, in some users, trigger behavior resembling that of patients with severe psychological disorders.

Composed of the leaves and flowers of *Cannabis sativa,* marijuana is the most commonly used hallucinogen. It achieves its psychedelic effects via its active ingredient delta-6-tetrahydrocannabinol (THC). In 1996, several drugs, including marijuana, were approved for limited medical use by Nevada, Arizona, Washington, and five other states. Although the treatment remains controversial, marijuana may alleviate pain in those suffering from AIDS and certain cancers. The drug also has helped some patients to regain appetite and endure otherwise unbearable medical regimens.

Hallucinogens are classified according to which of several neurotransmitters they most closely resemble in structure: acetylcholine, norepinephrine,

drug potentiation the effect of one drug to increase the effects of another

■ **concordance rate** the rate of agreement between a pair of twins for a given trait; a pair of twins is concordant for the trait if both of them have it or if neither has it

dopamine, or serotonin. For example, LSD resembles serotonin, which means that this drug exerts an agonist effect on neural synapses that use serotonin.

In their efforts to understand why people experiment with these and other psychoactive drugs, and why many drugs quickly lead to dependence and tolerance, researchers have uncovered many clues and formulated several theories. In the next section, we examine several of the leading models of addiction.

Models of Addiction

Theories about how people become addicted to drugs can be grouped into three general categories: biomedical models, reward models, and social learning models.

Biomedical Models: Addiction as Disease

Biomedical models of addiction view physical dependence as a chronic brain disease caused by the biological effects of psychoactive drugs (Leshner, 2001). The simplest model maintains that addicts inherit a biological vulnerability to physical dependence (Miller & Giannini, 1990). Researchers point to evidence from studies comparing drug abuse among identical and fraternal twins. Such studies compare the **concordance rate,** or rate of agreement, of physical dependence among monozygotic (MZ) and dizygotic (DZ) twins. A pair of twins is concordant for the trait—in this case, drug addiction—if both of them have it or if neither has it.

Although concordance studies suggest that genes play a role in physical dependence on many psychoactive drugs, researchers are cautious in interpreting the results from such studies. Even in rare studies in which MZ twins who have been raised in different environments are compared and found to have a high concordance rate, it is impossible to completely rule out possible confounding effects due to other variables. Moreover, twin studies do not pinpoint the specific gene or genes that might promote physical dependence.

Another biomedical model points to altered neurochemistry as the basis for both physical and psychological dependence. According to the *withdrawal-relief hypothesis,* drug use serves to restore abnormally low levels of dopamine, serotonin, and other key neurotransmitters (Giannini & Miller, 1989). In support of this hypothesis is evidence that depression, anxiety, low self-esteem, and other unpleasant emotional states are associated with neurotransmitter deficiencies. By elevating the release of presynaptic dopamine, drugs such as cocaine and the amphetamines restore neural functioning *and* produce a sense of psychological well-being.

For most of the twentieth century, the withdrawal-relief model was based primarily on evidence from opiate addiction. As explained earlier, opiates suppress the brain's natural production of endorphins. By doing this, heroin and other opiates trigger dependence. The first receptor-based theory of addiction, the opiate model was quickly adopted as the basic biomedical model for addiction to all drugs that induce physical dependence. Nicotine acts on acetylcholine receptors, amphetamine and cocaine act on catecholamine receptors, and barbiturates presumably act on receptors for gamma-aminobutyric acid. In each case, addiction might involve the same sequence of receptor adaptation to an artificial source as occurs with opiate addiction. One glaring exception to the opiate receptor theory as a general model, however, is alcohol, which does not appear to act on specific receptors.

The opiate receptor/withdrawal-relief model was appealing because the idea that addicts need more of their drug to relieve physical distress made their intense determination to obtain drugs seem understandable, a rational response to their withdrawal sickness. However, the model does not explain why addicts begin taking a drug in sufficient dosages and with enough frequency to develop physical dependence in the first place. A second problem with this model is its inability to explain why many users suffer a relapse, even long after withdrawal symptoms have subsided.

Reward Models: Addiction as Pleasure Seeking

Researchers looking for an explanation for the initial motivation for repeated use have focused on the pleasurable effects of psychoactive drugs. The impetus for this shift in thinking stems from several bodies of research, including animal studies of brain reward circuits and the recent epidemic of cocaine abuse (Lyvers, 1998).

The Brain's Reward System

While attempting to locate the sleep-control system in the brainstems of laboratory rats, James Olds and Peter Milner (1954) accidentally stimulated the septal area of the hypothalamus. To their surprise, the rats refused to leave the area of their cages in which they had been stimulated.

All major drugs of abuse, including nicotine and the other stimulants, overstimulate the brain's reward system, which also becomes active when a person engages in pleasurable behaviors that promote survival, such as eating or having sex. With the use of stimulants, this circuit goes into overdrive, repeatedly activating the neurons until the drug leaves the body. Given the choice between psychoactive drugs that put this circuit into overdrive and other, more mundane pleasures, physically dependent animals and human addicts will often choose the former. Rats allowed to press a lever to electrically stimulate their reward systems have been observed to do so up to 7,000 times per hour (Figure 8.3, page 324).

Figure 8.3

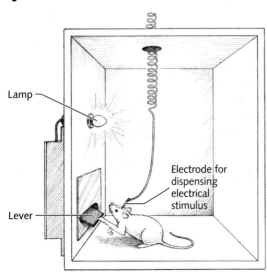

Lamp

Electrode for dispensing electrical stimulus

Lever

Intracranial Self-Stimulation
Whenever the small lamp on the panel is lit, pressing the lever will cause an electrical stimulus to be delivered to the reward system of the rat's brain. Using this experimental arrangement, rats have been observed to lever-press at rates faster than one response per second.

Evidence for Reward Models

According to the reasoning of reward models, addiction may best be understood as being motivated by pleasure seeking (Withers, Pulvirent, Koob, & Gillin, 1995). Cocaine, alcohol, nicotine, and other psychoactive drugs may induce physical dependence because they increase the availability of dopamine in the brain, putting the reward system into overdrive (Thompson, 2000).

Further evidence for the reward system link in addiction comes from the fact that people who are physically dependent on one substance are more likely to be addicted to others as well. Smokers, for example, consume twice as much alcohol as nonsmokers and are 10 to 14 times more likely to abuse alcohol (Leutwyler, 1995). In addition, although the number of smokers has dropped dramatically, it is unchanged among those who are physically dependent on alcohol. This pattern also holds for other drugs of abuse. In 1995, an estimated 13.6 percent of adult American smokers used illicit drugs, compared with only 3 percent of nonsmokers (Leutwyler, 1995).

Because use of tobacco, as well as alcohol and marijuana, has been found to play a pivotal role in the development of other drug dependencies and high-risk behaviors, these drugs are often referred to as **gateway drugs**—that is, they "open the door" to experimentation with other chemical substances (Gerstein & Green, 1993). In a nationwide survey of high school seniors, Richard Clayton and Christian Ritter (1985) found that cigarette smoking and alcohol use were the most powerful predictors of marijuana use for both girls and boys.

Shortcomings of the Reward Model

Despite its seeming logic, the reward model does not provide the final answer. Although it is true that cocaine, heroin, and other drugs with the greatest potential for addiction evoke the most powerful euphoria, marijuana and several other psychoactive drugs that are not considered physically addictive also produce feelings of well-being (Jones, 1992). In contrast, tobacco, which is now regarded as highly addictive and as difficult to abstain from as cocaine or heroin (Kozlowski, Appel, Fredcker, & Khouw, 1982), induces a euphoria that is hardly on the same scale as that elicited by cocaine (Jarvis, 1994).

Reward models by themselves are also unable to explain why drug use continues even when unpleasant side effects occur—that is, why cocaine addicts continue to use the drug despite feelings of anxiety, agitation, and even convulsions (Withers et al., 1995) or why alcohol or heroin abusers do not abstain despite the nausea and vomiting they experience. Terry Robinson and Kent Berridge's (2000) two-stage theory, known as the *incentive-sensitization theory* of addiction, provides a rationale for this behavior. In the first stage, the origi-

■ **gateway drug** a drug that serves as a stepping-stone to the use of other, usually more dangerous, drugs

nal good feelings from drug use prevail; in the second stage, drug use becomes an automated behavior. Repeated drug use sensitizes the brain's dopamine-serotonin reward systems to drug-related cues. Thus, even though pleasure may not increase, the systems continue to respond to the cues because they have become conditioned stimuli that evoke dopamine release and craving.

In support of their theory, Robinson and Berridge note that sensitization of the dopamine-serotonin systems, which mediate motivational responses to other incentives such as money, may explain the tendency of former addicts to engage in substitute compulsive behaviors such as gambling. There is also considerable scientific evidence that drug-induced sensitization of dopamine neurons does occur (Lyvers, 1998; Self & Nestler, 1995).

Social Learning Models: Addiction as Behavior

Shortcomings in the reward and biomedical models have led to a movement away from disease models of addiction. Although psychoactive drugs do indeed trigger neurochemical changes, and research does point to hereditary risk factors in dependence, there is good reason to view addiction as a *behavior* that is shaped by learning as well as by social and cognitive factors. For instance, smokers "learn" to smoke in a variety of situations—while socializing with friends, after eating a meal, and so forth. Through conditioning, the pleasurable physiological effects of nicotine, together with other rewarding aspects of social situations, transforms these situations into powerful triggers for smoking. Furthermore, the outcome of treatment for drug abuse is strongly influenced by the presence of social support, the user's employment, and the presence of effective skills for coping with the stress of withdrawal (Brown, Myers, Mott, & Vik, 1994; Miller, Westerberg, Harris, & Tonigan, 1996).

A person's identification with a particular drug may also play a key role in both the initiation and the maintenance of an addiction. Seeing oneself as a heavy drinker or smoker, for example, may lead to the adoption of a certain lifestyle that makes quitting the drug a monumental task involving a new sense of self (Walters, 1996). Thus, a drinker whose social network revolves entirely around the neighborhood bar may find it especially hard to stop drinking.

Conversely, people, especially young people, may be protected against drug use by family, school, religion, and other conventional social institutions. According to this *social control theory,* the stronger a young person's attachment to any social institution, the less likely he or she will be to begin using drugs (or to break *any* social norms). The closely related *peer cluster theory* maintains that peer groups are strong enough to overcome the controlling influence of family, school, or religious values. Data from the Asian Student Drug Survey of ninth- and twelfth-grade students in California showed that peer cluster theory was more strongly supported than social control theory. However, the fact that teens who professed strong moral beliefs and positive feelings about school were less likely to use drugs (unless their immediate peer cluster

■ **blood alcohol level (BAL)**
the amount of alcohol in the blood, measured in grams per 100 milliliters

consisted of drug users) can be construed as support for a protective effect (Nagasawa, Qian, & Wong, 2000).

With this theoretical background to addiction in place, let us turn to two of the most common addictions: alcohol and nicotine dependence.

Alcohol Use and Abuse

Classified as a depressant, alcohol, or more accurately *ethyl alcohol* (ethanol), slows the functioning of the central nervous system in a manner similar to tranquilizers such as Valium. When you drink an alcoholic beverage, approximately 20 percent of the alcohol is rapidly absorbed from the stomach directly into the bloodstream. The remaining 80 percent empties into the upper intestine, where it is absorbed at a pace that depends on whether the stomach is full or empty. Drinking on a full stomach delays absorption up to about 90 minutes.

Once alcohol is absorbed, it is evenly distributed throughout body tissues and fluids. Roughly 95 percent of the absorbed alcohol is metabolized in the liver at the rate of about 10 milliliters (one-third ounce) of 100 percent ethanol per hour. In other words, it takes an average-sized adult about 1 hour to metabolize the amount of alcohol contained in a 1-ounce glass of 80 proof liquor (about 40 percent ethanol), a 4-ounce glass of wine, or a 12-ounce bottle of beer (Julien, 2001). Drinking at a faster pace results in a larger amount of alcohol remaining in the bloodstream and eventually intoxication.

The amount of alcohol in the bloodstream is your **blood alcohol level (BAL).** In most states, a blood alcohol level of 0.08 grams percent (g%) constitutes legal intoxication (*grams percent* is the number of grams of ethanol contained in 100 milliliters blood). A person who attempts to drive an automobile with a BAL above this amount can be charged with driving while under the influence of alcohol. A typical college student would need to consume only one standard drink an hour for every 30 to 35 pounds of body weight to reach an illegal BAL level. Table 8.1 illustrates the relationship between body weight and driving impairment. Because of individual differences in tolerance for alcohol, however, these figures are only an approximation. Some people develop a higher tolerance and are able to drink larger amounts of alcohol before becoming obviously impaired. For others, however, intoxication may occur with blood alcohol levels as low as 0.03 or 0.04 g%. Because women generally weigh less than men, they tend to have a lower tolerance for alcohol. Women also produce less of the enzyme *alcohol dehydrogenase,* which breaks down alcohol in the stomach. As a result, after consuming the same amount of alcohol, women have a higher blood alcohol content than men, even allowing for differences in their body sizes.

Table 8.1

Estimating Blood Alcohol Level

Number of Standard Drinks in One Hour

Weight	1	2	3	4	5	6	7	8	9	10
100	.029	.058	.088	.117	.146	.175	.204	.233	.262	.290
120	.024	.048	.073	.097	.121	.145	.170	.194	.219	.243
140	.021	.042	.063	.083	.104	.125	.146	.166	.187	.208
160	.019	.037	.055	.073	.091	.109	.128	.146	.164	.182
180	.017	.033	.049	.065	.081	.097	.113	.130	.146	.162
200	.015	.029	.044	.058	.073	.087	.102	.117	.131	.146
220	.014	.027	.040	.053	.067	.080	.093	.106	.119	.133
240	.012	.024	.037	.048	.061	.073	.085	.097	.109	.122

Caution	Driving Impaired	Legally Drunk

To use this chart, find the number closest to your body weight in pounds in the left margin. Each of the columns to the right represents a specific number of standard drinks. Where the columns and rows intersect represents the approximate BAL. Next, multiply the number of hours since you began drinking by 0.015 (the rate at which alcohol is metabolized). Finally, subtract this product from the number from the table. For example, suppose you weigh 120 pounds and have three drinks in 2 hours: Moving across from 120, your initial BAL would be 0.073 g%. Subtracting from that number .030 g% [which is 2 (hours) multiplied by 0.015%] would yield a BAL of 0.043.

Source: *A Primer of Drug Action*, 9th ed. (p. 96), by R. M. Julien, 2001, New York: Worth.

The short-term effects of alcohol are dose-dependent. At blood alcohol levels ranging from about 0.01 to 0.05 g%, a drinker usually feels relaxed and mildly euphoric. As the level increases to 0.10 g%, memory and concentration are dulled, and reaction time and motor functioning are significantly impaired. At 0.10 to 0.15 g%, walking and fine motor skills become extremely difficult. By 0.20 to 0.25 g%, vision becomes blurry, speech is slurred, and walking without staggering is virtually impossible. The drinker is noticeably drunk and may lose consciousness. Death may occur at a BAL of 0.35 or more. These physical effects contribute to several hundred thousand alcohol-related accidents and crimes annually.

A Profile of Alcohol Abusers

As Figure 8.4 shows, about 51 percent of adults in the United States are classified as current drinkers (defined as having at least one drink during the preceding month). Of these, about 15 percent are binge drinkers (five or more drinks on one occasion in the past 30 days), and about 5 percent are heavy

Figure 8.4

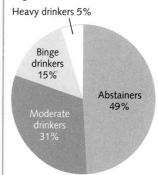

Heavy drinkers 5%
Binge drinkers 15%
Abstainers 49%
Moderate drinkers 31%

Alcohol Use among U.S. Adults by Type of Drinker About 51 percent of adults in the United States are classified as current drinkers and 49 percent are abstainers. Among those who drink, 15 percent are classified as binge drinkers (five or more drinks on one occasion during the past month) and 5 percent are heavy drinkers (five or more drinks on the same occasion on 5 or more days during the past month). **Source:** Preliminary results from the 1997 National Household Survey on Drug Abuse by the U.S. Department of Health and Human Services, 1998, Washington, DC: U.S. Government Printing Office.

drinkers (five or more drinks on the same occasion on 5 or more days over the past month) (U.S. Department of Health and Human Services, 1998). Most drinkers do so responsibly and do not develop a substance abuse problem. However, as many as 10 to 14 million Americans are estimated to have serious alcohol problems and about 7 million are dependent on alcohol (Thompson, 2000). The prevalence of the various categories of drinking behavior varies by age, gender, education level, ethnicity, and culture. Adults between 21 and 39 years of age have the highest rates of drinking, but the 18 to 25 cohort has the highest rates of binge and heavy drinking (USDHHS, 1998). Alcohol use among adolescents age 12 to 17 dropped substantially after the legal age for purchasing alcohol was increased to 21 in most states. In 1979, before these laws were put in place, fully 50 percent of those in this age group used alcohol; by 1992, however, only 1 out of 5 reported using alcohol (USDHHS, 1998).

Compared with women, significantly more men are current drinkers, binge drinkers, and heavy drinkers (USDHHS, 1998), and most are between 25 and 44 years of age (Weisner, Greenfield, & Room, 1995). Approximately 30 to 50 percent of drinkers meet the criteria for major depression, 33 percent have a coexisting anxiety disorder (social phobias being most common in men, agoraphobia in women), 14 percent have antisocial personalities, and 36 percent are addicted to other drugs (Julien, 2001).

Despite the fact that college campuses began to be inundated with alcohol education programs in the 1980s, studies indicate that most U.S. college students use alcohol (Marlatt, Baer, & Larimer, 1995) and that nearly one-quarter of college students can be classified as heavy, or problem, drinkers (Kim, Larimer, Walker, & Marlatt, 1997). When heavy episodic, or binge, drinking is considered, these rates rise to nearly one-half of all students. In 2000, a survey by the Harvard School of Public Health found that 44 percent of college students are binge drinkers and 74 percent say they binged in high school.

The prevalence of drinking also varies by ethnic and cultural background (USDHHS, 1998). In the United States, alcohol addiction rates are extremely low among the Amish, Mennonites, Mormons, and Orthodox Jews (Trimble, 1996). Furthermore, European Americans have higher rates of drinking than African-Americans, Asian-Americans, or Hispanic-Americans. African-Americans also have fewer heavy drinkers than European Americans and Hispanic-Americans. Contrary to popular stereotypes, African-American high school students have the lowest reported use rates for virtually *all* psychoactive drugs (Johnston et al., 1999).

Although the specific causes of ethnic and cultural group differences in risk are not known, certain people in these groups may be at higher or lower risk because of the way they metabolize alcohol. One study of Native Americans, for instance, found that they are less sensitive to the intoxicating effects of alcohol (Wall, Garcia-Andrade, Thomasson, Carr, & Ehlers, 1997). People who "hold their liquor" in this way may therefore lack (or ignore) warning signals that ordinarily make people stop drinking. Asian-Americans, on the other hand, may be less prone to alcohol abuse because they have genetically lower levels of *aldehyde dehydrogenase,* an enzyme used by the body to metabolize alcohol (Suddendorf, 1989; Thomasson & Li, 1993). Without this enzyme, toxic substances build up after a person drinks alcohol and cause flushing, dizziness, and nausea.

Several recent studies suggest that teen drinking is especially damaging to the brain. Although researchers once thought that the brain is fully developed by age 16 or 17, significant neurological development continues at least until age 21. Heavy drinking at a young age may impair that development.

The Impact of Alcohol Consumption

Alcohol affects all parts of the body. At the most basic level, because cell membranes are permeable to alcohol, alcohol enters the cell and disrupts intracellular communication. Alcohol also affects genes that regulate cell functions such as the synthesis of dopamine, norepinephrine, and other important neurotransmitters.

Alcohol and the Body

Although alcohol abuse has been implicated in a number of physical problems and diseases, such as cancer of the liver, this section describes only the major ones.

Alcohol and the Brain The craving that some people develop for alcohol, the adverse reactions that occur during withdrawal, and the high rate of relapse all are due to biochemical changes in the brain brought on by long-term use of alcohol. Even after decades of study, however, researchers still do not know exactly how alcohol promotes alcohol abuse or dependency. Alcohol appears to have major effects on the hippocampus, a brain area associated with learning, memory, emotional regulation, sensory processing, appetite, and stress (see Chapter 3). It does so by breaking down into products called *fatty acid ethyl esters,* which inhibit neurotransmitters in the hippocampus that are strongly associated with emotional behavior and cravings. Dopamine transmission, in particular, appears to be strongly associated with the rewarding properties of alcohol, nicotine, opiates, and cocaine. Investigators have focused on nerve-cell structures known as dopamine D2 receptors (DRD2), which influence the activity of dopamine. Mice with few of these receptors show low interest in and even aversion to alcohol (Maldonado et al., 1997).

Alcohol abuse also indirectly affects other parts of the brain. For example, it may interfere with the body's absorption of thiamin, one of the B vitamins. The absence of thiamin may contribute to **Korsakoff's syndrome,** a neurological disorder characterized by extreme memory difficulty, including the inability to store new memories.

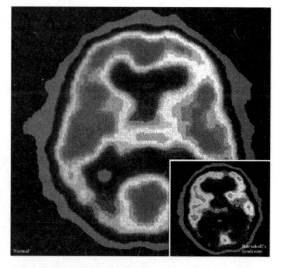

Korsakoff's Syndrome
These PET scans show brain activity in a normal patient (left) and a patient suffering from Korsakoff's syndrome (right inset). The frontal lobes are seen at the bottom center of each scan; the darker areas represent low metabolic activity. In a PET scan, low metabolic activity in response to thought-provoking questions indicates problems with memory and other cognitive functioning. Courtesy Dr. Peter R. Martin from *Alcohol Health & Research World,* Spring 1985, 9, cover.

■ **Korsakoff's syndrome** an alcohol-induced neurological disorder characterized by the inability to store new memories

■ **fetal alcohol syndrome (FAS)**
a cluster of birth defects that include facial abnormalities, low intelligence, and retarded body growth caused by the mother's use of alcohol during pregnancy

Alcohol and the Immune and Endocrine Systems Chronic alcohol use weakens the immune system, damages cellular DNA, interferes with normal endocrine system development, and disrupts the secretion of growth hormone, which may cause a variety of other endocrine changes. Alcohol abuse has been linked to decreased testosterone levels in men, leading to impotence and decreased fertility. In women, menstrual disturbances, spontaneous abortions, and miscarriages increase with the level of alcohol consumption. Alcohol may also decrease estrogen levels in women, which may partly explain the association between alcohol and increased risk of breast cancer (Wolfgan, 1997).

Alcohol and the Cardiovascular System Alcohol promotes the formation of fat deposits on heart muscle, which lowers the efficiency of the heart and contributes to cardiovascular disease. It also increases heart rate and causes blood vessels in the skin to dilate, resulting in a loss of body heat. Furthermore, chronic use may increase blood pressure and serum cholesterol and accelerate the development of atherosclerotic lesions in coronary arteries. Although women are susceptible to alcohol-related heart damage at lower levels of alcohol consumption than men, heavy use of alcohol erases the gender differential in susceptibility to chronic heart disease: Both men and women who abuse alcohol are equally likely to suffer a fatal heart attack before age 55 (Hanna, Defour, & Elliott, 1992).

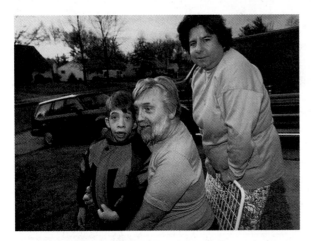

Fetal Alcohol Syndrome
If a woman drinks heavily during critical periods of fetal development, she puts her unborn child at risk of having fetal alcohol syndrome. Besides the malformed facial structures seen here, the child is also likely to be mentally retarded. These foster parents took on the task of raising this FAS child, despite known problems.
© David H. Wells/Corbis

Alcohol and the Gastrointestinal System Excessive use of alcohol contributes to stomach inflammation and the formation of gastrointestinal ulcers. Severe inflammation of the liver (*hepatitis*) and the replacement of normal liver cells by fibrous tissue (*cirrhosis*) are two common chronic diseases caused by alcohol abuse. Cirrhosis of the liver is an irreversible disease that causes approximately 26,000 deaths each year in the United States.

Alcohol and Pregnancy Alcohol freely crosses the placenta of pregnant women, making alcohol a potent teratogen. Alcohol levels in a developing fetus quickly become the same as those of a mother who drinks. Pregnant women who drink during critical stages of fetal development place their infants at risk of developing **fetal alcohol syndrome (FAS).** FAS causes severe birth defects, including low intelligence; microcephaly (small brain); mental retardation; retarded body growth; facial abnormalities such as malformed eyes, ears, nose, and cheekbones; and congenital heart defects.

The behavioral, psychological, and social effects of alcohol are just as dangerous as its physical effects, as the next section will explain.

Psychosocial Consequences of Alcohol Use

As blood alcohol level initially rises, many drinkers feel cheerful, self-confident, and more sexually responsive. As levels continue to rise, however, higher-order cognitive functions are disrupted, including planning, problem solving, and self-awareness. Furthermore, by focusing the drinker's attention on the immediate situation and away from any possible future consequences, alcohol impairs judgment and facilitates urges that might otherwise be resisted (see Chapter 6). This alcohol-induced sense of confidence and freedom from social constraints is known as **behavioral disinhibition.** Too often, the result of this condition is increased aggressiveness, risk taking, or other behaviors the individual would normally avoid.

Alcohol also makes it difficult for the drinker to interpret complex or ambiguous stimuli, partly because drinkers have a narrower perceptual field; that is, they find it harder to attend to multiple cues and easier to focus on only the most salient ones (Chermack & Giancola, 1997). In a recent study, Antonia Abbey, Tina Zawacki, and Pam McAuslan (2000) invited 176 unacquainted male and female college students (88 male–female pairs) to converse for 15 minutes after consuming either alcoholic or nonalcoholic drinks. Participants in the alcohol conditions received a dose of 80-proof vodka mixed with tonic calculated to induce a peak blood alcohol level of 0.04 percent. Some of the participants were deceived—told they were drinking alcohol when they weren't or told they were not drinking alcohol when they were. The 0.04 percent dose was selected because it was high enough to produce cognitive deficits, yet low enough for participants who were given alcohol but told they were drinking only tonic water to be deceived. Following a 10-minute absorption period, a breathalyzer test was administered, and the male–female "couples" conversed for 15 minutes. Trained observers coded the participants' behavior for two types of cues: (1) hints about dating availability and signs of potential sexual interest and (2) attentive cues, which were more ambiguous signals possibly indicating friendliness or sociability, rather than sexual interest. Afterward, participants completed a variety of questionnaires assessing their own behaviors as well as those of their conversation partner.

The results indicated that both men and women who drank alcohol perceived their partners and themselves as behaving more sexually and more disinhibited than did those who did not drink. The effects were somewhat stronger in males, perhaps confirming social stereotypes about intoxicated behaviors being more acceptable in men. However, the effects of alcohol consumption depended on the type of cue being evaluated. Intoxicated participants exaggerated the meaning of dating availability cues and *ignored* the meaning of ambiguous attention cues. Thus, alcohol allows people to concentrate on

■ **behavioral disinhibition** the false sense of confidence and freedom from social restraints that results from alcohol consumption

salient cues that fit their current beliefs (or hopes) and disregard more ambiguous cues that do not.

These results have implications for college prevention programs. Most students realize that intoxication is dangerous, although this does not necessarily keep them from drinking heavily (Norris, Nurius, & Dimeff, 1996). As the researchers note, "two drinks are enough to affect perceptions of disinhibition and sexuality. Students who feel sexy and uninhibited are at risk for having sex with someone they do not know well, having unprotected sex, feeling comfortable forcing sex on someone, or being the victim of forced sex." Health psychology's challenge is to make students take these risks seriously, rather than feeling that they are invulnerable (see Chapter 6). One suggestion offered by the researchers is that students could watch videotapes simulating risky situations and discuss them in mixed-sex groups. "Hearing the other gender's perceptions of the actors might help them realize they may not always understand their opposite sex companion's motives and intentions."

Alcohol-induced cognitive impairments are especially destructive during adolescence, perhaps because even low doses can impair the judgment of young teens who are already distracted by the ongoing psychological, physiological, and social challenges of puberty. For instance, high school students and college students who use alcohol, compared with their nondrinking counterparts, tend to have more sexual partners and to be less likely to use condoms (Lowry et al., 1994; MacDonald, Zanna, & Fong, 1996). A recent survey of 50,000 U.S. high school students compared teenagers who had used alcohol six or more times in the past 30 days with their counterparts who never or rarely used alcohol. The more frequent drinkers were absent from school nearly four times more often, more likely to ride in a car with a driver who had been drinking, nearly three times as likely to engage in antisocial behaviors such as stealing and vandalizing property, and more than twice as likely to be sexually active (Lammers, Ireland, Resnick, & Blum, 2000).

Excessive alcohol use has been associated with a variety of other social problems, including difficulties in interpersonal relationships, school failure, and various types of violence, including homicides, assault, robbery, suicides, and spousal abuse (Wolfgan, 1997). Half of all people convicted of rape or sexual assault were drinking before the commission of their crimes (Crowell & Burgess, 1996; Seto & Barbaree, 1995). Drinking also increases the chances of being a victim of crime. About half of all sexual assault victims report that they were drinking alcohol at the time of the assault (Abbey, McAuslan, & Ross, 1998). Remember, however, that these correlations do not prove that alcohol *causes* aggression or crime (see Chapter 2). Most crimes are committed by people who are *not* alcohol abusers, and most alcohol abusers are not criminals.

Alcohol contributes to violence not only by loosening restraints due to behavioral disinhibition but also by increasing a person's sensitivity to pain and frustration. Under the influence of alcohol, people are more sensitive to electric shocks and react with more aggression to frustration than when they are sober. In addition, brain imaging studies show that repeated heavy use of alcohol, stimulants, and other drugs disrupts frontal lobe activity, which impairs decision making and planning and lowers a person's normal threshold for violence. In a recent study, Antoine Bechara and his colleagues (2001) had alcohol abusers participate in a laboratory gambling task. One-third of the participants showed no decision-making impairment when playing the game. In contrast, approximately one-fourth of the participants performed almost exactly as patients with frontal lobe damage do on the same task (Grant, Contoreggi, & London, 2000), invariably opting for a small, immediate payoff in the game even when that strategy proved unprofitable in the long run. These results suggest that alcohol users who show impaired decision-making ability are at heightened risk for becoming addicted.

At the worst extreme, alcohol abuse may lead to death—of the person who has been drinking and/or innocent bystanders. In fact, over 40 percent of all traffic fatalities and a substantial proportion of drownings, falls, and other fatal accidents are related to alcohol-impaired cognitive and behavioral functioning, making alcohol consumption the fifth leading cause of death in the United States, the leading cause of death for people under age 45, and (after AIDS) the leading contributor to death among young people (Liu et al., 1997). Furthermore, among men, those who drink heavily are roughly twice as likely to die before age 65 than those who do not drink. Among women, the number of heavy drinkers who die before age 65, as compared to nondrinkers, is even larger (National Institute on Alcohol Abuse and Alcoholism, 2001).

Factors Contributing to Alcohol Dependence

In the late 1950s, the American Medical Association first described the symptoms of *alcoholism*. Although the term is still widely used, its ambiguity has led experts to prefer the more descriptive *alcohol dependence* and *alcohol abuse*. Like any form of drug dependence, **alcohol dependence** involves the use of the drug in order for the person to function normally. The symptoms include the development of tolerance; excessive time spent obtaining, consuming, or recovering from the use of alcohol; reduction of important activities due to drinking; and continued drinking despite knowledge that alcohol is causing a physical or psychological problem (American Psychiatric Association, 1994).

As is true for other psychoactive drugs, a defining feature of alcohol dependence is the presence of a withdrawal syndrome when consumption is ceased or reduced. The *alcohol withdrawal syndrome* consists of a cluster of symptoms that include nausea, sweating, shaking ("the shakes"), hypertension, and anxiety. In severe cases, these symptoms coalesce into a neurological state called **delirium tremens**—or the DTs.

Alcohol dependence is often closely related to **alcohol abuse,** which is characterized by the *Diagnostic and Statistical Manual of Mental Disorders* (DSM-IV) as a maladaptive drinking pattern in which at least one of the

■ **alcohol dependence** a state in which the use of alcohol is required for a person to function normally

■ **delirium tremens (DTs)** a neurological state induced by excessive and prolonged use of alcohol and characterized by sweating, trembling, anxiety, and hallucinations; a symptom of alcohol withdrawal

■ **alcohol abuse** a maladaptive drinking pattern in which drinking interferes with role obligations

following occurs: recurrent drinking despite its interference with role obligations; continued drinking despite legal, social, or interpersonal problems related to its use; and recurrent drinking in situations in which intoxication is dangerous.

Various factors have been implicated in explaining why certain people are more likely than others to abuse alcohol. No single factor or influence, however, completely explains the origins of alcohol dependency or abuse.

Genes and Alcohol Dependence

There is now substantial evidence that alcohol dependency is at least partly genetic, although it does not seem that a single, specific gene causes this disorder. Instead, some people may inherit a greater tolerance for the aversive effects of alcohol as well as a genetically greater sensitivity to the pleasurable effects (Devor, 1994). Both tendencies may be factors in early excessive drinking, leading to dependence. Consider the evidence:

- Researchers have located a gene in some alcohol abusers that alters the function of the dopamine receptor called DRD2. Genetic variation in DRD2 may influence concentrations of and responses to synaptic dopamine. This gene is also found in people with attention deficit disorder, who have an increased risk for alcohol dependency (Cook et al., 1995).

- When either the mother or father of a male child is alcohol-dependent, the son is significantly more likely to later abuse alcohol himself (Cloninger, Bohman, Sigvardsson, & von Knorring, 1985). In fact, for males, alcoholism in a first-degree relative is the single best predictor of alcoholism (Plomin, Defries, McClearn, & McGuffin, 2001). Interestingly, in contrast to the results of studies on male children of alcohol abusers, those from twin and adoption studies on female children of alcohol abusers have provided weaker evidence for the role of heredity (McGue, 2000).

- Adopted children are more susceptible to alcohol dependency if one or both of their biological parents was alcohol-dependent (Wood, Vinson, & Sher, 2001).

- Identical twins have nearly twice the concordance rate for alcohol abuse or dependency. This is true whether the twins were raised together or apart and whether they grew up in the homes of their biological parents or adoptive parents. A study of monozygotic and dizygotic twins revealed that when one MZ twin was dependent on or abused alcohol, in 76 percent of the cases, the other MZ twin also showed signs of alcohol addiction (Kendler, Preschott, Neale, & Pedersen, 1997).

- Alcohol's anxiety-relieving effects may also be enhanced among children of alcohol absuers (Sayette, 1993). People who are less sensitive to alcohol's effects may be at a relatively high risk for alcohol dependence because they lack the feedback mechanisms that signal overconsumption (Wolfgan, 1997).

- The personalities of those most likely to abuse alcohol have several common traits, each of which is, at least in part, genetically determined. These traits include a quick temper, impulsiveness, intolerance of frustration, vulnerability to depression, and a general attraction to excitement (Kaplan & Johnson, 1992).

Based on such evidence, researchers have estimated the *heritability* of alcohol dependency or abuse to be about 0.357 for males and 0.262 for females. (Recall that heritability refers to the variation in a trait, in a particular population, in a particular environment, that can be attributed to genetic differences among the members of that group. Heritability refers to *group* rather than *individual* differences in a trait. It does not indicate the degree to which genes determine the likelihood of a trait in a particular person.)

Even if additional genetic factors in alcohol dependence are identified, however, it is unlikely that heredity can explain all cases of alcohol dependence. In fact, another view is that the *lack* of genetic protection may play a role. Like fat and sugar, alcohol is not readily found in nature, and so genetic mechanisms to protect against alcohol dependence may not have evolved in humans as they frequently have for protection against naturally occurring threats such as bacteria, viruses, and other pathogens (Potter, 1997).

Gene–Environment Interactions

Current models of the origins of alcohol dependency emphasize the interaction of environmental and genetic factors (for example, Cloninger, 1987). Certain person–environment combinations may mutually reinforce each other and lead to substance use or interact in such a way as to constrain use (Hawkins, Catalano, & Miller, 1992). In one study, students between 12 and 15 years old were tested over a 3-year period, as were their parents and siblings (Bates & Labouvie, 1995). The participants were presented with a list of 53 alcohol-related problems and asked to indicate how many times each had happened to them. They were asked, for example, how many times they got into fights, neglected responsibilities, experienced memory loss, or were unable to complete their homework because they were under the influence. Each participant also completed a variety of scales assessing sensation seeking, impulsiveness, need for achievement, and the quality of interpersonal relationships. Person–environment combinations that included impulsiveness, disinhibition, deviant peer group associations, and low parental control acted as catalysts for alcohol use. Conversely, high educational goals and parental control were protective factors in preventing alcohol and substance experimentation (Bates & Labouvie, 1995).

Other studies have found that the parents of alcohol-dependent children are more likely to be less educated and of lower socioeconomic status than are the parents of offspring who are not problem drinkers. These parents, according to their children, also tended to be less supportive and to be involved in

behavioral undercontrol a general personality syndrome linked to alcohol dependence and characterized by aggressiveness, unconventionality, and impulsiveness; also called deviance proneness

negative emotionality a state of alcohol abuse characterized by depression and anxiety

tension-reduction hypothesis an explanation of drinking behavior that proposes that alcohol is reinforcing because it reduces stress and tension

less-than-ideal marriages (Hunt, 1997). Lynne Cooper, Robert Pierce, and Marie Tidwell (1995) also found that although neither paternal nor maternal drinking problems consistently predicted substance use among adolescent offspring, chaotic and unsupportive family situations were strongly predictive of early alcohol consumption.

Alcohol, Temperament, and Personality

Research studies that link temperament and personality to alcohol dependence provide another clear indication of the interaction of nature and nurture. A person's temperament is determined in part by heredity and in part by upbringing. Age also plays a role, with adolescents and young adults being more vulnerable to the alcohol-abusing aspects of temperament than those in other seasons of life.

Researchers no longer attempt to identify a single "alcoholic personality," focusing instead on specific personality traits that appear to be linked to alcohol dependence. One such trait is a temperament that includes attraction to excitement and intolerance of frustration (Brook, Cohen, Whiteman, & Gordon, 1992; Kaplan & Johnson, 1992). A second is **behavioral undercontrol** (also called *deviance proneness*), characterized by aggressiveness, unconventionality, overactivity, and impulsive behavior. A third is **negative emotionality,** which is characterized by depression and anxiety (Sayette & Hufford, 1997). Marked by such traits, high-delinquent teens show consistently elevated levels of use-related problems. Antisocial pathology apparently fosters problem substance use (Stice, Myers, & Brown, 1998).

Alcohol and Tension Reduction

One of the most influential behavioral explanations of drinking behavior, indeed of all addictive behaviors, is the **tension-reduction hypothesis.** According to this model, alcohol and other addictive drugs are reinforcing because they relieve tension, in part by stimulating the central nervous system to release neurotransmitters that calm anxiety and reduce sensitivity to pain (Parrott, 1999). Although many people, including those who treat alcohol abuse and those who are dependent upon alcohol, believe that some people may cope with stress by drinking, evidence for the tension-reduction hypothesis is mixed. One difficulty with this hypothesis is that although anxiety level may decrease early in a drinking bout, both anxiety and depression levels often *increase* thereafter (remember alcohol is a depressant) (Nathan & O'Brien, 1971). Thus, the model may explain why a bout of drinking *begins,* but it does not explain why it continues.

Social-Cognitive Factors

For some, alcohol abuse may stem from a history of drinking to cope with a variety of life events or overwhelming situational demands. Alcohol may help some people cope defensively with difficult environments by altering their thought processes. Jay Hull's *self-awareness model* (1987) proposes that alcohol distorts information processing, making the drinker's thinking more superficial and less self-critical. By focusing attention away from thoughts such as "I'm no good at anything," alcohol may allow some people to feel better about themselves. In other words, people may drink to avoid self-awareness. A similar, *self-handicapping model* proposes that some drinkers use alcohol as an excuse for personal failures and other negative outcomes in their lives ("I was drunk"). Both models highlight the importance of the social context in which drinking occurs, as well as the drinker's expectancies regarding the drug's effects.

Alcohol and Context Marilyn Senchak, Kenneth Leonard, and Brian Greene (1998) questioned college students to determine the frequency of drinking in different social contexts. Participants were asked, "With whom do you usually or most frequently drink?" The typical social drinking context endorsed by college students was strongly related to their level of alcohol consumption and their individual personalities. Those who preferred large social contexts involving both men and women tended to be heavier drinkers, as well as less depressed and more outgoing, than were those who preferred smaller, mixed-sex contexts.

Although men and women were equally likely to drink in large, mixed-sex groups, women were more likely than men to drink in small, mixed-sex groups. Men who drank in same-sex groups (whether large or small) reported more frequent drunkenness than men in small, mixed-sex groups did. This suggests that men who drink heavily may seek out social contexts in which this behavior will be tolerated.

The riskiest drinking context, particularly for men, was either large, mixed-sex groups or small, same-sex groups, but perhaps for very different reasons. Drinking in a large, mixed-sex group was associated with low depression and a socially outgoing (extraverted) personality. The second style, drinking in small, same-sex groups, seemed to indicate more introverted individuals (especially men) drinking in response to negative internal states. Other researchers have made a similar distinction between two types of heavy drinkers, one influenced by sensation seeking (perhaps as part of an active student lifestyle) and another influenced by personal problems (Brennan, Walfish, & AuBuchon, 1986; Fondacaro & Heller, 1983). One important implication of such studies is that the interaction of individual characteristics and social drinking contexts may be important in predicting heavy drinking.

A recent study shows that members of fraternities and sororities drink more heavily than other students, dubbed the *Greek effect* by the researchers (Sher, Bartholow, & Nanda, 2001). To find out if heavy college drinking predicted similar behavior later, the researchers surveyed students again 3 years

■ **alcohol expectancies**
individuals' beliefs about the effects of alcohol consumption on behavior, their own as well as that of other people

after graduation. The results showed that post-college drinking was more moderate once students were removed from a social environment that supported heavy drinking.

Alcohol and Expectations As is true of all psychoactive drugs, alcohol's impact depends not only on the dose but also on the circumstances under which the drug is taken, the user's personality, mood, and **alcohol expectancies** regarding the drug's effects. People who believe they have received alcohol behave just like those who have imbibed, whether or not they have (Leigh, 1989). In one study, people drove more recklessly in a driving simulator when led to believe they had just consumed alcohol (McMillen, Smith, & Wells-Parker, 1989).

Personal beliefs and expectations about alcohol use influence drinking behavior in another way as well. In a 5-year study conducted at fifty-six public schools in upstate New York, Lawrence Scheier and Gilbert Botvin (1997) found that adolescents' beliefs about their peers' alcohol use and attitudes predicted their own alcohol use. Those who were certain that many of their friends drank regularly—and enjoyed doing so—were more likely to begin using alcohol themselves. As another example, people who believe that alcohol promotes sexual arousal become more responsive to sexual stimuli if they believe they have been drinking (Abrams & Wilson, 1983). The impact of alcohol expectancies on drinking behavior is explored more fully in the Reality Check on pages 340–341.

Treatment and Prevention of Alcohol Dependency

Most problem drinkers receive outpatient rather than inpatient intervention, and most are able to quit drinking without formal intervention (McMurran, 1994). The treatments generally involve the use of drugs or therapy, or some combination of the two.

Factors that appear to influence the willingness of a person to enter treatment for alcohol dependence include gender, age, marital status, and ethnicity. Among women, factors that predict entry into treatment include being older and unmarried and having a lower level of education, employment, and income. For men, factors that predict entry include having experienced alcohol-related social consequences, being older, and belonging to an ethnic minority (Wolfgan, 1997). Although evaluations of the effectiveness of self-help groups are limited (Sayette & Hufford, 1997), drinking-related beliefs, readiness and motivation to change, and social support for abstinence are important predictors of the success or failure of treatment.

Drug Treatment
The extensive efforts of researchers to understand the physiological mechanisms by which alcohol affects the brain have led them to uncover a number

of pharmacological treatments for alcohol dependency. Medications include *detoxification* agents to manage alcohol withdrawal, alcohol-sensitizing agents to deter future drinking, and anticraving agents to reduce the risk of relapse.

As noted, many people who are dependent on or abuse alcohol also suffer from clinical depression. Antidepressants that increase levels of serotonin by inhibiting its reuptake at synapses are sometimes used to treat those in the early stages of abstinence from alcohol. The best known of these is *fluoxetine* (Prozac). Some researchers believe that deficiencies of serotonin may cause alcohol craving (Anton & Kranzler, 1994). Other researchers have taken a different approach, focusing instead on the role of dopamine in alcohol dependency. As you'll recall from our discussion of the reward model, alcohol and other drugs induce dependence because they increase the availability of dopamine, which puts the brain's reward system into overdrive. By treating alcohol dependency with drugs that block the release of dopamine, they decrease the reinforcing aspects of drinking alcohol (Thompson, 2000). *Naltrexone,* an opiate antagonist that reduces alcohol's reinforcing properties in the brain, was approved in 1995 by the FDA for the treatment of alcohol dependency.

Aversion Therapy

Researchers generally agree that treatment of alcohol dependence is more successful when drugs are combined with behavioral and psychological therapy. One such method, **aversion therapy,** associates a nauseating drug such as *Antabuse (disulfiram)* with drinking, with the goal of getting the patient to avoid alcohol. Antabuse treatment interferes with the metabolism of alcohol, causing an accumulation of acetaldehyde. Although the drug does not reduce cravings for alcohol, if the patient takes a single drink within several days of ingesting Antabuse, a variety of unpleasant effects occur, including nausea, sweating, racing heart rate, severe headaches, and dizziness.

The logic behind the use of Antabuse stems from learning theory. Drugs like this, which produce sickness when a person drinks, are designed to produce a *conditioned aversion* to alcohol. When taken daily, Antabuse can result in total abstinence (Julien, 2001). A major problem, however, is patient compliance. Many people simply stop taking the drug on a regular basis, which dramatically reduces its effectiveness (Gessner & Gessner, 1992).

Because of compliance problems with Antabuse, some therapists prefer to conduct aversion therapy trials in a controlled, clinical setting. In this Pavlovian conditioning technique, the client is given a drink of alcohol, followed by an *emetic drug,* which induces vomiting within a short period of time. By carefully timing the interval between the drink and the emetic drug, the latter functions as an unconditioned stimulus and becomes associated with the taste, smell, and act of taking a drink of alcohol. These stimuli thus become conditioned stimuli and trigger the unpleasant reaction of nausea.

■ **aversion therapy** a behavioral therapy that pairs an unpleasant stimulus (such as a nauseating drug) with an undesirable behavior (such as drinking or smoking), causing the patient to avoid the behavior

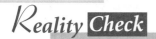

Alcohol Expectancies

Alcohol's behavioral effects stem not only from its impact on brain functioning but also from the drinker's expectations. To gain some insight into your alcohol expectancies, indicate whether you agree or disagree with each item below based on your own personal opinion, belief, and/or experience regarding the consumption of two or three drinks of alcohol. If an item is always or sometimes true, check *Agree*. If an item is never true, check *Disagree*.

OPINIONS ABOUT AND EXPERIENCES WITH ALCOHOL

Agree   Disagree

_____   _____   1. Drinking makes the future seem brighter.

_____   _____   2. Alcohol seems like magic.

_____   _____   3. I feel more coordinated after I drink.

_____   _____   4. If I'm feeling restricted in any way, a few drinks make me feel better.

_____   _____   5. Alcohol makes me more interesting.

_____   _____   6. Having a few drinks is a nice way to celebrate special occasions.

_____   _____   7. Drinking is pleasurable because it's enjoyable to join in with people who are enjoying themselves.

_____   _____   8. Drinking makes me feel good.

_____   _____   9. Some alcohol has a pleasant, cleansing, tingly taste.

_____   _____   10. Drinking adds a certain warmth to social occasions.

_____   _____   11. After a few drinks, I am sexually responsive.

_____   _____   12. I often feel sexier after I've had a few drinks.

_____   _____   13. I am more romantic when I drink.

_____   _____   14. I'm a better lover after a few drinks.

_____   _____   15. I enjoy having sex more if I've had some alcohol.

Agree   Disagree

_____   _____   16. If I'm feeling restricted in any way, a few drinks make me feel better.

_____   _____   17. After a few drinks it is easier to pick a fight.

_____   _____   18. Drinking makes me feel flushed.

_____   _____   19. I feel powerful when I drink, as if I can really influence others to do as I want.

_____   _____   20. Drinking increases male aggressiveness.

_____   _____   21. If I have a couple of drinks it is easier to express my feelings.

_____   _____   22. A few drinks make it easier to talk to people.

_____   _____   23. When I'm drinking, it is easier to open up and express my feelings.

_____   _____   24. Drinking gives me more confidence in myself.

_____   _____   25. A few drinks make me feel less shy.

_____   _____   26. Alcohol enables me to fall asleep more easily.

_____   _____   27. Alcohol helps me sleep better.

_____   _____   28. Alcohol decreases muscular tension.

_____   _____   29. Alcohol can act as an anesthetic, that is, it can deaden pain.

_____   _____   30. Alcohol makes me worry less.

Scoring: Each group of five items measures a different global expectancy about alcohol's effects. Items 1–5 measure the belief that alcohol is a global, positive transforming agent; 6–10, the expectation that alcohol enhances physical and social pleasure; 11–15, the belief that alcohol enhances sexual experience and performance; 16–20, the belief that alcohol increases power and aggression; 21–25, the expectation that alcohol increases social assertiveness; and 26–30, the expectation that alcohol reduces tension. Your score on each subscale can range from 0 to 5, with higher scores representing a stronger expectancy that alcohol has the stated effect. Research studies have found that alcohol expectancies are strongly correlated with drinking practices and are, in fact, better predictors than demographic variables such as socioeconomic status, gender, and ethnicity. One study (Brown, 1985) found that the best ex-

pectancy predictor for heavy drinkers (who frequently drink to the point of sickness) was social and physical pleasure (items 6–10), whereas the most powerful expectancy predictor for problem drinkers (heavy drinkers who also experience trouble with authorities such as driving while under the influence) was tension reduction (items 26–30).

Sources: "Expectations of Reinforcement from Alcohol: Their Domain and Relation to Drinking Problems," by S. A. Brown, M. S. Goldman, A. Inn, and L. Anderson, 1980, *Journal of Consulting and Clinical Psychology, 48,* p. 422; "Expectancies versus Background in the Prediction of College Drinking Patterns," by S. Brown, 1985, *Journal of Consulting and Clinical Psychology, 53,* pp. 123–130.

Relapse Prevention Programs

Because of the unusually high rate of relapse in alcohol dependence (roughly 60 percent a year following treatment), many treatments, while helping the person to remain alcohol-free, focus on enabling the person to deal with situations that tempt relapse. When faced with a situation such as a cocktail party at which other people are happily imbibing, many former drinkers may become physically aroused and begin to crave alcohol. Many relapse prevention programs therefore emphasize gaining stimulus control over such situations that may precipitate a return to drinking (Marlatt & Gordon, 1985).

One form of relapse prevention is based on the gradual *extinction* of drinking triggers. Treatments have been developed in which drinkers are repeatedly exposed to alcohol-related stimuli, such as the aroma of their favorite drink, but they are not allowed to drink. With repeated exposure over a number of sessions, the patients' initially powerful physical and psychological conditioned responses diminish (Monti, Rohsenow, Rubonis, & Niaura, 1993).

Many relapse prevention programs also incorporate *coping* and *social-skills* training, or CSST, which helps "inoculate" drinkers by teaching specific strategies for coping with high-risk situations without the help of alcohol. Such situations typically involve social pressure, negative emotions such as anger and frustration, and communication difficulties. Inoculation focuses on improving the person's assertiveness, listening skills, and ability to give and receive compliments and criticism and on enhancing close relationships (Foxhall, 2001). In addition, the recovered drinker is taught skills that permit him or her to abstain in drinking situations. *Drink refusal training* entails the modeling and rehearsal of skills needed to turn down offers to drink.

Self-Help Groups

One of the most widely accepted nonmedical efforts to deal with alcohol dependence is Alcoholics Anonymous (AA). AA's 12-step approach recognizes the biochemical model of alcohol abuse and suggests a belief in a higher power to battle what is viewed as an incurable disease. Its theory is that "once an alcoholic, always an alcoholic," and it disagrees entirely with the belief that alcoholics can be reformed into moderate, responsible drinkers. As of 2001, AA counts more than two million members worldwide.

Self-help groups such as AA generally involve group discussions of members' experiences in recovering from alcohol abuse. Members benefit by connecting with a new, nondrinking network and sharing their fears and concerns about relapse. Another self-help group, Rational Recovery, offers a nonspiritual alternative to treating alcohol dependence.

Preventing Alcohol Problems

Alcohol prevention researchers target individual drinkers as well as the social environments in which drinking occurs. Preventive treatments therefore aim to change attitudes about drinking, strengthen coping skills, or restructure environments to reduce the risk of alcohol-related problems.

Most alcohol abuse and dependency prevention programs stem from one of two theoretical perspectives: *wellness theory* and *problem behavior theory*. Wellness theory proposes that healthy behavior is a "conscious and deliberate approach to an advanced state of physical and psychological/spiritual health" (Ardell, 1985, p. 2). Young people who generally have a sense that their worlds are coherent and understandable, who feel confident that they have the skills necessary to meet life's demands, and who feel a commitment to themselves and to their lives generally adopt a health-enhancing lifestyle (Antonovsky, 1990). In contrast, problem behavior theory suggests that drug use, early sexual activity, truancy, and other risky behaviors often occur together as a syndrome and trigger other problems later in life (Jessor, 1987).

Eleanor Kim and her colleagues (1997) questioned a random sample of college freshmen to determine whether drinking was part of an isolated group of unconventional social behaviors (as problem behavior theory suggests) or more accurately understood as part of a more general health or wellness orientation. The results supported the problem behavior theory. The healthy behavior choices made by those who abstained from alcohol, light-moderate drinkers, binge drinkers, and heavy drinkers showed clear trends when other health behaviors were examined.

Prevention programs are often most effective when they target children and adolescents, before they have succumbed to the habit. To this end, many primary prevention strategies have been put in place. Among those that have proved at least partly effective are health education classes that realistically delineate the potential hazards of drug use, strict enforcement of drunk-driving laws, higher prices of alcohol and cigarettes, harsher punishments for those who sell (or make available) alcohol and cigarettes to minors, and education classes that inform parents of the hazards of various drugs and improve parent–child communication.

As noted earlier, peer culture is a major social influence on drug use. Several primary prevention programs, including the Alcohol Misuse Prevention Study (AMPS), are based on correcting faulty reasoning about peers' drug use and improving social skills in targeted groups. The AMPS was designed to help preadolescent students resist social pressures leading toward alcohol consumption. For instance, role-playing exercises allow students to practice declining alcohol, marijuana, and other drug offers in various social situations. Should students actually encounter such situations, they will have behavioral and cognitive *scripts* for declining the drug offer. The program's beneficial effects have been shown to persist through grade 12 (Wolfgan, 1997).

Since the Drug Free Schools and Communities Act of 1986, most elementary and secondary schools have included some classroom programming aimed at preventing drug use. Does it work? So far, the results have been mixed (Smith, 2001). A recent longitudinal study evaluated the effectiveness of middle school social influence programs that teach children to resist peer pressure and try to change their perceptions that teen use of drugs is widespread. Sadly, the researchers found no difference in drug use in these schools compared with control schools (Peterson, Kealey, Mann, Marek, & Sarason, 2000). Results such as these suggest that psychologists' understanding of substance abuse prevention is far from complete and that much more research is needed. The most promising new research takes a systems approach (see Chapter 2), recognizing that a person's choice to use drugs is the result of many interrelated environmental factors and contexts.

Realistically, however, health psychologists recognize that as long as drugs are available and are not perceived as serious threats to health, many young people will try them and many will eventually abuse them. Following this line of reasoning, one strategy is to delay the young person's experimentation as long as possible. Doing so will increase the odds that he or she is realistically informed about the hazards of the drug and has the cognitive maturity to avoid the faulty reasoning that often leads to drug abuse. The younger a person is when he or she starts drinking, the more likely he or she will be to abuse or become dependent on alcohol. One study sponsored by the National Institutes of Health found that people who began drinking before they turned 15 were four times more likely to become alcohol abusers than were those who started drinking at the legal age of 21. Other studies have documented that underage drinkers also get into more trouble at home and school and are more likely to be sexually active. In contrast, every year drinking alcohol is delayed, the risk of becoming alcohol-dependent decreases by 14 percent.

Tobacco Use and Abuse

Along with caffeine and alcohol, nicotine is one of the three most widely used psychoactive drugs. Native to the New World, the tobacco plant is first represented in history on a Mayan stone carving dated from A.D. 600 to 900, and tobacco smoking is first mentioned in Christopher Columbus' log books for his legendary voyage of 1492.

Figure 8.5

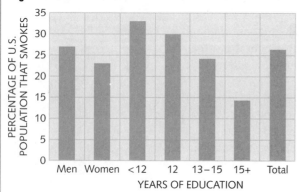

Who Smokes?

Smoking is most prevalent among men and people with less than a high school education. Overall, 50 million adults in the United States, about one in every four, currently smoke. Clearly, the nation failed to meet the national health goal set by the Healthy People 2000 project of limiting smoking to 15 percent of the population by the year 2000.

Sources: *Reducing Tobacco Use: A Report of the Surgeon General— 2000,* by D. Satcher, 2000, Washington, DC: U.S. Department of Health and Human Services; "Tobacco Smoking," by N. E. Grunberg, J. J. Brown, and L. C. Klein, 1997, in A. Baum, S. Newman, J. Weinman, R. West, and C. McManus (Eds.), *Cambridge Handbook of Psychology, Health, and Medicine* (pp. 606–610), Cambridge, UK: Cambridge University Press.

Prevalence of Smoking

Cigarette smoking in the United States peaked in the early 1960s, when approximately half of all adult American men and one-third of adult women smoked. From the late 1960s until the mid-1990s, the total number of smokers declined steadily—to about 25 percent of all American adults, evenly divided among women, men, whites, and blacks (Grunberg, Brown, & Klein, 1997). However, the decline was not evenly distributed, with most of the decrease occurring among upper socioeconomic status (SES) groups and men. Lower-SES individuals continued to smoke, and the prevalence of smoking among women increased sharply. Today, smoking is most prevalent among men, young adults 25 to 44 years of age, and people with less than a high school education (Figure 8.5).

Smoking rebounded among U.S. and Canadian teenagers during the late 1990s, reversing the 30-year trend of declining incidence and prevalence (Brooke, 2000). In 1999, about 23 percent of North American high school seniors classified themselves as daily smokers—up nearly 25 percent since 1990 (Johnston, Bachman, & O'Malley, 1999). Across all grades, nearly 34 percent of all high school students use cigarettes (Centers for Disease Control and Prevention, 2000). Cigarette smoking is also on the rise among college students. Nancy Rigotti, Jae Lee, and Henry Wechsler (2000) of Harvard University's School of Public Health surveyed 15,000 students at 116 U.S. and Canadian colleges in 1993, 1997, and 1999. The results showed that 28 percent of college students were current smokers in 1999, up from 22.3 percent in 1993. The study found increased rates of cigarette smoking among all students regardless of age, sex, race, type of college, or region of the country. This increase reflects a 32 percent increase in smoking among high school students between 1991 and 1999. Cigar use ranked second, with 8 percent of students reporting they had smoked a cigar within the past 30 days. Some health experts speculate that the rise in smoking among college students may be because this older group has largely been ignored by anti-tobacco health campaigns.

Smoking has also become increasingly prevalent in Asian countries such as China, where 70 percent of men (but only 10 percent of women) smoke, and Japan, where 35 percent of the population smokes (Coleman, 1997; Schwartz & Pomfret, 1998). In developed countries as a whole, it is estimated that tobacco is responsible for 24 percent of all male deaths and 7 percent of all female deaths (Peto et al., 1996). Equally troubling is the fact that smoking rates are skyrocketing in developing countries such as Kenya and Zimbabwe, causing the World Health Organization to predict that by the year 2025, 7 out of every 10 tobacco-related deaths will occur in developing countries, where many people are uninformed about the dangers of smoking (WHO, 2000).

Still, the news is not all bad. The most recent "Surgeon General's Report on Tobacco Use Among High School Students" (CDC, 2000) found that although smoking increased among twelfth graders between 1991 and 1999 (39.6 percent to 42.8 percent, respectively), smoking rates dropped 17 percent among high school freshmen, perhaps indicating that teen smoking rates have peaked (see Figure 8.6). The report also found that the smoking rate for African-American high school students dropped from 22.7 percent to 19.7 percent, markedly lower than the rate among European American students (38.6 percent).

Physical Effects of Smoking

Cigarette smoking is the single most preventable cause of illness, disability, and premature death in this country and in much of the world. In the United States alone, it is estimated that 435,000 people a year die from smoking-related illness—more than the combined number of deaths from murders, suicides, AIDS, automobile accidents, alcohol and other drug abuse, and fires (Grunberg et al., 1997).

The death rate for smokers is 70 percent higher than for nonsmokers (Liese & Franz, 1996). Of the nearly half million Americans who die each year due to smoking, 82,000 die from noncancerous lung diseases, 112,000 from lung cancer, 30,000 from cancers of other body organs, and 200,000 from cardiovascular disease (Julien, 2001). To put this in perspective, consider that roughly half of all deaths due to cardiovascular disease, lung cancer, and emphysema (*chronic obstructive pulmonary disease, or COPD*, a progressive disease that results in severely diminished lung capacity and respiratory volume) are smoking related. It is estimated that each cigarette smoked reduces life expectancy by 14 minutes. An adult who has smoked two packs of cigarettes a

Figure 8.6

Smoking among U.S. High School Students
Although adult smoking decreased sharply over the past 25 years, especially among people with more years of education, it made a partial comeback among U.S. teens during the 1990s. Still, researchers are hopeful that this trend has peaked and that the Healthy People 2010 objective of fewer than 1 in 5 high school students as smokers will be met.

Sources: "National Alternative Youth Risk Behavior Survey," Centers for Disease Control and Prevention, October 28, 2000, www.cdc.gov/nccdphp/dash/yrbs/; *Monitoring the Future: National Results on Adolescent Drug Use*, by L. D. Johnston, P. M. O'Malley, and J. G. Bachman, 2001, Bethesda, MD: National Institute on Drug Abuse.

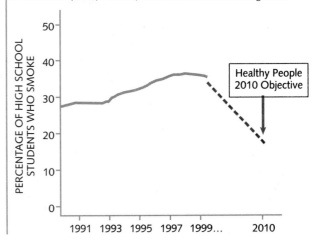

By one estimate, tobacco companies need to recruit 2 million new smokers every year to replace those who have died or finally quit smoking (Lynch, Bonnie, & Nelson, 1995).

day (40 cigarettes) for 20 years can expect to lose about 8 years of his or her life.

Each time a person lights up, 4,000 different chemical compounds are released. It is these chemicals that—while they provide pleasure and energy—cause disease and eventually death. For example, the nicotine in cigarette smoke contributes to the development of cardiovascular disease by activating specific neural receptors, which in turn causes an increase in heart rate and blood pressure and the constriction of arteries, all symptoms that lead to heart disease. The presence of nicotine also causes serum cholesterol levels to rise, hastening the formation of artery-blocking atherosclerotic lesions.

Cigarette smoke leads to bronchial congestion by increasing the production of mucus in the throat and lungs while simultaneously damaging the hairlike *cilia* that line the respiratory tract. This leads to higher-than-normal incidence rates of bronchitis, emphysema, and respiratory infections.

The link between smoking and cancer is no longer a matter of debate. Benzo[a]pyrene (BPDE), a chemical in cigarette smoke, has been identified as a causative agent in lung cancer (Denissenko, Pao, Tang, & Pfeifer, 1996). BPDE damages a cancer suppressor gene, causing a mutation of lung tissue. Smoking is also a factor in cancers of the mouth, larynx, stomach, pancreas, esophagus, kidney, bladder, and cervix (Newcomb & Carbone, 1992).

Given the same lifetime exposure to tobacco smoke, the risk for developing lung cancer is 20 to 70 percent higher in women than men at every level of exposure, indicating that women are more susceptible to the carcinogens in tobacco. Women who smoke during pregnancy are more likely to miscarry or to have low-birth-weight infants and infants who die from sudden infant death syndrome (Byrd, 1992). Because cigarette smoke reduces the delivery of oxygen to the developing person's brain, the resulting *fetal hypoxia* can cause irreversible intellectual damage. Schoolchildren whose mothers smoked during pregnancy have lower IQs and an increased prevalence of attention-deficit hyperactivity disorder (ADHD) (Milberger, Biederman, Faraone, Chen, & Jones, 1996).

Smoking Effects Disguised as Aging

Health experts are discovering that a number of disorders once believed to be the normal consequences of aging are, in fact, caused by long-term smoking and other behavioral pathogens. For example, some of the mental decline observed among elderly persons may be caused by tobacco-related bleeding in the brain ("silent strokes") that goes unnoticed. Laura Launer and her colleagues at Erasmus University Medical School in the Netherlands conducted a meta-analysis of four European studies of 9,223 people aged 65 and older. The participants (22 percent of whom were smokers, 36 percent former smokers, and 42 percent nonsmokers) were tested once and then again 2 years later on short-term memory, attention, and simple mathematical calculations. All three groups showed a decline in cognitive performance over the 2-year period, but the decline was by far the greatest among smokers. Former smokers showed slightly greater decline than nonsmokers did, but the difference was not statistically significant (Launer & Kalmijn, 1998).

Secondhand Smoke

The hazards of smoking extend beyond the direct risks to the smoker. Secondhand smoke contains an even higher concentration of many carcinogens than smoke inhaled directly from a cigarette. According to a 1996 study of more than 10,000 nonsmokers conducted by the Centers for Disease Control (Domino, 1996), nearly 9 out of 10 nonsmoking Americans are exposed to environmental tobacco smoke (ETS, or *secondhand smoke*). The study reported measurable levels of *cotinine* (a chemical the body metabolizes from nicotine) in the blood of 88 percent of the nonsmokers. The presence of cotinine is proof that a person has been exposed to, and absorbed, tobacco smoke.

It is estimated that 4,000 Americans die each year from lung cancer caused by ETS. Nonsmokers who are regularly exposed to secondhand smoke are 20 to 70 percent more likely to die from cardiovascular disease than those who are not so exposed (Wells, 1994). Children who live with smokers have a significantly higher prevalence of pneumonia, ear and nasal infections, and the skin disorder eczema. Female nonsmokers whose husbands smoke stand a 1.32 greater chance of developing lung cancer than do nonsmoking wives of nonsmoking husbands.

Why Do People Smoke?

To understand why people smoke, we need to consider each of the major stages of smoking behavior: initiation, maintenance, cessation, and relapse (Grunberg et al., 1997).

Initiation

Initiation of drug use often occurs through social contacts, independent of the physiological effects of the drug. With the exception of cocaine and amphetamines, initial use of many psychoactive drugs is often unpleasant. As a result, a period of experimentation typically precedes the development of regular drug use, thus suggesting that factors other than physical effects are important in the initiation and maintenance of drug use until dependence develops.

Advertising is a powerful influence. In the United States, for example, *Joe Camel*—who once ranked second only to Mickey Mouse in face recognition among American schoolchildren—has been superseded by the Camel Kids passing out free packs of cigarettes at clubs. In a clever twist of this once highly effective advertising campaign, Sonia Duffy and Dee Burton showed kindergarten through twelfth-grade Chicago students two currently used

Between 1987 (when Joe Camel was first introduced by R. J. Reynolds) and 1997, Camel's share of the teenage cigarette market increased from less than 3 percent to over 13 percent. Is it any wonder that in 1997 the Federal Trade Commission accused Reynolds of targeted appeals to teenagers?

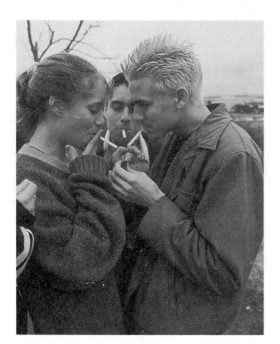

Social Influences on Smoking
Whether a teenager smokes depends to a large extent on whether his or her friends also smoke. Although peer influence is a major factor in determining tobacco use or abuse, the reverse is also true: Adolescents tend to select friends who have similar interests and habits. © Grantpix / Photo Researchers, Inc.

antismoking messages: "Smoking kills" and "Smoking causes lung cancer, heart disease, emphysema and may complicate pregnancy." The messages were either plain, printed messages or featured a Joe Camel–like cartoon character leaning nonchalantly against a sign bearing the message. All of the cartoon messages received higher ratings of importance and believability than the plain ones (cited in Azar, 1999).

Role modeling and peer influence also lead many teenagers to start smoking (Leventhal & Cleary, 1980). Athletes and celebrities who smoke create the image that smoking is linked with success, beauty, and even sexual arousal. One study reported that image, smoking among friends, relaxation, and pleasure were the reasons most often cited for smoking among 11-year-olds (Stanton, Mahalski, McGee, & Silva, 1993). Adolescents whose parents, older siblings, and friends smoke are also more likely to start smoking themselves, whether or not the parent expresses a positive attitude toward smoking (Chassin, Presson, Todd, Rose, & Sherman, 1998). In contrast, among adolescents whose parents and close friends do not smoke, smoking is rare (Moss, Allen, Giovino, & Mills, 1992).

In light of the evidence linking social influences with the initiation of smoking, the U.S. Surgeon General has concluded that situational factors are more important than personality factors in explaining why people start smoking. Nevertheless, a number of *vulnerability factors* differentiate teens who are more likely to become dependent on nicotine and other psychoactive drugs. These factors are quite diverse, vary from person to person, and even change from time to time. Smoking is especially prevalent among those who feel less competent and less in control of their future, and who perceive a lack of social support (Camp, Klesges, & Relyea, 1993). In addition, rebelliousness, a strong need for independence, and perceptions of benefits such as weight control, increased alertness, and stress management are also linked to smoking initiation.

Teenagers who smoke are twice as likely as nonsmokers to have had sexual intercourse, three times as likely to drink alcohol, and seventeen times more likely to experiment with marijuana (USDHHS, 1995). They are also more likely to feel alienated from school, to engage in antisocial behavior, to have poor physical health, and to feel depressed (Kandel & Davies, 1996).

Maintenance

Once a person has begun to smoke, a variety of psychological, behavioral, social, and biological variables contribute to making it difficult for him or her to abstain. For one, adolescents who smoke also believe that their behavior is only temporary—when asked, they often report they will no longer be smoking in

5 years and that the long-term consequences of tobacco will not affect them. For another, adolescents are oriented toward the present, so warnings of the long-term health hazards of cigarette smoking generally are not sufficient to deter smoking, especially in the face of social pressures to smoke.

Biologically, there no longer is any doubt that heavy smokers are physically dependent on nicotine. Support comes from evidence that laboratory animals will learn difficult new behaviors in order to self-administer nicotine, suggesting that the drug has powerful properties as a reinforcer. Nicotine stimulates the sympathetic nervous system and causes the release of catecholamines, serotonin, corticosteroids, and pituitary hormones (Grunberg, Faraday, & Rahman, 2001). In addition to these effects, nicotine induces relaxation in the skeletal muscles and, as noted earlier in the chapter, stimulates dopamine release in the brain's reward system (Nowak, 1994). Needless to say, this makes cigarette smoking a highly reinforcing behavior.

Genes and Smoking Evidence of a genetic component in why smokers continue to smoke comes from a large meta-analysis of twin studies, which estimated a 60 percent heritability for smoking (Heath & Madden, 1995). More recently, researchers have reported that smokers and nonsmokers differ in a gene that influences physiological responses to dopamine. Specifically, they have found a connection between smoking and the gene for a *dopamine transporter*—a protein that "vacuums up" dopamine after it has been released by a neuron. In one study, Caryn Lerman and her colleagues (1999) found that people with one form of the gene (the "9-repeat allele") were less likely to be smokers than people with other forms of the dopamine transporter gene. Other studies have linked the 9-repeat allele to increased levels of dopamine, indicating reduced efficiency at removing excess dopamine compared with those who inherit other forms of the gene. Sue Sabol and her colleagues at the National Cancer Institute have found that former smokers were more likely than current smokers to have the 9-repeat allele, indicating that this gene may boost people's ability to quit smoking.

Stress, Smoking, and the Brain's Reward System For many smokers, coping with stress is a key psychological factor in their habit. Kent Hutchinson and his colleagues at Oklahoma State University studied the relationship among endogenous opiate peptides (EOPs) (neurotransmitters that activate the brain's dopamine reward pathways), nicotine (which activates EOPs), and stress (Hutchinson, Collins, Tassey, & Rosenberg, 1996). Male smokers were randomly assigned to one of two drug conditions (EOP blocker versus placebo) and one of two stress conditions (stress versus no stress). Men in the EOP blocker condition received 50 mg of naltrexone, the opiate antagonist that prevents EOPs from activating the brain's dopamine reward pathways.

■ **nicotine-titration model** the theory that smokers who are physically dependent on nicotine regulate their smoking to maintain a steady level of the drug in their bodies

All the men were first allowed to smoke one cigarette in order to make sure they started at the same level; then they were not permitted to smoke for the first 90 minutes of each of four experimental sessions (to allow the naltrexone to be absorbed). During each session the participants worked on two computer-based slot machine programs. One paid off key presses with nickels on a variable-ratio schedule of reinforcement. The other paid off key presses in credits that could be exchanged for puffs on a cigarette.

During the experiment, participants were permitted to smoke only by earning points on the slot machine task. Participants in the stress condition were paid an extra $2.50 to perform a difficult math problem. The catch was that $0.25 was deducted for each incorrect answer.

The combination of naltrexone and the stress of the mental arithmetic increased the number of key presses for cigarette puffs. The administration of naltrexone apparently prevented the brain's EOPs from activating the brain's dopamine reward pathways. The result was that smokers worked harder to earn cigarette puffs to offset the effects of the opiate antagonist.

Results such as these suggest that long-term smokers may smoke in order to maintain a constant level of nicotine in their bloodstream. A series of studies by Stanley Schachter and his colleagues (1977) provide support for the **nicotine-titration model.** Schachter discovered that smokers smoke roughly the same amount day after day. When they are unknowingly forced to switch to lower-nicotine brands, they compensate by smoking more cigarettes, inhaling more deeply, and taking more puffs (Schachter, 1978). In addition, Schachter discovered that nicotine metabolism varies with the smoker's level of stress, providing a physiological explanation for why smokers tend to smoke more when anxious. When a smoker feels stressed, more nicotine is cleared from the body *unmetabolized,* forcing the smoker to smoke more to get his or her usual amount of nicotine.

Closely related to the idea of the nicotine-titration model, the *affect management model* proposes that smokers strive to regulate their emotional states (Tomkins, 1966). Accordingly, *positive affect smokers* are trying to increase stimulation, feel relaxed, or create some other positive emotional state. In contrast, *negative affect smokers* are trying to reduce anxiety, guilt, fear, or other negative emotional states.

In support of the affect management model, researchers have uncovered a link between nicotine use and depression, naturally leading to questions of whether one causes the other or whether some third factor contributes to both. A recent longitudinal study of high school students suggests that smoking and depression have a reciprocal effect, triggering a vicious cycle of smoking and negative mood (Windle & Windle, 2001). Every 6 months over the 18-month study, students completed questionnaires assessing depression and cigarette smoking, in addition to variables such as temperament, parents' smoking behavior, family dynamics, delinquent activity, and friends' alcohol

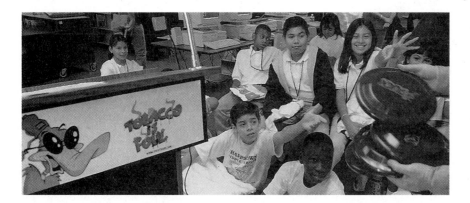

Antismoking Campaigns for Young People
Students at Sharpstown Middle School reach for frisbees after watching Texas Department of Health officials kick off a tobacco prevention advertising campaign in Houston. The campaign, featuring an animated duck and developed with the help of teenagers across the state, is being funded by money from the Texas tobacco settlement. AP/Wide World Photos

and drug use. The results showed that teens who were heavy smokers at the beginning of the study were more likely than those who smoked less to report symptoms of depression. In addition, students who had persistent symptoms of depression at the start of the study were more likely than other students to increase smoking, even when other factors were taken into consideration.

Prevention Programs

Because it is so difficult for ex-smokers to remain nicotine-free, health psychologists have focused a great deal of their energy on efforts at primary prevention of smoking. However, because several older generations began smoking before prevention became the focus, smoking cessation programs are still an important part of the health psychologist's work, as you will learn in the next section.

Some of the prevention strategies identified by health psychologists, which have been more or less effective in reaching their goal, include educational programs in schools, public health messages, bans of tobacco advertising, increasing tobacco taxes, and campaigns to ban smoking in public places. In this section, we discuss some of the major prevention strategies.

Information Campaigns

The most successful antismoking campaigns provide nonsmoking peer role models that shift people's overall image of what behaviors are acceptable and valued (Azar, 1999). Kim Worden and Brian Flynn (1999) followed more than 5,000 children in Vermont, New York, and Montana; half the children participated in a school-based antismoking intervention program and were exposed to a variety of radio and television commercials featuring nonsmoking role models, while the others only participated in the school program. Instead of focusing on the health hazards of smoking, the commercials featured teens who were enjoying life without smoking, who demonstrated how to refuse a cigarette, and who emphasized that most kids today don't smoke and don't approve of smoking. Four years later, children in the intervention group were less likely to smoke than children who participated only in the school program.

In another study, Cornelia Pechmann and Chuan-Fong Shih (1999) tested the effectiveness of 196 antismoking ads on seventh- and tenth-grade California students. Out of seven different types of antismoking ads, only three were effective in reducing the teenagers' desire to smoke. Two of the successful ads showed peers who think smokers are misguided and young people choosing not to smoke; the third ad showed how smokers endanger family members through secondhand smoke.

Antismoking Campaigns and Ethnic Minorities

Antismoking campaigns have been less effective among ethnic minorities, perhaps partly because tobacco companies have targeted a disproportionate amount of advertising toward minority communities, especially the African-American and Hispanic-American communities. African-American men have the highest smoking rates among the major racial/ethnic groups in the United States (Borum, 2000). They also have the highest rates of death due to lung cancer—six times that of European American men (see Chapter 10). African-American women, however, smoke at about the same rate as females in the general population.

Overall, Hispanic men smoke at about the same rate as non-Hispanic men, while Hispanic women smoke somewhat less than non-Hispanic women and Hispanic men (Escobedo & Remington, 1989). Acculturation partly explains these smoking patterns. Traditional Hispanic culture frowns upon smoking in women but not in men. In an unhealthy twist, the generally less rigid American gender roles have meant that smoking rates among more acculturated Hispanic-American women in the United States are higher than those among less acculturated women.

Although the U.S. government does not routinely collect comparable statistics for Asian-Americans or Native Americans, numerous local surveys of specific groups have estimated that approximately 28 percent of Native American men and 35 percent of Native American women smoke. One Hawaiian survey reported smoking rates of 25 percent for those of Filipino descent and 21 percent for those of Japanese descent, compared with 29 percent for Native Hawaiians (Chung, 1986). As with other minority groups, however, there is considerable variation across Native American subgroups. Some groups, such as Northern Plains and Alaskan Native Americans, have higher-than-average smoking rates (ranging from 42% to 70%), while others, such as Native Americans in the Southwestern United States, have much lower rates (13% to 28%). And men who recently emigrated from Southeast Asia have among the highest smoking rates of any ethnic group in the United States (Chen, 1994).

Increasing Aversive Consequences

The most successful primary prevention programs involve increasing the aversive consequences of smoking. For example, increasing the tax paid on cigarettes is quite effective. Consider the experience of Canadian smokers, whose cigarette tax has increased 700 percent since 1980. When a pack of cigarettes cost more than five dollars, many teenagers thought twice about smoking (Brown, Kane, & Ayres, 1993). According to the U.S. Centers for Disease Control, increasing the tax paid per pack of cigarettes by 10 percent reduces smoking by about 4 percent (Brown et al., 1993). The impact is the sharpest among teenagers, who have less disposable income and are in the age group most vulnerable to smoking behavior.

As another example, teens caught smoking, possessing, or buying tobacco products in Broward County, Florida, must appear in court with their parent or guardian and watch a video on the dangers of smoking. The judge also orders either a $25 fine or a day of community service picking up cigarette butts around public buildings. Underage offenders who fail to comply with the sentence may also lose their drivers' licenses. So far the tactic seems to be working. A survey of 402 offenders and their parents or guardians showed that nearly one-third of the teens reported using less tobacco than they did before their citation, and 15 percent had not used tobacco at all (Chamberlin, 2001).

Another way to increase the immediate aversive consequences is to legislate change in the workplace, such as by imposing smoking bans. Today, 81 percent of American universities prohibit smoking in public areas and 21 percent prohibit smoking in residence halls (Baillie, 2001). The success of such programs is mixed. Banning smoking from the work environment appears to be most helpful for those who have low habit strength, a desire to quit, and other social supports for their efforts (Borland, Owen, & Hocking, 1991).

Inoculation

Most effective for deterring smoking in adolescents have been "inoculation" programs that teach practical skills in resisting social pressures to smoke. Because smoking generally begins during the junior high and high school years, primary prevention programs are typically conducted in schools before children reach their teens.

The most successful inoculation programs are based on a *social learning model,* which focuses on three variables that influence teenage smoking behaviors: social pressure to begin smoking, media information, and anxiety. One successful 10-week program conducted by Gregory Botvin (1980) included both informational and skills components. In the informational component, a health expert discussed the physical effects of smoking and how to think critically about tobacco advertising. In the skills component, students practiced asserting their decision not to smoke, even when encouraged by their peers to "light up" at parties, while waiting at the bus stop, and in other situations where smoking is likely to occur. A similar peer-led program designed to build skills to counteract social pressure to smoke resulted in lower smoking incidence rates among the intervention group, both immediately and at a 2-year follow-up (Murray, Richards, Luepker, & Johnson, 1987).

Another program, designed by Richard Evans (1993), used films, role playing, and rehearsal to help the teens improve their social skills and refusal skills. In the films, same-age models were depicted encountering and resisting social pressure to smoke. The students also role-played situations, such as when someone is called "chicken" for not trying a cigarette. The students were instructed to give responses such as "I'd be a real chicken if I smoked just to impress you." After several sessions of "smoking inoculation" during the seventh and eighth grades, these students were only half as likely to start smoking as were those in a control group at another school, even though the parents of both groups had the same rate of smoking.

The U.S. Public Health Service is banking on the success of an inoculation program that brings children and parents together, teaching parents better parenting skills and children problem-solving and other skills. The families and their 10- to 14-year-old children attend separate skill-building training sessions and then meet weekly for supervised family activities such as role-playing and joint problem solving. The children's sessions focus on goal-setting, stress management, communication, responsibility, and resisting peer pressure. The parents' sessions focus on learning how to express affection, set rules, and encourage desirable behaviors. The goal is to enhance family functioning in general and specifically to give children the skills they need to reject substance abuse.

Preliminary results from a study of 33 middle schools have been encouraging. Children in the families that received the intervention waited longer to use tobacco, alcohol, and marijuana than control children. Four years into the study, the experimental group was 35 percent less likely to be smoking, 40 percent less likely to drink excessively, and 56 percent less likely to use marijuana. Even participants who did start smoking or drinking did so less frequently than control group members (Clay, 1999).

Cessation Programs

Since 1977, the American Cancer Society has sponsored the annual Great American Smokeout, in which smokers pledge to abstain from smoking for 24 hours. For many smokers, the Smokeout has been a first step in successfully quitting tobacco for good. The percentage of smokers who said they participated increased from 18 percent in 1995 to 26 percent in 1996.

It is estimated that over 3 million deaths have been prevented as a result of people either quitting smoking or not beginning in the first place.

Smoking cessation programs generally fall into two categories: those based on an addiction model and those with cognitive-behavior approaches

(Lichtenstein & Glasgow, 1997). Programs based on an addiction model of smoking emphasize the pharmacological properties and habitual behavior engendered by nicotine (Henningfield, Cohen, & Pickworth, 1993). Cognitive-behavioral models focus on motivation, conditioning, and a variety of other psychological processes designed to help smokers better understand the stimuli that trigger smoking (Lando, 1986). Intervention is aimed at helping the smoker develop coping skills to gain stimulus control over smoking triggers and to cope with anxiety, stress, and other emotions without smoking.

Addiction Model Treatments

A variety of pharmacological replacement therapy programs have been developed for smokers, including transdermal nicotine patches, nicotine gum, and inhalers. These *nicotine replacement programs* have helped millions of smokers in their efforts to quite smoking. Once available only as expensive prescription drugs, most are now available over the counter.

People who smoke continuously day in and day out are good candidates for *transdermal nicotine patches,* which have become the most common pharmacological treatment for smoking. Worn during the day, the bandagelike patches release nicotine through the skin into the bloodstream. Users are able to gradually reduce the daily dose in a series of steps that minimize withdrawal symptoms and help ensure success in remaining smoke-free (Fiore, Smith, Jorenby, & Baker, 1994; Wetter, Fiore, Baker, & Young, 1995).

However, nicotine patches are only moderately successful as a stand-alone treatment for smoking. One study reported an abstinence rate advantage of only 17 percent over a non-nicotine placebo patch after a year of follow-up (Tonnesen, Norregaard, Simonsen, & Sawe, 1991). A meta-analysis of 17 studies of the nicotine patch revealed an initial abstinence rate of 27 percent for subjects wearing an active patch, compared with 14 percent for subjects with a placebo patch. After 6 months, the active patch resulted in a 22 percent abstinence rate, compared with 9 percent in the placebo groups.

Like all pharmacological treatments, the effectiveness of nicotine gum varies with the strength of the smokers' dependency on nicotine and his or her particular smoking habits. Available since 1984, nicotine gum appears to be most helpful for smokers who tend to smoke many cigarettes in a short period of time—after work, say. Nicotine gum may be most effective when used as part of a comprehensive behavioral treatment program (Hall, Herning, Jones, Benowitz, & Jacob, 1984). Some researchers believe that the relief of withdrawal symptoms and cravings is largely a placebo effect rather than a pharmacological effect of the actual nicotine in the gum (Gottlieb, Killen, Marlatt, & Taylor, 1987). Still, it is estimated that nicotine gum produces only half the abstinence rate of transdermal patches (Hughes, 1993).

The most recent intervention is the nasal inhaler, a plastic tube filled with 10 mg of nicotine that smokers can "puff" on 2 to 10 times a day. A double-blind, placebo-controlled clinical trial of the nicotine inhaler allowed

■ **satiation** a form of aversion therapy in which a smoker is forced to increase his or her smoking until an unpleasant state of "fullness" is reached

participants to use the inhaler for 3 months, followed by 3 months in which subjects reduced the number of uses by 25 percent. A 1-year follow-up showed that 15 percent of the inhaler group continued to refrain from smoking, compared with 5 percent in the control group.

Recognizing the possible biochemical common ground of nicotine and alcohol addiction, researchers are experimenting with new medications for treating addiction. *Isradipine,* a drug that has proved helpful in controlling alcohol cravings, also appears to affect dopamine levels in the brain. Similarly, *bupropion* (Zyban), a powerful antidepressant, may curb nicotine cravings by mimicking tobacco's ability to increase brain levels of dopamine (Leutwyler, 1995). Like many other pharmacological discoveries, Zyban's efficacy in treating nicotine addiction was discovered by accident. Researchers knew that depression was a common symptom of nicotine withdrawal, and so began experimenting with antidepressants to alleviate addiction rather than depression.

Cognitive-Behavioral Treatments for Smoking

Given the importance of modeling, reinforcement, and principles of learning in the development of drug abuse, it makes sense that health experts rely on a number of cognitive and behavioral techniques to help people quit smoking. As with its use in treating alcohol dependence, *aversion therapy* involves pairing unpleasant consequences with smoking in order to condition an aversion to smoking. In one of the most frequently used techniques, smokers increase their usual smoking rate until the point of **satiation,** an unpleasant state of "fullness." One variation involves *rapid smoking,* in which a smoker periodically is asked to smoke a cigarette as fast as he or she can. Rapid smoking and satiation are both designed to associate nausea with smoking. Aversion strategies have also used electric shock and nausea-inducing drugs. For many smokers, aversion therapy is an effective way to begin to quit (Kamarck & Lichtenstein, 1985).

Smoking Cessation Programs for Ethnic Minorities and by Gender

Health organizations are beginning to realize that no single approach to smoking cessation is likely to work with all smokers. Interventions need to be targeted to specific groups, especially in order to take into account cultural traditions, values, and gender. For instance, women have more difficulty quitting smoking than men, and nicotine replacement therapy is less effective in women than in men, possibly because women may be more responsive to non-nicotine stimuli associated with smoking (see Byline Health). There is also evidence that Hispanic-American smokers appear to be more perceptive of social cues than are smokers from other groups (Nevid, 1996). This includes the positive connection between smoking and socializing with friends, as well as the

Men Cite Nicotine, Women Say Social Intangibles Are behind Urge to Smoke
Beth Azar

Nicotine clearly drives a man's desire to smoke, but it may be less of a catalyst for women, according to research by psychologist Kenneth Perkins, Ph.D.

That's not to say that nicotine isn't important for women, he says. Rather, he has found that the external pleasures of smoking, such as holding and smelling a cigarette, seem to be more important to them. In contrast, nicotine, more so than external factors, seems to influence men's smoking the most.

These findings may have implications for smoking-cessation programs that hope to help women. Several studies find that female smokers have a harder time quitting than men do, particularly with nicotine replacement therapies, indicating that other techniques may be needed.

"Women appear to be less sensitive to different doses of nicotine than men," says Perkins, professor of psychiatry at the University of Pittsburgh. For example, if he asks smokers to use a nasal spray with varying doses of nicotine or a placebo, women can't tell the difference—even between nicotine and no nicotine. Men, in contrast, can tell the difference even between different doses of nicotine, says Perkins.

This phenomenon, he says, may result from a general inability of women to perceive their own physiological activity, as found in several studies by psychologist James Pennebaker, Ph.D., of the University of Texas at Austin. In a laboratory environment women are less able than men to perceive physiological changes such as increased blood pressure, heart rate, or blood glucose levels, finds Pennebaker.

However, women are just as good as men if asked to observe the same physiological functions in context. For example, if women are exercising or watching a scary movie they are just as sensitive as men to heart rate fluctuations.

Women appear to be more perceptive to contextual and social cues than to internal cues, says Perkins. So, in terms of smoking, women likely pay more attention to the sight and smell of a cigarette than to the dose of nicotine they're receiving from the cigarette.

In his studies with the nicotine nasal spray, he's stripped the experience of nicotine from the context of smoking. For men, it doesn't matter as much. They feel as comfortable and relaxed in response to nicotine they sprayed into their noses as they do when they're smoking. For women, these positive effects occurred only when they smoked cigarettes, not when they used the nasal spray.

"It can't only be the nicotine that women are responding to," says Perkins. "Women to some extent are reacting positively to the way they take nicotine in through smoking."

Perkins isn't saying that women don't become dependent on nicotine, he emphasizes. Both nicotine and non-nicotine factors are related to smoking for men and women. But nicotine appears to be less important for women while non-nicotine factors are more important.

Such a finding is significant for treatment. If nicotine replacement therapy is all people are relying on, women will get short-changed, says Perkins.

Exercises

1. The results of scientific studies must, of course, be replicated before they are accepted. Can you think of another way of testing the hypothesis that men and women have different sensitivities to nicotine and social cues connected to smoking? (*Hint:* Design an experiment that doesn't use a nasal spray to deliver nicotine but instead manipulates a social or contextual cue related to smoking.)

2. Assuming that the gender differences found in these studies are reliable, how might you design a smoking cessation intervention targeted at women? At men?

Source: *American Psychological Association Monitor*, January 1999, p. 15.

negative connection between their smoking and setting a bad example for their children. It makes sense, then, that appropriate interventions in helping Hispanic-Americans quit smoking would be to teach them how to politely refuse a cigarette, and to provide antismoking messages that incorporate concerns about modeling, secondhand smoke, and other negative social consequences of smoking.

In one example of the development of a culturally sensitive smoking cessation program, Jeffrey Nevid and his colleagues (1996) organized an 8-week "Si, PUEDO" ("Yes, I Can") intervention in a predominantly Hispanic community in New York City. The intervention incorporated videotaped vignettes of Hispanic actors remaining smoke-free in a variety of social situations. In addition, deep-seated cultural values such as *machismo* (masculinity), *familiarismo* (responsibility to family), and *respeto* (respect for self and others) were used to convey antismoking messages.

Are Smoking Cessation Programs Effective?

There have been relatively few randomly controlled studies examining the effectiveness of smoking cessation programs for adolescents. The conventional wisdom seems to have been that teens are not going to quit smoking until they're older, so why bother? A recent review of 17 adolescent smoking cessation studies that included control groups indicated that, on average, about 21 percent of teenagers in such programs quit smoking (Sussman, Simon, & Stacy, 1999). Six months later, however, this figure dropped to 13 percent. For comparison purposes, about 11 percent of people who attempt to quit smoking on their own, without an intervention, are able to do so (Carpenter, 2001). The programs that were most effective were those that:

- enhanced teen's intrinsic and extrinsic motivation to quit through the use of rewards and education targeted at reducing their ambivalence about quitting.
- were tailored to adolescents' developmental needs (rather than those that make superficial changes to adult programs) and made intervention programs fun.
- provided social supports to help teens persevere and avoid relapse.
- showed teens how to make use of community resources for remaining nicotine-free.

Research studies involving adult smokers have found that smoking treatment programs are most useful when two or more methods are used together. For example, treatment programs that combine behavioral methods with nicotine replacement are more effective than either approach used alone (Cinciripini, Wallfisch, Hague, & Van Vunakis, 1996; Levesque, Prochaska, & Prochaska, 1999).

Whichever combination of techniques is used, Edward Lichtenstein and Russell Glasgow (1997) of the Oregon Research Institute argue that quitting smoking is determined by three individual factors: motivation to quit (including persistence despite withdrawal symptoms and stress), level of physical dependence on nicotine, and barriers to or supports in remaining smoke-free. As depicted in Figure 8.7, the three factors interact. The extent of a smoker's physical dependence, for example, will certainly influence both readiness to quit and persistence motivation. The presence of a smoking spouse, workplace smoking bans, a child pressuring a parent to quit, and other barriers and supports may also influence motivation.

James Prochaska (1996b) suggests that many smoking cessation programs dilute their effectiveness by targeting multiple behaviors and failing to recognize that different smokers have different needs. Prochaska proposes, instead, that planned interventions be organized according to each smoker's stage of quitting. His transtheoretical model outlines six stages of behavior change: precontemplation, contemplation, preparation, action, maintenance, and termination. Smokers in the precontemplation stage, for example, are often defensive and resistant to action-oriented programs. They often are demoralized by previous failures to quit smoking and consequently are put off by information campaigns condemning their unhealthy behavior. Historically, health experts considered such people as unmotivated or not ready for therapy. Prochaska, however, would suggest that treatment for people at this stage include reassurance that becoming a nonsmoker—like becoming a smoker in the first place—is not something that happens overnight. Rather, there are stages in its development, and many smokers who attempt to quit are not successful the first time.

Figure 8.7

Factors in Smoking Cessation

According to this model, readiness motivation is the primary, proximal causal factor in determining whether a person makes a serious attempt to quit. Social and environmental supports or prompts, such as a workplace no-smoking policy, increases in the price of tobacco, persistent reminders from one's child to stop smoking, or a physician's advice can also affect readiness motivation.

Source: "A Pragmatic Framework for Smoking Cessation," by E. Lichtenstein and R. E. Glasgow, *Psychology of Addictive Behaviors,* 1997, *11*(2), pp. 142–151 (Figure 1).

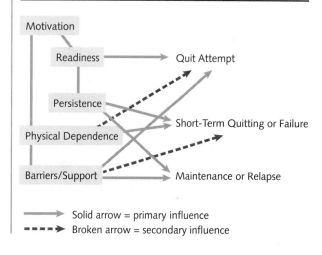

The stage approach appears to have three advantages over traditional, nonstage interventions. First, it generates a much higher rate of participation. When free smoking clinics are provided by health maintenance organizations (HMOs), only about 1 percent of subscribers participate. In two home-based interventions involving 5,000 smokers each, Prochaska and his colleagues recruited smokers to stage-matched interventions. Using this approach, the researchers generated remarkably high participation rates of 82 to 85 percent (Prochaska, Velicer, Fava, & Laforge, 1995).

A second strength of stage-based interventions is a dramatic improvement in the number of participants who complete the treatment (the retention rate of participants). A meta-analysis of 125 nonstage smoking cessation programs revealed an average retention rate of only about 50 percent (Wierzbicki & Pekarik, 1993). Remarkably, Prochaska and his colleagues have reported nearly 100 percent retention rates when treatment is individualized according to a stage approach.

Figure 8.8

**Percentage of Abstinent Former Smokers, by
Stage of Quitting**
The amount of progress former smokers make in remaining abstinent is directly related to the stage they were in at the start
of the intervention. Smokers in the precontemplation phase
display the smallest amount of abstinence from smoking over
18 months, whereas those in the preparation stage show the
most progress in 6-, 12-, and 18-month follow-ups.

Source: "Revolution in Health Promotion: Smoking Cessation as a Case
Study," by J. O. Prochaska, 1996, in R. J. Resnick and R. H. Rozensky (Eds.),
*Health Psychology through the Life Span: Practice and Research Opportuni-
ties* (pp. 361–375), Washington, DC: American Psychological Association.

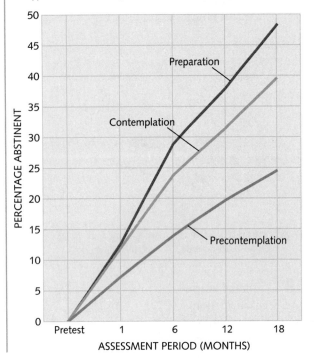

The third advantage is the most important: The
amount of progress participants make in remaining smoke-free is directly related to the stage they
were in at the start of the interventions. This *stage effect* is illustrated in Figure 8.8, which shows that
smokers in the precontemplation phase display the
smallest amount of abstinence from smoking over
18 months, whereas those in the preparation stage
show the most progress in 6-, 12-, and 18-month
follow-ups. As discussed in Chapter 2, stage-based
interventions proceed in a gradual series of steps,
with the reasonable goal of helping smokers advance
one stage at a time.

Relapse: Back to the Habit

Unfortunately, only a small percentage of people
who quit remain smoke-free for very long. Although
70 percent of adult smokers claim they want to quit,
fewer than 1 in 10 is able to do so, and as many as 80
percent of smokers who quit smoking relapse within
1 year (Leutwyler, 1997).

Many factors are involved in relapse, the most
fundamental being the severity of withdrawal symptoms and craving (Killen, Fortmann, Kraemer, &
Varady, 1992). Ex-smokers also may experience extremely unpleasant side effects, which are immediately eliminated by a return to smoking. For example, some ex-smokers gain weight (perhaps because
of slower metabolism, increased preference for
sweet-tasting foods, or substituting quantities of
food for cigarettes), have difficulty sleeping, are more
irritable, and find it difficult to concentrate (Grunberg, 1986).

Another factor in relapse is the strength of previously conditioned associations to smoking (Killen et al., 1992). Smoking behaviors, as well as nicotine's
physiological effects, become conditioned to a variety of environmental stimuli.
Many ex-smokers relapse in the face of an irresistible urge (conditioned response) to smoke in certain situations or environments—for example, with that
first cup of coffee in the morning or after a meal.

Because of this dismal prognosis for ex-smokers, smoking relapse has received considerable research attention in recent years. A working conference
sponsored by the National Institutes of Health (NIH) took a first step in ad-
dressing the relapse problem by encouraging health experts to adopt a "stages

of change" model in developing programs to prevent relapse. For example, rather than encouraging ex-smokers to attend an occasional follow-up session reminding them of the hazards of smoking, the NIH group encouraged training in relapse-prevention strategies much earlier in the stages of quitting.

Summing Up

Substance Use and Abuse

1. Millions of Americans use illicit drugs, alcohol, and cigarettes every day. The combined health hazards and costs of drug use and abuse are incalculable. During pregnancy many drugs will cross the placenta and act as teratogens to adversely affect fetal development.

2. Drugs affect behavior by influencing the activity of neurons at their synapses. Some (agonists) do so by mimicking natural neurotransmitters, others (antagonists) by blocking their action, and still others do so by enhancing or inhibiting the reuptake of neurotransmitters in the synapse.

3. Drug addiction is a pattern of behavior characterized by physical and psychological dependence, the development of tolerance, and the presence of an abstinence or withdrawal syndrome when the drug is not available.

4. Psychoactive drugs act on the central nervous system to alter emotional and cognitive functioning. Stimulants such as caffeine and cocaine increase activity in the central nervous system and produce feelings of euphoria. Depressants such as alcohol and opiates reduce activity in the central nervous system and produce feelings of relaxation. Hallucinogenic drugs such as marijuana and LSD alter perception and distort reality.

Models of Addiction

5. Biomedical models propose that physical dependence is a chronic disease that produces abnormal physical functioning. One aspect of these models is based on evidence that some people inherit a biological vulnerability toward dependence on certain drugs. The withdrawal-relief hypothesis suggests that drugs deplete dopamine and other key neurotransmitters. Another model proposes that psychoactive drugs are habit-forming because they overstimulate the brain's dopamine reward system.

6. Reward models suggest that the pleasurable effects of psychoactive drugs provide the initial motivation for repeated use. All major drugs of abuse, including nicotine and the other stimulants, overstimulate the brain's reward system.

7. Shortcomings in the biomedical and reward models of addiction were the impetus for social learning models, which view addiction as shaped by learning and by other social and cognitive factors.

Alcohol Use and Abuse

8. Alcohol depresses activity in the nervous system, clouds judgment, and is linked to a variety of diseases. Alcohol is also involved in half of all traffic accidents. Genes play a role in alcohol dependence, especially in men. The sons of alcohol-dependent parents are more likely to tolerate alcohol and develop problem drinking themselves. Psychosocial factors such as peer pressure, a difficult home environment, and tension-reduction may contribute to problem drinking.

9. Individuals marked by behavioral undercontrol and negative emotionality are especially prone to alcohol dependence. As is true of all psychoactive drugs, alcohol's impact depends in part on the user's personality, mood, past experiences with the drug, and expectations regarding its effects. Alcohol abuse is continued drinking that becomes linked with health problems and impaired functioning. Alcohol dependence is an abnormal state of physical dependence characterized by loss of control over drinking behavior. Alcohol dependence is generally accompanied by tolerance.

10. Alcohol treatment usually begins with detoxification from alcohol under medical supervision. Counseling, psychotherapy, and support groups such as AA also may help. Pharmacological treatments for alcohol dependence include aversion therapy, which triggers nausea if

alcohol is consumed. Antidepressants such as Prozac may help reduce alcohol cravings.

Tobacco Use and Abuse

11. Cigarette smoking is the single most preventable cause of death in the Western world today. A stimulant that affects virtually every physical system in the body, nicotine induces powerful physical dependence and a withdrawal syndrome. Social pressures most often influence the initiation of smoking.

12. Most people start smoking in their teenage years. Once a person begins smoking, a variety of psychological, behavioral, social, and biological variables contribute to make it difficult to abstain from nicotine. Researchers have reported a connection between smoking and the gene for a dopamine transporter—a protein that "vacuums up" dopamine after it has been released by a neuron.

13. According to the nicotine-titration model, long-term smokers may smoke in order to maintain a constant level of nicotine in their bodies. Smoking prevention programs that focus on refusal skills and other inoculation techniques prior to the eighth grade may be the best solution to the public health problems associated with smoking.

14. The most successful antismoking advertisements provide culturally sensitive nonsmoking peer role models that shift people's overall image of what behaviors are "normal" and valuable within one's peer group.

15. No single treatment has proved most effective in helping smokers quit smoking. Most programs have an extremely high relapse rate. Modern treatments for smoking deal with psychological factors through relapse prevention and physiological factors through nicotine replacement.

Key Terms and Concepts

drug abuse, p. 314
drug use, p. 314
blood-brain barrier, p. 315
teratogens, p. 316
agonist, p. 317
antagonist, p. 318
drug addiction, p. 318
physical dependence, p. 318
withdrawal, p. 318
drug tolerance, p. 319

psychological dependence, p. 319
psychoactive drugs, p. 319
drug potentiation, p. 321
concordance rate, p. 322
gateway drug, p. 324
blood alcohol level (BAL), p. 326
Korsakoff's syndrome, p. 329
fetal alcohol syndrome (FAS), p. 330
behavioral disinhibition, p. 331
alcohol dependence, p. 333

delirium tremens, p. 333
alcohol abuse, p. 333
behavioral undercontrol, p. 336
negative emotionality, p. 336
tension-reduction hypothesis, p. 336
alcohol expectancies, p. 338
aversion therapy, p. 339
nicotine-titration model, p. 350
satiation, p. 356

Health Psychology on the World Wide Web

Web Address	Description
http://www.monitoringthefuture.org/	The University of Michigan's ongoing study of the behaviors, attitudes, and values of American secondary school students, college students, and young adults.
http://www.health.org/	The National Center for Substance Abuse Prevention.
http://www.tobaccofreekids.org	The National Center for the Tobacco-Free Campaign.
http://www.niaaa.nih.gov	The National Institute on Alcohol Abuse and Alcoholism.
http://www.pitt.edu/~ejb4/min	The Minority Health Network (MHNet), an excellent information source for individuals interested in the health of ethnic minorities.

Critical Thinking Exercise

Alcohol Consumption and Aggression

Now that you have completed Chapter 8, take your learning a step further by testing your critical thinking skills on this scientific reasoning exercise.

Psychologists have long recognized a two-way association between alcohol consumption and violent or aggressive behavior. Not only may drinking alcohol promote increased aggressiveness, but being the victim of aggression may lead to excessive alcohol consumption. What might account for this two-way relationship? Could it be biologically, psychologically, or socially based? Although psychologists do not yet have all the answers, new research is providing important insights into this problem. This exercise examines the topic of alcohol consumption and aggression. The first set of questions requires you to think critically and independently about this topic. Answer the following questions on your own.

1. Is it possible that alcohol might encourage aggression or violence by exerting a direct effect on the body, for example, by weakening brain mechanisms that normally restrain impulsive behaviors such as aggression? As a researcher, how could you test this hypothesis in an ethical, socially acceptable manner?

2. Some scientists believe that alcohol may promote aggressive behavior in some people by impairing information processing, causing, for example, a narrowing of attention, or misjudgment of social cues. As a researcher, how might you test this hypothesis?

3. A third hypothesis is that alcohol consumption might promote aggression because people expect it to. As a researcher, how might you test the impact of social and cultural expectancies on aggression?

Now go to the following Web site to complete this exercise: http://www.niaaa.nih.gov

4. Compare your answers to questions 1, 2, and 3 to the information provided by the National Institute on Alcohol Abuse and Alcoholism. What actual research evidence supports the direct-effects hypothesis? The information-processing hypothesis? The social and cultural expectancies hypothesis?

4

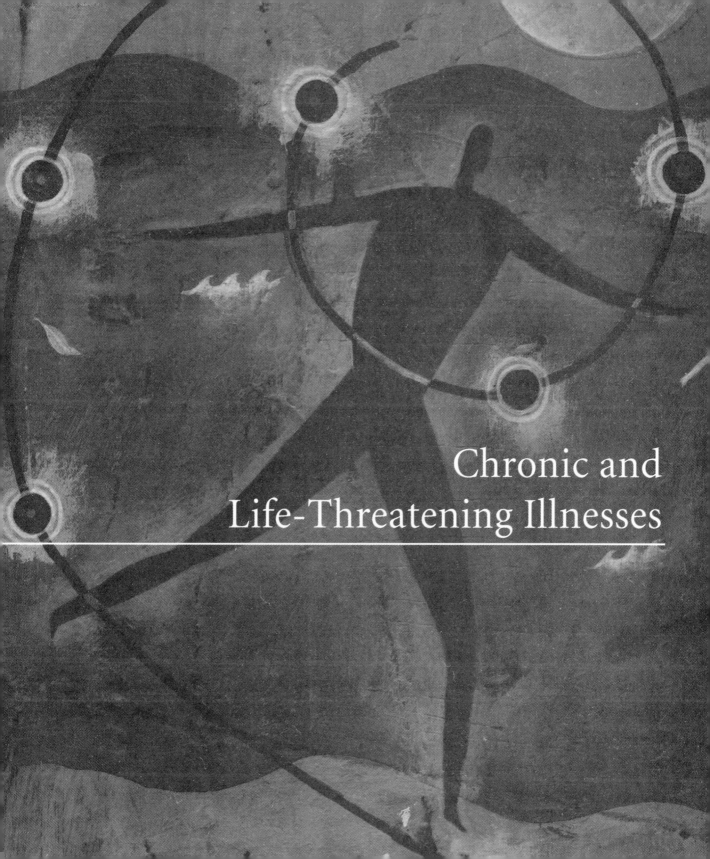

Chronic and
Life-Threatening Illnesses

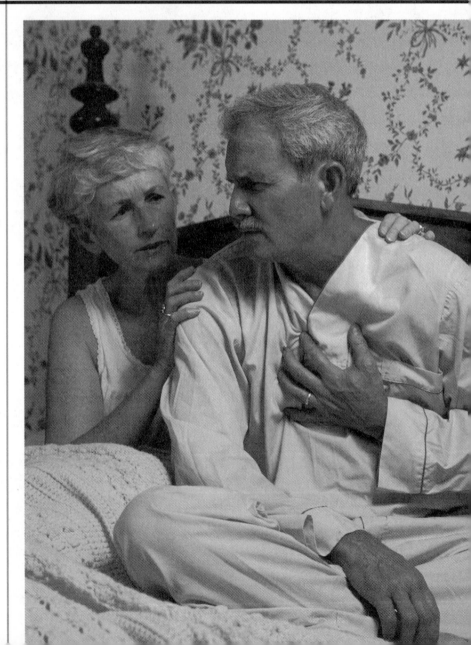

9

Cardiovascular Disease and Diabetes

On the evening of April 10, 1997, Bryan McIver, M.D.—a dedicated young endocrinologist at the Mayo Clinic—was driving to his laboratory to check on an experiment he had been conducting. He thought nothing of the mild case of indigestion he'd been feeling since having dinner with some friends. The dinner was curry, and mild stomach acidity was something he often experienced, so it seemed like a normal night.

When he arrived at the hospital at 11:42 P.M., he again felt some discomfort in his chest, but he ignored it. Walking past the emergency room 3 minutes later, things changed dramatically, and in his words ". . . the world went blank . . . and I died."

What happened was a sudden and complete blockage of one of his heart's main coronary blood vessels. Within seconds, Dr. McIver's heart floundered into the chaos of ventricular fibrillation. In this state, the rhythmic muscular contractions of the heart fall out of sync and blood is no longer pumped to the body. Almost immediately, his blood pressure dropped to zero, the oxygen supply to his brain was cut off, and he passed into unconsciousness.

When the brain doesn't have oxygen, it begins to die within about 3 minutes. After 6 minutes, brain death occurs, and there is almost no chance for recovery. This would almost certainly have happened to Dr. McIver had his heart attack happened a minute earlier as he strolled through the darkened parking lot or a minute later once he'd reached the seclusion of his laboratory. Miraculously, his collapse occurred in the hospital corridor, just a few feet from the emergency room.

Dr. McIver hardly fit the typical profile of a cardiac patient. He was a 37-year-old nonsmoker with no history of high blood pressure, vascular disease, or diabetes. Although one grandmother had died of a stroke (in her 80s), his family is generally long lived.

To be sure, McIver had some risk factors. For one, he was born and raised in Scotland, a country that has one of the highest rates of cardiovascular disease in the Western world. For another, he rarely exercised and had a high-stress job. Although he was not overweight (6-foot-1 inch, 197 pounds), his cholesterol level of 204 mg/dl was a bit above the recommended level of 200 mg/dl or lower. And his LDL cholesterol (the bad kind) of 149 mg/dl was also higher than the recommended ideal (less than 130 mg/dl). Even so, less than one month before his heart attack, Dr. McIver had been given a clean bill of health during a thorough physical exam. He was told only to try to exercise a bit more and lose a pound or two. Yet here he was, being resuscitated from the near-death experience of a massive heart attack.

Following standard procedure to normalize his cardiac rhythm, the doctor administered a series of electrical shocks to defibrillate Dr. McIver's heart back to a normal rhythm. When this failed, he injected a series of medications. Approximately 18 minutes after Dr. McIver's collapse, his heart rhythm and blood pressure returned to normal.

Although he continues his high-pressure work as a medical researcher, he's taken steps to improve his coronary risk factor profile to ensure that he lives a long, healthy life. Many others, however, are far less fortunate. This is why coronary disease remains the number one cause of death in the United States and many other developed countries.

This chapter will examine the biological, psychological, and social risk factors in two major chronic illnesses: cardiovascular disease (including high blood pressure, stroke, and heart disease) and diabetes. Although some of the risk factors in these diseases are beyond our control, many reflect lifestyle choices that are modifiable. Since each of these disorders involves the circulatory system, let's first review how the heart and circulatory system should work, then take a look at what goes wrong when each of these diseases strikes.

The Healthy Heart

As you'll recall from Chapter 3, the cardiovascular system comprises the blood, the blood vessels of the circulatory system, and the heart. About the size of a clenched fist and weighing only about 11 ounces, the heart consists of three layers of tissue: a thin outer layer, called the *epicardium;* a thin inner layer, called the *endocardium;* and a thicker middle layer, the heart muscle itself, or *myocardium* [derived from the Greek roots *myo* (muscle) and *kardia* (heart)]. The myocardium is separated into four chambers that work in coordinated fashion to bring blood into the heart and then to pump it throughout the body. Like all muscles in the body, the myocardium needs a steady supply of oxygen and nutrients to remain healthy. And the harder the heart is forced to work to meet the demands of other muscles in the body, the more nutrients and oxygen it needs.

In one of Mother Nature's greatest ironies, the heart's blood supply comes not from the 5 or more quarts of blood pumped each minute through its internal chambers of the heart but rather from two branches of the aorta (the major artery from the heart) lying on the surface of the epicardium. These left and right *coronary arteries* branch into smaller and smaller blood vessels called arterioles until they become the capillaries that supply the myocardium with the blood it needs to function. (See Chapter 3 for a diagram of the heart and the flow of blood through it.)

Cardiovascular Diseases

When the blood supply from the coronary arteries is interrupted or impeded beyond a critical point, the chance of cardiovascular disease developing increases substantially. About 60 million Americans suffer from some kind of disorder of the heart and blood vessel system, collectively referred to as **cardiovascular disease (CVD).** Leading all diseases

▓ **cardiovascular disease (CVD)** disorders of the heart and blood vessel system, including stroke and coronary heart disease (CHD)

▓ **coronary heart disease (CHD)** a chronic disease in which the arteries that supply the heart become narrowed or clogged; results from either atherosclerosis or arteriosclerosis

▓ **atherosclerosis** a chronic disease in which cholesterol and other fats are deposited on the inner walls of the coronary arteries, reducing circulation to heart tissue

in killing about 950,000 people (40 percent of all deaths) a year in the United States, cardiovascular disease appears in many guises, including stroke and **coronary heart disease (CHD),** a chronic illness in which the arteries that supply the heart become narrowed or clogged and cannot supply enough blood to the heart (National Center for Health Statistics, 2000). Before discussing the biological, social, and psychological factors that contribute to the onset of these diseases, we need to describe their underlying physical causes: atherosclerosis and arteriosclerosis.

The Causes: Atherosclerosis and Arteriosclerosis

Most cases of CVD result from a vascular (blood vessel) disease in which the smooth inner walls of the coronary arteries (*endothelium*) develop tears that don't heal properly. As blood rushes into the heart, it expands, straining the flexible coronary arteries lying on its surface. Just at the moment of peak expansion, a blast of high-pressure blood squirts through, creating even more strain. These two sources of strain almost inevitably injure the coronary arteries, leading to microscopic tears, or *lesions,* in the epithelium. When the endothelium is damaged, lipoproteins (especially LDL cholesterol) seep into the lining of the blood vessel. As is their custom, the body's scavenging *macrophages* attack and ingest the LDL. These macrophages, stuffed full of LDL, form a fatty streak over the damaged lining of the blood vessel. The resulting scar tissue becomes a "Band-Aid" on the arterial wall.

Arterial lesions generally heal without complication. However, when lesion repair continues over an extended period of years, the macrophages become so burdened with fat that they can no longer digest it. Gradually the repairs break down, more macrophages are drawn in, and the expanding scar tissue signals the presence of **atherosclerosis.** In this disease, the linings of the arteries thicken as deposits of macrophages stuffed with LDL, abnormal cells, and other cellular debris accumulate over the lesion. As this accumulation of cellular debris, called an *atherosclerotic plaque,* develops, the arterial passageways become narrowed, or *occluded,* and the flow of blood through the coronary arteries is impeded (Figure 9.1).

Figure 9.1

Atherosclerosis
Atherosclerosis is a common disease in which cholesterol and other fats are deposited on the walls of coronary arteries. As the vessel walls become thick and hardened, they narrow, reducing the circulation to areas normally supplied by the artery. Atherosclerotic plaques cause many disorders of the circulatory system. How atherosclerosis begins is not clear; possibly, injury to the artery causes scavenger macrophages to attack cholesterol deposits.

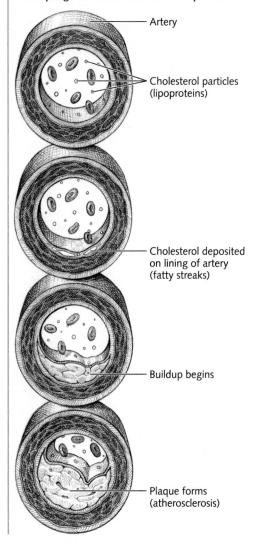

Artery

Cholesterol particles (lipoproteins)

Cholesterol deposited on lining of artery (fatty streaks)

Buildup begins

Plaque forms (atherosclerosis)

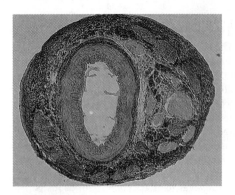

Arteriosclerosis
In arteriosclerosis, the coronary arteries lose their elasticity and are unable to expand and contract as blood flows through them. © J & L Weber/Peter Arnold

Coronary artery lesions do not necessarily lead to CVD. Indeed, such lesions have been found in children as young as 2 or 3 years of age. And by the late twenties, most people have developed coronary artery lesions, usually without symptoms. Although plaques tend to develop in most people in their thirties and forties, these plaques will not threaten their health—at least not until age 70 or older. Those not so fortunate, like Dr. McIver, may develop damaging plaques as early as their twenties or thirties—or even younger.

Closely related to atherosclerosis is **arteriosclerosis,** or "hardening of the arteries." In this condition, the coronary arteries lose their elasticity, making it difficult for them to expand and contract (imagine trying to stretch a dried-out rubber band). This makes it even harder for them to handle the large volumes of blood needed during physical exertion. In addition, a blood clot is much more likely to form in, and block, a coronary artery that has lost its elasticity due to arteriosclerosis.

The Diseases: Angina Pectoris, Myocardial Infarction, and Stroke

Left unchecked, atherosclerosis and arteriosclerosis may advance for years before a person experiences any symptoms. Such was the case with Dr. McIver. Once the process gets underway, however, any one of three diseases is likely to occur.

The first begins with a gradual narrowing of the blood vessels. Any part of the body that depends on blood flow from an obstructed artery is subject to damage. If the narrowing affects arteries in the legs, a person may experience leg pain while walking. When the arteries that supply the heart are narrowed with plaques, restricting blood flow to the heart—a condition called *ischemia*—the person may experience a sharp, crushing pain in the chest, called **angina pectoris.** Although most angina attacks usually pass within a few minutes without causing permanent damage, ischemia is a significant predictor of future coronary incidents.

Angina attacks typically occur during moments of unusual exertion, because the body demands that the heart pump more oxygenated blood than it is accustomed to handling—for example, when a casual runner tries to complete a 26-mile marathon. Angina may also occur during strong emotional arousal, exposure to extreme cold or heat, or even when sleeping. In one study, mental stress during daily life, including feelings of tension, frustration, and sadness, more than doubled the risk of ischemia in the subsequent hour (Gullette, Blumenthal, Babyak, & Jiang, 1997).

The second, much more serious cardiac disorder occurs when a plaque ruptures within a blood vessel, releasing a sticky mass that can further reduce

■ **arteriosclerosis** also called "hardening of the arteries," a disease in which blood vessels lose their elasticity

■ **angina pectoris** a condition of extreme chest pain caused by a restriction of the blood supply to the heart

blood flow or even obstruct it completely. Within seconds of the complete obstruction of a coronary artery, a heart attack, or **myocardial infarction (MI),** occurs and a portion of the myocardium begins to die (an *infarct* is an area of dead tissue). Unlike angina, which lasts only a brief time, MI involves a chronic deficiency in the blood supply and thus causes permanent damage to the heart.

The third possible manifestation of cardiovascular malfunction is a **stroke,** or cerebrovascular accident. Strokes affect 500,000 Americans annually, claiming 150,000 lives each year. They are the third leading cause of death, after myocardial infarctions and cancer. The most common type of stroke (*ischemic stroke*) occurs when plaques or a clot, an obstruction in an artery servicing that part of the brain, blocks the flow of blood to an area of the brain.

The effects of stroke may include loss of speech or difficulty understanding speech, numbness, weakness or paralysis of a limb or in the face, headaches, blurred vision, and dizziness. Strokes usually damage neural tissue on one side of the brain, with a resulting loss of sensation on the opposite side of the body. Remarkably, an estimated 11 million U.S. adults each year (4 percent of the population) have "silent strokes"—damage to tiny clusters of cells inside the brain that causes no obvious symptoms—that are never detected until, over time, memory losses, dizziness, slurred speech, and other classic stroke symptoms begin to occur.

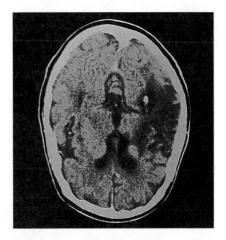

Stroke Damages the Brain
This CT scan of the brain of a 70-year-old stroke victim shows that when blood flow to the brain is blocked, cells in the brain may be destroyed. The darkened area on the right shows where brain tissue has died because of an inadequate blood supply. The lack of blood may be due to an obstruction in a cerebral artery or to the hemorrhaging of a weakened artery wall. The result is paralysis or weakness on the left side of the body (since the tissue destroyed is on the right side of the brain).
© Mehau Kulyk/Science Photo Library/Photo Researchers

Diagnosis and Treatment

Medicine has made great strides in diagnosing and treating cardiovascular disease in recent years. Although CVD was once a "silent killer" with seemingly no warning signals, health care providers now have an array of techniques for detecting its precursors, atherosclerosis and arteriosclerosis, early in their development. And while a heart attack was once an almost certain death sentence, in many cases today patients can be successfully treated with medication or with such techniques as angioplasty, bypass surgery, or even a heart transplant.

Diagnostic Tests

The most commonly used test of cardiac health is an **electrocardiogram (ECG or EKG),** in which electrodes attached to key points on the body measure the electrical discharges given off by the heart as it beats. A graphic representation of the discharges can reveal patterns of abnormal heart rhythms (*arrhythmia*), although in many cases abnormalities are not apparent unless the heart is stressed. When this is suspected, an *exercise electrocardiogram,* or stress test, may be administered while the person runs on a treadmill.

▪ **myocardial infarction (MI)** a heart attack; the permanent death of heart tissue in response to an interruption of blood supply to the myocardium

▪ **stroke** a cerebrovascular accident that results in damage to the brain due to lack of oxygen; usually caused by atherosclerosis or arteriosclerosis

▪ **electrocardiogram (ECG or EKG)** a measure of the electrical discharges that emanate from the heart

■ **coronary angiography** a diagnostic test for coronary heart disease in which dye is injected so that x-rays can reveal any obstructions in the coronary arteries

Although stress tests are more sensitive than standard EKGs, they are far from perfect—as many as 25 percent of people with coronary heart disease produce normal stress test results. If a problem is suspected, doctors may also fit patients with a portable 24-hour EKG unit that continuously records heart activity as they go about their normal activities.

Another scanning technique, the *echocardiogram,* uses the sound reflection or echo of sound waves bounced against the chest to create an image of the heart. This image can reveal damage to the myocardium, the presence of tumors or blood clots, valve disorders, and even weakened regions of arteries where blood-filled pouches called *aneurysms* have formed.

Coronary angiography is the most accurate means of diagnosing coronary heart disease. First developed in the 1940s and 1950s, angiography is now a routine procedure in cases in which a stress test has revealed possible coronary heart disease. A small cardiac catheter (a thin, flexible tube) is threaded through an artery (typically in the groin) into the aorta, and from there into a coronary artery that is suspected to be blocked with plaque. Dye is injected through the catheter so that the artery becomes visible when x-rays are taken, revealing the extent of the blockage. Patients remain awake and only partially sedated during the procedure.

Coronary Angiography
In this method of diagnosis, a small cardiac catheter is threaded through an artery into the aorta, then to the coronary artery suspected of blockage. The dye injected through the catheter enables the surgeon to x-ray the artery (upper left) and locate the blockage. © Greenlar/ The Image Works

Treatments

Depending on the severity of the problem, the coronary disease patient may be given medication to treat or prevent cardiac malfunction or may have to undergo surgery.

Cardiac Medications Several types of drugs may be used to treat CHD. These include *nitroglycerine,* which increases the blood supply to the heart and stabilizes the heart electrically; *beta-blockers* and *calcium-channel blockers,* which lower blood pressure and reduce the pumping demands placed on the heart; *vasodilators,* which expand narrowed blood vessels; and *anticoagulants,* which help prevent the formation of blood clots. If a heart attack is diagnosed within the first few hours of its occurrence, a common practice is to give an intravenous infusion of a *thrombolytic agent* to quickly dissolve any blood clots.

Medication is also used to help lower the serum cholesterol levels of people who are unable to do so by diet and exercise. However, some of these drugs pose other health hazards (such as being carcinogenic) and are prescribed only as a measure of last resort in patients with an extremely high risk of myocardial infarction (Brody, 1996a).

Cardiac Surgery If angiography reveals substantial blockage in one or more coronary arteries, several surgical treatments may be recommended. In **coronary artery bypass graft (CABG)** surgery, an incision is made in the patient's breastbone and a small piece of a vein is removed from elsewhere in the body (typically a leg but also an arm or the chest) and grafted around the region of a blocked or narrowed artery. The bypass allows blood to circumvent the blockage and flow more freely to the undernourished section of myocardium. Bypass surgery is typically recommended when blockages are severe and when the patient has not responded to other forms of treatment.

Another surgical intervention is **coronary angioplasty.** In this procedure, commonly called *angioplasty,* a catheter is threaded into a leg artery up into a blocked coronary artery, and a balloon at the tip is then inflated to "squash" the plaque against the wall of the blood vessel. The balloon is then deflated and the catheter removed. In most cases, a fine metallic mesh tube called a *stent* is inserted into the artery to reduce the likelihood that it will become narrowed again. In other cases, an *atherecotomy* is performed and blockages are surgically removed or destroyed by laser, a rotating blade, or a diamond-studded drill.

First used successfully in 1977, angioplasty helps clear obstructed arteries in 90 to 95 percent of cases. It is less costly than bypass surgery, avoids the added hazards of open-heart surgery, and is associated with a shorter recovery period. Like CABG, it relieves symptoms of ischemia and improves the quality of life for most patients. However, up to 40 percent of arteries opened by angioplasty close up again within 6 months (Comarow, 2000). To improve the odds, a promising new technique supplements angioplasty by bombarding plaque with tiny radioactive pellets that inhibit scar tissue that could result in new blockages.

Although medication and surgical procedures have been fairly successful in prolonging life in heart patients, some medical researchers are taking an entirely different approach that attempts to get around the fact that the heart, unlike other muscles, does not regenerate after it is damaged. In a recent study, researchers damaged the hearts of rabbits to mimic the scar tissue of a myocardial infarction. They then transplanted embryonic muscle cells from the rabbits' powerful leg muscles into the diseased portions of the myocardium. Compared to control animals that received no further treatment following their MI, rabbits that received transplants improved noticeably in cardiac performance (O'Neill, 1998). Still in the earliest stages of development, this experimental treatment may someday restore function to human hearts damaged by myocardial infarctions.

■ **coronary artery bypass graft (CABG)** cardiac surgery in which a small piece of a healthy vein from elsewhere in the body is grafted around a blocked coronary artery, allowing blood to flow more freely to a portion of the heart

■ **coronary angioplasty** cardiac surgery in which an inflatable catheter is used to open a blocked coronary artery

Risk Factors for Cardiovascular Disease

Despite medicine's ever-expanding arsenal of techniques for the detection and treatment of coronary heart disease and stroke, cardiovascular disease is still the leading cause of death worldwide. Although the mortality rate from CVD has decreased in the United States and other affluent countries (Figure 9.2), it has increased in Eastern Europe and the developing world (Huston, 1997). Still, more than 4,000 people in the United States suffer a heart attack every day of the year. Let's take a look at who is likely to develop CVD, and why.

The Framingham Heart Study

What causes plaque to form in the coronary arteries? Why do the coronary arteries of some people escape the buildup of scar tissue while those of others become obstructed at a young age? Research has identified a number of risk factors that are linked to CVD. Much of this knowledge comes from the Framingham Heart Study, one of the most celebrated epidemiological studies in the history of medicine. When the study began in 1948, the mortality rate due to cardiovascular disease in the United States was 146.2 cases per 100,000 people. This rate increased to a peak of 220.3 cases per 100,000 in 1963 and has dropped steadily ever since. In 1996, the most recent year reported, it reached a low of 87 cases per 100,000 (Brink, 1998). Much of the credit for this dramatic improvement in mortality rates is due to "healthy heart" initiatives that stem from the Framingham study. The results of this remarkable study have undoubtedly extended the lives of millions.

Before Framingham, epidemiologists studied disease by examining medical records and death certificates. Framingham set a new standard for epidemiological research by inaugurating the concept of studying the health of living persons over time. This landmark study used a *prospective design* that included 5,209 healthy people in the small town of Framingham, Massachusetts.

Figure 9.2

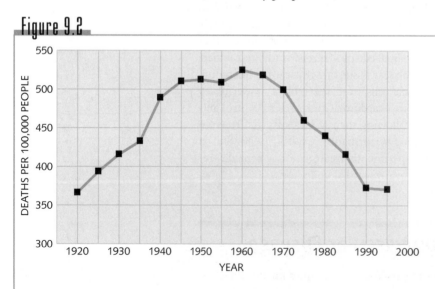

Annual U.S. Cardiovascular Disease Mortality
Although the mortality rate from CVD has decreased in the United States and other affluent countries, it has increased in Eastern Europe and the developing world. In Europe, for instance, the CVD mortality rates range between 981 and 1,841 per 100,000 people. In Southeast Asia and the Western Pacific, CVD mortality rates are as high as 3,752 and 3,527 per 100,000 people, respectively (WHO, 2000).

Sources: *Health, United States, 2000,* by National Center for Health Statistics (www.cdc.gov.net/); *The World Health Report, 2000,* by World Health Organization, 2000, Annex Table 3, pp. 164–169.

The plan of the original researchers was to follow the subjects for 20 years to see what factors—demographic, biological, and/or psychological—predicted the development of cardiovascular disease. Although more than half of the original study group has died, the study has continued with researchers now also collecting data from the children of the original participants.

Researchers chose Framingham because it was a stable community that included a mix of people of Polish, Italian, Irish, Jewish, English, Greek, and French-Canadian descent. Unfortunately, the town had few minorities in 1948, and the study is largely of white people of European ancestry. Today researchers are recruiting African-Americans, Hispanic-Americans, Native Americans, and Asians and Pacific Islanders from Framingham and nearby communities to create a more representative sample.

Every 2 years, the original participants received a complete physical exam that included an electrocardiogram (EKG), blood pressure test, and more than 80 separate medical tests (their children have exams every 4 years). In addition, each participant completed a battery of psychological tests and health questionnaires. The researchers asked questions about the participants' level of anxiety, sleeping habits, nervousness, alcohol and tobacco use, level of education, and their typical response to anger.

The Framingham study has identified two basic categories of *risk factors* for CVD: *uncontrollable risk factors* such as family history, age, and gender; and *controllable risk factors*, such as obesity, hypertension, cholesterol level, and tobacco use.

Uncontrollable Risk Factors

A number of risk factors result from genetic or biological conditions that are beyond the individual's control.

Family History and Age

Family history strongly predicts CVD. This is especially true for those who have a close male relative who suffered a heart attack before age 55 or a close female relative who had a heart attack before age 65. Advancing age is also a risk factor for CVD. Indeed, approximately one-half of all CVD victims are over the age of 65.

Gender

The risk of cardiovascular disease also rises sharply in men after age 40. Except in women who smoke cigarettes, the risk of CVD remains low until menopause, when, as we will explain, it begins to accelerate. However, the risk is still much higher among men until about age 65. In fact, men have roughly the same rate of CVD as women who are 10 to 15 years older (U. S. Bureau of the Census, 2000). The lifetime risk of death from CVD in men is 50 percent;

in women it is 30 percent. This gender difference explains in part why women live longer than men do. In all developed countries and most developing countries, women outlive men by as many as 10 years. Recall that in the United States, life expectancy at birth is currently about 79 years for women and 72 years for men.

Some experts believe that the gender difference in CVD mortality may be caused by differences in the sex hormones: testosterone and estrogen. Testosterone has been linked with aggression, competitiveness, and other behaviors that are thought to contribute to heart disease. Coincidentally, testosterone levels increase during early adulthood, just when the difference in mortality between men and women is at its peak. Some researchers therefore attribute the spike in mortality to "testosterone toxicity" (Perls & Fretts, 1998).

Testosterone also increases blood levels of LDL cholesterol and decreases HDL cholesterol, promoting an unhealthy ratio of "bad" to "good" cholesterol that places men at greater risk of coronary heart disease and stroke. Estrogen, on the other hand, lowers LDL cholesterol and increases HDL cholesterol, perhaps by regulating the activity of the liver enzymes involved in cholesterol metabolism. Estrogen also neutralizes *oxygen free radicals*—unstable cellular chemicals that have been implicated in vascular damage and aging. Estrogen levels, therefore, may protect premenopausal women against the development of CVD. The risk of CVD development changes when women become estrogen-deficient at the time of natural menopause. This explains in part why treatment with estrogen after menopause reduces a woman's risk of dying from cardiovascular disease by 50 percent or more (Massey, Hupp, Kreisberg, Alpert, & Huff, 2000).

Menstruation might also be a factor in the gender difference in CVD mortality. Because of the monthly shedding of the uterine lining, premenopausal women have approximately 20 percent less blood in their bodies than do men, with a resulting lower concentration of iron ions. Iron is essential for the formation of oxygen free radicals, and lower iron could lead to a lower rate of cardiovascular disease and other age-related diseases in which oxygen radicals play a role. Interestingly, men who frequently contribute blood tend to have lower levels of LDL cholesterol and atherosclerosis, perhaps for the same reason (Perls & Fretts, 1998).

Although women may be at lower risk for CVD than men, heart disease takes the lives of more American women than any other cause, affecting one of about every three women (as opposed to one in eight for breast cancer). Still, many women—and their doctors—believe that breast cancer is the biggest threat to their health, despite the fact that CVD takes the lives of five times as many women as breast cancer (Figure 9.3). This may explain why men who complain of chest pain are more likely to be referred for heart diagnostic tests than women and why women are less likely to receive cholesterol-lowering drugs than men, despite having similar blood levels of cholesterol (Fischman, 2000).

Figure 9.3

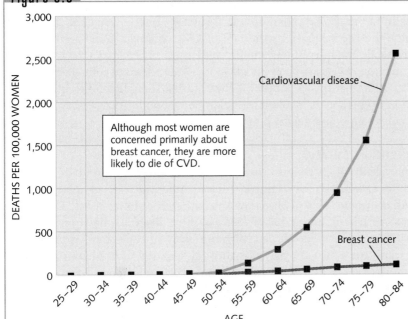

Although most women are concerned primarily about breast cancer, they are more likely to die of CVD.

Mortality Rates for Cardiovascular Disease and Breast Cancer in Women by Age

Although women may be at lower risk for CVD than men, heart disease takes the lives of more American women than any other cause, affecting one of about every three women.

Source: *Health, United States, 1997,* by National Center for Health Statistics, 1999. Washington, DC: U.S. Government Printing Office.

Men and women also differ in their prognosis for recovery following a heart attack. Compared to men, women are twice as likely to die following a heart attack. Among survivors, women are more likely to suffer a second heart attack and more likely to die after bypass surgery than men are.

Several factors may explain these differences. For one, women with cardiovascular disease tend to be older than their male counterparts. In addition, cardiovascular disease tends to be recognized sooner in men than in women, perhaps reflecting the medical bias that cardiovascular disease is more of a male problem. Until recently, women have been underrepresented in clinical studies of CVD. As a result, the gold standard in diagnosing and treating CVD is based on male physiology, and complaints of chest pain in women may not be taken as seriously by women or their doctors as such symptoms are in men.

Studies have also shown that men receive more aggressive diagnostic and treatment procedures than do women (Ayanian & Epstein, 1997). Men are twice as likely to be referred for coronary angiography and bypass surgery. As John Ayanian and Arnold Epstein have suggested, the gender difference in mortality may mean either that women are not being treated aggressively enough or that men are being treated too aggressively.

Some researchers have recently questioned whether the gender-CVD relationship is truly biological in nature. If so, then we would expect that the size of the gender gap in heart disease would be the same throughout history. However, such is not the case. Until about 1920, men had a 20 percent higher mortality from CVD (Nikiforov & Mamaev, 1998). Over the next four decades, the gap widened as the rate of CVD among middle-aged men *increased* while the rate among middle-aged women *decreased*. Today, middle-aged men are twice as likely to die from CVD as women in the same age bracket. Although this cohort effect suggests that something other than (or in addition to) biology is involved in the gender gap in heart disease, researchers have not yet pinpointed what it might be.

Race and Ethnicity

The prevalence of CVD also varies across racial and ethnic groups. Compared to white Americans, for example, African-Americans are at increased risk and Asian-Americans and Hispanic-Americans are at lower risk (CDC, 2001). African-Americans are about 75 percent more likely to die from coronary heart disease and about 60 percent more likely to suffer strokes than white Americans are. Heart disease mortality rates in 1997 for African-American women, ages 45 to 64, were twice the rate of white women of the same age, even after adjustments were made for differences in body mass index and other risk factors (National Center for Health Statistics, 1997).

Economic factors have been suggested as a possible cause of ethnic and racial differences in CVD. People of low socioeconomic status (SES) tend to have more total risk factors for cardiovascular disease, including high-fat diets, smoking, and stressful life experiences such as racial discrimination (Gillum, Mussolino, & Madans, 1998; Stunkard & Sorensen, 1993). As noted in Chapter 1, African-Americans are disproportionately represented among lower socioeconomic groups. African-Americans generally have the same risk factors for CVD as European Americans, but at a higher level that begins during childhood (Winkleby, Robinson, Sundquist, & Kraemer, 1999).

Lack of exercise may also be a factor. As a group, affluent people tend to exercise more, perhaps because they have more free time, can more easily afford exercise equipment, or may be better informed about the hazards of sedentary living. European American women, for example, are two to three times as active as African-American women during leisure time (Nevid et al., 1998).

It is natural to wonder whether ethnic and racial differences in risk of cardiovascular disease would exist if disparities in education, family income, and disease risk factors for CVD were controlled for. Investigators have found that even then, ethnic and racial groups have different morbidity and mortality rates (Krieger, Rowley, Herman, Avery, & Phillips, 1993). In one study, Marilyn Winkleby and her colleagues (1998) compared CVD risk factors among groups of African-American, Hispanic-American, and European American women. Regardless of their ethnic background, low-SES women had elevated risk factors compared to high-SES women. However, after education and family income were controlled for, African-American and Hispanic-American women still had more risk factors than European American women. These findings strongly indicate that both ethnicity and socioeconomic factors are involved in determining an individual's risk of developing CVD.

Some researchers believe that differences in psychosocial stressors are partly to blame for racial and ethnic disparities in CVD (Macera, Armstead, & Anderson, 2001). Single-parent households are a case in point. In many African-American neighborhoods, which are often segregated from the general population and of low socioeconomic status, female-headed families are the primary residential and family unit (Jargowsky, 1997). For example, a 1990 study of urban neighborhoods in which at least 40 percent of the households fell below the poverty line found that nearly 75 percent of African-American families were female headed. These women are more likely to die of coronary disease, perhaps as a result of the high levels of stress associated with raising a family without a partner (Leclere, Rogers, & Peters, 1998).

Another stressor that may produce racial and ethnic differences in CVD mortality rates involves limited access to and use of health care, as well as preferential medical treatment. As noted in Chapter 6, there are vast differences among ethnic groups in the availability of affordable health care. Furthermore, African-Americans—male or female—are less likely than white males to receive aggressive treatments such as bypass surgery and angioplasty. This double standard of care may be due to many factors, including, of course, discrimination, which causes some minority patients to mistrust health care (Peterson, 1997).

Controllable Risk Factors

Although uncontrollable risk factors cannot, by definition, be changed, they do not necessarily doom a person to death by heart attack. Knowing one's inherent risk profile is an important step in reducing the risk of CVD, however, because it allows high-risk individuals to minimize their total risk profile by changing those things they *can* control. Even with a family history of heart disease, for example, a person can control his or her blood pressure, eat a healthy diet, maintain a normal body weight, and thus reduce overall risk. Doing so can reap huge benefits. For instance, the Chicago Heart Association Detection Project evaluated the health outcomes for men between ages 18 and 39, men between 40 and 59, and women between ages 40 and 59 years. Younger men in the "low risk" category (those with the healthiest lifestyles) had a life expectancy 9.5 years longer than other men in their age group. For healthy men aged 40 to 59 years, life expectancy was extended by 6 years. For women in the "low risk" category, life was extended by 5.8 years (Stamler et al., 1999).

■ **hypertension** a sustained elevation of diastolic and systolic blood pressure (exceeding 140/90)

Hypertension

Blood pressure is the force exerted by blood as it pushes out against the walls of the arteries. When pressure is too high, it can damage the vessels and lead to atherosclerosis. Once pressure climbs past 120/80, the risk of cardiovascular disease begins to rise. But the condition is not called **hypertension** until it consistently exceeds 140/90.

Depending on the degree of elevation in blood pressure, one of several types of medication is typically prescribed. Diuretics work by decreasing the amount of fluid in the body. Beta-blockers cause the heart to beat more slowly and less forcefully, thus decreasing pressure in the arteries. Calcium channel-blockers decrease the work of the heart and relax blood vessels. Vasodilators also relax blood vessels. Some newer medications act on neural regions that control blood pressure. All these medications are effective, assuming that the right medication is given for the right problem. Also, it is not uncommon for doctors to try different medications before finding the one that works best.

Before the Framingham study, physicians believed that blood pressure increased as a natural consequence of aging. A rule of thumb had been that normal systolic blood pressure was equal to one's age plus 100. Thus, a 65-year-old was considered normal if his or her systolic pressure was as high as 165. We now know that a pressure this high more than quadruples the risk of stroke.

Although most cases of high blood pressure are classified as *primary,* or *essential, hypertension,* meaning that the exact cause is unknown, several possible causes have been suggested. At a biological level, for example, the more forceful heartbeats of a person with high blood pressure may be caused by additional fluid in the body due, perhaps, to a high salt diet or an increased stiffness of the arteries. Researchers tend to agree, though, that hypertension does not have a single cause but is the result of the interaction of biological, psychological, and social factors. Obesity, lack of exercise, dietary salt, and excessive stress can produce hypertension in biologically predisposed people. Hypertension is also related to anxiety and anger, especially in middle-aged men. In a major longitudinal study, researchers measured anxiety, anger symptoms, expression of anger, and blood pressure in middle-aged and older men. An 18- to 20-year follow-up revealed that men 45 to 59 who scored high on a standardized measure of trait anxiety were twice as likely to develop hypertension (Markovitz, Matthews, Kannel, Cobb, & D'Agostino, 1993).

One indicator that heredity may play a role in hypertension is the fact that the prevalence of hypertension varies widely among racial and ethnic groups. For instance, approximately 35 percent of African-American men have high blood pressure, compared with about 24 percent of European American men (American Heart Association, 1999). This may be due to the fact that obesity and diabetes—both of which contribute to hypertension—are also more common among African-Americans (Wing & Polley, 2001).

Although genes may create a biological predisposition to hypertension, heredity alone cannot explain the widespread variation in the prevalence of hypertension among different ethnic and cultural groups. For example, although hypertension is more prevalent among African-Americans than among European Americans, it is even more common among lower-SES African-Americans than among middle-SES African-Americans (Harburg, Erfurt, & Haunstein, 1973). A number of researchers have proposed that the greater exposure to social and environmental stressors among lower-SES African-Americans, rather than genetic differences, may result in excessive sodium retention by the kidneys (Anderson, Balon, Hoffman, Sinkey, & Mark, 1992). Sodium retention causes blood vessels to constrict, with a corresponding rise in blood pressure.

Some investigators have suggested that the higher rate of hypertension among African-Americans might reflect greater **cardiovascular reactivity (CVR)** to stress—especially the stress of racial discrimination—in the form of larger increases in heart rate and blood pressure and a greater outpouring of epinephrine, cortisol, and other stress hormones (Krieger & Sidney, 1996). Several studies have found that African-American college students react to racially provocative movie scenes and discussions of racist topics with increased blood pressure (Armstead, Lawler, Gorden, Cross, & Gibbons, 1989; McNeilly et al., 1996). Other investigators have failed to confirm reports showing a correlation between greater CVR and racism among African-Americans. In a recent study, Carolyn Fang and Hector Myers (2001) asked African-American and European American college students to view film excerpts depicting neutral, anger-provoking (but nonracist), and racist situations. The anger-provoking and racist film clips triggered greater increases in blood pressure than the neutral film clips in both African-American and European American men. However, the racist clips did not elicit greater CVR than the anger-provoking (but nonracist) clips in either group of men.

These inconsistent findings may occur because of the presence of other factors, including past experience with racial discrimination and variations in socioeconomic status. In a series of studies, Nancy Krieger and her colleagues reported that low-SES African-American men displayed greater cardiovascular reactivity to racial stressors than high-SES African-American men *or women*. The low-SES men also reported significantly greater firsthand experience with racial prejudice (Krieger & Sidney, 1996; Krieger, Sidney & Coakley, 1998). Taken together, the findings of these studies suggest that racial discrimination probably does contribute to CVD risk in many African-Americans; the degree to which it contributes depends at least in part on an individual's gender and socioeconomic status.

Obesity

Excess body weight increases a person's risk of hypertension and all cardiovascular disease, in part because of its association with high cholesterol. The risk of excess fat depends somewhat on how the fat is distributed. The so-called apple-shaped person, with excess fat in the midsection (the "beer belly"), has the greatest risk of cardiovascular disease. This may be because such people

cardiovascular reactivity (CVR) an individual's characteristic reaction to stress, including changes in heart rate, blood pressure, and hormones

■ **hypercholesterolemia** a genetic disease in which people have a chronically elevated level of cholesterol in their bloodstream

also tend to have lower levels of HDL cholesterol than pear-shaped people, who carry excess weight in the hips, buttocks, and thighs. Differences in where body fat is distributed may also help to explain why men have higher rates of CVD than women, at least until menopause. Men are much more likely than women to be "apples."

Cholesterol Level

As we explained in Chapter 7, cholesterol is a waxy substance produced by the liver and also found in animal fats, certain oils, and egg yolks, but not in vegetables or vegetable products. It is a critical component of cell membranes and is most common in the blood, brain tissue, liver, kidneys, adrenal glands, and the fatty myelin sheaths that surround nerve fibers (see Chapter 3). Cholesterol is also one of the main ingredients of atherosclerotic plaque.

Doctors have known for years that people with a genetically high level of cholesterol—a chronic disease called **hypercholesterolemia**—also have a high rate of cardiovascular disease, beginning at a young age. People with cardiovascular disease also tend to have high cholesterol levels. Before the Framingham Heart Study, however, there was no prospective evidence that excess dietary cholesterol was a coronary risk factor. The Framingham Heart Study found that people with low serum cholesterol rarely developed cardiovascular disease, whereas those with high levels had a high risk.

In another long-term study, researchers reported that cholesterol level at age 22 accurately predicted incidence of coronary heart disease, stroke, and mortality in the future (Klag et al., 1993). The study's participants were separated into groups based on their total serum cholesterol. Those with levels that placed them in the top 25 percent (209 to 315 mg/dl) were seven times more likely to develop cardiovascular disease and twice as likely to die of a heart attack as those with the lowest levels of serum cholesterol (118 to 172 mg/dl).

How High Is Too High? Today, health experts generally consider that a blood cholesterol level lower than 200 milligrams per deciliter (mg/dl) is associated with a low risk of cardiovascular disease. A level of 240 or greater doubles the risk.

Total cholesterol is only part of the story, however. As noted in Chapter 3, a more complete picture comes from comparing the relative amounts of *high-density lipoprotein (HDL), low-density lipoprotein (LDL),* and *triglycerides* (also called *very-low-density lipoprotein, or VLDL*). Even people with low levels of total cholesterol are at increased risk if these proportions are faulty.

Some studies have suggested that regular consumption of antioxidant nutrients (agents believed to promote health by reducing the buildup of cell-damaging waste products of normal metabolism), such as vitamin E, beta-carotene, selenium, and riboflavin (which are plentiful in fruits and vegetables), may also prevent cardiovascular disease. Antioxidants neutralize oxygen free radicals and prevent them from causing the oxidation of LDL cholesterol (Stampfer, Rimm, & Walsh, 1993). Oxidation would otherwise lead to injury, scarring, and the buildup of fatty plaque in the blood vessel walls. In one

Recall from Chapter 3 that low-density lipoprotein, or LDL, is the so-called bad cholesterol; high-density lipoprotein, or HDL, is the so-called good cholesterol.

longitudinal study, researchers found that men with the highest levels of antioxidants had a two-thirds lower risk of cardiovascular disease than those with the lowest levels (Morris, Kritchevsky, & Davis, 1994). However, antioxidants may be effective primarily in people who are free of coronary heart disease. In a recent randomized placebo-controlled trial of more than 9,000 women and men with a history of CHD, taking a daily vitamin E supplement did not reduce myocardial infarction or mortality any more than did a daily placebo (Hoffman, 2000).

Research also suggests that moderate alcohol consumption may lower total cholesterol and raise HDL levels. Consider the French Paradox: Mortality rates from cardiovascular disease are markedly lower in France than in other industrialized countries, despite the fact that the French people eat more rich, fatty foods; exercise less; and smoke more (Hackman, 1998). Studies suggest that the French may suffer less cardiovascular disease because of their regular consumption of red wine, which contains natural chemical compounds called *flavonoids* (see Byline Health on pages 384–386). Scientists think biologically active flavonoids lower the risk of cardiovascular disease in three ways: reducing LDL cholesterol, boosting HDL cholesterol, and slowing platelet aggregation, thereby lessening the chances of a blood clot forming (Hackman, 1998).

Despite this interesting possible relationship between moderate wine consumption and a healthy heart, the issue remains controversial. We *do* know that excessive alcohol consumption increases the risk of suffering an MI. Much additional research is needed before we can conclude that the benefits of moderate alcohol consumption outweigh the potential risks.

How Low Is Too Low? A number of studies have raised concerns about the wisdom of following a diet that is extremely low in fat and cholesterol. There is evidence that men with extremely low serum cholesterol levels have higher-than-normal rates of accidental death and suicide (Jones, Johnson, Robinson, & Ybarra, 1998) and are more likely to commit (or be the victim of) homicide (Cummings & Psaty, 1994).

How could low serum cholesterol correlate with increased rates of violent death? One possibility is that low cholesterol contributes to depression. In one study, researchers found that male psychiatric patients with a serum cholesterol level below 160 were three times more likely to suffer from clinical depression than those with higher cholesterol levels (Morgan, Palinkas, Barrett-Connor, & Wingard, 1993).

The low-cholesterol/violent death relationship continues to be debated. Some researchers believe that some other factor, such as smoking or low socioeconomic status, may be related to both low cholesterol and violent death. Or there may be some overarching pathway by which cholesterol increases aggression (Jacobs, Muldoon, & Rastam, 1995). Although no definitive explanation has been offered for the relationship between low cholesterol and increased mortality rates, many health experts are rethinking the standard recommendation to lower cholesterol at all costs.

Paradox or Not, Cholesterol in France Is on the Rise

Jane E. Brody

Americans, famous for wanting their cake and eating it too, were delighted to learn that even though French foods seem to be rich in fat, much of it artery-clogging saturated animal fat, the French are not nearly as likely to be cut down in midlife by heart attacks. This intriguing phenomenon is called the French Paradox, and it has drawn comment, criticism and speculation for much of this decade.

But the latest treatise on the subject, published in a recent issue of *The British Medical Journal*, suggests the paradox may not be so paradoxical after all. Rather, the authors maintain, it is only a matter of time before the fatty French diet exacts its coronary toll. These scientists, Malcolm Law and Nicholas Wald, specialists in preventive medicine at St. Bartholomew's and the Royal London School of Medicine and Dentistry, point out that for decades until 1970, the French ate much less animal fat and had significantly lower blood cholesterol levels than did Britons, who were in no better shape than Americans.

But as the French diet grew richer, French cholesterol levels did too.

"Only between 1970 and 1980 did French values increase to those in Britain," the authors noted, adding that since only about 1 percent of men die of heart disease before age 50, it takes decades of exposure to a high-fat diet to exact this toll.

Though the new British report is the most thorough analysis of this "time-lag hypothesis," it has been put forward before as an explanation for French diet and health. Dr. Marion Nestle, chairwoman of the department of nutrition at New York University, noted several years ago that it was not until 1985 that French consumption of fat caught up to that of Americans.

In an interview, Dr. Nestle said, "There's been a steady increase in fat consumption in France over the last 20 years as the French diet has become more Americanized." She noted that the French were now eating more meat and fast foods, snacking more, eating fewer regular relaxed meals, exercising less, and drinking less wine than in the past. And, predictably, they are getting fatter.

Wait a few more decades, Dr. Nestle predicted, and the French will no longer enjoy a coronary death rate that is less than half that of Americans.

Still, even if the French did not reach American levels of fat consumption until recently, something still seems to have been protecting their hearts. How else could they have gotten away with their apparent penchant for eggs, butter and cream, not to mention patés and rich cheeses full of saturated fat and cholesterol?

Several health experts, commenting on the report by Dr. Law and Dr. Wald, have offered possible explanations that could prove helpful to Americans seeking to lower their risk of heart disease without forgoing all the pleasures of dietary fat.

Learning from the French

Dr. Meir Stampfer and Dr. Eric Rimm of the Harvard School of Public Health stress in their commentary that coronary disease is not due to any single factor and that preventing it cannot result from only one adjustment in living habits, like eating less saturated fat. Although they do not dismiss the idea that time will take its toll on the French heart, they cite several other differences in dietary habits between the French and Britons (and, by extension, Americans) that studies strongly suggest play an important role in heart disease. For example:

Alcohol "Law and Wald may be too quick to dismiss the role of alcohol as a partial explanation," the Boston researchers wrote. Many studies have shown a strong relationship between an increased intake of alcohol and a lower level of cardiac deaths. Alcohol raises blood levels of protective HDL cholesterol, which helps rid arteries of fatty deposits. Red wine in particular, the favored beverage in France, contains chemicals that lower the risk of blood clots that could touch off a heart attack. Also important may be the pattern of alcohol consumption. In France wine is drunk slowly with meals.

"The evidence of benefit from moderate consumption of alcohol is very, very strong, and it seems to be strongest when alcohol is taken with meals on a moderate, regular basis as opposed to weekend bingeing or alcohol consumed alone," Dr. Stampfer said in an interview. Moderate consumption means a daily limit of two glasses of wine for men and one glass for women.

Fiber The French consume two to three times more fiber from whole grains and grain products than do Britons and Americans.

These cereal fibers have been linked in at least three major studies to a decreased risk of heart disease, most recently this month in a study of nearly 69,000 middle-aged nurses published in the *Journal of the American Medical Association*. Each increase of five

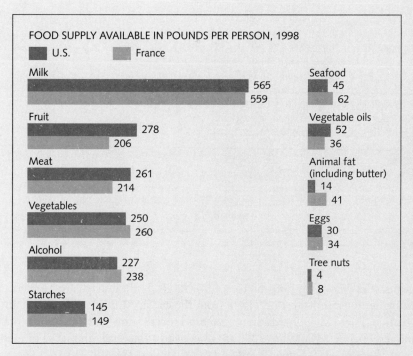

FOOD SUPPLY AVAILABLE IN POUNDS PER PERSON, 1998

■ U.S.   ■ France

Food	U.S.	France
Milk	565	559
Fruit	278	206
Meat	261	214
Vegetables	250	260
Alcohol	227	238
Starches	145	149
Seafood	45	62
Vegetable oils	52	36
Animal fat (including butter)	14	41
Eggs	30	34
Tree nuts	4	8

What exactly do the French eat and drink? Pretty much what Americans eat and drink. Although these figures represent the availability of certain foods, they can be interpreted to indicate people's food preferences. Clearly, the present diets of France and the United States reveal more similarities than differences.

grams a day of cereal fiber (the amount in a half-cup of bran-flake cereal) was associated with a 37 percent decrease in coronary risk among these women. Similar associations were found in the Iowa Women's Study and in men in the Health Professionals Follow-Up Study.

Nuts The French eat about twice as many nuts as Americans do. Several studies that followed tens of thousands of men and women in this country showed that "even modest amounts of nuts were associated with a markedly lower risk of coronary heart disease, a benefit greater than would be predicted from their effects on serum cholesterol," Dr. Stampfer said. The fat in nuts is the unsaturated kind that lowers the level of harmful LDL cholesterol. "Ironically, many health-conscious Americans have been avoiding nuts because they are high in fat," he noted. Over all, for the last 30 years, the French intake of heart-sparing polyunsaturated fat has been nearly twice that in Britain, Dr. Stampfer and Dr. Rimm noted.

Folate When Americans visit France or dine in fancy French restaurants in this country, they tend to eat rich, fancy foods. "But the French people don't eat fancy foods day to day," Dr. Stampfer said. "They eat many more fruits and vegetables," including those that are rich in a B-vitamin called folate (or folic acid), which has been associated with a decreased risk of heart disease. Good sources of folate include dark green leafy vegetables and orange juice.

Glycemic Load Frequent consumption of foods that quickly raise the level of sugar in the blood has been linked to an increased risk of developing heart disease and diabetes. When blood sugar rises, insulin is released to process it, which stimulates the production of a harmful form of triglycerides, a known coronary risk factor. In general, whole foods and minimally processed grains (including pasta, which is made from crushed as opposed to finely ground semolina wheat) produce a low glycemic load, while sweets, pastries, white bread and potatoes produce a high glycemic load. Americans who snack on sweets and refined carbohydrates raise their glycemic load and, in turn, their risk of heart disease.

Cheese and Foie Gras Dr. Serge Renaud, research director at France's National Institute of Health and Medical Research, maintains that there is something different about the fats in duck and goose liver and in cheese that makes them less damaging and possibly even protective of the heart. His evidence in part comes from the heart of foie gras country, the Gascony region of southwest France, where the coronary death rate among middle-aged men is about half that of the rest of France. He has said that "goose and duck fat is closer in chemical composition to olive oil than it is to butter and lard." What, if anything, may be special about the fats in cheese is now under study.

Portion Size Rich foods or not, the French simply eat less than Americans do. French portion sizes tend to be a third to a half of American portions, and until recently, the French sat down to eat leisurely meals three times a day and rarely ate between meals, Dr. Nestle said. French visitors to America are typically aghast at the amount of food piled on plates in American restaurants and homes. The French are more gourmets than gluttons, as evidenced by the difference in obesity rates: 30 percent here versus 8 percent there.

Despite their dietary advantages, the French still get heart disease. Dr. Dean Ornish, cardiac specialist at the University of California at San Francisco, has pointed out that while "heart attacks are less frequent in France, they are still the leading cause of death there."

And as Dr. Nestle noted, French habits are changing, and not for the better. Children are now given soft drinks, not wine, to drink; wine consumption over all has dropped to about half of former levels; snacking is now commonplace, more and more family meals are coming from pizza parlors and McDonald's and more people are driving to big markets to shop instead of walking to local groceries.

As she and others have said, it is only a matter of time.

Source: *New York Times,* Personal Health (June 22, 1999).

Exercises

1. What is the "French Paradox"? How might the "time-lag hypothesis" explain this paradox?

2. What other dietary habits may help protect the French against CVD?

3. With the increasing Americanization of French food habits, would you expect their rate of CVD eventually to parallel that of the United States?

Thus, it appears that both high and low levels of cholesterol are associated with higher overall death rates. Data from the classic Multiple Risk Factor Intervention Trial (MRFIT) study reported a mortality rate for men with total cholesterol below 140 or above 300 as being nearly twice as high as that of men with cholesterol levels between 180 and 220 (Stamler et al., 1999).

Tobacco Use

We now know that smoking more than doubles the chances of having a heart attack and is linked to one of every five deaths due to coronary heart disease. Smokers have twice the risk of having a stroke and are less likely to survive an MI than are nonsmokers.

On the positive side, within 2 years after a person has quit smoking, the elevated risk of CVD associated with smoking decreases to almost the level of those who have never smoked (American Heart Association, 1999).

Psychosocial Factors in Cardiovascular Disease

Puzzled by the fact that many of their patients were *not* obese, middle-aged men with elevated cholesterol, cardiologists decided that they must be overlooking something. So they broadened their search for risk factors that might help explain the discrepancy. This section will focus on three of their findings: Type A behavior, hostility, and stress and social support.

The Type A Personality

Cardiologists have long suspected that certain personality traits are linked to cardiovascular disease, and in the late 1950s, cardiologists Meyer Friedman and Ray Rosenman began to study personality traits that might predict coronary events (Friedman & Rosenman, 1959). They found a coronary-prone behavior pattern that included competitiveness, a strong sense of time urgency, and hostility, which they labeled **Type A.** In contrast, people who are more relaxed and who are not overly pressured by time considerations tend to be coronary disease-resistant. This they called **Type B** behavior.

In the 1960s and 1970s, literally hundreds of epidemiological studies supported the association between Type A behavior and risk of future CVD in both men and women. Most impressive was the Western Collaborative Group study. At the start of the experiment, the men, ranging in age from 39 to 59 years, were free of cardiovascular disease. By the end of the $8\frac{1}{2}$-year prospective study, those who had been labeled Type A were more than twice as likely as Type B men to have developed cardiovascular disease (Rosenman et al., 1975). Soon after, data from the Framingham Heart Study depicted a similar relationship for women (Haynes, Feinleib, & Kannel, 1980). Studies such as these led a review committee of the National Heart, Lung, and Blood Institute to conclude that Type A behavior was an independent risk factor for CVD.

In an effort to explain this relationship, researchers have focused on physiological differences between Type A and Type B people. Among their findings: Type A people have more rapid blood clotting and higher cholesterol and triglyceride levels under stress than their Type B counterparts (Lovallo & Pishkin, 1980). Type A people also often display greater autonomic arousal (see Chapter 3), elevated heart rate, and higher blood pressure in response to challenging events (Jorgensen, Johnson, Kolodziej, & Schreer, 1996). In relaxed situations, both types are equally aroused. When challenged or threatened, however, Type A people are less able to remain calm. This pattern of "combat ready" hyperreactivity is most likely to occur in situations in which Type A persons are subjected to some form of feedback evaluation of their performance (Lyness, 1993).

Recently, a secondary cluster of traits combining depression with high levels of anxiety—both of which are independently linked to CVD—has been observed in Type A individuals (Frasure-Smith, Lesperance, & Talajic, 1995). Depression appears to be particularly lethal, as shown by a 12-year Centers for Disease Control study (Anda et al., 1993). Depressed people were more vulnerable to CVD, even after the researchers controlled for differences in age, gender, smoking, and other CVD risk factors. Moreover, depressed people have four times the risk of recurrence of a heart attack compared to MI survivors with no depressive symptoms (Frasure-Smith, Lesperance, Juneau, Talajic, & Bourassa, 1999).

Type A Friedman and Rosenman's term for competitive, hurried, hostile people who may be at increased risk for developing cardiovascular disease

Type B Friedman and Rosenman's term for more relaxed people who are not pressured by time considerations and thus tend to be coronary-disease resistant

Figure 9.4

Type A Behavior and Hostility

When provoked, Type A students retaliated against their instigators by choosing higher shock intensities. Type B students were less likely to show this tendency to retaliate. Note that the numbers representing shock intensity are arbitrary numbers; the students read their own meaning into each level of intensity.

Source: "Coronary-Prone Behavior Pattern and Interpersonal Aggression," by C. S. Carver and D. C. Glass, 1978, *Journal of Personality and Social Psychology,* 36, pp. 361–366.

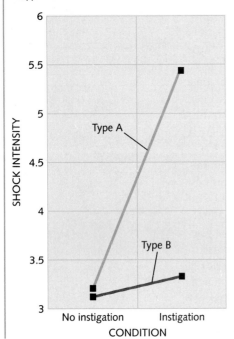

Narrowing It Down: Hostility and Anger

Believing that the Type A syndrome was too global, researchers began to analyze the three component behaviors (hurriedness, competitiveness, and hostility) to determine whether one or more of these components might more accurately predict cardiovascular disease. They already suspected that competitiveness and time efficiency were not nearly as dangerous as hostility.

In a classic study, Charles Carver and David Glass (1978) attempted to learn whether Type As and Type Bs responded differently to anger-provoking situations or interruptions in their efforts to reach a goal. A Type A or a Type B student was placed in a room with an actor hired by the experimenters. In the first part of the experiment, the actor and the student were asked to solve a difficult wooden puzzle in a short period of time. In the *instigation condition,* the actor disrupted the student's attempts at the puzzle and made insulting comments about his or her performance (for example, "I don't know what's taking you so long; it's not that difficult!"). In the *no instigation* condition, the actor did not interact at all with the student.

In the second phase of the study, the student was required to "teach" the actor a concept by delivering an electric shock whenever the actor made an incorrect response (no actual shocks were delivered). The student was free to choose which of 10 shock intensities would be delivered each time the actor made an error.

Figure 9.4 presents the results of this experiment. In the instigation condition, Type A students chose significantly higher shock intensities than did Type B students. However, in the no instigation condition, both types administered about the same level of shock. These results suggest that when provoked or prevented from reaching a goal, Type As have a more hostile reaction than do Type Bs.

In another study, Neil Grunberg, Stacey Street, Jerry Singer, and I (Straub, Grunberg, Street, & Singer, 1990) asked Type A and Type B students to play a competitive board game over the telephone, allegedly against another student, whose actual game moves were carefully scripted by the experimenter. Type A students played the game much more aggressively than did their Type B counterparts, doing everything they could to prevent their opponents from winnning or even temporarily gaining an advantage in the game. They did so even when their hostile "blocking" actions caused them to lose money.

Hostility

Results such as these have led researchers to focus more closely on hostility as the possible "toxic core" of Type A behavior. Hostility has been characterized as a chronic negative outlook that encompasses feelings (anger), thoughts (cynicism and mistrust of others), and overt actions (aggression). As such, it is considered an attitude that is generally longer in duration than specific emotions that trigger short-lived strong physical arousal. With hostility, as with other attitudes, it's not so much *what* is said as *how* it is said (Kop & Krantz, 1997). Erika Rosenberg and her colleagues (1998), for example, showed that the facial expression for contempt was significantly related to hostility and defensiveness (defined as the tendency to deny the existence of undesirable traits in oneself).

Redford Williams and his colleagues at Duke University administered a questionnaire and interview assessment called the Cook-Medley Hostility Scale (Ho Scale) to a large group of coronary patients. They found a striking correlation between patients' scores on the questionnaire and the severity of blockage in their coronary arteries. Hostile patients had significantly more severe coronary artery blockages than did less hostile patients (Williams, 1996).

In another study, epidemiologist Richard Shekelle and his colleagues (1983) reviewed the hostility scores of middle-aged men who had earlier participated in a study of Type A behavior. He found that high hostility—but not designation as Type A—accurately predicted a patient's risk of suffering a fatal heart attack as well as his risk of dying at an early age from other stress-related diseases. The hostility–CVD relationship remained significant even when other risk factors (such as smoking, high serum cholesterol, and family history) were controlled for.

As compared to high blood pressure or smoking, how strong an effect does hostility have on coronary risk? A relatively recent study indicates that hostility is nearly as poisonous. As Figure 9.5 shows, people with the highest scores on the Ho Scale are more than 1.5 times as likely to suffer an acute MI as are people with the lowest scores (Barefoot, Larsen, von der Lieth, & Schroll, 1995). The comparable risks for hypertension are 3.1 (untreated) and 2.0 (treated); smoking 30 g of tobacco per day, 2.8; anger, 2.66; highest versus lowest quartiles of plasma cholesterol, 2.8 (Whiteman, Fowkes, & Deary, 1997).

Some researchers have speculated that hostility may underlie the relationship between CVD and several seemingly uncontrollable risk factors, including gender, age, and possibly ethnicity. For example,

Figure 9.5

Hostility and Heart Attacks

Even after other risk factors (such as hypertension and smoking) are controlled for, the highest scorers on a hostility scale are more than 1.5 times as likely to suffer an acute MI as are the lowest scorers. Similarly, people with untreated hypertension are 3.1 times as likely to suffer an acute MI as are people without hypertension. For treated hypertension, the relative risk drops to 2.0. Compared to nonsmokers, those who smoke 30 g of tobacco per day have a relative risk of 2.8. Angry people are 2.66 times as likely to have an acute MI as are nonangry people. And, of course, elevated plasma cholesterol has a risk factor of 2.8.

Sources: "Hostility, Incidence of Acute Myocardial Infarction, and Mortality in a Sample of Older Danish Men and Women," by J. C. Barefoot, S. Larsen, L. von der Lieth, & M. Schroll, 1995, *American Journal of Epidemiology, 142*, pp. 477–484; "Hostility, Cigarette Smoking and Alcohol Consumption in the General Population," by M. C. Whiteman, F. G. R. Fowkes, I. J. Deary, & A. J. Lee, 1997, *Social Science and Medicine, 44*, pp. 1080–1096.

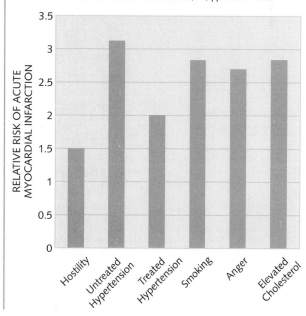

In a controversial study, researchers noted a correlation between the estimated hostility scores of U.S. cities and the incidence of CVD. Philadelphia had the highest hostility score and the highest incidence of cardiovascular diseases (Huston, 1997). What other factors might explain this result?

men have a higher incidence of CVD than do women; they also tend to be more hostile. Interestingly, Karen Matthews has provided evidence that male children also have higher hostility scores than their female peers (Matthews, Owens, Allen, & Stoney, 1992). Both hostility scores and incidence of CVD increase after people reach age 40 (Colligan & Offord, 1988). Furthermore, African-American men, who have an extremely high incidence of CVD, score higher on standard hostility tests than do African-American women and white men (Scherwitz, Perkins, Chesney, & Hughes, 1991).

Although hostility is related to CVD mortality, its status as an independent risk factor for cardiovascular disease continues to be debated (Smith & Gallo, 2001). For instance, hostility is also related to other behaviors that promote CVD, including obesity, hypertension, alcohol and tobacco use, negative life events, and little social support (Siegler, Peterson, Barefoot, & Williams, 1992). These relationships, which suggest that hostility is not an *independent* risk factor for CVD, have caused researchers to narrow their investigations to specific components of hostility—such as anger.

Anger

Just as health psychologists narrowed their focus from Type A behavior to hostility, a number of researchers have recently begun to focus on one specific component of hostility—the anger associated with an aggressively reactive temperament—as an even better predictor of heart disease (Miller et al., 1996; Whiteman et al., 1997).

Can a sudden burst of anger lead to a heart attack? The movies, soap operas, and folk wisdom would lead us to believe so—and it can happen. But how often? Actually, not so frequently, but often enough to cause concern. By one estimate, 20 percent of fatal myocardial infarctions occur in response to an angry outburst (Ferroli, 1996). In the massive Atherosclerosis Risk in Communities (ARIC) study, 256 of the 13,000 middle-aged participants had heart attacks. Janice Williams and her colleagues at the University of North Carolina found that the people who scored highest on an anger scale were three times more likely to have a heart attack than those with the lowest scores. People who scored in the moderate range on the anger scale were about 35 percent more likely to have a heart attack. This elevated risk was true even after taking into account the presence of other risk factors such as smoking, diabetes, elevated cholesterol, and obesity (Williams et al., 2000).

Indeed, strong negative emotions such as anger may be as dangerous to the heart as smoking, a high fat diet, or obesity. In one study, Harvard University researchers interviewed MI survivors, ages 20 to 92, for information about their emotional state just before their heart attacks. The researchers devised a seven-level anger scale ranging from calm to very angry to enraged. The results revealed that heart attacks were more than twice as likely to occur in the 2 hours that followed an episode of anger than at any other time. The largest jump in risk occurred at level 5 anger (enraged), in which the person is very angry and tense, with clenching fists or gritting teeth. Arguments with family members were the most frequent cause of anger, followed by conflicts at work and legal problems (Hilbert, 1994).

However, the anger that generates a heart attack may have been preceded by countless such episodes, reflecting a maladaptive pattern of coping with stress that has developed over a lifetime. In a massive longitudinal study, Duke University researchers studied the long-term effects of anger responses among lawyers divided according to their anger and hostility levels. Over the course of the 25-year study, researchers found a roughly equivalent rate of death due to coronary disease in Type A and Type B personalities. But when they adjusted for hostility and anger, they found that the hostile and angry lawyers were dying at seven times the rate of the nonhostile and nonangry lawyers—in both Type A and Type B personalities (Williams, 1989).

Suppressed, or inhibited, anger may be as hazardous to health as expressed anger. James Pennebaker (1992) has developed a general theory of inhibition that is based on the idea that to hold back one's thoughts or feelings requires work that, over time, results in low levels of stress that can create or exacerbate illness. In support of this theory, cardiac patients who deny their anger or frustration are 4.5 times more likely to die within 5 years than are other cardiac patients (Bondi, 1997). Suppressed anger was an even stronger predictor of mortality than elevated cholesterol level or cigarette smoking.

Why Do Hostility and Anger Promote Cardiovascular Disease?

Given that an angry, hostile personality predicts an increased risk of cardiovascular disease, how do these traits work their damage? Several theoretical models have been proposed. These models differ in their relative emphasis on biological, psychological, or social factors. This section describes the various models, then concludes with health psychology's biopsychosocial explanation of how hostility and anger contribute to cardiovascular disease.

Psychosocial Vulnerability

Some theorists maintain that hostile adults lead more stressful lives and have low levels of social support, which, over time, exert a toxic effect on cardiovascular health. In support of this *psychosocial vulnerability hypothesis,* researchers have found that chronic family conflict, unemployment, social isolation, and job-related stress have all been linked to increased risk of CVD (Kop, Gottdiener, & Krantz, 2001).

The Work Environment The work environment can be an important source of satisfaction—or stress. As we saw in Chapter 5, jobs associated with high productivity demands, excessive overtime work, and conflicting requirements accompanied by little personal control tend to be especially stressful. Assembly-line workers as well as those who wait tables and perform similarly stressful jobs are, in fact, more susceptible to coronary disease (Bosma, Stansfeld, & Marmot, 1998). In addition, workers who feel they have been promoted too quickly or too slowly, those who feel insecure about their jobs, and those who feel that their ambitions are thwarted are more likely to report stress and to show higher rates of illness, especially coronary disease (Taylor, Repetti, & Seeman, 1997).

Researchers have also found that especially complex jobs (jobs that make mental demands that require skill and training) may promote coronary disease, especially among hostile, hurried workers. Complex jobs may cause susceptible individuals to manifest Type A behavior because they elicit the impatience and hurriedness that is characteristic of the Type A person (Schaubroeck, Ganster, & Kemmerer, 1994).

Social Support As we saw in Chapter 5, coping with stressful events is especially difficult when an individual feels cut off from others. William Ruberman found that 3 years after surviving an acute myocardial infarction, those with a combination of high stress and social isolation had four times the death rate of people with low stress and strong social support (Ruberman, Weinblatt, Goldberg, & Chaudhary, 1984).

Living alone after suffering a heart attack is also associated with a higher risk of a recurrence of CHD (Case, Moss, Case, McDermott, & Eberly, 1992). Redford Williams (1996) found that coronary disease patients who were unmarried and/or had no one with whom they could share their innermost concerns were three times more likely to die in the next 5 years than patients who had a confidante—a spouse or a close friend.

Other researchers have reported a similar, elevated rate of coronary death among women who perceive little support either in the workplace or at home (Kawachi et al., 1994). They suggest that stress accompanied by social isolation and feelings of subordination are independent risk factors for coronary heart disease. This relationship held true even after the researchers controlled for other traditional risk factors such as hypertension, total serum cholesterol, obesity, and smoking.

Social Networks Having a reliable and dependable social network also provides protection against death due to coronary disease. Dwayne Reed and his colleagues from the Honolulu Heart Program interviewed a large sample of men about their relationships with relatives and coworkers and their memberships in religious and social organizations. Each person's score was based on the amount of contact he had in each area. The researchers found that risk of coronary disease was inversely related to the size of each man's social network. That is, the men who reported the largest social networks had the least disease (Reed, McGee, Yano, & Feinleib, 1983).

For those who have a large social network during their work years, retirement can represent a major disruption in that network. Ward Casscells and his colleagues interviewed the families of men who had died within 24 hours of the onset of coronary disease symptoms and an equal number of men chosen from the same neighborhood and age group who had the disease but did not die (the control group). After adjusting for age and previous history of coronary disease, they found that the relative risk of having a fatal heart attack was 1.8, or nearly twice as high, in those men who had recently retired compared to those who were still working (Cascells et al., 1980).

The Health Behavior Explanation

We have seen that hostility, anger, job strain, and social isolation may affect health directly. Some researchers believe that they may also have an indirect effect on health. For example, people with poor support may not take care of themselves as well as those who have someone to remind them to exercise, eat in moderation, or take their medicine. Similarly, a person with a cynical attitude may perceive health-enhancing behaviors such as following a low-fat diet and active lifestyle as unimportant while ignoring health warnings regarding smoking and other health-compromising behaviors. Hostility and anger have also been linked with excessive alcohol and caffeine consumption, greater fat and caloric intake, elevated LDL cholesterol, lower physical activity, greater body mass, hypertension, sleep problems, and nonadherence to medical regimens (Miller, Smith, Turner, Guijarro, & Hallet, 1996).

Psychophysiological Reactivity Model

Many researchers believe that stress, hostility, and anger act slowly over a period of years to damage the arteries and the heart. When we vent our anger, our pulse quickens, the heart pounds more forcefully, and blood clots more quickly. In addition, blood vessels constrict, blood pressure surges, and blood levels of free fatty acids increase. Our immunity also changes as adrenaline, cortisol, and other stress hormones suppress the activity of disease-fighting lymphocytes.

To pinpoint the physiological bases of hostility, researchers studied hostile men and women who were harassed while trying to perform a difficult mental task. The stress caused an unusually strong activation of the fight-or-flight response in these people and, when challenged, they displayed significantly greater cardiovascular reactivity in the form of larger increases in blood pressure and greater outpourings of epinephrine, cortisol, and other stress hormones (Kop & Krantz, 1997).

Interestingly, nighttime cardiac response is normal in hostile people, suggesting the reaction is not innate but rather a direct response to daytime stressors. Hostile people apparently have a lower threshold for triggering their fight-or-flight response than do nonhostile people (Williams, 2001).

The Biopsychosocial (Mind–Body) Model

As in other areas of health-compromising behavior, health psychologists have combined the insights of these models to provide a biopsychosocial (mind–body) explanation for how hostility and anger contribute to cardiovascular disease. This model suggests that in order for a chronic disease such as CVD to develop, a person must first have a physiological predisposition. This is determined by family history of CVD and previous health history (other diseases, poor diet, tobacco use, and so on). Whether or not CVD develops then depends on a variety of psychosocial factors in the person's life, including the level of stress from the work and home environments, the availability of social support, and whether the individual is hostile or angry. Hostile cognitive-emotional states are expected to lead to antagonistic and aggressive behaviors that produce interpersonal conflict and hostility from others, which, in turn lead to a reduction in social support, more negative effect, and artery-damaging cardiac reactivity. Thus, hostile attitudes create a self-fulfilling prophecy for the mistrusting, hostile person by producing a hostile environment.

Fortunately, most people can minimize the health-compromising effects of hostility. Although changing one's personality is not easy, hostility can be countered with efforts to control reactions, abort hostile reactions, and treat others as you would have them treat you. (See Reality Check.)

Reducing the Risk of Cardiovascular Disease

Heart attacks have become a widespread problem in industrialized countries in the last 50 years or so. Why? Perhaps because fast-food chains are everywhere, smoking is on the rise among some groups, the number of obese adults is one-third of the population and rising, and exercise machines rust in garages or serve as handy clothes racks.

Although epidemiological research has provided a wealth of information that should help us prevent cardiovascular disease—limit fat intake, quit smoking, lose excess weight, and get regular exercise—we persist in making heart-unhealthy choices. Some researchers believe that our poor decisions are made by brains that were shaped to cope with an environment substantially different from the one our species now inhabits (Nesse & Williams, 1998). On the African savanna, where our species originated, those who had a tendency to consume large amounts of usually scarce fat were more likely to survive famines that killed their thinner companions. Those with a rapid-fire fight-or-flight reaction had a clear advantage in hunting and reacting to hostile threats and were more likely to survive and pass on these traits to their offspring. And we, their descendants, still carry these evolved urges and hostile tendencies.

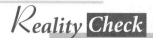

Test Your Hostility and Level of Suppressed Anger

Research studies have shown that if you're angry at the world, you'd best let the world know—but in a civil way that does not lead to an artery-threatening hostile outburst. How many of the following early warning signs of suppressed anger can you detect in yourself?

- trouble falling or staying asleep
- large chunks of time spent thinking about problems
- loneliness
- frequent headaches
- teeth clenching or grinding
- comments made by other people about your bad temper
- unwillingness of other people to tell you things they think might upset you
- opinions of other people that you are stubborn or opinionated.

HOSTILITY AND SUPPRESSED ANGER QUESTIONNAIRE

To get a general idea of how hostile you tend to be, answer the following questions.

1. When in the express checkout line at the supermarket, do you often count the items in the baskets of the people ahead of you to be sure they aren't over the limit?

2. When an elevator doesn't come as quickly as you think it should, do your thoughts quickly focus on the inconsiderate behavior of the person on another floor who's holding it up?

3. Do you frequently check on family members or coworkers to make sure they haven't made a mistake in some task?

4. When you are held up in traffic do you quickly sense your heart pounding and your breath quickening?

5. When little things go wrong, do you often feel like lashing out at the world?

6. When someone criticizes you, do you quickly begin to feel annoyed?

7. If an elevator stops too long on a floor above you, are you likely to pound on the door?

8. If people mistreat you, do you look for an opportunity to pay them back, just for the principle of the thing?

9. Do you frequently find yourself muttering at the television during a news broadcast?

If you answered yes to four or more questions overall, your hostility level is probably high. Redford Williams (1996) has suggested that becoming more trusting is the antidote to cynical hostility and anger. He offers the following tips for becoming less hostile:

- Admit to a friend that your hostility level is too high and let her or him know you are trying to reduce it.
- When cynical thoughts come into your head, yell "Stop!" (silently, if you are in public).
- Try to talk yourself out of being angry. Reason with yourself.
- Distract yourself when you're getting angry. For example, pick up a magazine from the rack if you're kept waiting in a supermarket checkout line.
- Force yourself to be quiet and listen when other people are talking.
- Learn how to meditate, and use this skill whenever you become aware of cynical thoughts or angry feelings.
- Try to become more empathetic to the plight of others.
- When someone is truly mistreating you, learn how to be effectively assertive rather than aggressively lashing out.
- Take steps to increase your connectedness to others, thereby countering the tendency of hostile people to ward off social support.
- When people wrong you, forgive them.
- Volunteer to help others less fortunate than yourself.
- Learn to laugh at your hostile tendencies.
- Engage in regular exercise.
- Get a pet. People who have pets seem to live longer and be healthier, perhaps because animals, especially dogs, are so affectionate and undemanding. Unlike many people, pets give much more than they get.
- Learn more about the core teaching of your chosen religion. A central principle of the major world religions is to treat others as we would have them treat us.
- Pretend that this day is your last. Your hostile tendencies will come into perspective.

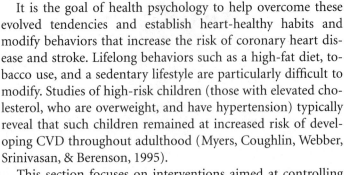

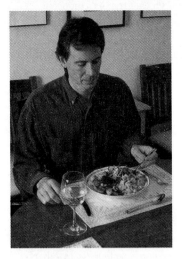

It is the goal of health psychology to help overcome these evolved tendencies and establish heart-healthy habits and modify behaviors that increase the risk of coronary heart disease and stroke. Lifelong behaviors such as a high-fat diet, tobacco use, and a sedentary lifestyle are particularly difficult to modify. Studies of high-risk children (those with elevated cholesterol, who are overweight, and have hypertension) typically reveal that such children remained at increased risk of developing CVD throughout adulthood (Myers, Coughlin, Webber, Srinivasan, & Berenson, 1995).

This section focuses on interventions aimed at controlling hypertension, reducing elevated serum cholesterol, and reversing atherosclerosis. The most serious behavioral risk factor in CVD, cigarette smoking, was discussed in Chapter 8.

Controlling Hypertension

For every one-point drop in diastolic blood pressure, which measures the pressure between heartbeats, there is an estimated 2 to 3 percent reduction in the risk of a myocardial infarction (Massey et al., 2000). Interventions aimed at lowering high blood pressure typically begin with pharmacological treatment. However, because hypertension is often symptomless, many patients fail to comply with a prescribed medication regimen.

Changing behavior can also go a long way toward lowering blood pressure (Shapiro, 2001). For example, lowering sodium intake can bring about significant improvement in blood pressure readings. Many people with hypertension are sodium-sensitive, meaning that excess sodium raises their blood pressure. Since there is no test for sodium-sensitivity, almost everyone with hypertension should restrict dietary sodium to 2,000 mg per day.

Numerous studies have shown that regular aerobic exercise can help lower the resting blood pressure of people with hypertension. It can also improve a person's cholesterol profile by increasing HDL cholesterol and reducing the ratio of total serum cholesterol to HDL cholesterol. Even when exercise fails to reduce hypertension or improve a person's lipid profile, it conveys a heart-protecting benefit: Physically fit hypertensives with elevated cholesterol actually have a lower overall risk of CVD than unfit individuals who have normal blood pressure and cholesterol (Blair et al., 1989).

Reducing excess body weight can also help a person gain control over hypertension. As noted in Chapter 7, the most effective way to lower body mass index is to combine exercise with a healthy diet. Dieting alone often leads to an undesirable loss of muscle mass as well as fat. Furthermore, people tend to quickly regain weight that is the result of dieting alone.

Even if a person has had a heart attack, these preventive behaviors can play an important role in controlling the negative effects of CVD. For example,

Risk Reduction—and Preventing Recurrences
Regular exercise and good nutrition have been shown to be significant factors in reducing risk of having a CVD episode. They are also valuable for those who have had a heart attack or a stroke. At top, a former heart-attack victim (center) saw his illness as a wake-up call and changed his life. He now has the highest karate level in his area. The person above is reducing his cholesterol and other fats with a vegetarian diet and a glass of wine.
© Dion Ogust / The Image Works; © Syracuse Newspapers / Randi Anglin / The Image Works

exercise improves the heart's ability to pump blood to working muscles as well as the muscles' ability to extract and make use of oxygen from the blood. Neil Oldridge (1988) conducted a meta-analysis of studies involving over 4,000 heart attack patients. The results showed that 25 percent fewer patients who participated in cardiac rehabilitation exercise programs died from cardiovascular disease.

Reducing Cholesterol

Health experts recommend keeping cholesterol intake to a maximum of 300 mg per day (for example, an average egg yolk contains about 215 mg of cholesterol and a 3 ounce piece of liver contains about 331 mg of cholesterol). They also caution that the primary factor in raising serum cholesterol is *not* eating excess cholesterol in foods but in consuming too much saturated fat (more than 10 percent of your total daily calories). Saturated fats raise serum cholesterol by signaling the body to manufacture fewer LDL receptors, which help the liver to remove cholesterol from the body.

The major sources of saturated fats are animal fats, butter fat, tropical oils, and heavy hydrogenated oils. Monounsaturated and polyunsaturated fats such as those contained in olive and canola oil are a much healthier choice. Although they have just as many calories as saturated fats, they help lower serum cholesterol and improve the HDL/LDL cholesterol ratio. Monounsaturated fats are preferable since they lower LDL cholesterol without affecting protective HDL cholesterol levels. Polyunsaturated fats lower total cholesterol by lowering both LDL and HDL cholesterol. Although health psychologists agree that reducing the saturated fat content of your diet is beneficial, they disagree about whether the fat should be replaced by monounsaturated fat or by carbohydrate. When saturated fat is replaced by carbohydrate, the reduction in LDL cholesterol is often accompanied by an increase in triglycerides (common fats found in the bloodstream that are derived from fats and carbohydrates in food) and a reduction in HDL cholesterol. However, when monounsaturated fats are substituted for saturated fats, the same degree of LDL cholesterol lowering often occurs, with less or no change in triglyceride or HDL levels. A Mediterranean-type diet, rich in fruits and vegetables, whole grains, olive oil and other monounsaturated fats, fish, and moderate consumption of red wine, has been associated with a reduction in the risk of CVD that is independent of its effect on LDL-cholesterol (Massey et al., 2000). Eating more fiber, fruits, vegetables, and grains also has a cholesterol-lowering effect, perhaps by binding with acids that cause cholesterol to be pulled from the bloodstream.

It is important to note that there is great individual variability in the response of serum cholesterol to diet. Unfortunately, at this time it is impossible to predict who will respond to dietary changes and who will not. Generally speaking, a trial period of 3 to 6 months is needed to determine whether diet will be effective in altering a person's cholesterol profile.

Reversing Atherosclerosis

We have seen that behaviors such as smoking and eating a diet high in saturated fat can promote the development of cardiovascular disease. Recent evidence indicates that we can actually *reverse* the development of CVD by modifying these and other controllable risk factors. Vincent Maher and his colleagues studied the effects of lowering LDL cholesterol and increasing HDL cholesterol in a group of male CHD patients, who averaged 62 years of age and had elevated serum cholesterol levels and a family history of heart disease (Maher, Brown, Marcovina, Hillger, & Zhao, 1995). The patients were placed on a modified diet that limited their daily intake of saturated fat to less than 30 percent of total daily calories and were then assigned to one of three treatment groups. Patients in two of the groups were given different cholesterol-lowering medications. A third control group received a placebo.

The results showed that the combination of a low-fat diet and cholesterol-lowering medication had the most beneficial effects. Men in *both* drug groups achieved a significant improvement in their HDL/LDL ratios compared to those in the placebo group. Even more important, the combination of a healthier diet and cholesterol-lowering medication reduced the occurrence of subsequent angina and other coronary events by slowing (and in many cases, reversing) blockages in the patients' coronary arteries. Results such as these have led researchers to conclude that lowering cholesterol levels may reduce an individual's risk of CVD by as much as 25 to 35 percent (Massey et al., 2000).

In another study of CHD patients, Dean Ornish of the University of California, San Diego, combined stress management, aerobic exercise, relaxation training, smoking cessation, and an even more restrictive diet (less than 10 percent of total daily calories from saturated fat) in a comprehensive intervention program for CHD patients. The intervention consisted of a 1-week intensive residential training program followed by 12 months of regular follow-up meetings. A control group of CHD patients was given standard advice about exercise, diet, smoking, and stress reduction but left to make changes on their own. At the end of a year, the treatment group showed less severe angina and, most spectacularly, significant reversal of atherosclerosis (Ornish et al., 1990).

However, the Ornish program is very demanding, and it is not clear which aspect was most responsible for the remarkable results. A less daunting 8-week program combining stress management and moderate aerobic exercise reported a significant reduction in angina and decreased use of medication among patients awaiting bypass surgery. By the end of the second month, half the patients no longer needed surgery (Bundy, Carroll, Wallace, & Nagle, 1998).

After CVD: Preventing Recurrences

Most people who survive a myocardial infarction recover well enough to resume near-normal lives within a few weeks or months. However, they remain high-risk individuals and need to make lifestyle adjustments in order to improve their chances of living a long life and avoiding a recurrence of CHD. In addition to quitting smoking, reducing dietary cholesterol, losing excess weight, exercising regularly, and keeping blood pressure within a healthy range, CHD survivors may need assistance in managing their levels of stress and controlling anger and hostility.

Many stroke victims are not so lucky. Extensive paralysis of one side of the body prevents them from resuming anything like a normal life. However, with a lot of work and social support from their family and friends, some do return to a near-normal existence. Like those with coronary heart disease, they can make lifestyle adjustments that will increase their longevity.

Managing Stress Following a Cardiovascular Episode

A heart attack or stroke can cause substantial distress to both the patient and his or her family members. While many patients make a complete recovery and are able to resume most of their previous activities, some remain psychologically impaired for a long time. A major goal of many recent intervention programs is to deal with the approximately one-third of the patients who experience significant stress, anxiety, or depression lasting more than 1 year after their hospitalization (Bennett & Carroll, 1997).

In one program, Nancy Frasure-Smith and Raymond Prince (1989) assigned nurses to contact post-MI patients regularly during the year following their heart attacks to evaluate whether they were experiencing stress. When a patient indicated that stress was indeed a problem, the nurse instigated what he or she considered the appropriate stress-reduction procedure. In some cases, this simply entailed talking through the source of stress with the patient; in more serious instances, patients were referred to other health professionals such as a psychologist, social worker, or cardiologist. Over the course of the 7-year study, patients in the stress-management group had significantly lower rates of cardiac mortality and morbidity compared to control patients, who received standard post-hospitalization contact.

Controlling Hostility and Anger

A number of studies have reported positive effects of CVD interventions directed at reducing Type A behavior and hostility. These interventions are based on two premises:

1. Hostile people are more likely to encounter stress, which increases the prevalence of atherosclerosis-promoting experiences involving anger.

2. Hostile people are less likely to have stress-busting resources such as social support, partly as a result of their antagonistic behavior.

Intervention studies focus on helping hostile people gain control over their angry emotions. In the typical program, the psychologist first attempts to gain insight into the triggers of anger-inducing incidents by having participants self-monitor their behavior. Next, he or she develops strategies to help the person cope with such aggravation—for example, by avoiding especially stressful situations such as rush hour traffic and controlling their reactions, perhaps by counting to 10 before reacting to a provoking incident. As the person is increasingly able to cope with problem situations, the psychologist turns to a more cognitive intervention, so that the person can learn to challenge cynical attitudes and modify unrealistic beliefs and expectations about life.

The efficacy of these interventions has been supported in dozens of studies. In the largest study to date, called the Recurrent Coronary Prevention Program (RCPP), patients were randomly allocated to a treatment program, while others received the usual care and attended group meetings directed at problems associated with coronary disease and its management. The treatment program used a wide range of cognitive and behavioral techniques to help patients reduce environmental triggers for their hostility and to modify their hurried, competitive behavior and cynical thought processes. After nearly 4 years of the RCPP intervention, hostility, hurriedness, and cynicism were significantly lower in treatment patients but unchanged in control patients. In addition, the risk of a second heart attack was significantly lower in treatment patients than in control patients. Most important, total cardiovascular mortality rates were reduced by 50 percent in treatment patients, with the greatest reduction being among those who showed the most change in their toxic behavior (Friedman, Thoresen, & Gill, 1986). Clearly, psychological interventions can reduce antagonistic behavior patterns and can lead to a reduction in cardiovascular risk.

Clinical health psychologists have used a variety of other strategies to help individuals cope with anger. One effective strategy is relaxation training, which was discussed in Chapter 5 as an effective means of coping with stress. Another method involves teaching angry persons new social and communication skills in which they learn to be more civilly assertive and to become aware of other people's cues that would normally provoke anger in them. Teaching participants to avoid provocative situations and to take themselves less seriously are also common goals of anger-intervention programs.

Jerry Deffenbacher and Robert Stark (1992) have demonstrated the efficacy of anger-control interventions. Using a combination of progressive relaxation, deep breathing, imagery, and cognitive restructuring, people who learned these skills experienced significant reductions in anger compared with those in a no-treatment control group.

Diabetes

■ **diabetes mellitus** a disorder of the endocrine system in which the body is unable to produce insulin (Type I) or is unable to properly utilize this pancreatic hormone (Type II)

One of the most important risk factors for the development of CVD is **diabetes mellitus,** which involves the body's inability to produce or properly use insulin, a hormone that helps convert sugar and starches from food into energy. There is no cure for diabetes and its cause remains a mystery, although both heredity and lifestyle factors appear to play roles. Currently, about 6 percent of the U.S. population has diabetes, making the disease the third most common chronic illness in this country and the seventh leading cause of death.

Prevalence rates for diabetes vary markedly around the world: The disease is absent or rare in some indigenous communities in developing countries in Africa, the Eastern Mediterranean, and the Western Pacific, while prevalences of 14 to 20 percent have been reported among some Arab, Asian Indian, Chinese, and Hispanic-American populations (World Health Organization, 2000). As Figure 9.6 shows, in the United States, African-Americans, Hispanic-Americans, and Native Americans are at higher risk for adult-onset diabetes than European Americans, Asian-Americans, and Cuban-Americans (USDHHS, 2000).

Types of Diabetes

As shown in Table 9.1 (page 402), there are two basic types of diabetes: juvenile-onset diabetes (called insulin-dependent diabetes mellitus or Type I diabetes), and adult-onset diabetes (called non-insulin-dependent diabetes mellitus or Type II diabetes). Type I diabetes, which first appears in childhood (usually between 5 and 6 years of age) or later during adolescence, is an autoimmune disease in which the person's immune system attacks the insulin- and glucagon-producing *islet cells* of the pancreas (Roberts, 1998). In a healthy person, the opposing actions of these hormones help regulate the blood level of the sugar glucose. Glucagon stimulates the release of glucose, causing blood sugar levels to rise, and insulin decreases blood sugar levels by causing cells to take up glucose more freely from the bloodstream. Without functioning islet cells, the body is unable to regulate blood sugar levels and the individual becomes dependent on insulin injections. The symptoms of Type I diabetes, which include excessive thirst and urination, craving for sweets, weight loss, fatigue, and irritability, are largely the result of the body's inability to metabolize glucose for energy, which forces it to begin feeding off its own fats and proteins.

Type II diabetes—a milder form of the disease that usually appears after age 30—is found in more than 90 percent of all people

Figure 9.6

Death from Diabetes in the United States, 1997
Diabetes takes a greater toll on some ethnic groups than others, especially African-American, Hispanic-American, and Native American. Among all U.S. adults, 75 deaths per 100,000 population were related to diabetes in 1997. The *Healthy People 2010* target is to reduce this number to 45 or fewer deaths per 100,000 people.

Source: *Healthy People 2010,* by Centers for Disease Control and Prevention (www.health.gov/healthypeople/).

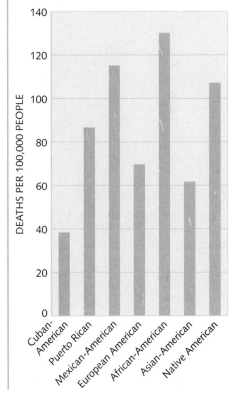

Table 9.1

Characteristics and Risk Factors of Type I and Type II Diabetes

Type I	Type II
Autoimmune disorder in which insulin-producing cells of the pancreas are destroyed	Chronic illness in which the body fails to produce enough or to properly use insulin
Peak incidence occurs during puberty, around 10 to 12 years of age in girls and 12 to 14 in boys	Onset occurs after age 30
	Affects more women than men
Accounts for 5–10% of all cases of diabetes	Accounts for 90–95% of all cases of diabetes
Symptoms may mimic flu, including excessive thirst, frequent urination, unusual weight loss, extreme fatigue, and irritability	Symptoms include any of the Type I symptoms and blurred vision, frequent infections, cuts that are slow to heal, tingling or numbness in hands or feet
Requires insulin injections	Requires strict regimen of diet and exercise
Affects women and men equally	
Higher prevalence among European Americans than other ethnic groups	**Who Is at Greater Risk?**
	People over age 45 with a family history of diabetes
Who Is at Greater Risk?	People who are overweight
Children of parents with Type I diabetes	Women who had gestational diabetes or who had a baby weighing 9 pounds or more at birth
Siblings of people with Type I diabetes	People who don't exercise regularly
	People with low HDL cholesterol or high triglycerides
	African-Americans, Native Americans, Hispanic-Americans, Asians, and Pacific Islanders
	People of low socioeconomic status

with diabetes. It results from *insulin resistance* (a condition in which the islet cells of the pancreas fail to make enough insulin) and/or an insensitivity to insulin caused by a decrease in the number of insulin receptors in target cells. The symptoms of Type II diabetes include frequent urination, irregular menstruation, fatigue, slow healing of cuts and bruises, dryness of the mouth, and pain or cramps in the legs, feet, and fingers. Type II diabetes is more common among women, overweight people, members of certain ethnic groups, and those of low socio-economic status. *Gestational diabetes* is a temporary form of insulin resistance that usually occurs about halfway through a pregnancy as a result of the mother's inability to produce sufficient insulin. Gestational diabetes usually goes away after the baby's birth, but women who have had gestational diabetes have a greater risk of later developing Type II diabetes, as do women who gave birth to babies weighing 9 pounds or more at birth.

In both types of diabetes, two types of blood sugar problems can develop: *hypoglycemia* (blood sugar level that is too low) and *hyperglycemia* (blood sugar level that is too high). An estimated 50 to 75 percent of individuals with diabetes develop one or more long-term health complications as a result of their body's inability to regulate blood sugar (Talbot, Nouwen, Gingras, Belanger, & Audet, 1999). Elevated levels of glucose, for instance, cause the walls of arteries to thicken, accelerating the development of atherosclerosis and cardiovascular disease. Men with diabetes are also twice as likely to develop hypertension and CHD as men without the disorder. Women with diabetes have 3 to 7 times the risk of developing CHD as women who do not have diabetes. Because unregulated glucose levels in the blood can damage the retinas of the eyes, diabetes is also the leading cause of blindness among adults (people with diabetes are 17 times more likely to go blind than those without the disease). Diabetes is also associated with increased risk of kidney disease, cancer of the pancreas, and damage to the nervous system that may cause memory impairments (especially among older adults) and loss of sensation or pain in the extremities. In severe cases of poor circulation and loss of sensation in the extremities, amputation of the toes or feet may be required (Everhart & Wright, 1995).

Causes of Diabetes

As with other chronic illnesses, diabetes may be caused by multiple factors, including viral or bacterial infections that damage the islet cells of the pancreas, an overactive immune system, and genetic vulnerability. Nutritional "Westernization," which includes a diet high in fat and processed foods as well as total calories, also may be a contributing factor in diabetes, especially within racial and ethnic groups that follow such diets, for example, African-American females (Christoffel & Ariza, 1998). Increased television watching associated with reduced physical activity and poor nutrition may also contribute to Type II diabetes in young people (Rosenbloom, Joe, Young, & Winter, 1999).

Stress has also been suggested as a precipitating factor in both Type I and Type II diabetes, especially among individuals with a strong family history of the disease (Dougall & Baum, 2001; Lehman, Rodin, McEwen, & Brinton, 1991). People who have already been diagnosed with diabetes, as well as those at high risk for the disease, also react to laboratory and environmental stressors with abnormally greater changes in their blood glucose levels than do people not at risk for diabetes (Surwit & Williams, 1996). Following the *diathesis-stress* model of disease (see Chapter 4), some investigators have suggested that abnormal blood sugar responses to challenging events (a symptom of an overreactive sympathetic nervous system), in conjunction with long-term exposure to high levels of stress, may be a *direct* path in the development of diabetes (Esposito-Del Puente et al., 1994). Indirectly, stress may also promote the development of diabetes by adversely affecting the individual's diet, level of compliance with treatment regimens, and tendency to exercise (Balfour, White, Schiffrin, Dougherty, & Dufresne, 1993; Harris & Lustman, 1998).

Treatment of Diabetes

Fortunately, most people with diabetes can control their disease through lifestyle modifications—by changing their diet, regulating their weight, and exercising regularly, for example—and, in some cases, with daily injections of insulin. The goal of treatment is, of course, to keep blood sugar at a stable, healthy level. The medical community is currently debating whether both types of diabetes should be treated in the same way, including medication for precise glucose control, or differently, with Type II diabetes focusing on diet (reducing sugar and carbohydrate intake and keeping the total number of calories consumed each day within a narrow range), weight control, and exercise and Type I requiring insulin management (Feifer & Tansman, 1999). In practice, a combination of treatments is used with Type II diabetes, depending on the severity of the individual case and the effectiveness of dietary and exercise modifications.

Health Psychology and Diabetes

The knowledge, beliefs, and behavior of patients strongly affect their ability to manage their disease and its impact on every domain of their health (Feifer & Tansman, 1999). This makes the health psychologist's role in the care and treatment of people with diabetes particularly important, as underscored by the standards of treatment recommended by the American Diabetes Association (ADA). The ADA standards focus on lifestyle, cultural, psychological, educational, and economic factors in addition to medication (ADA, 1997); they also emphasize that *self-management* is the cornerstone of treatment for all people with diabetes. As a result, psychologists are increasingly becoming involved in the primary care of people with diabetes (Feifer & Tansman, 1999). This section discusses psychologists' various roles in treating diabetes.

Promoting Adjustment to Diabetes

A patient who receives a diagnosis of diabetes may experience a range of emotions, including shock, denial, anger, and depression (Jacobson, 1996). Helping patients accept their diagnosis is the first step in promoting self-management of diabetes. Consider the case of Beatrice, a 64-year-old African-American woman with a 20-year history of hypertension and a 4-year history of Type II diabetes. Beatrice reported feeling anger at her initial diagnosis. Over the next few months, she began exhibiting symptoms of depression and anxiety, and her already poor glucose control got even worse (Feifer & Tansman, 1999). Using *rational-emotive therapy,* psychologists challenged Beatrice's negative perceptions about her disease and helped her to feel better about herself, manage her moods, and deal with her self-care tasks on a day-to-day basis. As her acceptance of the disease and the once seemingly overwhelming tasks of self-management improved, Beatrice ultimately gained much stronger control over her blood sugar levels.

Illness Intrusiveness Even after they have accepted their diagnosis, many patients with diabetes continue to struggle with **illness intrusiveness,** which refers to the disruptive effect of diabetes on their lives. Illness intrusiveness can adversely affect an individual's well-being in at least two ways: directly, when the condition interferes with valued activities and interests, and indirectly, as a result of reduced perceptions of personal control, self-efficacy, and self-esteem (Devins, Hunsley, Mandin, Taub, & Paul, 1997). One study found that illness intrusiveness was strongly correlated with symptoms of depression among a large sample of Canadian Type II diabetes patients (Talbot et al., 1999). However, research has shown that having strong social support and good personal coping resources—along with high self-esteem, a sense of mastery, and feelings of self-efficacy in the face of adversity—are associated with fewer depressive symptoms in people with diabetes (and, for that matter, those with lung cancer or cardiovascular disease) (Penninx et al., 1998).

To help those without the support or resources needed to cope with diabetes, psychologists design interventions to reduce diabetes intrusiveness on daily living (such as teaching people to redefine personal priorities in order to increase participation in enjoyable activities and restructuring their irrational expectations regarding the intrusiveness of the disease), as well as interventions aimed at mobilizing social support and improving personal coping skills.

Blood Glucose Awareness Another problem of diabetes patients is often a poor understanding of the disease and its symptoms. One study found that more than 50 percent of patients with diabetes had inaccurate beliefs about blood glucose levels, including the symptoms of hypoglycemia and hyperglycemia (Gonder-Frederick, Cox, Bobbitt, & Pennebaker, 1989). As a result, the patients often overlooked or missed some potentially serious symptoms, and overreacted to other, irrelevant ones. Health psychologists have reported impressive results from *blood glucose awareness training*—in which patients learn to gauge their blood sugar levels from environmental cues (such as time of day or ongoing activity), physical symptoms (such as nausea and dryness of mouth), and mood (such as fatigue and irritability). Through such training, which is similar in many ways to biofeedback training, most people with diabetes can learn to reliably recognize various cognitive and behavioral indicators of different blood glucose levels (Cox, Gonder-Frederick, Julian, & Clarke, 1994). Compared to untrained control patients, patients trained in blood glucose awareness have achieved other health benefits:

illness intrusiveness the extent to which a chronic illness disrupts an individual's life by interfering with valued activities and interests and reducing perceptions of personal control, self-efficacy, and self-esteem

- Improved glucose control and fewer long-term health complications
- Fewer automobile and other accidents resulting from states of hypoglycemia
- Fewer hospitalizations for blood sugar level abnormalities

Treating Diabetes-Related Psychological Disorders

People with diabetes tend toward feelings of depression, especially during the early stages of adjusting to the disease. Psychologists have also found that diagnosable clinical disorders such as major depression, anxiety, and eating disorders are more prevalent among adults with diabetes than they are in the general population (Katon & Sullivan, 1990). Prevalence rates for major depressive disorder, for example, which range from 5 to 25 percent in the general population, have been found to range from 22 to 60 percent among those with diabetes (Gavard, Lustman, & Clouse, 1993; Talbot et al., 1999).

The physical and emotional demands placed on the individual with diabetes, including strict compliance to a complex treatment regimen of daily self-monitoring of blood glucose levels, preparing special meals, and taking medication, can be difficult and frustrating. This task is made all the more challenging when the individual suffers from unusual psychosocial distress or a psychological disorder. Many research studies have found an association between the presence of psychological disorders and poor compliance (Littlefield et al., 1992). With depression, for instance, self-care tasks such as daily monitoring of glucose levels or preparation of special foods may seem futile or too difficult to accomplish. Many health professionals have suggested that individuals with diabetes should have psychosocial evaluations at some point during their medical treatment, preferably soon after the time of diagnosis (King, Peragallo-Dittko, Polonsky, Prochaska, & Vinicor, 1998). Health psychologists who are involved in the primary care of people diagnosed with diabetes are in a good position to refer them to appropriate clinical psychologists, if needed (Feifer & Tansman, 1999).

Managing Weight and Stress

Effective weight management is particularly important for patients with diabetes because it improves the body's ability to regulate glucose, and thereby reduces the need for medication. Using a mind–body approach that combines nutrition, education, low-calorie diets, and regular exercise, weight-loss programs often produce substantial weight loss among people with diabetes. As with all weight-loss programs, however, the main problem has been in maintaining the loss (Bradley, 1997; Wing, 1993). Too often, people with diabetes relapse to unhealthy dietary practices and sedentary lifestyles, and quickly regain the weight they lost.

The importance of exercise to diabetes patients has been confirmed in studies regarding the prevention of Type II diabetes. One prospective study of male alumni of the University of Pennsylvania found that physically active men had the lowest incidence of Type II diabetes over a 15-year period (Helmrich, Ragland, Leung, & Paffenbarger, 1991). This protective effect remained even after the researchers controlled for other major diabetes risk factors, including obesity, hypertension, and family history of the disease.

Equally important is stress management. In people with diabetes, reactions to stress strongly influence whether and how well they follow a particular regimen. For example, stress may begin the vicious cycle of overeating, poor control over diabetes, more stress, and overeating. Thus, there are good reasons to expect stress management to be of value in diabetes management. Relaxation training and other stress management techniques appear to be beneficial for many individuals with diabetes, especially those who are experiencing considerable stress, which researchers believe disrupts their management of the disease.

Increasing Compliance with Treatment Regimens

Health psychologists have approached the issue of compliance in two ways: by seeking to identify factors that predict compliance or noncompliance and by developing interventions to improve compliance with different aspects of a treatment regimen. Research studies indicate that compliance with diabetes treatment regimens cannot be predicted from sociodemographic factors such as age, gender, ethnicity, or personality (Goodall & Halford, 1991). As with other health conditions in which lifestyle components such as diet and exercise are critical, several factors contribute to noncompliance. First, patients with diabetes may perceive prescribed treatment as recommended and discretionary rather than mandatory, and fail to comply. Adding to this is most certainly a *gradient of reinforcement.* The person newly diagnosed with diabetes often feels no ill effects—severe medical complications of diabetes may not arise for a decade or more—and may find his or her current lifestyle too enjoyable to change. Social and environmental circumstances are also factors in poor compliance, as is the complexity of a lifelong regimen of self-care (Landis et al., 1985). During periods of unusual stress or social pressure to behave in unhealthy ways, for instance, dietary and exercise compliance often decreases among those with diabetes (Goodall & Halford, 1991).

Working from the transtheoretical model discussed in Chapter 6 (page 262), health psychologists might try to get diabetes patients to comply with a treatment regimen by helping them cycle through the stages of precontemplation, contemplation, preparation, action, and maintenance. For example, the psychologist would almost certainly tell an obese woman newly diagnosed with Type II diabetes to lose weight. However, since she probably does not feel sick, she sees no reason to change from her delicious high-calorie, high-carbohydrate diet (precontemplation). To move her to the stage of contemplation, he or she would try to explain the connection between diet and diabetes (she perceives a link, but she isn't ready to give up her favorite foods). Further education and support for change (family members are enlisted to help her modify her diet, for instance) may nudge the patient into the stage of preparation (she knows she will diet), and then to action (the patient works hard at dieting). Finally, during the maintenance stage (working to avoiding relapse to unhealthy eating habits), she is likely to benefit from interventions that focus on how to maintain the treatment regimen in the face of circumstances that undermine it (such as unusual stress or social pressure to eat unhealthy foods). For example, maintenance interventions for Beatrice, who abandoned her medical regimen each time she encountered a stressful life event, involved exercises to promote stress management and improve her communication coping skills. The general topic of why certain people are more likely to delay making healthy lifestyle changes and seeking health care is discussed in Chapter 12.

Enhancing Communication and Increasing Social Support

Empowering individuals with diabetes (or any chronic illness) to actively participate in decision making in their treatment regimen has a variety of benefits. Among these are an increased perception of control, enhanced doctor–patient communication, greater confidence in prescribed treatment regimens, and improved compliance. In one study, diabetes patients who were taught to be more assertive in acquiring knowledge about the disease and using that information to negotiate treatment decisions with their physicians showed significant increases in their perceived self-efficacy, regulation of blood glucose, and satisfaction with their treatment regimen (Greenfield, Kaplan, Ware, Yano, & Frank, 1988). Case in point: Beatrice, whom we met earlier, had received from her physician basic information about living with diabetes. She was too intimidated, however, to discuss her fears, self-care needs, and difficulty complying with her treatment regimen. She did, however, discuss these issues with her psychologist, who used assertiveness training to prepare Beatrice to approach her doctor to resolve these issues, which she later did.

The problems of managing diabetes extend beyond the individual to members of his or her family, who may react in ways that adversely (or favorably) affect the patient. Family therapy is often helpful in this regard. Therapy often begins with education about diabetes, what must be done to achieve control, and how the behaviors of family members affect the individual's control. This can be particularly important in the management of Type I diabetes in children and adolescents. Parents, for example, may become overly protective of a teenager newly diagnosed with diabetes, unnecessarily restricting activities and promoting a sense of helplessness in their son or daughter. Family therapy directed at improving communication and conflict resolution among family members has been demonstrated to improve diabetes control among children who perceive deficiencies in these areas in their families (Minuchin, Rosman, & Baker, 1978). Research studies also indicate that when parents are actively involved in their son's or daughter's diabetes management (such as helping with blood glucose monitoring), greater control over the disease is the result (Andersen, Ho, Brackett, Finkelstein, & Laffel, 1997).

Summing Up

The Healthy Heart

1. The cardiovascular system consists of the blood, the blood vessels of the circulatory system, and the heart. The heart consists of three layers of tissue: a thin outer layer, called the *epicardium;* a thin inner layer, called the *endocardium;* and a thicker middle layer, the heart muscle itself, or *myocardium.* The myocardium is separated into four chambers that work in coordinated fashion to bring blood into the heart and then to pump it throughout the body.

Cardiovascular Diseases

2. Cardiovascular diseases (CVD), which include coronary heart disease (CHD) and stroke, are the leading causes of death in the United States and most developed countries.

3. Cardiovascular disease results from atherosclerosis, a chronic disease in which coronary arteries are narrowed by fatty deposits and plaques that form over microscopic lesions in the walls of blood vessels, and arteriosclerosis, or hardening of the arteries.

4. When the arteries that supply the heart are narrowed with plaques, restricting blood flow to the heart (*ischemia*), the person may experience heart pain, called angina pectoris. When severe atherosclerosis or a clot causes a coronary artery to become completely obstructed, a heart attack, or myocardial infarction (MI), occurs and a portion of the myocardium begins to die. A third possible manifestation of cardiovascular malfunction is a stroke, which occurs when a blood clot obstructs an artery in the brain.

5. Medicine has made great strides in diagnosing and treating heart disease. Diagnostic techniques include EKG monitoring and coronary angiography. Treatment interventions include medications for controlling blood pressure, cholesterol level, and preventing blood clots and cardiac surgery in the form of coronary artery bypass grafts and balloon angioplasty.

Risk Factors for Cardiovascular Disease

6. The Framingham Heart Study, a prospective study of cardiovascular disease that has collected data for over half a century, has identified a number of coronary risk factors.

7. The uncontrollable risk factors for CVD include family history of heart disease, age, gender, and ethnicity. The risk of cardiovascular disease increases with age, is much higher among men than women, and varies across racial and ethnic groups. Economic and social factors have been suggested as the cause of racial and ethnic variation in CVD.

8. The major controllable risk factors for CVD are hypertension, smoking, and elevated serum cholesterol. Most cases of high blood pressure are classified as essential hypertension, meaning that the exact cause is unknown.

9. Cholesterol levels that are too high promote the development of atherosclerosis; among men, extremely low cholesterol levels may be associated with increased mortality due to suicide and violent death.

Psychosocial Factors in Cardiovascular Disease

10. Characterized by a competitive, hurried, hostile nature, the Type A behavior pattern has been linked to increased risk of CVD. Researchers now point to hostility and anger as the toxic core of Type A behavior.

11. Several theoretical explanations have been proposed to explain the relationship between a hostile, angry personality and cardiovascular disease. The psychosocial vulnerability model maintains that hostile people have more stressful life events and low levels of social support, which, over time, have a toxic effect.

12. The health behavior model proposes that hostile people are more likely to develop cardiovascular disease because they tend to have poorer health habits than less hostile people.

13. The psychophysiological reactivity model maintains that frequent episodes of anger produce elevated cardiovascular and neuroendocrine responses that damage arteries and contribute to coronary disease.

14. Combining the insights of other models, the biopsychosocial (mind–body) model suggests that in order for CVD to develop, a person must first have a biological predisposition toward it. Whether or not CVD develops depends on a variety of psychosocial factors in the person's life, including stress, the availability of social support, and the person's temperament.

Reducing the Risk of Cardiovascular Disease

15. Lifestyle modifications can significantly reduce a person's risk of cardiovascular disease. Interventions for

hypertension include reducing weight, limiting salt and alcohol intake, and increasing exercise. Eating more fiber, fruits, vegetables, and grains and less cholesterol and saturated fat can reduce serum cholesterol levels and improve the ratio of HDL cholesterol to LDL cholesterol.

After CVD: Preventing Recurrences

16. Comprehensive interventions that combine stress management, aerobic exercise, relaxation training, and low-fat diets may even reverse the development of cardiovascular disease.

17. Interventions for hostility help people gain control of environmental triggers for their anger and learn to modify their negative emotions and cynical thought processes. Reducing hostility can substantially reduce the risk of future ischemia in cardiac patients.

Diabetes

18. Diabetes mellitus is a chronic disease in which the body is unable to produce or properly use the hormone in-sulin. Diabetes can develop in either childhood (Type I) or adulthood (Type II), with Type I diabetes generally involving more serious health complications and the need for daily insulin injections. Many individuals with diabetes also benefit from lifestyle modifications that include a strict regimen of diet and exercise.

19. Health psychology's role in diabetes has included studying factors in adjusting to the disease, such as psychological distress, personal coping skills, and social support, as well as factors that affect compliance with treatment regimens. Many individuals with diabetes also suffer from psychological disorders, including major depression, anxiety, and eating disorders.

20. Health psychologists are increasingly becoming involved in the primary care of diabetes, assisting those with diabetes with interventions aimed at promoting adjustment to the disease through reducing illness intrusiveness, increasing weight control and stress management, enhancing communication, and increasing compliance with complex treatment regimens.

Key Terms and Concepts

cardiovascular disease (CVD), p. 368
coronary heart disease (CHD), p. 369
atherosclerosis, p. 369
arteriosclerosis, p. 370
angina pectoris, p. 370
myocardial infarction (MI), p. 371
stroke, p. 371

electrocardiogram (ECG or EKG), p. 371
coronary angiography, p. 372
coronary artery bypass graft (CABG), p. 373
coronary angioplasty, p. 373
hypertension, p. 380
cardiovascular reactivity (CVR), p. 381

hypercholesterolemia, p. 382
Type A, p. 387
Type B, p. 387
diabetes mellitus, p. 401
illness intrusiveness, p. 405

Health Psychology on the World Wide Web

Web Address	Description
http://www.amhrt.org/	Web site of the American Heart Association.
http://www.heartinfo.com	Heart Information Network.
http://www.diabetes.org	Web site of the American Diabetes Association.
http://www.cdc.gov/diabetes/	The Centers for Disease Control and Prevention's Web resources for diabetes.
http://www.nhlbi.nih.gov/index.htm	The National Heart, Blood, and Lung Institute Web site has information on a number of heart-related issues, including links to African-American cardiovascular health resources.

Web Address	Description
http://www.healthnet.org/programs/procor	Information relating to cardiovascular health in the developing world.

Critical Thinking Exercise

Hostility, Depression, and Heart Disease

Now that you have completed Chapter 9, take your learning a step further by testing your critical thinking skills on the following practical problem-solving exercise.

Although everyone feels angry from time to time, when everyday anger turns destructive, it can have a variety of unhealthy effects. In addition to reducing the overall quality of your life, uncontrolled anger can damage relationships and make you feel as though you're at the mercy of an unpredictable force.

Hostility and anger may also directly affect the health of your heart. In a recent study, Duke University researchers asked patients with *ischemia* to wear wireless heart monitors for 48 hours. The patients were also asked to keep a diary of their emotions—sadness, tension, frustration, happiness, and feeling in control—during the same time period. The researchers found that patients who had stressful feelings were twice as likely to have a bout of ischemic pain an hour later as patients who didn't have stressful feelings.

In another, long-term prospective study of medical students at Johns Hopkins University, researchers found that those experiencing depression were, on average, twice as likely to develop cardiovascular disease or suffer a heart attack 15 years later. Other studies examining the effects of depression on the heart have found that people who already have heart disease are up to eight times more likely to develop *ventricular tachycardia*—a dangerous heart arrhythmia—than heart disease patients who are not depressed.

The effect of positive emotions on the heart is also a subject of research. One ongoing study at the Institute of Heart-Math has reported that feelings of love and gratitude in coronary patients may actually make the beating of the heart more uniform and consistent. This change is similar to the "relaxation response"—a state that is physiologically the opposite of the "fight-or-flight" response, in which blood pressure is reduced and blood flow is increased to the heart.

The American Psychological Association's Web site includes an outstanding series of essays called "Psychology and Everyday Life," which offers solid, direct advice based on the latest research on hostility and the heart. It also discusses strategies for anger management, such as cognitive restructuring. As part of this exercise, check out this information at the following Web address and then prepare answers to the questions that follow:

http://www.apa.org/pubinfo/anger.html

1. In what ways is anger like other emotions? In what ways is anger unique?

2. What are the common triggers of anger? How often does a typical person become angry? Who tends to become angry more often?

3. What do researchers believe to be the causes of an "anger-prone" temperament? (In your answer, be sure to touch specifically on biological, social, and psychological factors in anger.)

4. Researchers believe that hostility is one of several emotions that force the heart to work overtime and, over time, may promote the development of heart disease. For example, hostility may increase blood clotting and the levels of sugar and fats in the blood. Physiologically, what other emotion-induced changes may account for this relationship between hostility and heart disease?

5. How can cognitive restructuring be used to help anger-prone individuals gain control of their anger? What are several other strategies for keeping anger and hostility under control?

10 Cancer

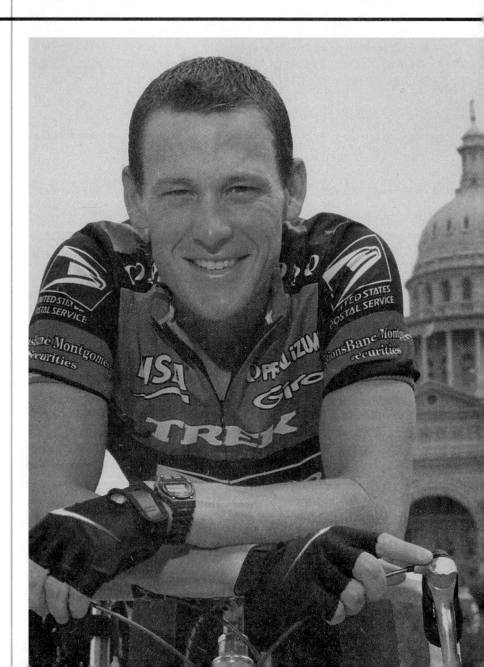

A thletes learn to live with aches and pains, so professional cyclist Lance Armstrong wasn't worried when his right testicle became swollen. He was riding well and winning races, and so he wrote it off as some "physiological male thing," or a minor injury from sitting on an unpadded bike saddle day after day. When his testicle swelled to 3 times its normal size and he began coughing up blood, he agreed to have a checkup. The immediate diagnosis was testicular cancer. The news went from bad to worse when additional tests revealed that the cancer had already spread to his lungs and his brain. When a childhood friend asked what Lance's chances were, a doctor told him "Well, your friend is dead."*

Lance chose not to believe this dismal prognosis. With the help of his mother, teammates, and friends, he began to attack his cancer with the same focus and fierce competitive spirit he used in bike races. He became a student of cancer, absorbing every relevant book, magazine, and journal article he could find. At every turn he made informed choices that bolstered his confidence in his treatment as well as his sense of control over what was happening to his body. So, instead of the standard radiation therapy for brain tumors, Lance chose surgery because it was less likely to affect his central nervous system and balance on a bicycle. He also elected to undergo four cycles of the most aggressive, 5-day-a-week regimen of chemotherapy (treating cancer with chemicals).

The treatment was a mighty struggle, as he kept losing weight no matter how much he ate. Moreover, he always felt weak, and he couldn't shake his fatigue, despite sleeping more than ever. However, he refused to stay in bed. "Do you have a gym here?" he asked a disbelieving nurse, who arranged access to a stationary bike.

A few weeks after completing treatment, Armstrong received a clean bill of health and set out to resume his life as a professional athlete. This too proved to be a struggle. "I was physically recovered but my soul was still healing. I was entering a phase called survivorship." And that he did! Four years later, Lance had won the Tour de France (a 3-week, 2,290-mile bike race that many consider the most grueling sporting event in the world) three times. Along the way, he passed the 5-year milestone of being cancer-free, met the love of his life, and started a family. Today, Lance says that cancer was "the best thing that ever happened to me . . . it forced me to survey my life with an unforgiving eye. . . . I don't know why I got the illness, but it did wonders for me, and I wouldn't want to walk away from it. Why would I want to change, even for a day, the most important and shaping event in my life?"

Although Lance Armstrong's story is inspirational, not all sufferers of life-threatening chronic diseases such as cancer cope in such a positive, constructive manner. Nor is every victim able to mobilize the social support of family and friends. And, of course, not every type of cancer can be cured. This chapter will examine the various biological, psychological, and social processes that influence a person's risk of developing cancer and the course of the disease once it gets started. We will also look at the various biomedical, psychosocial, and alternative treatment regimens that are available and the ways in which people cope with the disease. Although many types of cancer are life threatening, the good news is that in many cases, it can be controlled, even cured, especially when detected early.

---

*All quotes from Armstrong, L. (with Sally Jenkins). (2000). *It's not about the bike: My journey back to life.* New York: Putnam.

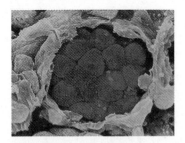

A Malignant Tumor
This scanning electron micrograph shows a tiny lung tumor (center) filling an alveolus (one of the air sacs that make up the lungs). The individual cancer cells are coated with microscopic, hair-like structures known as microvilli. © Moredun Animal Health Ltd/Science Photo Library/ Photo Researchers, Inc.

▩ **cancer** a set of diseases in which abnormal body cells multiply and spread in uncontrolled fashion forming a tissue mass called a tumor

▩ **metastasis** the process by which malignant body cells proliferate in number and spread to surrounding body tissues

▩ **carcinoma** cancer of the epithelial cells that line the outer and inner surfaces of the body; includes breast, prostate, lung, and skin cancer

▩ **sarcoma** cancer that strikes muscles, bones, and cartilage

▩ **lymphoma** cancer of the body's lymph system; includes Hodgkin's disease and non-Hodgkin's lymphoma

▩ **leukemia** cancer of the blood and blood-producing system

What Is Cancer?

The second leading cause of death in the United States, **cancer** is not one disease but a set of more than 100 related diseases in which abnormal body cells multiply and spread in uncontrolled fashion forming a tissue mass called a *tumor*.

Not all tumors are cancerous. *Benign* (noncancerous) tumors tend to remain localized and usually do not pose a serious threat to health. In contrast, *malignant* (cancerous) tumors consist of renegade cells that do not respond to the body's genetic controls on growth and division. To make matters worse, malignant cells often have the ability to migrate from their site of origin and attack, invade, and destroy surrounding body tissues. If this process of **metastasis** is not stopped, body organs and systems may be damaged, and death may result. Although some malignant cells remain as localized tumors and do not automatically spread, they do pose a threat to health and should be surgically removed.

Types of Cancer

Most of the more than 250 types of cancers can be classified as one of four types:

- **Carcinomas** attack the *epithelial cells* that line the outer and inner surfaces of the body. The most common type of cancer, carcinomas account for approximately 85 percent of all adult cancers. They include cancer of the breast, prostate, colon, lungs, pancreas, and skin. Affecting one out of every six people in the United States, skin cancer is the most common (and most rapidly increasing) type of cancer in America (Greenlee, Hill-Harmon, Murray, & Thun, 2001).

- **Sarcomas** are malignancies of cells in muscles, bones, and cartilage. Much rarer than carcinoma, sarcomas account for only about 2 percent of all cancers in adults.

- **Lymphomas** are cancers that form in the lymphatic system. Included in this group are *Hodgkin's disease,* a rare form of lymphoma that spreads from a single lymph node, and *non-Hodgkin's lymphoma,* in which malignant cells are found at several sites. Approximately 60,000 new cases of lymphoma are diagnosed each year, of which 90 percent are non-Hodgkin's lymphoma.

- **Leukemias** are cancers that attack the blood and blood-forming tissues, such as the bone marrow. Leukemia leads to a proliferation of white blood cells in the bloodstream and bone marrow, which impair the immune system. Although often considered a childhood disease, leukemia strikes far more adults (an estimated 25,000 cases per year) than children (about 3,000 cases per year).

Figure 10.1

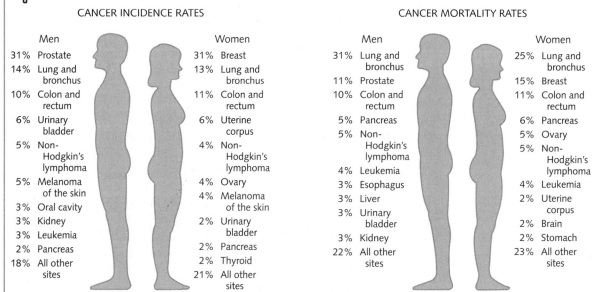

Estimated New Cancer Cases and Deaths by Type and Gender, 2001
Although the breasts in women and the prostate in men are the leading sites of new cases of cancer (left), lung cancer continues to be the leading cause of cancer deaths in both men and women (right).

Source: "Cancer Statistics, 2001," by R. T. Greenlee, M. B. Hill-Harmon, T. Murray, & M. Thun, 2001, *CA, A Cancer Journal for Clinicians, 51*, 15–36.

Cancer Susceptibility

The question of who is likely to get cancer is a difficult one. There are many types of cancer—from breast cancer to skin cancer to leukemia—and many individual factors, such as gender, age, and ethnic background, that affect susceptibility. For example, although overall a higher percentage of men (43.48 percent) develop cancer than women (38.34 percent), women are more likely to develop any cancer before age 60. As Figure 10.1 shows, although women are more commonly diagnosed with breast cancer and men with prostate cancer, lung cancer is the top killer of both genders (Greenlee et al., 2001). Whether and where cancer strikes also vary with age. As is true for many other chronic diseases, the older people become, the greater their chances of developing and dying of cancer. But in the United States cancer is also the second leading cause of death (after accidents) among children between 1 and 14 years of age. The most common cancers in this age group are leukemias, tumors of the nervous system, lymphomas, soft-tissue sarcomas, and tumors of the kidney (Greenlee et al., 2001). In young adults between 15 and 34 years of age, the leading sites of cancer are somewhat different in men and women. For women in this age group they are breast, cervix (uterus), and brain cancer as well as leukemia and non-Hodgkin's lymphoma. For men in this age group they are brain, colon and rectum, and soft-tissue cancer as well as leukemia and non-Hodgkin's lymphoma.

Variations in the distribution of cancers by race and ethnicity add to the complexity of cancer's epidemiology. For instance, African-Americans have the highest *incidence rates* for cancer overall—60 percent greater risk than Hispanic-Americans and Asian-Americans—primarily because of high rates of lung and prostate cancer among men. Between 1990 and 1997, cancer incidence rates decreased slightly among European Americans, Hispanic-Americans, and Native Americans, while remaining relatively stable among African-Americans and Asian/Pacific Islander Americans (Ries et al., 2000).

Not only are African-Americans more likely to develop cancer, they are also about 33 percent more likely to die of the disease than are European Americans, and more than twice as likely to die of cancer as Asian/Pacific Islanders, Native Americans, and Hispanic-Americans. Between 1990 and 1997, cancer *mortality rates* decreased significantly among European Americans, African-Americans, and Hispanic-Americans, while remaining relatively stable among Asian/Pacific Islanders and perhaps increasing among Native Americans (Ries et al., 2000).

As we noted in Chapter 1, several variables contribute to ethnic differences in chronic disease incidence and mortality, and cancer is no exception. Among these variables are socioeconomic status, knowledge about a specific disease and its treatment, and attitudes toward the disease. Many researchers believe that these factors affect access to health care and compliance with medical advice and, in doing so, contribute to the differences in cancer rates among ethnic groups (Meyerowitz, Richardson, Hudson, & Leedham, 1998). As we have seen, access and compliance are linked to numerous health behaviors that influence disease vulnerability and survival time once the disease process begins.

If we look at specific cancers, the picture becomes somewhat clearer. Consider breast cancer. Although white women are more likely to develop breast cancer than African-American women, African-American women are more likely to die of the disease. There are two possible reasons for this. First, African-American women historically have been less likely to perform regular breast self-examination and to obtain mammograms (a form of x-ray that allows for early detection of breast cancer), the two most effective means of early detection (Murray, 1999). Things are changing, however. The latest estimates of mammography screening among adult women in the United States show that health education campaigns are beginning to pay off: A higher percentage of African-American women have had a mammogram within the past 2 years than their European American counterparts (American Cancer Society, 2001).

A second reason for ethnic and racial differences in breast cancer is that African-Americans and other minorities tend to have less access to health insurance and health care facilities and greater distrust of the medical establishment, which may be perceived as insensitive and even racist. For these reasons, they are less likely to receive regular screenings that could improve their chances of surviving the cancer. This explains why cancer of all types is generally diagnosed in later (usually more serious) stages in African-Americans than it is in white Americans.

Ethnic differences in diet, tobacco use, and other risk factors for cancer also play a role in group differences in mortality rates. For example, African-Americans tend to smoke more and consume fattier diets than other Americans, two behaviors implicated in many forms of cancer. As another example, although Asian-Americans have lower all-cause mortality rates than white Americans, their mortality rates for stomach cancer—which is strongly influenced by diet—are much higher (Greenlee et al., 2001).

Another factor in the higher cancer mortality rates among African-American men and women is a poorer prognosis once diagnosed. African-Americans are *less* likely than European Americans to be diagnosed with cancer at a localized (nonmetastasized) stage, when the disease generally is more easily and successfully treated. Furthermore, African-Americans have lower 5-year relative survival rates than European Americans for most cancers *at every stage of diagnosis* (Greenlee et al., 2001).

Are We Winning the Battle against Cancer?

Although researchers have been successful in learning how to prevent, and even cure, some forms of cancer, the disease continues to increase in incidence and prevalence throughout the world (see Figure 10.2 on page 418). This increase is due in part to improved methods of diagnosis and more widespread efforts at early detection. Cancer mortality rates have also been steadily increasing in the United States throughout this century, rising from 64 out of every 100,000 Americans in 1900 to 200 out of every 100,000 at the end of the twentieth century (National Center for Health Statistics, 2000). What accounts for this discouraging trend? Are we losing the battle against cancer?

Many possible reasons have been offered for the rise in cancer mortality. The first is based on somewhat positive achievements. Because other chronic diseases, especially cardiovascular disease, have declined, people are living longer. However, since the risk of cancer increases with age, these longer-living people are more likely to die from this disease.

Other reasons for the increase in cancer mortality are less encouraging. Among these are a dramatic increase in cancers stemming from AIDS (see Chapter 11); an increase in exposure to the sun, pesticides, and other environmental **carcinogens** (agents that cause cancer); and the ever-increasing rise in smoking-related deaths, especially among women (Leiss & Savitz, 1995).

Despite this dismal news, many experts see reasons for optimism about cancer trends. For one, some studies show that a person's chances of recovery from cancer have increased from 1 out of every 2 to 3 out of 5. Another reason is that among men and women under 55 years of age, cancer mortality is *decreasing*. It is only when people of all ages are grouped together that the

■ **carcinogen** a cancer-causing agent such as tobacco, ultraviolet radiation, or environmental toxin

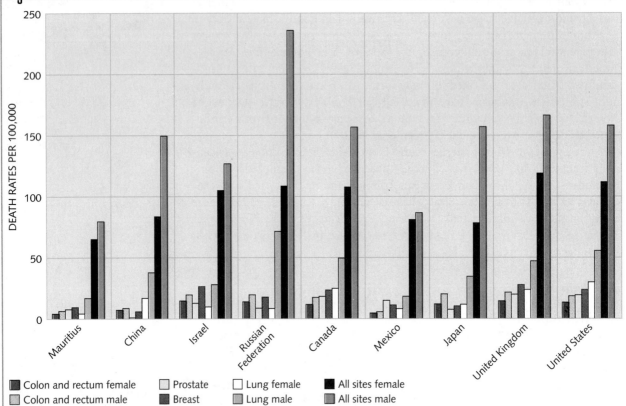

Cancer around the World for Selected Sites and Countries
As these age-adjusted death rates per 100,000 people reveal, there is considerable variation in the incidence of various types of cancer around the world. Considering all sites
combined, for example, incidence rates among men vary from as high as 237 per
100,000 in the Russian Federation to as low as 80 per 100,000 in the African nation of
Mauritius. Throughout the world, women have lower rates of cancer than men when all
sites are combined. This gender disparity, however, is much larger in some countries
(Japan, for instance) than others (for example, Mexico).
Source: Mortality Database. World Health Organization, 1999 (www.who.int/whosis/mortl).

increase in mortality is apparent. Much of the decrease is due to the large
number of men who have quit smoking—death rates among men are dropping more rapidly than for women, who have been slower to quit and whose
lung cancer morbidity continues to rise (Greenlee et al., 2001).

Finally, the optimism of health experts is based on the knowledge that
something can now be done to prevent or, if needed, treat many forms of
cancer. For example, researchers continue to find that the causes of most
cancers are avoidable. In fact, almost all of the increase in cancer mortality

rates since 1950 can be attributed to an increase in the rate of lung cancer, whose cause is most frequently related to lifestyle. And for those who are stricken, more than ever before, a cure may be possible. In 1900, very few people diagnosed with cancer survived more than a year or two. By the end of the century, the survival rate improved steadily so that today about half the individuals who are diagnosed with all types of cancer survive 5 years or longer (Greenlee et al., 2001). Several cancers that had grim prognoses only a few decades ago can often be cured today, including most skin cancers, testicular cancer, some forms of lymphoma, bone cancer, and kidney cancer and leukemia in children. Added to those who have been cured are millions more "survivors" than ever before—people who continue to battle their disease every day.

Most important, recent studies indicate that lifestyle changes and improved detection have contributed to declines in the rates of new cancer cases, which will eventually lead to reduced mortality rates. A report jointly issued by the National Cancer Institute, the Centers for Disease Control, and the American Cancer Society indicates that the overall cancer incidence rate—the number of new cases per 100,000 people per year for all cancers combined—declined an average 0.8 percent per year between 1990 and 1999 (Ries et al., 2000). The incidence of newly diagnosed cancers among African-Americans also fell during this period, reversing a 20-year trend.

What Causes Cancer?

Despite the enormous variation in cancer by site, gender, age, and ethnicity, a number of general theories of how all forms of cancer begin have been advanced. The theories share the common belief that cancer begins as a result of a virus or a genetic mutation. In some individuals, the disease process is then advanced by genetic, immune, behavioral, and/or psychosocial factors that cause the abnormal cells to proliferate until a tumor develops.

Viruses and Genetic Mutations

As with many human diseases, viruses cause some types of cancer. Beginning with the 1910 discovery that a sarcoma in chickens is caused by an airborne virus that is transmitted from bird to bird, researchers began a massive search for cancer-causing human viruses. Although at least five known forms of cancer are attributed to viruses, they account for only about 15 percent of all human cancers (Purves & Orians, 2000). Most cancers are caused by genetic mutations that gradually accumulate over a period of years. This is why most cancers develop in older people.

mutagen a substance such as a carcinogen that causes mutations in a cell's genetic code

oncogenes genes that stimulate cellular growth and division

suppressor genes genes that prevent the proliferation of malignant cells by acting as a brake on cellular growth and division

At least two lines of evidence link cancer with genetic mutations. First, cancer is an inherited property of cells. Once a cancer cell begins multiplying, all its daughter cells are also cancerous. Second, most carcinogens such as x-rays, pesticides, tobacco smoke, and food chemicals are also **mutagens** (agents that cause mutations to a cell's genetic code).

Most researchers believe that repeatedly exposing parts of the body to environmental carcinogens can trigger mutations. Of the more than 100 trillion cells that make up an adult human, certain ones must divide, at just the right time, for the individual to remain healthy. Normally, cells divide only when the genes on the cell's DNA instruct them to do so. These instructions are subject to a careful system of genetic checks and balances that ensure that each of the body's organs and tissues maintains a size that is appropriate for the body's overall well-being. When the DNA is damaged, faulty processes occur in the genes that normally regulate when and how rapidly new cells are produced. **Oncogenes** (from the Greek word *onkos*, meaning "mass," as in a tumor) stimulate cellular growth and division. In contrast, **suppressor genes** act as brakes on cell division, preventing the runaway proliferation of cells and the development of tumors.

As long as oncogenes and suppressor genes function normally, there is a precise balance between the growth-promoting and growth-inhibiting processes in the cell. But when either gene is disabled by a mutation, the cell's reproductive processes can begin to spin out of control. In cancerous cells, activated oncogenes force an overproduction of growth factors while the inhibitory messages of suppressor genes are absent because the suppressor gene is inactive (Weinberg, 1996). Like a speeding locomotive with a stuck throttle and no engineer to pull the brakes, this runaway cell division leads to a malignant tumor.

Because most cancers develop slowly, biomedical researchers have been able to precisely map the oncogenes and suppressor genes that malfunction at each stage in certain cancers.

The "Two-Hit" Hypothesis

Most cancers arise when a cell accumulates a number of genetic mutations, usually over a period of many years, even decades. Eventually, the abnormal cell no longer responds to genetic controls on growth and reproduction. As the cancerous cells appear in increasing numbers, a tumor is formed.

The "throttle" and "brake" analogy for oncogenes and suppressor genes, respectively, is somewhat oversimplified. This is because there are many oncogenes and suppressor genes, only some (or none) of which may be active at a given time in a given cell. To further complicate matters, about 10 percent of all cancers are clearly inherited. Some people are born with genetic mutations that directly promote excessive growth in certain cells (Trichopoulous, Li, &

Figure 10.3

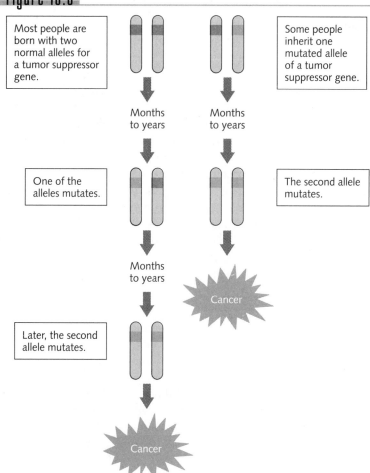

Most people are born with two normal alleles for a tumor suppressor gene.

Months to years

One of the alleles mutates.

Months to years

Later, the second allele mutates.

Cancer

Some people inherit one mutated allele of a tumor suppressor gene.

Months to years

The second allele mutates.

Cancer

The "Two-Hit" Hypothesis
Two copies of a mutation are normally needed to deactivate a tumor suppressor gene. People with an inherited predisposition are born with one copy (allele) already mutated, and so need only one other mutated gene to develop cancer.

Hunter, 1996). Such cases are extremely rare, however, accounting for perhaps 5 percent of cancer deaths. Far more common are general inherited traits such as fair skin, which increases susceptibility to skin cancer, or a physiological inefficiency in the way the body eliminates certain carcinogens.

Most people are born with two normal copies (*alleles*) of each gene, including suppressor genes. In inherited cancer, people are born with one mutated copy of a suppressor gene. Compared to those who inherit two normal copies of the gene, they are at greater risk of developing the malignancy regulated by this particular gene because only one additional mutation must occur. In contrast, a person with no family history of cancer must have two mutations before the malignancy develops. This "two-hit" hypothesis, which is outlined in Figure 10.3, explains why inherited cancers tend to strike much earlier in life.

■ **immunocompetence** the overall ability of the immune system, at any given time, to defend the body against the harmful effects of foreign agents

■ **immune surveillance theory** the theory that cells of the immune system play a monitoring function in searching for and destroying abnormal cells such as those that form tumors

Stress, Immunocompetence, and Cancer

With recent advances in *psychoneuroimmunology* (PNI), researchers are paying more attention to psychological factors—in particular, the role of stress—in the development of cancer. As you'll recall from Chapter 4, PNI researchers study the relationships among the mind, the body, and immunity (Overmier & Gahtan, 1998). **Immunocompetence**—the immune system's ability, at any given time, to mount an effective defense against disease and the harmful effects of foreign agents—depends on many factors, including the individual's overall health, the nature of the health-threatening disease or foreign agent, and the presence of stress.

The most commonly measured components of the immune system are the immune cells, the leukocytes or white blood cells (see Chapter 3, page 107), which work collectively to mount a response against "non-self" (external) invaders. Researchers are able to measure the levels of T cells, B cells, and NK (natural killer) cells in the body by collecting blood or saliva samples. They are also able to measure the strength of immune functioning by analyzing the effectiveness of these cells in attacking tumors or antigens.

How Stress Affects Immunity

How might stressful events promote the development of cancer? According to the **immune surveillance theory,** cancer cells, which develop spontaneously in the body, are prevented from spreading and developing into tumors by NK cells and other agents of the immune system. In other words, immune cells constantly patrol the body for abnormal cells, which they hunt down and kill. However, when the immune system is overwhelmed by the number of cancer cells or weakened by stress or some other factor, the immune system's surveillance system is suppressed and cancer may develop (Holland & Lewis, 1996).

Research has generally supported the immune surveillance theory. For example, mice who were exposed to stressful light conditions had significantly higher rates of tumors than a control group. That is, nearly 80 percent of the mice exposed to the stressful, flashing light developed tumors. Tumor growth in the other mice occurred more slowly and in fewer animals.

Research has also found that stress affects specific immune cells. Research has generally supported the immune surveillance theory. For example, studies have found that women with breast cancer typically have lower T and NK cell counts and activity levels than healthy women. Lower levels of immune activity are also linked to decreased cancer survival times, as well as to greater (and faster) cancer recurrence (Delahanty & Baum, 2001).

In humans, stressful events—excessive exercise, exams, divorce, bereavement, caring for a terminally ill relative, environmental catastrophes, unemployment, and occupational stress, for example—have been shown to affect immune functioning (Herbert & Cohen, 1993). Like the rats, humans show reduced activity of key immune cells—including NK cells and T cells—when confronted with such chronic stressors. For example, in one study, medical students exhibited a weakened immune response—reduced NK cell activity, alterations in T cell populations, and decreased *cytokine* production—during exam periods (Kiecolt-Glaser et al., 1986). Cytokines are hormonelike substances released by lymphocytes that instruct NK cells and cytotoxic T cells to kill tumor cells. The most extreme effects were observed in students with the highest levels of overall life stress, loneliness, or a tendency to overreact to stressful events (Kiecolt-Glaser et al., 1984; Workman & La Via, 1987).

Like exams and catastrophic events, stressful relationships can also take a toll on immune functioning. In one study, recently separated or divorced women and men had lower percentages of circulating NK and helper T cells than a comparison group of married persons (Kiecolt-Glaser & Glaser, 1989). Among married couples, chronic marital conflict has been linked to higher levels of distress and weakened antibody response (Malarkey, Kiecolt-Glaser, Pearl, & Glaser, 1994). Even loving relationships can become stressful and adversely affect immune functioning, as when a person is responsible for the long-term care of an elderly or sick relative. For instance, Janice Kiecolt-Glaser and her colleagues have found lower percentages of total lymphocytes and helper T cells and higher levels of the antibodies for various viruses in people who care for a relative with Alzheimer's disease (Kiecolt-Glaser, Dura, Speicher, Trask, & Glaser, 1991).

Researchers have also studied the effects on immune function of short-term stressors but have not found that they cause any long-term damage. Generally, stresses caused by challenging computer tasks, mental arithmetic, electric shock, and loud noise produce increases in the numbers of circulating NK cells and a decrease in the ratio of helper T to suppressor T cells. However, the response to stress is rapid, occurring as soon as 5 minutes after the onset of stress (Herbert & Cohen, 1994), and, in most cases, the cells return to prestress levels within 15 minutes after the stressor has ended.

Stress and DNA Repair

Prolonged stress also might promote cancer by impairing the body's ability to repair errors that take place during cell division. DNA must be accurately replicated with every cell division. The price of errors can be great—malignancies, even death.

Fortunately, although DNA replication is not perfectly accurate and the DNA of nondividing cells may be damaged by environmental agents, cells normally have DNA repair mechanisms that "proofread" each replication and correct any errors they detect. In one such mechanism, an enzyme removes mismatched chemical bases in the genetic code and replaces them with correct matches. When this mismatch repair system is not working properly, people become susceptible to a variety of diseases, including the skin disease *xeroderma pigmentosum*. Those who suffer from this disease lack the mechanism that normally repairs damage caused by ultraviolet radiation, and thus exposure to sunlight nearly always triggers skin cancer (Purves & Orians, 2000).

This repair system may be impaired by several factors, one of which is persistent or extreme stress. In one study, two groups of rats were exposed to a chemical carcinogen in their food. One group was subjected to an acute environmental stressor and, compared to unstressed control animals, the stressed rats showed significantly reduced levels of the enzyme that removes the mismatches (Glaser et al., 1985).

In summary, although there is a growing body of evidence that various types of stress trigger immune changes, researchers have not yet identified at precisely which point these changes increase disease susceptibility. Indeed, immune responses of stressed persons generally fall within normal ranges (Bachen, Cohen, & Marsland, 1997).

When disease does strike a stressed person, it is possible that such factors as age, family history, and the presence of an already compromised immune system (as occurs in autoimmune disorders) might be interacting with stress and immune response to determine health outcome. For example, we know that immune functioning declines with age—as indicated by decreases in NK cell activity and antibody production—and so stress would naturally have more significant consequences for an older person with an already compromised immune system.

Risk Factors for Cancer

It is interesting to speculate about the number of cancer cases that would arise naturally in a population of otherwise healthy people who completely avoided all environmental carcinogens. By one estimate, epidemiologists suggest that less than 25 percent of all cancers would develop anyway as a result of uncontrollable genetic and biological processes (Trichopoulos et al., 1996). In most cases of cancer, controllable factors such as smoking and diet play the most important role.

This section examines a number of risk factors for cancer. Although risk factors increase a person's chance of developing cancer, not every person with those risk factors will develop the disease. Many people with one or more risk factors never develop cancer, whereas others who develop the disease have no known risk factors (see Reality Check).

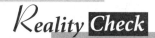 *Measuring Your Risk of Cancer*

Although health experts have not yet been able to write an equation that accurately predicts who is most likely to develop specific cancers, they have identified a number of lifestyle and background factors that are correlated with increased risk. To get a rough estimate of the magnitude of these factors in your risk profile, answer "yes" or "no" to the following American Cancer Society questions.

___ 1. Has a member of your immediate family had cancer, excluding basal and squamous skin cancers?

___ 2. Do you or does any member of your immediate family have a history of pre-cancerous growths?

___ 3. Are you 45 years of age or older?

___ 4. Do you currently smoke or use other tobacco products, such as smokeless tobacco or snuff? Or are you a former smoker, having smoked regularly for at least a year or more?

___ 5. Are you overweight?

___ 6. Do you drink two or more alcoholic drinks daily?

___ 7. Have you had a history of severe sunburns, even back in childhood? Do you enjoy sunbathing and often sunbathe without sunscreen lotion?

___ 8. Do you watch your fat intake, making sure not to consume more than 30 percent of your total caloric intake in the form of dietary fat?

___ 9. Do you follow a diet rich in fruits, vegetables, and dietary fiber?

___ 10. Do you generally avoid foods that are smoke-, nitrite-, or salt-cured?

___ 11. Do you limit your alcohol intake to fewer than two drinks per day?

___ 12. Do you use sunscreen protection (SPF value of 15 or higher) when you go out in the direct sun for longer than a few minutes?

___ 13. Do you protect your skin from overexposure to the sun by wearing protective clothing?

___ 14. Do you avoid use of all tobacco products?

___ 15. Do you exercise regularly and take generally good care of your health?

___ 16. Do you get regular health checkups and follow recommended cancer screening guidelines, given your age and family history, such as Pap smears, prostate cancer screening tests, clinical breast exams and mammography, and digital rectal exams?

___ 17. If you are a woman, do you regularly examine your breasts for lumps? If you are a man, do you regularly examine your testicles for lumps?

___ 18. Do you limit your exposure to environmental hazards such as asbestos, radiation, and toxic chemicals?

___ 19. Do you avoid tanning salons and home sunlamps?

___ 20. Is your diet rich in sources of essential vitamins and minerals?

Scoring: "Yes" answers to questions 1–7 are associated with an increased cancer risk. "Yes" answers to questions 8–20 are associated with a lower cancer risk. Although no particular score translates into a precise risk estimate, the more "yes" answers to questions 1–7 and the fewer "yes" answers to questions 8–20, the greater your overall cancer risk. Examine your responses carefully and ask yourself which risk factors you can change to help improve your chances of remaining cancer-free.

The National Cancer Institute offers software, called the "breast cancer risk tool," to estimate a woman's personal risk of developing breast cancer, first within the next 5 years, and then over the course of a lifetime. The program bases its estimates on six questions: a woman's age, the age at which she began menstruating, the age at which she gave birth to her first child, the number of breast cancers in her mother and sisters, the number of breast biopsies she has had, the biopsy results, and the woman's race. The software can be obtained by calling (800) 4-CANCER or from the institute's Web site at http://cissecure.nci.nih.gov/ncipub/subjects.asp (then click on "breast").

Tobacco Use

As you'll recall from Chapter 8, smoking is the most preventable cause of death in our society. The American Cancer Society estimates that in 2000 about one in every five deaths in the United States was caused by tobacco use.

Of these, 175,000 were the result of cancer, making tobacco the single most lethal carcinogen in this country (American Cancer Society, 2001).

Smoking is responsible for nearly 90 percent of lung cancers. (Recall that benzo[*a*]pyrene [BPDE], a chemical in cigarette smoke, has been identified as a causative agent in lung cancer. BPDE damages a cancer suppressor gene, causing a mutation of lung tissue.) For male smokers, lung cancer mortality rates are about 23 times higher than those of nonsmokers; for women, the rates are 13 times higher (American Cancer Society, 2001). For unknown reasons, female smokers are more likely than male smokers to develop lung cancer (The Society for the Advancement of Women's Health Research, 1998).

Especially troubling is what appears to be an epidemic of lung cancer in women (Brody, 1998b). In 1964, when the Surgeon General's first report on the hazards of smoking was published, men were six times as likely as women to die of lung cancer. Today, the American Cancer Society estimates that each year 67,000 women will be diagnosed with lung cancer, just 26,100 fewer women than men. Looked at another way, women today have a five times greater incidence of smoking-related cancer than women born at the turn of the twentieth century.

Smoking is also linked to cancers of the mouth, pharynx, larynx, esophagus, pancreas, uterine cervix, kidney, and bladder. In addition, there is mounting evidence that smoking may contribute to breast cancer, a cause of great concern considering the recent rise in smoking rates among women. In one prospective study that followed healthy women over a 6-year period, researchers found that women who smoked were 1.26 times more likely to die of breast cancer than were women who had never smoked. Among those who smoked two packs or more each day, the relative risk rose to 1.74, whereas those who smoked half a pack or less had a relative risk of only 1.19. In addition, women who started smoking before age 16 were 60 percent more likely to die from breast cancer than those who started after age 20 (Calle, Miracle-McMahill, Thun, & Heath, 1994).

As this study shows, whether smoking will result in malignancy depends on a number of factors, including the number of cigarettes smoked per day, the cigarettes' tar content, and, most important, the duration of the habit. Starting to smoke at a very young age multiplies the risk substantially.

Passive Smoking

Passive smoking, or environmental tobacco smoke (ETS), has significant health consequences for nonsmokers. Although constant exposure to ETS—in the workplace or at home—causes much less lung cancer than active smoking does, the Environmental Protection Agency estimates that about 3,000 lung cancer deaths occur each year in the United States due to passive smoking (Healthink, 2001). The most compelling evidence comes from the Nurses' Health Study, a prospective study of 121,701 women begun in 1976. All women were between age 35 and 55 years at the start of the study. They completed a baseline questionnaire in 1980, recording medical history, health behaviors (including hazards such as exposure to ETS), and subsequent questionnaires every 2 years, updating histories and behaviors. In a recent report, nurses who said they were regularly exposed to ETS had a 91 percent higher relative risk of a heart attack or death, compared to nurses who were not regularly subjected to smoke (Ishibe et al., 1998). Looked at another way, second-hand smoke is a risk factor on the order of outdoor air pollution or household exposure to the radioactive gas radon (Trichopoulous et al., 1996). These sobering statistics have launched numerous legislative efforts to ban smoking in public places.

Cigars and Smokeless Tobacco

In recent years, cigars, cigarillos, and smokeless tobacco have become increasingly popular. Especially trendy among younger adults is "dipping snuff." In this practice, tobacco is placed between the cheek and gum and nicotine (along with a number of other carcinogens) is absorbed through the tissue that lines the mouth. Nationwide, about 7 percent of men 18 to 24 years of age and about 20 percent of male high school students use smokeless tobacco (Shapiro, Jacobs, & Thun, 2000).

Many cigar aficionados and users of smokeless tobacco are not aware that these products contain the same deadly carcinogens as cigarettes. Neither is a safe substitute for cigarettes. Both lead to powerful dependence, addiction, and serious health consequences, including cancers. Oral cancer, for example, occurs much more frequently among users of smokeless tobacco and cigars than among those who do not use tobacco. In fact, compared with nontobacco users, cigar smokers have four to ten times the risk of dying from laryngeal, oral, or esophageal cancers. Likewise, men who smoke three or more cigars a day have a 7.8 times higher risk of lung cancer compared to nonsmokers; for men who inhale, the risk is 11 times higher (Shapiro et al., 2000).

Diet and Alcohol Use

Only diet rivals tobacco smoke as a cause of cancer, accounting for nearly the same number of deaths each year (Trichopoulous et al., 1996). Diet is a primary factor in as many as one-third of all cancer deaths (Brody, 1998c). A number of dietary factors can affect cancer risk, including the types of foods you eat, how the food is prepared, the size of your portions, whether you eat a balanced diet, and your overall caloric balance.

Although little is known about the mechanisms by which specific foods convey their health-related effects, we generally know which foods people should avoid and which they should eat in abundance if they want to minimize their risk of getting cancer. Foods to avoid are animal (saturated) fat in general

■ **carotenoids** light-absorbing pigments that give carrots, tomatoes, and other foods their color and are rich sources of antioxidant vitamins

and red meat in particular, which are linked to a number of specific cancers, including cancer of the colon, rectum, and prostate. Healthy foods include many vegetables, fruits, and legumes (such as beans and peas) and carbohydrates such as whole grains (brown rice and whole-wheat bread, as opposed to processed or refined "white" flours and grains). Good fats are unhydrogenated fats that come primarily from plant sources. Coffee (caffeinated or decaf) and some artificial sweeteners can be consumed in moderation.

Cancer-Causing Foods

The cancers that have been most directly been linked to foods are those that affect the cells that line bodily tissues, including those in the lungs, colon, bladder, stomach, and rectum, and, to a lesser degree, the uterus, prostate, breasts, and kidneys (Henderson et al., 1990; Whittemore et al., 1995). It comes as no surprise that these cancers are most prevalent in cultures noted for high-fat diets, such as the United States. The average American obtains an estimated 36 to 41 percent of his or her total calories from fats. (Recall from Chapter 7 that the recommended daily limit is no more than 30 percent of calories from fats.)

Evidence linking saturated fat to breast cancer is mixed. Cross-cultural studies have found that Japanese-American women are more likely to develop breast cancer when they live in the United States and consume a high-fat American diet (Wynder, Fujita, & Harris, 1991). The traditional soy-rich Asian diet may partially explain the normally low risk of breast, uterine, and other hormone-related cancers in Asian women. Soy products contain plant estrogens that enhance health when used in place of meats. On the other hand, data from the Nurses' Health Study, as well as a meta-analysis of research studies of more than 300,000 women, found *no* conclusive link between dietary fat and breast cancer (White, 1999). More research is needed before we can draw any definitive conclusions about the relationship between dietary fat and breast cancer.

Cancer-Fighting Foods

Foods that may play a protective role against some cancers do so by blocking carcinogenic processes in body cells. For example, *antioxidants* such as vitamins A and C may buffer against the cell-damaging activities of free radicals (see Chapter 3).

Especially beneficial are dark green, yellow, and orange vegetables that are rich in **carotenoids,** light-absorbing pigments found in certain plants. Carotenoids are responsible for the color of carrots, tomatoes, pumpkins, broccoli, cauliflower, brussels sprouts, citrus fruits, and strawberries. One carotenoid, *beta-carotene,* traps the light absorbed by plant leaves and is broken down by the body as a rich source of vitamin A. Vitamin A is essential in maintaining the health of the cells that line the lungs and stomach. Diets that include five to nine servings daily of foods that are rich in beta-carotene are linked to reduced risk of cancer of the lung, stomach, colon and rectum, and, to a smaller degree, the breasts, bladder, and pancreas. Cooked tomato products, which are rich in the carotenoid *lycopene,* may reduce the risk of prostate cancer (Brody, 1998c).

Other studies have found that diets rich in fruits, vegetables, and fiber may offer some protection against colon and rectal cancers, most likely because they promote rapid removal of cancer-causing wastes from the body (Steinmetz, Kushi, Bostick, Folsom, & Potter, 1994). In a massive study of Seventh-Day Adventists, George Fraser (1991) found that people who ate fruit at least twice a day had one-fourth the risk of developing lung cancer as those who ate fruit less than three times a week. Participants who ate fruit three to seven times each week had about one-third the risk of developing lung cancer.

Data from the Nurses' Health Study reveal that premenopausal women who consumed five or more servings per day of fruits and vegetables were 23 percent less likely to develop breast cancer than those who ate fewer than two servings per day (Zhang et al., 1999). Although this level of protection appears to be modest, we should remember that the link between obesity and breast cancer is very strong (see Chapter 7), and eating a lot of fruits and vegetables helps to maintain a healthy weight level.

Researchers are studying many other foods as possible weapons against cancer. Some have reported highly significant negative correlations (-0.75 in men and -0.67 in women) between fiber-rich cereal consumption and the incidence of colorectal cancer (Rosen, Nystrom, & Wall, 1988). Other protective foods include garlic, onions, and leeks (which contain a compound called *allium* that may protect against breast cancer), and *selenium*-rich foods such as fish, liver, garlic (garlic has both allium and selenium), eggs, and whole grains (which may reduce the risk of prostate cancer). The newest anticancer candidates are green tea, olive oil (which may reduce the risk of breast cancer when used to replace other fats), and foods rich in Vitamin D and calcium (which may reduce both breast and colon cancer). Table 10.1 on page 430 summarizes the sources of several anticancer food candidates and their possible benefits.

Alcohol

Although moderate consumption of alcoholic beverages may reduce the risk of cardiovascular disease (see Chapter 9), excessive drinking, especially among tobacco users, has been shown to be a major risk factor for cancer of the upper respiratory and digestive tracts. In addition, bacterial infections and immune-mediated skin disorders are more severe and frequent among heavy drinkers (Antony et al., 1993; Higgins & duVivier, 1994).

Alcohol may also contribute to breast, colorectal, and liver cancer. Women who consume two or more alcohol-containing drinks a day have at least a 25 percent greater risk of developing breast cancer than women who do not use

Table 10.1

Foods That May Prevent Cancer*

Substance	Source	Possible Health Benefit
Garlic	Garlic powder, cloves, supplements	May have antioxidant properties that protect against breast and stomach cancer
Flavonoids	Red wine, grapes, apples, cranberries	May reduce the risk of lung and colorectal cancer
Lycopene	Tomatoes, red peppers, watermelon	May have stronger antioxidant properties than beta-carotene that protect against several cancers, including prostate cancer
Beta-carotene	Dark yellow and orange fruits, leafy dark green vegetables, apricots, pumpkins, carrots, spinach, and squash	Associated with reduced risk of cancer of the lung, stomach, colon and rectum, and, to a smaller degree, the breasts, bladder, and pancreas
Selenium	Liver, mushrooms, garlic, fish	Believed to increase the antioxidant effects of vitamin E and protect against prostate cancer
Isoflavones	Beans, grains, soy products	May reduce the risk of breast and prostate cancer
Indoles	Cruciferous vegetables such as broccoli, brussels sprouts, and cabbage	May reduce the risk of several forms of cancer

*This table lists several dietary substances that *may have* anticancer properties. At present, however, none of these properties has been definitively supported by research. As further research is conducted, some of the substances may prove to be ineffective and/or dangerous when taken in high doses.

alcohol (Diez-Ruiz, et al., 1995). Alcohol-related cirrhosis is a frequent cause of liver cancer and may place the immune system in "overdrive," even when no threat (other than excessive alcohol) is present.

However, we must be cautious in drawing conclusions about alcohol and immunocompetence. This is because people who abuse alcohol may also suffer from poor nutrition and sleep deprivation and be exposed to other pathogens that may compromise their health.

Physical Activity

New research indicates that lack of physical activity may be a risk factor for certain cancers. One prospective study of men with colon cancer, men with rectal cancer, and healthy men found that the more sedentary a man's job, and the longer he had worked at that job, the greater his risk of colon cancer (Vena et al., 1985). More recently, researchers have similarly reported an inverse relationship between overall physical activity levels and the risk of colon cancer in both women and men (White, Jacobs, & Daling, 1996). These results suggest that a sedentary lifestyle is indeed a risk factor for colon cancer, one of the leading causes of cancer mortality.

Regular physical activity—either work-related or recreational—may also protect against breast cancer. For example, Suzanne Shoff and her colleagues found that physically active women who had lost weight since they were 18, or had gained only minimal amounts of weight, were only half as likely as their inactive counterparts to develop breast cancer after menopause (Shoff et al., 2000). A recent review of research studies investigating exercise and breast cancer reported reductions in breast cancer rates ranging from 12 percent to 60 percent among physically active women (Gammon, John, & Britton, 1998). The most compelling evidence comes from the Nurses' Health Study, which reported that women who exercised 7 hours or more per week were 20 percent less likely to develop breast cancer than women who exercised less than 1 hour per week (Rockhill et al., 1999). Walking, the most frequently reported exercise, was as effective in protecting against cancer as more strenuous forms of exercise. More important than exercise intensity in decreasing risk was a sustained history of exercising.

Family History

Although less than 5 percent of all cancers are inherited, genetic vulnerability can interact with other risk factors to increase an individual's risk of cancer (Ellenhorst-Ryan, 1997). For example, approximately one-third of the 175,000 women diagnosed with breast cancer each year in the United States have a family history of the disease, that is, are genetically vulnerable to the disease (Esplen, Toner, Hunter, Glendon, Butler, & Field, 1998). Evidence again comes from the Nurses' Health Study, which found that the daughters of women diagnosed with breast cancer before age 40 were more than twice as likely to develop breast cancer, as compared to women whose mothers had no history of the disease. The daughters of women with breast cancer after age 70 were one and a half times more likely to develop breast cancer. Participants who had a sister with breast cancer were more than twice as likely to develop this cancer themselves; when both mother *and* sister were diagnosed with breast cancer, the risk increased to two and a half times (Colditz et al., 1993).

The genetic predisposition toward breast cancer appears to be caused by mutations in one of two genes that are involved in repairing damage to cellular DNA: *BRCA1* (breast cancer gene 1) and *BRCA2* (breast cancer gene 2). As many as 500,000 women in the United States (from all sociocultural groups) are estimated to be **carriers** of one or both of these genes (that is, they have both a normal and a mutant form of a particular gene). Women who have mutations in these genes, causing them to malfunction, have a 56 percent to 87 percent lifetime chance of developing breast cancer (Mayo Clinic Health Oasis, 2000).

It is important to remember, however, that only a small percentage of all breast cancer cases are inherited. The vast majority (nearly 95 percent) are linked to a combination of genetic and nongenetic risk factors. In one massive study, researchers found that only 5.9 percent of the British women diagnosed with breast cancer before age 36 had a BRCA1 or BRCA2 mutation (Stratton,

carrier in genetics, a person who carries both a normal and a mutant version of a gene; a carrier may pass on a mutation that may lead to a disease in his or her offspring, even though the disease is not present in the carrier

Buckley, Lowe, & Ponder, 1999). Among women who had breast cancer between the ages of 36 and 45, only 4.1 percent had one of the mutations. Extrapolating from these figures, the researchers estimate that 1 in 900 people in the healthy general population carries a mutation in BRCA1 and about 1 in 800 carries a mutation in BRCA2.

Because most cases of breast cancer are caused by nongenetic factors, the absence of the mutation does not guarantee that a woman will not develop breast cancer. Other risk factors include obesity, age at menarche, exercise, smoking, diet, use of oral contraceptives, the presence of other diseases of the breast, radiation exposure, and use of alcohol.

Both men and women can inherit and pass on defective BRCA genes. Families in which breast cancer is inherited typically demonstrate the following characteristics:

- Breast cancer in two or more close relatives, such as a mother and two sisters.
- Early onset—often before age 50—of breast cancer in family members.
- History of breast cancer in more than one generation.
- Cancer in both breasts in one or more family members.
- Frequent occurrence of ovarian cancer.
- Ashkenazi (Eastern and Central European) Jewish ancestry, with a family history of breast and/or ovarian cancer (researchers have identified two BRCA1 mutations and one BRCA2 mutation that are particularly prevalent in this group).

Other forms of cancer are also linked to mutant genes. One example is basal cell carcinoma, the most common (and usually localized) form of skin cancer (Gailani et al., 1996). Another example is ovarian cancer, which is linked to damage to the BRCA2 gene. BRCA2 is also believed to play a role in cancer of the prostate, pancreas, and larynx (Smith, 1998). Men who carry this mutant gene are nearly twice as likely as noncarriers to develop prostate cancer by age 80.

Environmental and Occupational Hazards

For the past two decades, no subfield of cancer epidemiology has identified as many new carcinogens as that concerned with environmental toxins (Willett, Colditz, & Mueller, 1996). The list of potential hazards ranges from the sun to low frequency electrical and electromagnetic fields emanating from power lines and cell phones to fluoride in drinking water to proximity to nuclear plants and landfills.

Naturally, the degree of cancer hazard posed by these risks depends on the concentration of the carcinogen and the amount of exposure to the toxin. However, even low-dose exposure can represent a significant public health hazard when a large segment of the population is involved.

■ **melanoma** a potentially deadly form of cancer that strikes the melatonin-containing cells of the skin

Toxic Chemicals

Various chemicals show definite evidence of being carcinogenic. Among these are asbestos, vinyl chloride, and arsenic. In addition, some researchers believe that chlorine-containing organic compounds found in some household cleaning and pest-control products may increase the risk of breast cancer and, possibly, other hormone-related cancers. Although the popular media has focused on the dangers of pesticides such as DDT, the very low concentrations found in some foods are generally well within established safety levels and pose minimal risks.

Environmental toxins in the air, soil, and water are estimated to contribute to about 2 percent of fatal cancers, mainly of the bladder and the lungs. Although long-term exposure to high levels of air pollution—especially by smokers—may increase the risk of lung cancer by as much as 50 percent, this pales in comparison to the 2,000 percent increased risk caused by heavy smoking itself.

Although a few studies have linked water chlorinating and fluoridation with bladder cancer, most experts believe that the potential health risk is small and is outweighed by the greater danger of the spread of diseases such as cholera and typhoid fever by germs in uncholorinated water (Trichopoulous et al., 1996). Moreover, fluoride in drinking water is an effective agent in preventing tooth decay.

Radiation

Beginning in the 1960s, a well-tanned complexion was fashionable. However, many people burn rather than tan, and we now know that the only long-term effect of sunburn is skin cancer. In those days, when skin-protective sunscreens were generally unknown, sunbathing was especially risky. Is it any wonder that 40 to 50 percent of all Americans who reach 65 develop skin cancer (ACS, 2001)? Although tanning oil companies market sunscreen as often today as their more traditional tan-promoting lotions, skin cancer is the most common and most rapidly increasing type of cancer in the United States.

High-frequency radiation, ionizing radiation (IR), and ultraviolet (UV) radiation are proven carcinogens. Ultraviolet B rays, which can damage DNA, cause more than 90 percent of all skin cancers, including **melanoma,** a potentially deadly form of cancer that forms in skin cells. A number of researchers believe that the overall frequency of sunburns during childhood is a key factor in melanoma. This explains why people who tan rather than burn have a lower incidence of melanoma (Leffell & Brash, 1996). Another factor in the rising trend in skin cancer is the thinning of the earth's ozone layer, which filters skin-damaging ultraviolet (UV) radiation.

Given the evidence that the sun's ultraviolet rays can cause cancer, why do so many people continue to bask in the sun? In the most extensive study of sunbathers to date, researchers interviewed sun worshippers at California

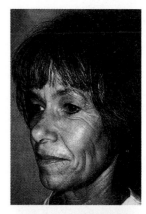

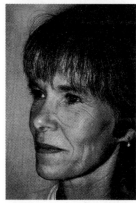

The Hazards of Sunbathing Despite its clear link to skin cancer, sunbathing continues to be popular, especially among people willing to take risks to improve their appearance. These photos of identical twins make the effects of tanning—and smoking—obvious, even to those who ignore messages about the health hazards of radiation from the sun. Sixty-year-old Gay Black (top) spent many hours in the sun and at one time was also a smoker. Her twin, Gwen Sirota (bottom), did neither. AP/Wide World Photos

beaches to determine the factors that influenced their decision to lie in the sun (Keesling & Friedman, 1987). Those with the deepest tans (who also reported spending the largest amounts of time in the sun) were least knowledgeable about skin cancer. They also were more relaxed, more sensitive to the influence of peers who valued a good tan, tended to take other risks, and were more focused on their appearance.

Others have no choice regarding exposure to radiation because of their occupation, for example. High-dose IR can affect virtually any part of the body, but especially the bone marrow and the thyroid gland. Radiation exposure can increase lung cancer risk, especially among tobacco users.

Non-ionizing, or low-frequency, radiation (such as that arising from microwaves, radar screens, electricity, and radios) has not been shown to cause cancer. Another common fear—living near a nuclear plant—is largely unfounded. In a massive 35-year study of over 40 million people, researchers compared cancer death rates of Americans who lived near nuclear plants with cancer death rates of people who lived in counties that had no nuclear sites. No differences were found in the two groups (Jablon, Hrubec, & Boice, 1991). Similarly, although toxic wastes in dump sites can threaten health through air, water, and soil pollution, most community exposures involve very low dose levels and do not pose serious health threats.

Occupational Carcinogens and Pollution

People whose work involves exposure to certain chemicals have long been known to be at greater risk of developing cancer than others. Work-related cancers mostly affect the lung, skin, bladder, and blood-forming systems of the body (Trichopoulous et al., 1996). For example, those who work with asbestos, chromium, and chromium compounds are much more likely than other workers to develop lung cancer. Workers exposed to benzene, a solvent used in making varnishes and dyes, are at high risk for developing leukemia.

Other substances now known to be carcinogenic include diesel exhaust and radon. In recent years, however, strict control measures in the workplace, at least in the developed world, have reduced the proportion of cancer deaths caused by job-related carcinogens to less than 5 percent. Unfortunately, such control measures generally lag behind the pace of industrialization in developing countries, and so job-related cancers are likely to increase in these countries.

Personality

As early as the second century, the Greek physician Galen (A.D. 131–201) proposed that melancholic individuals were cancer prone (see Chapter 1). Centuries later, researchers continue to wonder whether certain personality types are more likely to develop cancer (Smith & Gallo, 2001). For instance, belief in the connection between personality or stress and the development of breast cancer is widespread. This belief is reflected in media reports on health issues; for example, in 1997 *Self* magazine reported that "hostile arguing may compromise a woman's immune function" (McAuliffe, 1997).

Given the discussion of the impact of stress and coping styles on health in Chapter 5, you should not be surprised that specific personality dispositions have been linked with cancer development, psychological adjustment, survival, and recurrence. But we have to be careful before leaping to this conclusion. As we've seen before, it is difficult to determine whether psychosocial factors such as cognitive style or mood are *causes* or *consequences* of chronic diseases such as cancer.

Suppose researchers find that people who are often angry develop cancer more often than others do. Can you conclude that this trait causes cancer? The answer, clearly, is "no." Most studies of cancer and personality have compared cancer patients with healthy control subjects. Although the inference is that personality differences between the groups *preceded* and even caused the disease, definitive proof is extremely difficult. Isn't it possible that being diagnosed with a serious illness could itself trigger anger and other mood alterations rather than vice versa? And, of course, chemotherapy, radiotherapy, and other biomedical interventions may induce physiological changes that directly alter mood as well. Before we can conclude that the mind can cause cancer, however, we need evidence from prospective research studies that investigate psychosocial factors in a large sample of healthy people over a period of years.

Patrick Dattore and his colleagues did just that. In a massive prospective study, they compared scores from the Minnesota Multiphasic Personality Inventory (MMPI) that had been obtained from a group of patients several years *before* cancer was detected with the personality profiles of a control group (Dattore, Shontz, & Coyne, 1980). Those who subsequently developed cancer differed from the disease-free control subjects in two ways: They were more likely to suppress their emotional reactions to events, and they *reported* less depression.

To test the relationship between personality type and cancer, Hans Eysenck and other researchers conducted two major prospective studies (Eysenck, Grossarth-Maticek, & Everitt, 1991; Grossarth-Maticek, Eysenck, Pfeifer, Schmidt, & Koppel, 1997). At the beginning of the studies, the participants were designated as one of four personality types on the basis of their responses to personality questionnaires. Over the next decade, the researchers compared the causes of death among the four personality types. In both studies, cancer was the top killer among people who had difficulty expressing emotion and tended toward hopelessness in response to stress. Cardiovascular disease was the leading cause of death for people who were easily frustrated, had short tempers, tended to blame others for their stress, and tended toward hostile, angry responses. The third type was a mixture of the first two personalities, and the fourth type had a positive, trusting outlook. Neither the third nor fourth type was especially vulnerable to either cancer or heart disease.

Type C (cancer-prone) personality a passive, uncomplaining person who tends to repress emotions and may be prone to developing cancer

The Type C Personality

These and other studies led researchers to describe the **Type C (cancer-prone) personality.** Cancer-prone individuals were hypothesized to be passive, uncomplaining, and compliant and to have difficulty expressing their emotions. As nurses, oncologists, and other health care professionals have long noted, cancer patients tend to be "nice people" (Holland & Lewis, 1996).

A number of researchers have begun focusing on suppression and denial of emotions as the toxic core of the Type C personality. Brian Esterling and his colleagues (1994) found that subjects who scored high on a personality test that measured repression showed reduced immunocompetence, as indicated by higher levels of herpes virus antibody. This relationship was significant even after controlling for medication use and a range of other health practices.

Depression has also received considerable attention as a personality disposition that may contribute to cancer, although the results are somewhat mixed (Cohen & Herbert, 1996). In a 20-year study of men who completed the MMPI in 1957, those with higher depression scores had twice the risk of dying of cancer two decades later (Perskey, Kempthrone-Rawson, & Shekelle, 1987) compared to their nondepressed counterparts.

Depression has also been linked with more rapid progression of tumors (possibly due to lower NK cell activity) and shorter survival time among patients diagnosed with breast cancer (Cohen & Herbert, 1996; Levy, 1985). A prospective study by researchers at the National Institute on Aging analyzed the case histories of women and men over age 70. Ten years into the study, the cancer rate among those who had been diagnosed as chronically depressed—*after* accounting for age, sex, smoking, and other habits—was 88 percent higher than for nondepressed participants (Penninx et al., 1998).

Despite these compelling findings, critics have questioned the validity of the link between an emotionally unexpressive, depressed personality style and cancer because these studies have not always been successfully replicated. In fact, some studies have not been able to establish *any* link between cancer and personality type, depressed or otherwise (Zonderman, Costa, & McCrae, 1989). Furthermore, several studies have reported that depression *does not* place people at increased risk for either cancer incidence or cancer mortality (Kaplan & Reynolds, 1988; Zonderman et al., 1989).

Why the inconsistency in results? One possibility is that research on the role of depression in cancer has generally focused on cancer as a generic disease. It is possible that a greater focus on particular disease sites may clarify the relationship between specific personality dispositions and specific cancers (Cohen & Herbert, 1996).

A recent meta-analysis examined the relationship between personality and other psychosocial factors and breast cancer (McKenna, Zevon, Corn, & Rounds, 1999). The researchers found only a moderate association between the development of breast cancer and the tendency to use denial or repression in coping with life stressors, recent experiences of separation and loss, a history of stressful life experiences, or a personality style characterized by conflict avoidance. The remaining hypothesized psychosocial contributors to breast cancer received little statistical support. These findings, therefore, fail to support many of the popular assumptions regarding the influence of personality or psychological factors on the development of breast cancer.

Any link between emotional depression/suppression and other personality characteristics and cancer is also subject to the influence of other factors such as occupation and health attitudes and behaviors. It is important to show, for example, that the relationship is not due to the fact that people who gravitate toward occupations involving possible exposure to toxic chemicals and other carcinogens are also more likely to be depressed—or that depressed people tend to "let themselves go" by smoking more, eating a fatty diet, and in other ways increasing their health risk.

The safest conclusion we can draw at this point is that the link between specific personality traits and cancer is *suggestive* but inconclusive. Additional research is needed, but to be convincing, future prospective studies must do more than merely establish (or fail to establish) correlations between certain traits and the development of cancer. As several researchers have argued, they should attempt to pinpoint the *mechanisms* by which such factors lead to the development of malignancies (Linkins & Comstock, 1988).

Cancer Prevention and Treatment

As with other chronic illnesses, health psychologists are especially interested in helping prevent cancer. Recall from Chapter 6 that *primary prevention* includes measures designed to combat an illness (including its risk factors) before it develops. In contrast, *secondary prevention* includes measures to identify and treat an illness early, with the aim of stopping or reversing the problem; and *tertiary prevention* includes measures to contain damage once a disease has progressed beyond the early stages. Strategies at all three levels of prevention are employed in the fight against cancer.

Primary Prevention: Modifying Cancer-Promoting Behaviors

The best way to control cancer is, obviously, to prevent it from ever developing. Although there is no guaranteed way of preventing cancer, there are some things people can do to reduce the risk. As we've seen, controllable behaviors—using tobacco, eating a fatty diet, exposing the skin to the sun's ultraviolet rays, and moving through life in a hopeless, depressed manner, for example—play a major role in most cancers.

Factors Affecting Primary Prevention

According to the *health belief model* (HBM) discussed in Chapter 6, whether individuals will adopt a health-protective behavior depends on their perception of their *susceptibility* to the health threat, the *severity* of the threat, the *benefits* of the proposed health action for mitigating the threat, and whether they can overcome perceived *barriers* to the health behavior.

The use of sunscreen is a good example of how the HBM works. Researchers have found that perceived susceptibility to skin cancer is positively associated with intentions to protect the skin from the sun (Jones & Leary, 1994; Mahler, Fitzpatrick, Parker, & Lapin, 1997). Perceived severity, however, does not seem to predict sun protection efforts (Lescano & Rodrigue, 1997). Perceived barriers (such as the belief that "sunscreen is messy") and weak self-efficacy ("it's too much of a hassle") strongly predict weak or nonexistent sun protection intentions and behaviors (Carmel, Shani, & Rosenberg, 1994; Jackson & Aiken, 2000). Another factor in sunscreen use is peer influence. In general, teenagers and young adults hold strongly positive attitudes toward sunbathing, based in part on their perception that a tanned appearance is attractive and, ironically, healthier (Fritschi, Green, & Solomon, 1992; Leary & Jones, 1993). However, whether they will protect themselves with sunscreen is powerfully influenced by whether their friends regularly use sunscreen (Banks, Silverman, Schwartz, & Tunnessen, 1992; Wichstrom, 1994). Their behavior is also influenced by image norms for attractiveness and style, set by celebrities and by the entertainment and fashion industries. Indeed, adolescents' concerns with how they present themselves to the world are highly predictive of a wide range of health behaviors, including the use of sunscreen (Leary, Tchividjian, & Kraxberger, 1994).

Primary Prevention Messages

How might we persuade people to carry out a simple, cancer-protective behavior, such as using sunscreen, consistently? A first step might be to deliver a persuasive message designed to elicit this behavior (see Chapter 6). *Prospect theory* suggests that how people respond to messages depends on how these messages are framed. Health messages can be framed either in terms of potential gains (advantages or benefits) or in terms of potential losses (disadvantages or costs). An example of a gain-framed message is, "If you use sunscreen, you will increase your chances of keeping a healthy, supple, and attractive skin all your life." In contrast, a loss-framed message might state, "If you do not use sunscreen, your skin will age prematurely and you will increase your chances of developing skin cancer and dying early."

Two important factors in whether a gain-framed or loss-framed message is likely to be more effective are perceived risk and the type of health behavior being promoted—that is, whether it is a prevention behavior or a detection behavior (Salovey, Rothman, & Rodin, 1998). Prospect theory suggests that people avoid taking risks when they are focusing on potential gains but are more willing to take risks when they are focusing on potential losses. Since prevention behaviors (such as using sunscreen) provide a positive outcome— they lower an individual's vulnerability to a future health behavior (skin cancer)—they are perceived as involving little or no current risk. Detection behaviors (such as mammograms and prostate exams), on the other hand, may reveal that something is wrong with an individual's health and so are perceived to be very risky. Following this line of reasoning, we would expect the performance of prevention behaviors to be facilitated best by gain-framed messages and detection behaviors by loss-framed messages.

A Yale University study compared the effectiveness of four differently framed messages (two gain-framed and two loss-framed) in persuading beachgoers to obtain and use sunscreen (Detweiler, Bedell, Salovey, Pronin, & Rothman, 1999). Each participant completed a questionnaire assessing his or her sunscreen attitudes and intentions, once prior to and again after reading two gain- or loss-framed brochures regarding sunscreen use. The gain-framed messages focused either on attaining a desirable outcome ("Use sunscreen to help your skin stay healthy") or not experiencing an undesirable outcome ("Use sunscreen to decrease your risk of getting skin cancer"). Loss-framed messages were also phrased in two distinct ways: attaining an undesirable outcome ("Without sunscreen you increase your risk of developing skin cancer") or failing to attain a desirable outcome ("Without sunscreen you cannot guarantee the health of your skin"). On returning his or her completed questionnaires, each participant was given a coupon that could be redeemed half an hour later for a free sample of SPF 15 sunscreen.

As predicted by prospect theory, the results showed that participants who read either of the two gain-framed brochures, compared with those who read either of the loss-framed brochures, were significantly more likely to redeem their coupon for sunscreen and expressed the intent to repeatedly apply sunscreen while at the beach and use sunscreen with an SPF of 15 or higher.

Secondary Prevention: Early Diagnosis

When cancer does develop, its impact on health frequently can be minimized through early detection and treatment. Although early detection can prevent death and perhaps reduce treatment time, there may still be months or years of painful or uncomfortable treatment. This is because cancer develops over time, as neoplastic cells grow into tumors that metastasize to surrounding

Figure 10.4

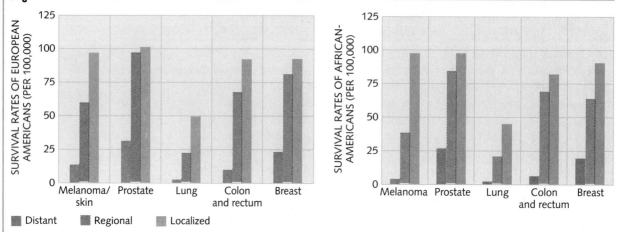

■ Distant ■ Regional ■ Localized

Five-Year Relative Survival Rates by Race and Stage at Diagnosis
Five-year relative survival rates are commonly used to monitor progress in the early
detection and treatment of cancer. This includes all survivors, whether in remission,
disease-free, or under treatment. *Localized* refers to a malignant tumor confined entirely
to the organ of origin. *Regional* refers to a malignant tumor that has extended beyond
the limits of the organ of origin into the surrounding organs or tissues, involves regional
lymph nodes by way of the lymphatic system, or is both extended beyond the organ of
origin and involves the regional lymph nodes. *Distant* refers to a malignant cancer that
has spread to parts of the body remote from the primary tumor either by direct extension
or by metastasis to distant organs and tissues, or via the lymphatic system to distant
lymph nodes. The earlier the detection, the greater is the likelihood that the tumor will
be localized; thus survival increases markedly the earlier the cancer is diagnosed.
Source: Surveillance, Epidemiology, and End Results (SEER) Program, by National Cancer Institute
(search.nci.nih.gov/).

tissues. As Figure 10.4 shows, detecting this process early on, before malignant
cells have gained a strong foothold, can dramatically improve a person's
chances of survival. Unfortunately, as many as 30 percent to 50 percent of people with noticeable cancer symptoms delay 3 or 4 months before seeking medical attention (Singer, 1988).

Techniques of Secondary Prevention
Some types of cancer—for example, breast and cervical cancer—do not have
immediately obvious symptoms. For this reason, the American Cancer Society
and National Cancer Institute have advocated increased screening for breast
and cervical cancer, which together cause 14 percent of all cancer deaths.
Because 90 percent of breast tumors are first detected through breast self-

examination (BSE), women are advised to conduct a BSE regularly, at least once a month. Between 20 and 40 years of age, all women should have a clinical breast examination by a physician every 3 years. After age 40, they should have annual clinical exams and mammograms.

Two other highly effective techniques for detecting breast cancer are *thermography* (a procedure in which breast abnormalities are identified from uneven patterns of skin temperature) and *computed tomography,* or CT, scans (a diagnostic test in which a computer combines information from multiple x-rays to pinpoint breast abnormalities). Although these procedures are costly, they may be warranted when other tests are inconclusive. Health experts believe that following this schedule of screening could reduce cancer mortality by 25 to 40 percent (White, Urban, & Taylor, 1993).

Cancer experts also recommend that men perform regular testicular self-examinations. Testicular cancer is the leading cause of death from malignant tumors among 20- to 34-year-old men (about 10 percent), accounting for about 1 percent of all cancer mortalities in men. Many of these deaths could have been prevented by early detection. Although chances of full recovery are excellent if a solid tumor is caught early on, nearly half of all cases of testicular cancer are not diagnosed until the malignancy has spread to surrounding tissues. Five-year survival rates are better than 95 percent when the cancer is treated while it remains localized (Nicholson & Harland, 1995).

For those with family histories of cancer, genetic screening has become a useful method of early detection. A simple blood test can now detect genetic mutations linked to an increased risk of many types of cancer. Such tests, however, have raised a host of ethical and practical questions (see Byline Health on page 442). On the practical side, many laboratories administering these tests do not follow the admittedly vague and inadequate regulatory controls that help ensure the validity of genetic tests. And some labs market tests to physicians, obstetricians, and primary care providers who lack expertise in medical genetics.

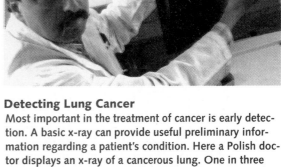

Detecting Lung Cancer
Most important in the treatment of cancer is early detection. A basic x-ray can provide useful preliminary information regarding a patient's condition. Here a Polish doctor displays an x-ray of a cancerous lung. One in three persons in Poland is a smoker, contributing to an annual national consumption of 90 billion cigarettes and increasing the number of smoking-related illnesses. © 1996 Piotr Malecki / Liaison Agency

The more significant problem has to do with the ethics of genetic testing and the knowledge it provides. If you were fated to develop cancer, would you want to know? What would you do if the results came back positive? Providing people with a diagnosis of an untreatable disease raises concerns, especially when dealing with children, who may not fully understand the implications of the tests. Others fear that children identified as carriers of serious diseases will be discriminated against. A related concern is the real possibility that

Choosing to Test for Cancer's Genetic Link

Jane E. Brody

In June, after completing treatment for an early breast cancer, I sought genetic counseling. I opted to have my blood tested, to find out whether my cancer might have been inherited, the result of a mutation in one of the two known tumor suppressor genes, BRCA-1 and BRCA-2.

Because my mother died at 49 of ovarian cancer, which is sometimes also due to mutations in these genes, I wanted all the information I could get. That way, I could decide how best to protect my own health and the health of my blood relatives, particularly my brother and his three children and my sons and their future offspring.

Just by being the descendant of Ashkenazi Jews whose ancestors came from Russia, there is one chance in 50 that I am a carrier for one of three mutations in these genes. And since my mother developed ovarian cancer at a young age, and I myself have had breast cancer, the odds of my having a mutated gene are greatly increased: to between 20 percent and 30 percent.

Although I have long followed early detection guidelines for both breast and ovarian cancer, I now know that there is more that I can do to assure that I do not get another cancer— especially one more likely to be fatal than the cancer I already had.

But not every woman with a history like mine has chosen to be tested, often for good reasons.

The ability to test for genetic abnormalities that greatly increase a woman's risk of developing breast or ovarian cancer has created new and potentially lifesaving options. But it has also raised a host of new concerns for women with a family history of these cancers, including medical insurance, employment discrimination, emotional distress, and strains on personal or family relations.

Many Choices Possible Three women I know, all of whom are also Ashkenazi Jews, have chosen different paths. Eva, who developed both ovarian and breast cancer just after menopause, said she and her 28-year-old daughter have decided not to be tested for the BRCA mutations for now. The results, she said, would not change their current behavior.

Eva said even if the results were positive, her newly married daughter would not undergo surgery to have her breasts and ovaries removed. She would rather not have to worry about a genetic albatross at this stage of her life. But she has already begun regular checkups, including annual mammograms, so that should a cancer develop, it might be detected at a curable stage.

Natalie, thus far healthy in her late 50s, has a strong family history of breast cancer: several relatives have had the disease. But she is not going to be tested, she said, "because I don't think I could handle it emotionally if I turned out to have the gene."

Ellie, in her mid-40s, lost her mother to breast cancer, diagnosed when her mother was 43, and has been riddled with anxiety about the disease since childhood. Other relatives have had cancer, including two cousins, one of whom died young of breast cancer. Both cousins carried BRCA mutations.

Ellie would like to be tested, too, but she is currently between jobs, and she is afraid that the discovery of an abnormal gene could jeopardize her future employment opportunities, as well as her ability to obtain affordable health insurance. Instead, she is trying to alleviate her anxiety and protect her health by following a more conservative course, having frequent checkups for the cancers associated with BRCA mutations.

Ellie made this decision after a two-hour session with a genetic counselor at Memorial Sloan-Kettering Cancer Center in New York. With the counselor, she constructed a family tree, showing how a genetic propensity for cancer might have been passed to her by her mother or father.

insurance companies will deny coverage to individuals who have a predisposition toward developing a particular disease.

Proponents of genetic testing argue that parents should be allowed to have their children tested so they can make informed decisions about treatment. And in cases where there is a family history of cancer, testing that rules out the presence of a genetic disorder can be a source of relief.

The counselor carefully reviewed all the pros and cons of genetic testing, which is done on a small blood sample. But he did not pressure Ellie to have the test. Instead, he outlined an exam schedule for her to follow in case she is at unusually high risk: She is to have manual breast examinations, by a doctor two to four times a year, perform monthly self-examinations and have annual mammograms to check for breast cancer.

In addition, the counselor recommended that Ellie undergo an ultrasound examination twice a year, and have a blood test for a gene marker called CA-125, to check for ovarian cancer. Beginning at age 40, he said, she should also have a colonoscopy every three to five years to check for colon cancer, which may also be more common in bearers of mutated BRCA genes.

Before the counseling session, Ellie said, she dealt with the anxiety created by her mother's experience with breast cancer "by keeping my head in the sand." But after learning of her cousin's death, and her sister's decision to have her breasts and ovaries removed while they were still healthy, Ellie said, she immediately began following the counselor's advice and made appointments for breast, ovary, and colon exams.

A Personal Strategy For my part, I sought counseling with my mind already made up: if there was a reasonably good chance that I had inherited a greatly increased cancer risk, I wanted to know that as soon as possible. Medical insurance and job security were not an issue in my case, and I have worried about getting ovarian cancer my entire adult life and have undergone annual examinations of my ovaries for more than 10 years.

I am still awaiting the results of the test. But I have already decided that if I test positive for a BRCA mutation, I will have my ovaries removed. At age 58, they are not doing me much good anyway, and I have just learned that the surgery can now be done through a laparoscope, with two tiny incisions and no overnight hospital stay.

I will not, however, have my breasts removed, I decided, especially since I have already had breast cancer, and know that in a postmenopausal woman it can be detected early and treated effectively with proper surveillance. Also, I am now taking tamoxifen, an anti-estrogen shown last year to cut a woman's breast cancer risk in half, though it is still not known if this protection extends to women with mutated BRCA genes.

I was surprised to learn that it would be wise to pay more attention to my colon, which at my age I should be doing anyway. And, if I have a mutated gene, my brother might also have inherited it, and at age 54 should have annual prostate examinations.

In tracing my family's medical history in preparation for my counseling session, I learned that my mother's father died at 60 of prostate cancer and that a maternal uncle also had the disease. These cancers increase the likelihood that a mutated gene runs in the family.

Some Words of Caution But before any woman found to have a mutated gene undergoes prophylactic surgery, the gene test should be repeated. Mistakes have been made by commercial laboratories, and even the best laboratories can be wrong some of the time. Also, keep in mind that the gene test is not perfect. Even if both BRCA genes are fully tested, some women may have an abnormal gene that is not detected by the current test.

Finally, beware of false reassurance. Even if you are not found to have inherited a mutated gene, you can still get breast cancer and you should continue with regular checkups. Keep in mind that more than 90 percent of breast cancers are not hereditary. And if you do choose to have prophylactic surgery, that too will not offer perfect protection: it will reduce the risk of breast and ovarian cancer by more than 90 percent, but it cannot totally eliminate that risk. Regular checkups are still in order.

Source: *The New York Times,* August 17, 1999.

Exercise
From the biopsychosocial perspective, what are some of the pros and cons of the ability to test for genetic abnormalities? Be sure to specify the individual biological, psychological, and social factors.

Early Detection and Delay Behavior

Despite the overwhelming evidence that early detection and treatment are the keys to increasing the chances of surviving certain types of cancer, many people refuse to perform routine exams on themselves. Similarly, they ignore early warning signs and delay seeking help. Table 10.2 on page 444 summarizes the percentage of adults in the United States who follow

Table 10.2

Prevalence of Cancer Screening among Five Racial and Ethnic Groups

Cancer Screening	European American	African-American	Hispanic-American	Native American	Asian/Pacific Islander
Prostate test (proctoscopy) within the past 5 years	30.4%	28.2%	22.4%	27.6%	
California*					24.3%
Hawaii*					40.7
Colorectal test	18.2	20.3	14.2	12.3	
California*					2.6
Hawaii*					23.8
Mammogram within past 2 years	73.7	76.1	63.5		
Alaska*				93.5	
Hawaii*					80.7
Cervical/uterine test within past 3 years	84.7	91.1	80.9	90.5	
Hawaii*					84.2

*Indicates state-specific prevalence estimates available for the corresponding race-ethnic group.
Source: Behavioral Risk Factor Surveillance System, Surveillance Summary Report, 2000. National Center for Chronic Disease Prevention and Health Promotion, Centers for Disease Control and Prevention.

recommended screening schedules for cancer of the prostate, breasts, colon and rectum, and cervix.

Many reasons have been offered for the failure of people to fully comply with the medical community's recommendations for preventive cancer screening. In the case of breast cancer (which has a high rate of compliance), some women may be fully aware of their susceptibility to the disease and recognize its seriousness but not feel confident that they can correctly perform a breast self-exam. Many women also express concerns about the safety and discomfort of mammography. Finally, many believe that treatments are ineffective and therefore see no reason to screen (especially if a sister, mother, or friend died following unsuccessful treatment). Some health experts are convinced that until a really effective treatment for breast cancer is found, it is doubtful that self-examination and mammography will be more widely practiced (Fallowfield, 1997). With the growing success of lumpectomies (surgery that removes only the tumor but leaves healthy breast tissue alone), laser imaging to obliterate tumors without scars, and other treatments for breast cancer, however, there is reason to be optimistic that self-screening will increase (Christiano, 2000).

Another factor in compliance is perceived vulnerability to the disease. In one study, nearly 75 percent of the women questioned did not perceive themselves as vulnerable to breast cancer (Fulton et al., 1991)—and only 30 per-

Table 10.3

Caution: Seven Warning Signs of Cancer

Remembering the word *Caution* will help you identify the most common warning signs of cancer. Although some of these symptoms can be caused by less serious conditions, you should definitely see a doctor to rule out cancer as the cause. Most important, don't wait until you feel discomfort or pain. In their early stages of development, most cancers do not cause pain.

C	Change in bowel or bladder habits.
A	A sore that does not heal.
U	Unusual bleeding or discharge.
T	Thickening or lump in the breast or any part of the body.
I	Indigestion or difficulty swallowing.
O	Obvious change in a wart or mole.
N	Nagging cough or hoarseness.

Source: American Cancer Society, 2001.

cent of those who did feel vulnerable felt the seriousness of their risk to be high. Among a group of people in a high-risk colon-cancer registry, those who opted for genetic testing were more worried that they would develop the disease than those who decided not to be tested (Codori et al., 1999).

People also delay seeking medical attention because they do not realize they should do so; in its earliest stages of development, cancer is usually not painful. Many symptoms may, in fact, be so minor as to go unnoticed until a lump, a change in the appearance of a mole, or a sore that refuses to heal becomes obvious (see Table 10.3). Even then, many people wait to seek attention until they feel discomfort or pain.

A final factor in delay behavior is anxiety. Women who seek out genetic screening for breast cancer, for example, tend to have moderately high levels of cancer-related distress (Lerman et al., 1999). Those who are depressed, together with those with extremely high (or low) levels of anxiety, are the least likely to seek testing.

In summary, research studies indicate that patients who seek medical attention in the face of early warning signs of cancer tend to be knowledgeable about cancer, have moderate levels of anxiety, and perceive some vulnerability to the disease (McCaul, Branstetter, Schroeder, & Glascow, 1996). Unfortunately, fear of a cancer diagnosis seems to paralyze some patients into inaction or denial that they may be vulnerable to a serious disease.

Modifying Delay Behavior

What can be done to promote greater screening and prompt medical attention when symptoms are detected? Among the many methods that have been tried are the use of fear-inducing advertising campaigns, educational programs, and external rewards.

For some cancers and some people, persuasive messages and informational campaigns may be all that is needed. For instance, male college students who listened to a taped message about testicular cancer or read a brochure about testicular self-examination were significantly more likely to perform a self-exam during the ensuing month than were control subjects (Brubaker & Fowler, 1990).

Two other simple attempts at increasing self-exams involve the use of periodic prompts informing a person that it is time to perform a self-exam and providing rewards for doing so. Several campaigns have reported that the use of reminder postcards or telephone calls ("Remember to practice a breast self-examination this month") produced modest increases in compliance with breast self-exam recommendations (Mayer & Frederiksen, 1986). Another study reported modest increases in screening when an extrinsic reward (a $1 lottery ticket or silver dollar) was offered for each breast self-exam.

Overall, however, public health campaigns and small-group interventions such as these have met with mixed success. Increasingly, health psychologists believe that customized appeals, using messages that fit patients' needs and knowledge, are most likely to encourage people to be screened. For example, Rosalind Dorlen and her colleagues have used James Prochaska's *stages of change* model (see Chapter 6) to design appeals focused on the motivational stages of African-American women, who have historically had low rates of mammography (Murray, 1999). Women were categorized as

- *Precontemplators*—who have never had a mammogram and who have no plans to have one in the coming year.
- *Contemplators*—who have never had a mammogram but plan to have one sooner or later.
- *Women of action*—who have had one or more mammograms and who may or may not have one in the next year.
- *Women of maintenance*—who have had one or more mammograms and definitely plan to have one in the coming year. (This, of course, is the most desirable motivational stage.)

Based on a woman's stage of motivation, Dorlen and her team vary their health appeal so that the message fits the recipient. For precontemplators, for example, it is "How small is the head of a pin? Not too small for a mammogram to find." This type of message highlights the diagnostic power of the test. For contemplators, the message is "Small is better. Think small, think mammogram," with a focus on prevention. And for women of maintenance, the message is "Looking out for little things is smart. Keep on getting mammograms," with the focus on continued upkeep and vigilance.

Health psychologists are also working with health care providers to make screening pleas more culture-focused, with the aim of encouraging more ethnic minorities to seek cancer care. Hispanic women, for example, are less likely to have heard of Pap smears (tests for cervical cancer) than African-American or white women, and fewer African-American and Hispanic women than white women understand that they should be tested annually (cited in Rabasca, 1999). In Hawaii, health psychologists are testing a new community-based intervention designed to encourage native Hawaiian women to seek cancer screening more consistently. The intervention centers on the altruistic Hawaiian concept of *kokua,* or "helping others without expecting help in return." The intervention brings together groups of native women to discuss the benefits of mammography and Pap smears. Afterward, participants are urged to share their new knowledge with their mothers, sisters, aunts, and friends. So far, among 600 randomly selected native women, cancer screening rates have increased substantially (Rabasca, 1999).

In another approach to culture-focused interventions, Regina Otero-Sabogal and her colleagues at the National Cancer Institute are conducting a randomized controlled trial of individualized health messages targeted at low-income, multiethnic women in Alameda County, California. Each woman in the intervention group will receive a personalized health letter written in her native language, incorporating health themes that reflect her ethnicity and personal barriers to having Pap smears or mammograms (for example, lack of knowledge, fear, and economic factors). Individualized health messages will be sent to the participants every 6 months during the 3-year study and will include information about where and when to schedule a screening appointment. Three months after the letter, community health care workers will call the participants (cited in Rabasca, 1999).

Interventions such as these may represent health psychology's greatest contribution in modifying delay behavior. By educating people about the importance of assuming responsibility for all aspects of health, including taking swift action when symptoms are detected, health psychologists will be leading the way for future generations to promote health for all people.

Secondary and Tertiary Prevention: Treatment Options

Until recently, the treatment options for most forms of cancer were severely limited, and cancer was often a death sentence. Today, there are many effective treatment options that have reduced death rates from most types of cancer, including surgery, chemotherapy, radiation therapy, and combination regimes such as those that involve both bone marrow transplantation and radiation therapy.

Surgery

The oldest form of cancer treatment, surgery generally offers the greatest chance for cure for most types of cancer. Approximately 60 percent of cancer

■ **immunotherapy**
chemotherapy in which
medications are used to
support or enhance the
immune system's ability to
selectively target cancer cells

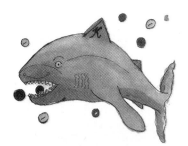

When child psychologist
Elizabeth King was diagnosed
with cancer, her son created a
story and illustration about a
character named "kemo shark,"
who swam around in his
mother's body eating cancer
cells and sometimes healthy
ones by mistake, causing her to
get sick. When King completed
her treatment, she developed
her son's story into a children's
comic book and funded the
nonprofit organization
KIDSCOPE to raise money to
distribute the book at no cost.
(See www.kidscope.org. —
Courtesy of KIDSCOPE;
Concept by Mitchell
McGraugh.)

patients have some form of surgery, which is usually recommended to achieve one or more of the following goals.

■ *Diagnostic* surgery is used to obtain a tissue sample for laboratory testing in order to confirm a diagnosis and identify the specific cancer. A procedure to remove all or part of a tumor for diagnostic tests is called a *biopsy.*

■ *Preventive* (or prophylactic) surgery is performed to remove a growth that is not presently malignant but is likely to become so if left untreated. This type of surgery is used for precancerous conditions such as polyps (normally benign growths of tissue) in the colon. Sometimes preventive surgery is used to remove an organ when people have an inherited condition that makes development of a cancer likely. For example, as noted earlier in Byline Health, women with a very strong family history of breast cancer and/or genetic testing results that show a mutation of the BRCA1 or BRCA2 genes may consider mastectomy (breast removal).

■ *Staging* surgery is used to determine the extent of disease. In *laparoscopy* a tube is passed through a tiny incision in the abdomen to examine its contents and remove tissue samples. A similar procedure to view the inside of the chest is called *thoracoscopy.*

■ *Curative* surgery involves the removal of a tumor when the tumor appears to be localized and there is hope of taking out all the cancerous tissue. Curative surgery is considered primary treatment of the cancer.

■ *Restorative* (or reconstructive) surgery is used to restore a person's appearance or the function of an organ or body part. Examples include breast reconstruction after mastectomy or use of bone grafts or *prosthetic* (metal or plastic) bone or joint replacements after surgical treatment of bone cancer.

Chemotherapy

Chemotherapy is the use of medicines to treat cancer. While surgery and radiation therapy destroy or damage cancer cells in a specific area, chemotherapy can destroy cancer cells that have spread, or metastasized, to parts of the body far from the original, or primary, tumor. This is because *systemic drugs* travel through the bloodstream to reach all areas of the body.

Depending on the type of cancer and its stage of development, chemotherapy can be used to cure cancer, to keep the cancer from spreading, to slow the cancer's growth, to kill cancer cells that may have spread to other parts of the body from the original tumor, or to relieve symptoms caused by the cancer. In one of the newest forms of chemotherapy, **immunotherapy,** medications are used to enhance the immune system's ability to selectively target cancer cells. A promising form of immunotherapy involves the use of *monoclonal antibodies* (laboratory-produced antibodies that target single antigens on the surface of cancer cells) to ensure the accurate imaging and destruction of tumor cells (Purves & Orians, 2000).

About 50 anticancer drugs are in use today. Although a single drug can be used to treat cancer, generally anticancer drugs are more powerful when used in combination. This strategy allows drugs with different actions to work together to kill more cancer cells and reduces the chance that the patient will develop a resistance to one particular drug.

Anticancer drugs are made to kill fast-growing cells; however, because these drugs travel throughout the body, they can affect normal, healthy cells. The normal cells most likely to be affected are blood cells that form in the bone marrow and cells in the digestive tract, reproductive system, and hair follicles. Some anticancer drugs can also damage cells of the heart, kidneys, bladder, lungs, and nervous system.

The most common side effects of chemotherapy are nausea and vomiting, hair loss, and fatigue. Less common side effects include bleeding, infections, and anemia. Although side effects are not always as bad as expected, their reputation makes chemotherapy an anxiety-provoking treatment.

Radiation Therapy

All cells, cancerous and healthy, grow and divide. But cancer cells grow and divide more rapidly than many of the normal cells around them. Radiation therapy (also called *radiotherapy*) uses special equipment to deliver high doses of x-rays, gamma rays, or alpha and beta particles to cancerous tumors, killing or damaging them so that they cannot grow, multiply, or spread. Although some normal cells may be affected by radiation, most appear to repair themselves and recover fully from the effects of the treatment. Unlike chemotherapy, which exposes the entire body to cancer-fighting chemicals, radiation therapy affects only the tumor and the surrounding area.

An estimated 350,000 cancer patients receive radiation therapy each year, more than half of all cancer cases. It is the primary treatment for cancer in almost any part of the body, including head and neck tumors, early-stage Hodgkin's disease and non-Hodgkin's lymphomas, and cancers of the lung, breasts, cervix, prostate, testes, bladder, thyroid, and brain. Radiation therapy also can be used to shrink a tumor prior to surgery (so that it can be removed more easily) or after surgery to stop the growth of any cancer cells that remain.

Like chemotherapy, radiation is often associated with side effects, including temporary or permanent loss of hair in the area being treated, fatigue, loss of appetite, skin rashes, and loss of white blood cells. On the positive side, thousands of people have become cancer-free after receiving radiation treatments alone or in combination with surgery or chemotherapy.

Alternative Treatments

Many cancer patients have tried one or more alternative treatments. Among these are aromatherapy, biofeedback, meditation, music therapy, prayer and spiritual practices, yoga, t'ai chi (an exercise-based form of "moving meditation"), art therapy, massage therapy, and herbal treatment. Although alternative therapies are generally unproven and have not been scientifically tested, many *can* be used safely along with standard biomedical treatment to relieve symptoms or side effects, to ease pain, and to improve a patient's overall quality of life. The safest approach is to carefully evaluate any form of treatment in terms of its claims and the credentials of those supporting the treatment, and then to talk to your doctor about any method under consideration. Alternative treatments for cancer will be discussed more fully in Chapter 14.

Coping with Cancer

Life-threatening chronic diseases such as cancer create unique stresses for both victims and their families. Cancer is a dreaded disease, which most people realize can be intensely painful and lead to disability, disfigurement, or death. As patients' expectations of survival have increased, so has the need for psychosocial supports aimed at restoring, or maintaining, quality of life. Health psychologists are helping focus attention and resources on enabling patients and their families to cope with the numerous adverse effects of cancer treatment.

Although research on the emotional and behavioral responses of cancer patients to surgery has been limited, studies consistently show high levels of anxiety both before and after an operation. Compared to patients who are undergoing surgery for benign conditions, cancer surgery patients have higher overall levels of distress and slower rates of emotional recovery. In one study, cancer patients had significantly greater feelings of crisis and helplessness for as long as two months after discharge from the hospital (Gottesman & Lewis, 1982).

Consider *bone marrow transplantation (BMT)*, which has developed over the past 25 years from an experimental treatment of last resort into a routine therapy for a variety of cancers, including leukemia and Hodgkin's disease (Andersen & Golden-Kreutz, 1997). The target of BMT, the bone marrow, is first destroyed with high-dose chemotherapy and, possibly, whole body radiation. After the marrow is removed, healthy replacement bone marrow is transplanted from a donor.

BMT patients and their families are faced with a number of stressors: a life-threatening disease; finding a compatible donor; and toxic treatment with painful, unpleasant, and potentially fatal side effects. The possible side effects include hair loss, skin disorders, infertility, infection, prolonged hospitalization (often in an isolation ward), and liver disease. Added to these stresses are the uncertainty of survival, feelings of dependency associated with long-term care, and the ongoing necessity of making difficult decisions at a time of extreme emotional turmoil. It is no surprise that many patients feel a profound sense of helplessness, loneliness, and depression (Andersen & Golden-Kreutz, 2001).

Even when cancer treatment is successful and the disease is in remission, the fear, stress, and uncertainty do not go away. The threat of recurrence looms, for some patients for the rest of their lives. In fact, the distress associated with cancer recurrence is generally even greater than that following the initial diagnosis (Thompson, Andersen, & DePetrillo, 1992).

Cancer survivors also face emotional trauma related to their experiences. Consider the case of a 40-year-old cancer survivor who received a bone marrow transplant for his leukemia. Two years later, the patient still had flashbacks of receiving radiation treatment whenever he heard the sound of an electric generator. Colors that reminded him of the hospital environment frequently triggered chills, sweating, and nausea. And he refused to allow his family to bring a Christmas tree into the house because the pine smell reminded him of a hospital disinfectant. About 13 percent of BMT patients have similar reactions and are diagnosed with *post-traumatic stress disorder* (PTSD) (see Chapter 4).

To help such patients, researchers at the Ruttenberg Cancer Center have developed a 10-session, trauma-focused intervention that teaches patients relaxation techniques and cognitive coping strategies to control PTSD symptoms (Smith, Redd, DuHamel, Vickberg, & Ricketts, 1999). The intervention is currently being tested in a randomized clinical trial in which patients receiving the intervention are assessed before the intervention, 1 week after the intervention, and 3 months later, to ascertain whether the program has reduced PTSD symptoms.

Health psychologists are also investigating ways to help breast cancer survivors cope with the aftermath of chemotherapy. Although most women cope well during treatment, a significant number feel distressed, sad, and fearful about their futures after the treatment. These feelings are often made worse by the fatigue that customarily follows a regimen of anticancer drugs—fatigue that causes some to worry that the disease is returning. Feelings such as these argue for regular interventions that educate cancer patients about what's normal following treatment, and for health psychologists to use their skills to improve the quality of life of cancer patients. Unfortunately, many health insurance providers do not distinguish between mental illness and psychosocial interventions for cancer patients. As a result, many patients find that anxiety is not covered by their health care insurance.

Longitudinal studies show, however, that for most patients the emotional crisis of diagnosis and treatment lessens as time passes, treatment ends, and recovery begins (Andersen & Golden-Kreutz, 1997).

Personality and Coping

Although the link between personality traits and the development of cancer is tenuous, research has shown that personality does predict how well a person copes with cancer. For instance, in a recent study of women treated for early-stage breast cancer within the prior year, researchers found that the strongest concerns were fear of recurrence, pain, and death. Harm from treatment, financial problems, and body-image concerns caused moderate worry, while concern about rejection was minimal. Younger women had stronger sexual and partner-related concerns than older women (Spencer et al., 1999).

Cancer victims who psychologically "give in"—who are unwilling to fight the disease—have a much poorer prognosis than those who maintain a "fighting spirit" (Giedt, 1997). For example, in one 15-year study of women with breast cancer, this spirit was associated with a significantly lower mortality rate than denial, helplessness, or even stoic acceptance (Greer, 1991). In a sense, then, *poor* adjustment and nonacceptance of the diagnosis are *positive* traits for cancer victims.

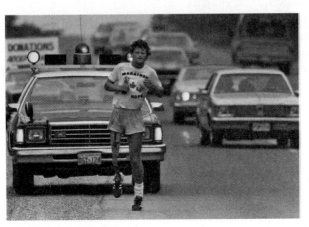

True "Fighting Spirit"
Canadian Terry Fox's refusal to be defeated by cancer has inspired several generations. In this photo, Terry, who lost his right leg to cancer, runs along a highway just before reaching the halfway mark in his cross-Canada run. Terry ran coast-to-coast on an artificial limb to raise money to fight the killer disease. © Bettmann/Corbis

Further evidence for the role of coping in cancer adjustment is provided from a study of women with newly diagnosed breast cancer (Stanton & Snider, 1993). Using a prospective design, the researchers demonstrated that patients who relied on a *disengaged* coping style experienced significantly greater psychological distress than those who coped in a more *engaged* manner. Other researchers have found that an optimistic disposition at the time the cancer is diagnosed is associated with an active, engaged coping style and less psychological distress over time (Carver, Pozo, Harris, Noriega, & Scheier, 1993). In one study of breast cancer patients, those who scored very low on a measure of dispositional optimism at the time of diagnosis experienced greater symptoms of anxiety and depression and relied more often on avoidant, emotion-focused coping than did their more optimistic counterparts (Epping-Jordan et al., 1999). Interestingly, in this study younger age was also predictive of greater anxiety and depression, *but only at the time of diagnosis.* The researchers suggest that relative to older women, younger women may experience higher levels of distress when the disease is diagnosed because they have more intrusive thoughts about their cancer. Younger and older women did not differ in their adjustment over the course of treatment and recovery, however. At 3 and 6 months after diagnosis, symptoms of anxiety and depression tended to occur only in those who continued to be troubled by persistent, intrusive thoughts about their illness.

Knowledge, Control, and Social Support

Considering the stress associated with being treated for cancer, most patients display remarkable physical and psychological resilience. Having access to information, perceiving some degree of control over treatment, and being able to express emotions while feeling supported by others are important factors in adjusting to cancer treatment.

Knowledge and Control

Health psychologists have made considerable progress in understanding the psychological reactions of patients to cancer treatment and the types of interventions that are effective in assisting their adjustment. They have found, for example, that procedural information (such as how the surgery, radiation, or chemotherapy regimen will be administered, as well as what the patient can expect before and after treatment) has wide-ranging benefits. Among these are fewer negative emotions, reduced pain, and briefer hospitalization (Johnston & Vogele, 1993).

Also beneficial are interventions that focus on preventing patients from feeling helpless during their treatment. Even something as simple as encouraging patients to make choices about the hospital environment can improve a patient's well-being (Patenaude, Hirsch, Breyer, & Astbury, 1990). For this reason, patients often are encouraged to decorate their room with pictures, photographs, and other personal items from home.

Social Support and Emotional Disclosure

Key to any effective intervention is providing cancer patients with emotional support and an opportunity to discuss their fears about the disease and its treatment (Andersen & Golden-Kreutz, 1997). For example, women with metastatic breast cancer who were allowed to discuss their fears showed an 18-month increase in survival (Spiegel, Bloom, Kraemer, & Gottheil, 1989). Similarly, men and women with melanoma who met regularly with a support group showed increased survival rates and reduced recurrence after 5 to 6 years, as compared to control patients who received standard biomedical treatment (Fawzy et al., 1993).

A more recent study examined the importance to patients of being able to actively process and express the emotions involved in coping with a life-threatening illness. The participants were recruited within 20 weeks after completing primary treatment (surgery, chemotherapy, radiation) for breast cancer. Over the next 3 months, women who expressed their emotions about cancer had fewer medical appointments for cancer-related health problems and reported significantly lower stress levels compared with their less expressive and less socially receptive counterparts (Stanton et al., 2000). The researchers suggest that by openly expressing one's fears—for instance, a loss of perceived control—"one may begin to distinguish what one can and cannot control [in order] to channel energy toward attainable goals, and to generate alternate pathways for bolstering control." They also suggest that repeated expression of emotions may decrease negative emotions and the physiological arousal that comes with them, leading cancer patients to believe that their situation is not as dire as originally thought and to derive some benefit from their adversity. Other studies have reported that experimentally inducing individuals to write or talk about stressful experiences can enhance physical and psychological health (Pennebaker, Mayne, & Francis, 1997; Smyth & Pennebaker, 2001).

A spouse or significant other provides an important source of social support for many cancer patients. When this relationship is perceived as solid and

For many cancer patients, there is a wide gap between optimal care and the care they actually receive. A report from the Institute of Medicine's National Cancer Policy Board, for instance, found that physicians often fail to recognize signs of depression and other long-term psychological effects of cancer and its treatment (Rabasca, 1999).

supportive, the patient's physical and emotional well-being benefits greatly. For example, cancer patients who are married tend to survive the disease better than unmarried persons (Pistrang & Barker, 1995). This is due in part to the fact that married patients—often because of nagging by their spouse—generally detect cancer and other diseases at an earlier stage of development, and they are more likely to seek early treatment.

The benefits of social support extend beyond marriage. Women and men who feel "socially connected" to a network of caring friends are less likely to die of all types of cancer than their socially isolated counterparts (Reynolds & Kaplan, 1990).

Social Support and Other Systematic Interventions

Other, more systematic interventions focus on improving the ability of patients to cope with their anxiety and stress during and immediately following cancer treatments. For example, Nancy Fawzy and her colleagues (1993) evaluated cancer recurrence and survival in patients suffering from malignant melanoma. For 6 weeks following surgery, half the patients attended weekly group meetings that centered on health education, stress-management skills, and social support. The others (the control group) did not attend any such meetings. A 6-year follow-up revealed that the intervention group had significantly better survival rates than the control group did.

Other studies have demonstrated that specific interventions are most effective at certain times. For example, one group of researchers divided breast, colon, lung, and uterine cancer patients into two groups: one that began a group intervention soon after entering the study and the other after 4 months (Edgar, Rossberger, & Nowlis, 1992). At the start of the study, both groups were measured on depression, anxiety, illness worry, and perceived personal control; follow-up measures were taken at 4-, 8-, and 12-month intervals. The intervention consisted of five 1-hour sessions that focused on developing coping skills, using such techniques as goal setting, problem solving, cognitive reappraisal, and relaxation training, and providing workshops on health-care resources. Coping improved for all patients, but the greatest reduction in stress levels occurred in the group whose intervention began 4 months after being diagnosed with cancer. According to the researchers, patients' needs shortly after being diagnosed with cancer are probably quite different from their needs a few months later, after the emotional shock of the situation has been overcome.

Psychoneuroimmunology and Holistic Medicine

Health psychologists have made considerable progress in developing cognitive-behavioral interventions in comprehensive cancer care. For adults, they have focused on pain relief, control of aversive reactions to treatment (such as nausea during chemotherapy), and enhancement of emotional well-being. For children, they have focused on increasing treatment compliance and reducing suffering (Redd & Jacobsen, 2001. Among the most widely used interventions are hypnosis, progressive muscle relaxation with guided imagery, systematic desensitization, biofeedback, and cognitive distraction. In this section, we describe two of the more common techniques: guided imagery and systematic desensitization.

Many of these interventions stem from the relatively new field of *psychoneuroimmunology (PNI)* (see Chapter 4). PNI researchers believe that the risk for many diseases, including cancer; the course that a particular disease follows; and the remission and recurrence of symptoms are all influenced by the interaction of behavioral, neuroendocrine, and immune responses.

In recent years, the PNI model has been integrated into the practice of **holistic medicine.** Rather than treating only the disease, holistic medicine incorporates physical, mental, emotional, and spiritual techniques to treat each person as a functioning whole (Giedt, 1997).

Guided Imagery

Guided imagery draws on patients' psychophysiological reactions to the environment to help them optimize physiological activity in various body systems and thus relieve pain or discomfort. For example, a patient who views an impending surgery as a life-threatening trauma may exhibit hypertension, cardiac arrhythmia, and other health-compromising responses prior to surgery. Conversely, a patient who looks forward to the same operation as a life-saving event is more likely to remain relaxed before, during, and following treatment.

In guided imagery, the therapist uses one or more external devices to help the patient relax and then form clear, strong, positive images to replace the symptoms. Effective images draw on several sensory modalities, including vision, hearing, touch, and even smell or taste and may be stimulated by taped music, sounds of nature, verbal suggestions, pictures of objects or places, aromas from scented candles, or a variety of other devices (Naparstek, 1994).

Guided imagery begins with the patient assuming a comfortable position, either lying down or sitting, with eyes closed or open. After taking several slow, deep breaths, the person begins a process of systematically attending to any areas of bodily tension, which are then relaxed. A variety of techniques may be used to assist relaxation, including progressive muscle relaxation, biofeedback training, or autogenic training. Several of these were described in earlier chapters.

Once a relaxed state is reached, the person visualizes a safe, peaceful place and strives to make the image as clear and intense as possible by focusing on sights, sounds, smells, and other sensory aspects of the moment. At this point, the patient follows taped suggestions (or a nurse or therapist's verbal suggestions) and forms a mental image of a symptom, such as pain or nausea. The patient then imagines the symptom changing. For example, the "red," fiery pain changes to a cool shade of blue; queasiness is expelled from the body with each exhalation.

■ **holistic medicine** treatment of the "whole person" that incorporates physical, mental, emotional, and spiritual components

■ **guided imagery** the use of one or more external devices to assist in relaxation and the formation of clear, strong, positive images

■ **systematic desensitization** a form of behavior therapy, commonly used for overcoming phobias, in which the person is exposed to a series of increasingly fearful situations while remaining deeply relaxed

After a few minutes of focusing on the altered symptom (sometimes describing its changed appearance to the nurse or therapist), the patient is instructed to relax, breathe deeply, and return to the peaceful place. After several sessions, which may last only 5 or 10 minutes, most patients are able to perform imagery without assistance.

Bellaruth Neparstek (1994), a psychologist who has used guided imagery with countless patients, suggests that imagery is beneficial for several reasons.

- The body reacts similarly to sensory events, whether they are real or imagined.
- Imagery triggers a state of relaxed concentration that enhances the person's sensitivity to health-promoting images.
- Using imagery gives the patient an increased sense of control and a decreased sense of helplessness over stressful aspects of disease or treatment.
- Guided imagery may also work through the *placebo effect*. People who believe that imagery and relaxation have the potential to improve their health may, in fact, experience physiological changes that enhance the ability to fight disease.

Systematic Desensitization

After several sessions of chemotherapy, nearly one-third of all patients begin to feel nauseated in anticipation of an upcoming treatment session. Many health psychologists consider this *anticipatory nausea* to be a form of classical conditioning, in which events leading up to treatment (such as driving to the hospital and sitting in the waiting room) function as *conditioned stimuli*, becoming linked to the powerful physiological reactions elicited as *unconditioned responses* by the cancer drug (see Chapter 1).

Health psychologists have learned that incorporating guided imagery into **systematic desensitization** effectively counters this classically conditioned side effect of chemotherapy. In this form of behavior therapy, commonly used to help people overcome phobias, the person is gradually exposed to increasingly fearful stimuli or situations, while remaining deeply relaxed. In one study, Gary Morrow and his colleagues (1992) trained a group of oncologists and nurses to use desensitization with cancer patients. The patients were then randomly assigned to one of two treatment groups (one conducted by a psychologist and one conducted by a nurse) or to a control group that received no intervention.

In the first stage, cancer patients established a hierarchy of difficult moments related to an approaching chemotherapy session, such as awakening on the morning of treatment, driving to the hospital, and sitting in the treatment room. After instruction in several relaxation-inducing techniques, the patients used guided imagery to visualize each moment in the hierarchy while remaining in a relaxed state. As they gradually worked their way up from the least threatening image to the most threatening image, the patients were *reconditioned* to feel relaxation rather than anxiety and nausea.

Both treatment groups experienced a substantial decline in the duration of their nausea following treatment. In contrast, the control group's nausea actually lasted 15 hours *longer* than ever, perhaps as a result of additional classical conditioning. In follow-up studies, Morrow and his colleagues have found that the benefits of desensitization often increase over time. Like athletes who gradually improve in their visual imagery skills, many patients report much less nausea and vomiting over time as they improve their control over their anxiety in anticipating treatment. For those that don't improve, failure may be related to a nocebo effect (recall from Chapter 1 that this is an adverse effect of a placebo). That is, patients who report that such interventions are not helpful generally reported an initial distrust of the intervention's effectiveness.

The intervention studies we have discussed provide substantial evidence that psychosocial factors can influence a cancer patient's response to treatment and, quite possibly, the course of recovery (or the likelihood of recurrence). Those studies that have reported longer survival for cancer patients are especially vivid demonstrations of the value of such interventions.

Summing Up

What Is Cancer?

1. Cancer is the second leading cause of death in the United States. It is actually more than 100 different but related diseases. They result from the uncontrolled multiplication and spread of body cells that form tumors.

2. Four general types of cancer are carcinomas, lymphomas, sarcomas, and leukemias. Carcinomas are cancers of the epithelial cells, which line the outer and inner surfaces of the body. Lymphomas are cancers of the lymph system. Sarcomas are cancers that develop from muscle, bone, fat, and other connective tissue. Leukemias are cancers of the blood and blood-forming system.

3. Cancer defies a simple description because its occurrence varies with gender, age, ethnicity, and race. Although the risk of several types of cancer has declined dramatically, overall cancer mortality rates increased steadily throughout the twentieth century. Lifestyle changes, improved detection, and reduced smoking have contributed to declines in rates of new cancer cases.

What Causes Cancer?

4. Although some cancers are caused by viruses, most are caused by genetic mutations that gradually accumulate over a period of years. Most carcinogens are also mutagens that damage DNA. In cancerous cells, activated oncogenes force an overproduction of growth factors while inhibitory messages, which are normally specified by suppressor genes, are absent.

5. A person with no family history of cancer must have two mutations before the malignancy develops. This "two-hit" hypothesis explains why inherited cancers tend to strike much earlier in life.

6. According to the immune surveillance theory, cancer cells are prevented from spreading by agents of the immune system that constantly patrol the body for abnormal cells. Prolonged stress may compromise the immune system and allow malignant cells to spread. Reduced immunocompetence has been demonstrated following exams, divorce, bereavement, unemployment, and occupational stress.

7. Persistent stress may impair a cell's ability to repair DNA, although age, family history, and the presence of an already compromised immune system might also play a role in the person's health.

Risk Factors for Cancer

8. The leading risk factor for cancer is smoking. Cancers of the mouth, pharynx, and esophagus are linked to all forms of tobacco use, including smokeless tobacco and cigars. Passive smoking has significant health consequences for nonsmokers.

9. Diet is a factor in as many as one-third of all cancer deaths. Fatty diets promote cancer of the colon, prostate, testes, uterus, and ovary. Excessive intake of salt, sugar, and alcohol may increase the risk of certain types of cancer. Diets that include plenty of fruits, vegetables, and whole grains may play a protective role against some cancers. Regular exercise may also be a protective factor for certain cancers. Alcohol use, especially among tobacco users, is a major risk factor for cancer.

10. Some forms of cancer are inherited. Women who carry the mutated BRCA1 gene and who have a strong family history of breast cancer have up to a 90 percent lifetime risk of developing the disease. Most cases of breast cancer, however, are caused by nongenetic factors.

11. Research has linked a variety of environmental factors to cancer, including ultraviolet light, toxic chemicals, and occupational carcinogens.

12. Personality factors have also been linked to cancer. A pattern of traits, including a hopeless attitude, depression, and the suppression of emotion, may be related to the development of cancer. Nonacceptance of cancer as a death sentence and a "fighting spirit" appear to be positive traits that tend to prolong survival among cancer patients.

Cancer Prevention and Treatment

13. When cancer does develop, its impact on health can nearly always be minimized through early detection and treatment. Advances in genetic screening, mammography, CT scans, and other detection technologies have dramatically improved the survival rates for many types of cancer. Many people fail to heed early warning signs of cancer.

14. Biomedical treatments for cancer include surgery, chemotherapy, and radiation therapy. Surgery generally offers the greatest chance for cure for most types of cancer. Chemotherapy is used to destroy fast-growing cancer cells that have spread to parts of the body far from the primary tumor. Unlike chemotherapy, radiation therapy affects only the tumor and the surrounding area.

15. Many cancer patients try one or more alternative treatments (such as meditation, biofeedback, or herbal treatments) to relieve side effects and to improve their overall quality of life.

Coping with Cancer

16. Cancer and cancer treatment create unique stresses for both patients and their families. Even when treatment is successful, the threat of the disease's recurrence looms.

17. A variety of psychosocial interventions have been used to assist patients in coping with cancer. Effective interventions enhance patients' knowledge about what to expect from treatment, increase the perception of control over their lives, and offer a supportive social environment in which to share fears and concerns.

18. Interventions that provide health education and teach specific skills for solving problems and managing stress are also beneficial to patients' well-being. Guided imagery and systematic desensitization have been proved to be effective interventions in helping patients control the side effects of chemotherapy and other cancer treatments.

Key Terms and Concepts

cancer, p. 414
metastasis, p. 414
carcinoma, p. 414
sarcoma, p. 414
lymphoma, p. 414
leukemia, p, 414
carcinogen, p. 417

mutagen, p. 420
oncogenes, p. 420
suppressor genes, p. 420
immunocompetence,
   p. 422
immune surveillance
   theory, p. 422

carotenoids, p. 428
carrier, p. 431
melanoma, p. 433
Type C (cancer-prone)
   personality, p. 436
immunotherapy,
   p. 448

holistic medicine,
   p. 455
guided imagery, p. 455
systematic desensitization,
   p. 456

Health Psychology on the World Wide Web

Web Address	Description
http://www.arc.com/cancernet/cancernet.html	The National Cancer Institute.
http://www.cancer.med.umich.edu/prostcan/prostcan.html	The University of Michigan's prostate cancer Web site.
http://www.microweb.com/clg/	Links to breast cancer Web sites.
http://www.cancer.org/	The American Cancer Society.

Critical Thinking Exercise

False Claims for Health Products On Line

In June 1999, the Federal Trade Commission (FTC) launched a new program to combat fraudulent health products on the World Wide Web and alert consumers, who increasingly are using the Internet as a major source of health information, to be especially skeptical.

The FTC estimated that more than 22 million Americans had searched on line for health and medical information as of December 1998 (Galewitz, 1999). Overall, 29 percent of Americans use the Internet for medical information, with 70 percent doing so without the knowledge of their primary care physicians.

Consumers most frequently search for information regarding cancer, followed by heart disease. An estimated 25 percent of those who use the Internet as a medical resource join an on line support group.

But the FTC also has evidence that consumers too often come up with less-than-credible medical advice on line. In several widely publicized cases, companies have used the Internet to make unsupported claims about a cure for arthritis made from beef tallow; a shark cartilage remedy to treat cancer and AIDS/HIV; and magnetic therapy devices that can alleviate high blood pressure and liver disease. Some companies even attempt to advertise products on line that have been declared unsafe by the Food and Drug Administration (FDA) and banned in drugstores. So far, the FTC has tracked down about 800 sites that advertise questionable disease cures. Particularly troubling is that some manufac-

turers use the Web to post seemingly credible scientific research about their product. But the average consumer browsing the Internet has no way of determining the quality of this evidence.

The Association of Cancer Online Resources (ACOR), which runs many of the Internet's cancer list servers, recently took steps intended to keep out bad health information from reaching its subscribers, more than 36,000 cancer patients and caregivers. Whenever a company posts a claim about a cancer cure, members of ACOR challenge them to offer scientific proof.

The Department of Health and Human Services is encouraging people to use the federal consumer health information gateway at www.healthfinder.gov as a reliable resource. The FDA has its own site — www.fda.gov — that consumers can search for additional information.

In this exercise you are asked to explore these two Web sites and then answer the following questions.

1. What is Med Watch? State its four goals.

2. In the legal sense, what is a "dietary supplement"? How are dietary supplements regulated?

3. Are advertisements for dietary supplements regulated by the FDA?

4. Does the FDA analyze the content of dietary supplements?

5. What kinds of claims can, and cannot, be made on the labels of dietary supplements?

11

HIV and AIDS

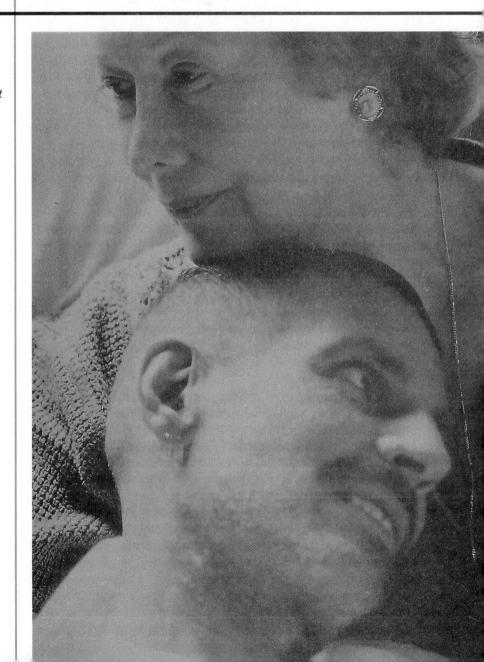

*M*ercy Makhalemele—a 23-year-old woman from Durban, South Africa—discovered that she was HIV-positive when she became pregnant with her second child. She had always been faithful to her husband of 5 years and simply couldn't understand how she had contracted the virus. Fearing what might happen if her husband and employer found out, Mercy kept her secret for almost a year. When she finally realized that her husband must have been the source and confronted him with the news, he became violent, beating her and pushing her against a hot stove that badly burned her wrist. Then he threw her out of the house, refusing to admit that he had given her the virus. Later, he stormed into the shoe store Mercy managed, shouting in front of coworkers and customers that he wanted nothing to do with someone with AIDS. Mercy was fired later that day.[1]

Mercy's experience is not an isolated story. AIDS has become the world's fourth leading cause of death and the number one killer in sub-Saharan Africa, where in 2000 it claimed 3 million lives and affected as many as one out of every three people (World Health Organization, 2000). In most African towns, however, asking whether AIDS is common will lead to a quick denial. The social stigma attached to AIDS is so strong that few will admit to being HIV-positive. Those who do come forward are shunned.

AIDS arouses such passion because it is associated with two highly taboo subjects: sex and death. The shame that AIDS victims feel and the treatment they receive from their neighbors, coworkers, and even family members is the greatest barrier in the battle to stop the spread of the dis-

ease. Even when AIDS testing is available, many Africans don't want to know if they have the virus. Those who know they have the disease are ashamed and afraid to admit it, so they act as if nothing is wrong, which often contributes to the spread of the disease. Similarly, many AIDS victims do not go to the clinics because they are too ashamed to be seen there, even though early treatment can prolong survival and dramatically improve the quality of life among those who are infected.

This tendency to "blame the victim" for his or her plight is not confined to developing countries. Many Americans also believe that AIDS patients are being punished for their immorality (Herek & Capitanio, 1997). Because of fears about AIDS and because many people link drug abuse and homosexuality to AIDS, patients and their families typically feel stigmatized. Afraid that disclosing their illness will lead to rejection by friends, neighbors, and coworkers, some may withdraw and become secretive. In so doing, they cut off the social support that can play a vital role in their survival.

Although AIDS is a newly discovered disease, some health experts believe that it actually may be thousands of years old. AIDS has become a global problem only recently because of the dramatic increase in mobility of most of the world's population, which has allowed the disease to spread from continent to continent. Although the initial panic created by the outbreak of the HIV virus has subsided somewhat in developed countries, where early screening and aggressive new drug treatments have given cause for hope, in developing countries the picture is bleaker than ever. Worldwide, an estimated 36 million people had HIV as of August 2001.

[1]Mercy Makhalemele's story is adapted from S. Daley, 1998, *Dead Zones: The Burden of Shame.*

■ **AIDS (acquired immuno-deficiency syndrome)** a life-threatening disease caused by the human immuno-deficiency virus in which the body's CD4 lymphocytes are destroyed, leaving the victim vulnerable to opportunistic diseases

■ **HIV (human immunodeficiency virus)** the retrovirus that causes AIDS; it injects its genome into lymphocytes, so that it reproduces when the cells are activated

This chapter takes a thorough look at the AIDS epidemic. We begin by examining the origins of the virus that causes AIDS, its impact on the body, and how the virus is spread. Next, we take up the question of how AIDS is treated. Because researchers generally believe that the development of a cure is unlikely in the near future, we'll examine how the spread of AIDS can be prevented through both medical and psychosocial interventions. The chapter concludes with a discussion of health psychology's role in the design and implementation of intervention programs to help AIDS patients, partners, and family members cope with their crisis.

The AIDS Epidemic

AIDS is an acronym for **acquired immunodeficiency syndrome,** a life-threatening disease caused by the **human immunodeficiency virus (HIV).** The virus attacks the body's immune system and leaves it vulnerable to infection. As HIV sickness develops into full-blown AIDS, its victims usually develop infections that would otherwise be handled with relative ease if their immune systems were not compromised. In this way, AIDS increases its victims' vulnerability to *opportunistic infections,* such as pneumonia and certain cancers, because the virus preys on their weakened immune systems.

A Brief History of AIDS

In the late 1970s, unrecognized cases of what we now know to be AIDS began to appear. Although no one knows exactly how the AIDS virus affected the first human, it appears to have originated in west central Africa, spreading quickly through Cameroon, the Democratic Republic of the Congo, Uganda, and neighboring countries. HIV is one of a family of primate viruses similar to a harmless virus found in certain subspecies of chimpanzees and green monkeys.

In February 1999, researchers from the University of Alabama found that a virus carried by the *Pan troglodyte troglodyte* chimpanzee, which was once common in west central Africa, was almost identical to HIV (Gao et al., 1999). The researchers claimed that these chimpanzees were the source of HIV and that the virus at some point crossed from chimpanzees to humans, perhaps when an unlucky animal handler was bitten, and gradually spread through the human population. It is not clear, however, that these chimpanzees are the original source of HIV because it is so rare that they are infected with the virus. It remains possible that both chimpanzees and humans were infected from a third, as yet unidentified, primate species.

Patient Zero

Whatever the origins of HIV, the role of international travel in its spread through the population is underscored by the case of "Patient Zero," a Canadian flight attendant named Gaetan Dugas, whose job and sexual habits made him a potent carrier for spreading HIV. Analysis of the early cases of AIDS showed that a large number of the infected individuals had either direct or indirect sexual contact with Gaetan Dugas. These cases could be traced to several different American cities that were frequent stops on the flight attendant's travel itinerary, suggesting that a single transmissible agent—like Dugas—was probably a key factor in the first wave of the disease.

The disease was first noticed in humans in 1980, when 55 young men (including Dugas) were diagnosed with a cluster of similar symptoms with an unknown cause. The symptoms were indicative of **Kaposi's sarcoma,** a rare cancer that attacks the cells that line blood vessels and is usually found only among the elderly. Epidemiologists suspected that the cause of the unexpected illness was a weakened immune system. Since most of the first reported victims were gay men and intravenous (IV) drug users, it appeared that the cause of the disease was a microorganism that was transmitted sexually or through the exchange of infected blood.

The Centers for Disease Control (CDC) finally tracked down Gaetan Dugas in 1982, a year after they published the first report on the disease. Dugas freely disclosed his sexual habits. Unaware that he had infected scores of homosexual men, Dugas estimated that he had as many as 250 sexual contacts in a typical year, even boasting that over 10 years, he'd easily had 2,500 sexual partners (Shilts, 1987). Although he refused to believe that he was the original carrier, Dugas cooperated by providing the names and telephone numbers of as many of his previous sexual partners as he could remember. By April 1982, epidemiologists were certain that 40 of the first gay men diagnosed with AIDS could be linked to Dugas: 9 in Los Angeles, 22 in New York City, and 9 in several other American cities. The odds that these connections were coincidental were infinitesimally small.

In 1983, the National Institutes of Health (NIH) in the United States and the Pasteur Institute in France simultaneously concluded that a new virus was the probable cause of the disease. In March 1984, Gaetan Dugas died. One month later the U.S. Department of Health announced that it had isolated a new virus—HIV.

The Spread of AIDS

During the last half of the 1980s, AIDS began to threaten the general population. Once limited mostly to white gay men, AIDS began surfacing among other ethnic groups. In January 1991, AIDS claimed its 100,000th victim. Public fear escalated when in November of that year basketball legend Magic

■ **Kaposi's sarcoma** a rare cancer of blood vessels serving the skin, mucous membranes, and other glands in the body

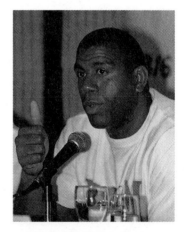

AIDS Awareness
On November 7, 1991, NBA superstar Earvin "Magic" Johnson stunned the world by announcing that he was HIV-positive. Because of Johnson's fame and the esteem and affection his fans felt for him, this statement was a major factor in increased AIDS awareness both in the United States and around the world. AP/Wide World Photos

Table 11.1

Regional HIV/AIDS Statistics and Features, December 1998

Region	Adults & children living with HIV/AIDS	Adults & children newly infected with HIV	Adult prevalence rate[1]	Percentage of HIV-positive adults who are women	Main mode(s) of transmission[2]
Sub-Saharan Africa	22.5 million	4.0 million	8.0%	50%	Hetero
North Africa & Middle East	210,000	19,000	0.13%	20%	IDU, Hetero
South & South-East Asia	6.7 million	1.2 million	0.69%	25%	Hetero
East Asia & Pacific	560,000	200,000	0.068%	15%	IDU, Hetero, MSM
Latin America	1.4 million	160,000	0.57%	20%	MSM, IDU, Hetero
Caribbean	330,000	45,000	1.96%	35%	Hetero, MSM
Eastern Europe & Central Asia	270,000	80,000	0.14%	20%	IDU, MSM
Western Europe	500,000	30,000	0.25%	20%	MSM, IDU
North America	890,000	44,000	0.56%	20%	MSM, IDU, Hetero
Australia & New Zealand	12,000	600	0.1%	5%	MSM, IDU
Total	33.4 million	5.8 million	1.1%	43%	

[1]The proportion of adults (15 to 49 years of age) living with HIV/AIDS in 1998
[2]MSM (sexual transmission among men who have sex with men), IDU (transmission through intravenous drug use), Hetero (heterosexual transmission)

Sources: National Institute of Allergy and Infectious Diseases (NIAID), June 2000, HIV/AIDS statistics (www.niaid.nih.gov/factsheets/aidsstat.htm). UNAIDS, December 2000, Report on the global HIV/AIDS epidemic (www.unaids.org/wac/2000).

Johnson announced that he was HIV-positive. This furor increased even more in February 1993, when tennis player Arthur Ashe died of AIDS contracted through a blood transfusion during heart surgery. But no cure was yet in sight; prevention was still the only weapon against AIDS as it claimed its 200,000th victim in 1993. The disease continued to grow exponentially, reaching 400,000 cases by 1994, with increased incidence among women and still no effective drugs.

As the millennium approached, however, there was some cause for optimism bounded by continued concern. While new anti-HIV drugs were finally proving to be effective, they weren't available to everyone who needed them, and, worldwide, the AIDS **pandemic** was spiraling out of control (see Table 11.1). In 2000, 5.3 million people were newly infected with HIV, making a total of 36.1 million people living with AIDS. Of these, 1.4 million were children under 15 years of age (World Health Organization, 2001).

pandemic a worldwide epidemic such as AIDS

The Epidemiology of AIDS

As you learned in Chapter 2, the first step in fighting and preventing a chronic disease like AIDS is taken by epidemiologists, who investigate the factors that contribute to its prevalence and incidence in a particular population. Keeping track of the distribution of AIDS by demographic traits is a difficult job because of the fluidity of the disease. However, it is most prevalent among certain populations.

In the United States, the AIDS epidemic has taken the greatest toll on young men, particularly African-Americans and Hispanic-Americans. At the beginning of 2000, 79 percent of the persons living with AIDS in the United States were men, 77 percent were between the ages of 35 and 64, and 21 percent were women (up from 15 percent in 1998). Very few young people have reported having AIDS—1 percent of those between the ages of 0 and 20—even though they make up 21 percent of the total population (Centers for Disease Control and Prevention, 2001). This last figure may be misleading, however, due to the long incubation period associated with the HIV virus. Many AIDS victims who are now in their twenties undoubtedly were infected while still in their teens.

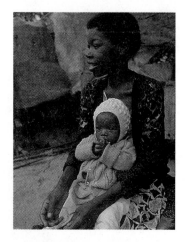

AIDS Is Out of Control in Africa
In Africa, more than 50 percent of women aged 15 to 25 are HIV-positive. This native of Kitwe, Zambia, is 27 years old. Her husband has already died of AIDS, and she has been diagnosed as HIV-positive. © A. Ramey/Stock Boston

Gender

Although in 1999 only 21 percent of AIDS victims in the United States were women, the rate of AIDS among women is increasing, and at a faster rate than that of men (Schneider, 2001). Women represent 40 percent of newly reported cases nationwide (and up to 60 percent in some inner cities) (Greiger-Zanlungo, 2001). Furthermore, women account for 25 percent of AIDS cases among adolescents and young adults (13 to 24 years of age). In some American cities, AIDS is the number one cause of death for young women.

These statistics are sobering, but the situation elsewhere in the world is much worse. Throughout Africa, more than 50 percent of women aged 15 to 25 are HIV-positive (in some countries this figure rises above 60 percent) (UNAIDS, 2000). In fact, globally, girls and women are 50 percent more likely than boys and men to contract HIV (UNAIDS, 2000). What accounts for this gender difference? One reason is that women are often less able to protect themselves from HIV, because they often are subordinate to men in intimate relationships (Ickovics, Thayaparan, & Ethier, 2001). Women who use illegal drugs are likely to use a needle only after their male counterparts have used it. They also have less control over whether a condom will be used during sexual intercourse.

Another reason is that more of the virus is found in ejaculate than in vaginal and cervical secretions. After intercourse, the infected lymphocytes in semen may remain in the vagina and cervix for many days, thus giving the virus more time to infect the woman. In contrast, secretions from an HIV-positive (HIV+) vagina and cervix are easily washed from the penis. Male-to-female

Figure 11.1

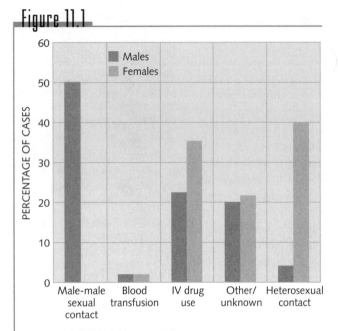

AIDS Cases by Exposure Category

The rate of AIDS among women is increasing at a faster rate than that among men. One reason is that male-to-female transmission of AIDS is far more common than female-to-male transmission. Another is that women are less in control of the decision of whether to use a condom. A third is that women generally use IV needles after their male partners.

Sources: *Health, United States,* by National Center for Health Statistics, 1998, Hyattsville, MD: United States Government Printing Office; *HIV/AIDS Surveillance Report, 9,* by Centers for Disease Control and Prevention (CDC), 1998, www.cdc.gov/hiv.

transmission of HIV through vaginal intercourse is far more common than is female-to-male transmission (Allen & Setlow, 1991) (see Figure 11.1).

Another difference between women and men is that on average, HIV levels in women are about half that of men with similar lymphocyte counts. Women progress to AIDS at a lower overall viral load than men (Farzadegan et al., 1998). These findings suggest the need for gender-based specificity in HIV/AIDS treatment, such as the need for lower cut-off points for determining drug treatment regimens. When this is done, women have the same rate of disease progression as men (Greiger-Zanlungo, 2001).

Sadly, among many impoverished young women, the risk of HIV infection is linked to sex that is used to obtain food and shelter or to support a drug habit. These women are much less likely to practice safe sex (Allen & Setlow, 1991).

Demographic Patterns

Worldwide, at least three large-scale patterns of HIV transmission have been identified. The first pattern is found in North America and Western Europe, where the most commonly affected groups are gay men and IV drug users. The second pattern includes sub-Saharan Africa and the Caribbean, where HIV and AIDS are commonly found in heterosexuals, equally distributed among men and women. The third pattern involves areas where HIV-infection rates are still relatively low and there are no specific lines of transmission. This pattern is found in Asia, Eastern Europe, North Africa, and some Pacific countries.

AIDS occurs among all races and ethnic groups. At the beginning of 2000 in the United States, 41 percent of AIDS cases were among African-Americans, 38 percent were European Americans, 20 percent were Hispanic-Americans, nearly 1 percent were Asian/Pacific Islanders, and less than 1 percent were Native Americans (Centers for Disease Control and Prevention, 2001). Figure 11.2 shows the devastating effect AIDS has had on the minority populations in the United States: Of the non–European Americans who are infected, 64 percent are African-Americans and 32 percent are Hispanic-Americans.

Ethnic and racial differences in rates of HIV transmission are thought to reflect sociocultural differences in drug use and the acceptance of homosexual and bisexual practices. For example, in impoverished minority communities, drug users commonly share needles; of course, when they share with HIV-positive drug users, they become infected themselves and expose their sexual partners. Intravenous drug use is therefore considered a cause of roughly 45 percent of AIDS cases among both African-Americans and Hispanic-Americans, whereas only 17 percent of AIDS cases among whites are linked to shared needles.

The initial spread of the HIV virus among IV drug users and gay men in the United States and other Western countries is believed to have occurred because these are relatively small, closed populations in which an individual is more likely to be exposed to the virus repeatedly. For many years, three out of four cases of AIDS were reported among the gay male population. Although rates among IV drug users and heterosexuals are increasing, gay men remain the largest group of AIDS sufferers. In 1998 alone, 16,642 AIDS cases were reported in gay men, compared with 11,070 in intravenous drug users and 6,735 in men and women who acquired HIV heterosexually (CDC, 2001).

In Africa, Asia, and other parts of the world where IV drug use and homosexuality are relatively uncommon, however, AIDS primarily strikes heterosexuals and both women and men in equal numbers.

Globally, heterosexual transmissions far outnumber all other sources of HIV transmission. Once it was understood how HIV was transmitted, the gay community in the United States led the fight to promote "safe sex." Many gay men limited their sexual partners, avoided anal intercourse, and began using condoms to protect themselves. Unfortunately, there is alarming evidence that younger gay men are beginning to revert to the risky sexual behavior that was prevalent before the AIDS epidemic initially struck (Kalichman, Nachimson, Cherry, & Williams, 1998).

Current Trends

When AIDS was first detected in 1980, fewer than 100 Americans had died of the disease. Less than 20 years later, more than 580,000 Americans had been diagnosed with AIDS, more than 360,000 had died from it, and AIDS had become the second leading killer of Americans between 25 and 44 years of age, second only to accidents.

The AIDS epidemic is spinning out of control. According to the World Health Organization (WHO), by the very beginning of 2001 the number of people living with HIV had grown to 26.1 million, 10 percent more than just 1 year earlier. In most nations, the number of people diagnosed with AIDS is doubling every 6 to 12 months. Worldwide, 11 people are infected every minute. Ten percent of these are under age 15.

The global death toll from AIDS continues to rise, totaling 3 million people in 2000 alone. AIDS is a still-emerging epidemic, with a death toll that has risen every year since the first reported cases. Even more alarming is that we can only guess how many people have been exposed to HIV and are therefore

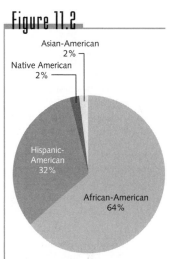

Figure 11.2

AIDS and Ethnicity in the United States
Although in absolute numbers AIDS occurs far more often among white Americans, it has taken a disproportionately greater toll on African-Americans and Hispanic-Americans. Although these groups make up only 12 and 8 percent of the population, respectively, together they represent 96 percent of all non–European American cases of AIDS.

Source: Centers for Disease Control and Prevention (CDC). *HIV/AIDS Surveillance Supplemental Report, 2001, 7. Characteristics of persons living with AIDS at the end of 1999.* Atlanta, GA: Department of Health and Human Services.

The Better Half Got the Worse End
Sheryl Gay Stolberg

The headlines last week trumpeted the good news: Deaths from AIDS had dropped 19 percent in the United States, continuing a decline first reported in May. The disease, it appears, has turned a corner in this country, changing from a death sentence into a chronic, treatable illness.

As the Centers for Disease Control and Prevention declared, "We have entered a new era in the HIV epidemic." Yet in the fine print of the government's statistics was a less cheerful tale. Between 1995 and 1996, deaths of women decreased by just 7 percent, as against 22 percent in men. And while the number of deaths dropped 28 percent for whites, the drop was 10 percent for blacks and 16 percent for Hispanic victims. The turnaround, in other words, has primarily benefited white men.

"The good news is that death rates are starting to fall," said Dr. Helene Gayle, who directs the AIDS program at the disease control centers. "The bad news is that the people who are having the least benefit from prevention efforts and better therapies are women and minorities." The trends are particularly troubling for women, who account for 20 percent of the AIDS population and are joining the nation's roster of cases faster than men. Most infected women are also minorities, and most are poor and uneducated. And their chances for survival are worse than for men, for reasons that have nothing to do with biology. When women get the same treatments as men, they fare just as well. But research has found that even when women are properly diagnosed, they are less likely than men to be placed on antiviral therapy.

One study, published in 1994 in the *Journal of the American Medical Association*, tracked 768 women and 3,779 men for 15 months. It found that women were 33 percent more likely to die than men who were comparably ill when they entered the study. In women, twice as often as in men, death was the first sign that HIV was progressing. Women, it was clear, were waiting longer than men to receive treatment. "It's definitely a tale of two cities, two communities," said Dr. Kenneth H. Mayer, director of the Brown University AIDS program.

The reasons for this are complex and have as much to do with socioeconomics and culture as with gender. Homosexual men, who account for the majority of men with AIDS, are often politically active, with strong networks of support. But many women with AIDS, experts say, do not know even one other woman infected with HIV. "Women, especially women of color, don't have the time or the money or the energy to be surfing the Internet to know what the new and improved latest treatment is," said Dr. Janet Mitchell, the head of the Department of Obstetrics and Gynecology at Interfaith Medical Center in Brooklyn. "They tend overwhelmingly to be mothers. They don't have that leisure to make AIDS the only focus in their life."

The CDC reports that while AIDS is now the second leading cause of death for American women aged 25 to 44, it is the leading cause of death for African-American women in that age group. In 1994, the centers reported that black women were almost 15 times more likely than white women to test positive for HIV. Black women are also more likely to shy away from AIDS

carriers who can spread the virus without being aware of doing so. One alarming estimate of the number of HIV carriers suggests that the number of reported AIDS cases is only the tip of the iceberg. This comes from the routine testing of military applicants: About 1 in 800, or 0.12 percent, were found to be HIV+ in January 1997. Extrapolating from this to the general population suggests that as many as 5 million Americans may be HIV+ (Cox, 1997).

Sadly, the battle against AIDS has not been won anywhere. More than 95 percent of all HIV-infected people live in the developing world, which is also where 95 percent of all AIDS deaths have occurred (WHO, 2001). In 1998 alone, sub-Saharan Africa was home to 70 percent of newly infected HIV victims and 80 percent of all AIDS deaths—2 million Africans (5,500 a day).

treatment, said Dr. Mitchell. "Communities of color tend to see Western medicine as an alternative and to see naturalistic, holistic approaches as what they will try first," she said. "If that fails, then maybe they'll say, 'Well, all right, Doc, I'll take your pills.'"

In a sense, the AIDS gender gap reflects the history of women with AIDS, a history in which women have always lagged behind men. AIDS made its first appearance in the United States in 1981 in homosexual men, who are now reaping most of the benefits of early prevention and education efforts. It was not until several years later that women began turning up with AIDS in large numbers. Some experts say it is to be expected that deaths in women will peak later in the epidemic.

Theresa McGovern, the legal director of the HIV Law Project in Manhattan, holds a different view. She blames the federal government for the disparity. "Ever since the beginning of this epidemic," she complained, "women have been overlooked." Ms. McGovern noted that it was not until 1993, after her group brought suit, that the Centers for Disease Control expanded its official list of AIDS-related illnesses to include ailments that are particular to women, such as cervical cancer and

chronic yeast infections. And even now, many doctors fail to recognize these conditions as signs of HIV infection. Moreover, it has only been four years since the National Institutes of Health began permitting women of childbearing age to participate in the early phases of AIDS clinical trials. Today, women account for 16 percent of the patients in government-financed AIDS studies, according to Dr. Anthony Fauci, director of the National Institute for Allergy and Infectious Diseases.

There are some efforts to close the AIDS gender gap. The Bristol-Myers Squibb Foundation, the charitable arm of the pharmaceutical company, recently gave $220,000 to the American Foundation for AIDS Research to establish the first national program to recruit and keep women in clinical trials. The foundation is giving the money to 12 community groups to study ways to overcome obstacles that keep women from enrolling in research, such as lack of day care or transportation. But Dr. Arthur Amman, who heads the AIDS research foundation, does not expect change in the numbers anytime soon. The statistics just released, he said, do not fully reflect the impact of protease inhibitors, the new drugs that have revolutionized AIDS treatment. "After

we see the impact of the protease inhibitors," he said, "the gap is going to get even bigger."

Perhaps just as troubling as the new numbers, Amman and others say, is the false impression they have left with the public. "You are reading in the paper that the epidemic is over," said Ms. McGovern, the legal aid lawyer, "and yet we are still watching these women die."

Source: *The New York Times,* July 20, 1997.

Exercises

1. Based on the material in the text and this article, what are some of the biological, psychological, and social factors in the AIDS gender gap?

2. What role can health psychology play in closing the gender gap? (Hint: Which of the factors identified above might be corrected through a primary or secondary prevention intervention?)

3. What can be done to get women to participate more actively in combating the AIDS epidemic? In their own treatment?

4. What can be done to encourage the research and health care establishments to close the AIDS gender gap?

Symptoms and Stages: From HIV to AIDS

HIV infects mostly lymph tissues, where *lymphocytes* develop and are stored. Recall from Chapter 3 that lymphocytes are immune cells that help prevent cancer and other chronic illnesses by controlling cell growth. They also guard against infection by producing antibodies. HIV invades and destroys a type of lymphocyte called the T cell (also called a CD4 cell), which is a crucial player in the immune response because it recognizes harmful microbes and signals B cells to begin producing antibodies. It also coordinates the release of natural killer (NK) cells.

■ **retrovirus** a virus that copies its genetic information onto the DNA of a host cell

■ **genome** all of the DNA information for an organism; the human genome consists of approximately 3 billion DNA sequences

How HIV Progresses

HIV is classified as a **retrovirus** because it works by injecting a copy of its own genetic material, or **genome,** into the DNA of the T cell (the host cell). Like all viruses, HIV can replicate only inside cells, taking over their machinery to reproduce. However, only HIV and other retroviruses incorporate their own genetic instructions into the host cell's genes.

The infected DNA may remain dormant in the chromosome of the host lymphocyte for a period of time. Eventually, however, the infected lymphocyte is certain to become activated against another virus or some other foreign substance. At that point, it divides, replicating HIV along with itself. As infected cells continue to divide, vast numbers of HIV particles emerge from the infected host and invade other lymphocytes.

Healthy human blood normally contains approximately 1,000 T cells per cubic milliliter. Despite the fact that HIV is reproducing in an infected person's body, this level may remain unchanged for years following HIV infection. Then, for reasons that biomedical researchers are still struggling to understand, T cell levels begin to decline and the immune system grows steadily weaker. Eventually, the victim is left with few functional immune cells and is unable to mount an effective defense against cells harboring HIV, HIV itself, and other invading microorganisms.

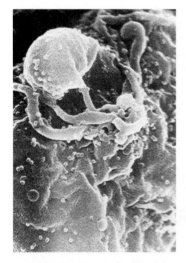

The AIDS Virus
Close-up view of the AIDS virus. HIV is classified as a retrovirus because it destroys lymphocytes by injecting a copy of its own genetic material into the host cell's DNA.
© John Chiasson / Liaison Agency

The Four Stages of HIV

HIV progresses through four stages of infection, which vary in length from person to person (see Figure 11.3). During the first stage, which lasts from 1 to 8 weeks, the immune system destroys most HIV and so people experience only mild symptoms that are similar to those of many other illnesses. Some victims develop a mild illness, with swollen lymph glands, sore throat, fever, and, in some cases, a skin rash. These symptoms are often so mild they go unnoticed; if noticed, they are not remembered.

The second stage, which may last for months or years, appears to be a period of latency because the person has no obvious symptoms except perhaps for swollen lymph nodes, which may go unnoticed. HIV is far from inactive during this period. In fact, during stage 2, as T cell concentration falls, HIV is constantly being replicated. Within 5 years, 30 percent of infected people move to stage 3, when T cells are further reduced, immune function is impaired, and opportunistic infections occur. Among the most common opportunistic infections are Kaposi's sarcoma (a cancer of blood vessels that causes purplish spots in the skin, mouth, and lungs), lymphoma, parasitic gastrointestinal infections, and *pneumocystis carinii pneumonia (PCP).* Caused by a parasite that infects the lungs, this type of pneumonia is the cause of death in 60 percent of AIDS victims.

During stage 4, the number of T cells drops from a healthy count of 1,000

Figure 11.3

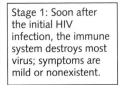

Stage 1: Soon after the initial HIV infection, the immune system destroys most virus; symptoms are mild or nonexistent.

Stage 2 (latency period): The T cell concentration falls and HIV concentration rises; accompanied by symptoms such as swollen lymph nodes.

Stage 3: As T cells are further reduced, immune function is impaired, and opportunistic infections occur.

Stage 4: Finally, almost all natural immunity is lost and full-blown AIDS occurs.

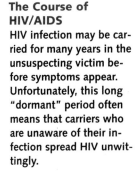

The Course of HIV/AIDS
HIV infection may be carried for many years in the unsuspecting victim before symptoms appear. Unfortunately, this long "dormant" period often means that carriers who are unaware of their infection spread HIV unwittingly.

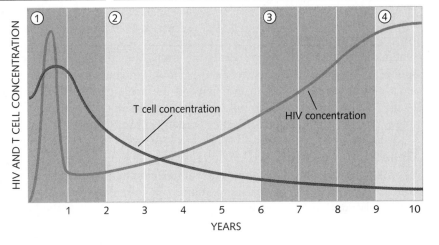

to 200 or less per cubic milliliter of blood and almost all natural immunity is lost. At this point, HIV has developed into full-blown AIDS. As T cell levels drop below 100, the balance of power in the immune system shifts to favor the invading virus. HIV levels soar, and microorganisms that the immune system normally would destroy easily begin to proliferate. Without treatment, death generally occurs within a year or two.

The Neurological Impact of AIDS

HIV affects many body systems, including the central nervous system. When HIV migrates to the brain and attacks brain cells, it triggers a variety of emotional and cognitive problems in half of all HIV-positive patients. In most cases, these disturbances involve forgetfulness, inability to concentrate, general confusion, and language impairment. In the later stages of AIDS, patients may display signs of depression, paranoia, and hallucinations that signal the **AIDS dementia complex,** a progressive cognitive deterioration that involves more substantial memory loss and confusion as well as shifts in personality. This complex may be caused by the dramatic loss of brain cells that accompanies the HIV infection. Researchers comparing samples of tissue from the brains of people who died from AIDS with those who died from other causes found a 40 percent lower density of neurons in the HIV group (Everall, Luthert, & Lantos, 1991).

"What HIV has done is tap into the most fundamental aspect of the immune system, and that is its immunological memory. It's the perfect mechanism for the virus to ensure its survival. Perfect because the virus lies silent inside cells that are programmed to do nothing but sit and wait. Their only job is to store a record of the germs they encounter, keeping the body prepared for the next time it sees them." (Haney, 2001, p. 11-A)

■ **AIDS dementia complex** an AIDS-related syndrome involving memory loss, confusion, and personality changes

Physiological Factors in the Progression of AIDS

Biomedical researchers have long been puzzled by the unpredictability of AIDS. The period from diagnosis of full-blown AIDS until death may be as short as several months or as long as 5 years. Furthermore, the average time from HIV infection to AIDS is about 10 years, although a lucky 5 percent of HIV-positive people live more than 15 years. Several factors are thought to play a role in the prognosis of AIDS.

Immunocompetence

One factor in a patient's prognosis is the strength of the initial immune response. HIV progresses much more slowly among patients whose immune systems mount strong lymphocyte activity in the acute stage of HIV sickness (stage 2). This strong defense apparently helps preserve the body's later ability to produce the T cells that target HIV (Bartlett & Moore, 1998).

Genetic Vulnerability

As with many chronic diseases, genetic vulnerability may also affect the rate at which AIDS develops. For viruses to attain their full impact on cells, they require collaboration from the body, which in the case of AIDS is the existence of the protein receptor to which HIV particles bind. AIDS researchers suspect that some people have genes that protect against the development of this receptor. Indeed, it appears that 1 percent of people of Western European descent inherit a gene from both parents that blocks the development of the receptor, giving them apparent immunity to HIV infection. Another 20 percent inherit the protective gene from only one parent and, while not immune to HIV, display a much slower progression of symptoms. Researchers have also found racial and ethic differences in responsiveness to anti-HIV drugs, suggesting the importance of considering a person's genetic profile prior to treatment (Mays et al., 2001).

Psychosocial Factors in the Progression of AIDS

After HIV exposure, the pace at which clinical symptoms begin to appear and the severity of illness at all stages of the disease vary tremendously. Poor nutrition, drug use, repeated HIV exposure, and other viral infections can all accelerate the progression of the disease. As with other diseases, however, epidemiologists have discovered that even after these physical risk factors are accounted for, there is still a tremendous amount of unexplained variability in the course of AIDS.

Stress and Negative Emotions

Health psychologists have investigated a number of psychosocial factors that influence the course of HIV infection and AIDS. Stress, negative emotions, and social isolation may influence the pace at which the disease progresses, perhaps by altering hormonal and immune environments that affect the resistance of host cells to the invading virus (Cohen & Herbert, 1996). Several researchers have reported that negative beliefs about the self, a pessimistic outlook, and chronic depression are all linked with a decline in T cells and a more rapid onset of AIDS among HIV-infected individuals (Burack et al., 1993; Segerstrom, Taylor, Kemeny, Reed, & Visscher, 1996). Similarly, HIV-infected African-American, Haitian, and Caribbean women who had a pessimistic outlook showed lower natural killer cell activity and T suppressor cell level, resulting in reduced immunity (Byrnes et al., 1998). HIV-infected individuals who maintain hope and are able to find meaning in their struggle tend to show slower declines in T cell levels and are even less likely to die (Bower, Kemeny, Taylor, & Fahey, 1997).

As is true of cancer victims, AIDS patients who deny their diagnosis may experience a more rapid development of AIDS-related symptoms. George Ironson and colleagues (1994) studied the progression of AIDS symptoms in a group of HIV-positive men who participated in a behavioral intervention program. At the start of the study all the men were asymptomatic. Two years later, those who refused to accept their **seropositive** status—that is, that they tested HIV-positive—showed a greater decline in T cells; decreased lymphocyte response to *phytohemagglutinin* (PHA), an antigen-triggering substance used to test immunocompetence; and other symptoms not seen in the positive-thinking patients.

Several researchers have suggested that the relationship between denial and AIDS may be part of a larger syndrome of emotional inhibition, which, as we saw in Chapter 10, has been linked to more rapid development of cancer and other chronic illnesses. For example, gay men who hide their sexual orientation deteriorate more rapidly following HIV infection than do men who more openly express their sexual identity (Cole, Kemeny, Taylor, Visscher, & Fahey, 1996).

Not all studies have found a positive relationship between negative emotions and changes in T cell counts, AIDS onset, or mortality rates (Kessler et al., 1991). In fact, some evidence indicates the opposite—that HIV-positive men who refuse to accept their diagnosis actually survive *longer* than those who accept their fate more readily (Reed, Kemeny, Taylor, Wang, & Visscher, 1994). Moreover, a meta-analysis of 34 studies found little evidence that negative emotional states such as depression, anxiety, or anger promote sexual behaviors that increase an individual's risk for contracting or transmitting HIV (Crepaz & Marks, 2001).

Why are the results of AIDS research studies inconsistent? One problem is that many of the studies measured stress, depression, or self-reported feelings of social support only at the *start of the study*. However, feelings of stress and depression are not static emotions; they may differ from one day or month to the next, depending on events in a person's life. Comparing the results of studies of different people with different statuses and at different times in their lives could be misleading.

seropositive the state of testing HIV-positive, indicating infection by the AIDS virus

For example, an HIV-negative person and an HIV-positive person respond differently to the loss of an intimate partner to AIDS. One study showed that during bereavement, HIV-positive men were more depressed, under greater stress, and more likely to use tranquilizing sedatives than HIV-negative bereaved men (Martin & Dean, 1993). In another study, researchers followed a group of 100 gay men up to 1 year before and 1 year after losing a partner to AIDS (Mayne, Acree, Chesney, & Folkman, 1998) and studied their high-risk sexual behaviors, such as unprotected anal intercourse, during the period of bereavement. Unprotected anal intercourse was relatively infrequent (2% to 5%) among HIV-negative participants prior to the death of their partner. This risky behavior increased to nearly 14 percent at 4 and 6 months after their partner's death and then returned to pre-bereavement levels by 12 months. Among HIV-positive men, 11 to 20 percent of participants engaged in unprotected anal intercourse prior to losing their partner. This dropped to between 4 and 7 percent at 2 to 6 months after their loss, and then increased to 31 percent by 12 months following the death of their loved one.

The researchers suggest that following the loss of a partner to AIDS an HIV-positive individual may feel more vulnerable and have an increased sense of his or her own mortality. This may promote greater adherence to health-promoting behaviors such as avoiding high-risk sexual activity. An uninfected survivor may experience survivor's guilt or, alternatively, relief after the stress of prolonged caregiving, possibly triggering an increase in more reckless behavior.

Research studies of how psychosocial factors such as outlook, social support, and stress affect the course of AIDS are at the cutting edge of health psychology. In addition to improving a person's chances of surviving HIV infection, the results of these studies will help us to gain a greater understanding of the interaction of biological, psychological, and social factors in health and disease and thus to refine our understanding of the connections between mind and body.

Stress and Social Support

Social support is also a factor in the progression of HIV sickness and AIDS. In one study, patients who tested positive for HIV were followed for 5 years. Those who reported greater isolation and less emotional support at the start of the study showed a significantly greater decline in T cells over the course of the study than those who reported feeling more socially connected (Theorell et al., 1995). In another study, Margaret Kemeny and her colleagues (1994) reported that HIV-positive men who recently lost an intimate partner to AIDS showed increased blood levels of *neopterin*, an indicator of more rapid disease progression, as well as a reduction in lymphocyte proliferation.

Lack of social support may cause AIDS to develop more quickly partly because it leaves those who are HIV-positive less able to cope effectively with stressful life events. In a prospective study of stressful life events, social support, coping, and AIDS that began in 1990, Jane Leserman and her colleagues

(2000) studied 82 HIV-infected gay men every 6 months. The participants reported the number of stressful events in their lives, their styles of coping with stressful events, and their satisfaction with the social support available to them. The researchers also measured blood levels of T cells, as well as serum levels of cortisol and other stress hormones.

Although none of the HIV-positive men had any AIDS symptoms at the start of the study, one-third of them have thus far exhibited some symptoms. For every increase in the number of stressful life events—equivalent to one severely stressful event (a death in the family or the loss of a job, for instance) or two moderately stressful events (illness in the family or strained relations with the boss, for example), the risk of AIDS doubled. The risk of AIDS has also doubled for every significant decrease in the average score on the satisfaction with social support scale, every increase in the use of denial as a coping strategy, and every 5 mg/dl increase in the level of serum cortisol.

Given the health benefits of having a strong social network, it is particularly tragic that AIDS is often a stigmatizing condition, and many of its victims lose friends and companions. Interestingly, at least one study suggests that pet ownership can provide a buffer against the isolation-induced depression that can accompany AIDS. Judith Siegel and her colleagues surveyed more than 1,800 gay and bisexual men, 40 percent of whom were HIV-positive and 10 percent of whom had already developed AIDS (Siegel, Angulo, Detels, Wesch, & Mullen, 1999). As other studies have found, men with AIDS, particularly those with the lowest levels of satisfaction with their social networks, showed markedly higher levels of depression than did HIV-positive men without AIDS and HIV-negative men in a control group. But whereas men with AIDS without pets were 300 percent more likely to report symptoms of depression than men without AIDS, men without AIDS who owned a pet were only 50 percent more likely to report symptoms of depression. The benefits of owning a dog or cat were strongest for men who felt the closest attachment to their pets, sleeping in the same room as their pets, for instance, and petting them frequently.

How HIV Is Transmitted

When AIDS was first reported in 1980, stories spread rapidly about the different ways in which AIDS is transmitted. Although some of the stories were true, many were false and aroused fear unnecessarily in the general public. A healthy dose of fear can be a good thing, especially for those who engage in high-risk behaviors. But, as we've seen, too much fear is not very helpful when you are trying to make logical decisions about health-related behaviors. As with all serious illnesses, it is important to know how HIV is actually transmitted, and how it is *not* transmitted.

Present in high concentration in the blood and semen of HIV-positive individuals, the virus can enter the body through any tear in the skin or mucous membranes, including those not visible to the human eye. HIV is transmitted

■ **hemophilia** a genetic disease in which the blood fails to clot quickly enough, causing uncontrollable bleeding from even the smallest cut

primarily through the sharing of virus-infected lymphocytes in bodily fluids—blood, semen, vaginal and cervical secretions, and breast milk. Fortunately, however, HIV is less easily transmitted than most other less deadly viruses (like malaria, for instance). Without a supportive environment of blood, semen, or the cytoplasm of a host cell, the virus quickly dies.

By studying groups of people who engage in risky behaviors, epidemiologists have gained a good understanding of how AIDS is spread. Research studies of high-risk groups have revealed that certain sexual behaviors (such as anal intercourse) and drug-related activities (such as needle sharing) are by far the primary means by which AIDS is spread.

Another route of infection involves a transfusion of infected blood. In the early years of the AIDS epidemic, HIV spread rapidly through transfusions of infected blood to victims of **hemophilia,** a genetic disease in which the blood does not clot quickly enough and the person suffers uncontrollable bleeding. Since 1985, however, blood banks have been screening all donor blood for HIV antibodies, and the risk of contracting HIV through transfusion has all but disappeared, accounting for only about 2 percent of all AIDS cases in the United States (Schreiber et al., 1996). According to the Centers for Disease Control, the chances of infection via blood transfusion are about 1 in 420,000 units of blood.

Children are usually infected through exposure to white blood cells from the mother's blood that pass through the placenta during labor and birth. Worldwide, it is estimated that one in four offspring of HIV+ women are so infected. Another 10 percent become infected after birth via breast feeding.

In a study of pregnant women in Florida, Ted Ellerbrock and his colleagues (1992) identified the key risk factors that predicted seropositive status. In order of importance they were as follows: being African-American, having sexual intercourse with a high-risk partner, having more than two sexual partners, and being a user of crack cocaine. As you will see later in this chapter, the association between AIDS and being a member of a minority group may be due to a number of factors, including lower socioeconomic status, gender stereotypes, and attitudes about sexual behavior. The link between crack cocaine and AIDS probably exists because unprotected sex with multiple high-risk partners often accompanies drug use.

Although the risk of accidental infection is very low, the possibility of patients being infected with HIV by doctors, dentists, and health care professionals became a public fear in 1991, when a Florida dentist with AIDS was reported to have infected six patients during office procedures (Ciesielski, 1992). The dentist had accidentally stuck himself with a needle, and then used that needle to inject anesthetics into his patients. To prevent such accidents from occurring, dentists and other health care workers today exercise caution around hypodermic needles. They have safety devices, such as a needle covered by a retractable sleeve that slides forward to cover the needle after an injection, that reduce the number of accidental needle-stick infections.

The chances of being infected through casual transmission (without sexual contact or sharing a needle with an infected person) are also very low. Some of the ways in which AIDS is *not* transmitted include

- donating blood; needles are discarded after a single use.

- exposure to airborne particles, contaminated food, or insect bites. There is no evidence that HIV can be transmitted through casual contact, coughs, or sneezes. To date, no family member or other caregiver has contracted HIV as a result of caring for an AIDS victim. Studies on insects indicate that they do not reproduce HIV.

- shaking hands, drinking from the same cup, engaging in superficial closed-mouth kissing, hugging, and sharing drinking fountains, public telephones, or toilets.

- sharing a work or home environment. As long as blood or genital secretions are not exchanged, family members and coworkers are unlikely to be infected through any form of casual contact. Studies on medical personnel who have been caring for AIDS patients since 1981 have consistently shown that there has been no spread of AIDS through casual contact.

Intervention Strategies for AIDS

In the absence of an effective HIV vaccine, psychosocial interventions are the only means of battling AIDS. Health psychologists play a number of roles in the battle against AIDS, including counseling people about being tested for HIV, helping individuals modify high-risk behaviors, helping AIDS patients cope with emotional and cognitive disturbances, and conducting bereavement therapy for those in the last stages of the illness, their family, and their friends.

Psychosocial Interventions

Since the beginning of the AIDS epidemic, many different interventions have been implemented. The earliest programs targeted high-risk groups such as gay males or IV drug users, using behavior modification and educational interventions to try to change attitudes and behaviors. Programs at the high school and college level have typically focused on increasing knowledge of AIDS and promoting safe sex. Mass media campaigns have emphasized awareness of how AIDS is transmitted—and they have been quite successful: By 1987, nearly all U.S. adults were aware of AIDS and more than 90 percent could correctly state the primary modes by which HIV is transmitted (Coates, Stall, & Hoff, 1990). Despite a slow beginning, AIDS education and other intervention programs skyrocketed during the late 1980s and 1990s, paced initially by the efforts of the gay community in the United States. As a result, public awareness of AIDS increased and a corresponding reduction in risk-related behaviors occurred, accompanied by a sharp decline in the number of new cases of HIV infection. Let's take a look at the theories on which the intervention programs are based and then at some of the interventions that are effective in reducing HIV/AIDS risk-related behavior.

The Basis for Psychosocial Interventions

Many of the theoretical models described in Chapter 6 have been used to predict whether and when people will change a risky health-related behavior. As a result, they often form the basis for HIV/AIDS intervention programs. First, we discuss the usefulness of these models in predicting behavior; in the next section we describe some of the interventions based on them.

Social cognitive theory, which suggests reciprocally determined relationships among environmental events, internal processes, and behavior (Bandura, 1997), has served as the framework for a number of interventions (Kalichman, Carey, & Johnson, 1996; Kalichman & Hospers, 1997). Three factors addressed by this model appear to be particularly important in successful intervention programs: *perceived social norms* regarding peer acceptance of HIV risk-reducing behaviors; *self-efficacy beliefs* controlling one's own thoughts, emotions, and behaviors in order to avoid unsafe behaviors; and *social skills*, the ability to respond assertively in negotiating risky behaviors. This was demonstrated by Seth Kalichman and his colleagues (1998), who found that gay men who practice high-risk behaviors also score lower on measures of perceived safer sex norms, safer sex self-efficacy, and social skills.

The health belief model—based on the idea that beliefs predict behavior—has achieved modest success in predicting condom use, the number of sexual partners, and knowledge of partners' past sexual history among a variety of high-risk groups (Abraham, Sheeran, Spears, & Abrams, 1992; Aspinwall et al., 1991). The theory of reasoned action, which also considers the person's attitude toward complying with other people's views, has achieved greater success, probably due to the influence of social norms on sexual activity of many at-risk populations, including teenagers (Schaalma, Kok, & Peters, 1993; Winslow, Franzini, & Hwang, 1992). As noted earlier, researchers have consistently found that people with more favorable attitudes toward condoms, as well as those who believe their friends are supportive of condom use, are more likely to engage in protected sex (Jemmott, Jemmott, Spears, Hewitt, & Cruz-Collins, 1992).

Support for stage models comes from evidence that certain individuals may profit more than others from a specific intervention. For example, younger, less knowledgeable individuals tend to benefit from educational interventions that close gaps in knowledge about how AIDS is transmitted, while older individuals in certain high-risk groups may be more likely to profit from interventions that stir them into preventive action.

In a recent investigation of the structure of beliefs about condom use, Dolores Albarracin and her colleagues interviewed a large, multiethnic sample of HIV-negative heterosexual males and females (Albarracin et al., 2000). Four psychosocial themes were analyzed for their ability to predict consistent condom use among heterosexual adults during vaginal sex. The themes investigated were the participants' beliefs that condom use: 1) provides effective *protection* from AIDS and other *sexually transmitted diseases (STDs)*, including herpes, hepatitis B, chlamydia, and HPV (human papilloma viruses); 2) is compatible with their *self-concept* concerning responsible sexual behavior; 3) either contributes to or takes away from their sexual *pleasure*; and 4) would have a negative impact on their *interaction* with their sexual partner. The results showed that the more closely condom use conformed to a person's self-concept and the less condoms were perceived as de-

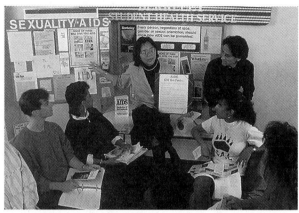

Education Should Begin at a Young Age
In the absence of a vaccine, preventing HIV infection remains our best weapon against AIDS. Throughout the world, educational campaigns are the major means of primary prevention.
© James D. Wilson / Woodfin Camp and Associates

creasing sexual pleasure, the more positive were the attitudes toward condom use. There was an association between intentions/behavior and all four areas examined: protection, self-concept, pleasure, and social interaction; but the association was much stronger with self-concept and pleasure.

Educational Programs

Educational programs and media campaigns are most likely to be effective when messages are adapted to the target group. One study, for example, compared the impact on African-Americans of an AIDS risk-reduction message delivered by white broadcasters with the same message delivered by African-American women that focused on culturally relevant themes, such as cultural pride and family responsibility (Kalichman, Kelly, Hunter, Murphy, & Tyler, 1993). Two weeks after watching the taped message, the African-American participants who had viewed the culturally relevant tape reported more concern and fear about AIDS than participants who had viewed the standard tape. They also reported either engaging or intending to engage in more preventive behaviors, such as being tested for HIV.

However they are delivered, all educational messages have one thing in common—to make people aware of AIDS and how to prevent it. There are a number of simple precautions that will protect against AIDS and other STDs. Obviously, abstaining from both drugs and sex or maintaining a monogamous sexual relationship with an uninfected partner are still the safest ways to prevent AIDS and other STDs. For those who are sexually active, it is important to limit the number of partners in the *sexual network,* range of sexual activities, and the extent of *sexual mixing* with people from other sexual networks (Catania, Binson, Dolcini, Moskowitz, & van der Straten, 2001). If a person has sex or shares a drug needle with someone who is HIV-positive, he or she may become a carrier of the virus. If the person then has sex or shares a drug needle with two other people, each of whom has sex or shares needles with two other people, it becomes obvious that the initial infection has the potential to spread to hundreds of other victims.

Health experts also offer the following specific precautions:

- Stay sober (alcohol and many other drugs lower inhibitions and increase the likelihood of high-risk behaviors).
- Avoid anal intercourse (the thin lining of the rectum makes this the most hazardous form of sex for transmitting HIV).
- Be selective in choosing partners. Avoid sexual contacts with people who are known to engage in high-risk sexual or drug-use behaviors.
- Use latex condoms during vaginal, anal, and oral sex. These barriers block nearly all sexually transmitted microorganisms, including HIV. Doctor-prescribed and fitted vaginal diaphragms or cervical caps that block semen and spermicides that paralyze sperm (and lymphocytes) are also advisable.
- Build caring, meaningful relationships with those with whom you are intimate.
- Never share hypodermic needles, razors, cuticle scissors, or other implements that may be contaminated with another person's blood or bodily fluids.
- Do not pay attention to rumors about AIDS. Donate blood to your local blood banks and encourage your healthy friends to do so. Doing so will help ensure the availability of an uncontaminated blood supply.
- Do not be lulled into a sense of complacency about AIDS and STDs by media reports about treatment breakthroughs. At present, there is no cure for AIDS.

Mass Screening and HIV Counseling

While education is important, it is often not enough. Many AIDS prevention programs now provide those at risk of HIV/AIDS with information about their current health status and about how AIDS is transmitted. Such programs began appearing in the early 1980s. In the most ambitious screening program to date, 110 million Japanese citizens were tested, resulting in the detection of 1,700 seropositive cases and 400 cases of full-blown AIDS (Gilada, 1991). HIV screening and basic counseling are also the primary preventive interventions in most state and federal programs.

People being screened for HIV benefit from interventions that help reduce their anxiety over testing positive. In a series of studies by Michael Antoni and his colleagues (2000), gay men were randomly assigned to intervention and control groups several weeks *before* HIV screening. Those in the intervention group participated in a multifaceted program that included aerobic exercise, relaxation training, and cognitive therapy aimed at modifying self-defeating attitudes. Each participant's psychological status and immunocompetence was assessed several times before and after receiving the results of screening. Among men who tested positive for HIV, those in the intervention group reported significantly lower anxiety and depression than those in the control group. They also displayed significantly stronger immune functioning, including increases in the levels and activity of CD4 cells and NK cells.

Are such counseling programs effective in reducing risky behaviors? The evidence is mixed, at best. One study of African-American inner-city teenagers randomly assigned some subjects to an AIDS risk-reduction group and the rest to a control group (Jemmott, Jemmott, & Fong, 1992). Those in the intervention group received educational materials and participated in workshops on high-risk behaviors conducted by African-American adults. Compared to control subjects, the teens in the intervention group reported greater condom use, fewer instances of intercourse, fewer sexual partners, and fewer instances of anal intercourse.

Health psychologists have also developed interventions to counteract the reality that many sexual encounters, especially with new partners, are emotionally intense, rushed, and not conducive to clear thinking and negotiating about safe sex (Miller, Bettencourt, DeBro, & Hoffman, 1993). The goal of such interventions is therefore to teach young men how to exercise self-control in sexual relationships and young women how to resist coercive sexual pressure. For example, intervention participants have been asked to use mental imagery to visualize risky sexual encounters that result in HIV infection. When coupled with role-playing exercises, modeling, and feedback, this type of intervention can be highly effective in giving young people the skills needed to avoid high-risk behaviors (van der Velde & Van der Pligt, 1991).

Unfortunately, successful interventions are more often the exception than the rule. Over an 18-month period, researchers compared HIV-risky behaviors in women who voluntarily sought HIV testing and counseling at four urban clinics and women who used other clinic services, such as physical examinations or vision tests. Although women in the counseling group were more concerned about AIDS than women in the comparison group, the two groups did not differ in the prevalence of HIV-risky behaviors. Both groups engaged in high-risk sexual behaviors, including having unprotected intercourse with partners of uncertain or high risk (Ickovics et al., 1998). Why is HIV counseling not automatically effective in changing high-risk sexual behaviors? One reason is that a person—even one who knows all about AIDS—must feel capable of controlling his or her risk-related behaviors in specific situations. Increasingly, health psychologists recognize that modifying sexual behaviors is a complex process involving two people with different agendas and different attitudes toward safe sex practices. For example, they have found that they cannot assume that both partners are equally empowered to consent to sex and to make decisions about risk. Many women report that in their first sexual experience (and too often, in subsequent experiences) their male partner coerced them to have intercourse (Bor, 1997). And although the female partner often is held responsible for ensuring the use of a contraceptive, she may not be empowered to insist that her male partner use a condom.

Research to date has shown a strong association between perceived *self-efficacy* and the prevalence of high-risk behaviors. For example, self-efficacy is linked to greater condom use among college students (Wulfert & Wan, 1993), gay men (Emmons et al., 1986), African-American teenagers (Jemmott et al., 1992), and Hispanic-American women (Nyamathi, Stein, & Brecht, 1995). In addition, gay men who have strong feelings of self-efficacy also tend to have fewer sexual partners and to be better informed about the sexual history of those with whom they are intimate (Wulfert, Wan, & Backus, 1996).

In another study of female college students (aged 17 to 23 years), those who scored high on self-efficacy regarding safe-sex practices were most likely to engage in AIDS-preventive behavior. These women also were least likely to deny their AIDS risk (Yzer, Fisher, Bakker, Siero, & Misovich, 1998). Along these lines, a five-city study of predominantly African-American women aged 15 to 34 years showed that those who consistently practiced safe sex were more likely to talk with others about condoms and felt more confident in their ability to negotiate condom use with their sexual partners (Stark et al., 1998).

Researchers have also found a relationship among self-efficacy, outlook on life, and the tendency to engage in high-risk sexual behaviors. A recent study showed that among sexually active inner-city minority adolescents (aged 15 to 18 years), those who were more optimistic were also more confident of their ability to practice safe sex (such as using a condom). Optimists also were more aware of and concerned about the dangers of unsafe sex (Carvajal, Garner, & Evans, 1998). Pessimists, on the other hand, were less concerned about the potential danger of unsafe sex, perhaps because they felt they had less to lose than their more optimistic counterparts. Furthermore, the pessimists' lack of feelings of self-efficacy led them to believe that there was nothing they could do to avoid those dangers, or the behaviors.

And finally, in a longitudinal study of heterosexual women, those who avoided unprotected intercourse had more favorable attitudes toward condoms and had a greater internal locus of control regarding their health. That is, they felt more personally responsible for protecting their bodies against HIV infection (as well as other health threats) than did women who more often had unprotected intercourse (Morrill, Ickovics, Golubchikov, Beren, & Rodin, 1996).

All these results suggest that the frequency of unprotected sex can be dramatically reduced with a few steps: Help people to improve their outlook on life, their feelings of self-efficacy, and their sense of personal control and encourage them to talk more openly about safe sex.

Promoting Disclosure of HIV-Positive Status

Because of fears about AIDS, and because the disease is commonly associated with homosexuality and IV drug use, HIV-positive people often feel ashamed and conceal their status. Many don't even tell their immediate family (Mansergh, Marks, & Simoni, 1995).

Most HIV/AIDS interventions have focused on preventing infection in at-risk uninfected persons. There have been few reported interventions aimed at preventing risky behaviors in people who have tested positive for HIV. By current estimates, of the 900,000 people in the United States infected with HIV, over 70 percent remain sexually active *after* they test positive for the virus (CDC, 1999; Kline & VanLandingham, 1994).

Withholding one's HIV-positive status from a partner obviously prevents that person from making an informed decision about sexual behavior and may result in the transmission of the virus to that person and others. Lying about one's HIV status or past sexual history or failing to volunteer the information is far too common. The results of one survey revealed that many college students would lie about their sexual history in order to obtain sex (Cochran & Mays, 1990).

Christine De Rosa and Gary Marks explored whether preventive counseling at the time of HIV diagnosis was associated with greater self-disclosure of HIV status to sexual partners. Among a sample of seropositive men, the researchers found that men who were counseled to disclose their status were more likely to do so than men who were not counseled. HIV-positive partners who disclose their HIV status are also more likely to engage in safer sexual practices (DeRosa & Marks, 1998).

Legal Issues

Regardless of how those who have tested seropositive feel about their responsibilities as carriers of HIV, AIDS is having a wide and varied effect on legal systems throughout the world. In the United States, scores of AIDS-related laws have been enacted in recent years. These laws are designed to protect the rights of HIV-positive people as well as those who are disease free. For example, many states have passed confidentiality laws that prohibit disclosure to anyone of *another* person's HIV status. Laws such as these have been passed because of the risks of discrimination that accompany AIDS. Antidiscrimination laws in the workplace and in housing are examples of this type of legislation.

As of June 2000, AIDS-related criminal statutes in the United States vary from state to state. In some states, persons who engage in activities that transmit or are likely to transmit any sexually transmitted disease (STD) are guilty of a Class C misdemeanor. In others, any person who exposes another to HIV through unprotected sexual activity or use of a hypodermic needle is guilty of a felony, when the infected person knows he is infected, has not disclosed the information, and has acted with specific intent to infect the other person. The thorny issue of AIDS and the law is explored further in the Critical Thinking Exercise at the end of this chapter.

Cognitive-Behavioral Stress Management

One of health psychology's roles in the AIDS pandemic is helping people who are HIV-positive to live with the infection. Several comprehensive intervention programs have been tested with seropositive patients. Many of these programs have been effective in improving the emotional and physiological well-being of HIV-positive individuals. In one, a team of social workers, psychologists, spiritual counselors, and patients meet weekly to discuss skills in managing depression, grief, anger, fear of dying, and other issues. Educational lectures and discussions focus on a variety of topics, including the legal rights of seropositive patients, stress management, and safer sex practices (Morokoff, Holmes, & Weisse, 1987).

A recent study evaluated the effectiveness of a 10-week cognitive-behavioral stress management (CBSM) intervention in reducing stress among seropositive men (Antoni et al., 2000; Cruess et al., 2000). Men who were randomly assigned to the experimental (intervention) condition participated in 10 weekly $2^1/_2$ hour meetings, which included both stress management and relaxation training components. The stress management portion focused on helping the men to identify cognitive distortions in their thinking and use cognitive restructuring to generate more rational appraisals of everyday stressors (see Chapter 5); it also taught them techniques to improve their coping skills, be more assertive, manage their anger, and make greater use of social support. Through group discussions and role-playing exercises, the men also learned to share experiences and disclose their fears and to apply various stress management concepts. The relaxation portion included progressive muscle relaxation training, meditation and abdominal breathing exercises, and guided imagery (see Chapter 10).

The results showed that the men who participated in the CBSM intervention reported significantly lower post-treatment levels of anxiety, anger, total mood disturbance, and perceived stress compared to the men who were assigned to an untreated control group (Figure 11.4). Moreover, those in the intervention group also displayed less norepinephrine output and significantly greater numbers of T-cytotoxic lymphocytes 6 to 12 months later.

Interestingly, men participating in CBSM also experienced significant increases in testosterone levels. Diminished levels of testosterone, which seems to cause decreased muscle mass, have been documented in HIV-infected men; these decrements appear to become more pronounced as the disease progresses to AIDS (Christeff et al., 1996).

Figure 11.4

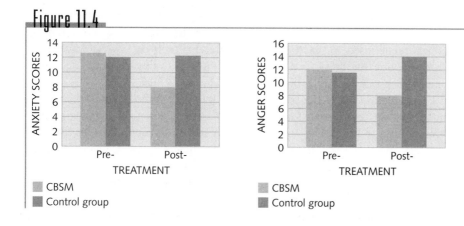

Pre- and Post-CBSM Treatment Anxiety and Anger in HIV-Positive Men

Prior to the intervention, men assigned to CBSM showed mood and anxiety scores similar to those men assigned to the control condition, as measured by scores on the *Profile of Mood States.* Following the intervention, CBSM participants reported significantly lower post-treatment anxiety and anger than their control group counterparts.

Source: "Cognitive-Behavioral Stress Management Intervention Effects on Anxiety, 24-Hour Urinary Norepinephrine Output, and T-Cytotoxic/Suppressor Cells over Time among Symptomatic HIV-Infected Gay Men," by M. H. Antoni, D. G. Cruess, S. Cruess, S. Lutgendorf, M. Kumar, G. Ironson, N. Kliomas, M. A. Fletcher, and N. Schneiderman, 2000, *Journal of Consulting & Clinical Psychology, 68*, pp.31–45.

How might CBSM lead to these beneficial physiological changes in HIV-seropositive individuals? One mechanism proposed to explain the effects of CBSM on immune functioning in these cases is based on the finding that norepinephrine levels tend to be elevated in HIV-infected people. As we saw in Chapter 3, elevated norepinephrine associated with arousal of the sympathetic nervous system may inhibit proliferation of lymphocytes in the body's immune response. This is, of course, particularly important for persons who are already plagued with decreased numbers of lymphocytes due to AIDS. CBSM may help sustain lymphocyte levels by moderating the individual's epinephrine response to challenging situations. The researchers also suggest that changes in cognitive coping strategies during the intervention or specific self-care behaviors (for example, better diet, more exercise) may contribute to elevated testosterone levels during CBSM. They also suggest that the intervention may have led to an increased sense of mastery over the disease itself. This is supported by other studies that have reported higher testosterone levels among the winners (versus the losers) in specific laboratory tasks (Bernhardt, Dabbs, Fielden, & Lutter, 1998).

Because of the inherent interactive nature of cognitive, affective, behavioral, and social elements of stress responses, it appears that the most effective way to "package" stress management interventions for HIV-infected persons may be a multimodal CBSM program (Antoni & Schneiderman, 2001).

Those who test positive may also need counseling and other interventions to help them cope with a wide array of problems over the course of the illness, including pain management, adherence to complicated medical regimens, and facing the possibility of death.

Communitywide Interventions

Intensive, coordinated, communitywide interventions have proved to be the best way not only to educate people about HIV and its modes of transmission but also to change social norms that influence sexual behavior. The most massive communitywide AIDS prevention program to date was implemented in San Francisco in 1982. The *San Francisco Model* involves seven different organizations chosen to reach people at different levels of risk (Coates, 1990). These include the mass media, schools, family planning centers, drug abuse clinics, health care organizations, and churches and clubs.

Each organization developed an educational program on how HIV is transmitted that was appropriate for its clientele. At each site, classes, videos, and models were used to teach safer sex practices. In addition, mass-media motivational messages and social action groups focused on increasing awareness of high-risk behaviors and reducing the social stigma attached to HIV-positive persons.

The comprehensive program proved immediately successful. At the start of the program, 60 percent of the sample reported engaging in high-risk behavior. By 1987, this figure had dropped to 30 percent. The continuing success of the program indicates that HIV/AIDS interventions need to strike on several fronts. Effective interventions are those that

- target high-risk behaviors among at-risk individuals.
- teach specific skills to reduce risk (such as proper condom use and needle cleaning).
- promote interpersonal assertiveness and other communication skills necessary to initiate and maintain lower-risk sexual relationships.
- address social and cultural norms that surround sexual activity.
- focus on improving self-esteem and feelings of self-efficacy regarding how to practice safer sex.
- address faulty, even "magical" thinking regarding HIV transmission and personal vulnerability.
- involve coordinated, community-level education.

Psychosocial Barriers to AIDS Interventions

Despite massive efforts to educate the public and discourage high-risk behaviors, condom use remains startlingly low. In a nationwide survey, Charles Catania and his colleagues found that only 17 percent of heterosexuals with multiple sexual partners always used a condom. Fully 38 percent reported *never* using condoms. Among heterosexuals who engaged in anal intercourse, 71 percent never used a condom and only 19 percent always did (Catania et al., 1992). And surveys reveal that although gay men are generally well informed about AIDS, heterosexual adolescents and other high-risk groups are not. Among single, pregnant inner-city women, for example, researchers have found an alarmingly high level of ignorance about AIDS or the sexual history of their partners (Hobfoll, Jackson, Lavin, Britton, & Shepherd, 1993).

Media depictions of sexual encounters, which almost never include the awkward search for and fumbling with a condom, do little to promote AIDS interventions aimed at promoting safe sex. This is particularly damaging for teenagers, who acquire a *script* of how things are supposed to progress and attempt to follow that script during their first intimate experiences (see Chapter 6). If a condom is not in the script, is it any wonder they will feel awkward in introducing one?

A number of studies have also found that misconceptions about sexual behavior in general, and HIV/AIDS in particular, are far too common. For example, Janet St. Lawrence (1993) found that nearly one-third of the sample of African-American teenagers she surveyed believed that they could prevent HIV infection simply by avoiding sex and other high-risk behaviors with people who "look like they have AIDS."

Another surprisingly common example of faulty reasoning about HIV/AIDS is the belief that the danger of HIV infection depends on the depth of the relationship with the HIV-positive person. This line of thinking causes many people to worry needlessly about casual contact with HIV-positive coworkers and strangers but to behave recklessly in their intimate behaviors with people they know more intimately (Nemeroff, 1995).

A closely related example of faulty AIDS/HIV thinking is the tendency of some people to feel that they are somehow less vulnerable to infection than others are. As explained in Chapter 6, these examples of *optimistic bias* and *perceived invincibility* surely contribute to the tendency to underestimate the risk that results from casual, unprotected sex; needle sharing; and other high-risk behaviors. Anna Kline and Jennifer Strickler's (1993) study of women in drug treatment programs is quite revealing. Although more than 76 percent of the women were IV drug users, 66 percent never used condoms and 47 percent had no knowledge of their sexual partners' HIV status; in addition, more than 84 percent thought they were unlikely to contract AIDS.

AIDS Complacency

Ironically, a significant impediment to AIDS prevention programs is the success of recent advances in treatment, which has brought new hope and optimism for HIV-infected people but at the cost of greater public complacency regarding the dangers of the disease. Widespread news of AIDS treatment breakthroughs has led to premature claims that HIV is more of a chronic than a life-threatening illness and that a complete cure is on the horizon. In addition, as you'll learn in the next section, anti-HIV drugs have become increasingly successful in reducing the concentrations of HIV in the infected person's body, suggesting to some that people under treatment may be less infectious.

As noted in Chapter 6, theories of health behavior emphasize that how people perceive their risk of getting a disease determines whether they will adopt

Diversity and Healthy Living

Sociocultural Factors and AIDS Prevention

Researchers have found that social and cultural factors play an important role in determining a woman's risk-related sexual behavior. For example, Adeline Nyamathi and her colleagues at UCLA found that among African-American and Latina women, self-esteem was linked with both the extent and quality of social support, which in turn was linked to active rather than avoidant coping strategies (Nyamathi, Stein, & Brecht, 1995). That is, women with strong social support believed in trying to handle and control a problem rather than putting it out of their minds or laughing it off. Active copers were also less likely to have a history of sexually transmitted disease (STD) and less likely to engage in risky behaviors that might lead to AIDS. Risky behaviors included using IV drugs, using noninjection drugs, having sex for money or drugs, and having a history of STD.

The researchers also found several differences between the ethnic groups. African-American women were more likely than Latina women to report a history of STDs, to use noninjection drugs, and to have multiple sexual partners. However, Latinas who were highly acculturated—immersed in the mainstream culture—were more likely than either African-American women or their less acculturated Latina counterparts to be IV drug users.

Many women in both ethnic groups used condoms infrequently, but for very different reasons. Among African-American women, lower self-esteem was associated with more perceived barriers to condom use. Among Latina women, however, *social resources* predicted lower condom use. The researchers suggest that this unexpected relationship reflects the traditional sociocultural and religious norms among Hispanics that forbid or strongly discourage the use of condoms. An earlier study found that less acculturated Latina women are less likely to carry and use condoms but are also less likely to report multiple sexual partners than their more acculturated counterparts (Marin et al., 1993).

Nyamathi's group also explored the participants' self-reported reasons for not using condoms consistently with their main sex partner. The perceived barriers to condom use fell into three categories. First, either the woman or her partner disliked the use of condoms. Second, either or both believed that protection (from AIDS and other STDs) was unnecessary. The third category, which reflected social and educational deficiencies as well as lifestyle hardships, included such things as the woman's fear of getting beaten up by her partner, not knowing how to use a condom, and feeling powerless to discuss safe sex with sexual partners.

The results of this study point to important cultural differences in why people practice, or do not practice, AIDS-

healthy behavior (Kalichman, 1998; Rosenstock, Strecher, & Becker, 1994). So, if they now perceive a reduced threat of HIV/AIDS, they—at least some groups—are more likely to engage in high-risk sexual behaviors. A recent study showed that gay and bisexual men who practiced high-risk sexual behaviors, such as unprotected anal intercourse, were more likely to endorse beliefs that new AIDS treatments reduce risks for HIV transmission (Kalichman et al., 1998). They also tended to be younger and less educated than were men who avoided unprotected anal intercourse. Believing that new treatments reduce HIV "infectivity" apparently made high-risk sexual behaviors seem less risky.

In another example of AIDS complacency, researchers have found that women involved in casual sexual relationships are 11 times more likely than women in more committed relationships to maintain safer sexual behavior over time. Women in committed relationships were more likely to engage in riskier sexual behaviors (Morrill et al., 1996). Although knowing one's partner,

preventive behaviors. They also suggest that immersion in the mainstream culture may be a mixed blessing for some ethnic minorities. Although higher acculturation is generally associated with more active coping and greater social resources, it may also be linked with more drug use and more risky behaviors leading to AIDS. Less acculturated Latinas, for example, may be *more* responsive to cultural proscriptions against the use of drugs and promiscuous behavior. The study also points to the need for culturally specific interventions to promote HIV-preventive behaviors. For example, enhancing the self-esteem of impoverished African-American women would give them the strength to require their partners to use condoms. Breaking down cultural barriers to condom use through family and community education would benefit Hispanic-American women.

A recent study comparing African and European HIV-positive women living in France points to another psychosocial barrier in how some women of color adjust to HIV/AIDS illness (Bungener, Marchand-Gonod, & Jouvent, 2000). In structured interviews, the researchers found that European women were more willing to disclose their HIV-positive status to both family and friends than African women. While 73 percent of the European women had informed a sister or brother of their seropositive status and 60 percent had informed their mothers or fathers, only 40 percent of the African women had informed a sib-

ling and only 16 percent had informed their mothers or fathers. Other researchers have also reported this difficulty in disclosing HIV status among African-American women (Bedimo, Bennett, Kissinger, & Clark, 1998). These findings suggest that women of African ancestry may benefit from counseling and other psychological interventions aimed at helping them resolve issues related to disclosure, in order to fully mobilize their networks of social support.

For men, gender-role beliefs and cultural values also play an important role. For example, some more traditional Latino men believe that sex is an uncontrollable urge in a man, that men have certain sexual rights, and that sexual excitement without ejaculation is harmful (Marin & Gomez, 1992). These beliefs could induce men to pressure women for sex. In a recent random survey of Latino adults (Marin, Gomez, Tschann, & Gregorich, 1997), researchers found that men who endorsed traditional gender-role beliefs about the uncontrollability of sexual impulses reported more coercive behaviors in their sexual relationships. Similar studies have found that nonminority college men who are sexually aggressive hold more traditional gender-role beliefs than those who are not sexually aggresive (Spence, Losoff, & Robbins, 1991). They also report lower self-efficacy in using condoms during the heat of passion or when under the influence of drugs or alcohol.

and his or her sexual history, is fundamental to safe sex, letting one's guard down over time may lead to trouble.

Reward Value of High-Risk Behaviors

Researchers have found that some individuals engage in risky sexual behavior because the risk makes the behavior more exciting and pleasurable. In a survey of HIV-negative gay and bisexual men, Jeffrey Kelley and Seth Kalichman (1998) found that the subjective reinforcement value (pleasure) of unprotected anal intercourse more strongly predicted condom use than perceived vulnerability to infection. The emotional meaning of having unprotected sex, including sexual fantasies and trust of one's partner, may also be a factor in why some individuals do not practice safe sex. Current condom use messages are neutral in tone, cognitively focused in their appeal, and oriented to disease prevention rather than to the positive or affective benefits of safe sex. In the future, HIV interventions may need to seek more explicitly to lessen the reinforcement value of high-risk sexual practices and increase the perceived value of safe sex.

Changing behavior is difficult enough, but maintaining that change poses a special problem. Among other things, relapse has been linked to depression as well as alcohol and substance abuse. For example, people who are otherwise conscientious in minimizing their risk profile often become less inhibited when under the influence of alcohol and other drugs (Gordon & Carey, 1996).

Medical Interventions

Until very recently, HIV infection was almost always a progressive, fatal disease. Medical interventions focused almost exclusively on treating the pneumonia and other opportunistic diseases that resulted from immune failure, not on eliminating (or even controlling) the rapidly replicating HIV virus. Today, however, scientists have a much better understanding of how the virus behaves in the body; they also have a number of potent weapons at their disposal. Several tests directly monitor levels of the virus in the body, thus giving doctors a more accurate means of determining how well a treatment regimen is working. In addition, several new classes of drugs have made it possible to treat HIV aggressively, improving overall health and dramatically increasing chances of survival.

As you'll recall, when our bodies are host to an invading virus, the immune system produces antibodies to fight off the infection. With many diseases, there are visible symptoms that signal the presence of an infection. Not so with the HIV virus. In the early years of the epidemic, the absence of symptoms prevented doctors from diagnosing AIDS until after an HIV positive patient had contracted one of the opportunistic diseases that commonly kill those with compromised immune function. Then, in 1993, researchers developed the *enzyme-linked immunosorbent assay (ELISA),* a blood test that enabled them to identify people who were seropositive for the HIV virus by detecting HIV antibodies in bodily fluids. Another test, called the Western blot test, analyzes blood proteins to confirm a positive ELISA test. In May 1996 the Food and Drug Administration approved the first of several reliable home testing systems for HIV.

Once they have determined that HIV has infected a person, doctors continue to monitor levels of the virus in the patient's blood because these levels strongly predict the pace at which AIDS develops. By doing so, they are able to modify ineffective treatments before immune failure results and the invading virus gets the upper hand. Viral levels of HIV are measured by *viral-load assays,* which measure copies of HIV RNA in a milliliter of plasma (the cell-free part of blood).

The HAART Regimen

Today's optimum treatment regimen is *highly active antiretroviral therapy,* or *HAART* for short. HAART involves multiple anti-HIV drugs that prevent the virus from replicating within host cells. Multiple drugs are used so that if one proves ineffective, the second (or third) may provide the needed insurance. In addition, HIV tends quickly to become resistant to drugs that do not completely suppress its replication. Because no single drug has been able to completely suppress the virus, any one drug may quickly lose its effectiveness if used in isolation, often within a matter of weeks.

One of the most commonly used drugs in the HAART regimen is **zidovudine (AZT)**. Introduced in 1983, AZT is one of a class of drugs called *reverse transcriptase inhibitors* because it blocks replication of the HIV virus by inhibiting the enzyme reverse transcriptase that HIV needs to reproduce itself. AZT reduces AIDS symptoms, increases T cell levels, and may prolong the patient's life. Unfortunately, however, many patients on AZT experience a variety of side effects, including anemia, which requires frequent blood transfusions; reduced white blood cell formation, which increases the risk of other infections; headaches; itching; and mental confusion. In addition, AZT's effectiveness wears off as the virus becomes resistant to it (Kinloch-de Loes et al., 1995). For this reason, AZT is often combined with a promising new group of anti-HIV drugs called *protease inhibitors,* which attack HIV at a different phase of its life cycle (Deeks, Smith, Holodniy, & Kahn, 1997). This combination of drugs has reduced HIV to undetectable levels in some patients (Balter, 1996).

Clinical trials of HAART have been quite promising. Recent studies of HIV+ patients at San Francisco General Hospital and Johns Hopkins University Hospital reported that 50 percent of patients given HAART therapy reached the treatment goal of only 500 HIV per milliliter—some within 6 weeks of beginning treatment. Although a 50 percent success rate would be considered disappointing in the treatment of many serious diseases, for HIV it represents a 100 percent improvement from just a few years ago. In some patients, HAART appears to stop HIV replication completely, giving health experts hope that treatment will work indefinitely.

One drawback of HAART, however, is that the regimen is difficult to follow, making adherence a challenge. Patients often must take 16 or more anti-HIV pills a day, some with food and some on an empty stomach, according to a precise schedule that can challenge even the most motivated and highly organized patient. Patients who are homeless, confused, or lacking in social support find such a regimen almost impossible to adhere to. Another drawback is that many AIDS patients simply can't afford it. The average cost of a year's treatment on the HAART regimen is $10,000 to $15,000. Even in the affluent developed countries where such care is available, many people lack the financial wherewithal or health insurance coverage necessary to cover such costs—and, of course, the countless impoverished people in undeveloped countries have little hope of effective treatment (Kolata, 1998).

Slowing the development of AIDS in developing nations (where 90 percent of those infected with HIV live) is a top priority for researchers. By one estimate, making the aggressive HAART treatment protocol available worldwide

■ **zidovudine (AZT)** the first anti-AIDS drug

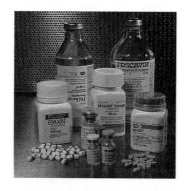

AIDS Intervention
Over the last few years, AIDS patients have been required to take a large variety of pills each day, on a very strict timetable. However, with research advances, more streamlined pharmacological regimens have been used and have been equally effective. © Gary Retherford/Photo Researchers, Inc.

would cost $36.5 billion. The inequities in HIV treatment and prevention hit children the hardest. In some parts of Africa, for example, four out of every ten children lose at least one parent to AIDS before age 15—and every day 1,600 babies are born with HIV. To help stop the transmission of HIV to infants, the United Nations AIDS agency began a program of prenatal care, AZT, and delivery assistance to women in 11 of the world's poorest nations. In the face of mounting evidence that HIV also passes to a child through breast milk, the program helps infected mothers find safe alternatives to breast feeding.

Other New Approaches

Another new approach to treating HIV stems from evidence that HIV particles are sometimes able to survive drug therapy by attaching to nondividing CD4 cells and remaining in a dormant state. Dormant HIV particles are ignored by the immune system because they are "invisible." Normally, when a virus infects a cell, the cell displays pieces of the virus, or antigens, on its surface. If something causes the nondividing cells to become active, the virus "awakens" and begins replicating once again. The experimental treatment involves drugs that purposely activate nondividing cells, causing them to become visible to the body's immune system, which is then able to mount a defense. The strategy carries a heavy risk: If the immune system is too weak, rallying more HIV particles to replicate may backfire and give HIV a firmer stranglehold.

Other AIDS researchers are attempting to develop new ways to restore immunocompetence in HIV-infected people. Clinical trials are under way in which patients are given low doses of *interleukin-2*, a drug that forces immature stem cells to mature into virus-fighting T lymphocytes and antibody-producing cells that target HIV. Another experimental technique harvests a small sample of immune stem cells from an HIV patient, nurtures their growth in the laboratory, and then returns them (in larger numbers and stronger form) to the patient's body.

A Preventive Vaccine

Given the capacity of HIV to become integrated in a host cell's DNA, prospects for a true cure that would detect and destroy every HIV-infected cell in the body appear bleak (Haney, 2001). Is there an alternative? A number of biomedical researchers are searching for a vaccine to prevent HIV infection. One of the major stumbling blocks is the enormous variability of HIV. Some researchers estimate that in an infected person with replicating HIV, more than 10 billion new viruses are made every day. New strains are constantly appearing; even if a vaccine is developed that proves effective against one strain, it may provide no protection against other strains. A second difficulty is the unusual life cycle of HIV. The rapid speed with which the virus infects CD4 cells and the long life of infected cells make the prospects for an effective protective vaccine quite unlikely.

Another possible approach is to develop a treatment to minimize and control the impact of HIV on the body. By controlling the replication of HIV, the onset of AIDS may be delayed. Some researchers are hopeful of developing a treatment that will completely block one of the many steps in the HIV life cycle (see Figure 11.5). In so doing, the virus may be stopped dead in its tracks. Scientists at the University of Montana are following a promising line of research that may lead to an AIDS control vaccine. They have developed antibodies in mice that attack HIV just as the virus begins to fuse to host cells. When the antibodies were injected into samples of HIV, the antibodies destroyed 23 of 24 strains of the virus (Gainetdinov & Caron, 1999).

Although biomedical researchers are quick to point out that there still is no "cure" for AIDS, the advances in treatment that have been achieved since late 1995 are unparalleled in the history of medicine. Before this time, "treatment" for HIV patients consisted almost entirely of making patients as comfortable as possible as they prepared to die. Today, the use of reverse transcriptase inhibitors, protease inhibitors, and the "AIDS cocktail" approach of HAART has increased hope that AIDS will someday become a manageable chronic disease—much like diabetes—rather than a terminal illness and that AIDS patients may look forward to a long, productive life (Chartrand & Seidman, 1996). The annual number of U.S. deaths among people with AIDS declined for the first time in 1996, dropping approximately 25 percent (CDC, 1998).

Figure 11.5

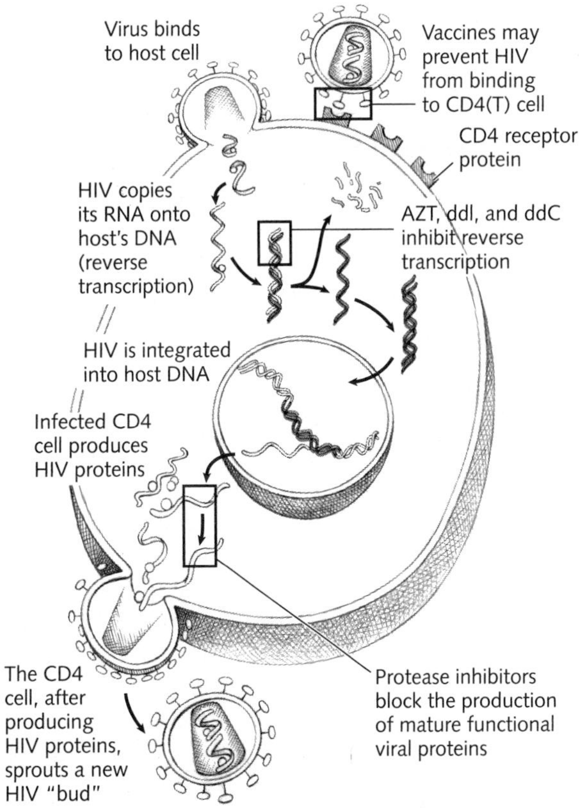

Strategies to Combat HIV Reproduction
Doctors have a number of potent anti-HIV drugs at their disposal. These widely used drugs block specific steps in the HIV life cycle.

Coping with HIV and AIDS

Chronic illnesses such as AIDS can have a dramatic impact on the individual as well as on family, friends, and caregivers. Those who have AIDS often find themselves isolated from social support networks as coworkers, neighbors, and even family and friends withdraw from them. Early studies suggested that psychological and emotional difficulties were common, with as many as one-half of AIDS patients having diagnosable psychological

HIV infection is a highly stigmatizing disease because it is difficult to conceal as the disease progresses, it is disruptive to the person's life and relationships, and it can cause physical disfigurement as part of its degenerative course. AIDS-related stigmas result in discrimination, prejudice, and isolation and are a major factor in limiting social support and assistance for coping with HIV.

American Psychological Association. Public Interest Directorate. Major HIV/AIDS topics and issues (www.apa.org/pi/aids).

and emotional disorders (Selwyn, 1986). However, most of the studies involved only gay men, making it difficult to rule out the impact of other variables (such as social stigma) on the individual's adjustment to the disease. Moreover, recent studies have indicated that the rates of persistent psychological disorders among AIDS patients are no different from those associated with other life-threatening diseases (Bor, 1997).

Impact on the Individual

When testing reveals the presence of infection, the person faces the challenges of coping with the stigma of AIDS, acknowledging the possibility of dying young, and developing strategies for minimizing the impact of the disease on his or her physical and emotional health (Siegel & Krauss, 1991). Ironically, with advances in biomedical technology, the fear of developing symptoms may actually be magnified. New tests are now able to reliably forecast when symptoms will probably appear.

When the challenges and fears associated with AIDS become overwhelming, victims may suffer depression and suicidal thinking, especially those who feel a withdrawal of family and social support; those who lose their jobs; or those who become disfigured as a result of the disease's progression or treatment. In a large national sample of HIV-infected women and men, John Fleishman and Barry Fogel (1994) found that more than 40 percent of those with AIDS were diagnosed with depression. Other researchers have found a 36-fold increase in suicide among men diagnosed with AIDS (Mazurk et al., 1988).

Not all patients who test HIV-positive develop psychological problems. Some may actually feel a sense of relief when the diagnosis finally ends a lengthy period of uncertainty about symptoms. And many long-term AIDS survivors are optimistic and resilient, which may give their immune systems a boost in combating the disease. AIDS patients who avoid self-blame for their plight and who maintain a sense of personal control over their ability to manage the disease are less likely to become depressed or anxious or show other signs of poor psychological adjustment (Benight et al., 1997; Rotheram-Borus, Murphy, Reid, & Coleman, 1996). They also show a lower norepinephrine-to-cortisol ratio, a stress hormone profile that indicates a healthier physiological response to everyday stressors (Benight et al., 1997).

As with other chronic illnesses, AIDS patients who use active coping strategies to solve their problems and maintain an upbeat outlook tend to fare much better than those who distance themselves physically or emotionally from their plight (Fleishman & Fogel, 1994). Active coping measures that have proved effective in reducing AIDS-related stress reactions include seeking information and social support (Siegel, Raveis, & Karus, 1997) and taking an active role in one's medical treatment regimen (Baum & Posluszny, 1999; Siegel & Krauss, 1991).

A number of researchers have studied long-term AIDS survivors in an effort to identify behavioral factors that might promote longevity (LaPerriere et al., 1990; Patterson, Shaw, Semple, & Cherner, 1996; Solomon, 1991). Three factors, in particular, seem to distinguish long-term survivors from those who succumb more quickly.

- *Maintaining physical fitness by engaging in regular exercise.* A number of researchers have reported that aerobic exercise interventions bolster immunocompetence in AIDS patients by preventing declines in level and activity of NK cells (LaPerriere et al., 1990). These interventions also help prevent the dramatic weight loss and other telltale signs of disease that often accompany the later stages of AIDS (Lox, McAuley, & Tucker, 1996).

- *Keeping an upbeat, positive outlook.* AIDS progresses more rapidly among patients who are chronically depressed, leading to significantly shorter survival times (Patterson et al., 1996).

- *Avoiding social isolation.* In fact, having a large social network is strongly correlated with longevity among AIDS patients (Patterson et al., 1996).

Impact on Family Members and Caregivers

Since the first reported cases of AIDS, the disease has been viewed as a social problem whose effects extend beyond the individual. Until recently, however, there has been relatively little empirical research on the impact of AIDS on family members and other relations. The absence of family-related research has helped perpetuate the myth that most AIDS victims are gay men who are not connected to families (Bor, 1997). Newer research has prompted a broader definition of "family" to include members of the extended family as well as same-sex partners.

Research into the effects on families is lacking because AIDS poses several unique problems. First, in most cases, AIDS changes the family structure and roles, often reversing standard developmental patterns. For example, children may die before their parents. When parents die, many young children and grandparents are forced to become caregivers at a time when they would normally expect to be in a more dependent role themselves (Bor & Elford, 1994). Second, AIDS places the additional burden of the disease's social stigma on its victims and their families. Uninfected family members may find their friends shying away from or even harassing them. And the social rejection may persist even after the AIDS victim has died.

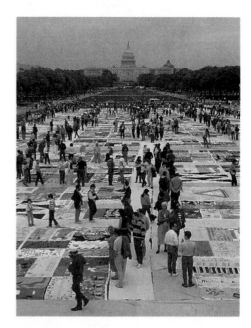

The National AIDS Quilt
HIV-positive individuals who remain socially connected fare better than those who feel shunned or isolate themselves. The National AIDS quilt, shown here in Washington, D.C., is being transported around the country to increase AIDS awareness and to prompt people to provide social support to sufferers. © A. Reininger/Woodfin Camp and Associates

AIDS can have a profound impact on a surviving partner. Most common is the fear of loneliness and, for those who are HIV-positive themselves, a fear of dying with no one to care for them. Anger at their partner's "abandonment" by dying first is also common. Even for partners who are not infected, the fear of being "tarnished" by having shared a relationship with an infected partner may cast a long shadow, making it difficult for the survivor to establish new relationships (Bor, 1997).

Caregivers

AIDS also has a powerful impact on health care providers and caregivers, many of whom have concerns about being infected themselves. Despite the relatively low risk, anxiety about working with AIDS patients persists and may lead to unusual occupational stress and burnout.

It is estimated that about 3 percent of the entire adult population in the United States has provided informal care to a person living with HIV or AIDS (Turner, Catania, & Gagnon, 1994). Although women predominate in most caregiving situations, many AIDS caregivers are men caring for other men (Turner et al., 1994). On average, caregivers devote over 20 hours per week solely to providing care. Almost two-thirds experience at least one chronic physical symptom; the most common are severe backaches and headaches.

The biggest factor in the impact of caregiving on a person's health is the length of the patient's illness. Those who act as caregivers for a long time and who rate their patient's health as very poor are less likely to report good health than those who have been providing care for a short time to a person living with AIDS or HIV in comparatively good health. This is true regardless of the nature of care-related activities or the amount of time devoted to caregiving each day (Wight, LeBlanc, & Aneshensel, 1998).

At present, no cure for AIDS exists and the disease continues to infect people throughout the world. Health psychologists play an important role in battling the HIV pandemic. In the early years, psychologists were key players in designing and implementing primary and secondary prevention efforts to reduce the spread of HIV and to help those who were HIV-positive cope with their illness. These efforts included interventions to reduce risky behaviors for AIDS and to help those who were HIV-positive adhere to complex treatment regimens. More recently, health psychologists have teamed up with immunologists and other scientists to study how psychosocial factors such as beliefs about AIDS and disclosing HIV status, perceived social support, coping style, and possible symptoms of anxiety and depression influence the course of HIV infection and its progression to AIDS. Based on the growing evidence from these investigations, psychologists are designing interventions that not only improve the quality of life of HIV-positive persons but also increase the odds of their long-term survival.

Summing Up

The AIDS Epidemic

1. The first cases of acquired immunodeficiency syndrome (AIDS) in humans appeared in 1980, when 55 young men (most of whom were gay or intravenous drug users) were diagnosed with a rare form of cancer. During the last half of the 1980s, AIDS began to threaten the general population.

2. In the United States, the AIDS epidemic has taken the greatest toll on young men, particularly African-Americans and Hispanic-Americans. Today, however, the number of new cases of AIDS among women in the United States—particularly African-American women—is increasing faster than among men. For a variety of biological, economic, and sociocultural reasons, women are more vulnerable to HIV infection and tend to contract the virus at a younger age and lower HIV viral load levels.

3. In other parts of the world, AIDS affects men and women equally, and heterosexual sex is the most common mode of transmission. Ethnic and racial differences in rates of HIV transmission are thought to reflect sociocultural differences in drug use and the acceptance of homosexual and bisexual practices.

Symptoms and Stages: From HIV to AIDS

4. HIV is transmitted primarily through the sharing of virus-infected lymphocytes in bodily fluids—blood, semen, vaginal and cervical secretions, and breast milk.

5. High-risk behaviors that promote HIV infection include having unprotected sex with multiple partners, using IV drugs, and sharing needles. HIV may also be transmitted from an infected mother to her unborn child during pregnancy, as well as from mother to child during breast-feeding.

6. The chances of casual transmission of AIDS without sexual contact or IV drug use are very low. The best ways to guard against HIV infection are limiting sexual partners, choosing partners carefully, and avoiding sexual contacts with those who are known to engage in high-risk behaviors.

7. AIDS is caused by the human immunodeficiency virus (HIV), a retrovirus that causes host cells to reproduce the virus's genetic code. In doing so, HIV destroys CD4 cells, progressively reduces immunocompetence, and leaves its victims vulnerable to a host of opportunistic infections.

8. HIV affects many body systems, including the central nervous system. When HIV migrates to the brain and attacks brain cells, it triggers a variety of emotional and cognitive problems in half of all HIV-positive patients.

9. HIV sickness progresses through four stages, which vary in length from person to person. The average time from HIV infection to AIDS is about 10 years, although 5 percent of HIV-positive people live more than 15 years. HIV progresses much more slowly among patients whose immune systems mount strong lymphocyte activity in the acute stage of HIV sickness.

10. Approximately 1 percent of people of Western European descent inherit a gene from both parents that prevents the virus from binding to host cells, giving them apparent immunity to HIV infection.

11. Health psychologists have investigated a number of psychosocial factors that influence the course of HIV infection and AIDS. Stress, negative emotions, and social isolation may influence the pace at which the disease progresses, perhaps by altering hormonal and immune environments that affect the resistance of host cells to the invading virus. However, not all studies have found a positive relationship between negative emotions and changes in CD4 cell counts, AIDS onset, or mortality rates.

Intervention Strategies for AIDS

12. In the absence of an effective HIV vaccine, psychosocial interventions are among the few means of battling AIDS. Health psychologists play a number of roles in the battle against AIDS, including counseling people about being tested for HIV, helping individuals modify high-risk behaviors, helping AIDS patients cope with emotional and cognitive disturbances, and conducting bereavement therapy for those waiting to die, their families, and their friends.

13. AIDS prevention programs include educational and media campaigns as well as focused intervention programs designed to reduce risky sexual and drug use behaviors. Because of the inherent interactive nature of cognitive, affective, behavioral, and social elements of stress responses, the most effective way to "package" stress management interventions for HIV-infected persons appears to be a multimodal program.

14. Although AIDS prevention programs have had some success, many barriers to prevention remain. Misinformation, feelings of personal invulnerability, cultural norms, and personal resources are all factors in the success (or failure) of AIDS prevention measures.

15. HIV screening is readily available in most developed countries, but complacency or fear of knowing prevent some people from seeking out their HIV status. Many people who do know their serostatus avoid telling their partners and relatives.

16. The most widely used screening test for HIV is the enzyme-linked immunosorbent assay (ELISA), which detects HIV antibodies in bodily fluids. Until recently, HIV infection was almost always a progressive, fatal disease. Today, however, doctors have a number of potent weapons that allow many people to live with asymptomatic HIV seropositivity for years. Aggressive drug treatment regimens such as highly active antiretroviral therapy (HAART) combine protease inhibitors with reverse transcriptase inhibitors such as zidovudine (AZT) to interrupt the replication of HIV.

Coping with HIV and AIDS

17. Chronic illnesses such as AIDS can have a dramatic physical and psychological impact on the individual as well as on family members, friends, coworkers, and caregivers. The main problems faced by AIDS victims are adjusting to the possibility of dying young and coping with heightened anxiety and depression. Family members and friends must also cope with the social stigma of the disease, often even after their loved one has died.

18. Health psychologists have designed a variety of psychosocial interventions to help people cope with AIDS. These include exercise, active coping exercises, and relaxation training.

Key Terms and Concepts

AIDS (acquired immunodeficiency syndrome), p. 462
HIV (human immunodeficiency virus), p. 462

Kaposi's sarcoma, p. 463
pandemic, p. 464
retrovirus, p. 470
genome, p. 470

AIDS dementia complex, p. 471
seropositive, p. 473
hemophilia, p. 476
zidovudine (AZT), p. 491

Health Psychology on the World Wide Web

Web Address

http://www.aaas.org/science/aidslink.htm

http://www.cdc.gov/hiv/

http://www.thebody.com/index.shtml

Description

AIDS links of the American Association for the Advancement of Science.

The Centers for Disease Control and Prevention's clearinghouse for HIV/AIDS prevention information.

An award-winning collection of HIV/AIDS resources covering a wide range of health and legal issues.

Critical Thinking Exercise

AIDS and Confidentiality

Despite the laudable intention of antidiscrimination laws, health care professionals often find themselves in a conflicted position. While not wishing to betray a patient's confidential medical condition, they are bound by a "duty to warn" in order to protect others. Historically, this has entailed the reporting and tracking of people with a variety of contagious diseases. In fact, public health laws have often mandated this duty as a check on reckless behavior that may pose a health threat to other people or to society in general.

And what about the rights of health care workers? In 1992, a surgical technician, who was accidentally cut by a scalpel during a postoperative procedure, was awarded a $102,000 judgment against the patient—who failed to disclose that she was HIV+. In response to cases such as these, some states have passed laws that allow health care professionals to be told when one of their patients has tested positive for HIV.

AIDS-related criminal laws are also becoming increasingly common. For example, a person who has been assaulted by another person can obtain a court order forcing the assailant to submit to AIDS testing. And when people who are HIV+ knowingly engage in sex or needle sharing without informing their partners, they can be prosecuted criminally in some states for "assault with a deadly weapon." Case in point: In October 1991, Alberto Gonzalez of Oregon became the first person in the United States to be convicted on assault charges for knowingly passing HIV to his girlfriend. As another example, in September 1992 a Colorado jury ordered United Blood Services of New Mexico to pay $6.6 million to a woman who contracted AIDS from blood donated by an HIV+ client of the company. Cases such as this raise the possibility that if a person died of AIDS after being infected by his or her sexual or drug partner, the partner could be charged with manslaughter.

In this exercise you are asked to think about some of the complex legal and ethical issues raised by AIDS as you prepare answers to the following questions.

1. Should insurance companies be allowed to require AIDS tests of new customers? Should they be permitted to refuse to offer coverage to those infected with the disease? Explain why you feel as you do.

2. Where does an HIV+ patient's right to confidentiality end and a nurse or doctor's duty to warn begin? Can you think of a situation in which the rights of the individual are superseded by those of society?

3. What responsibility does an HIV+ woman or man have toward any prospective children he or she might have?

4. Does a patient have the right to know that a doctor or dentist is HIV+/AIDS infected? Do health care workers always have the right to know that a patient is HIV+/AIDS infected?

5. Do state licensing boards have an obligation to block HIV+/AIDS-infected people from practicing medicine?

5

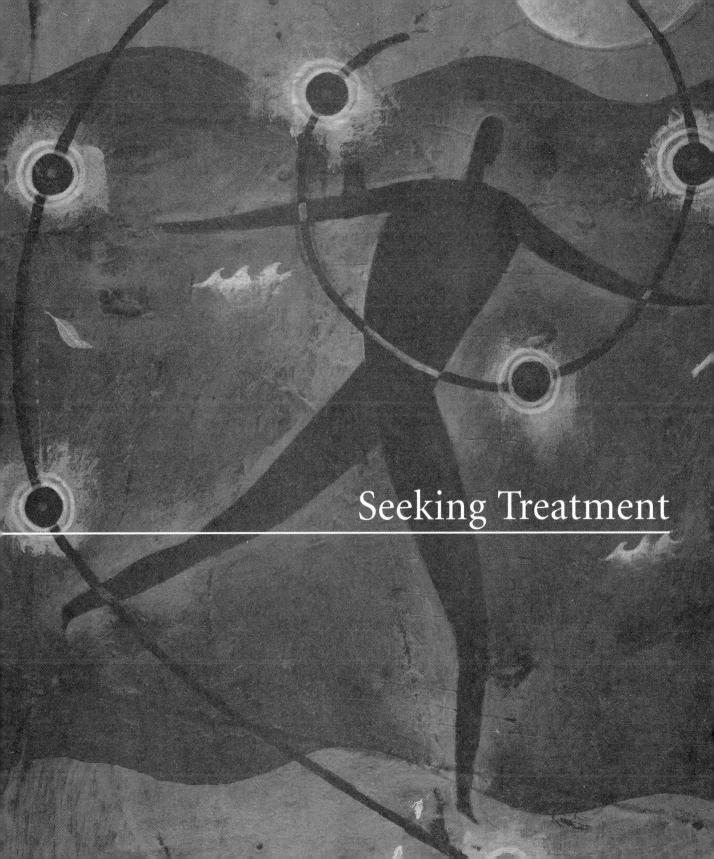

Seeking Treatment

12

Health Care and Patient Behavior

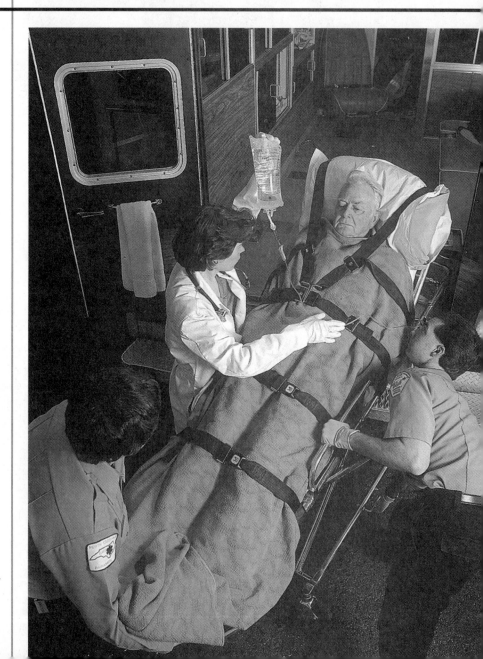

Even though the event happened 25 years ago, it is as vivid in my mind today as it was on that unusually warm afternoon in April when one of my fraternity brothers was nearly blinded. Taking a break from studying for finals, Bruce (not his real name) bounded through the lobby of our fraternity house where a bunch of us were watching the Detroit Tigers battle the St. Louis Cardinals in a spring training baseball exhibition game. "Anybody want to play handball?" Bruce asked. I declined, as did everyone but Chris. "I'll play," he said, "but only for about half an hour. I've got a chemistry final tomorrow."

The rest of us turned our attention back to the game and thought nothing more about handball until about 45 minutes later, when a worried-looking Chris came through the door with a woozy Bruce leaning heavily on him for support. It was easy to see that Bruce had somehow been hurt, and, before anyone spoke a word, I could see that his left eye was discolored and growing puffy. "What happened?" we asked in unison.

"Bruce took a handball squarely in the eye," Chris said. "I wanted to take him right over to the health center, but he refused."

"It's nothing," Bruce said shakily. "I'll probably have a black eye tomorrow, but I'll be fine. Just get me some ice and a couple of aspirin."

As Bruce stretched out on a couch, somebody ran for the ice and aspirin. The rest of us looked at one another doubtfully. As the minutes passed, Bruce's eye was looking angry and red, and the swelling was already starting to force his eyelid closed. And he was clearly in pain, wincing with every word he spoke. Vision was not something to mess around with, even if you were trying to keep up a stoic front for a bunch of college buddies. Especially if, like Bruce, you were hoping one day to become an airline pilot.

For all of these reasons, we knew what we had to do. In less than five minutes we had phoned Campus Safety, the Health Center, and Bruce's parents. Following their instructions we drove Bruce to the emergency room at County Medical Hospital, paced by a police cruiser with siren blaring and lights flashing. Half an hour after being hit by the handball, Bruce was rushed into the operating room, where a board-certified surgeon sutured his ruptured eyeball and saved his vision.

■ **illness behavior** people's responses to physical symptoms, including their recognition and interpretation of the symptoms

■ **sick role behavior** people's responses to being diagnosed with a particular disease or health condition

Why was Bruce reluctant to seek medical care? Why wasn't the pain in his eye sufficient to sound the alarm that his health was in jeopardy? To help explain the reasons that people are reluctant to seek treatment, we shift our focus from *primary* prevention to *secondary* prevention, that is, from actions designed to prevent a disease or injury to actions intended to identify and treat an illness early in its course (see Chapter 6).

Sooner or later, each of us comes into contact with a health care provider and the health care system. In most cases, these encounters are brief, perhaps involving a visit to the doctor because of the flu. In other cases, they involve more extended contact, such as a hospital stay following surgery, recuperating in a rehabilitation center following an accident, or living in an extended-care facility.

What role do social and psychological factors play in determining a patient's overall response to health care? This chapter explores this question by considering the relationships between patients and the health care system. There is mounting evidence that social and psychological factors have both a direct and an indirect impact on people's responses to health care. For one thing, they strongly influence when and how people decide they are sick. For another, people's confidence in their health care providers influences their satisfaction with treatment as well as how they respond to it. For a third, the extent and quality of communication with health care providers indirectly influences almost every aspect of health care, including how patients decide when they need medical attention, why some people choose to ignore health-related symptoms, and why some people carefully follow their provider's instructions while others do not.

We begin by describing the two stages health psychologists use to describe how people deal with medical symptoms: illness behavior and sick role behavior (Kasl & Cobb, 1966). **Illness behavior** refers to the ways in which people respond to physical symptoms. This includes whether they recognize the symptom and how they interpret that symptom—as normal aches and pains or as a sign of major illness. **Sick role behavior** refers to how people behave once they have recognized a symptom and interpreted it as a potential illness.

Illness Behavior

How and when does a person decide that she or he is sick? At what point does a nagging headache, upset stomach, or other symptom become serious enough that a person seeks medical attention? At any given moment, perhaps one out of every four people in the population has a health condition that is potentially treatable. However, the presence of symptoms is not always sufficient to force people to seek health care (Cameron, Leventhal, &

Leventhal, 1993). Why do some individuals keep up their normal activities even in the face of undeniable symptoms that something is wrong, while others take time off at the slightest symptoms? Are these individual differences stable *traits* or are they merely responses to specific situations?

People fail to recognize potentially serious medical symptoms for many reasons. Some avoid seeing a doctor because they believe that their symptoms are not serious and all that is needed is a day or two of rest, perhaps an over-the-counter medication, or some other form of self-care. Others avoid the use of health services because they lack health insurance or are afraid they can't afford it. Others may be fearful that their symptom *is* a sign of a serious condition, and their inaction is a result of denial. Finally, some people may avoid medical care because they are suspicious of the health care system and doubt its ability to treat their condition effectively.

Psychological Factors

The criteria that people use to recognize and interpret symptoms vary enormously. However, certain broad psychological factors play an important role in the process.

Attentional Focus and Symptom Recognition

One relatively stable psychological factor that influences people's awareness of physical symptoms is **attentional focus.** People who have a strong *internal focus* on their bodies, emotions, and overall well-being are more likely to detect symptoms—and to report them more quickly—than are people who are more *externally focused* (Pennebaker & Epstein, 1983). People who are socially isolated, bored with their jobs, and live alone are more likely to be internally focused, whereas people with more active lives are subject to more distractions that keep their minds off their own problems.

The relationship between attentional focus and symptom recognition is supported by evidence that momentary situational factors have a substantial impact on whether a symptom is registered. People tend to become more aware of physical sensations when they are bored than when they are deeply involved in a task. For example, they are far less likely to cough in response to a tickle in their throats during exciting parts of a movie than during boring parts (Pennebaker, 1980). Similarly, injured athletes often play through the pain, focusing only on the game. In situations such as these, the distractions of external events may temporarily overshadow internal symptoms.

Attentional Focus and Coping Strategies

Attentional focus also determines how people cope with health problems and other stressful events. When threatened with an aversive event, individuals referred to as **sensitizers** (also called *monitors*) actively monitor the event and

attentional focus a person's characteristic style of monitoring bodily symptoms, emotions, and overall well-being

sensitizers people who cope with health problems and other aversive events by closely scanning their bodies and environments for information

■ **repressors** people who cope with health problems and other aversive events by ignoring or distancing themselves from stressful information

their reaction to it; others, called **repressors** (also called *blunters*), avoid and psychologically blunt their reactions to such events (Miller & Nuessle, 1978). Sensitizers are people who cope with health problems and other aversive events by closely scanning their bodies and environments for information. Beyond the world of health care, sensitizers also seem to be more strongly affected by daily hassles. As we'll explain later, sensitizers also prefer high levels of information about their health in medical contexts and seem to fare better when it is provided.

The distinctive characteristics of sensitizers are not visible when stress is low or absent; they become most apparent when the sensitizer is confronted with potentially high levels of stress (Wardle, Pernet, Collins, & Bourne, 1994). For example, when confronted with the prospect of a potentially major or life-threatening illness, sensitizers report significantly greater physiological and behavioral distress and dysfunction, are slower to recover, and exhibit greater treatment side effects (Lerman et al., 1996; Schwartz, Lerman, Miller, Daly, & Masny, 1995).

In contrast, repressors tend to ignore or deny health-related information. They seem to look at life through rose-colored glasses, coping with negative events without bother or irritation and often by defending themselves from unwanted thoughts or unpleasant mood states. As we discussed in Chapter 5, research with different stressors suggests that avoidant-type strategies are often maladaptive over time (Roth & Cohen, 1986; Suls & Fletcher, 1985) and may be associated with a variety of long-term health effects, including more rapid cancer progression (Epping-Jordan, Compas, & Howell, 1994). These adverse effects are most evident when efforts to ignore the stressor fail and the individual resorts to more extreme defensive attempts, such as denial (Foa, Riggs, & Gershuny, 1995).

Repressing may create an especially powerful reluctance to seek medical screening procedures, which are typically oriented toward detecting serious illnesses. For some people, the distress of thinking about the possibility of disease creates a barrier to noticing symptoms (Millar & Millar, 1995). And for many of them, avoiding a screening test is the easiest way of coping with anxiety.

Outlook on Life

Whether a person is generally an optimist or a pessimist also influences the reporting of symptoms (Scheier & Bridges, 1995). People who have a generally positive outlook on life generally report fewer symptoms than do people who see the world darkly. Those in a good mood also consider themselves as healthier and feel less vulnerable to future illness than do people in bad moods (Leventhal, Hansell, Diefenbach, Leventhal, & Glass, 1996; Salovey, O'Leary, Stretton, Fishkin, & Drake, 1991). This may be a cognitive rather than a physiological phenomenon, however. Research on *state-dependent memory* reveals that people who are in a bad mood tend to think of illness-related memories more easily than people in a good mood (Croyle & Uretsky, 1987).

Illness Representations

How people react to symptoms is also heavily influenced by their personal views of health and illness, called **illness representations** (or *schemas*). Illness representations influence health in a variety of ways. One way is by influencing people's preventive health behaviors. Another is by affecting how they react when symptoms appear.

Researchers have studied several components of how an illness is represented. As explained below, each component by itself can substantially affect the individual's motivation to seek medical care.

1. *Identity* of the illness, including its label and symptoms. There appears to be a symmetrical bond between a disease's label and its symptoms. Thus, a person who has symptoms will seek a diagnostic label for those symptoms; a person who has been diagnosed (labeled) will seek symptoms that are consistent with that label. In a vivid example of this symmetry, Linda Baumann, Linda Cameron, Rick Zimmerman, and Howard Leventhal (1989) found that research participants who were told that they had high blood pressure were more likely than others to report symptoms commonly associated with this illness, such as tightness in the chest, jittery feelings, and so forth. This was true regardless of whether they really were hypertensive. Another example of the impact of labels on symptom recognition is *medical student's disease.* As many as two-thirds of aspiring physicians imagine that they themselves have symptoms of diseases they have studied (Mechanic, 1978).

2. *Causes*—external factors such as infection or injury, or internal factors such as genetic predisposition. For example, a student who interprets her tension headache as a by-product of cramming for an exam will probably react quite differently from the student who labels the same symptoms as signs of a brain tumor.

3. *Timeline,* including the duration and rate of the disease's development. For example, four out of ten patients being treated for hypertension believe that their condition is *acute,* that is, short in duration, caused by temporary agents, and not a serious threat to long-term health. In contrast, *chronic illnesses* are long in duration, caused by multiple factors, and represent potentially serious threats to long-term health. Patients who believe their illness is acute often drop out of treatment earlier than those who believe it to be chronic (Meyer, Leventhal, & Gutmann, 1985).

4. *Consequences,* including its physical, social, and economic impact. People are far more likely to ignore symptoms that minimally disrupt their daily lives (such as minor muscle soreness following a strenuous workout)

illness representation how a person views a particular illness, including its label and symptoms, perceived causes, timeline, consequences, and controllability

■ **comorbidity** the simultaneous occurrence of two or more physical and/or psychological disorders or symptoms

than they are to ignore symptoms that have a serious disruptive effect (such as a severe muscular strain that prevents a laborer from earning a paycheck).

5. *Controllability,* that is, beliefs regarding whether the illness can be prevented, controlled, and/or cured (Leventhal et al., 1997). People who view their disease or condition as incurable may skip appointments, neglect treatment, or even behave in self-destructive ways because they feel helpless and hopeless.

Note that the key to these components is the person's *perception* of the symptoms rather than the actual facts about the disease. How you react to a stomachache, for example, depends on whether you think it was caused by too much to eat or by some internal, uncontrollable factor.

Psychological Disturbances and Symptom Reporting

Whether people recognize health symptoms and/or interpret them as worthy of medical attention is also affected by emotional instability (formerly called neuroticism), which encompasses a number of specific traits, including self-consciousness, the inability to inhibit cravings, vulnerability to stress, and the tendency to experience anxiety, depression, and other negative emotions (Costa & McCrae, 1985). People who are anxious and those who score low on tests of emotional stability tend to report more physical symptoms, perhaps because they tend to exaggerate the seriousness of minor complaints that others are more likely to ignore (Larsen, 1992).

People who score low on tests of emotional stability may also suffer more actual symptoms than others *because of their anxious nature* (Gramling, Clawson, & McDonald, 1996). Support for this latter explanation comes from evidence that nearly two-thirds of people who visit doctors for common physical complaints such as nausea, dizziness, or aches and pains in various parts of the body are actually suffering from anxiety or depression (Malt et al., 1997). That is, symptoms of psychological or emotional disorders are sometimes misattributed to physical problems (Simon, Gater, Kisely, & Piccinelli, 1996).

It is estimated that as many as one-third of all hospitalized patients also suffer from diagnosable psychological disorders, as compared with 2 to 4 percent in the general population (Katon & Sullivan, 1990). This suggests that there is substantial **comorbidity** of psychological and physical disorders (Cohen & Rodriguez, 1995), meaning that both physical and psychological symptoms and disorders often occur simultaneously in some people. And indeed, psychological disorders such as anxiety or depression can predispose physical disorders through biological, behavioral, cognitive, and social pathways (see Figure 12.1). For example, depression might trigger poor health practices, such as alcohol abuse, and a general apathy regarding treatment regimens. Anxiety and depression can also lead to an excessive focus on bodily symptoms.

Figure 12.1

Psychological Disorders, Physical Disorders, and Illness Behavior
Psychological disorders can predispose physical disorders and illness behavior via a number of biological, behavioral, cognitive, and social pathways. Among these are stress-induced physiological arousal, abuse of alcohol, an excessive focus on bodily symptoms, and social isolation. For example, depression might lead to alcohol abuse, which could result in a variety of physical disorders such as cirrhosis of the liver.

Source: Adapted from "Pathways Linking Affective Disturbances and Physical Disorders," by S. Cohen and M. S. Rodriguez, *Health Psychology*, 1995, *14*, 374–380.

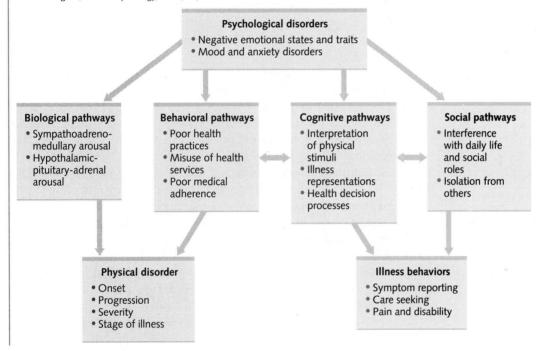

Sociocultural Factors

How people interpret symptoms is further influenced by sociocultural factors such as prior experience and expectations. For example, people who have a personal or family history of a particular medical condition tend to become *less* panicky or concerned about familiar symptoms than do those with no prior personal or family history of the condition, at least for minor medical conditions (Jemmott, Croyle, & Ditto, 1988). However, for more serious conditions—such as cancer—they are likely to react strongly to symptoms they've seen in stricken family members.

Prior experience can be either good or bad. On the positive side, it leads to increased accuracy, as when experienced parents calmly seek medical care for their second child, who exhibits a symptom familiar from their first child's younger days (Turk, Litt, Salovey, & Walker, 1985). On the negative side, experience may cause us to overlook or misinterpret symptoms. A good example is the tendency of many older adults to mistakenly assume that unusual fatigue, muscle weakness, or memory losses are merely symptoms of aging rather than signs of disease (Leventhal & Prohaska, 1986). Another example of experience gone awry is when busy workers mistakenly attribute physical symptoms of disease to the temporary effects of stress (Cameron, Leventhal, & Leventhal, 1995). This tendency to attribute symptoms to nondisease sources is particularly noticeable in the early stages of many diseases, when symptoms are most likely to be mild, slow to develop, and ambiguous (Benyamini, Leventhal, & Leventhal, 1997).

People also often exaggerate expected symptoms while ignoring or not detecting unexpected symptoms. In a classic study, Diane Ruble (1972) told one group of women that they were within 1 or 2 days of beginning menstruation and told another group that their periods were not due for 7 to 10 days. In fact, they were all about one week from beginning their periods. The first group reported significantly more psychological and physical symptoms of premenstruation than did the latter group, who did not expect their periods for another week or so. Although Ruble's findings indicate that *premenstrual syndrome (PMS)* may result not only from physical changes but also from a woman's beliefs, the results do not mean the women did not experience actual symptoms. Rather, they suggest that women who believe themselves to be premenstrual may overstate naturally fluctuating bodily states. Similarly, women who believe that most women experience unpleasant premenstrual changes are more likely to recall and amplify their own premenstrual changes than women who perceive PMS as an unusual complaint (Marvan & Cortes-Iniestra, 2001).

Another factor that influences our response to ambiguous sensations is the location of the symptoms. Symptoms that are readily apparent, such as those involving the face or the eyes or that are in some way disfiguring, tend to be regarded as more serious and provoke the seeking of treatment sooner than do symptoms involving the legs or trunk of the body (Eifert, Hodson, Tracey, Seville, & Gunawardane, 1996). Surveys of college students reveal that they are more reluctant to seek medical care for private body parts, such as the genitals, or those that are "stigmatized," such as the anus, than body parts perceived as especially critical to good health, such as the heart or blood (Klonoff & Landrine, 1993).

No less important in influencing our response to symptoms is the perceived severity of the symptom. In general, painful and incapacitating symptoms, as well as symptoms that are perceived as more serious, are more likely to prompt the person to seek care. Intermittent symptoms are less likely than persistent symptoms to trigger illness behavior. Even minor symptoms may provide care-seeking if the symptoms are persistent.

Sick Role Behavior

Recognizing a symptom or set of symptoms does not automatically lead to health care. Several demographic and sociocultural factors play important roles in determining sick role behavior, that is, whether a person will take the next step and seek professional help.

Age and Gender

In general, the very young and the elderly use health services more often than do adolescents and young adults (USDHHS, 1995). As any parent well knows, children develop many different infectious diseases as their immune systems are developing; therefore, they need general checkups, vaccinations, and regular health services. But as you will see in Chapter 15, the school years are among the healthiest of the entire life span, meaning that both the frequency of illness and the need to visit physicians declines steadily throughout late childhood, adolescence, and young adulthood. Health services begin to increase again in middle age and late adulthood as a result of the increasing prevalence of chronic, age-related diseases (see Figure 12.2).

Age also influences how people attribute the symptoms they detect and thus what they decide to do about them. For example, as adults grow older they increasingly tend to blame their age for mild symptoms that gradually appear, while sudden severe symptoms are more likely to be attributed to illness (Leventhal & Diefenbach, 1991). When symptoms are attributed to age, many people—especially the middle aged—tend to delay the seeking of health care.

Figure 12.2

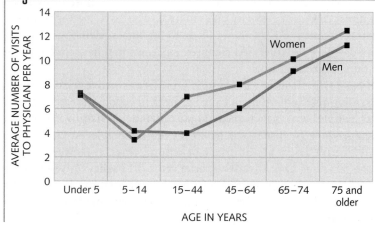

Age, Gender, and Physician's Contacts

In general, young children and older adults are more likely than adolescents and young adults to use health services. Starting in adolescence, women contact their physicians more than men do.

Source: *Healthy People 2000 Review, 1994,* by United States Department of Health and Human Services (USDHHS), 1995, Washington, DC: U.S. Government Printing Office.

Older people, however, are more likely to seek prompt care for ambiguous symptoms, perhaps due to intolerance of uncertainty.

Another factor in using health services is gender. Beginning in adolescence and continuing throughout adulthood, women are more likely than men to report symptoms and to use health services (Baum & Grunberg, 1991; Fuller, Edwards, Sermsri, & Vorakitphokatorn, 1993). This difference is due in large part to pregnancy and childbirth. New mothers are staying in the hospital about half a day longer than they did in the mid-1990s, when insurance companies cut childbirth stays to 24 hours and sparked outcries about "drive-by deliveries" (CDC, 1999). However, the male–female difference in physician contacts during early adulthood cannot fully account for the gender difference. Even when medical visits for pregnancy and childbirth are not counted, women still visit their physicians more often than do men.

Men often dodge the doctor, even when faced with potentially serious problems. Large-scale surveys conducted by CNN and the National Center for Health Statistics revealed the following (Papas, 1999):

- More than one-third of the sample of men wouldn't go to a doctor immediately even if experiencing severe chest pains (34 percent) or shortness of breath (37 percent), two possible signs of a myocardial infarction.
- Fifty-five percent of the women had undergone a cancer screening in the past year, mostly for cervical or breast cancer. Only 32 percent of the men sampled had been checked for cancer, mostly of the prostate gland.
- The women were more conscious than the men of taking care of their health and more likely to perceive that they had a medical need. Men were less likely than women to report having unmet medical needs (18.7 percent compared to 22.9 percent).

Why are women more likely than men to seek health care? One possible reason is that women are exposed to more illness. They are more likely to be involved in direct care of the elderly and children, who have the highest incidence of illness. Women also are more likely to be nurses, elementary school teachers, and day-care providers. As a consequence, women have an increased risk of becoming ill themselves.

Research has further found that women are more sensitive to their internal bodily symptoms than are men, causing them to report more symptoms (Pennebaker, 1982). Until they are older, many men delay visiting the doctor because they perceive themselves as healthy, even invincible. At age 25, the average male doesn't worry about injury or chronic disease. However, many women of the same age have already experienced a pregnancy and so may be more aware of the fragility of perfect health. This explanation does not imply that women get sick more often than men do, merely that they are more likely to notice and report any symptoms they experience. Furthermore, traditional gender roles mandate that men—"the stronger sex"—should not succumb to pain and discomfort.

Others believe that the gender difference in the seeking of health care is due to social factors. For instance, women visit doctors more than men because their health care tends to be more fragmented. For a routine physical exam, most men are "one-stop shoppers." That is, they visit a general practitioner or nurse practitioner who is able to perform most, if not all, of the needed tests. In contrast, a woman may need to visit three or more specialists or clinics for a thorough checkup: an internist for her physical, a gynecologist for a Pap smear, a mammography specialist to screen for breast tumors, and so forth. According to some, this fragmentation is yet another indication that Western medicine is male-biased and not well structured to meet women's basic needs (Rosenthal, 1993).

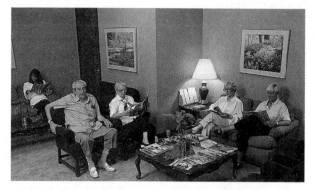

Women, the Elderly, and Sick Role Behavior
In general, women are more likely than men to seek health care. Furthermore, women over 65 are more likely than younger women to seek health care. Although the doctor's waiting room shown here is fairly empty, this is more the exception than the rule. Most people will spend anywhere from 15 minutes to 2 hours waiting to see their doctors.
© A. Ramey/Stock Boston

Socioeconomic Status

Socioeconomic status (SES) predicts both symptom reporting and the seeking of health care. High-income people generally report fewer symptoms and better health than do low-income people (Kaplan & Keil, 1993). However, when high-SES people do get sick, they are more likely to seek health care. This may explain why low-SES people are overrepresented among those who are hospitalized. People in lower-SES groups tend to wait longer before seeking treatment for their symptoms, making it more likely that they will become seriously ill and require hospitalization. In addition, people with lower family incomes are more likely to use outpatient clinics and hospital emergency rooms for medical care, probably because they are less likely to have health insurance and regular physicians than their financially advantaged counterparts (Flack et al., 1995). This explains why morbidity and mortality are highest among people at the lowest-SES levels.

The high cost of health care is not the only reason for SES differences in the use of health services. One surprising finding is that as a group, economically disadvantaged people tend to see themselves as less likely to develop serious illnesses than their financially advantaged counterparts (Rundall & Wheeler, 1979). Another is that there simply are not as many medical services available for people with low incomes. These two factors are made all the more troubling because, as we have seen throughout this book, low-income people generally have more health problems and health-damaging habits than do those who are better off.

■ **lay referral system** an informal network of family members, friends, and other nonprofessionals who offer their own impressions, experiences, and recommendations regarding a set of bodily symptoms

Culture and Ethnicity

Cultural factors and ethnicity also influence the way in which people respond to physical symptoms. Some cultures encourage a strong reaction to symptoms, while others socialize group members to deny pain and keep their symptoms to themselves (Sue & Zane, 1995). In one study, researchers compared the overall functioning of chronic back pain sufferers in six different countries (Sanders et al., 1992). American patients reported the greatest overall suffering and disruption of daily activities, followed in order by Italian, New Zealand, Japanese, Colombian, and Mexican patients.

Cultural factors also influence a person's tendency to seek treatment. People who hold illness beliefs that conflict with Western medicine are less likely to seek conventional care and more likely to rely upon a **lay referral system**—an informal network of family members, friends, and other nonprofessionals who offer their own impressions and experiences regarding a set of symptoms (Burnam, Timbers, & Hough, 1984). In response to a set of symptoms, a member of the referral system might help interpret a symptom ("My niece had a growth like that, and it turned out to be nothing at all") or give advice about seeking treatment ("Jack waited until his cancer had metastasized and it was too late to treat. You'd better call your doctor right away"). They may also offer specific recommendations, such as saying that RICE—rest, ice, compression, and elevation—is just the ticket for your sore ankle.

Several researchers have studied ethnic and cultural variations in the lay referral system. They have found, for example, that ethnic groups differ widely in the degree to which they believe that human intervention in health outcomes is possible, or desirable. Christians and Jews, for example, have historically been distinguished from other groups in their belief in *activism*—that people not only can but should influence health because natural events are controllable. Other groups attribute disease to nonphysical factors (Landrine & Klonoff, 1994). In such cases, people may be more inclined to employ non-Western practices for treatment (see Chapter 14). This poses an interesting problem for Western health care providers, since the closer a patient's cultural background or ethnicity is to that of Western physicians, the more the patient's *reported* symptoms will approximate those that are recognizable as signs of disease.

A related cultural factor in determining the likelihood of a person's seeking treatment for a particular symptom is upbringing. People whose parents paid close attention to physical symptoms and sought regular health care may be more likely to do the same. Conversely, those whose parents were suspicious of doctors and more likely to rely on self-care or some form of alternative treatment may be more likely to carry that suspicion with them.

Attributions

Many people are motivated to determine the causes of events, including health outcomes. This is especially true when outcomes are unexpected and disruptive. Thus, people routinely generate hypotheses about the causes of their symptoms, particularly when the symptoms are highly salient and potentially serious (Cacioppo, Andersen, Turnquist, & Petty, 1986). In one study, 95 percent of a sample of women with breast cancer had formed a causal attribution for their cancer—for example, genetic vulnerability, poor diet, or use of an estrogen supplement. The causes were not always based on medical facts but on the need to have a cause (Taylor, Lichtman, & Wood, 1984).

But these attributions often are inaccurate, even among people who are well educated. For example, Elizabeth Klonoff and Hope Landrine (1994) reported that some college students believe that certain illnesses, such as AIDS, are caused partly by sin, God's will, or another nondisease factor. Less dramatically, the students tended to attribute certain illnesses—such as hypertension and migraines—to emotional causes and others—such as colds and flu—to infection. This is significant because the perceived cause of an illness may influence whether a person seeks treatment. For example, if an illness is attributed to emotional causes, a person might be less likely to seek treatment; if the disease is attributed to an infection, she or he might be more likely to seek treatment.

Seeking Treatment

When we talk about seeking treatment, we can categorize most people into the "normal use" classification and place the others into two broad categories: delayers and overusers. Health psychologists have investigated the reasons for these two extremes of behavior.

Delay Behavior

Do you or someone you know sometimes avoid thinking about health care until a *serious* need arises? Do you tend to ignore symptoms for as long as possible in the hope that they will disappear? Clearly, for medical emergencies such as heart attacks, getting help as quickly as possible is of the utmost importance. Although other chronic diseases and conditions may not present this kind of minute-by-minute urgency in survival, seeking timely care when symptoms first appear can make the difference between dying from the disease or condition and catching it when it may still be treatable. For example,

■ **delay behavior** the tendency to avoid seeking medical care because symptoms go unnoticed *(appraisal delay)*, sickness seems unlikely *(illness delay)*, professional help is deemed unnecessary *(behavioral delay)*, the individual procrastinates in making an appointment *(scheduling delay)*, or the perceived benefits of treatment do not outweigh the perceived costs *(treatment delay)*

beginning treatment for certain types of cancer while it is still localized and before it has metastasized to other areas of the body often makes the difference between a long, full life and one that is shortened prematurely.

Despite the seemingly obvious benefits of seeking care when symptoms first appear, many people ignore their symptoms and do not seek medical help. This is called **delay behavior.** For example, despite seemingly overwhelming evidence of the need for immediate medical attention for myocardial infarction, sufferers frequently wait hours before admitting their chest pain is serious; patients who feel lumps in their breasts or testicles sometimes postpone a visit to a doctor for months. Why do people delay seeking medical attention for such serious conditions?

In one analysis of factors in delay behavior, Martin Safer and his colleagues (Safer, Tharps, Jackson, & Leventhal, 1979) described five stages in the decision-making process for seeking medical care; at each stage, a person can exhibit delay behavior (see Figure 12.3). The model predicts that people will avoid seeking medical care because symptoms go unnoticed *(appraisal delay)*, sickness seems unlikely *(illness delay)*, professional help is deemed unnecessary *(behavioral delay)*, the individual procrastinates in making an appointment *(scheduling delay)*, or the perceived benefits of treatment do not outweigh the perceived costs *(treatment delay)*.

What determines the amount of delay during each stage? During the appraisal delay stage, the sensory prominence of the symptoms is the most important factor. Interviews with patients seeking care at hospital clinics indicated that patients delayed less when they were in pain or bleeding. Myocardial infarction patients who stopped to research their symptoms by consulting books and other sources delayed more than five times as long as patients who did not research their symptoms. Initial pain led to a short delay, whereas talking with others about one's symptoms resulted in a significantly longer delay (Matthews, Siegel, Kuller, Thompson, & Varat, 1983).

In the illness delay stage, other factors, such as previous experience with the symptoms, also came into play. Patients who had

Figure 12.3

Stages of Delay in Seeking Medical Attention

The delay model proposed by Martin Safer and colleagues shows that noticing symptoms does not automatically lead to treatment. People have to make a concerted effort to take each step, so it's possible for intervening factors to interrupt the process.

Source: "Delay in Seeking a Cancer Diagnosis. Delay Stages and Psychophysiological Comparison Processes," by B. L. Anderson, J. T. Cacioppo, and D. C. Roberts, *British Journal of Social Psychology*, 1995, *34*, 33–52.

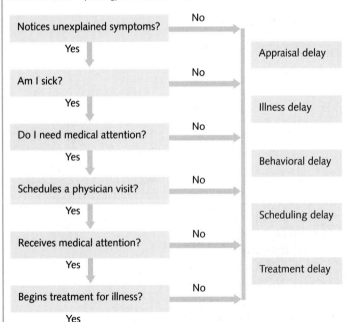

previously experienced similar symptoms were more likely than those who experienced symptoms for the first time to delay seeking medical attention. For example, with *carpal tunnel syndrome,* a nerve disorder caused by repetitive motion, the symptoms may come and go over a long period of time, and so people tend to ignore them. Only when the symptoms (numbness in the fingers and shooting pain up the arm) become persistent will the person start moving through the stages. In addition, patients who spent more time thinking about their symptoms and imagining the consequences of being sick were more likely to delay seeking medical attention.

In the last three stages, delay was longest for patients who were more concerned about the cost of treatment, had little pain, and were doubtful that their symptoms could be cured. The association between not feeling pain and delaying medical care is unfortunate because pain is not a major symptom in the early stages of a number of chronic diseases, including cancer, hypertension, and diabetes.

Overusing Health Services

At the opposite extreme are people who misuse health services by seeking care when they do not have a diagnosable health condition. The magnitude of this problem for the health care system is revealed in a startling statistic: Physicians estimate that as much as two-thirds of their time is taken up by people with problems that are either medically insignificant or the result of emotional disturbances (Miranda, Perez-Stable, Munoz, Hargreaves, & Henke, 1991).

Hypochondriasis

Why do some people visit their physicians when there is no real need? A commonsense explanation is that such people suffer from **hypochondriasis,** or the false belief that they have a disease when they do not (see Diversity and Healthy Living on pages 518–519). Most people with hypochondriasis experience vague or ambiguous symptoms that they exaggerate and misattribute to disease. They also may have an exaggerated fear of contracting a disease, even in the face of information that nothing is, in fact, wrong and that there is no real danger. An underlying factor in many cases of hypochondriasis appears to be *neuroticism* (emotional instability), a state of emotional maladjustment that encompasses a number of specific traits, including self-consciousness, the inability to inhibit cravings, vulnerability to stress, and the tendency to experience anxiety, depression, and other negative emotions (Costa & McCrae, 1985).

Is this commonsense view of hypochondriasis correct? Or are all people who report imaginary symptoms feigning illness, or **malingering,** in order to derive **secondary gains,** that is, whatever benefits they can from sick role behavior? Generally speaking, people suffering from hypochondriasis amplify vague or ambiguous symptoms that are, in fact, benign into excessive worry

hypochondriasis the condition of experiencing abnormal anxiety over one's health, often including imaginary symptoms

malingering making believe one is ill in order to benefit from sick role behavior

secondary gains the "rewards" associated with sick role behavior, including increased attention, the ability to rest, freedom from responsibility, and so forth

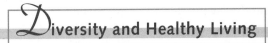

Chronic Fatigue Syndrome

Katie Lucas was so exhausted that she could barely get out of bed or perform even the simplest physical or mental task. "I remember one occasion having to take out a calculator to subtract 12 from 32," she said. "That's pretty bad." In Atlanta, Wilhelmina Jenkins was unable to complete her doctoral training in physics due to chronic fatigue that made thinking and writing all but impossible. "All they could recommend to me was changing my lifestyle—getting more rest," she said. "I tried every kind of change I could think of, and nothing helped; I just continued to go downhill."

Lucas and Jenkins suffer from **chronic fatigue syndrome (CFS),** a puzzling disorder suffered by an estimated 1 million patients in the United States, 80 percent of whom are women. In addition to persistent fatigue that lasts for months or longer, other symptoms of CFS include headaches, infections of unknown origins, and difficulties with concentration and memory (Ray, 1997). People afflicted with CFS are often so debilitated they are unable to carry out their normal, everyday activities. Making matters worse is the widespread view that they are not really sick but are merely malingerers whose symptoms are self-induced to gain attention, sympathy, or release from overwhelming responsibilities.

The cause of CFS has been much debated; the majority of patients report that it began with an apparent infection, and a significant number state that they were under considerable stress at the time (Komaroff & Buchwald, 1991). Because there is no diagnostic test for CFS and no known treatment, some doctors believe the condition is actually a form of hypochondriasis, or even a **hysterical epidemic** caused by modern culture. Throughout history, *hysteria* has served as a physical manifestation of distress—a form of expression, if you will, for people who otherwise are unable to verbalize their problems. First described in women during the late nineteenth century, hysteria involved puzzling physical disabilities—blindness or paralysis, for example—that Sigmund Freud believed to be the result of emotional conflicts. Many historians and sociologists believe that hysteria was really a "Victorian disorder," a female reaction to sexual repression and limited career opportunities, which all but disappeared with the advent of feminism. Along with those who have *recovered memories* of childhood trauma and abuse or suffer from *Gulf War syndrome* or *dissociative identity disorder* (formerly called multiple personality disorder), CFS "victims," say the critics, are merely manifesting contemporary signs of hysteria (Showalter, 1999).

There is evidence, however, that those who consider CFS to be a form of hysteria or hypochondriasis are probably wrong. For example, researchers at Johns Hopkins University have established a link between chronic fatigue and low blood pressure. Strapping CFS patients on a tilt table and then gradually moving them upright to a 70-degree angle, researchers found that at one point the patients' blood pressure drops suddenly from about 125 to 45,

■ **chronic fatigue syndrome (CFS)** a puzzling disorder of uncertain causes in which a person experiences headaches, infections of unknown origins, extreme tiredness, and difficulties with concentration and memory

■ **hysterical epidemic** the widespread attributing of bodily symptoms of stress to a particular disease that has become culturally fashionable

about their health. To find out whether hypochondriasis is linked with emotional maladjustment, Paul Costa and Robert McCrae (1985) administered to average adults the Emotional Stability Scale and the Cornell Medical Index, which assesses a broad range of medical symptoms. The results showed that adults who scored high on emotional instability averaged two to three times as many physical complaints as those who scored low on emotional instability. But does this prove that neuroticism causes hypochondriasis? As we have seen, correlational evidence such as this cannot pinpoint causality. Even if it could, we would be unable to discern the *direction* of causality. Mightn't it be possible that having many aches, pains, and illnesses causes an excessive preoccupation with one's health?

It is particularly unfair—and inaccurate—to denounce everyone who calls a health provider in the absence of indisputable physical symptoms, because stress and anxiety often create a number of physical symptoms that may re-

immediately triggering CFS symptoms. By boosting the patient's water and salt intake and providing pressure-elevating medication, researchers have been able to help about 75 percent of the CFS patients. Other researchers have found that administering low doses of the stress hormone hydrocortisone, known to be in short supply in many people with CFS, boosts energy, mood, and activity level (Rutz, 1998). The research also indicates that a high percentage of CFS patients suffer from a persistent viral infection and immune system dysfunction and that treatment of these problems can alleviate some of the symptoms (Ablashi et al., 2000; Pall, 2000). Evidence such as this is helpful to frustrated patients, who have frequently been told by doctors who can find nothing wrong with them that they are imagining their symptoms.

The role of psychological factors in CFS, however, continues to be debated. Some experts suggest that CFS and depression have a common cause because of similar symptoms such as fatigue. Others have pointed to differences between the two disorders. For example, weight loss, suicidal thinking, guilt, and low self-esteem are all less common in CFS than in depression, while flu-like symptoms, muscle weakness and pain, and fatigue are more common.

The time course of CFS varies from patient to patient, with some experiencing rapid improvement and full recovery, while others worsen over time and/or experience repeated cycles of relapse and remission (Hinds & McCluskey, 1993). Because there is no generally accepted drug treatment for CFS, treatment usually involves managing the symptoms and engaging in moderate activity. Cognitive-behavioral interventions designed to increase tolerance of symptoms and to modify maladaptive illness beliefs have also been effective in some patients (Sharpe et al., 1996). The disorder can be so debilitating, unresponsive to traditional medical regimens, and frustrating that some CFS sufferers turn to various forms of alternative and fringe medicine. In the Midwest, one nurse suffering from CFS actually took her own life with the help of Dr. Jack Kevorkian (Showalter, 1999).

Because the debate appears to be shifting from whether the symptoms of disorders such as CFS are real—those affected are definitely sick, according to an increasing number of experts—some health experts question whether there is any point in continuing the search for specific, organic causes. Simon Wessely, professor of psychological medicine and director of the Chronic Fatigue Syndrome unit at King's College in London, believes that doing so is a disservice to patients: "Doctors have been searching for the Holy Grail to explain these syndromes for the last 150 years without success. . . . If a patient is told the problem is due to a permanent deficit in the immune system or a persistent virus or chronic disability of the nerves or brain, this just generates helplessness and the patient becomes a victim," he said. "And if you say the problem is psychological, this generates anger on the part of patients who don't regard psychological ills as legitimate. Looking for any single cause misses the point. Regardless of how or why they may have started, these syndromes are multifactorial, like heart disease" (Brody, 1999a).

semble the symptoms of a biologically based disorder (Miranda et al., 1991). For example, excessive worry and anxiety (perhaps about upcoming exams) often disrupt sleeping and concentration, trigger a bout of diarrhea and nausea, suppress appetite, and result in a state of general agitation (Pennebaker, Burnam, Schaeffer, & Harper, 1977).

Somatization

Some researchers use the term **somatization** to refer to the translation of emotional distress into physical symptoms when there is no apparent biological cause for these symptoms (Cummings, 1991). The most frequently cited symptoms include backaches, chest pain, heart palpitations, abdominal pains, chronic headaches, unusual allergies, chronic malaise, and hyperventilation (Quill, 1985). Nearly any physical symptom can appear at any age in both women and men, but somatization is particularly likely during stressful

■ **somatization** the translation of emotional distress into physical symptoms when there is no apparent biological cause for these symptoms

transitional times in life—for example, the beginning of college, marriage, the birth of a child, unemployment, and retirement. Research consistently demonstrates that somaticizers account for between 30 and 60 percent of all outpatient physician visits (Cummings, 1991) and that a typical somaticizer consumes up to nine times more in health care costs than the average person (Smith, 1994).

The Health Care System

The World Health Organization defines a health care system as *all activities whose primary purpose is to promote, restore, or maintain health* (WHO, 2000). Formal health services, including the professional delivery of personal medical services by physicians, midwives, nurses, and technicians, are clearly within these boundaries, as is the use of all medication, whether or not prescribed by a provider. So is home care of the sick, which is how an estimated 70 to 90 percent of all sickness is managed. By this definition, health care systems today are one of the largest sectors in the world economy, with global spending an estimated $2,985 billion, or nearly 8 percent of the world gross domestic product (WHO, 2000).

The resources devoted to health care systems are very unequally distributed throughout the world, and not in proportion to the distribution of health problems. For instance, 84 percent of the world's population live in low- and middle-income countries, which account for only 11 percent of global health spending (4 percent of gross domestic product in those countries), despite the fact that these countries bear 93 percent of the world's disease burden (see Chapter 2).

In both rich and poor nations, health needs today are very different from those of 100 or even 50 years ago. Expectations of access to some form of health care continue to increase, as do demands for measures to protect individuals against the financial cost of poor health. People today also turn to health systems for a much more diverse array of problems than before, that is, not just for pain relief or the treatment of debilitating diseases and conditions, but also for information on nutrition, substance use, child-rearing, and countless other issues. Still, at the heart of the modern health system is the hospital.

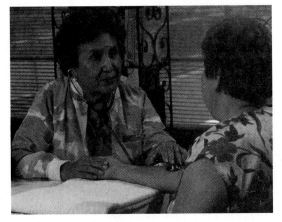

Home Care
The cost of health care accounts for nearly 8 percent of the world gross domestic product. Home care services across the world account for the majority of this cost. For example, this Native American practical nurse cares for this elderly woman at home. © Bob Daemmrich / The Image Works

The Administrative Structure of the Modern Hospital

There are about 6,000 registered hospitals in the United States, admitting over 34 million people as patients each year (AHA, 2001); these include community and municipal hospitals, Veterans Administration (VA) hospitals, and psychiatric hospitals. Many hospitals now specialize, for example treating only acute diseases or trauma that results from injury. This shift in focus is due in large part to economic pressure to reduce the high cost of hospitalization. As Figure 12.4 shows, by a huge margin, the largest piece of the health care "pie" is the cost of hospitalization.

The modern hospital has a complex, hierarchical administrative structure. At the top is usually a board of trustees, consisting of community and business leaders charged with overall policymaking, long-range planning, and fundraising. Directly below the trustees are the hospital administrators and medical staff, each group with its own line of authority. The administrative staff deals with the everyday matters of keeping the hospital running smoothly—keeping patient accounts, ordering supplies, purchasing equipment, and maintenance, for example. The medical staff, which includes the physicians and the nurses, is responsible for medical treatment. In most American hospitals, physicians are not employees of the hospital. Rather, they are employed in private practice or affiliated with a managed care plan and provide services at the hospital for their patients through these sources. Most receive salaries from the managed care plan or bill patients individually.

The Nursing Staff

Nurses are the backbone of the health care system, and the demand for their services continues to outstrip their supply. Of primary interest are the registered nurses (R.N.s), who are either nurse practitioners or clinical nurse specialists. *Nurse practitioners* have completed bachelor's and master's programs in nursing as well as training in primary care. They often work with physicians in private practice, seeing their own patients and providing all routine medical care, including prescribing treatments for various illnesses and conditions. *Clinical nurse specialists* specialize as health care providers in an area of practice such as cardiac or cancer care, pediatrics, gerontology, or mental health.

Nurses are in a unique position among medical staff. Although employed by the hospital, they are also considered to be physicians' assistants. These multiple roles sometimes create conflicting demands, such as when a doctor orders an expensive diagnostic test for a patient but the hospital administration wants to discourage use of the test as a cost-containment strategy.

Nursing is a stressful occupation for several reasons. First, nurses may also feel tension stemming from conflict between their own professional goals and

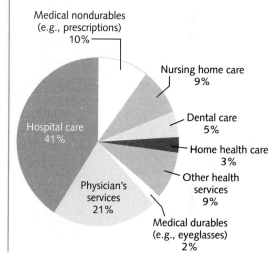

Figure 12.4

The Health Care "Pie"
Out of every dollar spent on health services in the United States, nearly 42 cents go to pay for hospitalization. Small wonder that economic pressures have dramatically reduced the average length of a hospital stay from about 8.3 days in 1965 to around 5 days in 1998 (AHA, 1999). Health psychologists believe that if more efforts were placed on promoting health and preventive care, the need for expensive hospitalization would be dramatically reduced (NCHS, 1995).

Sources: *Hospital Statistics,* by AHA, 1999. Chicago: American Hospital Association; *Health, United States, 1994,* by National Center for Health Statistics (NCHS), 1995. Hyattsville, MD: U.S. Public Health Service.

Medical nondurables (e.g., prescriptions) 10%

Nursing home care 9%

Dental care 5%

Home health care 3%

Other health services 9%

Medical durables (e.g., eyeglasses) 2%

Physician's services 21%

Hospital care 41%

those of physicians and hospital administrators. Although both nurses and physicians work from a *cure orientation* in which they seek to restore patients to good health, nurses also work from a patient *care orientation*. That is, while their primary goal is to heal patients, an equally important goal is to make the healing process as humane as possible. Although they do care about the patients, hospital administrators have a *core,* or *institutional orientation,* in which they are concerned primarily with ensuring the smooth flow of services, keeping the physical facilities of the hospital well maintained, and so forth. Caught in the middle, nurses are especially prone to conflict, dissatisfaction, and a high rate of turnover.

Second, nurses may suffer stress from the conflict between their high level of medical training and low involvement in decision making. For example, they are not allowed to administer medication, although their experience often makes it obvious when it is needed. Third, nurses often struggle with monumental issues, such as balancing their medical oath to "do no harm" with requests from dying patients to assist them in committing suicide. One *New England Journal of Medicine* study showed that 19 percent of nurses who care for the dying had engaged in *euthanasia* or assisted suicide (Scanlon, 1996). Seven percent had done so on their own, without a physician's request. These conflicts, along with the numerous other stresses of working with sick people, place nurses at high risk of *burnout*—an occupational hazard characterized by emotional and physical exhaustion, a loss of meaningfulness in one's work, and an increasingly depersonalized and cynical attitude toward patients (see Chapter 4). One explanation of burnout is that the hurried, fast-lane pace of the modern hospital, coupled with the pain of watching patients suffer, forces burned-out nurses to psychologically distance themselves from their clients and from their career (Parker & Kulik, 1995).

The Changing Health Care System

As medical costs have skyrocketed, the American health care system has undergone many changes. Walk-in clinics, *extended care facilities,* and home help services, for example, handle an increasing proportion of smaller emergencies and long-term care for those who are not seriously ill. Extended care facilities include convalescent homes, nursing homes, and other facilities for patients with chronic illnesses or disabilities that prevent them from living on their own. In addition, *rehabilitation centers* treat those who are recovering from specific conditions, such as stroke, spinal cord injuries, head injuries, and degenerative diseases, while *psychiatric hospitals* offer long-term care for people diagnosed with psychological disorders such as schizophrenia. Finally, *hospices* provide both institutional and home health care for those who are terminally ill.

Managed Care

The most dramatic cost-containment strategy is the increasing prominence of *health maintenance organizations (HMOs)* and other forms of **managed care**—health care that seeks to control costs by eliminating waste and unnecessary procedures and by providing economically sound treatment guidelines to hospitals and doctors. Under a managed care system, each patient is assigned a *primary care physician,* who manages his or her treatment by acting as a gatekeeper to determine when referrals to specialists within the system are warranted. About one in five insured Americans now belongs to a managed care program. Another type of managed care plan, the *preferred provider organization,* or *PPO,* groups together a network of hospitals and physicians who pool their resources to minimize costs and discount their fees to members.

One concern about managed care is that medical decision making is being taken out of the hands of doctors and patients and shifted to insurance companies and other third-party providers. Although this keeps costs down, critics complain that it also eliminates the patient's right to choose his or her own doctor or hospital—for example, to stay with the doctor who's been treating the family for years.

Another concern is that the medical care provided by HMOs may not be of the same quality as that provided by private physicians. One study found that, compared to fee-for-service patients, HMO patients tended to have less expensive tests prescribed for them, were less likely to be admitted to a hospital, and, when admitted, were discharged sooner (Miller & Luft, 1994). We have to be careful in generalizing from such results, however. Managed care programs vary greatly in their policies and quality of care, so it's a good idea to shop around and ask careful questions of providers before selecting a plan.

A large number of American adults are dissatisfied with their managed care programs. A 1998 U.S. News/Kaiser Family foundation study reported that two-thirds of Americans have had some problem with the system and that 75 percent were worried about facing health care problems in the future.

Clearly, the health care system is in flux. Politicians, economists, and medical professionals are all looking for solutions to the health care problem. At the core of the problem is the high cost of medical care. This is why HMOs have become so popular. Thanks to managed care, more companies can afford to provide benefits to employees and runaway health care costs have been somewhat contained.

The High Cost of Health Care

Why does health care cost so much? One reason is that under the old "fee-for-service model," doctors and hospitals had a financial incentive to throw every treatment option available at every illness or health problem. The more procedures they carried out, the greater their income. And patients, too, had few reasons to worry about the costs of their treatment since

■ **managed care** health care that seeks to control costs by eliminating waste and unnecessary procedures and by providing economically sound treatment guidelines to hospitals and physicians

third-party payment insurance programs allowed them to pass their bills straight to their insurers almost without regard to costs. When Medicare was enacted into law in 1965, the government seemed to be institutionalizing this "blank check" mentality in which most or all health care costs were covered by private insurers and federal programs. The result was escalating inflation of health care costs that made the American system the most expensive in the world. In 1980, for instance, Americans spent $247 billion on health care, or 8.9 percent of the gross domestic product (GDP). By 1995 that figure had risen to $988 billion, or 13.6 percent of the GDP, as compared to only 7 percent for Japan, 9 percent for Germany, and about 10 percent for Canada (Brink, 1998).

Another reason health care costs have skyrocketed is that many doctors say that fear of *malpractice suits* has forced them to practice *defensive medicine,* ordering possibly unnecessary diagnostic tests and procedures that serve primarily to protect them from legal action. Many health experts believe that the economics of health care make it inevitable that the American health care system will ultimately shift to some form of national health insurance program. Most European countries, as well as Japan and Canada, have national health insurance programs that ensure high-quality care for every citizen. In Canada, hospitals are funded almost entirely by the government, while physicians are paid on the basis of the specific services they provide. England has a national health insurance system in which hospitals are financed and run by the government, and physicians are either salaried or paid a flat fee based on the number of patients they treat. In contrast, the health care system in the United States traditionally has been a unique mixture of public, private nonprofit, and private for-profit hospitals, in which most physicians were compensated on a fee-for-service basis. This compensation does, however, come from a variety of sources, sometimes from insurance companies, sometimes directly from patients, and sometimes from government programs such as Medicare, Medicaid, or the Veterans Administration.

Still, national health care has its critics. Although the quality of care is generally excellent, critics point to some significant drawbacks, such as the potentially long wait for certain operations and other procedures. In England, when patients began to complain of inadequate access to doctors, more and more wealthy citizens began taking out private health insurance. And increasingly, many Canadian citizens cross the border into the United States in order to obtain certain health care services that are low priority in nationalized Canadian hospitals (Kaplan, 1993). Regardless of who provides health care—nurse or physician—and whether that care is covered under a fee-for-service or managed care system, the patient–provider relationship is a crucial factor in how effective and satisfying the care is.

The Patient–Provider Relationship

"I really don't have time to explain all this," Dennis Moore's physician said as he hurried away, and for the second time that day Moore saw red. Earlier that day Moore, a former army officer who had commanded a river gun boat in Vietnam, had also seen the red of his own blood as he urinated. He desperately needed answers to questions—"Why am I bleeding? Do I have cancer? Will I be alive in a year?"—but he was too frightened and angry to stick around and stormed out of his doctor's office. A week later he learned from a more responsive doctor that the bleeding came from ulcers in his colon and a noncancerous tumor.

The relationship between health care provider and patient is the backbone of all medical treatment. One reason is that 60 to 80 percent of medical diagnoses and treatment decisions are made on the basis of information that arises from the medical consultation process alone. Another is that patients and providers do not always share the same view of the effectiveness of the process. Too often, providers overestimate how well a consultation went and how likely it is that the patient will follow through on their advice. A third reason is that the quality of the patient–provider relationship plays an important role in promoting patient compliance with treatment instructions.

Factors Affecting the Patient–Provider Relationship

Research has demonstrated that the central elements of the patient–provider relationship are *continuity of care, communication,* and the overall *quality of consultations* (Sihvonen, Kayhko, & Kekki, 1989). The same principles apply to this relationship regardless of the provider (physician, nurse practitioner, or medical technician) or the health care system. Under the fee-for-service model, 78 percent of patients reported being "very satisfied with their doctors." Today, under managed care, only 54 percent of patients report this same level of satisfaction (Brink, 1998). One reason for this decrease in satisfaction is that half of all patients are convinced that treatment decisions—including which providers they can see and whether they will even have the opportunity to develop a long-term relationship with them—are based strictly on what their health plan will cover.

Provider Communication Problems

The information exchanged between doctor and patient during a consultation is often crucial to formulating diagnoses and in deciding on the course of treatment. Effective communication ensures that patients' symptoms and concerns are understood by their health care providers and that information and treatment instructions are accurately received and carried out by the patient.

Patients often leave a consultation dissatisfied due to a lack of information, poor understanding of medical advice, and the perception that they are unable to follow recommended treatment or advice (Weinman, 1997). And, as Dennis Moore's story illustrates, faulty communication about their condition and treatment is also a major source of anxiety for many patients. Ideally, health care providers listen carefully to patients, ask questions to ensure that patients understand their condition and treatment, and fully inform patients about every aspect of their care. In addition to the verbal messages patients and providers send, their nonverbal behavior often provides important information, for instance, regarding a patient's underlying emotional state or the doctor's level of interest and empathy with the patient.

Lack of information is a direct by-product of "too little time, too much to do." Many health care providers simply do not spend enough time with their patients. A United Hospital Fund study clocked "average physician speed" in New York City at 1.9 to 3.1 patients per hour (Zuger, 1998). Despite the use of complicated equations to balance waiting time, no-show rates, and average length of visit, on some days physicians move at breakneck speeds of 3.2, 4.7, even 5.3 patients per hour. It's no wonder that more than half of U.S. households changed doctors within the past 2 years, most citing dissatisfaction about the communication with their physicians (Fischman, 2000).

Research consistently shows that the more time physicians spend with their patients, the more satisfied the patients are, particularly when their doctors take some time just to chat. Moreover, people with high blood pressure, diabetes, ulcers, and arthritis are more likely to follow their treatment plans to a successful conclusion when they understand their care and have a voice in it. Faster doctors who see more patients each day have less satisfied patients, who are also less likely to be up-to-date on immunizations, mammograms, and other health-enhancing procedures and tests (Zuger, 1998).

Some health care providers also *miscommunicate* with patients by failing to listen carefully or treating them either like medical school faculty or children. An early series of studies by Phillip Ley (1988) analyzed the content of physicians' comments during their consultations in terms of complexity, clarity, and organization. The findings of these studies showed that far too often the medical information provided was too detailed or complex for patients to understand or retain and that patients and doctors frequently interpreted the same information in different ways. The same studies reported that 28 percent of general practice patients were dissatisfied with the consultations and treatment they received. Among hospitalized patients, dissatisfaction was an even higher 41 percent.

Why such poor communication skills in supposedly highly intelligent and skilled professionals? Several reasons. First, people generally are not chosen for medical training based on their social skills or communicative skills but on their technical expertise. Second, until relatively recently medical schools placed little emphasis on this type of training. Few providers, for instance, were trained to deliver bad news, and many—out of sheer ignorance or in response to time pressures—say things to patients and families that cause unnecessary emotional pain and may even reduce the effectiveness of treatment. There is clear evidence that *how* bad news is delivered influences how well the stress is handled and whether it fosters or hinders a person's ability to cope with the situation (Brody, 1999b).

The harm that stems from poorly delivered bad news can be long-lasting, even permanent. One *Journal of the American Medical Association* study reported that, even after months had passed, cancer survivors and their loved ones were able to recall what made getting the news more or less difficult. Many expressed persistent negative feelings about how the news was conveyed (Ptacek & Eberhardt, 1996). In the worst instances, providers seemed to adopt coping strategies to minimize *their* discomfort with delivering bad news and failed to realize what was needed to minimize their patients' and the patients' loved ones' trauma. What the patients wanted was to hear all available information about their condition; to have ample opportunity to vent their feelings and ask questions; to be informed about available support services, including support groups for family members; and to be given as much time with their providers as needed to fully understand the medical condition, its treatment, and the likelihood that treatment would be successful.

A third factor in poor communication is that providers vary in their attitudes and beliefs about their own role and the patient's role during consultations. In one study of 74 physician consultations, researchers reported that in nearly two-thirds of the cases the physician interrupted his or her patient's description of symptoms after only 18 seconds (Beckman & Frankel, 1984). Moreover, too many physicians also use highly technical jargon that patients can't understand or, at the other extreme, overly simplistic language better suited to a child. Some researchers have suggested that some providers use jargon-filled language to discourage patients from asking too many questions or to keep them from realizing that the provider is not certain about the patient's problem (Taylor, Lichtman, & Wood, 1984). Whatever the reason, patients may be left with limited or misleading information and possible feelings of helplessness.

Another problem is that like people everywhere, some health care providers hold prejudicial patient stereotypes. Several studies have reported that physicians provide less information to and are less supportive of African-American and Hispanic patients and patients of lower socioeconomic class than other patients in the same health care setting (Epstein, Taylor, & Seage, 1985). Patients who present themselves for treatment for certain disorders also seem to evoke more negative reactions from physicians. For example, psychological disorders such as anxiety or depression may provoke especially brief visits. There is also evidence that many physicians have negative perceptions of the elderly, which are made even worse when older patients have difficulty communicating. Is it any wonder that among patients aged 65 and older, only 54 percent state high confidence in their physicians (Haug & Ory, 1987)?

Sexism is also present in health care, making communication between male physicians and female patients, for example, sometimes less than perfect. A number of research studies demonstrate that female physicians demonstrate more proficient clinical performance than do their male counterparts, conducting longer office visits, asking more questions, and showing significantly more verbal and nonverbal support (Hall, Irish, Roter, Ehrlich, & Miller, 1994). As with many things, patients often are most comfortable communicating and interacting with health care providers who are of the same gender and similar in other ways to themselves.

Patient Communication Problems

Health care providers should not receive all the blame for miscommunications. Patients themselves often are uninformed and unprepared to communicate about sensitive health matters. For example, patients who are overly anxious may not process information efficiently, frustrating providers who feel they must repeat instructions unnecessarily. Moreover, a surprising number of patients give faulty information or mention the symptom of greatest concern in an almost off-hand manner, fearing either that doctors will not be fully forthcoming in telling the truth about serious conditions or that their fears may be confirmed.

Another factor in miscommunication is the differing educational and social backgrounds of patient and provider. Traditionally, physicians have been upper-middle-class white males. Their patients, however, reflect a much more heterogeneous group, often of lower SES and from different ethnic and cultural backgrounds. While the provider may think he or she is clearly explaining a problem, the patient may be reading a whole different meaning into the explanation. Research has shown that such misunderstandings are widespread and that patients with the most extensive and complicated health care problems are at greatest risk for misunderstanding their diagnoses, medications, and treatment instructions (Parker, 2000).

Other studies demonstrate that patients often have an incomplete or inaccurate understanding of the causality or seriousness of various medical conditions. One study reported that one in three patients believed their hypertension could be cured by treatment when, in fact, it can be managed only through medication and lifestyle changes (Roth, 1979). One factor in this type of medical misinformation is that health promotion and patient education information has traditionally been written at reading levels at or above the tenth grade. Such material clearly is not accessible to the millions of patients with lower-level reading skills. An obvious solution to this problem is the use of nonwritten materials in health education, using surrogate readers, and—most important—reshaping the health care system so that patients with low literacy levels have access to information.

Patient–provider misunderstandings are also more likely to occur when patients and providers come from different ethnic and cultural backgrounds. This was demonstrated in a recent study of Israeli doctors and Ethiopian immigrant patients that compared patient evaluations of health consultations with evaluations made by their doctors (Reiff, Zakut, & Weingarten, 1999). Physicians rated the health status of these patients and the effectiveness of their consultation significantly higher than did the patients. Low patient–provider agreement occurred mainly for illnesses with stress-related or culture-specific associations. Although immigrant patients who had been in their new homelands longer had somewhat greater agreement with their providers than did more recent immigrants, many continued to report symptoms and concerns that were culturally specific—and completely lost on their new doctors. One implication of this study is that including trained translators who are knowledgeable about the cultural backgrounds of immigrant patients can reduce medical misunderstandings and increase patient satisfaction.

Models of the Patient–Provider Relationship

Nearly half a century ago, Thomas Szasz and M. Hollender (1956) proposed three models of the doctor–patient relationship that parallel the prototypical styles of parent–infant, parent–adolescent, and adult–adult models of communication: *activity-passivity, guidance-cooperation,* and *mutual participation.* The traditional model of this relationship is a paternalistic one in which providers take the active, upper hand, essentially treating patients either as passive infants (activity-passivity) or as adolescents who, although older and more mature, still require a steady, mature hand to direct their health care (guidance-cooperation).

These paternalistic relationships were challenged by the consumer movement of the 1960s and 1970s that promoted a more active role for patients and mutual participation between provider and patients. Patients are becoming more assertive today, insisting that they be heard—and fully informed. They are "well-informed consumers" who insist on playing a more active role in the patient–provider interaction (Haug, 1994). This growing sense of shared responsibility is not universal, however, and is much more typical of health care systems in Western, developed countries. A recent study of Lebanese women's experiences with maternity care found that the vast majority accorded total trust to their physicians and rarely questioned their decisions regarding various procedures. When questioned, the women reported that many aspects of their care were intimidating and unsatisfactory. However, the extent of passivity and feelings of dissatisfaction varied with the participants' SES and the amount of psychosocial support they received throughout the process of childbirth. Higher SES levels and more extensive support were strongly associated with less passivity and greater satisfaction with treatment (Kabakian-Khasholian, Campbell, Shediac-Rizkaliah, & Ghorayeb, 2000).

The quality of the patient–provider relationship often takes a direct toll on health. Patients who are satisfied with their consultation, their provider's communicative style, and the overall patient–provider relationship are more likely to comply with treatment instructions once they return home. This was dramatically revealed in a recent study of adherence among patients with diabetes. Paul Ciechanowski and his University of Washington colleagues attempted to correlate treatment adherence among patients with diabetes with three categories of attachment (Ciechanowski, Katon, Russon, & Walker, 2001). Patients who showed *secure attachment* reported the highest levels of confidence and trust in their physicians. Patients who demonstrated *insecure attachment* reported less confidence and trust in their providers, either because they seemed too busy (*preoccupied attachment*) or simply unresponsive to their patients' needs and concerns (*dismissing attachment*). The results demonstrated that patient–provider attachment categories were useful predictors of compliance. Patients in the dismissing group had worse control of glucose levels than did patients in the secure and preoccupied subgroups. Patients in the dismissing group had even worse control of glucose levels if they rated patient–provider communications as poor. A follow-up study found that patients in the insecurely attached subgroups were less likely to see their primary care provider than those in the securely attached group.

It is easy to dismiss traditional, paternalistic providers as being ineffective and for promoting insecure relationships with their patients. Although many patients welcome their new, more active role in their health care, we must remember that people differ in their abilities and willingness to assume this type of role. It is true that patient lifestyle and adherence to treatment regimens are often determining factors in the outcome of health care treatment and that patients and providers today continue to debate where the responsibility for optimum care lies. However, overemphasis on patient responsibility can have the negative effect of making some patients feel responsible for conditions over which they have little or no control. Even when patients assume a relatively passive role in their relationships with providers, there are many things that providers and patients can do to ensure that their communication is smooth and clear. This is the topic of the next section.

Improving Patient–Provider Communication

Patient–provider relationships are improving for several reasons. Most importantly, health care providers increasingly realize that patients are more likely to follow instructions and respond well to treatment when their knowledge is recognized and incorporated into the treatment regimen. For example, chemotherapy patients often have a better sense of how to minimize the adverse side effects associated with certain medications than will a physician unfamiliar with their particular case. And doctors and patients alike increasingly recognize that lifestyle factors such as diet, smoking, and exercise are major risk factors for both illness and disability. In order to practice good medicine, doctors must treat these risk factors as well as physical symptoms, which requires the patients' cooperation.

In response to the growing awareness of the importance of good patient–provider communication, communication skills training is now regarded as a fundamental component of medical and nursing education. For instance, a 1999 survey of nurse practitioner programs identified the three most important curriculum topics as *primary care, health promotion/disease prevention,* and *effective patient–provider relationships/communication* (Bellack, Graber, O'Neil, Musham, & Lancaster, 1999). Communication training includes a focus on *active listening* skills in which providers echo, restate, and seek to clarify patients' statements to achieve a shared understanding of symptoms, concerns, and treatment expectations. It also includes training in developing good rapport with patients, through appropriate eye contact and other responses designed to acknowledge patients' feelings and to help them talk. In addition, providers receive instruction in how to communicate with patients about sensitive or difficult health topics, as well as in how to give bad news.

Interventions

A number of communication-enhancing interventions have been targeted at patients, especially those about to receive an important consultation. These interventions generally have focused on increasing patients' level of participation, specifically in order to ensure that their concerns are clearly heard and that they leave the consultation with a clear understanding of the information that has been provided (Weinman, 2001).

To help patients who are overly passive, Sheldon Greenfield and Sherrie Kaplan (1985) have developed a program of *assertiveness coaching* for patients waiting to see their physicians. The 20-minute intervention begins with a careful review of the patient's medical record. From this review, a psychologist helps the patient formulate a set of clear questions for the doctor. The psychologist also offers a brief pep talk, in which the patient is reminded that being assertive doesn't mean being aggressive. It means taking an active role and entering the doctor's office with a clear sense of one's goals. It means telling the doctor about feelings, fears, and symptoms without being hindered by embarrassment or anxiety.

Assertiveness coaching can pay huge dividends. By establishing a greater degree of control in their office visits, patients who have been coached obtain more information. Follow-up interviews reveal that 4 months later, they had missed less work, rated their overall health as better, and reported fewer symptoms than control patients who did not receive the assertiveness coaching.

The Internet and the Patient–Provider Relationship

When Julie Remery had a recent bout with the flu, she was coughing so badly one night that her husband Kevin nearly took her to the emergency room at 3 A.M. Instead, he logged onto their HMO's Web site and learned that the over-the-counter antihistamine Julie was taking could actually worsen phlegm and that switching to an expectorant might help. After picking up the recommended medication at a 24-hour pharmacy, he e-mailed his wife's doctor for an appointment the next day.

As this story illustrates, the Internet is becoming a major vehicle for health care. From approximately 7 million users in 1996, the number of people who regularly use the Internet to search for health care information climbed to 25 million in 1999 and had reached 37 million by May 2000 (Kassirer, 2000). Surveys of users indicate that most believe the Internet has made them better consumers of health information. In one survey, nearly half had urged a family member or friend to visit a doctor, changed their exercise or eating habits, or made a treatment decision for themselves as a result of their cyber search (Miller & Reents, cited in Kassirer, 2000). Patients who access authoritative medical information also visit emergency rooms and doctors' offices less frequently, cutting health care costs (Landro, 2001).

Information therapy, as it is sometimes called, may soon become part of every health care provider's training (Kassirer, 2000). Eventually, it is expected that physicians will treat minor health problems such as common low back pain, upper respiratory infections, and urinary infections by e-mail, just as they have previously done by telephone. Using patients' test results from reliable home monitoring equipment, physicians are expected to prescribe and adjust doses of drugs, send laboratory reports, and refer patients to other providers. Health care professionals will offer these services and health care insurers will cover them just as they cover medications, surgery, and other medical procedures.

Some experts caution that the patient–provider relationship may change in the wake of enhanced electronic communication, greater access to health and medical information on-line, and other changes in technology, but not necessarily for the better. For instance, e-mail, which can be an impersonal, mechanical encounter, has become an indispensable form of communication at a time when many consider direct patient–provider interactions to have become too sterile already. E-mail also lacks context, so the multiple clues during a face-to-face consultation are lost with on-line care. A patient's appearance, body language, and tone of voice, for instance, often are important cues used by skilled providers to assess the patient's physical and psychological well-being. If e-mail replaces some face-to-face interactions, providers will be in danger of developing even shallower relationships with their patients.

Hospitalization

When I was admitted to the hospital, I felt I was losing control of my life." These words describe the experiences of many patients who are hospitalized for surgery, radiation or chemotherapy, and other treatments for serious illnesses. Although the word *hospital* comes from the same root as the word *hospitality*, many patients don't find hospitals to be very hospitable places. This is because the psychological well-being of the patient is not a primary goal of modern health care (Friedman, 1992). Rather, its goals are to bring together all the necessary medical staff and equipment to cure people who are seriously ill and, in the process, to maximize efficiency. In fact, surveys from around the world consistently reveal that the single greatest stressor for health care providers is to be behind schedule (Zuger, 1998). And one of the surest ways to provoke physicians into anger is to force them to wait—for a piece of missing equipment, for a patient to fumble through a lengthy list of complaints, or for a needed procedure to be approved by a cost-conscious hospital administrator. For this reason, nearly every aspect of the health care environment, including hospital stays, is subservient to the need to avoid unnecessary delays.

Loss of Control and Depersonalization

Upon entering the hospital, patients feel they are being absorbed by what sociologist Erving Goffman (1961) described as a *total institution* that takes control of virtually every aspect of life. Hospitalized patients are expected to conform submissively to the rules of the hospital, including its schedule for eating, sleeping, and receiving visitors, and to make their bodies available for examination and treatment as their doctor orders. They have little or nothing to say about who can examine them, when examinations can take place, what they can wear, or when they receive their medications. Throughout their hospitalization, patients are expected to remain passive, cooperative, and uninvolved.

Besides loss of control, patients also often suffer from being treated as a nonperson, an insurance number, and a body to be medicated, watched, and managed. Being referred to as "the appendectomy in Room 617" calls attention to the fact that nearly every aspect of a patient's identity—other than his or her reason for being in the hospital—disappears. Sometimes this *depersonalization* is so complete that hospital staff converse among themselves in the patient's presence, ignoring the patient's questions and comments and using medical jargon designed to exclude the patient. Although intended to allow physicians and nurses to telegraph their conversations in order to convey a great deal of information quickly, this type of treatment leaves most patients feeling both helpless and anxious (Bennett & Disbrow, 1993).

In 1999, the average hospital stay was 5.0 days, down from 7.3 days in 1980. An increase in same-day surgery, new drug therapies, and cost-management controls account for the shorter average stay. The rate of hospitalization has also declined. In 1980, 168 of 1,000 Americans were hospitalized. That rate dropped nearly 30 percent to 122 per 1,000 population in 1990 and to 116 per 1,000 in 1999.

—National Center for Health Statistics, 2001

This one-dimensional, depersonalized view of patients is prompted not only by the need for efficiency but also by the need to reduce the daily stress of the hospital environment. The pressures of making decisions that have life-or-death implications for their patients and working in an environment with hazardous chemicals and patients with contagious illnesses may encourage hospital staff to emotionally distance themselves. And when patients do not respond to care, or die, depersonalization may help some to cope.

Factors Affecting Adjustment to Hospitalization

How a patient adjusts to the hospital experience depends on a variety of factors, including the nature of the health problem, the patient's age, the presence of emotional support, and the individual's cognitive style and coping strategies. For example, older adults generally find it easier to cope with chronic illnesses than do adolescents and younger adults, for whom "out of season" illnesses are unexpected and may seem particularly cruel (Holahan & Moos, 1982). Also, patients awaiting surgery who have already faced a similar operation (or undergone some kind of surgery) are generally less anxious than inexperienced patients (Kulik & Mahler, 1993).

Cognitive Style

Hospitalized patients may display a variety of adverse psychological symptoms, particularly if they engage in a self-defeating attempt to assign *blame* for their plight. As we have seen, some people are more likely to feel responsible for what happens to them. Others are more likely to assign responsibility externally—to other people, to bad luck, or simply to fate. Still others do not assign any kind of responsibility. What impact does this cognitive style have on how a patient adjusts to hospitalization? Do people who blame themselves for a serious illness, for example, wallow in guilt or self-hatred that delays their recovery and emotional adjustment? Do people who assign blame externally become bitter and angry, and thereby worsen their own prognosis?

Health psychologists have consistently found that the more patients dwell on assigning blame for their illnesses and other traumatic events—whether to themselves or to others—the more their emotional adjustment suffers (Downey, Silver, & Wortman, 1990). There is some evidence that seeking to blame others is the greater of the two "emotional evils," perhaps because it is harder to "forgive" others (as when injured, for example, by a drunk driver) than to forgive themselves (as when smoking or practicing unsafe sex leads to a serious health condition) (Kiecolt-Glaser & Williams, 1987; Taylor, Lichtman, & Wood, 1984).

Coping Strategies

How well a person adjusts to hospitalization and medical treatment depends on whether the patient tends to rely more on problem-focused or emotion-focused coping. As discussed in Chapter 5, *problem-focused coping* involves efforts that are intended to change some aspect of the stressor, whereas *emotion-focused coping* involves thoughts and actions intended to manage the distressing emotions that arise in the stressful encounter (Lazarus & Folkman, 1984).

People are fairly consistent in how they cope with stress, including the stress of being hospitalized. For some hospital situations, problem-focused coping is highly effective, as when a patient reports rising pain levels and the need for additional medication. In other situations, emotion-focused coping is more appropriate—for example, when a patient believes (rightly or wrongly) that his or her health problem cannot be changed, as when a pelvic fracture forces a patient to remain immobilized in traction.

A number of studies (for example, Altshuler & Ruble, 1989; Kliewer, 1991) have found that how a person appraises his or her ability to control the stressor predicts whether problem-focused or emotion-focused coping will be most adaptive. If control is perceived to be high, the use of problem-focused coping will result in lower psychological distress in children, adolescents, and adults facing a variety of illnesses and other traumatic events (Weisz, McCabe, & Dennig, 1994).

In the majority of situations, though, problem-focused, or active, coping strategies are more adaptive than emotion-focused, or avoidant, coping strategies. For example, the cancer patient who adopts a fighting spirit; who plans a course of action that includes dietary and exercise modifications; and who seeks emotional support from family, friends, and other cancer survivors is generally expected to do better than the patient who avoids thinking about his or her plight. Active coping—information gathering, seeking social support, and cognitive restructuring, for example—has often been linked to better self-esteem and better psychological adjustment in chronically ill adults (Hough, Lewis, & Woods, 1991).

Avoidant coping, on the other hand, is associated with fatalism, denial, helpless coping, and withdrawal from others, all behaviors that have been related to more depressed mood and distress (Hays, Turner, & Coates, 1992; Leserman, Perkins, & Evans, 1992). It is also generally associated with poorer individual adjustment to medical treatment in both children and adults, particularly in patients suffering from hypertension, diabetes, and rheumatoid arthritis (Causey & Dubow, 1992; Manne & Zautra, 1990; Moos, Brennan, Fondacaro, & Moos, 1990). For some medical conditions, however, avoidant coping may be an effective means of reducing the negative impact of a health threat. For example, while waiting for a blood test, patients who distract their thoughts rather than dwelling excessively on the possible discomfort they are about to experience often report lower levels of stress (Kiyak, Vitaliano, & Crinean, 1988). Similarly, avoidant coping through distraction has proven effective during dental surgery (Wong & Kaloupek, 1986).

For more serious conditions, such as cancer or HIV/AIDS, the answer is not a simple one. Some patients cope by actively confronting the situation and seeking up-to-date medical information and social support. Others cope by behaving defensively—for example, by abusing alcohol or other drugs or denying the problems at hand (Hays et al., 1992; Leserman et al., 1992).

In one study, researchers asked pediatric oncology patients, aged 7 through 16 years, and healthy control participants to complete measures of depressive symptoms, trait anxiety, and active and avoidant coping (Phipps & Srivastava, 1997). Oncology patients who scored higher on the use of avoidant-coping strategies such as blunting scored significantly lower on measures of depression and trait anxiety. In a 7-year prospective study of gay men at different stages of HIV/AIDS infection, researchers investigated the relationship between coping strategy and the progression of the disease (Mulder, de Vroome, van Griensven, Antoni, & Sandfort, 1999). The results revealed that avoidant coping predicted a lower rate of decline in several important markers for HIV infection, including the rate of decline of CD4 cell counts (see Chapter 3).

The researchers offer two possible explanations for the slower progression of HIV/AIDS among men who used avoidant coping. For one, because the active copers may have been experiencing more physical symptoms (and therefore had fewer CD4 cells/ml) at the time they completed the coping questionnaire, their deteriorating condition may have provided stronger motivation to take an active approach. Alternatively, it may be that avoidant coping is adaptive at the asymptomatic stage of HIV infection. Trying to avoid or withdraw from difficult situations and focus on other things may be an appropriate way to handle this life-threatening infection at an early stage. At least one other study has found that realistic acceptance during the early stages was associated with a faster progression of HIV/AIDS (Reed, Kemeny, Taylor, Wang, & Visscher, 1994).

In sum, for serious illnesses such as cancer and HIV/AIDS, the most effective coping strategy depends on where in the course of the disease the person is.

How Children Cope with Medical Procedures and Minor Injuries

Richard Lazarus' *three-stage model of coping* (see Chapter 5) has been applied to how children cope with acute events such as injury or an anticipated painful diagnostic test or medical treatment—as opposed to major life events such as death or chronic disease (Lazarus & Launier, 1978). The first stage of this model involves *appraisal* of the stressor, the second stage involves *encounter* with the stressor, and the third stage involves *recovery* from the stressor.

Most studies of how children cope with acute pain have focused on the encounter stage because children rarely appraise potentially harmful situations beforehand—or they would avoid them! In a recent study, 8-year-old boys and girls were asked to role-play four situations, each designed to assess what the children themselves would do and what they would suggest a friend should do when encountering acute pain (Peterson, Crowson, Saldana, & Holdridge, 1999). The situations involved hypothetical medical procedures (an injection or a blood test) and minor injuries (a bruise on the leg or a cut from a piece of glass).

The children's coping responses were coded into three categories: *proactive coping* (imagine you are someplace else doing something fun, take deep breaths, try to relax your muscles); *neutral coping* (sit still, be quiet, do what the nurse says); and *reactive coping* (yell, cry, hit the doctor). As Table 12.1 reveals, children were more likely to suggest reactive coping strategies for themselves and more proactive responses for friends. There were also differences in coping mechanisms for medical procedures and injuries. These results suggest that children are likely to use less effective coping strategies for themselves than they would recommend to a friend when confronting similar stressors. In this regard they are like adults, who recognize adaptive coping techniques such as relaxation and exercise and recommend them to friends, yet often engage in maladaptive coping behaviors such as smoking and the abuse of alcohol.

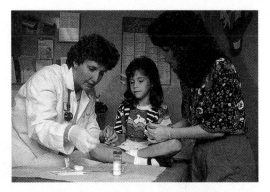

Children and Medical Procedures
In order to get children to undergo difficult or "scary" medical procedures, parents, nurses, and doctors should understand how the child appraises such situations. The parent and nurse here are working together to keep the child calm and focused. © William Campbell/Corbis Sygma

"Good" and "Bad" Patients

Ask any nurse to describe the "ideal patient" and the "patient from hell" and you are certain to receive a ready and consistent answer. In 1975, Judith Lorber identified three basic types of patients from the standpoint of hospital staff. Three out of every four patients are either "good" or "average" patients, in that they conform to the patient role in a passive, unquestioning, and cooperative manner. The difference between a good and an average patient is that average patients frequently have minor complaints that are easily handled and cause hospital personnel few

Table 12.1

Frequency of Children's Coping Responses

Situation	Response[a]		
	Proactive	Neutral	Reactive
Self	62	51	79
Other	105	30	15

[a]Each child can contribute to the analysis more than once.

Source: "Of Needles and Skinned Knees: Children's Coping with Medical Procedures and Minor Injuries for Self and Other," by L. Peterson, J. Crowson, L. Saldana, & S. Holdridge, *Health Psychology*, 1999, *18*(2), pp. 197–200.

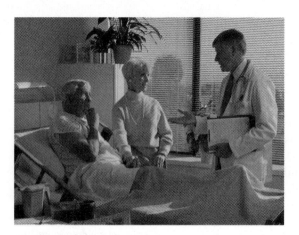

The Good Patient
Patients who adopt the "good patient" role are cooperative, attentive, and well-liked by medical staff. However, the good patient does not have to be passive, afraid to ask relevant questions or requiring physicians and nurses to explain procedures as they occur. © Walter Hodges/Corbis

problems. "Good patients" make even less trouble for hospital staff than average patients, perhaps for fear that complaining will cause the staff to mistreat them. It is no surprise that such patients are well liked by the medical staff.

About one out every four patients, however, is viewed as a "bad patient"—a patient who complains too much, becomes overly emotional, refuses to cooperate, and demands extra attention. The very young and the seriously ill are usually forgiven for being bad. However, those who are bad but not seriously ill are likely to be typecast as troublemakers.

What leads to these different hospital patient roles? One factor appears to be the manner in which a patient responds to the loss of control associated with hospitalization. Some patients are unable to suppress their needs for active involvement in their treatment, exhibiting angry **reactance** to depersonalization and the helplessness of being hospitalized. Reactance is an example of a more general process in which people who are deprived of their freedom become angry and attempt to assert themselves (Brehm, 1966). In contrast, "good patients" are more likely to display helplessness behaviors, characterized by their passivity and unquestioning acceptance.

Which behavior is best for the patient? Research has found that neither good nor bad patient behavior is necessarily adaptive (Taylor, 1979). Although good patients may receive a great deal of attention and be well liked by hospital staff, they may be less likely to try actively to improve their condition. They either ignore or do not report new pains or symptoms because they believe that they are unable to influence their recovery. In either case, they may be delaying their recovery. Similarly, because they feel helpless, they find it difficult to make decisions about their care. Again, they may delay their recovery.

Are "bad" patients any better off? It depends. Patients who respond to hospitalization with angry reactance may experience heightened secretion of stress hormones, which may delay recovery and even lead to other health problems. On the other hand, patients who are appropriately assertive in their medical care obtain numerous benefits, including reduced feelings of depersonalization and helplessness, higher self-esteem, and greater confidence in their treatment.

■ **reactance** the tendency of some patients to respond to the depersonalization and helplessness of hospitalization with anger and efforts to assert themselves

Preparing for Hospitalization

Facing surgery, chemotherapy, and many other invasive procedures is especially daunting for patients because it means confronting their vulnerability and mortality. Surgeons and anesthesiologists have an old saying: "The way a patient enters anesthesia is the way he or she will come out of it."

In other words, patients who approach treatment with an optimistic demeanor, confidence, and a sense of being in control often do better both during and after treatment than do highly anxious people who feel helpless and overwhelmed by the situation. For this reason, psychological interventions are increasingly used to prepare patients for stressful medical procedures.

The most effective interventions are those that increase patients' sense of *control* over their treatment and recovery. Although interventions often overlap in the types of control they emphasize, most can be categorized in terms of one of three types of control.

- *Informational Control*—interventions that focus on the particular procedures and/or physical sensations that accompany a medical treatment.
- *Cognitive Control*—interventions that direct the patient's attention to the positive aspects of a procedure (such as improved health) rather than on feelings of discomfort.
- *Behavioral Control*—interventions that teach techniques for controlling pain and speeding recovery during and after a medical procedure.

Increasing Information Control

One of the first psychologists to study the role of informational control in hospitalized patients was Irving Janis, who in 1958 studied fear levels in patients before and after surgery. Following a presurgery intervention, which involved analysis of patients' feelings, Janis categorized the patients according to the amount of fear, anxiety, and feelings of vulnerability they reported. After the surgery, Janis re-interviewed the patients to learn how well they had understood and followed the presurgery coping information they had received and to assess their postoperative emotional mood. The results showed that patients who displayed moderate levels of fear had the fewest postoperative emotional problems. Janis attributed these results to the realistic manner in which moderately fearful patients approached their operation. Their concern was appropriate to allow them to gather information about the procedure and to develop optimal defenses and coping strategies. Patients who were extremely fearful or nonfearful did not ask questions or gather information to prepare for the procedure, and were thus poorly equipped to cope with the pain or discomfort that followed the procedure. High-fear patients were too focused on their own emotions to process the preparatory information, while patients who initially reported low fears tended to become upset or angry after their surgery.

In a follow-up study, Janis examined the impact of a simple presurgery intervention on the recovery progress of patients. Patients in the intervention group were given information about possible unpleasant symptoms they might experience following surgery. Compared to a control group of patients who were given little information, the patients in the prepared group requested less pain medication, made fewer demands on the hospital staff, and recovered faster than those who received the usual information. They also reported greater satisfaction with their surgeon and hospital staff (Janis, 1958).

Since Janis' pioneering studies, many others have conducted research to determine the type of information that is most helpful to patients. Imagine that you are in the hospital for a minor operation that, although not dangerous, is likely to be followed by a painful recovery. What type of information would you want? Would you want a detailed description of the surgery (procedural information) and/or what you can expect to feel before, during, and after surgery (sensory information)? Sensory information allows you to make an accurate attribution for sensations that you actually do experience. If you are told, for example, that it is customary to feel nauseated for a few days following a particular medical procedure, you will not be surprised when you actually do feel sick to your stomach. More important, armed with accurate information beforehand you will not worry when the symptom appears. Unprepared, however, you might fear that your nausea is a sign that something has gone wrong, that you are not recovering properly. Procedural information, on the other hand, may reduce stress by giving patients an increased sense of control over what their bodies are experiencing. When procedures are expected and predictable, many patients develop greater confidence and become more relaxed.

The results of studies comparing the advantages of procedural and sensory information have been mixed. One reason for the inconsistency in findings is that researchers may define improvement differently. For example, some may use as their criterion the length of the hospital stay while others may use improvements in mobility, muscular strength, and other physical measures related to recovery or requests for pain medication as their standard. In a large-scale meta-analysis, researchers reported that although both procedural and sensory information are beneficial to patients preparing for stressful medical procedures, procedural information appears to help the greatest number of patients. In many instances, of course, providing both types of information produces the maximum benefits (Johnson & Vogele, 1993).

Interestingly, researchers have found that a patient's reaction to procedural or sensory information regarding a stressful medical procedure depends, in part, on his or her style of coping (Shipley, Butt, Horwitz, & Farbry, 1979). As you might expect, sensitizers tend to deal with stressful medical procedures with constant vigilance and anxious monitoring of the cues of discomfort, while repressors deny stress, actively suppress stressful thoughts, and do not appear to be anxious.

Researchers have also discovered that sensitizers welcome as much detailed information as they can get while they are awaiting stressful medical procedures, while repressors prefer to know as little as possible. In one study, women who were about to undergo diagnostic screening for cervical cancer were first classified as sensitizers and repressors on the basis of their self-reported desire for medical information (Miller & Mangan, 1983). Next, half the patients of each type were given extensive preparatory information about the procedures; the others were given minimal information. The patients who experienced the least physical discomfort during the exam (as measured by average heart rate before and after receiving the information and following the exam) were those who received the appropriate amount of information based on their preferences. See the Reality Check on pages 542–543 to determine whether you are a sensitizer or repressor.

Increasing Cognitive Control

Modeling—learning by watching others—is a widely used intervention for increasing cognitive control. In one study, researchers showed dental patients a videotape of a nervous dental patient who reduced his nervousness by learning to relax and communicate more effectively with the dentist (Law, Logan, & Baron, 1994). Patients with a self-reported need for control, who generally felt helpless during dental treatment, had the most beneficial response to the modeling intervention. Compared to control subjects, and those with a lower need for control, these patients reported significantly lower levels of pain, anxiety, and stress.

Another example of a cognitive control intervention is helping patients prepare for a medical procedure by controlling the focus of their attention. In one study, a group of surgical patients was taught to direct their attention away from worries about the discomfort of their upcoming surgery, focusing instead on its potentially positive outcomes (Langer, Janis, & Wolfer, 1975). Other surgical patients were randomly assigned to a comparison group that spent the same amount of time with a psychologist before their operation but focused only on general issues related to hospitalization. Those in the intervention group reported less anxiety and required fewer pain medications. They were also rated by hospital staff as dealing significantly better with their surgery than control patients.

A number of controversial cognitive control interventions incorporate *guided imagery,* in which patients rehearse instructions for mentally influencing the perception of pain, blood flow, immune functioning, and other "involuntary" processes that may influence their recovery. Although traditional Western medicine has considered these processes to be outside voluntary control, the growing body of psychoneuroimmunology research suggests that people can learn to alter them somewhat, and thus improve their chances for a speedy recovery (Pert, Dreher, & Ruff, 1998).

Cognitive control interventions encourage patients to redefine their role—from that of an immobile body being worked on to that of an active participant. Doing so may reap huge health benefits. Consider the effects of a cognitive control intervention on blood loss. Doctors have long been puzzled by the

Reality Check

Taking Charge of Your Health Care

Different people have different preferences for the type of health services they seek. Some want to know every little detail of their condition and treatment, while others prefer to know little or nothing. Some want to be actively involved in choosing specific treatment regimens and caring for themselves, while others want professionals to care completely for them.

Preferred Type of Health Care The following questionnaire asks for your opinions about different kinds of health care. For each of the following statements, decide whether you *agree* or *disagree* and check the column that best fits your opinion. Because each person is different, there are no "right" or "wrong" answers.

Agree   Disagree

___   ___   1. I usually ask the doctor or nurse many questions about what he or she is doing during a medical exam.

___   ___   2. Except for serious illness, it's usually better to take care of your *own* health than to seek professional help.

___   ___   3. I'd rather have doctors and nurses make the decisions about what's best for me than for them to give me a whole lot of choices.

___   ___   4. Instead of waiting for them to tell me, I usually ask the doctor or nurse immediately after an exam about my health.

___   ___   5. It is better to rely on the judgments of doctors (who are experts) than to rely on "common sense" in taking care of your own body.

___   ___   6. Clinics and hospitals are good places to go for help since it's best for medical experts to take responsibility for health care.

___   ___   7. Learning how to cure some of your illness without contacting a physician is a good idea.

___   ___   8. It's almost always better to seek professional help than to try to treat yourself.

___   ___   9. It is better to trust the doctor or nurse in charge of a medical procedure than to question what he or she is doing.

___   ___   10. Learning how to cure some of your illness without contacting a physician may create more harm than good.

___   ___   11. Recovery is usually quicker under the care of a doctor or nurse than when patients take care of themselves.

___   ___   12. If it costs the same, I'd rather have a doctor or nurse give me treatments than do the same treatments myself.

___   ___   13. It is better to rely less on physicians and more on your own common sense when it comes to caring for your body.

___   ___   14. I'd rather be given many choices about what's best for my health than to have the doctor make decisions for me.

___   ___   15. I avoid thinking about my health care until a health care need arises.

___   ___   16. I sometimes fail to pay attention to the instructions I receive from my health care provider.

___   ___   17. I have regular medical exams and have established a relationship with a primary health care provider who knows my health history.

___   ___   18. I make an effort to think about my health care needs and plan ahead to meet those needs.

19. To be honest, I sometimes ignore symptoms for as long as possible in the hope that they will disappear.

20. I lack the means of paying for health care and have not made arrangements in case I need medical services.

21. I sometimes give incomplete information on medical histories due to embarrassment, forgetfulness, or inattention.

22. I pay attention to any changes in my body and bring any symptoms to the attention of my primary health care provider.

23. I really don't know what I would do or where I would go in case of a medical emergency.

24. I often skip regular medical exams because I'm too busy.

25. I always follow my health care provider's instructions as closely as possible.

Scoring: The above statements provide an informal assessment of a person's preferences for more or less active participation and a more or less informed role in health-related decision making. People who prefer a more active, informed role tend to agree with the following statements: 1, 2, 4, 7, 13, 14, 17, 18, and 22.

Sources: Adapted from "Working with Your Doctor," by T. Ferguson. In D. Goleman & J. Gurin (Eds.), *Mind-Body Medicine,* 1996 (pp. 429–450). New York: Consumer Reports Books; *Health in the New Millennium,* by J. S. Nevid, S. A. Rathus, & H. R. Rubenstein, 1998 (pp. 659–660). New York: Worth.

When patients who desire an active role in their health care feel a sense of control over their treatment and know what to do, they generally experience a better outcome. Henry Bennett and Elizabeth Disbrow (1996) have developed a program to teach patients how to actively participate in their treatment. Although the program is geared toward surgical patients, it includes important lessons for anyone who is about to undergo an unpleasant or in other ways anxiety-provoking examination or procedure. Here are some of their suggestions for coaching yourself through such events.

Take the Procedure Seriously If you were about to compete in the Ironman Triathlon, you certainly would be

nervous, but you would prepare in order to ensure your chances of success. Being an active participant in treatment begins by channeling your anxiety into the design of your training plan. Gathering information about the procedures that will be used, what you can expect to feel, and any options you might have will help you approach the procedure with greater confidence.

Instruct Your Body Beforehand Give yourself mental instructions during the days before the procedures, just as an athlete does when "psyching" or visually preparing for a big event. The most direct mind–body approach is a specific instruction that helps you exert some control over physical responses that might affect recovery, such as muscle tension or blood flow. Some patients find it helpful to record their program on an audiotape for later playback.

Respect Your Coping Style Research has shown that patients cope best when their health care provider takes their coping style into consideration. Taking things a step further, you will cope best if you are aware of your own preferred way of coping with stressful situations. Are you a repressor, who prefers not to be overwhelmed with information or asked to make too many decisions? If so, don't worry about asking too many questions because you think it is expected of you. Conversely, if you are a sensitizer, acknowledge your need to feel a sense of control over the situation by asking your physician, nurses, and other staff members for as much information as you feel you need. Good hospitals and clinics are flexible and experienced enough to be able to meet the needs of both types of patients.

Be Assertive. Don't Accept a Treatment You Don't Want Once you know the kind of support that is most comfortable for you, don't wait passively for someone to give it to you. *Ask* for it. If you are not satisfied with a particular recommendation, seek another opinion. Don't feel pressured to blindly accept a medical regimen that doesn't feel right.

Insist on Being Heard Describe your symptoms, complaints, and concerns as fully and clearly as possible. Your health is at stake here, so don't hold back or cover up because of embarrassment or anxiety. By the same token, don't exaggerate your symptoms. If you feel that your provider is not giving you his or her full attention, or is cutting you off too quickly, say something like, "Doctor, if I may just finish. I want to make sure you have the full picture."

Lamaze training natural childbirth preparation designed to prepare prospective parents by enhancing their informational, cognitive, and behavioral control over the procedure

knowledge that two patients who undergo similar surgical procedures often lose very different (and unpredictable) amounts of blood. In a remarkable study, Henry Bennett and his colleagues randomly divided patients about to undergo spinal surgery into three groups for a 15-minute presurgery intervention (Bennett, Benson, & Kuiken, 1986). One group was told only about how the neural functioning of their spinal cords would be monitored during the operations. Another group was also taught how to relax their muscles as they entered anesthesia and again as they were waking up. Those in a third, *blood-shunting*, group were told, in addition to everything the other groups were told, the importance of conserving blood by trying to control their blood flow during surgery. To increase their confidence, they were reminded of how blushing, which reddens the face by increasing blood flow, can be triggered just by being embarrassed. Then they were told that their blood would "shunt" away from the site of surgery during the procedure. Remarkably, patients in the blood-shunting group lost an average of 500 cc less blood than those in either the control group or the relaxation group, where the average amount lost was nearly 1 full liter (900 cc).

Increasing Behavioral Control

Interventions designed to increase patients' behavioral control might include relaxation instructions, breathing exercises, and other techniques to reduce discomfort or speed recovery during or after a stressful medical procedure. Such interventions may provide patients with an even greater sense of control since they focus on actual tools to influence how the patient is feeling (Manyande et al., 1995).

In a classic study, anesthesiologist Larry Egbert and his colleagues at Massachusetts General Hospital told 46 patients awaiting abdominal surgery that they could relieve their postsurgical pain by relaxing the muscles surrounding the site of their incision (Egbert, Battit, Welch, & Bartlett, 1964). They also were given breathing exercises to reduce pain. As Figure 12.5 shows, during the days after their surgery these patients requested lower doses of morphine for pain relief and were discharged earlier than a control group of patients who did not participate in a behavioral control intervention.

Perhaps the most widely used psychological intervention designed to help prepare patients for a medical procedure is **Lamaze training,** which is designed to prepare prospective parents for natural childbirth. At the heart of the Lamaze technique is training that enhances the prospective mother's behavioral control over breathing and the muscles of the uterus, which push the baby out. Delivering mothers who are afraid tend to tighten their muscles, counteracting the natural rhythmic contractions of childbirth, which lengthens labor and makes it more painful.

Natural childbirth has become increasingly popular over the past few decades. In fact, most American obstetricians now recommend natural childbirth classes for prospective parents (Wideman & Singer, 1984). Many parents choose to avoid pain-reducing and tranquilizing drugs that cross the mother's placenta and harm their newborn child. Cross-cultural research reveals that women in cultures in which childbirth is anticipated with less fear and apprehension generally report shorter, less painful deliveries, indicating that inadequate psychological preparation may play a role in the difficulty that some mothers experience during labor.

Interventions aimed at increasing behavioral control are most beneficial for medical procedures in which the patient's participation can assist progress. In delivering a baby, for example, the mother-to-be clearly *can* do something to make things run more smoothly. Conversely, behavioral control interventions may be useless when medical procedures require that the patient remain still and passive. For example, cardiac catheterization and dental surgery both require that patients be inactive. There is little that the patient can do to make the procedures more pleasant or to assist the health care providers.

In summary, nearly any medical procedure can make a patient anxious, and undergoing surgery can be especially stressful. But research indicates that the more patients know about what to do and expect before, during, and after surgery, the more likely it is that the surgery will go smoothly and recovery will be rapid.

Figure 12.5

Emotional Support and Pain Medication
In this classic study of abdominal surgery patients, those who received encouragement, instruction in breathing exercises to control pain, and information about what they could expect to feel after the operation required less pain medication (morphine) in the days afterward.

Source: "Reduction of Postoperative Pain by Encouragement and Instruction of Patients: A Study of Doctor-Patient Rapport," by L. D. Egbert, C. Battit, E. Welch, and M. K. Bartlett, *New England Journal of Medicine*, 1964, *270*, 825–827.

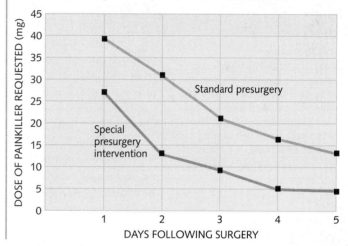

The Role of Health Psychology in Health Care Settings

The past several decades have seen promising developments in the field of psychological preparation of patients for medical procedures. Prior to 1975, the vast majority of interventions reflected the general belief that preparation should focus primarily on providing patients with procedural information and establishing trust between the medical staff and the patient (Vernon, Foley, Sipowicz, & Schulman, 1971). In the mid-1970s, however, the

Cancer patients at Delaware County Memorial Hospital in Drexel Hill, Pennsylvania, are offered an integrative approach to care. It includes an 8-week class that teaches mindfulness meditation and cognitive-behavioral strategies to reduce stress. Patients can also take advantage of a massage therapist and a free weekly yoga class. The psychologists may employ hypnosis to help people harness the strengths of the mind over the body's pain.
—(O'Connor, 2001)

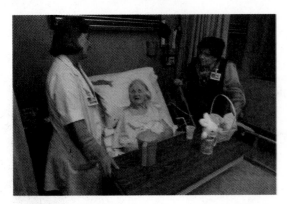

Collaborative Care
Today, the health care system is increasingly focused on collaborative care, the combined efforts of physicians, psychologists, and other health care people, such as this social worker talking with a nurse and her patient. © Mitch Wojnarowicz / The Image Works

■ **collaborative care** a cooperative form of health care in which physicians, psychologists, and other health care providers join forces to improve patient care

focus shifted toward greater use of modeling (e.g., Melamed & Siegel, 1975) and other procedures for teaching effective coping strategies (Zastowny, Kirschenbaum, & Meng, 1986). By the early 1980s, there was consensus that effective preparation should include the teaching of coping skills and patient involvement (Elkins & Roberts, 1983).

The important role of psychologists in improving physical health through enhancing treatment outcomes has now been firmly established. This has led to a significant increase in the number of psychologists working in general health care settings (Groth-Marnat & Edkins, 1996; Sweet, Rozensky, & Tovian, 1991). In fact, a growing number of medical residency programs are encouraging greater use of **collaborative care**, in which physicians, psychologists, and other health care providers join forces to improve patient care (Daw, 2001). Effective July 1, 2001, the Accreditation Council for Graduate Medical Education (ACGME) required that resident physicians in all specialties be taught to work with other professionals in order to provide the best and most cost-efficient patient care. The new guidelines also require that new physicians must be knowledgeable in the epidemiological and social-behavioral sciences and be able to apply this knowledge to patient care. Conversely, psychologists are increasingly being required to learn primary care so that both sides of the partnership know and understand the other's work.

If health psychology has one fundamental message regarding optimum health care, it is that health care is not achieved through defining the separate responsibilities of patients and health care providers, but through their harmonious interaction. In this era of managed care and mutual participation between patients and providers, each of us is being encouraged to assume a more active role in our health. Health psychology informs our understanding of this role through a growing body of research findings on sociocultural factors in illness behavior, patient–provider relationships, and styles of coping with health care treatment and hospitalization.

Summing Up

Illness Behavior

1. Detecting physical symptoms, interpreting their medical significance, and making the decision to seek health care (*illness behavior*) are each strongly influenced by psychological processes, including the individual's past experience, personality, culture, and gender, as well as by the individual's focus of attention and tendency to either monitor or repress health threats.

2. People who have a strong internal focus detect and report symptoms more quickly than people who are more externally focused. Sensitizers tend to monitor their

health more closely than do repressors. Consequently, repressors are more likely to cope with distressing medical symptoms by distancing themselves from unpleasant information.

3. Illness representations regarding the type of disease, its causes, time frame, consequences, and controllability also influence how people react to physical symptoms and whether they seek medical attention.

Sick Role Behavior

4. Social and demographic variables, such as prior experience, expectations, cultural norms, age, gender, and socioeconomic status, also influence both illness behavior and the steps a person takes once an illness has been diagnosed (sick role behavior).

Seeking Treatment

5. Health services may be underused or overused. Delay behavior may result from a failure to notice symptoms (appraisal delay), refusal to believe one is actually sick (illness delay) or needs professional help (behavioral delay), and so does not make an appointment (scheduling delay), or the belief that the benefits of seeking treatment are not worth the costs (treatment delay).

6. Some people may use health services when there is no real need because they are feigning illness (malingering) or falsely believe they have a disease when they do not (hypochondriasis). In others, bodily symptoms are an expression of emotional stress (somatization).

The Health Care System

7. There are many types of hospitals, each catering to particular health needs. Among these are extended care facilities, rehabilitation centers, psychiatric hospitals, and hospices.

8. As medical costs have risen, the health care system has undergone many changes. Among these is the advent of walk-in clinics and home help services, health maintenance organizations, preferred provider organizations, and other forms of managed care. One concern about managed care is that medical decision making is being taken out of the hands of physicians and shifted to insurance companies. Another concern is that managed care may not be of the same quality as that provided by private physicians.

The Patient–Provider Relationship

9. The relationship between health care provider and patient is the backbone of all medical treatment. The central elements of this relationship are continuity of care, communication, and the overall quality of consultations. Poor communication between health care providers and patients is common, given the time pressures of health care and the fact that providers generally are not chosen for medical training based on their social or communicative skills but on their technical expertise. Other factors in miscommunication include the attitudes and beliefs patients and providers have regarding their roles, as well as gender, cultural, and educational differences between providers and patients.

10. The traditional model of the patient–provider relationship is a paternalistic one in which providers take an active, upper hand, treating patients who essentially remain passive. This model was challenged by the consumer movement of the 1960s and 1970s that promoted a more active role for patients and mutual participation between provider and patients. The patient–provider relationship is important because patients who are satisfied with their provider's communicative style and with the overall quality of their relationship with their provider are more likely to comply with treatment instructions once they return home.

11. Communication skills training is now regarded as a fundamental component of medical and nursing education. Some experts worry, however, that the patient–provider relationship may change, but not necessarily for the better, in the wake of enhanced electronic communication, greater access to Internet health and medical information, and other changes in technology.

Hospitalization

12. One of the most persistent problems of hospitals is the depersonalization of patients as a result of a need for efficiency and the need of hospital staff to emotionally distance themselves from those who are very sick or dying.

13. How a patient adjusts to being hospitalized depends on a variety of factors, including the nature of the health problem being treated, the patient's age, the presence of emotional support, and the individual's cognitive style and coping strategies.

14. Although avoidant coping generally is associated with poor adjustment to most medical conditions, it may be helpful for situations such as waiting for a blood test or dental surgery, when distraction from excessive thinking about discomfort may reduce stress.

15. When a medical condition is perceived as being controllable, problem-focused coping is generally most beneficial. However, for uncontrollable conditions, such as when a parent is being treated for a chronic illness, emotion-focused coping is common.

16. Research studies reveal that children, like adults, often use less effective coping strategies for themselves than they would recommend to a friend when confronting similar stressors.

17. The so-called good patient enters the hospital thinking that the sick role involves passively accepting all facets of treatment. Conversely, "bad patients" are less cooperative and may display angry reactance in response to depersonalization and the helplessness of being hospitalized. Carried to an extreme, each of these patient roles may have negative health consequences.

Preparing for Hospitalization

18. Psychological interventions designed to restore or enhance control often improve adjustment to hospitalization and to stressful medical procedures. The benefits of preparatory information, relaxation training, modeling, and guided imagery training have all been documented.

Key Terms and Concepts

illness behavior, p. 504
sick role behavior, p. 504
attentional focus, p. 505
sensitizers, p. 505
repressors, p. 506

illness representation, p. 507
comorbidity, p. 508
lay referral system, p. 514
delay behavior, p. 516
hypochondriasis, p. 517

malingering, p. 517
secondary gains, p. 517
chronic fatigue syndrome, (CFS) p. 518
hysterical epidemic, p. 518

somatization, p. 519
managed care, p. 523
reactance, p. 538
Lamaze training, p. 544
collaborative care, p. 546

Health Psychology on the World Wide Web

Web Address	Description
http://www.ncqa.org	Web site of the National Committee for Quality Assurance (NCQA), which evaluates and accredits managed health care programs.
http://www.ahcpr.gov	The Agency for Health Care Research and Quality (AHRQ)—a government clearinghouse responsible for monitoring health care in the United States. The site also provides practical health care information, research findings, and data to help consumers, health care providers, insurers, researchers, and policymakers make informed decisions about health care issues.
http://nhic-nt.health.org	The National Health Information Center (NHIC)—a health information referral service. NHIC puts health professionals and consumers who have health questions in touch with those organizations that are best able to provide answers. NHIC was established in 1979 by the U.S. Department of Health and Human Services.

http://www.omhrc.gov

The Office of Minority Health Resource Center serves as a national resource and referral service on minority health issues by collecting and distributing information on a wide variety of health topics, including substance abuse, cancer, and heart disease.

Critical Thinking Exercise

Selecting a Health Care Plan

Now that you have read and reviewed Chapter 12, take your learning a step further by testing your critical thinking skills on the following practical problem-solving exercise.

Choosing a health care plan has a number of important consequences. Unfortunately, many people have little or no influence when it comes to selecting their health care. The plan offered by your college or employer is often the only "game in town," unless you are willing to research other plans on your own and, in most cases, pay higher insurance premiums.

To help prepare you to make an informed choice of health care services, gather information on at least two health care plans (including the one that currently provides your coverage, if appropriate). Then prepare answers to the following questions:

1. How much does coverage cost? Be thorough in totaling all typical charges, including regular insurance premiums, deductibles, charges for physician visits, prescription costs, and any other out-of-pocket expenses.

2. How much are costs likely to rise over the years? What is the plan's history of premium rate increases?

3. How much would you have to pay for hospitalization should you need major surgery? Are there annual or lifetime caps on some costs?

4. What services are covered under the plan? While all plans cover basic health care, some also cover dental care, mental health care, vision testing and eyeglasses, maternity benefits, and preventive care. Does the plan provide the kinds of coverage you think you will need?

5. Does the health care plan permit you to choose your own doctor, or are you limited to choosing from those on an approved list of physicians? What about referrals to specialists? Who decides whether a specialist's services will be covered and where you can go? If you choose to seek a second opinion or use a specialist who is not on the list, what additional charges will you have to pay?

13

Managing Pain

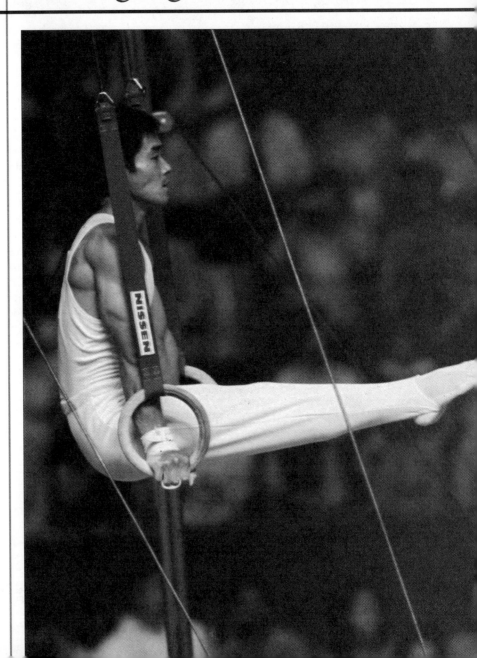

A grainy photograph from the 1976 summer Olympics shows six proud Japanese gymnasts during the gold medal ceremony. Second from the right stands a small, muscular man with a medal around his neck and an expression of triumph on his face. Unlike his four teammates, who stand rigidly at attention as their national anthem is being played, the man stands with his right leg slightly bent—as if he might be in pain. The man is Japanese gymnast Shun Fujimoto.

During the 1932 Los Angeles Olympic Games the Japanese gymnastics team finished dead last—a humiliating defeat that triggered a national mission to become an international gymnastic power. When the games resumed following World War II, the mission was finally fulfilled as the Japanese team won the gold medal in four consecutive Olympics: Rome, Tokyo, Mexico City, and Munich. However, going after their fifth straight title at the 1976 Montreal games the team appeared to be headed for defeat when Fujimoto, their star competitor, broke his kneecap while performing the floor exercise.

Blessed with incredible strength and a nearly perfect gymnastic physique, Fujimoto was a fierce competitor and team leader whose buoyant spirit and national pride had rallied his teammates many times in previous competitions.

But how could he continue? Although Olympic rules prohibited him from taking a painkiller, Fujimoto decided to stay in the competition and try to endure excruciating pain. "I did not want to worry my teammates," he recalled. "The competition was so close I didn't want them to lose their concentration with worry about me."

Fortunately, the next apparatus was the pommel horse—an event in which the knees are mostly locked in place. Unless he fell, the pain might be tolerable. Without notifying his coaches or teammates of his injury, Fujimoto completed a nearly flawless performance, receiving a score of 9.5 out of a possible 10.

The final event, however, would be more much more demanding. The high rings tests arm strength, but vital points can also be lost during the dismount, when the gymnast descends from a great height after a swinging routine that propels him or her into the mat at high velocity. "I knew when I descended from the rings, it would be the most painful moment," Fujimoto remembered. "I also knew that if my posture was not good when I landed I would not receive a good score. I must try to forget the pain."

After another nearly perfect routine, Fujimoto landed, smiled for the judges, held his position for the required amount of time, before his injured leg buckled beneath him. Incredibly, he received a score of 9.7, enough to propel his team to victory.

clinical pain pain that requires some form of medical treatment

Biological, psychological, and social factors contributed to Fujimoto's development as a gymnast, and those same factors played a role in his triumphant Olympic victory. The story also makes clear one of health psychology's most fundamental themes: that the mind and body are inextricably intertwined. Fujimoto's determination not to let his teammates down allowed him to overcome a painful injury, which, in other circumstances, would most certainly have been crippling.

The struggle to understand pain—what causes it and how to control it—is a central topic in health psychology. Until recently, however, researchers knew next to nothing about this common, yet extraordinarily complex phenomenon. Moreover, medical schools did not spend much time covering the topic of pain. Over the past three decades, health psychologists have made considerable progress in filling in the gaps. In this chapter we discuss the components of pain; the ways in which it is experienced; how it is measured; and the biological, psychological, and social factors that influence the experience of pain. And we will take a look at how pain is treated within medicine and in the latest multidimensional interventions introduced by health psychology.

What Is Pain?

Few topics in health psychology are as elusive as pain. Pain is obviously a physical sensation—when we fall and scrape a knee, we feel a stinging sensation that has real, physical substance. Yet the pain of losing a loved one or ending a long-term relationship is more psychological than physical in nature, although often just as real. And sometimes pain is not altogether unpleasant. After a hard workout on the track, for example, I often feel a deep muscular fatigue that is most definitely physical, yet almost pleasant. This chapter focuses on **clinical pain,** that is, pain that requires some form of medical treatment. Let's begin by considering how many of us suffer pain and how often.

Epidemiology of Pain

Few people manage to get through life without experiencing pain now and then. Several major epidemiological studies reveal just how common pain is. One massive study reported that 82 percent of New Zealanders had experienced significant pain in one or more sites, with the majority reporting more than one life-disrupting pain episode. Women reported more pain than men did, and the prevalence of pain increased with age (James, Large, Bushnell, & Wells, 1991).

Most people experience an average of three to four different kinds of pain each year. According to the *Mayday PainLink Report* (2000), 40 million Americans suffer from long-lasting pain caused by lower back problems, arthritis, cancer, repetitive stress injuries, migraine headaches, and other conditions. Moreover, pain is the most common reason that people seek medical treatment. According to the same report, 17 percent of all people suffer from long-lasting pain, and 75 percent of these had sought medical treatment during the past year.

Pain obviously has devastating effects on individuals; it also has a high social cost. One national survey revealed that more than 550 million workdays are lost each year because of long-lasting pain (Turk & Nash, 1996). People spend millions of dollars each year on medications to help them cope with pain caused by headaches, muscle strains, colds, and influenza. Add to this the costs of surgery, hospitalization, disability compensation, and lost income, and the annual costs of long-lasting pain may reach as high as $100 billion. No other class of health problems even approaches this level of impact.

Components of Pain

Perhaps more so than any other everyday experience, pain clearly illustrates the biopsychosocial (mind–body) model. This model distinguishes among the biological mechanisms by which painful stimuli are processed by the body: the subjective, emotional experience of pain; and the social and behavioral factors that help shape our response to pain (Fordyce, 1988).

Let's consider a specific example to illustrate how these components come together to create the experience of pain when you strike your thumb with a hammer. First, you have the physical sensation of pain—an immediate, sharp stab of pain as your grip on the hammer slips and you strike your thumb. Next, you become angry and frustrated with your clumsiness and, depending on the severity of your injury, your loss in dexterity. If the pain persists, behavior changes may occur. You may avoid using your aching hand. Your hand becomes weak from inactivity, and you may begin to depend on others for assistance.

Thus, *pain* involves our total experience in reacting to an unpleasant event, an experience shaped by biological, psychological, and sociobehavioral forces, which, in turn, reflect our genetic legacy, previous experiences, personality, and coping resources (Kroner-Herwig et al., 1996).

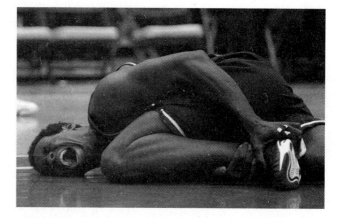

Components of Pain
Pain obviously has a strong physical component, as the face of Chris Webber of the Sacramento Kings clearly reveals. It also has emotional and psychological components; because the shot that landed him on his ankle won the game for his team, Chris's pain is probably somewhat more bearable, as the joy of winning overshadows the pain. © AFP/Corbis

acute pain sharp, stinging pain that is short-lived and usually related to tissue damage

Significance and Types of Pain

Despite the discomfort and stress it can cause, pain is essential to our survival. Stick your toe into hot bath water, and the stinging sensation causes you to immediately jerk your foot out of the water. A nagging pain that radiates down your arm prompts a visit to your doctor to rule out possible cardiovascular disease. Thus, although pain can be excruciating, it is also highly adaptive. Along with your pulse rate, blood pressure, and body temperature, pain is a vital sign that reveals a great deal about your body. Pain sounds a warning that something's wrong and alerts you to try to prevent further physical damage.

Not feeling pain is hazardous to your health. Actor-director Christopher Reeve can't feel pain below his neck, which poses many dangers. Reeve (like other quadriplegics) can't feel the numbing pain that may signal that he needs to shift the position of his arms to improve blood flow or that a spot on his back is being rubbed raw by his wheelchair. He doesn't feel the pain of a stomachache or the gripping pain of a muscle cramp in his toes. That's why, every day, he relies on others to exercise his muscles, check his skin, and perform many other checks to keep him healthy and safe (Farrington, 1999).

The adaptive value of pain is also illustrated by the unlucky few who are born with *congenital insensitivity to pain,* a genetic disorder that makes them almost completely insensitive to pain (Brand & Yancey, 1994). Although they are able to distinguish other tactile sensations, including temperature and pressure, pain is simply not in their realm of experience. Children born with this disorder have no motivation to steer clear of hot stoves or sharp objects and often, susceptible to accidents, do not live to adulthood.

Types of Pain

In general, researchers divide pain into two broad categories: acute pain and chronic pain. **Acute pain** is sharp, stinging pain that is usually localized in an injured area of the body. Although acute pain can last from a few seconds to several months, it generally subsides as normal healing occurs. Examples include a burn, a fracture, an overused muscle, or pain after surgery. Another type of acute pain is *acute recurrent pain,* in which episodes of discomfort are interspersed with periods in which the individual is relatively pain-free. Periodic migraine headaches are of this type.

Sometimes, however, acute pain doesn't go away. Frances Keefe (1982) has suggested that when acute pain persists beyond the time of normal healing, people enter a *prechronic stage.* According to Keefe, this time is critical because it determines whether the sufferer actually overcomes the pain or develops a sense of helplessness that may lead to a lifelong battle with pain. In such cases, pain no longer serves a useful biological purpose as a warning signal. Instead, the pain itself is the problem and has become a health-damaging force (Bonica, 1990). This is the case for the millions who suffer some degree of chronic pain that has no detectable organic cause (or an organic cause inconsistent with the magnitude of the pain reported) and that has endured past a 3-month point of healing (Grant & Haverkamp, 1995).

Chronic pain may be continuous or intermittent, moderate or severe in intensity, and felt in just about any of the body's tissues. At least two types have been differentiated (Turk, 2001). *Chronic noncancer pain* is always present (chronic) but does not respond to treatment and is not life-threatening—for example, nagging lower back pain. In contrast, *pain associated with a malignant disease process* (such as that associated with cancer and rheumatoid arthritis) becomes more severe as the underlying medical condition worsens.

Chronic pain lowers the person's overall quality of life and increases his or her vulnerability to infection and thus a host of diseases. Pain also can cause other physical problems, such as when the pain of a headache leads to stomach upset.

Chronic pain can also take a devastating psychological toll, triggering lowered self-esteem, insomnia, anger, hopelessness, and many other signs of distress. Compared with acute pain patients, those with chronic lower back pain tend also to have higher rates of depression and personality disorders and are more likely to abuse alcohol and other drugs (Brewer & Karoly, 1992; Kinney, Gatchel, Polatin, Fogarty, & Mayer, 1993).

Hyperalgesia

Another challenge faced by those with chronic pain is that they may become even more sensitive to pain, a condition known as **hyperalgesia.** Hyperalgesia also happens when people are sick or injured, and may facilitate recovery by stimulating recuperative behaviors such as getting extra rest and following a healthy diet. The general body weakness and aches you get when you have the flu make up one example of this process.

Hundreds of experiments over more than 100 years have confirmed that hyperalgesia often occurs as a normal adaptation during sickness. In one study, rats that received injections of a drug that made them sick exhibited a significantly stronger behavioral response to a painful stimulus than did control rats (Wiertelak et al., 1994). In humans, most kinds of internal pain, from mild indigestion to the agony of certain kidney disorders, are accompanied by increased sensitivity in nearby tissues. In the 1890s, physiologists Henry Head and Mames MacKensie observed this phenomenon and proposed that signals from diseased parts of the body set up an "irritable focus" in the central nervous system that creates areas of enhanced pain sensitivity in nearby body parts. The fact that the increased sensitivity to pain occurs in otherwise healthy tissues strongly suggests that the signals originate in the central nervous system (Cervero, 2000).

■ **chronic pain** dull, burning pain that is long lasting

■ **hyperalgesia** a condition in which a chronic pain sufferer becomes more sensitive to pain over time

Measuring Pain

Because of its multidimensional and subjective nature, pain is not easily measured. Nevertheless, clinicians and researchers have developed a number of means of assessing pain: *psychophysiological measures, behavioral measures,* and *self-report measures.*

Psychophysiological Measures

There are no objective measures of pain, only subjective ones (Skevington, 1995). Not that clinicians and researchers haven't tried to find them. In fact, the problem of measuring pain set the stage for the very earliest *psychophysical studies* in the new field of psychology. These studies highlight the familiar *mind–body* (*psyche,* meaning mind; *physike,* meaning body) *problem:* How does conscious awareness derive from, and equate to, the physical sensations of the body?

One way to assess pain is to measure the specific physiological changes that accompany pain. For example, *electromyography (EMG)* assesses the amount of muscle tension experienced by patients suffering from headaches or lower back pain. Unfortunately, there have been no consistent results to suggest that the level of muscle tension accurately predicts pain (Chapman, 1984). Researchers have also carefully recorded changes in heart rate, breathing rate, blood pressure, skin temperature, and skin conductance, all indicators of *autonomic arousal* (see Chapter 3). Once again, however, the measures have generally not provided any consistent differences between people with and those without a specific type of pain such as a headache (Andrasik et al., 1982). Their failure may well be because pain is only one of many factors that contribute to autonomic changes; others include diet, attention, activity level, stress, and the presence of illness.

Behavioral Measures

Another way to measure pain is to look for signs of it in a patient's behavior. This can be done by relatives and friends of the patient or by health care professionals in structured clinical sessions.

Wilbert Fordyce (1976), a pioneer in pain research, has developed a pain behavior-training program. The researcher first asks the observer—say, the pain sufferer's roommate—to list five to ten behaviors that frequently signal the onset of a pain episode. For example, the observer might tally the amount of time the person spends in bed during an average day, the number of verbal complaints, or the number of requests for painkillers.

In clinical settings, nurses and other health professionals are trained to systematically observe patients' pain behaviors during routine care procedures. One frequently used pain inventory is the *Pain Behavior Scale,* which consists of a series of target behaviors, including vocal complaints, facial grimaces, awkward postures, and mobility (Feuerstein & Beattie, 1995). The patient is asked to perform various activities, such as walking across the room, touching the toes, and picking up an object from the floor while the observer rates the occurrence of each target behavior on a 3-point scale: "frequent," "occasional," and "none" (Ohlund et al., 1994).

Self-Report Measures

The most frequently used measures of pain are based on the patient's verbal or written report of his or her pain. Self-report measures can take one of three forms: *structured interviews* with a doctor or therapist; *rating scales* on which patients assign numerical values to various aspects of their pain; and *standardized pain inventories,* which assess several different dimensions of pain.

Structured Interviews

When a patient seeks treatment for pain, the health professional generally begins with a brief structured interview, which usually centers on such topics as

- When the pain started and precipitating event(s).
- How the pain has progressed and what treatments have been tried, including medications, surgeries, chiropractic, and acupuncture.
- What activities increase or decrease the pain.
- Changes in activity because of pain, including recreational activities, social activities, employment, and family responsibilities.
- How the patient responds to other people when pain is at its worst.
- How others, such as family members, react when the patient shows that he or she is in pain.

This information can provide the health professional with a clearer sense of the patient's coping resources, the overall impact of pain on the quality of his or her life, and what is needed for an effective intervention (Feuerstein & Beattie, 1995).

Pain Rating Scales

The simplest way to measure pain is to have patients fill out a questionnaire, assigning a numerical value to indicate their discomfort in a given situation. Pain rating scales may also be based on verbal report, in which the person chooses from a list the word that most accurately describes the pain. Rating scales are so easy to use that they are the preferred means of assessing pain in young children. The numerical scales also seem to be used in verbal reports.

Many clinicians also find it useful to have patients keep a *pain diary* in which they rate pain episodes over a period of time, along with daily events, medications, and so forth. Pain diaries paint a more accurate picture of an individual's pain than an isolated measurement because they reveal how constant the pain is, whether it follows a pattern, and how it is affected by various activities (Jensen & McFarland, 1993). However, pain diaries may not be appropriate for some patients because they may focus even more attention on the pain and thus interfere with treatment and recovery.

Pain Inventories

Some years ago, pain research pioneer Ronald Melzack developed a system for categorizing pain along three dimensions (Melzack & Torgerson, 1971). The first dimension, *sensory quality,* highlighted the tremendous variations that occur in the sensation of pain—it can be stabbing, burning, throbbing, or dull, to list only a few possibilities. The second dimension, *affective quality,* focuses on the many different emotional reactions that pain can trigger, such as irritation, fear, or anger. The final dimension is *evaluative quality,* which refers to the sufferer's judgment of the severity of the pain as well as its meaning, or significance. From this multidimensional model of pain Melzack derived the McGill Pain Questionnaire (MPQ), which has become the most widely used pain inventory today (Bradley, 1993).

Although the MPQ is most often used as an overall measure of discomfort, it is also helpful in identifying whether a patient tends to use sensory, affective, or cognitive labels to describe his or her discomfort. For example, people tend to use such terms as "throbbing" to describe the sensory dimension of pain and "tiring" to describe the affective dimension.

The MPQ reliably differentiates a number of pain syndromes. People suffering from headaches, for example, tend to choose the same pattern of words to describe their pain, while those suffering from lower back pain choose a different pattern (Melzack & Wall, 1988). However, the MPQ has been criticized for requiring subjects to make fine distinctions among very similar words. What, for example, is the difference between "beating" and "pounding" pain? The MPQ is also of limited usefulness for people for whom English is not the primary language, as well as for children under 12 years of age (Karoly, 1988).

Measuring the Fear of Pain

Chronic pain is what patients report fearing most about illness, even though many serious conditions, such as cancer in its early stages, may cause little or no pain. So controlling is pain that the fear of suffering is more stressful to many patients than the prospect of losing a limb or dying. By a huge margin, seeking relief from pain is the number one reason for requests for assisted suicide or euthanasia (Cherny, 1996).

For some patients, overwhelming fear becomes a major obstacle to treatment and recovery. To help clinicians identify such individuals, researchers have developed the Pain Anxiety Symptoms Scale (PASS), a 40-item questionnaire that measures fear of pain rather than pain itself (McCracken, Zayfert, & Gross, 1992). Using information from a patient's responses, the clinician is in a better position to develop an individualized treatment regimen that might include stress management, relaxation training, or other techniques to help reduce the patient's fear of pain.

■ **free nerve endings** sensory receptors found throughout the body that respond to temperature, pressure, and painful stimuli

The Physiology of Pain

As you slip on the icy sidewalk, you fall hard on your elbow. In the instant before you feel the pain, a cascade of biochemical and electrical reactions occurs. All sensory information, including pain, begins when *sensory receptors* on or near the surface of the body convert a physical stimulus—such as the pressure of striking the ground—into neural impulses. As the pressure of striking the ground activates the receptors in the skin covering your elbow, they stimulate neurons in the peripheral nervous system that relay the message to your brain. Only when the brain registers and interprets this neural input is pain experienced. What happens in between the stimulation of sensory receptors and the brain's interpretation is the subject of a great deal of exciting new research.

Pain Pathways

Unlike our other senses, pain is not triggered by only one type of stimulus—nor does it have a single type of receptor. Tissue injury isn't the only thing that will produce pain. The corneas of your eyes, for instance, are exquisitely sensitive. Almost any stimulus, from a speck of dust in the eye to the application of a bit too much pressure when inserting a contact lens, will be experienced as pain, even though the cornea suffers no damage. All of these stimuli trigger the pain response in the brain through different receptors.

Pain Receptors

The simplest sensory receptors for pain are the **free nerve endings.** They are found throughout the body, in the skin as well as in muscles (contributing to muscle cramps), the internal organs of the viscera (stomachaches), membranes that surround joints and bones (arthritic pain), and even the pulp of teeth (toothaches).

Although free nerve endings are the simplest sensory receptors, they are also the most poorly understood. What we do know is that they respond primarily to temperature change and pressure. They also respond to certain chemicals secreted in damaged body tissues. However they are aroused into

nociceptor (no-chi-SEP-tur) a specialized neuron that responds to painful stimuli

fast nerve fibers large, myelinated nerve fibers that transmit sharp, stinging pain

slow nerve fibers small, unmyelinated nerve fibers that carry dull, aching pain

action, it appears that free nerve endings begin a process that ends when the brain registers and interprets the sensation as pain. It is important to note, however, that free nerve endings *contribute to* rather than *create* the pain experience and that they are but one aspect of the complex process that is pain. For this reason, researchers refer to free nerve endings that are activated by noxious (painful) stimuli as **nociceptors.**

Another reason free nerve endings are not true pain receptors is that psychological factors such as whether we are paying attention to pain, our emotional state, and how we interpret a situation can affect whether pain is experienced. For example, during the excitement of the Olympics, Shun Fujimoto, whose knee injury we described at the beginning of the chapter, continued to compete without pain. Only after the competition, when his attention was not distracted, did he report discomfort. As another example, patients suffering from a variety of injuries and illnesses often report that their pain is strongest when they are feeling depressed and hopeless (Turk & Nash, 1996). When their emotions rebound, their pain is reduced.

Fast and Slow Fibers

The pain process begins when neural signals from free nerve endings are routed to the central nervous system via **fast nerve fibers** and **slow nerve fibers**. *Fast nerve fibers* are relatively large, myelinated neurons that conduct neural impulses at about 15 to 30 meters per second (myelin is the fatty coating on the axons of some neurons that increases the speed of neural transmission). *Slow nerve fibers* are smaller, unmyelinated fibers that conduct electrical impulses at about 0.5 to 2 meters per second.

The fast and slow fibers are the messengers for two pain systems in the brain: a *fast pain system* and a *slow pain system.* The fast pain system (involving the fast nerve fibers) appears to serve only the skin and mucus membranes; the slow pain system (involving the slow nerve fibers) serves all body tissues except the brain itself, which does not experience pain (Thompson, 2000). The fast pain system carries pain that is perceived as stinging and localized in one area, while slow nerve fibers signal dull, aching pain that is generalized throughout the body.

Strong mechanical pressure or extreme temperatures normally stimulate fast nerve fibers, while slow nerve fibers are typically activated by chemical changes that occur in damaged body tissues. These chemical changes lower the thresholds of both types of nerves, making them more responsive to further stimulation. This is why even the lightest touch on an injured area of skin can be extremely painful.

To get a feeling for the practical differences in the speed of the two pain systems, consider that slow fibers relaying a painful message from your foot could take as long as 2 seconds to reach the brain. In contrast, the faster fibers relay their messages up to 100 times faster. This explains a familiar experience.

Sticking your toe in unbearably hot bath water will stimulate the fast pain fibers, producing an immediate sharp pain. As we noted in Chapter 3, the message is carried from the skin to the spinal cord, where it is passed via a single interneuron to motor neurons that cause you to jerk your toe out of the water. But this highly adaptive *spinal reflex* is completed well before you experience the deeper, dull pain that really hurts. The uncomfortable delay you spend waiting once you're out of the bath for the pain to hit occurs because the slow pain system lags behind in getting its message to your brain.

After leaving the skin, the sensory fibers of the fast and slow pain systems group together as nerves to form *sensory tracts* that funnel information up the spinal cord to the brain. Both types of pain fibers enter through the back of the spinal cord, where they synapse with neurons in the **substantia gelatinosa** (Figure 13.1). In the spinal cord, the pain fibers link up with sensory nerves that carry touch, pressure, and limb movement sensations to the thalamus, the brain's sensory switchboard.

On its way to the thalamus, the fast pain pathway triggers neural activity in the reticular formation, which, as you may recall from Chapter 3, is the brain's mechanism for arousing the cortex in response to important messages and for

■ **substantia gelatinosa** the dorsal region of the spinal cord where both fast and slow pain fibers synapse with sensory nerves on their way to the brain

Figure 13.1

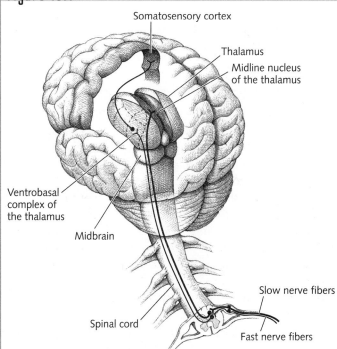

Somatosensory cortex

Thalamus

Midline nucleus of the thalamus

Ventrobasal complex of the thalamus

Midbrain

Spinal cord

Slow nerve fibers

Fast nerve fibers

Pain Pathways
The thinner line illustrates the pathway for fast, acute pain, which originates with fast nerve fibers in the spinal cord and projects to the somatosensory cortex. The thicker line illustrates the pathway for slow, chronic pain, which begins with slow nerve fibers in the spinal cord.

referred pain pain manifested in an area of the body that is sensitive to pain but caused by disease or injury in an area of the body that has few pain receptors

substance P a neurotransmitter secreted by pain fibers in the spinal cord that stimulates the transmission cells to send pain signals to the brain

enkephalins endogenous opioids found in nerve endings of cells in the brain and spinal cord that bind to opioid receptors

periacqueductal gray (PAG) a region of the midbrain that plays an important role in the perception of pain; electrical stimulation in this region activates a descending neural pathway that produces analgesia by "closing the pain gate"

reducing our awareness of unimportant stimuli. Once in the thalamus, incoming messages are routed to the *somatosensory area* of the cerebral cortex, the area that receives input from all the skin senses.

The amount of somatosensory cortex allotted to various regions of the body determines our sensitivity in that region. For example, even though your back has a much larger surface area than your face, there are many more sensory receptors in the skin of your face, and therefore more somatosensory cortex. This means, of course, that your face is capable of sensing weaker touch stimuli than is your back. The internal organs of the body are not mapped in the cortex in the same way as the skin. For this reason, although we can sense pain from the body's interior, it is much harder to pinpoint. In fact, visceral (internal) pain often becomes **referred pain,** in that it feels as though it originates on the surface of the body rather than in the body part in which the cause that produced the pain is situated. So reliable is this phenomenon that referred pain is often used to diagnose serious medical conditions. A patient complaining of pain in the shoulder, for example, is often scheduled for an EKG stress test because that type of pain often accompanies advanced heart disease.

The slow pain system follows roughly the same pathway as the fast system up the spinal cord to the brainstem (refer to Figure 13.1). In the brainstem, slow pain messages are reprocessed; from there they travel to the hypothalamus, the rear portion of the thalamus, and then to the amygdala of the limbic system. Although many details of these higher regions of the slow pain system have yet to be worked out, a widely held view is that they mediate our subjective experience of pain, including the means by which our emotions and motivational state modulate pain (Willis, 1995).

The Biochemistry of Pain

Like all neurons, those that carry pain messages depend on several types of chemical neurotransmitters to relay information across synapses. One neurotransmitter, called **substance P,** with another neurotransmitter called *glutamate,* continuously stimulates nerve endings at the site of an injury and within your spinal cord, increasing pain messages.

A third group of neurotransmitters called **enkephalins** (the smallest member of the brain's natural opiates, the endorphins) bind to receptors in the brain to deaden pain sensations. Through their synapses with slow fibers, enkephalin-containing neurons are believed to regulate how much substance P is released and, therefore, how much of the slow pain system's message is passed through to the brain. If substance P is not released, or if it is released in small quantities, an incoming pain message may be reduced or completely blocked.

What activates enkephalin neurons? The search for an answer to this question has led researchers to the **periaqueductal gray (PAG)** area of the midbrain. When this area is stimulated, pain is reduced almost immediately, with the analgesia continuing even after stimulation is discontinued (Kolb & Wishaw, 2001). So powerful is the analgesia that researchers have actually performed surgery on laboratory animals using no other anesthesia than electrical stimulation of the PAG (Reynolds, 1969). The PAG is also believed to be the primary site at which drugs such as morphine exert their analgesic effects. Even a miniscule amount of morphine will produce substantial pain relief if it is injected directly into cells of the PAG (Basbaum & Fields, 1984).

Thus, it appears that the brain is capable of "turning off" pain through a *descending neural pathway*—the PAG down to neurons in the substantia gelatinosa of the spinal cord. This descending pain control pathway uses the neurotransmitter *serotonin* to activate enkephalin-containing spinal neurons, which, in turn, inhibit pain information coming from substance P fibers (Figure 13.2).

But what turns on the pain-inhibiting cells in the PAG? The answer to this question was discovered by one of the pioneers of the field of psychoneuroimmunology. While still a graduate student, Candace Pert discovered that neural chemicals called *peptides* function as "information messengers" that affect the mind, emotions, the immune system, and other body systems simultaneously (Pert, Dreher, & Ruff, 1998). One of the peptides she identified was *endorphin* (meaning, *the morphine within*). As we noted in Chapter 3, endorphins are natural opioids powerful enough to produce pain relief comparable to that of morphine and other opiates (Julien, 2001).

It turns out that the PAG has numerous opiate/endorphin receptors. Endorphins produced in the brain and spinal cord act as neurotransmitters and inhibit pain by binding to receptors in the PAG and by acting on cells in the spinal cord and brainstem. The presence of endorphin in the PAG initiates the pain-relieving activity of the descending pathway.

The circumstances that trigger the production of endorphins are the subject of ongoing research. A variety of events have been demonstrated to increase the level of endorphins. One is stress. **Stress-induced analgesia (SIA)** refers to the pain relief that results from the body's production of endorphins in response to stress. A number of animal studies have confirmed that endorphins mediate stress-induced analgesia. In one study, rats exposed to extremely loud noises (the stressor) became relatively insensitive to pain for a minute or two afterward, as indicated by their unresponsiveness to a

■ **stress-induced analgesia (SIA)** a stress-related increase in tolerance to pain, presumably mediated by the body's endorphin system

Figure 13.2

The Pain-Inhibiting System

Neural activity resulting from stimulation of the midbrain's periaqueductal gray (PAG) activates inhibitory neurons in the spinal cord. These, in turn, act directly on incoming slow nerve fibers to block pain signals from being relayed to the brain. The slow nerve fibers contain substance P and glutamate. When the nerve fibers' release of substance P is inhibited, as it is here, the ascending pain signal is aborted (that is, prevented from traveling to the brain).

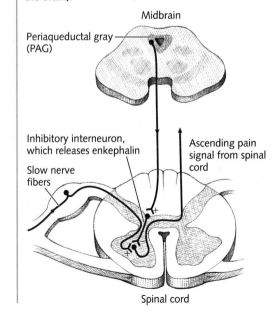

Midbrain

Periaqueductal gray (PAG)

Inhibitory interneuron, which releases enkephalin

Slow nerve fibers

Ascending pain signal from spinal cord

Spinal cord

■ **naloxone** an opioid antagonist that binds to opioid receptors in the body to block the effects of natural opiates and painkillers

normally painful stimulus (Helmstetter & Bellgowan, 1994). However, rats injected with an endorphin-blocking drug called **naloxone** before the noise did not show the stress-induced analgesia, showing once again that the pain-relieving effect depends on endorphins. Classified as an *opioid antagonist*, naloxone binds to opioid receptors in the body, blocking the effects of both naturally occurring (endogenous) opiates and artificial (exogenous) painkillers such as morphine. So powerful is naloxone in counteracting the effects of opiates that the drug is used as the primary treatment for narcotic overdoses. The effects of naloxone, however, are quite brief, lasting for only 15 to 30 minutes.

Similar neurochemical effects may account for the *placebo effect* in pain relief. As we discussed in Chapter 1, many research studies have demonstrated that one-quarter to one-third of people suffering pain receive significant relief simply by taking a placebo. A classic field study of dental pain (Levine, Gordon, & Fields, 1978) was the first to suggest that endorphins might mediate SIA and thus produce the placebo effect. Three hours after having a major tooth pulled (a painful moment, to say the very least), the researchers gave one-half of a group of dental patients a placebo. The remaining subjects received an injection of naloxone. One hour later, subjects who had received the placebo were injected with naloxone, and those who had received naloxone were injected with the placebo. After each injection, the participants were asked to indicate on a standard pain-rating scale the degree of pain they were experiencing.

What do you suppose happened? Under the "influence" of a placebo, patients should report some relief in their dental pain. This, in fact, is exactly what happened, which provides additional support for the validity of the placebo effect. But what do you suppose happened when the patients were under the influence of naloxone? Since naloxone blocks the effects of opiates, including the body's own endorphins, administering this drug provides a good test of the hypothesis that the placebo effect is mediated by endorphins. If this hypothesis is true, we would expect that under the influence of naloxone patients should report feeling *increased* pain compared to that reported during the placebo condition. This is exactly what happened, indicating that the placebo effect is at least partly the result of the body mustering its own mechanisms of pain relief. The most recent research shows that expectations for pain relief are necessary for a person to experience a placebo response (Price, 1999). As we'll see later in the chapter, some other nonmedical techniques for producing analgesia may also work because they trigger the release of endorphins.

A controversial *New England Journal of Medicine* study has cast doubt on the general belief that dummy pills and other sham treatments (placebos) help patients being treated for various medical conditions. Danish researchers Asbjorn Hrobjartsson and Peter Gotzche (2001) conducted a meta-analysis of 130 clinical trials from around the world, involving conditions that ranged from the common cold to seasickness to Alzheimer's disease. In most studies,

Figure 13.3

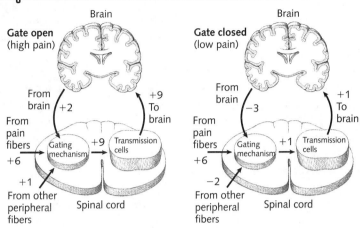

The Gate Control Theory of Pain

In Melzack and Wall's gate control theory, excitatory signals (pluses) tend to open the gate; inhibitory signals (minuses) tend to close the gate. The drawing on the far left—with a net of +9 excitatory signals—illustrates the conditions that might exist when the pain gate remains open and strong pain is felt. The drawing to the right—with a net of only +1—illustrates the conditions that might exist when the pain gate is closed as a result of strong inhibitory stimulation from the brain and peripheral nerve fibers. In both situations, strong pain signals arrive at the spinal cord from both fast and slow pain fibers, along with signals from other peripheral nerve fibers and the brain.

Source: *The Challenge of Pain,* by R. Melzack and P. D. Wall, 1988. New York: Basic Books.

in which patients were randomly assigned to either a placebo or no treatment, the placebo group fared no better than those who received no treatment. The exceptions were studies involving pain treatments in which patients reported how much symptoms bothered them, rather than those involving an objective measure such as blood pressure. Placebo patients in pain studies averaged a 15 percent reduction in pain.

Gate Control Theory

In the past, several theories have been proposed to explain pain perception. Most, however, fell short in accounting for all aspects of pain—biological, psychological, and social. In 1965, Ronald Melzack and Peter Wall outlined a **gate control theory** that overcame some of the shortcomings of earlier theories. Although the theory has received its share of criticism, it remains the dominant theory of pain today. And because it highlighted the significant role of psychosocial factors in pain, the theory has also played an important role in the history of health psychology (Turk, 2001).

The central idea of gate control theory is that the pain experience is not the result of a straight-through sensory channel that begins with the stimulation of a skin receptor and ends with the brain's perception of pain. Rather, incoming sensations that *potentially* signal pain are modulated in the spinal cord as they are conducted to the brain. They are also subject to modification under the influence of descending pathways from the brain.

The theory proposes the existence of a neural structure in the back of the spinal cord that functions like a gate (see Figure 13.3), swinging open to

gate control theory the idea that there is a neural "gate" in the spinal cord that regulates the experience of pain

increase the flow of transmission from nerve fibers or swinging shut to decrease the flow (Melzack & Wall, 1965, 1988). With the gate open, signals arriving in the spinal cord stimulate sensory neurons called *transmission cells,* which, in turn, relay the signals upward to reach the brain and trigger pain. With the gate closed, signals are blocked from reaching the brain, and no pain is felt.

What causes the spinal gate to close? Melzack and Wall (1988) suggested that the mechanism is found in the substantia gelatinosa of the spinal cord. As we saw earlier, both the small and large pain fibers have synapses in the substantia gelatinosa. Depending on which fibers are activated, the substantia gelatinosa, the "gatekeeper," will open or close the gates. Activity in the fast pain fiber system tends to close the gate, whereas activity in the slow pain fiber system tends to force the gate open.

To account for the influence of psychological processes such as attention, anxiety, and culture on the perception of pain, Melzack and Wall also described a *central control mechanism* by which a neural pathway that descends to the spinal cord from the brain can also shut the gate. Through this mechanism, anxiety or fear may amplify the experience of pain, while the distraction of other activities, such as athletic competitions, can dampen the experience of pain.

Let's see how well the gate control theory explains several familiar aspects of pain. While running outdoors last winter, I slipped on an icy patch and twisted my ankle. Fortunately, I was close to home and managed to limp to safety, all the while feeling stinging pain. According to the gate theory, the twisting of my ankle activated countless slow pain fibers, forcing the gate open and sending a painful message to my brain.

When I arrived home, I immediately took off my running shoe and began rubbing my swelling ankle. The temporary relief that I felt is an example of counterirritation, stimulating one area to reduce pain in another. Although well known to every school child (and aging, clumsy runners!), who instinctively rubs a sore spot, exactly why this method worked was unknown before the gate theory provided the answer. According to the gate theory, I felt relief because deep massage activated fast pain fibers, which in turn triggered activity in the substantia gelatinosa, which in turn closed the gate in my spinal cord and prevented the twisted ankle pain messages carried by the smaller pain fibers from reaching the brain.

Melzack (1993) now proposes that messages reaching the brain are further processed by a widely distributed network of brain neurons, which ultimately determine a person's perceptual experience. This network of cells also seems to operate even in the absence of sensory input, placing even greater emphasis on the role of the brain in triggering pain (as in the phantom limb sensation described on pages 568–569) as well as in reducing pain.

Besides presenting a coherent theory that organizes the many diverse aspects of pain, the gate control theory has led to several clinical techniques for controlling pain, including one that involves the artificial stimulation of the large pain fiber system. We look at this and other pain management techniques later in the chapter. First, however, let's take a closer look at some of the psychological and social factors that influence our perception of pain.

Psychosocial Factors in the Experience of Pain

The experience of pain is a complex, multidimensional phenomenon involving not only physical events but also psychological factors and the social learning processes that people acquire through family members and cultural learning. All pain patients are acting (and reacting) members of social groups. In this section we take a look at how such groups influence the experience of pain.

Age and Gender

Across a wide variety of measures, research studies reveal consistent age and gender differences in pain behavior. For example, older people generally are more vigilant than young people in monitoring their health status; they also see themselves as more vulnerable (Skevington, 1995). This may explain why there is a progressive increase in reports of pain and a decrease in tolerance to experimentally induced pain as individuals grow older (Clark & Mehl, 1971).

Age

Certain pains tend to increase in frequency with age, especially headaches, facial pain, and abdominal pain. In a survey of adults aged 25 to 74 years those over 56 were twice as likely as the 25- to 45-year-olds to have experienced two or more pain episodes during the previous month and three times as likely to have had five or more episodes (Mechanic & Angel, 1987). From the findings of another large survey, Michael von Korff and his colleagues (1995) estimate that by the age of 70, 34 percent of adults will have experienced significant facial pain; 40 to 50 percent will have had severe headache, abdominal, or chest pain; and 85 percent will have had substantial back pain.

Before we conclude that aging is inevitably accompanied by a world of pain, we do well to ask ourselves whether other factors, such as overall health, differences in socialization, and coping resources, might account for age-related differences in pain tolerance. As we have seen, it is very easy for researchers examining differences between groups of people (such as age cohorts) to overlook such factors. If we look at the study by David Mechanic and Ronald Angel more closely, we find that adults over age 65 who reported a greater sense of

Phantom Limb Pain

Sometimes people experience pain that has no apparent physical cause. One example is **phantom limb pain,** which is the experience of pain in an amputated arm or leg. Although most amputees experience phantom sensations of touch, pressure, warmth, cold, position, and movements, between 65 and 85 percent report phantom pain sufficiently severe to disrupt social and work activities for substantial periods of time (Williams, 1996). The pain may be occasional or continuous and is usually described as "cramping," "shooting," "burning," or "crushing."

Although phantom limb pain tends to persist even years after the stump tissues have healed, it usually improves over time. But the number of *trigger zones* may spread to healthy areas of the body. A touch or pressure in one of these spots may trigger pains in the phantom limb.

Phantom pain develops most often in patients who experienced pain in the limb for some time prior to amputation. It is much less common in those who lose a limb suddenly. In addition, phantom pain often resembles, in quality, the type of pain that was present before the amputation. Ronald Melzack describes a patient who had a painful wood sliver jammed under his fingernail at the time that he lost the same hand in an industrial accident. For years, the patient reported a painful splinter sensation under the fingernail of his phantom hand. Former United States Senator Bob Kerrey, who lost his right leg to a land mine in Vietnam, reportedly beat his phantom foot with a plastic bat to subdue painful spasms (Brownlee, 1995).

Phantom limb sensations are incredibly "real" in their vivid sensory qualities and precise location in space—so real that an amputee may try to step off the bed onto the phantom foot or pick up a telephone with a phantom hand. Even minor sensations of the missing limb are felt, such as a wedding ring on a phantom finger or a painful corn on a phantom foot. Amputees who suffer from Parkinson's disease may continue to perceive "tremors" like those that occurred in the missing limb before its amputation.

The Search for a Cause The underlying mechanisms of phantom limb pain remain a mystery. Historically, the search for the cause focused on single factors, such as damage to peripheral nerves or the patient being neurotic and imagining his or her pain. One explanation proposed that phantom pain resulted from the amputee's poor emotional adjustment to loss of the limb. Another suggested that damaged nerve fibers in the stump continued to send neural messages to the central nervous system that were interpreted as painful stimuli. A third explanation was that emotional memories are stored alongside sensory memories for the missing limb.

Recent studies have shed light on another possible mechanism in phantom limb pain—evidence that neurons in the brain rewire themselves to seek input from other sources after a limb is amputated. A team of researchers led by Michael Merzenich, a neuroscientist at the University of California at San Francisco, amputated the middle fingers from a group of adult owl monkeys. After the monkeys recovered, the researchers electrically stimulated the remaining fingers on each monkey's paw while recording electrical activity from the somatosensory area of the monkey's brains. Remarkably, Merzenich found that cortical neurons that originally fired in response to stimulation of the amputated finger responded every time he touched the remaining fingers of the monkeys' paws. The neurons had not responded to stimulation of these fingers before the amputation (cited in Ranadive, 1997).

In 1991, researchers at the National Institute of Mental Health expanded on Merzenich's findings. Working with macaque monkeys, the researchers severed the nerves that normally carried sensory information between the cortex and the arm, forearm, paw, and rear of the head. The team then stimulated various body parts and found that the part of the cortex that had previously responded to the arm and back of the head now responded when the monkeys' faces were stimulated.

■ **phantom limb pain**
following amputation of a limb, false pain sensations that appear to originate in the missing limb

overall well-being complained less about pain than those in other age groups. When questioned, those in the oldest age group were more likely to attribute physical symptoms to normal age-related changes. This finding supports the idea that pain perceptions are influenced by social comparisons with people in other reference groups. For example, adults who reported that their parents had experienced frequent, severe pain were themselves more likely to report substantial back, muscle, and joint pain.

At about the same time, Vilayanur Ramachandran, a neuroscientist at Scripps Research Institute, conducted experiments on human amputees who had lost a finger or a hand (Ramachandran & Rogers-Ramachandran, 2000). Blindfolding his patients, Ramachandran applied pressure to different parts of their bodies and discovered that several subjects reported phantom hand sensations as areas of their face were touched. Ramachandran suggested that his findings made sense because the cortical areas that once served the missing finger or hand are adjacent to those that serve the face. Perhaps neurons in these adjacent areas invade those areas left fallow because sensations are no longer received from the missing limb.

This idea of neural reorganization, or "rewiring," represents a radical shift in the way scientists view the brain. Historically, it was thought that there was a critical period in brain development, after which few changes occurred. Now, however, it is obvious that the brain exhibits a considerable amount of *plasticity* throughout life.

Treatment Phantom limb pain is a condition that is often extremely resistant to conventional pain therapies. One long-term study of over 2,000 amputees who were treated for phantom limb pain found that only about 1 percent experienced any lasting benefits, despite the use of a variety of treatments (Sherman, Sherman, & Parker, 1984). Among the treatments that have been tried, with varying degrees of success, are the fitting of prosthetic limbs, ultrasound, transcutaneous electrical nerve stimulation (TENS) (see page 578), anti-inflammatory and anticonvulsant drugs, and nerve blocks such as injections of local anesthetics into trigger points (Williams, 1996).

Recent discoveries about the brain's plasticity are giving researchers new insights into how to treat phantom limb pain, as well as other neural injuries. For instance, researchers have been observing patients with spinal cord injuries in which inflammation or pressure on the spine is blocking neural pathways. Left unchecked, spinal trauma such as this often leads to cortical reorganization similar to that observed in phantom limb sufferers. As the inflammation subsides and the patients recover, the researchers have used magnetic resonance imaging to compare the degree of recovery to the amount of cortical reorganization. The researchers have found that those who experienced *the least* amount of neural rewiring during their recovery were most likely to regain full functioning.

These findings have led to the suggestion that artificially preventing cortical reorganization could help patients recover from such spinal cord injuries. One approach involves the use of a drug that inhibits the glutamate levels in the brain. As we saw earlier, glutamate is a neurotransmitter that enables communication between neurons as they pass pain messages from an external stimulus, such as a blow to the hand, all the way to the brain. Similarly, after a spinal cord injury or amputation—when neurons suddenly stop receiving input signals from their neighbors—glutamate enables the abandoned neurons to connect with other neurons that will provide them with stimulation, thereby enhancing cortical reorganization.

Blocking glutamate receptors may prevent abandoned cortical neurons, which are no longer communicating with a missing limb, from forming new synapses with neurons linked to other parts of the body. When the blockage to the spinal cord subsides, the original cortical connections and functions remain intact. Research testing whether blocking glutamate receptors will also prevent neural reorganization in amputees (and thereby reduce phantom limb pain) is presently underway.

In the meantime, Ramachandran has devised a simpler therapy: a mirror box, which allows an amputee to "see" the phantom limb. For example, when James Peacock, a security guard whose right arm was amputated, slips his intact left arm into the box, mirrors make it appear as if his missing right arm is there as well. The box has provided the only relief Peacock knows from wrenching spasms in his phantom hand. "When I move my left hand," he says, "I can feel it moving my phantom hand" (Brownlee, 1995).

When pain tolerance is tested in the laboratory, the age-pain relationship is even murkier. With pressure, for example, pain tolerance appears to decrease with age; but if heat or cold is used, tolerance appears to increase with age (Woodrow, Friedman, Siegelaub, & Collen, 1972). The picture is complicated even further by the fact that age and gender have interactive effects in pain. Across the life span, age differences in pain behavior are much larger in men than in women (Woodrow et al., 1972).

Gender

Gender differences in health behavior are already apparent in adolescence, with boys being less likely than girls to seek medical care. Girls feel more vulnerable to illness, place a higher value on health, and accept more responsibility for their own health than do boys (Skevington, 1995). As adults, women are more likely to report medical symptoms to a doctor and to experience more frequent episodes of pain than are men (Muellersdorf & Soederback, 2000).

Gender differences extend to the types of pain most commonly reported by women and men (LeResche, 2000). Women seem to suffer more than men from migraines and tension headaches, as well as from pelvic pain, facial pain, and lower back pain (Breslau & Rasmussen, 2001). For other types of pain, however, men and women seem to suffer equally. Recent investigations of patients with *irritable bowel syndrome* (a common gastrointestinal disorder characterized by abdominal pain, diarrhea, and bloating), for example, have reported no significant differences in the experiences of men and women (Heckmann et al., 2001).

Gender and racial differences are also apparent in how the medical community responds to certain pain syndromes. In a study of medical consultations for a variety of complaints, Lois Verbrugge and Richard Steiner (1981) reported that women and men received similar treatment for chest and back pain. Overall, however, women consistently received 5 to 10 percent more prescription drugs for common complaints than did men. A more recent study asked primary care physicians to treat three hypothetical pain patients (with kidney stones, back pain, and sinusitis). For kidney stone pain, male physicians prescribed higher doses of a narcotic analgesic to European American patients than to African-American patients, while female physicians prescribed higher doses to African-Americans. For back pain, male physicians prescribed higher doses of painkillers to males than to females, while female physicians prescribed higher doses to females (Weisse, Sorum, Sanders, & Syat, 2001).

Researchers have found that certain analgesics provide greater and longer-lasting relief for women than they do for men, suggesting a possible gender difference in pain physiology. Jon Levine and his colleagues at the University of California, San Francisco, reported this unexpected finding while studying a new class of analgesics called *kappa-opioids,* which are chemically similar to morphine and heroin. Levine's team asked men and women who had just had wisdom teeth pulled to report their degree of pain as the original anesthesia wore off, and then every 20 minutes following an injection of a kappa-opioid. Although the women reported experiencing more pain immediately following their surgery, 20 minutes after receiving the opioid their pain had decreased to a significantly greater degree than it had for men (Gear et al., 1996).

Despite such findings, a number of researchers believe that the emphasis on differences between women and men is unwarranted and reflects stereotyped medical views about treating men and women rather than responses to specific symptoms (Skevington, 1995). The essential *similarity* of women and men is made clear in studies of gender differences in the experience of pain. Although some researchers have reported that females have a lower pain tolerance than males (Woodrow et al., 1972), others have found only trivial differences (Elton, Stanley, & Burrows, 1983). A recent meta-analysis reported that, on average, women *do* have lower pain thresholds than men but that the size of the difference is quite modest (Riley, Robinson, Wise, Myers, & Fillingim, 1998).

Moreover, the equivocal conclusions of many early studies of gender differences in pain may be the result of intervening social factors in how the experiments were conducted. This line of reasoning was explored in a study in which college students were exposed to a *cold pressor test* (Levine & DeSimone, 1991). This standard laboratory procedure involves immersing a subject's hand and forearm in a bath of icy water (2 degrees C) for several minutes. The male and female students were randomly and equally assigned to male and female experimenters. The results showed that women reported more pain than men did. More interesting was the fact that men reported significantly lower pain ratings to a female experimenter than to a male experimenter. However, there was no difference in the female students' self-reports of pain to experimenters of either sex. These and other researchers have suggested that gender differences reflect traditional sex roles, with men responding to female experimenters with a more stoic "macho" image (Fillingim, 2000).

Sociocultural Factors

Cultural and ethnic groups differ greatly in their response to pain, suggesting that different groups establish their own norms for both the degree to which suffering should be openly expressed and the form that pain behaviors should take. Research studies demonstrate that the sociocultural context also influences how pain is conceptualized, which, in turn, affects the relationship between pain patients and their health care providers. In one study, for instance, European Americans, Latinos, Puerto Ricans, and Polish Americans in New England and Puerto Rico participated in formal and informal interviews regarding their symptoms and treatment. In Puerto Rico, both providers and patients generally viewed chronic pain as a biopsychosocial experience. In New England, however, where the traditional biomedical view of mind–body dualism prevailed among virtually all health care providers, patients reported higher levels of stress and alienation in their relationships with their providers (Bates, Rankin-Hill, & Sanchez-Ayendez, 1997).

Sociocultural variations in the experience of pain are brought into sharp focus in the various religious rituals and rites of passage of many cultures. In Africa, for example, members of certain cultural groups walk on burning coals and pierce their flesh with spikes, with no visible evidence of pain. Stoicism

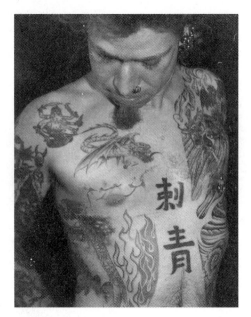

Psychosocial Influences on Pain
The experience of pain is shaped by the meanings we attach to events. In some cultures and religions, seemingly excruciating body piercing is perceived as benign and brings great honor. In many Western cultures today, body piercing and "branding" are not only acceptable behaviors but also are desirable in certain age and social groups. In New York's East Village, the brander heats thin bits of steel and presses them into the customer's flesh.
© Reuters/Peter Morgan/Archive Photos

brings high status, while expressions of pain bring shame because they are viewed as signs of cowardice. In contrast, the open expression of pain is encouraged and approved among some Mediterranean peoples (Burrows, Elton, & Stanley, 1979).

It is important to note that cultural differences in pain reactions are probably related to differences in *pain tolerance,* not to differences in *pain threshold.* Pain threshold, defined as the minimum intensity of a noxious stimulus that is perceived as pain, tends to be more strongly affected by physiological factors, whereas pain tolerance is more strongly influenced by psychological factors, such as expectations about an upcoming experience or the meaning attached to a certain type of pain.

Childbirth provides another vivid example of cultural variation in the experience of pain. Among Yap women in the South Pacific, childbirth seems to be treated as a run-of-the-mill activity that brings little pain. Expectant mothers continue their daily activities almost to the point at which labor pains begin, when they walk to a childbirth hut to deliver their child with the help of a midwife. After a very brief recovery period, the new mother resumes her normal schedule of activities. In sharp contrast to this matter-of-fact approach to having a baby is the experience of many Latina women (Scrimshaw, Engle, & Zambrana, 1983). In traditional Hispanic culture, childbirth is viewed as a cause for much greater worry. Even the Spanish word for labor, *dolor,* means sorrow or pain. As expected, researchers have found a significantly higher incidence of painful labor and delivery complications among Latina women than among Yap women (Scrimshaw et al., 1983).

Surveys of American adults suffering chronic lower back pain, postoperative dental pain, and other pain syndromes have shown differences in the level of pain reported by Americans of African, Hispanic, Asian, and European descent (Faucett, Gordon, & Levine, 1994). In addition, surveys of lower back pain sufferers in various countries reveal greater impairment among Americans, followed by Italians and New Zealanders, Japanese, Colombians, and Mexicans (Sanders et al., 1992).

However, as with age and gender differences, we should be cautious in interpreting cultural variation in reported pain. One reason is that cross-cultural studies often are criticized for lacking linguistic and semantic equivalence. For example, while English has at least four basic words to describe pain—ache, sore, hurt, and pain—the Japanese have three words for pain and the Thais have only two (Fabrega & Tyma, 1976), making it difficult to equate subjective pain reports across groups.

Moreover, as psychologists have long noted, studies of *within-group variation* have been far less popular than studies of *between-group variation.* That is, researchers—like people in general—are frequently victims of faulty reasoning that leads them to focus on the relatively few ways in which certain groups differ rather than on the greater number of ways in which they are the same. In a striking example of this, James Lipton and Joseph Marbach (1984) interviewed facial pain patients, comparing the self-reported pain experiences of African-Americans, Irish Americans, Italian Americans, Jewish Americans, and Latin-Americans. Only 34 percent of the participants' responses showed significant intergroup differences, while the remaining 66 percent exhibited similar responses from group to group. In fact, the researchers found much stronger evidence of *intraethnic variation* (individual variation within each group) than they did *interethnic variation.*

A final reason for being cautious in interpreting the results of cultural pain studies is that cross-cultural studies are correlational in design, making it difficult to rule out socioeconomic pressures, social support, coping resources, and other underlying factors.

Social Learning

In the mid-1980s, Australian labor unions fought for, and won, legislation providing paid leave for any worker suffering a *repetitive strain injury.* Over the next six months, the number of such cases skyrocketed, showing how a change in social context can influence people's experience of pain (Azar, 1998).

If social and cultural factors do affect the experience of pain, how do they exert their influence? Many health psychologists believe that social learning and social comparison play a critical role in determining an individual's future processing of the pain experience. An individual's earliest models for pain behavior are the family and his or her cultural group. Observing family members and other people in the reference group helps a person determine what pain behaviors are appropriate in a given situation. How will others react if I cry, for example, or ask for a medication to relieve my suffering?

The social environment shapes an individual's pain experience in yet another way. In some social and cultural groups, a person who grimaces or moans almost always receives attention from others. Such attention may serve as an operant reinforcer and increase the occurrence of open expressions of pain in the future. In other groups, open expressions of pain are either ignored (leading over time to their extinction) or received with hostility (leading over time to their suppression).

As with many behaviors, how we learn to respond to pain begins in childhood. Children whose parents disregard their pain behavior may grow up more stoic in their approach to pain than children whose parents pay undue attention to every minor ache and pain (Pennebaker, 1982). This process of socialization may explain the finding that firstborn children and only children may have a lower tolerance to experimentally induced pain (Sternbach, 1986). Compared to later-born children, these children's pain may get more attention from their parents because first-time parents are inexperienced and tend to panic when their first child is ill. Later, when they've learned what to expect, they typically give less reinforcement to pain behavior. On the other hand, children who have many siblings may complain *more* about pain, perhaps because they feel it's the only way they can compete with their brothers and sisters for parental attention.

Is There a Pain-Prone Personality?

Are there people who often have migraine headaches? Are they ambitious, orderly, a bit obsessive, and rigid in their thinking? This widely held stereotype of migraine sufferers begs the question of whether there is a *pain-prone personality*. To find out, researchers have used a variety of personality tests, especially the Minnesota Multiphasic Personality Inventory (MMPI). The MMPI contains 10 clinical scales, including scales that measure concern with body symptoms, depression, paranoia, social introversion, and other personality traits.

Both acute and chronic pain patients often show elevated scores on two MMPI scales: hysteria (the tendency to exaggerate symptoms and use emotional behavior to solve problems) and hypochondriasis (the tendency to be overly concerned about health and to overreport body symptoms). Chronic pain sufferers also tend to score high in depression (Low & Peck, 1987). In fact, depression is about three to four times more prevalent among lower back pain patients than it is among people in the general population (Sullivan, Reesor, Mikail, & Fisher, 1992).

Researchers have also attempted to determine whether any personality traits are consistently found among placebo responders, that is, people whose apparent pain is eliminated when they are given placebos as pain killers. Researchers have investigated locus of control, emotional dependence, introversion/extraversion, impulsivity, and many other traits that might correlate with responsiveness to placebos (Richardson, 1994). Unfortunately, the results of countless studies have revealed no consistent differences in placebo responders and nonresponders. For example, both extraversion and introversion have emerged in various studies as traits that predict placebo responsiveness (Richardson, 1997). Many researchers believe that the inconsistency in findings suggests that placebo responsiveness may not be an enduring *dispositional trait*. Rather, it is a *situational trait* that may be manifested in certain situations but not in others (Montgomery & Kirsch, 1996).

In general, some researchers believe that more telling than personality types are individual differences in how patients cope with serious health problems, including chronic pain. Pain researcher Dennis Turk and James Nash (1996) at the University of Washington have identified three subtypes of pain patients:

- *Dysfunctional patients* report high levels of pain and psychological distress, feel they have little control over their lives, and are extremely inactive.

- *Interpersonally distressed patients* feel they have little social support and that other people in their lives don't take their pain seriously.

- *Adaptive copers* report significantly lower levels of pain and psychological or social distress than those in the other two groups and continue to function at a high level.

Turk believes that tailoring treatments to match a patient's coping style will achieve better, longer-lasting results. In one study, Turk provided a comprehensive stress-management treatment to a group of patients with chronic jaw pain (Turk, Zacki, & Rudy, 1993). The program included an educational component, relaxation training, and a "bite plate" to help the patients learn to monitor muscle tension in their jaws. Although all the subjects reported lower levels of pain and psychological distress following the treatment program, most of those classified as dysfunctional patients relapsed within 6 months. In contrast, adaptive copers continued to report lower levels of pain that remained stable well past the 6-month follow-up. In a subsequent study, Turk and his colleagues added a cognitive therapy component to the standard stress-management program and tested its effectiveness on a second group of dysfunctional jaw pain sufferers. This time almost none of the subjects relapsed, and the pain improvements lasted well past the 6-month follow-up.

Treating Pain

The treatment of pain is big business. It is estimated that Americans consume between 10,000 to 20,000 *tons* of aspirin alone each year (Frank, Sperling, & Wu, 2000). There are two broad categories of pain treatment: medical interventions and nonmedical interventions, which include cognitive-behavioral treatments such as hypnosis and biofeedback. Although health care professionals once scoffed at most nonmedical treatments, the proven effectiveness of using psychological techniques with pain patients, as well as evidence that some—such as the placebo effect—work partly by mobilizing the body's physical system of analgesia, have increasingly led to the realization that there is no sharp dividing line between physical and nonphysical pain treatments.

In this section, we'll look first at the more well-known pharmacological, surgical, and electrical stimulation treatments, then at the psychological treatments now widely used in pain control. Finally, we'll take a close look at cognitive-behavioral therapy, an eclectic form of treatment that represents health psychology's contribution to pain management.

Pharmacological Treatments

For most patients, *analgesic* (pain-relieving) drugs are the mainstay of pain control techniques. Analgesics fall into two general classes. The first includes "central acting" *opioid drugs* such as morphine. The second category consists of "peripherally acting" *nonopioid* chemicals that produce their pain-relieving and anti-inflammatory effects at the actual site of injured tissue.

Opioid Analgesics

Formerly called *narcotics* (from the Greek word *narke,* which means numbness), the opioids are *agonists* (excitatory chemicals) that act on specific receptors in the spinal cord and brain to reduce either the intensity of pain messages or the brain's response to pain messages.

The most powerful and most widely used opioid for treating severe pain is morphine, which is administered orally, rectally, or by injection. After binding to receptors in the PAG, the thalamus, and cells at the back of the spinal cord, morphine produces intense analgesia and indifference to pain, a state of relaxed euphoria, reduced apprehension, and a sense of tranquility. Because of morphine's powerful effects, regular users predictably and quickly develop both tolerance and dependence, so quickly that doctor-prescribed doses of morphine sometimes have to be increased—to retain their effectiveness—from clinical doses of 50 to 60 milligrams per day to as high as 500 milligrams per day over as short a period as 10 days (Julien, 2001).

There is one drawback to the powerful effects of morphine, however. Its effectiveness makes it addictive, and therefore many physicians are reluctant to prescribe opioid analgesics and often *undermedicate* pain patients by prescribing doses that are too weak to produce meaningful relief from pain. So strong is the fear of causing pain patients to become addicted that many types of pain are inadequately treated (Hill, 1995) (see also Byline Health on pages 578–579).

One solution to the problem of undermedication has been *patient controlled analgesia*—giving responsibility for administering the pain-killing drugs to the patients. Today, some patients with severe, chronic pain have small morphine pumps implanted near sites of localized pain. Patients can activate the pump and deliver a small pain-relieving dose whenever they need it. Many postsurgical burn and cancer patients are fitted with morphine pumps connected to intravenous lines that allow them to do the same (Morey, 1998).

A recent alternative to the use of prescription opioids stems from the finding that many chronic pain patients have lower-than-normal levels of endorphins in their spinal fluid. Clinicians are experimenting with synthetic endorphins to boost their stores. In several promising studies, patients have reported excellent, long-lasting pain relief after receiving injections of a synthetic form of endorphin called *beta-endorphin* (Farrington, 1999).

A 2001 survey of Australian registered nurses found that there was "a clear knowledge deficit" in the management of pain in the elderly. For example, only 4 out of 10 nurses knew that it is unnecessary to avoid giving potent painkillers to frail elderly patients. Nurses who specialized in palliative care showed the greatest knowledge of treating older patients' pain.
—Sloman, Ahern, Wright, & Brown, 2001

Nonopioid Analgesics

The nonopioid analgesics include aspirin, acetaminophen, and ibuprofen, as well as indomethacin, phenylbutazone, ketorolac, ketoprofen, and naproxen. Also called **nonsteroidal anti-inflammatory drugs (NSAIDs),** these drugs produce several effects:

- Pain reduction without sedation (analgesia)
- Reduction of inflammation (anti-inflammatory effect)
- Reduction of body temperature when fever is present (antipyretic effect)
- Inhibition of platelet aggregation (anticoagulant effect)

Although aspirin is a highly effective analgesic for low-grade pain, many people cannot tolerate its side effects, which include heartburn and stomachache, ringing in the ears, thirst, and hyperventilation. As an alternative, they may take acetaminophen (Tylenol) or ibuprofen (Motrin), which are easier to tolerate.

NSAIDs relieve pain by blocking a chemical chain reaction that is triggered when tissue is injured. Consider sunburn pain. One of the chemicals produced at the site of the burn is called *arachidonic acid,* which the body converts into **prostaglandin,** the substance responsible for sunburn pain and inflammation. Prostaglandin also causes free nerve endings to become more and more sensitized as time passes. This is why the tissue injury that accompanies sunburn usually goes unnoticed while you are at the beach. Later that night, however, your skin is so sensitive that even a cool shore breeze is painful to your skin. In order to convert arachidonic acid into prostaglandin, an enzyme called cyclooxygenase, or COX, is needed. NSAIDs work their magic by blocking COX.

The newest class of NSAIDs, called *COX-2 inhibitors,* ease pain as effectively as aspirin and ibuprofen but with even less gastric distress. This new class of painkillers is good news for regular NSAID users, 107,000 of whom are hospitalized and 16,500 of whom die each year from gastrointestinal complications resulting from NSAID use.

Surgery, Electrical Stimulation, and Physical Therapy

For centuries, healers have used surgery in their attempts to relieve severe pain. Their reasoning made sense: If pain is a simple *stimulus-response* connection between peripheral pain receptors and the brain, why not simply cut, or lesion, pain fibers so that the messages don't get through? In their search, surgeons have tested the analgesic effects of lesions that disrupt incoming messages before they reach the spinal cord, as well as lesions placed higher in the "pain highway," such as in the brainstem.

Sometimes surgery is helpful. For example, destroying thalamic cells of the slow pain system has been demonstrated to alleviate some deep, burning pain,

■ **nonsteroidal anti-inflammatory drugs (NSAIDs)** aspirin, ibuprofen, acetaminophen, and other analgesic drugs that relieve pain and reduce inflammation at the site of injured tissue

■ **prostaglandin** the chemical substance responsible for localized pain and inflammation; prostaglandin also causes free nerve endings to become more and more sensitized as time passes

Amid New Calls for Pain Relief, New Calls for Caution

Sheryl Gay Stolberg

William Bergman knew how he wanted to die. "He wanted to be free of pain," said his daughter, Beverly, "and die at home with us." But when Mr. Bergman, an 85-year-old retired railroad detective from Hayward, Calif., contracted lung cancer last February, he got only half his wish. He died at home, his daughter said, but in miserable pain.

To experts in end-of-life care, it is a familiar tale: an elderly patient dies in intractable pain. But Bergman's daughter has set out to give this old story a different ending and in the process has touched off an intense debate about how best to improve the treatment of the dying.

With the help of the Compassion in Dying Federation, an Oregon group whose director helped legalize assisted suicide in that state, Ms. Bergman filed a complaint to the Medical Board of California, asking that her father's doctor be disciplined for failing to prescribe powerful narcotics that could have given relief to the dying man. The effort was unsuccessful. In August, the board wrote Bergman that while "pain management for your father was indeed inadequate," no disciplinary action would be taken.

Nevertheless, Bergman's complaint represents a new tack in the long-running campaign by patient advocates to improve care of the dying. For decades, doctors have worried that they might be disciplined, or even face criminal prosecution, for the aggressive use of morphine and other narcotics to control pain. Now, some advocates are trying to swing the pendulum in the other direction, by pressing authorities to punish doctors for not using pain medicine aggressively enough.

"It is clear that doctors can get into trouble for overprescribing; everybody knows that," said Dr. Joanne Lynn, president of Americans for Better Care of the Dying, a nonprofit group based in Washington. "We need a counterweight that you can also get into trouble for deliberately underprescribing."

So far, complaints to state medical boards about undertreatment of pain have been rare, said Dale L. Austin, deputy executive vice president of the Federation of State Medical Boards, which represents 69 licensing authorities around the nation. But Mr. Austin calls it "an up-and-coming issue."

In a survey conducted last year, [researchers] found that 8.1 percent of state medical board members questioned knew of doctors who had either been investigated or disciplined for undertreating pain. That was up from 5 percent in 1991.

It has been more than 4 years since the Supreme Court, in rejecting a constitutional right to die, noted that dying patients do have a right to the brand of medicine known as **"palliative care,"** which focuses on controlling pain and providing comfort. Many doctors and nurses say that patients

■ **palliative care** health care that focuses on easing pain and providing comfort, especially at the end of life

■ **counterirritation** analgesia in which one pain (for example, a pulled muscle) is relieved by creating another, counteracting stimulus (such as rubbing the site of the injury)

such as that experienced by some cancer patients, without altering the sense of touch or the more acute, stinging pain of the fast pain system. More often, however, surgery has unpredictable results and its effects are short-lived, perhaps because of the nervous system's remarkable regenerative ability that enables pain impulses to reach the brain via several alternative paths (Zimmerman, 1979). As a result, some pain patients have endured numerous "hit-or-miss" surgeries that provide only short-term relief, incurring substantial risk to their health, staggering medical bills, and untold suffering. And in some cases, patients actually experience *worse* pain due to the cumulative damage of repeated surgeries on the nervous system. For these reasons, surgery is rarely used to control pain today, and only as a last-ditch effort.

More effective than surgery is **counterirritation,** which involves stimulating one area of the body to reduce pain in another part of the body. For example, with **transcutaneous electrical nerve stimulation (TENS),** brief

who contemplate suicide might not do so if they were confident their pain would be adequately treated.

But studies show that patients routinely suffer pain that could be relieved, in part because of lingering fears among doctors about the consequences of prescribing narcotics too liberally.

In an attempt to ease those fears, many state licensing authorities have adopted new policies on pain management in recent years. California's guidelines, revised in 1994, are typical. They say that doctors will not be disciplined for prescribing powerful pain medications if they take a proper medical history, outline a treatment plan, obtain informed consent from their patients, monitor the use of the drugs, and keep detailed records. In May, the Federation of State Medical Boards published a similar set of model rules for its members to follow.

A similar chilling effect exists in states where doctors must write multiple prescriptions for controlled substances on a special pad—one copy for the doctor, one for the pharmacist, and one for state drug enforcement authorities, who monitor the prescriptions in an attempt to curb trafficking in illicit narcotics.

When Bergman was discharged from the Eden Medical Center in Castro Valley, Calif., his internist, Dr. Wing Chin, prescribed Vicodin, an oral analgesic that did not fall under the so-called triplicate requirement. Bergman's daughter said she asked for something stronger, but, records show, Chin said he could not immediately order anything stronger because he did not have his triplicate pad with him. Instead, Bergman was given an injection of a pain reliever and a skin patch that contained a narcotic.

Chin declined to be interviewed. But end-of-life care experts say the triplicate requirement, recently eliminated in New York, often keeps doctors from prescribing the most powerful narcotics.

"It is a huge deterrent," said Lynn. "You have to use the prescriptions in sequence. You can't put a pad in your office and a pad in your black bag and a pad in the hospital, and if they are stolen there is hell to pay. A lot of times, a doctor will try to substitute a less potent drug that doesn't require all this documentation." In any event, managing pain is a tricky business, and experts say standards may vary with each individual case.

"The problem with pain is that it is sometimes easy to manage—and sometimes very difficult," said Dr. Diane E. Meier, director of the palliative care program at Mount Sinai Medical Center in Manhattan. "It is easy to say that a doctor was incompetent. But that doctor might have been doing the best job humanly possible, and still fail."

Source: New York Times (nytimes.com, October 31, 1998).

Exercises

1. What is palliative care? Why is this form of care controversial?

2. You have been asked to debate the subject of palliative care. What points would you raise should you be asked to argue in favor of legislation mandating a patient's right to palliative care? What points would you raise if asked to argue against such legislation?

---

pulses of electricity are applied to nerve endings under the skin near the painful area. Alternatively, stimulating electrodes may be placed or implanted at the appropriate level of the spinal cord where nerve fibers from the painful area enter the back of the spinal cord. By adjusting the frequency and voltage of the stimulation, patients are able to self-administer treatment. If successful, TENS produces a feeling of numbness that overcomes the sensation of pain.

TENS yields excellent *local pain relief* for some chronic pain patients, particularly when stimulation is applied to regions of the body where touch and pressure sensitivity remains intact. A recent longitudinal study reported that a single trial of TENS produced significant pain relief in 64 percent of patients with different pain syndromes, including those caused by nerve injuries or damage to the spinal cord and those with no demonstrable cause (Kim & Dellon, 2001). Four years after the study, of those who had elected to have a

■ **transcutaneous electrical nerve stimulation (TENS)** a counterirritation form of analgesia involving electrically stimulating spinal nerves near a painful area

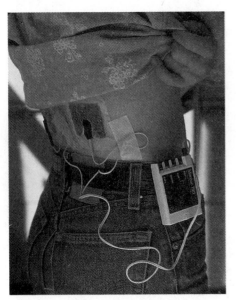

TENS

Back pain can be relieved with transcutaneous electrical nerve stimulation (TENS). Portable TENS machines help relieve the pain of thousands of sufferers. After the person logistically places the pads shown here on either side of the painful area, he or she can hook the small electrical conduit to a belt and continue with daily activities while pulses are delivered to the body. © Tom Lyle / The Stock Shop / Medichrome

permanent stimulator implanted, 21 percent rated their pain relief as excellent, 50 percent as good, and 29 percent as fair.

For more widespread and severe pain (such as that associated with some advanced cancers), another electrical form of analgesia, called *stimulation-produced analgesia (SPA)*, involves delivering mild electrical pulses through electrodes that are surgically implanted in the brain. Once again, patients self-administer treatment, determining when and how much stimulation is needed. SPA appears to work by stimulating endorphin neurons, which activate the body's natural system of analgesia. Accordingly, SPA electrodes are implanted in brain sites known to be rich in opioid receptors. Although SPA is expensive and entails the risk associated with brain surgery, many pain patients report that their pain seems to melt away. As an added benefit, SPA does not seem to disrupt the other senses, and there is no mental confusion as often occurs with opioid analgesia (Farrington, 1999).

People who are in pain, as well as those who are suffering disability as a result of disease, injury, or surgery, may also be referred to a physical therapist for assistance. *Physical therapists* are rehabilitation professionals who promote optimal health and functional independence through their efforts to identify, correct, or prevent movement dysfunction, physical disability, or pain.

Physical therapists typically create an individualized program of targeted exercises to improve the patient's muscular strength, flexibility, and coordination. Depending on the individual's needs, they may also concentrate on improving the patient's daily living skills, such as bathing, dressing, and cooking. Physical therapy often begins in the hospital and continues as long as needed.

Cognitive-Behavioral Therapy

Because no single pain control technique has proved to be the most effective in relieving chronic pain, many health care providers today use an *eclectic*, or "cafeteria," approach to helping their patients manage pain. This means that treatment is tailored to each individual case and that the patient is taught several pain-management strategies from which he or she may choose as needed.

One example of such a program is **cognitive-behavioral therapy (CBT),** an umbrella term for a variety of multidisciplinary interventions aimed at changing a person's experience of pain by changing his or her thought processes and behaviors (Grant & Haverkamp, 1995). CBT involves such strategies as distraction, imagery, relaxation training, exercising, and deep breathing.

CBT is rapidly becoming the dominant model for treating pain, being used by an estimated 73 percent of clinicians who treat chronic pain (Grant &

■ **cognitive-behavioral therapy (CBT)** a multidisciplinary pain-management program that combines cognitive, physical, and emotional interventions

Haverkamp, 1995). Although the specific components of CBT vary from one intervention to another, most programs

- Include an education and goal-setting component that focuses on the factors that influence pain and clarifies the client's expectations for treatment.
- Include cognitive interventions to enhance patients' self-efficacy and sense of control over pain.
- Teach new skills for responding to pain triggers.
- Promote increased exercise and activity levels.

Education and Goal Setting

CBT counselors often begin by giving patients a brief course that explains the differences between acute and chronic pain, the mechanisms of gate control theory, and the effects of depression, anxiety, lack of activity, and other controllable factors on pain. Patients are drawn into the educational phase by being encouraged to generate examples from their own pain experiences, perhaps by keeping a daily diary that records pain frequency, duration, and intensity; medication use; and hour-by-hour mood and activity levels. In addition to allowing both patient and counselor to review pain patterns without having to rely on the patient's memory, the diary almost always gives clients new insights into some of the factors that affect their pain experience. These insights are invaluable in promoting an increased sense of control over pain.

This phase is most useful for establishing specific goals for the intervention. As with any behavioral management program, goals need to be specific and measurable to prevent miscommunication and the development of unrealistic expectations. Goals also should be phrased in such a way as to downplay the common tendency to dwell on pain. For example, rather than "I would like to be able to resume my normal activities without feeling pain," a better goal is "I would like to take a brisk, 30-minute walk, four times a week."

Cognitive Interventions

Our attitudes and beliefs are powerful influences on our health. Faulty reasoning often contributes to poor health outcomes and interferes with treatment. As part of a pain-management program, *cognitive restructuring* challenges maladaptive thought processes and helps pain sufferers to redefine pain as an experience that is more manageable than they once believed (Philips, 1988). It is also directed at correcting the patient's irrational beliefs, which contribute to anxiety and amplify pain.

Health psychologists recognize a general pattern of cognitive errors in the thinking of chronic pain patients, including

- *Catastrophizing.* Many pain sufferers overestimate the distress and discomfort caused by an unfortunate experience (such as being injured).

- *Overgeneralizing.* Some pain victims believe that their pain will never end and that it will completely ruin their lives. As we have seen elsewhere, such *global* and *stable attributions* of a negative event often lead to depression and poorer health outcomes.

- *Victimization.* Some chronic pain patients feel that they have experienced an injustice that consumes them. Many are unable to get beyond the "Why me?" stage in dealing with their pain.

- *Self-blame.* In contrast, some chronic pain patients come to feel a sense of worthlessness because of their pain and may blame themselves for not being able to carry on their normal family and work responsibilities.

- *Dwelling on the pain.* Some pain sufferers simply can't stop thinking about their pain problem. They may repeatedly "relive" painful episodes and replay negative thoughts over and over in their minds.

Because negative beliefs and thoughts are obviously counterproductive to a successful treatment intervention, CBT therapists often use *rational-emotive therapy* (see Chapter 4) to challenge illogical beliefs. Another helpful technique has patients practice developing an *internal dialogue,* in which maladaptive pain thoughts are replaced with more positive and optimistic thoughts. Moreover, because many chronic pain patients have misconceptions or exaggerated fears about their pain and its treatment, simply providing accurate, realistic information often helps them to restructure their pain.

Cognitive Distraction Earlier, we described several situations in which painful events were either ignored (the injured athlete involved in an intense competition) or even perceived as benign (the person undergoing a religious ritual or rite of passage). Other examples come easily to mind: the soldier who is unaware of being wounded until after helping a friend reach safety and the seriously injured firefighter who ignores his or her own pain while rescuing an unconscious victim from a burning building.

Does this type of *cognitive distraction* have any *practical* usefulness in pain control? Many CBT therapists think so. Think back to the last time you visited the dentist to have a tooth filled. If your dentist's office is like mine, the treatment room is filled with numerous attention-getting stimuli. Music is piped in, colorful mobiles spin from the ceiling, and dreamy landscapes hang on soothing wallpaper. There's even a pile of stuffed animals sitting in the corner, in the direct line of vision of the unfortunate person sitting in the dental chair.

Do such things work? One study exposed dental patients to one of three conditions. One group listened to music during their dental procedure; another group listened to the music *after* receiving a verbal suggestion that the music might help relieve their pain and stress; a third group served as control subjects and received neither the suggestion nor the music. Compared to control subjects, patients in the two music conditions reported experiencing significantly less discomfort during their treatment (Anderson, Baron, & Logan, 1991). Music is also frequently used to help burn victims distract their attention from painful treatments, such as having wound dressings changed.

Imagery

A closely related pain-control technique that is often used with cognitive distraction is *imagery*. Designed to promote changes in a person's perceptions, imagery has two components: a mental process (as in imagining) and a procedure (as in *guided imagery*). Although imagery is often used synonymously with *visualization,* this is misleading: the latter refers only to seeing something in the mind's eye, while good imagery involves using all the senses.

Imagery is actually a form of self-hypnosis because it involves focused concentration and attention. Furthermore, it is incorporated into relaxation techniques that involve suggestions (for example, "Your hands are heavy") and into *mental rehearsal,* which helps prepare patients to undergo an uncomfortable medical treatment. By mentally rehearsing (imagining) surgery or a difficult medical treatment, patients can rid themselves of unrealistic fantasies and thus relieve the anxiety, pain, and side effects that are exacerbated by heightened emotional reactions.

In a typical intervention, the patient first learns a relaxation strategy. Then, while the patient is relaxing, the practitioner describes the treatment and recovery period in sensory terms, taking the patient on a guided imagery "trip." Practitioners are careful to be factual without using emotion-laden or fear-provoking words and to describe, where possible, the medical procedure in a positive way. The patient is also taught coping techniques such as distraction, mental dissociation, muscle relaxation, and abdominal breathing.

Like cognitive distraction procedures, imagery techniques are based on the concept that our attention and awareness have a limited capacity. According to this, pain is a stimulus that competes for attention with other stimuli in a person's internal and external environments (Morley, 1997). The purpose of the intervention is to teach patients to switch their attention from pain to other stimuli or to restructure their interpretation of their current focus of awareness. For example, a pain patient may be taught to construct a vivid, multisensory image, such as strolling through a lush meadow on a beautiful spring day, focusing intently on the sights, sounds, and smells of the meadow. The elaborated features of the image presumably compete with the painful stimulus and lower its impact.

How effective is imagery in controlling pain? As is true with hypnosis and relaxation training, imagery is most often used to supplement other techniques, so its effectiveness as a stand-alone treatment is based primarily on anecdotal evidence (Eccleston, 1995). The few published results that exist are almost uniformly positive. Thus far it seems that imagery works best with low to medium levels of pain intensity (Jensen & Karoly, 1991), especially those that are slow to develop and can be anticipated. Compared to untrained control subjects, patients who have been trained in the use of positive imagery may experience a number of benefits, including reduced anxiety and pain during dental procedures (Horan, Laying, & Pursell, 1976), use of fewer pain medications and reduced treatment side effects (Langer, Janis, & Wolfer, 1975), and increased pain tolerance to experimentally induced pain (Chaves & Barber, 1974).

Imagery is also a fundamental component of *Lamaze training*, the most widely used method of prepared childbirth in the United States (Wideman & Singer, 1984). Rather than being "natural childbirth" as it has been mistakenly described, the Lamaze method is "prepared childbirth" that provides an analgesic effect through cognitive and behavioral rather than chemical means. When my wife and I participated in Lamaze childbirth classes, we received extensive instruction in developing a *focal point*—an actual or imagined image (such as a photograph that holds great personal meaning) that she was to focus on in order to distract her attention away from labor pains. To be effective, the image has to be practiced, controllable, and easy to call up.

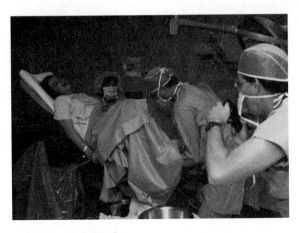

Painless Childbirth
Childbirth is feared as a painful event in some cultures more often than it is in others. Prepared childbirth—using the Lamaze method—is increasingly used in Western industrialized nations. Although "lack of medication" implies more pain, breathing exercises and psychological preparedness actually decrease the amount of pain felt by the mother-to-be. © Vince Streano/Corbis

However, many imagery studies have used only a handful of people and have not been replicated, leaving the effectiveness of imagery open to question. Still, there is enough evidence of a relationship between imagery and pain control that the Office of Alternative Medicine, part of the National Institutes of Health, has called for further and more precise investigation into imagery.

Reshaping Pain Behavior Consider the case of Mrs. Y, a 37-year-old office administrator who entered the University of Washington's pain-management program. For the past 18 years Mrs. Y has experienced constant lower back pain that allows her to get out of bed less than 2 hours a day. The rest of the time she spends reclining—either reading, watching TV, or sleeping. Although over the years Mrs. Y has had four major surgical procedures (including removal of a herniated disc and a spine fusion), her ability to function continues to deteriorate. At the time of admission to the hospital, she was taking four or five highly addictive opiate painkillers per day, despite the fact that x-rays and a complete physical examination revealed no evidence of any actual organic problem.

Although pain may initially be caused by an injury or underlying organic pathology, over time its expression is often maintained by social and environmental reinforcement. Like Mrs. Y, some chronic pain sufferers may not progress in their treatment because adhering to the role of a pain patient brings them a number of benefits, including plenty of solicitous attention from others, lots of rest, and freedom from daily hassles (such as work). One goal of many comprehensive treatment programs, therefore, is to modify pain behaviors, such as excessive sleeping, complaining about discomfort, and requests for pain medication (Morley, 1997). Stemming from a conditioning model (see Chapter 1), the intervention begins by identifying the events (stimuli) that precede targeted pain behaviors (responses) as well as the consequences that follow (reinforcers). Treatment then involves changing the *contingencies* between responses and reinforcers to increase the frequency of more adaptive ways of coping with discomfort.

In the case of Mrs. Y, reinforcing consequences (hospital staff attention, rest, and so on) were made contingent on desirable behaviors (such as walking or some other mild form of exercise) rather than on maladaptive pain behaviors such as complaining, dependence, and excessive requests for painkillers. To make the program work, family members—who tend to be overly attentive to signs of pain in their loved ones and thereby reinforce excessive rest and nonparticipation in normal family activities (Morley, 1997)—were also brought into the treatment program. They were taught to change their behavior toward their loved one in order to reduce pain behaviors and increase more positive ways of coping. As a result of the combined efforts of both hospital staff and family members, Mrs. Y's pain behaviors were quickly *extinguished.*

Evaluating the Effectiveness of Pain Treatments

Which approach to pain control works best? The answer seems to be, "It depends." In a study comparing cognitive-behavioral treatments with traditional physical therapy for pain control among patients with chronic lower back pain, researchers found evidence supporting both approaches (Heinrich, Cohen, Naliboff, Collins, & Bonnebakker, 1985). *Physical* functioning improved the most among patients who received physical therapy. In contrast, *psychosocial* gains were greatest among patients who received the cognitive-behavioral intervention.

The most effective pain-management programs are multidisciplinary programs that combine the cognitive, physical, and emotional interventions of CBT therapy with judicious use of analgesic drugs (Peat, Moores, Goldingay, & Hunter, 2001). The goals of such programs extend beyond the control of pain to restoring the patient's overall quality of life by decreasing the reliance on medication, restoring activity levels, and enhancing psychological and social well-being.

In studies with tension headache sufferers, for instance, biofeedback has proved to be about twice as effective as a placebo in reducing pain and slightly

Figure 13.4

Headache Relief Following Biofeedback and Relaxation Training
Both biofeedback and relaxation training are more effective than a placebo in relieving the pain of tension headaches. Across many studies, however, the greatest relief occurred when biofeedback and relaxation training were combined.

Source: "Pharmacological versus Non-Pharmacological Prophylaxis of Recurrent Migraine Headache: A Meta-Analytic Review of Clinical Trials," by D. A. Holroyd and D. B. Penzien, 1990, *Pain, 42,* pp. 1–13.

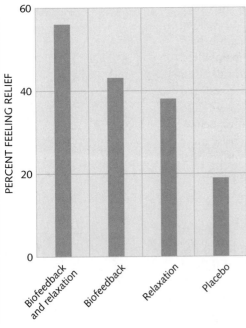

more beneficial than relaxation training. Recall from Chapter 5 that biofeedback is a technique for converting certain supposedly involuntary physiological responses into electrical signals and providing visual or auditory feedback about them so the person can learn to control those responses. As Figure 13.4 shows, however, the greatest relief was experienced by headache sufferers who received biofeedback *and* relaxation training in a combined treatment (Holroyd & Penzien, 1986). Until recently, it was generally believed that migraine headaches were caused by abnormally dilated blood vessels, so most were treated with drugs that work by constricting blood vessels. However, new research using neuroimaging devices that allow researchers to watch patients' brains during migraine attacks shows that people who are prone to migraines have abnormally excitable neurons in their brainstems (Bahra, Matharu, Buchel, Frackowiak, & Goadsby, 2001). This may explain why, for migraine headaches, biofeedback combined with relaxation training appears to be nearly as effective as conventional pharmacological treatments (Holroyd et al., 1995).

Most importantly, effective programs encourage patients to develop (and rehearse) a specific, individualized *pain-management program* for coping when the first signs of pain appear, as pain intensifies, and so forth. In doing so, patients learn to redefine their role in managing pain, from being passive victims to being active and resourceful managers who can *control* their experiences. The increased feelings of self-efficacy that follow from these steps are surely an important element in determining the patient's degree of pain and overall well-being (Keefe, Dunsmore, & Burnett, 1992).

Unrelieved pain has enormous effects on people, including slowing recovery in patients, creating burdens for caregivers and family members, and increasing costs to the health care system. Recently, a national organization that sets standards for health care programs underscored the psychological effects of pain by establishing new guidelines for the assessment and management of pain (Rabasca, 1999). Under the new guidelines, health care facilities (including nursing homes) are expected to

- Recognize that patients have a right to appropriate assessment and management of pain.
- Assess the existence, nature, and intensity of pain in all patients.
- Facilitate regular reassessment and follow-up.
- Educate staff about pain management and assessment.

- Establish procedures that allow staff to appropriately prescribe effective pain medications.

- Educate patients and their families about effective pain management. Relaxation training, imagery distraction, calming self-statements, massage, and exercise are recognized as effective nonmedical methods of managing pain.

Summing Up

What Is Pain?

1. Pain involves our total experience in reacting to a damaging event, including the physical mechanism by which the body reacts; our subjective, emotional response (suffering); and our observable actions (pain behavior).

2. Pain is categorized in terms of its duration as acute, acute recurrent, chronic noncancer, and pain associated with a malignant disease process. The first two types are temporary; the others are long-lasting.

Measuring Pain

3. Researchers have tried unsuccessfully to develop objective, psychophysiological measures of pain. Because of pain's subjective nature, however, they have had to rely on behavioral measures, structured interviews, rating scales, and pain inventories such as the McGill Pain Questionnaire.

The Physiology of Pain

4. Pain typically begins when free nerve endings in the skin called nociceptors are stimulated. The nociceptors relay this input to fast nerve fibers that signal sharp, acute pain, or slow nerve fibers that signal slow, burning pain. Pain signals travel from these peripheral nerve fibers to the spinal cord, and from there to the thalamus, a message sorting station that relays the pain message to your cerebral cortex, the reasoning part of your brain. The cortex assesses the location and severity of damage.

5. Endorphins and enkephalins produced in the brain act as neurotransmitters and inhibit pain by acting on cells in the substantia gelatinosa of the spinal cord and the periacqueductal gray region of the brain.

6. The gate control theory suggests that a pain gate exists in the spinal cord. The pain gate may be closed by stimulation of the fast pain fiber system, whereas activity in the slow-pain system tends to open the gate. The gate may also be closed by the brain's descending pathway.

Psychosocial Factors in the Experience of Pain

7. The experience of pain is subject to a variety of psychosocial factors. Although older people and women are more likely to report higher levels of pain than younger people and men, the relationships among pain, gender, and aging are complex. They also may reflect faulty reasoning that tends to exaggerate the relatively few ways in which age groups, women, and men differ, while ignoring the greater number of ways in which they are similar.

8. Cultural differences in pain reactions are probably related to differences in pain tolerance, rather than differences in pain threshold. Although some researchers have reported ethnic differences in pain, others have found much greater variation among individual members within an ethnic group than variation between ethnic groups.

Treating Pain

9. The most common biomedical method of treating pain is the use of analgesic drugs, including opioids such as morphine. These centrally acting drugs stimulate endorphin receptors in the brain and spinal cord. A less addicting class of analgesics, the nonsteroidal anti-inflammatory drugs (NSAIDs), produce their pain-relieving effects by blocking the formation of prostaglandins at the site of injured tissue. Electrical stimulation techniques, such as TENS, deliver mild electrical impulses to close the pain gate in the spinal cord.

10. Efforts to find a pain-prone personality have generally been unsuccessful. There is some evidence that chronic

pain patients have elevated scores on MMPI subscales for hysteria, hypochondriasis, and depression.

11. The most successful pain treatment programs are multidisciplinary and combine the use of analgesic drugs with eclectic cognitive-behavioral programs. These programs use a mix of techniques to develop individualized pain-management programs, including cognitive restructuring of pain beliefs, distraction, imagery, and relaxation training.

12. Behavioral interventions rely on operant procedures to extinguish undesirable pain behaviors, while reinforcing more adaptive responses to chronic pain.

Key Terms and Concepts

clinical pain, p. 552
acute pain, p. 554
chronic pain, p. 555
hyperalgesia, p. 555
free nerve endings, p. 559
nociceptor, p. 560
fast nerve fibers, p. 560
slow nerve fibers, p. 560

substantia gelatinosa, p. 561
referred pain, p. 562
substance P, p. 562
enkephalins, p. 562
periacqueductal gray (PAG), p. 562
stress-induced analgesia (SIA), p. 563

naloxone, p. 564
gate control theory, p. 565
phantom limb pain, p. 568
nonsteroidal anti-inflammatory drugs (NSAIDs), p. 577
prostaglandin, p. 577

palliative care, p. 578
counterirritation, p. 578
transcutaneous electrical nerve stimulation (TENS), p. 578
cognitive-behavioral therapy (CBT), p. 580

Health Psychology on the World Wide Web

Web Address	Description
http://www.painfoundation.org	Web site of the American Pain Foundation.
http://www.theacpa.org	The American Chronic Pain Association.
http://www.headaches.org/	Web site of the National Headache Foundation.
http://www.wellweb.com/pain/pain.htm	The Wellness Web's pain-management site.

Critical Thinking Exercise

Acupuncture Pain Relief

Now that you have completed Chapter 13, take your learning a step further by testing your critical thinking skills on this scientific reasoning exercise.

Several studies suggest that acupuncture can be effective in relieving pain in some individuals. In one such study, pain was induced in a group of volunteer subjects by electrically stimulating a tooth (Mayer & Price, 1976). Each participant was asked to report the degree of pain experienced before receiving an acupuncture pain-control treatment and again after receiving the treatment. The results showed that acupuncture increased the participants' pain thresholds (the intensity of electrical stimulation needed to trigger pain) by 27 percent.

In the second part of the study, each participant received an injection of naloxone, the opioid-antagonist that reverses any form of analgesia resulting from endorphin production. Under the influence of naloxone, patients reported *increased* pain levels comparable to pretreatment levels.

1. State the researchers' research hypothesis in your own words. Identify the independent and dependent variables.

2. How did the researchers test their hypothesis? Was it a valid test? What would be an appropriate control group for this study?

3. In the second part of the study, why were the participants injected with naloxone? What possible explanation of the results in the first part of the study were the researchers testing?

4. What do the findings of the second part of the study suggest regarding how acupuncture might work to relieve pain?

5. What might be an alternative explanation for the results of this study?

14

Complementary and Alternative Medicine

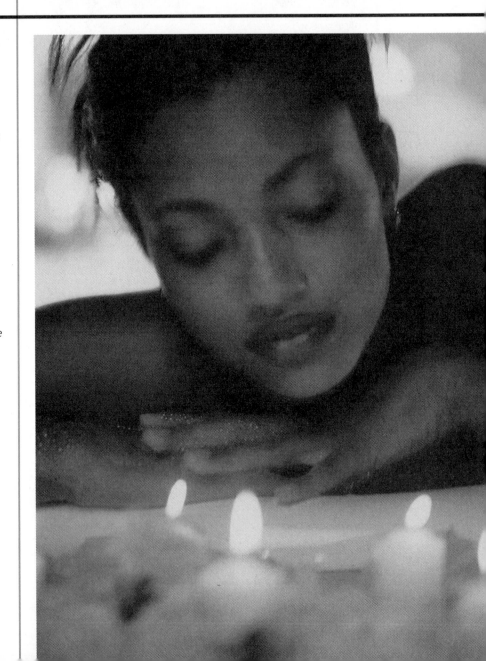

*I*magine that your vacation tour group is involved in a serious bus accident in a remote region. One member of your group has a deep cut in his arm that needs immediate attention. Another woman is delirious with pain and has a dangerously high fever. Unfortunately, you have no medical supplies and no cellular phone, and you haven't seen another vehicle on this desolate road all day. Fortunately, one of your traveling companions is a medical intern. Quickly taking charge of the seemingly hopeless situation, she cleanses your companion's wound with urine, sutures the edges together with safety pins, and suggests that the patient lick his wound to keep it moist as it heals. To treat the traveler with the high fever, she sterilizes the blade of a pocketknife with a lit match, cuts a vein in the woman's arm and drains about a cup of blood. Smiling as she finishes her work, the intern reassures your group that both "patients" will be fine.

This scenario sounds preposterous, doesn't it? It isn't. Just ask Michigan State physiology professor Robert Root-Bernstein, who explains that cleansing with urine and bloodletting are folk remedies that have been widely used throughout the world for hundreds, or even thousands, of years (Root-Bernstein & Root-Bernstein, 1997).

Staff at the National Institutes of Health estimate that less than one-third of the world's health care is delivered by allopathic, or biomedically trained, doctors and nurses. The remainder comes from self-care and nontraditional treatments. This may mean a trip to the acupuncturist, massage therapist, or chiropractor; on-line purchases of aromatherapy ingredients, herbal medicines, or megavitamins; or a daily hour of meditation.

A visit to any large bookstore reveals an abundance of books about nontraditional health care. Andrew Weil's books on alternative medicine continue to attract a huge audience, while holistic medicine guru Deepak Chopra's *Ageless Body, Timeless Mind* has sold more than 7 million copies since it was first published in 1993 (Ernst, 1996).

Celebrity accounts and personal testimonials on behalf of unconventional treatments contribute to the growing interest in such therapies. Perhaps best known was author and critic Norman Cousins' powerful description of his battle with an incurable illness. As you'll recall from the Critical Thinking Exercise in Chapter 5, Cousins attributed his successful recovery to his unconventional approach to healing: a program of massive doses of vitamin C and comedy movies. The success of his treatment led him to become a crusader for the view that "the hospital is no place for a person who is seriously ill" (Cousins, 1976). This grim warning took on new meaning in November 1999, when a scathing report by the National Academy of Sciences' Institute of Medicine indicated that medical errors kill 44,000 to 98,000 patients in United States hospitals each year, making these errors the eighth leading cause of death—ahead of highway accidents, breast cancer, and AIDS.

holistic medicine an approach to medicine that considers not only physical health but also the emotional, spiritual, social, and psychological well-being of the person

complementary and alternative medicine (CAM) the use and practice of therapies or diagnostic techniques that fall outside of conventional biomedicine

Despite the public's growing acceptance of nontraditional treatments, such methods are only slowly being integrated into "mainstream" medicine, if at all. In this chapter we take a careful look at unconventional health care, focusing on an *evidence-based analysis* (Spencer, 1999). This model assumes that nontraditional health interventions must be subjected to the same rigorous testing that traditional biomedical interventions are subjected to and that any alleged health benefits must have stood the test of standard scientific methodology.

What Is Complementary and Alternative Medicine?

Traditionally, the term *alternative medicine* has been used to identify a broad range of therapeutic approaches and philosophies that are generally defined as "treatments and health care practices not taught widely in medical schools, not generally used in hospitals, and not usually reimbursed by medical insurance companies" (NIH, 1998). A number of these approaches are also referred to as **holistic medicine,** which typically means that the practitioner considers the physical, mental, emotional, and spiritual needs of the whole client.

In earlier chapters, we discussed several relatively recent nontraditional therapies, including guided imagery, stress management, cognitive reappraisal, and other techniques that form the basis of health psychology interventions. In this chapter, we focus on nontraditional therapies that are commonly classified as alternative medicines: *acupuncture, mind–body therapies, chiropractic,* and *naturopathy.*

Establishing a Category for Nontraditional Medicine

Some "alternative" methods have been around far longer than antibiotic medicines, angioplasty, and other more recent biomedical therapies. For this reason, the term *alternative* hardly seems appropriate. A more appropriate term, recently coined by health care experts, is *complementary medicine,* which emphasizes that many "alternative medicines" are best used in conjunction with—rather than instead of—regular (or *allopathic*) medicine. For example, hypertension might be treated with a blood-pressure-lowering drug *and* relaxation training: the combined effect of the two interventions exceeds that of either the drug by itself or reduces the doses of the drug needed, thus minimizing any adverse side effects.

In this chapter, we will use the term **complementary and alternative medicine (CAM)** to refer to the range of health-promoting interventions and diagnostic therapies that may not be part of any current Western health care system, culture, or society (Spencer, 1999). Although these therapies all belong to the same category, they are not necessarily based on a common philosophy. In fact, they may have contradictory beliefs about the best way to heal. The Office of Alternative Medicine (OAM) at the National Institutes of Health has recently developed the classification scheme depicted in Table 14.1, which separates alternative medical health care practices into five major domains.

Navajo Healing
Complementary and alternative medicine (CAM) includes a wide variety of practices, some more or less accepted in Western civilization. Here a Navajo medicine person treats a patient with rocks and minerals, creating a sacred sand painting. © Martha Cooper/Peter Arnold, Inc.

Three Ideals of Complementary and Alternative Medicine

Despite the endless variety of alternative therapies, most forms of alternative medicine *do* share several features, which distinguish these interventions from traditional medicine. Most work from three fundamental ideals: to provide health treatment that is natural, that is holistic, and that promotes wellness.

Natural Medicine

For many people, the modern world has become too synthetic, too artificial, and too toxic. One person yearns for a closer connection to nature, another chooses to wear only "natural" cotton fibers, and a third grows her own herbs. This "back-to-nature" backlash is a fairly recent phenomenon. During most of

Table 14.1

Domains of Complementary and Alternative Medicine

Alternative medical systems	Complete health care systems that evolved independently of conventional biomedicine. Examples include traditional Oriental medicine, ayurveda, homeopathy, and medical systems developed by Native American, Aboriginal, African, Middle Eastern, and South American cultures.
Mind–body interventions	Techniques designed to affect the mind's capacity to influence bodily functions and symptoms. Examples include meditation, hypnosis, prayer, music and art therapy, and mental healing.
Biologically based therapies	Natural and biologically based interventions and products, often overlapping with conventional medicine's use of dietary supplements. Includes herbal and orthomolecular approaches, as well as special diets (e.g., Atkins, Ornish, Pritikin).
Manipulative and body-based methods	Using touch and manipulation with the hands as diagnostic and therapeutic tools. Includes chiropractic, osteopathy, and massage therapy.
Energy therapies	Focus either on energy fields originating within the body (biofields) or those from other sources (electromagnetic fields). Examples include Qi Gong, therapeutic touch, Reiki, and the use of magnets.

Source: National Center for Complementary and Alternative Medicine (http://nccam.nih.gov).

the twentieth century, the public seemed to have an undying faith in modern technology, science, and biomedicine.

Then, in the second half of the twentieth century evidence increasingly indicated that advances in health-related technology were not always healthy—and things began to change. Rachel Carson's 1962 book *Silent Spring* made the public aware of the potential harm of DDT, a chemical developed during World War II and introduced in the 1940s as a miraculous insecticide. After years of widespread aerial spraying of what was believed to be a harmless insecticide, Carson showed, and others confirmed, that the chemical was harming fish and birds by traveling up through the food chain. Ten years after Carson voiced her concerns, the U.S. government banned DDT and a growing public distrust of science was triggered.

Fueled by evidence of the hazards of DDT and other pesticides, artificial colors and sweeteners, the volatile chemicals given off by disposable diapers, and the environmental toxin du jour, the public's distrust of science has begun to extend to medicine. The growing popularity of CAM seems to indicate a growing desire for more "natural" treatments. Until quite recently, conventional medicine has done little to meet this apparent need. Indeed, as physician Steven Bratman (1997) notes: "Most medical doctors tend to feel an instinctive contempt for the very concept of 'natural' substances. The form of medicine they practice aims to correct nature's errors, guard against nature's dangers and supplement nature's weaknesses. To trust nature is not an ideal of conventional medicine."

Although the philosophy of a "natural" medicine inspires many CAM practitioners, it is a mistake to assume that all CAM therapists agree. Herbal therapy and massage certainly are natural, but some other popular alternative treatments are not. Consider chelation therapy. This controversial intervention involves injecting the synthetic chemical EDTA into the bloodstream as a treatment for angina and atherosclerosis.

Holistic Medicine

Complementary and alternative medicine also aims to avoid the narrow specialization of conventional biomedicine. As physician Patch Adams—a pioneer of holistic medicine—noted, "Treat a disease and you win or lose, treat the person and you win every time" (Adams & Mylander, 1998). Many patients seek out alternative care because they prefer to work with practitioners who will see (and treat) them as a whole person. Steven Bratman describes one extreme case of a man whose various symptoms eventually led to treatment by six medical specialists: a neurologist (for cognitive symptoms stemming from a stroke), an orthopedist (for bone degeneration), an ophthalmologist (for eye pain), a dermatologist (for skin lesions), a urologist (for bladder problems), a cardiologist (for heart valve leakage), and a dermatologist (for a skin rash). Until an elderly neighbor (who happened to be a retired general practitioner) realized that the seemingly independent symptoms were similar to the syphilis cases he had often seen 40 years earlier, no one suspected that a simple program of penicillin shots was all the man needed.

Specialization and fragmentation are predictable consequences of the analytical nature of biomedicine, which encourages doctors to focus on the fine details of the symptoms that each patient presents. As a backlash against the overspecialization of conventional medicine, many alternative practitioners broaden their analysis of each patient's complaints to examine diet, emotions, and lifestyle as well the specific symptoms of the disease or condition. This is especially true of traditional Chinese medicine, ayurveda, and homeopathy (a largely unproven system of so-called energy medicine developed in the nineteenth century by Samuel Hahnemann, which advocates such ideas as the "law of similars"—the most effective remedy for a particular disease is a minute quantity of the very substance that would trigger the disease's symptoms in a healthy person).

Promoting Wellness

Given Western biomedicine's historical focus on battling disease, it is understandable that the concept of wellness is too vague for medical science to rally around. Instead, biomedicine orbits around disease, while the primary focus of many alternative treatments is to strengthen the individual, even if the person currently has no serious symptoms.

Alternative practitioners believe that medication, surgery, and other mainstream interventions can fight illness but generally cannot produce an optimal state of healthy vitality. Indeed, although most medical interventions eliminate major symptoms, they often leave behind one or more adverse side effects, such as upset stomach or headache.

Many alternative treatments *do* make the person "feel like a million bucks," even if only temporarily. Acupuncture and massage therapy may produce feelings of relaxation; chiropractic generates a feeling of being energized. Whether these effects are due to positive suggestion, a placebo effect, or the patient's expectations doesn't matter—the patient still benefits. Furthermore, note CAM advocates, the same can be said of medication. Patients so strongly expect that certain treatments such as chemotherapy will make them feel ill that placebos trigger the same symptoms. While medication triggers expectations of illness, many alternative treatments connote a more pleasant, desirable state.

Complementary and alternative medicine is not so rigid that practitioners believe theirs is the only right way; many admit that both disease-focused and wellness-focused approaches are needed, depending on the circumstances. For many varieties of CAM, the concept of wellness is closely connected with belief in the existence of a "life energy" or "vital force," known as **vitalism.** In **traditional Oriental medicine,** as you'll recall from Chapter 1, the life force of *qi* (pronounced *chee* in Chinese and *kee* in Japanese) is believed to flow through every cell of the body. Acupuncture, herbal therapy, and other interventions supposedly restore vitality by correcting blockages, deficiencies, and isolated excesses of qi.

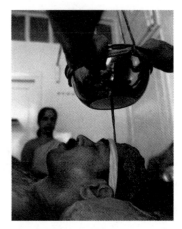

Ayurvedic Heat Treatments In ayurveda, the practitioner emphasizes treatment of the whole person, including diet, emotions, and lifestyle as well as the specific symptoms of the disease or disorder. The patient in this photo is receiving ayurvedic oils and massage to improve blood circulation at a clinic in New Delhi, India. John Moore / The Image Works

■ **vitalism** the concept of a general life force, popular in some varieties of complementary and alternative medicine

■ **traditional Oriental medicine** an ancient, integrated herb- and acupuncture-based system of healing founded on the principle that internal harmony is essential for good health

How Widespread Is Complementary and Alternative Medicine?

According to a recent report in the *Journal of the American Medical Association*, four out of ten Americans use some form of CAM (Jonas, 1996). Americans visited alternative therapy practitioners some 629 million times in 1997, a 47 percent increase over 1990, and spent approximately $27 billion out-of-pocket dollars on alternative therapies—just about as much as they spent on all physician services the same year (Hwang & Molter, 1998). Even holistic veterinarians for pets are cropping up! The most commonly reported alternative therapy is chiropractic, followed by massage therapy, herbal medicine, taking megavitamins, and meditation.

CAM appears to be used most often by 25- to 49-year-olds, primarily for back problems, anxiety, depression, and headaches. Asked why they chose an alternative treatment, respondents to one major survey said they believed that they could achieve faster results if they combined alternative and traditional medicine (72 percent did not tell their physician). Others said they simply wanted to try every available option to boost their health. Many reported that alternative practitioners were better listeners, and the respondents appreciated the extra time these practitioners were likely to give to them (Eisenberg et al., 1998).

Some researchers think that the statistics on the popularity of CAM are overblown. For example, another study (Druss & Rosenheck, 1999) reported that during 1996, an estimated 6.5 percent of the U.S. population used both CAM and conventional medical care; 1.8 percent used only CAM services; 59.5 percent used only conventional care; and 32.2 percent used neither. The different figures may be due to several factors. For one, the 1999 study included only questions on practitioner-based therapies. For another, unlike the earlier telephone survey, the 1999 study included non-English speakers and households without telephones. Because less educated and poorer individuals generally use fewer unconventional medical services than the general population, this may have affected the survey results (Paramore, 1997). The use of CAM is even more common throughout Europe and Asia. For example, between 20 and 50 percent of adult Europeans use CAM therapies; in the Netherlands and Belgium consumer surveys indicate usages as high as 60 percent (Fisher & Ward, 1994).

The use of unconventional medical therapies is increasing throughout the world. Even more important, the perceived effectiveness of CAM therapies seems to be increasing, among both the general public and traditional allopathic physicians. A meta-analysis of 12 separate surveys of physicians' perceptions of the effectiveness of CAM therapies, conducted throughout Europe and the Middle East, indicated that CAM therapies were considered to be at least moderately effective (Ernst, Resch, & White, 1995).

Medicine or Quackery?

Many of the same trends that led to the emergence of health psychology have also fueled increasing interest in alternative forms of medicine. These trends include increasing public concern about

- the costly and impersonal nature of modern medical care.
- adverse effects of treatment.
- the seemingly profit-driven nature of health care and medical research that ignores unpatentable (and unprofitable) treatment options, such as herbal medicines.

Ironically, the surge in popularity of CAM is also due, at least in part, to the success of Western biomedicine. Although people living in developed countries are less likely to die from infectious diseases such as smallpox, as average life expectancy has increased, so too have the rates of chronic diseases for which biomedicine has, as of yet, no cure. CAM therapies give people something else to try as they battle such diseases and strive to increase their *average health expectancy* (see Chapter 15).

Finally, the "doctor knows best" attitude, which has dominated patient–provider relations, seems to be giving way to a more activist, consumer-oriented view of the patient's role. This, coupled with the growing public distrust of the scientific outlook and a reawakening of interest in mysticism and spiritualism, has given strong impetus to the CAM movement.

What Constitutes Evidence?

CAM advocates and conventional physicians and scientists differ most in their views of what constitutes an acceptable research design and which kinds of evidence are needed to demonstrate effectiveness. Biomedical researchers demand evidence from controlled clinical trials, in which hypothesis testing and scientific reasoning are used to tease apart the individual pathogens that cause disease and isolate the treatments that are clinically effective in eradicating or controlling the pathogens (Spencer, 1999). CAM practitioners, whose therapies are based on a more holistic philosophy, claim that treatment variables cannot always be studied independently. A case in point is the testing of herbal remedies. Under the direction and regulation of the FDA, biomedical researchers developing new medications must isolate the active agent in a drug before it can be approved for human trials. But many practitioners of herbal medicine claim that certain tonics and combinations of plant medicines are effective precisely *because* of the interactions among the various substances. According to this view, any attempt to isolate one ingredient from another would render the treatment useless.

I've been told to see a chiropractor, to have my liver flushed out, and to drink hydrogen peroxide! My doctor muttered a nasty word when I said I planned to try alternative medicine. She told me it was all garbage. I'd believe her except for one thing: I'm in pain, and her treatments are not helping me.

—A lower back pain patient

As a result of such differences in perspective, many alternative practitioners are willing to endorse interventions even when the evidence backing their claims is far from convincing based on conventional standards of scientific reasoning. Health food stores, for example, have shelf after shelf of impressive-sounding literature that is largely unsupported. As always, one should keep this in mind when evaluating statements made by alternative practitioners (see Reality Check).

Biomedical researchers and CAM advocates also differ on the importance of pinpointing causation and isolating the mechanisms of how a therapy works. CAM advocates see this as an unproductive exercise. More important to them is finding a technique or medicine that works and helping people to improve their lives.

Finally, the two groups differ in their focus. Rather than just seeking to remove a pathogen or to "cure" a physical condition, as biomedical practitioners do, CAM therapists emphasize the overall quality of a patient's life, broadening their focus to include important psychological, social, emotional, and spiritual aspects. Consequently, many CAM studies appear unfocused, do not use hy-

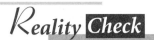

Reality Check

Patient, Heal Thyself . . . But Be Careful!

CAM guru Andrew Weil believes taking control of your daily lifestyle is the key to good health (Lemley, 1999). How many of Weil's lifestyle tips do you practice?

- Throw out all oils other than olive oil, all artificial sweeteners containing saccharin or aspartame, and all products containing artificial coloring.
- Keep flowers in your home.
- Eat whole grains.
- Substitute green tea for coffee or black tea.
- Do periodic "news fasts." Do not read, watch, or listen to the news for one day.
- Take vitamin C, 250 milligrams twice daily; vitamin E, 400 international units daily if you are under 40, 800 if you are over 40; selenium, 200 to 300 micrograms daily; mixed carotenes, 25,000 international units daily.
- Never drink any water that tastes of chlorine. Never use hot tap water for drinking or cooking.
- Buy or grow organically produced fruits and vegetables. Be wary of pesticide-laden strawberries, bell peppers, spinach, cherries, peaches, celery, apples, apricots, green beans, grapes, and cucumbers.
- Make a list of friends who make you feel more alive and happy. Spend time with one of them this week.

- Eat at least two meals of fish and two of soy protein weekly.
- Eat more garlic.
- Observe a moment of gratitude for your food before your meals, in any way that you find comfortable.
- For five minutes daily, sit quietly and observe your breathing.
- Volunteer for a few hours at a hospital or charitable organization.
- Reach out and connect with someone from whom you are estranged.
- Walk for exercise, building up to 45 minutes, five days a week.

Choosing an Alternative Practitioner Weil's critics argue that this litany of directives is based on evidence that is at best mixed, and at worst, faulty or nonexistent. Therefore, before you make any major change in your health-related lifestyle (other than avoiding documented pathogens, high-risk behaviors, and other hazards), it is a good idea to consult your family physician. You should also do some research on your own, perhaps by seeking out illness-related self-help groups, books on alternative treatments, and family or friends with similar needs. In addition, you should fully investigate the background and experience of any alternative health practitioner whom you are considering consulting and be aware of any licensing requirements in your state. Above all, be suspicious of anyone who makes grandiose claims that he or she can cure you or that you will never be sick again. Also steer clear of anyone who expresses hostility or derision toward conventional medicine. Good practitioners understand that every therapy has its limitations and may not be the best medicine for every patient, even those with the same symptoms. Above all, remember that you are in charge of the treatment process.

NIH's Office of Alternative Medicine and the Mayo Clinic offer several guidelines for people who are considering the use of complementary and alternative therapies:

- *Get the facts.* Seek out credible sources of information about the safety and effectiveness of treatment before trying it. Credible sources of information include the published findings of scientific research in peer-reviewed scholarly journals. Too many consumers fail to realize that if a neighbor says a treatment worked, that does not constitute proof.

- *Examine the practitioner's expertise.* Consumers should examine the background, qualifications, and competence of any health care practitioner. They may do so by contacting a local regulatory agency or the appropriate state licensing board. Many alter-

native therapies have national organizations that will direct consumers to the appropriate agencies and even provide referrals. Talking with those who have had experience with a practitioner, including other health practitioners and patients, is also a good idea.

- *Consider the service delivery.* NIH recommends a visit to the practitioner's office or clinic to determine how, and under what conditions, the treatment is given. The primary issue is whether the service delivery follows regulated standards for medical safety and care.

- *Consider the costs.* Many alternative treatments are not covered by health insurance. Checking with several practitioners to find out what they charge for a certain treatment will help the consumer determine whether costs are appropriate.

- *Consult your health care provider.* Both traditional and nontraditional health care practitioners agree that too many people seek alternative forms of treatment without informing their doctors. Doing so is dangerous, because some treatments may actually worsen medical problems. Or there may be a toxic interaction between prescription and natural remedies. Furthermore, even if a supplement or some other treatment is fundamentally safe, there remains the danger that the person has misdiagnosed the condition. Competent health care management requires knowledge of the "complete picture" of a person's treatment.

pothesis testing or large samples, and tend to rely more on verbal reports from patients. It is not surprising that the quality of CAM studies, as judged by Western scientists, is considered poor (Patel, 1987).

For example, the Office of Alternative Medicine and the National Institutes of Health recently convened a panel to evaluate the quality of research on acupuncture (NIH, 1998). They found that needle acupuncture was effective for postoperative pain, dental pain, chemotherapy-induced nausea and vomiting, and for the nausea associated with pregnancy. In addition, acupuncture produced fewer adverse side effects than many drugs do. Despite these conclusions, however, overall the panel found the literature to be "mixed" regarding outcomes, and in many cases determination was impossible because of poor study design.

Participant Selection and Outcome Measures

As noted in Chapter 2, scientists have established specific criteria for the proper design of a clinical trial. Besides the obvious need to use the scientific

■ **anecdotal evidence** research evidence based on informal case histories, in which there is little or no objective documentation regarding a patient's diagnosis or the effectiveness of a treatment

method, researchers must begin by selecting large, representative samples of research participants, grouped by gender, age, socioeconomic status, and similarity of medical condition. These people are then randomly assigned to groups so that each has an equal chance of either receiving or not receiving the treatment of interest.

For both practical and ethical reasons, however, randomized clinical trials sometimes present problems for medical researchers, especially for CAM researchers. Many CAM trials include too few people in a group to allow researchers to determine whether results are statistically significant or due to chance alone. Furthermore, CAM practitioners often find it difficult (or morally unacceptable) to persuade volunteers to participate in a study in which they may be "randomized" into a no-treatment control group. For this reason, CAM evidence is often based on informal case studies. This type of **anecdotal evidence,** based as it is on subjective opinions regarding diagnosis and treatment outcomes, does little to advance the credibility of certain unconventional treatments (see Critical Thinking Exercise on page 635).

Another weakness in CAM research is the use of incomplete, biased, or invalidated treatment outcome measures (Spencer, 1999). Many CAM studies rely on self-report. Although within certain guidelines, self-report can yield useful information, skeptics are naturally concerned about the truthfulness of self-report data. Answers can be influenced by the research participants' desire to please the researchers, to appear "normal," and even to persuade themselves that they are experiencing symptom relief. This criticism is made all the more important by the fact that CAM studies too often rely on single-outcome measures rather than on several different measures that might, or might not, provide converging lines of evidence. The NIH panel evaluating research on acupuncture, for example, concluded that there were few acceptable studies comparing the effectiveness of acupuncture with either placebo or sham controls and so encouraged future researchers to provide accurate description of protocols for the types and number of treatments, subject enrollment procedures, and methods of diagnosing outcomes (NIH, 1998).

Participant Expectancy and the Placebo Effect

Medical students are often taught the story of "Mr. Wright," a California cancer patient who, in 1957, was given only a few days to live. After hearing that scientists had discovered that a horse serum, called *Krebiozen,* might be effective against cancer, he begged his doctor to receive it. Reluctantly, the patient's physician gave Mr. Wright an injection. Three days later, the disbelieving doctor found that the patient's golf-ball-sized tumors "had melted like snowballs on a hot stove." Two months later, after reading a medical report that the serum was, in fact, a quack remedy, Mr. Wright suffered an immediate relapse and died.

Although many doctors dismiss this story as an anecdote, researchers have long recognized that part of medicine's power to heal is derived from the expectations both patients and practitioners bring to therapy. Whenever patients are treated for an illness or health condition, any improvement may be due to one of four explanations:

- The treatment may actually be effective.

- The illness simply improved on its own over time. This is true of most illnesses, including pain.

- The patient was misdiagnosed and in fact did not have an illness.

- Patients improve on their own simply because they think someone is doing something for them (**Hawthorne effect**) or because of some nonspecific effect, such as a positive attitude that the treatment will be beneficial (*placebo effect*).

As you'll recall from Chapter 1, a placebo is typically a sham treatment or physiologically inert substance that a physician administers to placate an anxious or persistent patient. Placebos have been shown to successfully treat a variety of conditions, including headache, anxiety, hypertension, cancer, and depression. By one estimate, placebos are about 55 to 60 percent as effective for controlling pain as active drugs such as aspirin and codeine (Talbot, 2000). One review of placebo-controlled studies of antidepressant drugs reported that placebos and genuine drugs were equally effective (Blakeslee, 1998). Placebos can work for years, reducing symptoms as long as the patient believes they will do so.

Who responds best to a placebo? Knowing that in any study from 30 to 70 percent of patients will respond positively to placebos, researchers have attempted to identify characteristics such as gender, personality, or attitude that predict which subjects are most likely to be "placebo responders." So far, their efforts have been unsuccessful (Spencer, 1999). However, one intriguing aspect of the placebo effect is that a person who responds well to one CAM therapy will most likely respond favorably to other CAM treatments or to that treatment for other problems. Discussing this phenomenon among acupuncture *responders,* medical researcher Steven Bratman (1997) notes, "It is as if some people have the words *acupuncture me* written on their foreheads in invisible ink."

Why do placebos work? Alternative explanations are that placebos may operate by decreasing anxiety (Evans, 1974) or through classical conditioning (Vincent & Furnham, 1997). According to the conditioning explanation, the medical treatments we receive over the course of our lives are like conditioning trials. The physician's white coat, the disinfectant smell of a waiting room, the prick of a needle, and the taste and texture of each pill that is swallowed function as *conditioned stimuli* (see Chapter 1). Over the years, as each stimulus is paired with the biological impact of active drug ingredients (and other therapeutic outcomes), expectations of improvement become stronger and stronger. Later, when given a pill without active ingredients, or some other

Hawthorne effect the phenomenon in which patients improve on their own simply because they think someone is doing something for them

sham treatment, we may still experience a therapeutic benefit as a *conditioned response* to the same medical stimuli.

Herbert Benson (1996) has suggested that "remembered wellness" is another conditioned factor in placebo responding. After any therapeutic intervention, he suggests, we have a memory of past events, which helps to trigger a beneficial physical response. According to Benson, the quieting of the mind and body that accompanies relaxation is a good way to access this remembered wellness. Indeed, as we noted in Chapter 5, relaxation has proved effective in reducing a variety of physiological responses, including muscle tension, heart rate, and blood pressure, and thus in treating anxiety, pain, headaches, and a number of other illnesses.

A closely related explanation is that placebos tap into the body's natural "inner pharmacy" of self-healing substances (Brody, 2000). As we discussed in Chapter 13, researchers strongly suspect that at least part of placebo-based pain relief occurs because placebos stimulate the release of endorphins, morphine-like neurotransmitters produced by the brain (Amanzio & Benedetti, 1999). Placebos may also reduce levels of cortisol, norepinephrine, and other stress hormones.

While any medical procedure—from drugs to surgery—can have a placebo effect, critics contend that CAM is entirely placebo-based. When conventional therapies fail to help, the acupuncturist, chiropractor, or herbalist presents a powerful belief system designed to give the suffering patient hope that help is available. Some critics note that placebos are not nearly as effective as they are believed to be. For example, as noted in Chapter 13, a controversial meta-analysis by Danish researchers found little evidence that placebos had powerful effects other than reducing patients' reports of pain and other subjective symptoms (Hrobjartsson & Gotzche, 2001). Other researchers contend, however, that the methodology from this study makes the results suspect, since meta-analysis pools data from unrelated health conditions and widely differing protocols (D. Moerman, personal communication, 2001).

It is ironic that biomedicine's insistence on rigorous standards of scientific "proof" of the efficacy of a new drug or alternative therapy may have actually provided the strongest testimony for the prevalence of the placebo effect. That is, "scientific proof" requires the use of a double-blind, randomized controlled trial (see Chapter 2). The method is based on the premise that if either the patient or the researcher knows which treatment is "supposed to work," it would indeed work. That is, the working assumption is that the placebo effect occurs routinely (Goldstein, 1999).

Safety Issues

Another concern about the use of alternative medical systems is that most such therapies are not backed by research that measures safety. For example, unlike drugs that are regulated by the U.S. Food and Drug Administration (FDA), herbal remedies are not monitored as an industry. Many people wrongly assume that over-the-counter products are safe, that they are not strong enough to do serious damage. However, some therapies may have dangerous side effects. Certain herbal preparations have been found to contain potentially harmful substances such as mercury, lead, and arsenic, although typically in small amounts.

Another safety concern is that people who rely on alternative treatments such as herbal medicine may delay or lose the opportunity to benefit from scientifically based treatment (Hwang & Molter, 1998). This strategy can be particularly dangerous, especially for high-risk individuals, such as pregnant women. For example, while small doses of the herbs ephedra and kava root are sometimes used in cold remedies, both are stimulants that can increase heart rate and cause shortness of breath, which may be hazardous to the developing fetus. Similarly, although small amounts of ginger are often used to quell morning sickness, larger amounts may be harmful, especially during the first three months of pregnancy, when the baby's major organs are developing rapidly (Lynne, 1999). For this reason, physicians recommend that pregnant women not take any medications or herbal remedies during their first trimester.

acupuncture a component of traditional Oriental medicine in which fine needles are inserted into the skin in order to relieve pain, treat addiction and illness, and promote health

Does It Work?

How good is complementary and alternative medicine? What works and what doesn't? In this section we will try to answer these questions for several of the most widely used alternative treatments: acupuncture, mind–body therapies, chiropractic, and naturopathic medicine.

Acupuncture

Acupuncture was first practiced during the Bronze Age in ancient China as part of an integrated system of healing that was founded on the principle that internal harmony is essential for good health (see Chapter 1). In the West, it was recognized only 100 years ago (Lytle, 1993). Although Asian-Americans have a long history with acupuncture, general interest in acupuncture in the United States did not increase until 1972, when a *New York Times* correspondent underwent an emergency operation in China and was later treated with acupuncture for complications. Since then, acupuncture schools have begun springing up and there are now about 12,000 acupuncturists in the United States.

An acupuncture session typically begins with the acupuncturist asking a series of questions concerning the patient's physical, emotional, and environmental background. The practitioner may then examine the patient's tongue, take

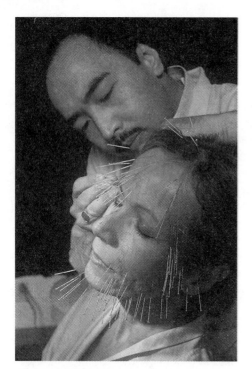

Acupuncture
Acupuncture, originally practiced in China only, has become increasingly popular throughout Western industrialized nations. It has proved most successful in treating pain, although practitioners contend that it rejuvenates the body. © J. P. Laffont/Corbis Sygma

his or her pulse, and/or palpate the abdomen. Based on the examination and detailed information about the patient's complaint, the acupuncturist formulates a plan for treating the patient. Treatment may involve inserting thin acupuncture needles superficially or as deep as one or more inches, depending on the particular site and the practitioner's style of treatment. Which of the approximately 2,000 acupuncture points are selected, along with the angle and depth of the needle insertion, varies with the symptom. Needles are sometimes twirled, heated, or electrically stimulated to maximize their effect. Acupuncturists often also incorporate herbal medicine and dietary recommendations in their treatment regimen—two other common components of traditional Oriental medicine.

In many instances, the effects of acupuncture are not immediate. Patients may not experience any improvement for a day or more or until they have undergone several treatments. With most chronic pain conditions, patients improve—if at all—after six sessions. More important, this improvement may last for weeks, months, or even years after treatment is discontinued.

How Is Acupuncture Supposed to Work?

The honest answer to this question is that no one really knows. Some advocates claim that acupuncture works by stimulating nerves, triggering the release of endorphins, or triggering skin resistance changes, but these explanations are nothing more than mere speculation.

Traditional acupuncturists believe that every part of the body corresponds to the whole, whether it's the ear or the sole of the foot. Classical acupuncture theory identifies 14 "lines of energy (qi)" on the body, called *meridians.* Most acupuncture points, believed to allow for corrections of blockages or deficiencies in qi, lie on these meridians. Treatment typically involves inserting one or more needles at a point at one end of a meridian to produce effects at the other end. Early researchers attempted to match the meridian lines with physical structures in the body, but they were unsuccessful.

But many conventional doctors, including those who practice acupuncture, find it hard to accept the concept of an invisible energy path, or qi, preferring instead to explain any treatment success as an example of the placebo effect. Others maintain that the pain of inserting acupuncture needles simply distracts the patient from his or her original pain, or that acupuncture triggers the release of the body's own natural painkillers (endorphins) and anti-inflammatory agents. None of these explanations, however, is widely accepted.

For a time, many acupuncturists latched onto an explanation that acupuncture works by affecting the electrical resistance of the skin. Some even use a *galvanometer*—a machine that measures skin conductivity—to pinpoint acupuncture sites where skin resistance is lower. However, because these devices are often unreliable, practitioners typically locate the points visually or by patient reactivity, that is, their sensitivity to pressure (Mclellan, Grossman, Blaine, & Haverkos, 1993).

Today, using tools such as functional magnetic resonance imaging (fMRI), researchers are probing the brain in search of specific acupuncture sites and effects. Comparing brain images of 12 chronic pain sufferers before and after acupuncture treatment (Hui et al., 2000), they have found that acupuncture needle manipulation at a point on the hand between the thumb and forefinger produced prominent decreases of neural activity in the nucleus accumbens, amygdala, hippocampus, and hypothalamus. These results suggest that acupuncture-induced analgesia may result from activation of descending pain pathways and other brain structures that modulate the perception of pain (see Chapters 3 and 13).

How Well Does Acupuncture Work?

Traditionally, acupuncture has been used to treat many different health conditions, including arthritis, asthma, athletic injuries, back problems, depression, headache, insomnia, sinusitis, stress, and even hemorrhoids. Use of acupuncture is also expanding to treat addictions and obesity and to assist recovery after surgery or stroke.

While acupuncture is often used for a wide range of medical conditions in China, in the United States its acceptance by allopathic physicians—if at all—is nearly always for the treatment of pain or addiction. Indeed, many chronic pain patients find some relief from acupuncture, escaping the adverse side effects that many prescription and nonprescription painkillers cause, including gastrointestinal bleeding and liver or kidney problems. Similarly, many substance abusers find relief from painful withdrawal symptoms through acupuncture.

Acupuncture is among the most heavily researched of the CAM therapies. Thousands of studies have been conducted, but many of them have been uncontrolled, have used sample sizes that were too small, or have been otherwise methodologically unsound.

As we saw in Chapter 2, the only scientific way to determine the effectiveness of interventions such as acupuncture is through controlled studies. But such studies are difficult to perform for several reasons: First, the highly individualized nature of acupuncture does not lend itself well to standardized tests. Acupuncturists themselves disagree about the appropriate acupuncture needle sites for a given medical condition. If you ask 10 acupuncturists to identify the appropriate needle sites for sinusitis, you are likely to get 10 different responses. Because some studies allow acupuncturists to choose their own points of stimulation, to control the number of sessions, and to use electrical stimulation if desired, it is very difficult for researchers to isolate independent variables or to compare study results.

A second problem is that researchers have had difficulty choosing appropriate nontreatment controls. For example, if the only reason an acupuncture treatment works is because the irritation of having needles stuck into the skin distracts the patient from the pain, then a placebo control must involve the same level of irritation. But in several trials where acupuncturists pretended to insert the needles into control subjects (by pressing the tubes that encase the needles onto their skin), most of the patients later reported that they could tell when the needles were actually inserted (Tashkin et al., 1985).

Double-blind controls, the mainstay of clinical trials, are even more problematic. Needles can be inserted at points that are inappropriate to a patient's health problem, making the patient blind to treatment, but the acupuncturist has to know whether the points are sham or real, so the study can't be double-blind. In one clever study, one acupuncturist diagnosed the patient's condition and another acupuncturist, who was unaware of the diagnosis, inserted the needles *where the first acupuncturist instructed.* In some patients, the needles were inserted into appropriate points that matched the diagnosis; in others, the needles were inserted into sham sites (Warwick-Evans, Masters, & Redstone, 1991).

Research trials that use sham acupuncture often show that it has some effect—in some cases, an effect as strong as genuine acupuncture (Fugh-Berman, 1997). Needless to say, the idea that stabbing patients at random points may be nearly as effective as using real acupuncture points is quite disturbing to acupuncturists who spend years memorizing the location of qi meridians and acupuncture points.

Yet another difficulty is that operational definitions of successful acupuncture treatments have been inconsistent at best, woefully vague at worst. In the case of addiction research, success has variously been defined as complete abstinence, decreased use, decreased cravings, diminished withdrawal symptoms, improved outlook, and increased productivity (Culliton, Boucher, & Bullock, 1999). Thus, one may report an intervention as successful because substance use decreased overall even though more than half the participants relapsed, while another may report similar findings as indicating a failed intervention. Such variations make it impossible to compare one study to another.

Acupuncture and Pain

An estimated 137 randomized clinical trials testing acupuncture's effectiveness on 10 painful conditions have been conducted. These studies provide evidence, although not statistically conclusive, that acupuncture provides *some* patients with *some* relief from painful conditions such as osteoarthritis (Dickens & Lewith, 1989), back pain (Coan, Wong, & Coan, 1980), migraine headaches (Vincent, 1989), painful menstrual cycles (Helms, 1987), tennis elbow (Brattberg, 1983), and postoperative dental pain (Richardson & Vincent, 1986).

One randomized controlled trial divided 50 patients with chronic lower back pain into two groups: an *immediate-treatment* group that received acupuncture right away and a *delayed-treatment group* that received its acupuncture several days later (Coan et al., 1980). The results showed that 83 percent of the immediate-treatment patients improved, experiencing, on average, half the pretreatment level of pain; only one-third of the delayed-treatment group improved immediately; and one-fourth got worse. Later, when the delayed-treatment group received acupuncture, 75 percent improved.

A meta-analysis of 14 controlled trials of acupuncture for chronic pain found that the results favored acupuncture (Patel, Gutzwiller, Paccaud, & Marazzi, 1989). Another meta-analysis of 51 controlled trials, however, found mixed results, leading the authors to conclude that the efficacy of acupuncture is not proved in the medical literature (ter Riet, Kleijnen, & Knipschild, 1990).

In a study to evaluate acupuncture's effectiveness in treating chronic migraine headaches, 30 patients received either real acupuncture or sham acupuncture (Vincent, 1989). Real acupuncture was significantly more effective in reducing pain and medication use than was sham acupuncture, and these effects lasted for over 1 year. However, in another study migraine patients were treated with either acupuncture or a placebo control. No statistically significant difference was found (Dowson, Lewith, & Machin, 1985). Again, the results are mixed.

Acupuncture has been tested in a number of studies of osteoarthritis pain, also with mixed results. In one retrospective study of acupuncture for knee joint pain, 75 percent of patients reported reduced pain (Zwolfer, Grubhofer, Cartellieri, & Sapcek, 1992). In a randomized, wait-list controlled trial, 29 patients with osteoarthritis of the knee reported significant pain reduction and increased joint mobility following acupuncture, as well as a $63,000 cost savings because they no longer needed surgery (Christensen, Iuhl, & Vilbeck, 1992). However, in two separate control trials comparing the effects of acupuncture and sham acupuncture, both were found to be equally effective (Eriksson, Lundeberg, & Lundeberg, 1991; Thomas, Eriksson, & Lundeberg, 1991).

Acupuncture and Addiction

Excluding 12-step programs, acupuncture is the most widely used CAM method for the treatment of substance abuse. It is especially useful in treating addiction to tobacco, alcohol, heroin, and cocaine. In fact, some drug courts mandate its use for the treatment of offenders (Culliton et al., 1999).

In 1985, the epidemic of crack cocaine use and an intensified search for a "magic bullet" to treat substance-abuse disorders led to formation of the National Acupuncture Detoxification Association (NADA). Since that time, NADA trainers have taught more than 4,000 acupuncturists, counselors, nurses, and physicians in the United States how to use acupuncture to treat substance abuse. As a result, there are now an estimated 700 to 1,000 chemical-dependency programs that use acupuncture for the treatment of addiction (Culliton et al., 1999).

Patients typically receive treatment in a group setting, seated in large chairs with arms and high backs to provide support. Soothing lighting, soft music, and herbal teas often accompany the session. Both ears are swabbed with alcohol, after which five $\frac{1}{2}$-inch sterilized disposable needles are placed into specific sites along the outer ear (auricular acupuncture). At the end of the 40-minute session the needles are removed.

In traditional biomedicine, substance-abuse intervention occurs in stages, with different drugs being used to help patients during withdrawal and rehabilitation and then for relapse prevention. In the earliest CAM interventions with substance abusers, acupuncture was initially used only during the detoxification stage in order to help patients cope with withdrawal. Today, however, its use often extends into the rehabilitation stage. The goals of acupuncture treatment include reducing the symptoms of withdrawal, including drug craving, keeping abusers in treatment programs, and continued abstinence from drug use.

As with other conditions, evidence regarding the effectiveness of acupuncture in treating substance abusers is mixed at best (Fugh-Berman, 1997). For example, by traditional methods, withdrawal from chronic use of prescribed opiate painkillers such as morphine or Demerol typically takes 3 to 6 months. In an uncontrolled trial involving electrical stimulation at ear acupuncture points, 12 of 14 chronic-pain patients (86%) were able to withdraw completely from narcotics within 2 to 7 days, apparently with few adverse withdrawal effects (Kroening & Oleson, 1985).

Similarly, two *controlled* studies on the treatment of alcohol recidivism—one with 80 patients and another with 54 patients—found that acupuncture treatment was more effective than sham treatment in reducing cravings for alcohol, drinking episodes, and treatment readmissions for detoxification (Bullock, Culliton, & Olander, 1989; Bullock, Umen, Culliton, & Olander, 1987). In the second study, these effects were maintained over a 6-month follow-up: The placebo group had more than twice the number of drinking episodes and readmissions to detoxification centers.

A recent 8-week Yale medical school study reported that acupuncture is an effective treatment for cocaine and heroin addiction (Avants, Margolin, Holford, & Kosten, 2000). The participants received individual and group counseling and were divided into three groups: an intervention group that received auricular acupuncture; a control group that received acupuncture in other points along the outer ear believed to have no treatment effect; and a second control group that viewed videotapes depicting relaxing images, such as nature scenes. Of those who received auricular acupuncture treatments along with counseling, 53.8 percent tested free of cocaine during the last week of the treatment and had longer periods of sustained abstinence, compared with 23.5 percent and 9.1 percent in the two control groups.

On the other hand, two recent studies of acupuncture treatment for cocaine addiction reported negative results (Bullock, Kiresuk, & Pheley, 1999). The first study randomly assigned 236 residential abusers to true, sham, or conventional treatment. The second applied true acupuncture to 202 randomly selected clients at three dose levels (8, 16, or 28 treatments). Overall, the true, sham, and conventional groups did not differ significantly on any outcomes, including abstinence, retention, and mood.

Despite the inconsistency of research evidence for acupuncture's effectiveness, acupuncture's success rate is among the highest of all alternative medical interventions and for some individuals it compares favorably with conventional treatments.

Dangers of Acupuncture

Acupuncture is generally considered quite safe because serious adverse effects are rare. Because disposable needles are used, there is little risk of infection, HIV transmission, or hepatitis. Occasionally, small bruises or bleeding may occur when a careless acupuncturist pierces a blood vessel.

As with all forms of CAM, one danger is that acupuncture patients may abandon conventional therapy and, in so doing, not receive a needed biomedical diagnosis or intervention. Although some alternative practitioners have been accused of discouraging their patients from using conventional treatment, this rarely seems to be the case with acupuncturists, who are generally quite respectful of conventional medicine (Brody, 1998).

Currently, 35 states and the District of Columbia have established clinical practice standards for acupuncturists. These are official statements from professional societies and government agencies that either describe how to care for patients with specific health conditions or illustrate specific techniques. Practitioners who have met these standards are "licensed" or "certified" by the *National Certification Commission for Acupuncture and Oriental Medicine.*

In 1996, the FDA classified acupuncture needles as a type of medical device, boosting the credibility of acupuncturists and increasing the likelihood that an insurance provider will pay for acupuncture treatments. Although the American Medical Association does not officially sanction acupuncture, more than 2,000 of the 12,000 acupuncturists in the United States are M.D.s. As another sign of growing recognition, the World Health Organization has identified some 50 diseases for which it considers acupuncture an appropriate treatment.

Mind–Body Therapies

The basic premise of mind–body therapies is that cognitive, emotional, and spiritual factors can have profound effects on one's health (McGrady & Horner, 1999). In this section, we'll examine three of the most popular mind–body therapies: hypnosis, relaxation and meditation (including tai chi and yoga), and spiritual healing.

Hypnotherapy

In Chapter 5, we discussed hypnosis as a means of treating stress-related problems. Hypnosis is even more often used to treat pain. Depending on the hypnotherapist, a variety of cognitive processes may come into play during a session of hypnosis, including focused attention, relaxation, imagery, expectation, and role-playing. The most salient feature of hypnosis is the *hypnotic trance,* which is a waking state of attentive and focused concentration in which the subject becomes detached from his or her surroundings and becomes absorbed by the hypnotist's *suggestions* that certain perceptions, thoughts, or behaviors will spontaneously occur.

Hypnosis has been used since antiquity, but its history in clinical medicine can be traced to James Braid, who in 1843 discovered that a person could be induced to fall into a state of "nervous sleep." After realizing that subjects in this state were unusually responsive to verbal suggestions, Braid named the phenomenon *hypnosis* after *Hypnos,* the Greek god of sleep. During the last part of the nineteenth century several prominent physicians, including Jean-Martin Charcot, James Esdaile, and Hippolyte-Marie Bernheim, began using hypnosis in their medical practices. It is reported that Esdaile performed numerous painless surgeries, including amputations, using hypnosis as the sole means of anesthesia. With the discovery of ether and other anesthetic drugs in the late nineteenth century, however, hypnosis fell into decline and has only recently experienced something of a revival in clinical medicine (Druckman & Bjork, 1994).

Hypnosis and Pain A typical hypnosis intervention for pain involves several overlapping stages.

- A prehypnotic stage in which the therapist builds rapport with the subject.
- The use of suggestions and imagery to induce relaxation and the focused attention of the hypnotic trance.
- The treatment stage, which may involve various kinds of suggestions and imagery to reduce the experience of pain.
- A "consolidation phase" that may incorporate *posthypnotic suggestions* to be carried out after the hypnosis session has ended.
- A posthypnotic stage, in which the patient is awakened, given additional instructions, and released. The hypnotherapist may also train the patient in self-hypnosis so he or she can practice the therapy at home.

Does Hypnosis Work? Hypnosis does not endow suggestible subjects with special powers. Physiologically, hypnosis resembles other forms of deep relaxation: a generalized decrease in sympathetic nervous system activity, a decrease in oxygen consumption and carbon dioxide eliminations, a lowering of blood pressure and heart rate, and an increase in certain kinds of brain-wave activity.

We all probably flow naturally in and out of hypnoticlike states all the time—for example, while watching a mind-numbing television program.

All of this suggests to health psychologists that hypnotic phenomena reflect the workings of normal consciousness (Spanos & Coe, 1992). Many researchers believe that people often move into trancelike states of focused concentration when they are under stress, such as when they are about to experience an uncomfortable treatment. During such moments, when a person in a position of authority issues an instruction, it may have as strong an effect as a posthypnotic suggestion. Support for this comes from the fact that those who are most likely to report pain relief from hypnosis also tend to be highly suggestible, fantasy-prone people and to be very responsive to authority figures. For example, when a physician distracts a child who is about to receive an injection or makes a statement such as, "This will feel like a little mosquito bite," the power of suggestion at this moment of focused concentration may very well help the child get through the difficult experience.

Relaxation and Meditation

As noted in other chapters, relaxation and meditation are related therapies that have proved successful in helping some patients cope with, and recover from, a number of medical conditions. In the most common variety of relaxation training, *progressive relaxation training (PRT)* subjects learn to divide their muscles into seven groups and then to tense and relax each group in turn. As their muscle control improves, practitioners learn to control several groups simultaneously and, finally, to monitor, tense, and relax all of their muscles at once.

Meditation is a process in which one tries to achieve greater "awareness without thought" (Fugh-Berman, 1997). Practitioners of *mindfulness meditation* learn to pay nonjudgmental, in-the-moment attention to changing perceptions and thoughts. Conversely, in *transcendental meditation* practitioners focus their awareness on a single object or on a word or short phrase, called a *mantra*.

In his classic experiment on relaxation, Herbert Benson (1993) fitted experienced practitioners of transcendental meditation with measurement devices to record changes in a number of physiological functions, including oxygen consumption—a reliable indicator of the body's overall metabolic state. After recording the participants' physiological state for a 20-minute baseline period during which they simply sat in a quiet resting position, Benson instructed the participants to begin meditating. The participants were not permitted to change their posture or activity; they simply changed their thoughts to maintain a meditative focus. Following the meditation period, which also lasted 20 minutes, the participants were instructed to return to their normal state of thinking. Compared to the premeditation period, the participants consumed significantly less oxygen while meditating (Figure 14.1, page 612). Other

In childhood, fantasizers had had at least one, but usually many, imaginary companions often drawn from storybook characters, real-life playmates who had moved away, and pets and toys whom they believed could talk. One of my subjects had seen the movie *Camelot* as a child and, for two years, imagined being the son of Arthur and Guinevere, commanding the King's court.
—Deirdre Barrett, hypnotherapist (2001)

Figure 14.1

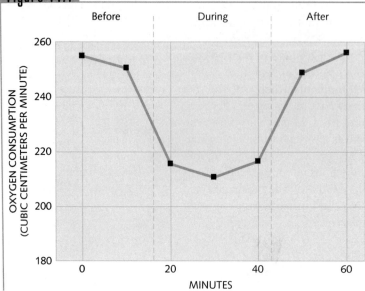

Oxygen Consumption during Transcendental Meditation
The body's metabolic rate, reflected in the amount of oxygen consumed, decreased significantly in experienced meditators when they switched from simply resting (before) to meditating (during); it rose when they stopped meditating (after).

Source: "The Relaxation Response," by Herbert Benson, 1993. In D. Goleman and J. Gurin (Eds.), *Mind–Body Medicine* (pp. 233–257). New York: Consumer Reports Books.

changes also occurred during meditation: Breathing slowed from a rate of 14 or 15 breaths per minute to approximately 10 or 11 breaths, and brain-wave patterns included more low-frequency alpha, theta, and delta waves—waves associated with rest and relaxation—and significantly fewer high-frequency beta waves associated with higher states of alertness. In addition, during meditation, the level of lactate (a chemical that has been linked to anxiety) in the participants' bloodstream decreased dramatically.

Relaxation, meditation, and other *physiological self-regulation* techniques are effective in helping to manage a variety of disorders (Gatchel, 2001). In one early study by Jon Kabat-Zinn (1982), 65 percent of the chronic-pain patients who spent 10 weeks in a mindfulness meditation program reported fewer overall symptoms, a significant improvement in mood, and a one-third or more reduction in their pain. Indeed, for patients with chronic lower back pain, relaxation training may be more effective than placebo medications or biofeedback (Stuckey, Jacobs, & Goldfarb, 1986). In another study, compared to a control group, patients who received a single hour of relaxation instruction the night before undergoing spinal surgery required less pain medication, complained less to nurses, and had shorter hospital stays (Lawlis, Selby, Hinnant, & McCoy, 1985).

Relaxation training and meditation have also proved effective in reducing the frequency of epileptic seizures. In one controlled clinical trial with epileptic patients, half the participants learned PRT; the other half first received a sham treatment, followed by PRT. The sham treatment had no effect, but PRT resulted in a 30 percent reduction in the average frequency of seizures in both groups. In another study, epileptic adults were divided into three groups: One learned to identify high-risk situations and apply PRT to them; the second received supportive therapy; and the third merely recorded how often they had seizures. Initially, only the first group showed a significant decrease in the frequency of seizures. In the second part of the study, both control groups were taught PRT—after which their seizure frequency decreased significantly (Dahl, Melin, & Lund, 1987).

Other researchers suggest that relaxation and meditation are no more effective than placebos in modulating physiological responses. Daniel Eisenberg and his colleagues (1993), for instance, performed a meta-analysis of research on the effects of relaxation, meditation, and biofeedback on blood pressure levels in patients with hypertension. As shown in Figure 14.2, compared with patients who received no treatment or a wait-list control group, patients receiving the CAM therapies showed a statistically (and clinically) significant reduction in both systolic and diastolic blood pressure. However, as compared with a credible placebo intervention (pseudo-meditation or sham biofeedback), the CAM therapies showed a smaller and neither statistically nor clinically significant blood pressure effect. The analysis also showed that no single CAM technique was more effective than any other in reducing blood pressure.

Tai Chi and Yoga Sometimes called "shadow boxing" or "moving meditation," **tai chi** originated in China hundreds of years ago and is a component of traditional Oriental medicine. A blend of exercise, dance, and concentration, the movements of tai chi are slow, circular, continuous, smooth, and controlled, and weight is shifted regularly from one foot to another. Groups of people concentrating on the rhythmical, dancelike movements of tai chi are a common sight throughout China.

Figure 14.2

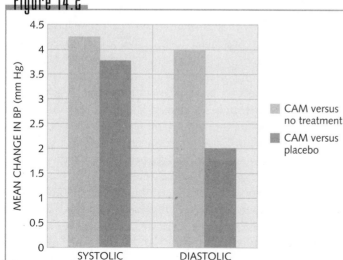

Relaxation Therapy and Hypertension
A meta-analysis of 26 control trials involving 1,264 hypertensive patients showed that CAM interventions based on relaxation training, meditation, and biofeedback were significantly more effective than no treatment in reducing systolic and diastolic blood pressure. Compared to credible placebo treatment, however, CAM interventions were much less effective; the difference between the treatments was statistically and clinically insignificant.

Source: Adapted from "Cognitive Behavioral Techniques for Hypertension: Are They Effective?" by D. M. Eisenberg, T. L. Delbanco, C. S. Berkey, T. J. Kaptchuk, B. Kupelnick, J. Kuhl, and T. C. Chalmers, 1993, *Annals of Internal Medicine, 118*, pp. 964–972.

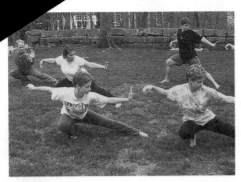

Tai Chi
A blend of exercise, dance, and concentration, tai chi movements are slow, controlled, and continuous. This component of traditional Oriental medicine is practiced by people of all ages and nationalities. Members of the Philosophy and Physical Taoism honors class at Western Kentucky University practice tai chi every Wednesday afternoon. © AP/Wide World Photos

Yoga, a Sanskrit word meaning "union," has strong ties with spiritual and mystical traditions originating in India, where it has been practiced for thousands of years. Yoga encompasses a global lifestyle, consisting of diet, meditation, and physical exercise (Christensen, 1996). The two primary forms practiced in the West are hatha yoga (physical postures and breathing) and raja yoga (relaxation and mental and spiritual mastery).

It is widely believed that yoga and tai chi provide some of the physical and psychological benefits of more strenuous exercise without straining the muscles or the cardiovascular system (Brown, Mucci, Hetzler, & Knowlton, 1989). One study found that elderly Chinese tai chi practitioners outperformed a group of sedentary, but otherwise matched, adults on three of five measures of physical strength and balance (Tse & Bailey, 1992). However, because the study failed to control for other types of exercise, the findings may merely reflect the difference between out-of-shape people and fit people.

This interpretation is borne out by another study that examined how tai chi influences recovery from stress. Ninety-six experienced tai chi practitioners were subjected to mental stress (arithmetic and other mental tests under time pressure in a noisy environment) and, at another time, emotional stress (watching a gruesome film). After each stress session, the participants were divided into four activity groups: tai chi, brisk walking, meditation, or reading, each of which was practiced for an hour. The results indicated that tai chi was not associated with any unique physiological benefits. For example, the heart rate and blood pressure of the tai chi practitioners were equivalent to these same indicators in the walkers. Furthermore, all four groups equally improved their mood and lowered their levels of stress hormones (Jin, 1992).

Although tai chi and yoga may offer no special advantages over other forms of relaxation and exercise and evidence of their effectiveness may have limited generalizablity because most studies failed to use randomized trials with a control group, they are growing in popularity, largely because health benefits *are* often demonstrated when comparing a participant's own pre- and post-intervention status. In one study of male physical education teachers, for example, a 3-month yoga intervention resulted in a significant reduction in systolic and diastolic blood pressure, heart rate, and respiratory rate and a decrease in autonomic arousal (Telles, Nagarathna, Nagendra, & Desiraju, 1993). Similarly, tai chi has been shown to promote cardiorespiratory functioning in elderly adults (Hennekens, 1996; Jin, 1992; Lai, Lan, Wong, & Teng, 1995) as well as to enhance positive mood effects and aerobic capacity (Zhuo, Shephard, Plyley, & Davis, 1998). Other studies have reported success in using yoga as an intervention in treating alcohol abuse (Nespor & Csemy, 1994), anxiety (Shannahoff-Khalsa & Beckett, 1996), cardiovascular disease (Schell, Allolio, &

yoga a movement-based form of relaxation and meditation that combines diet, physical postures, and breathing to promote physical and spiritual well-being

Schonecke, 1994), Type II diabetes (Divekar, Bhat, & Mulla, 1998), and osteoarthritis (Garfinkel, Schumacher, & Husain, 1994).

How Might Relaxation and Meditation Promote Health? Just how relaxation, meditation, yoga, or tai chi might work to promote health is the subject of ongoing debate. One suggestion is that the relaxation at the center of these therapies relieves stress, muscle tension, anxiety, and negative emotionality, all of which might exacerbate physical symptoms and increase a person's vulnerability to ill health. Indeed, one study of 25 healthy women found that regular practitioners of hatha yoga had fewer somatic complaints, lower excitability, reduced aggressiveness and emotionality, and greater life satisfaction than a matched group of non-yoga devotees (Schell et al., 1994).

Researchers also have suggested that relaxation and meditation may alter a person's emotional response to symptoms, such as pain. "I'm still in constant pain," notes one woman, who joined the pain reduction program at the University of Massachusetts after a bad fall left her with neck and back injuries and the chronic, painful condition called *fibromyalgia*. "Meditation makes the pain more bearable. I have less pain, muscles are more relaxed, and I have much better mobility" (Eisenberg et al., 1998). This makes sense, according to mind–body therapy advocates, because these techniques alter the way pain sufferers respond to painful sensations and the way they feel about them. Relaxation interventions often teach pain sufferers to reinterpret painful sensations, regarding them as "warm, even pleasant" rather than "burning and unpleasant" (Eisenberg et al., 1998).

Relaxation and meditation may also promote health by bolstering the immune system. In one study of 45 elderly people in independent living facilities, one group received relaxation training three times each week, another received social contact three times a week, and the third received no training or social contact. After one month, the relaxation group showed a significant increase in natural killer cell activity and the subjects reported feeling more relaxed. There were no significant changes in the groups that received social contact or no contact (Kiecolt-Glaser, Glaser, & Williger, 1985).

Transcendental meditators have also been found to have higher daytime levels of the serotonin metabolite 5-HIAA compared with controls, and these levels increase with meditation. Serotonin is a precursor of melatonin, a naturally occurring biochemical that promotes analgesia, lowers blood pressure and heart rate, and has an anti-stress, anti-insomnia effect. Health benefits such as these may help explain the findings of one remarkable study of elderly residents of nursing homes. The study randomly assigned the residents either to daily meditation or to no intervention. After 3 years, 25 percent of the nonmeditators had died, while *all* of those in the meditation group were still alive (Alexander, Langer, Newman, Chandler, & Davies, 1989).

Prayer and Spiritual Healing

As noted in Chapter 1, throughout history, religion and medicine have been closely connected as healing traditions. Indeed, throughout history spiritual and physical healing were frequently conducted by the same person. As Western biomedicine matured, however, the two traditions diverged. Rather than consulting a spiritual healer to cure infection and prevent disease, people began turning to vaccines, antibiotics, and the growing number of wondrous new weapons in the modern medical arsenal.

There are signs, however, that the wall between medicine and spiritual healing—which never was nearly as high in some countries as in the United States—is beginning to topple. Medical conferences and centers for research on spirituality and healing are cropping up at Harvard, Duke, and other top universities, and 61 out of 126 U.S. medical schools offered spirituality and health courses in 1999, up from only three schools just 5 years earlier (McVeigh, 1999). Moreover, one recent survey reported that 99 percent of family physicians agreed that "personal prayer, meditation, or other spiritual and religious practices" could increase the effectiveness of medical treatment (Yankelovich Partners, 1998).

The increasing popularity of fundamentalist Christianity, New Age beliefs, and alternative medicine has led to a renewed interest in possible links between spirituality and the healing process. Prayer and meditation are being used with increasing frequency in the treatment of many chronic diseases, including cancer (Primack & Spencer, 1996). And many are convinced of the efficacy of spiritual interventions. Anecdotal cases of tumor regression in response to prayer have been reported, as well as the effect of prayer in reducing anxiety (Dossey, 1993).

But is there scientific evidence to support this growing movement? Does spirituality promote health, as four of every five Americans believe (Matthews, 1997)? As is often the case with nontraditional interventions, the evidence is mixed. To be sure, there is evidence that faith and spirituality are *correlated* with health. A number of studies have reported that devotees of various religions—Catholic priests and nuns, Trappist monks, and Mormon priests—have lower illness and mortality rates than the general population. One study of mortality rates among nearly 4,000 Israelis reported that those living in orthodox religious communities were about half as likely as those living in nonreligious kibbutz settlements to have died over the 16-year course of the study (Kark et al., 1996).

A review of 27 studies found that, in 22 of them, frequency of attendance at religious services was associated with better health (Levin & Vanderpool, 1987). However, most of these studies were uncontrolled, making them vulnerable to mistaken interpretation and unable to pinpoint causation. An obvious case in point is that ill health may prevent many individuals from attending services in the first place. As another example, if religious people shared other health-promoting traits—say, they exercised as much as they worshipped or avoided smoking or excessive alcohol use—religion might have nothing to do with their improved health. Finally, it has been argued that women, who tend to be more religiously active than men, may in large measure account for the spirituality-longevity effect because women also tend to outlive the less religious members of the other gender (Sloan, Bagiella, & Powell, 1999). Several recent studies have attempted to rule out gender and other uncontrolled variables in the faith-health connection. One study of Californians reported that even after ruling out differences due to gender, ethnicity, age, and education, those who were religiously active were 36 percent less likely to die in any given year than their less religious counterparts (McCullough et al., 2000). In another study, researchers reported that those who rarely attended religious services were 1.87 times more likely to die during the 8-year study than were those who attended frequently (Hummer, Rogers, Nam, & Ellison, 1999). This difference was found even after the researchers controlled for the age, race, and gender of the research participants. The results of this study are depicted in Figure 14.3.

What accounts for the correlation between strong religious practices and longevity? At least three intervening factors remain strong candidates: *lifestyle, social support,* and *positive emotions.* First, those who are religiously active tend to smoke less, consume alcohol more moderately, eat less fat, be more active, and be less likely to engage in high-risk sexual behaviors than those in the general population (Sloan et al., 1999). Second, because religion tends to be a communal experience, those who are religiously active may benefit from more social ties than those in the general population. Throughout this book, we have seen the beneficial effects of social support on each domain of health. Third, religious activity may promote health by fostering more positive emotions, including an optimistic and hopeful worldview, a feeling of acceptance and personal control, and a sense that life itself is meaningful (Koenig & Larson, 1998).

Prayer

Despite the mounting correlational evidence that people who are religiously active are healthier, scientific evidence for the power of prayer in promoting health is virtually nonexistent (Fugh-Berman, 1997). No research to date supports the claim that any form of distant healing (intercessory prayer, mental healing, therapeutic touch, or spiritual healing) works. A recent

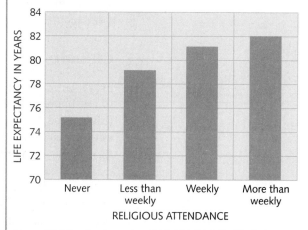

Figure 14.3

Religious Attendance and Life Expectancy
The results of this large national health survey conducted by the Centers for Disease Control and Prevention showed that religiously active people had longer life expectancies, even when the respondents' age, race, and gender were controlled for.

Source: "Religious Involvement and U.S. Adult Mortality," by R. A. Hummer, R. G. Rogers, C. B. Nam, and C. G. Ellison, 1999, *Demography, 36,* pp. 273–285.

meta-analysis of 23 clinical trials of distant healing that included random assignment of participants and placebo-based control groups reported that 13 of the studies (57 percent) yielded statistically significant effects, 9 showed no effect over control interventions, and 1 showed a negative effect. However, the methodological limitations of many of the studies made it impossible to draw definitive conclusions about the efficacy of distant healing (Astin, Harkness, & Ernst, 2000).

One widely cited study (Byrd, 1988) reported that prayer improved the cardiovascular status of 393 patients in a coronary care unit. However, the study was badly flawed. First, there were significant differences between the two control groups and the intervention groups. For instance, more than three times as many people in the control group came in with relatively serious conditions (for example, acute myocardial infarction, unstable angina), and more in the intervention group (prayer) came in with less serious or minor conditions (such as fainting or chest pain of unknown origin). Even more troubling, in this study the researchers made no distinction in outcome measures—death and cardiac surgery were both simply classed as "bad" outcomes. Of the 26 new problems, diagnoses, and other events, only 6 showed any difference between prayed-for patients and controls. On measures that couldn't be misinterpreted—death, for example, or days in the cardiac care unit after entering the study—prayer made no difference.

So what is the role of faith in the healing process? Richard Sloan and his Columbia University colleagues believe that doctors should remain cautious in "prescribing" faith (Sloan et al., 1999). "Linking religious activities and better health can be harmful to patients," they explain, "who already must confront age-old folk wisdom that illness is due to their own moral failure." However, they acknowledge that faith can help patients cope with illness. Although the scientific jury is still out on the connection between faith and healing, "respectful attention must be paid to the impact of religion on the patient's decisions about health care," they conclude.

Chiropractic

Therapeutic manipulation of the body dates from the beginning of recorded time: Hippocrates (fifth century B.C.) and Galen (second century A.D.), for example, used some form of it, and *bodywork* was common among physicians until the eighteenth century (Moore, 1993). The two most common forms of therapeutic manipulation today—*chiropractic* and *osteopathy*—are the only major forms of CAM originally developed in the United States.

The word *chiropractic* is derived from the Greek roots *cheir* (hand) and *praktikos* (done by). Its actual practice can be traced back to September 1895, when Daniel David Palmer, a magnetic healer in Iowa, supposedly cured a patient's deafness by realigning the man's spine. Two years later, Palmer founded the first school of chiropractic, based on his belief that the human body has an innate self-healing power and seeks a state of *homeostasis,* or balance. Imbalance was believed to be caused by *subluxations,* which are misalignments of bones within joints or abnormal movements that interfere with the flow of nervous impulses called *fixations.* By manipulating the bones, muscles, and joints, particularly in the spine, chiropractors work to improve the function of the neuromusculoskeletal system and restore homeostasis.

Although Palmer was enough of an ideologue to date things *BC* (Before Chiropractic) and *AC* (After Chiropractic), osteopathy is actually older. Andrew Taylor Sill, the allopathic physician who founded osteopathy, began teaching its principles in 1892, 3 years before Palmer's first chiropractic adjustment (Fugh-Berman, 1997). Although osteopathy is a more complete system of medicine (osteopaths can prescribe drugs, perform surgery, and do just about anything else M.D.s can do), chiropractic has always been more pervasive. Today, chiropractors provide over 90 percent of the manipulative therapy in the United States (Shekelle, Adams, & Chassin, 1992; Shekelle & Brook, 1991). Each year, between 3 and 10 percent of the U.S. population consult chiropractors (Eisenberg et al., 1993). In this section we will focus on chiropractic because it is more commonly practiced in this country.

Today, chiropractors are divided into two major groups, each of which has its own governing body. *Straight chiropractors* are traditionalists who continue to believe that subluxations cause pain and that manipulation is the best form of treatment. *Mixers* combine traditional manipulation along with a broad range of other CAM therapies, including massage, physical therapy, and nutritional therapy.

What to Expect during a Chiropractic Examination

Before performing any type of adjustment, the chiropractor will *palpate,* or feel, your vertebrae to detect misalignment of bones or muscular weaknesses. He or she may also test your reflexes to check neural functioning. X-rays may be taken to reveal any underlying joint problems that might interfere with treatment or be worsened by a chiropractic adjustment.

During a treatment, the chiropractor will adjust your joints one at a time, using a slight thrusting movement that moves a restricted joint just beyond its limited range of motion. You may be asked to lie on a padded table for a spinal adjustment or to sit or stand for an adjustment of the neck and other joints. Although the treatments are painless, it is not uncommon to hear joints crack during an adjustment.

What Is Chiropractic Used For?

Straight chiropractors maintain that chiropractic treatment can be beneficial for a wide range of ailments—from asthma to lower back pain to impotence.

Mixers, on the other hand, tend to recognize its effectiveness for a more limited range of conditions, especially acute lower back pain, headaches, and neck pain.

What Critics Say

The medical profession has been relentlessly hostile to chiropractors. As far back as 1910, Abraham Flexner's government report on medical education in the United States dismissed chiropractic without even the briefest consideration.

Critics charge that chiropractic treatments are useless because misaligned vertebra are common, harmless, and usually clear up on their own. Others question the premise that a sound nervous system is the foundation of overall health, pointing to quadriplegics, who often have healthy internal organs despite extensive nerve damage. Finally, some critics accept chiropractic treatment as effective for back pain but argue that it should be restricted to this disorder, since there is insufficient evidence to support its efficacy in treating other conditions.

Finally, critics note that some people use chiropractors as their primary care gatekeepers, a cause for concern since not all chiropractors are trained to diagnose all medical conditions. Moreover, chiropractic manipulation can cause severe damage to the body if there are fractures or tumors present.

Does It Work?

Despite such criticism, chiropractic remains very popular with the general public, forcing Congress, in 1974, to pass legislation requiring Medicare to pay for chiropractic services. In the same year, the NIH allocated $2 million to fund research on the effectiveness of chiropractic treatment. Although still considered a form of alternative medicine by many conventional doctors, chiropractic is gaining wider acceptance and is licensed in all 50 states. As another testimonial to the growing acceptability of chiropractic, the services of chiropractors generally are covered not only by Medicare and Medicaid, but also by about 85 percent of the major insurance plans (American Chiropractic Association, 1999).

Evidence for chiropractic's effectiveness in treating back pain has been accumulating since 1952, when a Harvard study reported that this was the most common reason for visiting a chiropractor and that one-fifth of back pain sufferers have used chiropractic successfully (Eisenberg et al., 1993). A 1974 retrospective study of back pain sufferers who had received workers' compensation found that those who received chiropractic treatment were as satisfied as and improved as much as their counterparts who opted for conventional medical treatment (Kane, Olsen, & Leymaster, 1974). A 1986 study of acute back pain patients found that three times as many patients were satisfied with their chiropractic care as with conventional treatment (cited in Cherkin, Deyo, Battie, Street, & Barlow, 1998).

Finally, a meta-analysis of 23 randomized controlled trials of chiropractic adjustment for lower back pain found that spinal manipulation was more effective than any comparison treatment (Anderson, Meeker, & Wirick, 1992). In another meta-analysis, researchers analyzed nine randomized, controlled trials that compared the effectiveness of manipulation with that of more conventional medical treatments for patients with acute lower back pain (Shekelle et al., 1992). The researchers concluded that spinal manipulation hastens recovery from acute, uncomplicated, lower back pain.

Research studies also show that chiropractic treatment may decrease the frequency and intensity of tension and migraine headaches and be beneficial in the treatment of otitis media (Froehle, 1996); hypertension (Crawford, Hickson, & Wiles, 1986); carpal tunnel syndrome (Feuerstein et al., 1999); some sports injuries (Jacchia, Butler, Innocenti, & Capone, 1994); and arthritis of the hip, wrist, or hand (Gottlieb, 1997).

Naturopathic Medicine

Naturopathic medicine aims to provide holistic, or whole body, health care by returning humans to their "natural state." This "back to nature" movement has been traced to German doctors such as Vincent Preissnitz (1799–1851), who balked at the harsh treatment used by medical doctors. While medical doctors were "treating" their patients with mercury, bloodletting, and other "modern cures," Preissnitz and other German "nature doctors" were taking patients for walks in the woods and recommending fasting to "detoxify the body," followed by a simple diet and the healing powers of fresh air, sunlight, and bathing in natural hot springs.

At about the same time, the *hygienic movement* was becoming popular in the United States. This movement, founded by Sylvester Graham (originator of the graham cracker), advocated a strict vegetarian diet, herbal treatments, and, naturally, an abundance of whole grains. Another dietary mogul who regarded conventional medicine as a fundamentally wrongheaded attempt to improve on nature through artificial means was John Harvey Kellogg, best known as the founder of Kellogg's cereal.

Benedict Lust (1869–1945), another advocate of natural treatments, coined the word *naturopath*. A German immigrant, Lust also opened the world's first health food store in New York City around 1920. From then until the start of World War II, naturopathic medicine was a popular alternative to conventional medicine. By the 1950s, however, the increasingly powerful American Medical Association, along with the discovery of penicillin and other potent antibiotics that were effective against many life-threatening diseases, forced naturopathy out of popularity.

Naturopathic medicine integrates herbal medicine, clinical nutrition, homeopathy, and sometimes other CAM therapies with modern medical methods of diagnosis and treatment. It also has three accredited medical

naturopathic medicine the system that aims to provide holistic health care by drawing from several traditional healing systems, including homeopathy, herbal remedies, and traditional Oriental medicine schools in the United States. Elements of naturopathic medicine therefore seem destined either to be absorbed into conventional medicine or to become a separate branch of it. Although naturopathic physicians are licensed to practice in only 11 states, the majority of other states allow them to practice in limited ways. Naturopathic practice is regulated by state law, and some insurance providers cover naturopathic health care.

Naturopathic Concepts

With the more recent "return to nature" movements, naturopathy has regained some of its earlier popularity. Modern naturopathy draws from several CAM traditions, especially herbal medicine, food supplement therapy, and dietary modification. Naturopaths follow seven basic principles: *help nature heal, do no harm, find the underlying cause, treat the whole person, encourage prevention, recognize wellness,* and *act as a teacher.* Each of these principles, of course, encompasses the three major ideals of CAM.

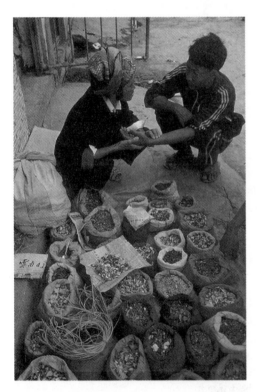

Herbal Medicines
Medicine sellers set up stalls in the open market to display the many herbs used to treat anything from a toothache to lower back pain to cancer. This seller is in Menghan, Yunnan Province, China. © Mike Yamashita / Woodfin Camp & Associates

Herbal Medicine

People have used plants to treat physical, mental, and behavioral conditions since the dawn of time, and all known cultures have ancient histories of folk medicine that include the use of herbs. This knowledge was often grouped into a collection called a *pharmacopoeia* or a *materia medica.* The ancient Greek and Roman cultures developed extensive pharmacopoeias (see Chapter 1). Until the thirteenth century, *herbology* was traditionally a woman's art in Europe. When the practice of healing was taken over by male-dominated medical schools as early as the thirteenth century, herbology lost favor and many women herbalists were prosecuted as witches.

In the United States, physicians relied on medicinal plants as primary medicines through the 1930s. In fact, botany was once an important part of the medical school curriculum. But during the second half of the twentieth century, the use of medicinal plants declined with developments in the ability to produce pharmaceuticals synthetically.

Today, most herbs are marketed as food supplements, since it is illegal for doctors to recommend an herb as a treatment for anything. Doing so is considered the same as prescribing an illegal drug. In practice, of course, herbs are widely used as treatments for numerous health conditions, with annual sales reaching the billions of dollars.

Types of Herbs Herbs can be prepared or marketed in different forms—as supplements, medicines, or as teas—depending on their intended use. Herbs can be used as tonics and remedies for virtually every known ailment and condition. Derived from the leaves, stems, roots, bark, flowers, fruits, seeds, and exudates (sap) of plants, herbs can be prepared in several ways, using either fresh or dried ingredients. Herbal teas can be steeped to varying strengths. Roots, bark, and other plant parts can be simmered into potent solutions called *decoctions*. Today, many herbs are also available in health food stores, pharmacies, and even groceries in the form of tablets and capsules. Highly concentrated alcohol-based herb extracts called *tinctures* are also popular.

Herbs play a central role in Chinese medicine, ayurvedic medicine, and Western herbal medicine (see Chapter 1). Western herbs are categorized in several ways. They may be grouped according to their potency. *Tonics*, or normalizers, have a gentle healing effect on the body, whereas *effectors* have potent actions and are used to treat illness. Herbs are also often grouped according to their effects on the body. These categories include anti-inflammatories, diuretics, and laxatives as well as other, lesser-known classes such as diaphoretics that promote perspiration and nervousness, which allegedly strengthen the nervous system. Herbs are also often grouped according to which of the body's systems they affect. The cardiovascular system, for example, is said to respond to ginkgo, buckwheat, linden, and other herbs claimed to strengthen blood vessels.

Do Herbs Work? Although roughly 25 percent of our pharmaceutical drugs are derived from herbs, physicians often believe that herbs are ineffective and potentially dangerous (McCarthy, 2001). Still, there is at least *some evidence* that plant-based medicines are effective in treating certain conditions. For example, researchers have found that the herb *Ma huang*, which contains the active ingredient *ephedrine*, can be effective in managing asthma (Ziment, 1988). As another example, ginger's proved anti-inflammatory and anti-rheumatic properties, coming from both human and animal trials, suggest that it may be effective in treating arthritis (Srivastava & Mustafa, 1992). As a third example, a recent large-scale meta-analysis has found that *capsaicin*, an extract from the cayenne pepper, is effective in relieving the pain of osteoarthritis (Zhang & Po, 1994).

On the other hand, the evidence for the effectiveness of some popular herbs is mixed, at best. For example, a meta-analysis of 26 controlled clinical trials (18 randomized, 8 double-blind) examined the effectiveness of the herb *echinacea*. Nineteen trials investigated whether a pure extract of the herb was more effective in preventing or curing infections (flu or cold) than a diluted mixture, four trials studied the herb's success in lessening side effects of cancer treatment, and three studied whether the herb affected immune function. Although the researchers found positive results for 30 of 34 treatment groups, once again most of the trials were of poor methodological quality and therefore questionable (Melchart et al., 1995).

Other studies have examined the effectiveness of herbal formulas in treating osteoarthritis. In one double-blind, placebo-controlled study, a combination of the herbs *Boswellian serrata, Curcuma longa, Withania somnifera,* and zinc resulted in a significant reduction in pain severity and disability in osteoarthritis patients (Kulkarni, Patki, Jog, Gandage, & Patwardhan, 1991). However, most of these herbs are unregulated and thus vary in potency and purity, making it difficult to generalize results.

Results such as these make it impossible to offer a definitive, across-the-board answer to the question "Do herbs work?". At present, the safest conclusion seems to be that certain herbs may be beneficial for certain conditions. In general, however, there simply is not enough good evidence that herbs work as well as many would like to believe. Furthermore, compared to the often-dramatic power of pharmaceutical drugs, herbs usually have fairly subtle effects. *Standardized extracts,* which have long been available in Europe and increasingly so in the United States, do seem to be more effective, perhaps because the dosages used are generally higher than those found in dried herbs.

Many advocates of herbal medicine claim that the presence of many different active and inactive ingredients, known and unknown, make botanical products safer and more effective than synthetic drugs. This is mostly speculation because there have been few clinical trials directly comparing herbs and pharmaceuticals in their effectiveness in treating specific diseases and conditions (Relman, 1998). Furthermore, advocates of herbal medicine typically neglect to mention the possible adverse side effects created by the lack of purity and standardization of some herbal products.

Food Supplement Therapy

The use of vitamins and food supplements is a second major emphasis of naturopathy and is perhaps the best known of all CAM treatments. Turn to nearly any popular magazine and you are sure to find at least one recommended supplement, such as vitamin E to deter atherosclerosis and prevent premature aging of the skin or folic acid to support the immune system.

As noted in Chapter 7, there is no longer any doubt that food supplements can have important health benefits. There is a large body of convincing research evidence that materials derived from foods can be effective in treating a number of diseases (Werbach, 1994). For example, niacin is effective in lowering cholesterol levels and glucosamine sulfate is effective in reducing the pain of arthritis. Moreover, food supplements often trigger fewer adverse side effects than do drugs of comparable effectiveness.

Food supplements are generally used in two ways: to correct dietary deficiencies (*nutritional medicine*) or in immense doses to trigger a specific therapeutic effect (*megadose therapy*). As nutritional medicine, they are useful in correcting fairly common deficiencies in many essential nutrients, including deficiencies in calcium, folic acid, iron, magnesium, zinc, and vitamins A, B6, C, and E. Although conventional biomedicine supports eating a balanced diet or, short of that, using nutritional medicine to correct deficiencies in vitamins and minerals, the use of megadose therapy is more controversial. Linus Pauling's famous recommendation to take 4,000 to 10,000 mg per day of vitamin C is a prime example. According to naturopaths, this huge dose—equivalent to eating 40 to 100 oranges per day, or 10 to 15 times the official recommended daily allowance (RDA)—is needed because the stresses of modern life and the effects of environmental toxins cause nutritional needs to increase beyond what a normal diet can provide. This claim remains controversial among nutritionists.

Dietary Medicine

Naturopaths have always believed that fruits, vegetables, nuts, and whole grains are "natural foods" and that any refinement of these foods reduces their natural vitality and health-promoting properties. In contrast, until quite recently conventional biomedicine has paid little attention to diet. Only in the past two decades have medical researchers begun to take seriously the idea that what people eat has a major impact on their health. As discussed in Chapter 7, the overwhelming evidence from large-scale epidemiological research has shown that diet plays a central role in preventing most of the major chronic diseases, including heart disease, strokes, and cancer of the breast, colon, and prostate.

Despite this agreement, naturopaths typically go well beyond conventional medicine's recommendations regarding diet. In addition to dramatically reducing consumption of meat and saturated fat, they decry the use of food preservatives, artificial fertilizers, pesticides, and the hormones used in modern farming. Instead, they recommend eating organic foods that are produced without these adulterations.

Another popular dietary concept in naturopathic medicine has to do with the idea of *food allergy* or, more accurately, *food sensitivity*. Diets based on avoiding "trigger" foods such as sugar, wheat, or dairy products are prescribed for many conditions, from arthritis to chronic fatigue (Wheelwright, 2001). When a food sensitivity is suspected, naturopaths typically place the patient on a highly restricted elimination diet of a small number of foods known to seldom cause allergic reactions. Rice, sweet potatoes, turkey, and applesauce are popular choices. If symptoms begin to clear up after several weeks on the restricted diet, foods are gradually added back into the diet, one at a time, while the patient keeps a journal of symptoms such as sneezing and headaches.

But even naturopaths disagree about the elements of a healthy diet. Proponents of *raw food theory,* a naturopathic concept dating back more than 100 years, believe that cooking foods destroys the "vital life force" (along with the vitamins, enzymes, and micronutrients) found in food. In contrast, the popular theory of *macrobiotics* condemns raw foods as unhealthy, considering them a cause of multiple sclerosis, rheumatoid arthritis, and other diseases. Macrobiotic nutritionists insist that all foods, including vegetables, should be cooked.

Do Dietary Modifications and Food Supplements Work? Epidemiological and experimental studies in animals and humans have provided substantial evidence that diet (in the form of foods or as supplements) can have a major effect on risk factors for certain diseases and the progression of disease. For example, over the past 10 years plant-based diets, dietary fiber supplementation, and antioxidant supplementation have become increasingly accepted treatments for managing cardiovascular disease. In fact, along with low-fat diets, aerobic exercise, and stress reduction, these treatments, which were at one time considered alternative therapies, are now considered either complementary or a part of standard medical practice for reducing risk of cardiovascular disease (Haskell, Luskin, & Marvasti, 1999).

Similarly, low-fat, high-fiber, basically vegetarian diets such as the *Pritikin diet* and the *Ornish diet* have been demonstrated to be effective in lowering blood glucose levels in people with diabetes. In one study, 60 percent of people with Type II diabetes on the Ornish diet no longer required insulin (McGrady & Horner, 1999). A number of epidemiological studies have also suggested a possible decrease in the prevalence of cancer in people who consume higher amounts of fruits and vegetables, perhaps due to their antioxidant effects (Primack & Spencer, 1999).

The value of food supplements, on the other hand, is not so clear. Certain supplements have been proved to be reasonably effective in treating certain conditions—for example, glucosamine sulfate for osteoarthritis, vitamin C for cold symptoms, and zinc for prostate enlargement. Despite these successes, however, megadose supplements rarely are as powerful as drugs, and supplement therapy alone usually is not adequate in managing serious health conditions.

Safety Concerns As with herbal medicines, the FDA cautions consumers that some unregulated dietary supplements may contain hazardous substances. For example, in January 1999, the FDA asked dietary supplement manufacturers to recall supplements that contained *gamma butyrolactone (GBL)*, which were sold via the Internet and in health food stores and health clubs. Marketed under such brand names as Blue Nitro, GH Revitalizer, and Revivarant, the popular supplement was supposed to build muscles, lower weight, and improve athletic and sexual performance. In fact, GBL contains a chemical also found in commercial floor strippers that affects the central nervous system; slows breathing and heart rate; and can lead to seizures, unconsciousness, and coma. GBL has been linked to one death and serious adverse effects in at least 54 other people (Schwartz, 1999).

As another example, contaminants in the once popular supplement L-tryptophan—touted as a pain reliever, a remedy for insomnia, and an antidepressant—caused a serious illness, *eosinophilia myalgia syndrome*. Some 30 people died in 1989 as a result of using this over-the-counter substance (Berge, 1998).

The FDA also warns against the use of certain herbs and food supplements by those who are also taking prescription medications. For instance, in a February 2000 public health advisory, the FDA cautioned that St. John's Wort had been found to reduce the effectiveness of the AIDS drug Indinavir by 57 percent (Piscitelli, Burstein, Chaitt, Alfaro, & Falloon, 2000). The FDA also cited a Zurich, Switzerland, study reporting that this popular herbal remedy for depression reduced levels of a transplant rejection drug (cyclosporin), increasing the odds, for example, that a heart transplant patient might reject a donated heart (Fugh-Berman, 2000).

What to Expect from a Visit to a Naturopath

Herbal medicines, food supplements, and dietary medicines we've discussed in this section are provided by naturopaths, who function as primary, preventive care doctors. A visit to a naturopath generally begins with a standard physical exam, possibly one that includes conventional blood and urine tests, and even radiology. Naturopaths will also spend considerable time recording the patient's medical history, focusing on the patient's lifestyle such as his or her diet, exercise, stress, and even emotional and spiritual issues.

After this initial examination, patient and naturopath work together to establish a treatment program. Usually, the program emphasizes noninvasive therapies and lifestyle changes such as eliminating unhealthy behaviors. The naturopath may then prescribe dietary changes, food supplements, and/or herbal medicine for any specific complaints. Depending on where the naturopath practices, conventional drugs, vaccinations, or even surgery may be recommended.

Does Naturopathy Work?

Diseases that are strongly affected by lifestyle and environment are among those for which naturopathic treatment is most often reported to be effective. For example, it has been used effectively to treat allergies, chronic infections, fatigue, arthritis, asthma, headache, hypertension, and depression, to name only a few conditions. In a typical case of hypertension, for example, a naturopathic doctor might prescribe a multifaceted treatment that includes dietary changes, vitamin and mineral supplements, herbal medicine, and lifestyle changes designed to reduce stress. For an arthritis sufferer, the regimen might include dietary modifications, herbal medicine, and massage.

Critics of naturopathic medicine raise several concerns. Chief among these is that unsuspecting consumers are flooded with inaccurate or deceptive information carrying extreme claims about the effectiveness of herbs. Herbal therapy is also criticized for being untested according to pharmaceutical standards. Herbalists reply that because herbs are natural products (and therefore cannot be patented), the extremely expensive testing required of pharmaceutical drugs is unlikely. Furthermore, debate continues over which part of an herb should be tested. Proponents point out that about 25 percent of today's prescription drugs are still at least partly derived from plants, that the modern pharmaceutical industry grew out of herbal medicine, and that many drugs—from the digitalis used to treat heart disease (derived from the foxglove plant) to morphine (from the opium poppy)—are still made from plant extracts. Another concern is safety. For this reason most herbalists recommend purchasing herbs

$\mathcal{D}$iversity and Healthy Living

Complementary and Alternative Medicine with the Very Young and the Very Old

In recent years there has been a rapid rise in the number of children and older adults receiving CAM treatments. The major reasons are word-of-mouth recommendations, fear of the side effects of medications, and the persistence of chronic conditions despite conventional medical treatments (Loo, 1999). The number of children receiving CAM treatments increased from approximately 2 percent in 1992 to 11 percent in 1994 (Spiegelblatt, 1994, 1995). Among the disorders being treated with CAM are pain, respiratory tract problems, ear infection, hyperactivity, enuresis, and gastrointestinal tract problems (Nyiendo & Olsen, 1988). Chiropractic is the most common form of CAM treatment used by children, followed by homeopathy, acupuncture, and naturopathy (Loo, 1999). Other CAM treatments used for children include touch therapy, osteopathy, and hypnosis.

Children The common cold is the most frequent acute illness throughout the world, with the typical preschooler averaging 4 to 10 colds per year. Ear infections and sinusitis are potentially serious complications of upper respiratory infections (URIs), and conventional biomedical treatments such as decongestants and antihistamines remain controversial and in most cases ineffective (Fireman, 1993; Luks & Anderson, 1996). Medications are frequently overprescribed and undoubtedly contribute to greater antibiotic resistance, higher health care costs, and the possible use of more dangerous medications such as steroids (English & Bauman, 1997).

The best-known alternative therapy for URIs—supplementation with vitamin C—originated in 1971, when Linus Pauling conducted a meta-analysis of four placebo-controlled trials of the antioxidant, concluding that vitamin C alleviates URI symptoms. More recent studies, however, indicate that the role of vitamin supplementation in preventing URIs remains unproven (Hamila, 1996, 1997).

Approximately two-thirds of all children will have had at least one ear infection (*acute otitis media,* or AOM) before age 3, typically treated with antipyretics and analgesics, oral decongestants, and antibiotics (Pichichero, 2000). In a recent prospective clinical study, researchers compared naturopathic remedies with conventional medicine in treating 103 German children between 1 and 11 years of age who were suffering from AOM. Naturopathic remedies were reported to be more effective in reducing pain and preventing relapses of AOM symptoms (Friese, Kruse, & Moeller, 1996). However, another randomized, double-blind, placebo-controlled study of 170 children (median age 4.2 years) reported that individually prescribed naturopathic remedies were largely ineffective in reducing symptoms or the use of antibiotics in URI (Lange de Klerk, Blommers, Kuik, & Bezemer, 1994).

Traditional Oriental medicine (TOM) has been used to treat bronchial asthma for centuries, and in some countries up to one-fourth of pediatricians believe in the effectiveness of acupuncture in treating asthma (Knipschild, 1994). In one double-blind, placebo-controlled study, 303 asthmatic children were assigned to three different herbal treatment groups, based on a TOM diagnosis of their symptoms. Compared to untreated control subjects, all of the herb-treated children experienced a greater improvement in their symptoms (including decreased production of histamine) (Hsieh, 1996). Attention deficit hyperactivity disorder (ADHD) is the most common neurodevelopmental disorder of childhood, with a prevalence rate between 2 and 11 percent (Shaywitz, Fletcher, & Shaywitz, 1997). Drug therapy is the most common form of treatment, usually involving the drug Ritalin (Greenhill, 1992). Partly because the etiology of ADHD remains unknown, a variety of CAM therapies have been tried, including herbal medicine, nutritional management, and acupuncture. For example, one clinical trial using Chinese herbs in the treatment of 66 children diagnosed with ADHD reported 84.8 percent effectiveness in improving attention and school performance and significantly reducing hyperactivity (Sun, 1994). Another randomized study found that Chinese herbal treatment was comparable to Ritalin in effectiveness but with fewer side effects (Zhang & Huang, 1990).

In a prospective, randomized, double-blind study conducted by NIH researchers, laser acupuncture was used in the treatment of ADHD in a small group of 7- to 9-year-old children (Loo, Naeser, Hinshaw, & Bay, 1998). Improvement in classroom behavior was reflected by significant decreases in the overactivity of five of the six children, according to teachers' assessments before and after treatment.

Elimination diets, megavitamin supplementation, and diets that focus on replacing trace elements are other popular forms of CAM therapy that have been used to treat ADHD. The *Feingold diet,* for example, eliminates food colors, artificial flavors, and highly processed foods from the ADHD child's diet, with mixed results in improving symptoms (Kien, 1990). One controlled study of fifty 7- to 12-year-old ADHD children, whose diagnosis was based on DSM-IV criteria, found a magnesium deficiency in blood and hair samples. The treatment group, who received a 200-mg daily supplement of magnesium for 6 months, showed an increase in the magnesium contents of their hair, which correlated positively with a significant decrease of hyperactivity (Starobrat-Hermelin & Kozielec, 1997). However, another double-blind, cross-over clinical trial found that megavitamins were ineffective in managing ADHD and had the added danger of potential toxicity to the liver (Haslam, Dalby, & Rademaker, 1984).

Another pediatric area in which there is growing interest in CAM alternatives to conventional treatment is immunization. Although vaccination is an essential component of pediatric well-child care and is required for entering school, the possibility of adverse side effects and the use of multiple-antigen vaccines are subjects of some controversy (Ellenberg & Chen, 1997; Robbins, 1993). A recent British survey reported that 21 percent of parents believed the risk of disease to be less than the risk of vaccination and would seek naturopathic treatment if any illness developed in their children (Simpson, Lenton, & Randall, 1995). Despite these beliefs, naturopathic vaccines are not yet supported by scientific data (Sulfaro, Fasher, & Burgess, 1994).

Although pediatric use of CAM in children continues to grow, scientific evidence remains sparse. As noted earlier, the scientific method is difficult to apply to holistic, individualized CAM therapies. For example, two children with the same diagnosis can easily be given the same standardized medication but are likely to receive different, individualized naturopathic or acupuncture treatments. Furthermore, despite the surprisingly large number of studies on the use of CAM in children, many of the studies have weak designs and other serious methodological flaws and cannot, therefore, be considered convincing evidence (Loo, 1999).

The Elderly Two chronic conditions striking many elderly people are Alzheimer's disease (AD) and osteoarthritis. AD is a degenerative disorder that alters memory, cognition, and behavior. In the United States, 10 percent of the elderly aged 65 and older have AD; up to 50 percent of those 85 and older have some form of the disease (Alzheimer's Association, 2000). In 1995, roughly 4 million individuals in the United States had AD, with the number estimated to triple by 2050 (Luskin et al., 2000).

In a survey of 101 physicians treating AD patients, 55 percent administered at least one CAM therapy to improve their patients' memory; 20 percent gave three or more treatments. These included vitamins (84%), health foods (27%), herbal medicines (11%), and home remedies (7%) (Coleman, Fowler, & Williams, 1995).

Gingko biloba extract (GBE) is a prevalent, legal, over-the-counter medicine in Europe. Although the FDA has not yet approved the extract, in the United States it can be purchased as a dietary supplement at health food and grocery stores. GBE has been tested in many randomized, placebo-controlled studies with patients showing moderate AD symptoms. One study reported that after 1 month of GBE or placebo treatment, attention, memory, and psychomotor ability all improved in the GBE group (Hofferberth, 1994). In another prospective, randomized, double-blind study, researchers reported that the GBE-based improvement in AD symptoms continued over a period of 24 weeks (Kanowski, Hermann, Stephan, Wierich, & Hoerr, 1996). A third study found that gingko increased the percentage of alpha brain waves, suggesting its role as a cognitive activator (Itil & Martorano, 1995). Finally, a meta-analysis of 25 randomized, placebo-controlled, double-blind studies confirmed that GBE was an effective form of treatment for early stage AD (Letzel, Haan, & Feil, 1996).

Osteoarthritis (OA) is the most common form of arthritis, involving a degenerative joint disease accompanied by inflammation, breakdown, and deterioration of cartilage in weight-bearing joints. Cartilage is the protein cushioning between the bones of joints; when damaged, it can cause severe joint pain, stiffness, and physical disability, making walking and other tasks of everyday living difficult. OA affects an estimated 16 million persons in the United States, mostly elderly women, and is the second leading cause of disability in adults 65 and over (West & Rink, 1997).

Although there is no known cure for OA, conventional treatment is aimed at pain relief and minimizing the disability caused by loss of joint mobility (Luskin et al., 2000). Common treatments include weight-loss programs, moderate aerobic exercise (for example, swimming or walking), physical therapy, use of mechanical support devices (for instance, canes, splints, or walkers), pain relievers (such as aspirin), and surgery (for example, arthroscopy or knee or hip replacement).

CAM therapies are widely used by OA patients. In 1982, the Arthritis Foundation estimated that $1.8 million had been spent on "unproven remedies" (Hawley, 1984). One Austrian survey of 100 OA sufferers found that 64 percent had used some form of "self-therapy" (including heat treatments and folk remedies) and that one-fourth had employed the services of CAM providers, primarily acupuncturists and chiropractors (Gray, 1985). Another survey found that of 384 OA patients surveyed, one-third used nontraditional treatments. A third survey found that CAM use was as high as 94 percent (Hawley, 1984).

rather than harvesting them in the wild. Plants have natural variations that can be misleading, and this has caused more than one death from a person's ingesting a toxic plant he or she believed to be a benign herb.

Looking Ahead: Complementary and Alternative Medicine in the 21st Century

Growing interest in CAM is viewed by some as one of several indications of a major paradigm shift in medicine and health care in the United States (Jacobs, 1999). One of the changes is a shift from the traditional view of the provider–patient relationship in which patients are willing, passive, and dependent to one in which patients are more activist health consumers. The new patient is more likely to demand and seek out accurate and timely health information on his or her own. As a result, the new patient no longer accepts his or her doctor's recommendations blindly and is more likely to be critical of traditional medicine and to consider (and use) alternative forms of treatment.

Armed with unprecedented access to health information from the World Wide Web, self-help books, and other media, today's patients are becoming more empowered to manage their own health. Turning to CAM practitioners is a predictable manifestation of this sense of empowerment—choosing your own treatment approach despite what your physician might suggest.

This assessment of changed patient behavior is supported by the results of a 1998 survey on the use of CAM published in the *Journal of the American Medical Association.* The sample of 1,035 patients (69 percent of whom responded to the mail survey) indicated that most who chose to use CAM did so because of a "congruence with their own values, beliefs and philosophical orientations toward health and life." In fact, most of the survey respondents reported using CAM not because they were dissatisfied with conventional medicine but rather because CAM was closer to their own beliefs about health. Only a small percentage of respondents (4.4 percent) reported using CAM as their sole source for treatment. For this reason, it may be more accurate to predict that alternative medicine will become more *complementary*—that is, a supplement, to allopathic medicine, rather than an alternative or replacement.

Among the demographic variables of respondents that predicted use of CAM were more education, poorer health status, a holistic orientation toward health, and a "transformational" change in health status that influenced their thinking. Fully 40 percent of the respondents reported that they had used some form of CAM during the preceding year for health conditions that included chronic pain (37 percent), anxiety and "other health problems" (31 percent), sprains/muscle strains (26 percent), addiction problems (25 percent), and arthritis (25 percent).

Even the government is jumping on the CAM bandwagon. The Dietary Supplement Health and Education Act of 1994 agrees that "consumers should be empowered to make informed choices about preventative health-care programs based on scientific studies relating to dietary supplements." More recently, the Health Coverage Availability and Affordability Act of 1996 (H.R. 3103) extends to consumers freedom of choice and greater access to food, drugs, medical devices, and procedures not yet approved by the FDA. In addition, an NIH panel of experts recently endorsed acupuncture for the treatment of some types of pain and nausea. And the NIH's Office of Alternative Medicine (OAM) is funding five research centers to explore mind–body interactions and numerous studies of dietary supplements, including the use of St. John's Wort for depression and of the amino acid glucosamine for osteoarthritis (Gillcrest, 1998).

Naturally, the alternative health care market contributes to this empowerment. The increase in the number of CAM providers is projected to be 88 percent between 1994 and 2010, whereas the increase in the number of physicians is projected to be only about 16 percent (Cooper & Stoflet, 1996). One market research company reported that in 1994, U. S. consumers spent more than $100 billion on various alternative health care products (Jacobs, 1999).

The Best of Both Worlds

In the end, no single approach to health care has all the answers; the search for the best solution to a medical condition often requires a willingness to look beyond one remedy or system of treatment. Already, many insurance companies cover certain alternative methods, including acupuncture. And conventional doctors are incorporating alternative therapies into their treatment regimens. The NIH estimates that more than half of all conventional physicians use some form of CAM themselves or refer their patients to such forms of treatment (NCCAM, 2001). As a result, there is a growing movement to provide CAM instruction as a regular part of medical school curriculum. Currently 63 medical schools offer elective courses in CAM (Spencer, 1999). A survey of American physicians' knowledge and use of, training in, and acceptance of CAM as legitimate yielded the range of attitudes summarized in Table 14.2, page 632. Diet and exercise, biofeedback, and counseling or psychotherapy were most often utilized.

Thus, health care in the United States is moving toward a more open-minded view of unconventional medicine. Even the American Medical Association (AMA) has shifted its views toward greater tolerance. As late as the mid-1970s, the AMA's official position was that "the fakes, the frauds, and the quackeries need to be identified, exposed, and, if possible, eradicated" (AMA, 1973).

Table 14.2

Percentage of Physicians (*n* = 176) Using Alternative Medicine and Classifying Various Treatments as Legitimate or Alternative

Treatment	Legitimate Medical Practice	Have Used in Practice	Alternative Medicine
Counseling/psychotherapy	97.2	30.8	12.4
Biofeedback	92.5	53.8	18.4
Diet and exercise	92.1	96.6	12.1
Behavioral medicine	91.5	58.9	16.8
Hypnotherapy	73.7	30.8	30.6
Massage therapy	57.5	35.1	42.0
Acupuncture	55.9	13.5	48.9
Chiropractic	48.9	27.2	45.7
Vegetarianism	45.9	22.2	53.3
Art therapy	39.1	12.9	42.4
Acupressure	38.4	12.9	52.6
Prayer	32.8	30.8	53.4
Homeopathic medicine	26.9	5.3	62.2
Herbs	22.6	6.9	67.7
Megavitamins	21.1	13.5	60.8
Oriental medicine	18.3	1.8	56.1
Electromagnetic applications	17.5	7.1	52.0
Native American medicine	16.9	3.5	60.1

Source: Adapted from "Physicians' Attitudes toward Complementary or Alternative Medicine: A Regional Survey," by B. M. Berman, B. K. Singh, L. Lao, B. Singh, K. S. Ferentz, and S. M. Hartnoll, 1995, *The Journal of the American Board of Family Practice, 8,* pp. 361–368.

By 1995, however, the AMA had substituted "alternative medicine" for "quackery" and passed a resolution encouraging its members to "become better informed regarding the practices and techniques of alternative or complementary medicine" (AMA, 1995). In November 1998, the prestigious *Journal of the American Medical Association* devoted its entire issue to the subject of alternative medicine. And where there once were none, there are now five peer-reviewed journals devoted to alternative medicine.

Still, caveat emptor, "let the buyer beware," is sound advice for consumers considering CAM therapies. Statutory requirements for the practice of CAM differ from state to state. Provider-practice acts for massage exist in 22 states. Licensure is now required in 25 states and the District of Columbia. Naturopathy practice acts exist in 12 states, although each state defines the scope of such practice differently (Spencer & Jonas, 1997).

The Politics of Medicine

The growing acceptability of CAM should not, however, be construed as an indication of its complete acceptance by the biomedical community. Both alternative and conventional medicine are guilty of discounting one another's approach to health care. Alternative practitioners tend to believe that everything conventional medicine says *must* be wrong, just as some physicians believe that everything opposed by the AMA must be quackery.

Partisanship and extremism are certainly roadblocks to rational thinking and barriers to good health care. It is probably safest to say that the truth lies somewhere in between the two viewpoints, that both conventional medicine and alternative medicine are mixtures of good and bad health practices. The best course is to be an informed consumer and to be skeptical about unsupported claims.

Clearly, the best result would be patients having access to the "best of both worlds." Following a conventional medical evaluation and discussion of conventional allopathic options, patients may choose a CAM consultation. But before doing so, the physician (according to Daniel Eisenberg, 1977), should

- Ensure that the patient recognizes and understands his or her symptoms.
- Maintain a record of all symptoms including the patient's own opinions.
- Review any potential for harmful interactions.
- Plan for a follow-up visit to review CAM effectiveness.

This approach is designed to help keep communication channels open between patient and provider so that the patient receives the most effective and safest treatment.

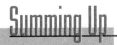

Summing Up

What Is Complementary and Alternative Medicine?

1. *Complementary and alternative medicine* (CAM) refers to the range of health-promoting interventions that fall outside of conventional, Western biomedicine. Most CAM practitioners work from three fundamental ideals: to provide health treatment that is natural, is holistic, and promotes wellness. The CAM movement has been around for many years, but it was eclipsed during most of the twentieth century by the success of biomedicine.

Medicine or Quackery?

2. Skeptics of CAM raise several concerns about unconventional treatments. Foremost among these concerns is that many CAM therapies have never been subjected to rigorous empirical scrutiny regarding their effectiveness or safety. When CAM studies are conducted, critics contend, the methods are often poor and conclusions questionable. Another concern is that people who rely on CAM therapies instead of conventional medicine may delay or lose the opportunity to benefit from scientifically based treatment.

3. For their part, alternative practitioners counter that it is often impossible to conduct the kinds of formal experiments that mainstream medical researchers are most comfortable with. For example, because many CAM therapies are based on a more holistic philosophy, its advocates claim that treatment variables cannot always be studied independently.

4. CAM skeptics also contend that when conventional therapies fail to help, the acupuncturist, chiropractor, or naturopathist presents a powerful belief system (Hawthorne or placebo effect) designed to give the suffering patient hope that help is available.

Does It Work?

5. Acupuncture was originally practiced as part of an integrated system of healing. Today, its use is sanctioned in the United States primarily for the treatment of pain and addiction.

6. The basic premise of mind–body therapies is that cognitive, emotional, and spiritual factors can have profound effects on one's health. Among the mind–body therapies are hypnosis, relaxation training and meditation (including tai chi and yoga), and spiritual healing.

7. Although hypnosis does not involve a unique state of consciousness, it may be effective in relieving pain in some patients. Those who are most likely to report pain relief from hypnosis also tend to be highly suggestible people and to be very responsive to authority figures.

8. Relaxation and meditation may also promote health by bolstering the immune system, reducing pain, and lowering stress hormones. Several studies have found that people who are religiously active are healthier and live longer than their less religious counterparts, perhaps due to differences in lifestyle, social support, and positive emotions.

9. Research studies also show that chiropractic treatment may decrease the frequency and intensity of tension and migraine headaches and be beneficial in the treatment of otitis media, hypertension, carpal tunnel syndrome, some sports injuries, and arthritis of the hip, wrist, or hand.

10. Naturopathic medicine aims to provide holistic, or whole body, health care by returning humans to their "natural state." Modern naturopathy draws from several CAM traditions, especially herbal medicine, food supplement therapy, and dietary modification.

11. Although roughly 25 percent of our pharmaceutical drugs are derived from herbs, physicians often believe that herbs are ineffective and potentially dangerous.

12. Regarding dietary treatments, there is substantial evidence from epidemiological and experimental studies on animals and humans that diet (in the form of foods or as supplements) can have a major effect on risk factors for certain diseases and the progression of disease.

Looking Ahead: Complementary and Alternative Medicine in the 21st Century

13. Growing interest in CAM is viewed by some as one of several indications of a major paradigm shift in medicine and health care in the United States.

Key Terms and Concepts

holistic medicine, p. 592
complementary and alternative medicine (CAM), p. 592
vitalism, p. 595

traditional Oriental medicine, p. 595
anecdotal evidence, p. 600
Hawthorne effect, p. 601
acupuncture, p. 603

tai chi, p. 613
yoga, p. 614
naturopathic medicine, p. 621

Health Psychology on the World Wide Web

Web Address	Description
http://odp.od.nih.gov/ods/	Web site of NIH's Office of Dietary Supplements, which tracks bona fide research on supplements from ginkgo biloba to melatonin.
http://nccam.nih.gov/	Web site of NIH's Office of Alternative Medicine.
http://www.pitt.edu/~cbw/altm.html	The Alternative Medicine Homepage.

Critical Thinking Exercise

Evidence or Anecdote?

Now that you have read and reviewed Chapter 14, take your learning a step further by testing your critical thinking skills on the following scientific reasoning exercise.

Surely almost all scientists, biomedical researchers, and those seriously interested in documenting the effectiveness of CAM would agree that, regardless of what theory health care practitioners wish to espouse, they cannot escape the obligation to support their claims with objective evidence. Despite frequent claims of abundant evidence for their pet therapy, some practitioners of alternative medicine offer little more than the claim itself, unsupported by objective and documented observations. To them, it seems, subjective belief in the treatment, if persuasive enough to the patient, should be adequate to support the claims.

When some CAM zealots provide "evidence," it is often in the form of an *anecdote*, a sort of case history, related by the patient or reported through the eyes of the practitioner. Anecdotal evidence *is* frequently found in the medical literature, in the form of case studies, to suggest the effectiveness of a treatment that has not yet been subjected to formal clinical trials. But in such cases, there is almost always meticulous documentation, including objective data, to *establish the diagnosis* before treatment begins and *to verify what actually happened* as an outcome measure of the effectiveness of the treatment. Consider the following example of an anecdote, offered by CAM guru Andrew Weil, in his *Eight Weeks to Optimum Health* (1999). In the first, a patient writes:

> Six years ago (I'm now twenty-seven) the doctors threw the ugly "C-word" at me and made it sound like a death sentence. (It was bone cancer.) They decided that they were the authorities and I was the victim and the only way was their way. I walked out of their offices never to return. I took up biking (about five hundred miles a week) and running (about sixty miles a week), and ate fresh fruit, juices, and whole grains . . . noth-

> ing else. Too bad more people out there won't acknowledge what a little self-determination and using one's subconscious can do to return a person to wholeness.

The patient goes on to say that he or she is now completely free of disease and hopes to help others discover alternative pathways to health and wholeness.

In the second example, Weil tells the story of a woman with an "unusual form of Parkinson's disease" which caused her to have frequent seizures. Following Weil's advice, she tried "acupuncture, yoga, massage, meditation," and finally "respiratory biofeedback," which eventually caused the seizures to stop.

To the critical thinker, these examples raise several questions: How do we know that these patients really had bone cancer and Parkinson's disease? And what really happened following the treatment?

To increase your awareness of the prevalence of unscientific thinking in the unconventional treatment "evidence" arena, find a current advertisement for a dietary supplement or other alternative treatment and then evaluate the quality of its supporting documentation. You should have no trouble finding material to work with. Check out any one of the many popular "natural health" magazines; alternatively, channel or Web surf until you find an appropriate television or Internet infomercial. Then answer the following questions:

1. What product is endorsed in the advertisement? Where was it advertised? To what group(s) of people is the product being targeted?

2. What is the nature of the supporting evidence for the product?

3. If the evidence is anecdotal, are objective data presented regarding the original, "pretreatment diagnosis" of patients and the outcome of the treatment?

4. Do you consider the evidence presented for the product to be credible and trustworthy? Explain your reasoning.

6

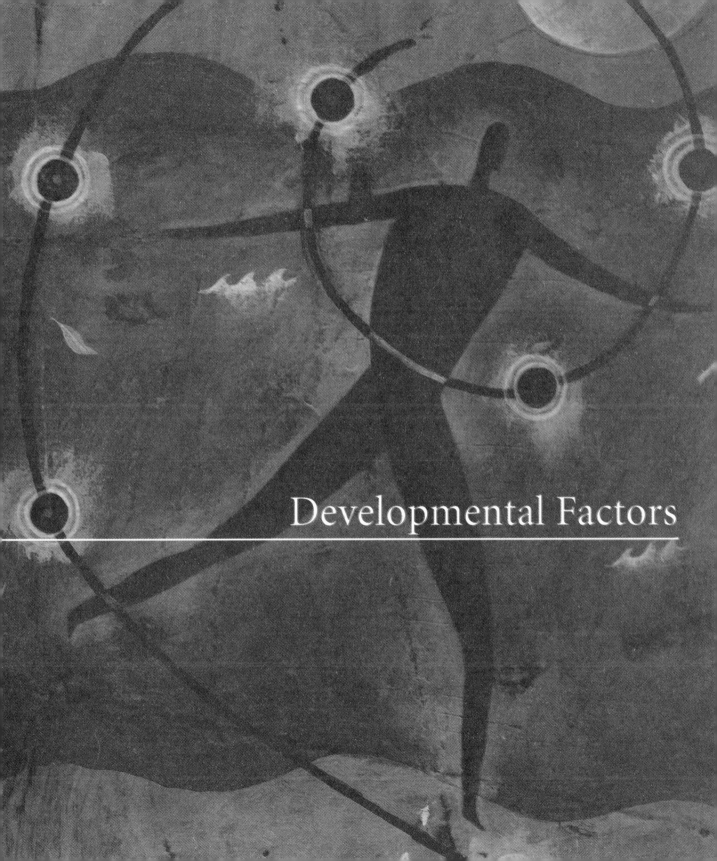

Developmental Factors

15

Health Psychology through the Life Span

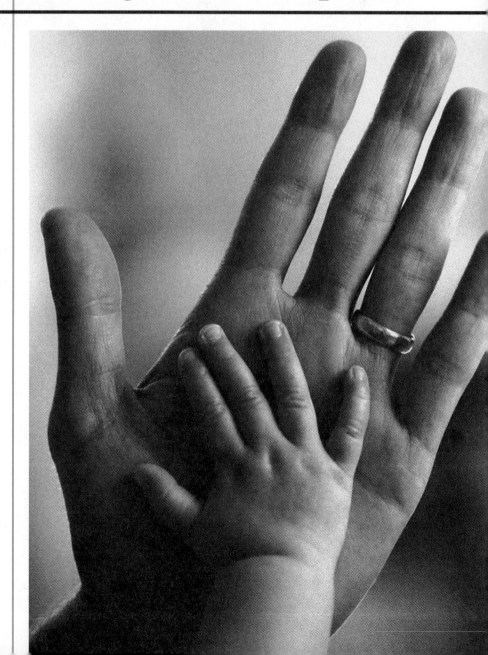

*I*t began in a relatively uneventful manner, as childhood health problems often do: soreness and swelling on the left side of 6-year-old Wyett's neck that seemed to appear overnight and wouldn't go away. An almost-casual visit to the family pediatrician revealed that the discomfort was due to swollen lymph glands yet did not seem to be a cause for alarm. Just to be safe, Wyett was referred to the university's pediatric hospital for a few more tests to rule out any (unlikely) serious health problems. After a morning of blood tests; physical examinations by a stream of nurses, doctors, and interns; and finally magnetic resonance imaging (MRI) of Wyett's neck, the now-worried parents were ushered into a small waiting room in the pediatric oncology wing of the hospital. There, the diagnosis hit full force: non-Hodgkin's lymphoma. Just as their son's life was beginning, it seemed to be in danger of ending.

Fortunately, Wyett and his family were not defenseless against a disease that only a few decades earlier would almost certainly have been fatal. A full biopsychosocial assault ensued, including state-of-the-art biomedical interventions that arrested the cancer, a healthy diet and exercise program, and relaxation training to ease the discomfort of chemotherapy and promote a positive outlook. In addition to his immediate family, Wyett's friends, classmates, primary care physician, and especially nurses provided extensive social support. Fourteen years later, Wyett is a healthy college junior who credits his survival to the powers of mind–body medicine.

At the other end of life's spectrum is Lucy Somerville Howorth of Cleveland, Mississippi, a centenarian, one of those 100-year-old "superstars" of aging fortunate enough not to have succumbed to life-threatening illnesses. Lucy's life began at the dawn of the last century, when most people still lived on rural farms and horses were the only means of transportation. Consider what she has witnessed in her time: two world wars, the Great Depression, Prohibition, the Spanish influenza pandemic that claimed more than 21 million people worldwide in one year—675,000 in the United States alone—and the rise and fall of communism. Lucy has seen transportation advance from the automobile to the airplane to the space shuttle; communication from the radio to television to the Internet. She has witnessed medicine's advance from the use of leeches for bleeding to MRIs, interferon, and laser-guided surgery. Through it all Lucy and other centenarians have persevered, some achieving fortune and fame, most living lives of relative anonymity.

Health psychologists are ideally suited to meet the challenges of dealing with and learning from the psychological and physiological problems facing people throughout the life span. A child with a life-threatening chronic illness presents especially intense stresses and coping challenges to both the child and his or her family. For the child, there is the pain and fear of chemotherapy, radiation, or surgical procedures and, of course, the threat of death; for the parents, the emotional toll of having a sick or dying child is often sufficient to trigger serious psychological and physiological symptoms in otherwise healthy individuals.

Health psychologists offer centenarians the ability to improve the quality of life for those who live in nursing homes, often victimized by senile dementia and physical frailty. They can also learn firsthand how people achieve long life. Besides benefiting from improvements in nutrition and public health, centenarians have their own secrets to long life. For example, Lucy Somerville Howorth attributes her *great age to heredity: "I guess I was blessed with the long genes," she says (Edelman, 1999, p. xii). Ivy Frisk points to lifestyle factors: "I lived a simple life and a clean life. And I worked like heck!" Philip Carret adds a bit more detail: "Don't worry, don't smoke, drink in moderation or not at all. And make as many friends as you can."*

In this chapter, we explore health psychology through the life span, focusing our attention on childhood, adolescence, and late adulthood. We will consider the origins of health-enhancing and health-compromising beliefs and behaviors in childhood and adolescence, the role of clinical health psychology in helping chronically ill children (and their families) cope with chronic illness and stressful medical procedures, the factors that speed up or slow down physical and psychological aging, and theories of why aging takes place at all.

Childhood and Adolescence

As you'll recall from Chapter 1, since the beginning of the twentieth century improvements in sanitation, housing, and medicine have resulted in a substantial shift in patterns of disease in the United States and other developed countries. This is especially true of diseases of childhood and adolescence. The introduction of widespread inoculation programs have to a large extent eradicated many diseases and have dramatically improved the general health of children in developed countries worldwide. It is important to remember, of course, that outside the developed world children are still at risk for infectious diseases that are no longer much of a problem in more affluent countries. Although a number of chronic diseases, genetic disorders, and other adverse health outcomes remain for which there are no cures, many of the most serious threats to the health of children and adolescents today are essentially preventable behavioral problems (Maternal and Child Health Bureau, 2000). Among these are inadequate diet; tobacco, alcohol, and drug use; automobile accidents; and early and unprotected sexual activity. In fact, such health-compromising behaviors are the major causes of both mortality and morbidity in childhood and adolescence (Maternal and Child Health Bureau, 2000). In this section, we examine some of these behaviors, first for childhood and then for adolescence.

Early Health Patterns

The early, formative years are particularly important for a child's health because they can set the pattern for the years to come. Fortunately, most children are healthy and grow rapidly during this period. Every year between the ages of 2 and 6, the typical child grows nearly 3 inches (7 centimeters) and gains about 4$\frac{1}{2}$ pounds (2 kilograms). These figures, however, are merely averages, and the range of healthy development is quite broad, particularly for height and body weight. Certain factors generally account for the differences in height. For example, children often are taller than their peers if they are well nourished, are rarely sick, have parents who are nonsmokers, live in urban areas, are firstborn, and are of African or northern European ancestry (Lowrey, 1986). Conversely, children may be shorter than average if they are malnourished, are frequently sick, are female of Asian ancestry, are of lower socioeconomic status, live in a rural area, have a mother who smoked during pregnancy, and are a third- or later-born child in a large family.

Compared to other stages of the life span, childhood for most children is uneventful in terms of overall health. In fact, during the school years children in developed nations are the healthiest of people of any age, being least likely to die or become seriously injured or ill. Among U.S. children ages 5 to 14, African-American children had the highest death rate in 1998 (29 per 100,000 children) and Asian/Pacific Islander children had the lowest death rate (14 per 100,000). As Figure 15.1 shows, unintentional injuries, birth defects, homicide,

Figure 15.1

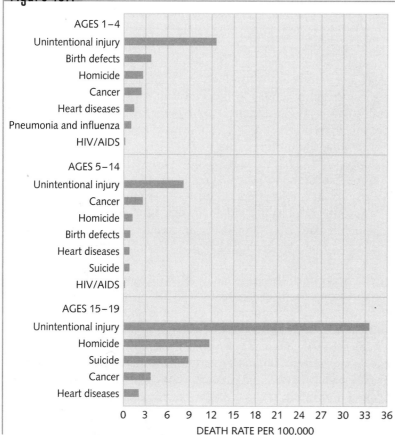

Leading Causes of Death in Children and Adolescents
In 1998 in the United States, 26,830 children and adolescents aged 1 to 19 died. By a large margin, injury was the major cause of death in all age groups. Since 1997, this represents a decrease of 3.4 percent among 1- to 4-year-olds and more than 4.3 percent among 5- to 14-year-olds. Although the death rate among adolescents increased during the mid- to late 1980s, it has decreased 19 percent since 1993. Note that the major causes of death among children and adolescents are external events such as injury and homicide.

Source: *Deaths: Final Data for 1998*, National Vital Statistics Reports, *48*(11), by S. A. Murphy, 2000. Hyattsville, MD: National Center for Health Statistics.

and cancer are the leading causes of death among children ages 1 to 4; between 5 and 14, unintentional injuries, cancer, and homicide are the leading causes of death; and for the 15- to 19-year-old group, unintentional injuries, homicide, and suicide are the leading causes of death (Childstats, 2001).

Child health varies by family income. Children living below the poverty line are less likely to be in very good or excellent health (68 percent) than children in higher-income families (86 percent) (Childstats, 2001). Males ages 5 to 17 are more likely than females in the same age group to have activity limitations due to illness, as are *low-birth-weight infants* (infants born weighing less than 2,500 grams, or about 5.5 pounds). The percentage of infants born with low birth weight has increased somewhat over the past 15 years, due in part to an increase in the number of twin and triplet births (MacDorman & Atkinson, 1999).

Childhood Nutrition

Within developed countries such as the United States, food is plentiful for most children, and variations in weight and height are more likely due to differences in genes than to differences in nutrition. Children are, however, susceptible to the risks of unhealthy eating habits. Where there is nutritional deficiency in developed countries, it is usually in the form of *iron-deficiency anemia,* caused by an inadequate supply of dark green vegetables, whole grains, eggs, and other foods with a high iron content. Although this problem is much more prevalent among low-income families (because less expensive foods tend to have a poor iron content), children of every socioeconomic class are at risk, due to their tendency to consume too many sugary and fatty foods. Besides promoting tooth decay—the most common disease of early childhood in developed countries—sugary foods fill up a small child too quickly, leaving no appetite for foods that contain vitamins, minerals, and other essential nutrients (Lewitt & Kerrebrock, 1998). As an example of the prevalence of unhealthy nutritional habits in children, by one estimate nearly 90 percent of U.S. preschoolers consume more than the recommended maximum daily amount of fat (30 percent of their daily calories) (Thompson & Dennison, 1994).

Children's food preferences—which often become adult food preferences—come partly from their parents, who set many expectations for the types of foods eaten, the frequency of meals, and so forth. Parents also use food—usually non-nutritious food such as candy or chocolate cake—as a reward to influence their children's behavior. For example, "If you eat your broccoli, you can have dessert." Although a learning theorist might applaud this effort to make a highly desired food (dessert) contingent on eating a less desired food (in order to reinforce eating the latter), many researchers have found that this coercive strategy is often counterproductive (Striegel-Moore, Silberstein,

& Rodin, 1986). Children often develop an even greater distaste for the target food, perhaps reasoning that "This food is so terrible that they have to bribe me to eat it!"

Childhood Obesity

The school years are, however, the time when obesity begins to become a serious health problem. Recall from Chapter 7 that the most objective measure of obesity is body mass index (BMI), which is determined by dividing a person's weight in kilograms by his or her height in meters squared. Using this statistical index, the cutoff for obesity at age 8 is a BMI of 18; at age 12, the threshold of obesity is a BMI of 23.

By this measure, it is estimated that between 20 and 30 percent of American children are obese, a figure that has risen steadily for the past four decades and parallels the incidence and prevalence of obesity among adults (Maternal and Child Health Bureau, 2000). These figures are, of course, troubling because of the many health risks associated with obesity. Obese children are at increased risk for a number of serious health disorders, including orthopedic and respiratory problems, diabetes, heart disease, and strokes (Eveleth & Tanner, 1991). And they often do not outgrow these problems. Obese adults, who were obese as children, report higher levels of stress and have more psychophysiological problems than adults whose obesity is of recent onset (Mills & Adrianopoulos, 1993).

Although genes may predispose a body type that is vulnerable to obesity, good health habits become increasingly important in overshadowing heredity's grip on body weight. As evidence, consider this: Children under age 3 with one obese parent are three times as likely as children with nonobese parents to become obese adults themselves. However, by age 10, the child's own body weight predicts the risk of obesity with far greater accuracy. Only 15 percent of normal-weight 10-year-olds who have one obese parent become obese adults themselves, while 64 percent of children who are obese at age 10 eventually become obese adults, even if neither parent was obese (Whitaker, Wright, Pepe, Seidel, & Dietz, 1997).

In the vast majority of cases, whether a particular child becomes obese depends on the interaction of several factors, including the following:

- *Body type.* Certain combinations of height, bone structure, and basal metabolism—all of which are strongly influenced by heredity—contribute to excess storage of body fat and an elevated BMI.

- *Television.* Watching TV promotes obesity in part because 60 percent of the commercials shown during Saturday morning cartoon shows are for foods. Of these commercials, about 51 percent are for sugary cereals; 22 percent, for candy and gum; and 11 percent, for cookies (Story & Faulkner, 1990). Since a typical child watches between 6 and 7 hours of television each day, in one year, children will literally be exposed to thousands of commercials for food products, almost all of them with high fat and sugar content. And the people depicted eating these foods are almost always slender, popular children, who appear to be having a great time because of their food choices (Ogletree, Williams, Raffeld, Mason, & Fricke, 1990). Television also promotes obesity by lowering metabolic rate. While glued to the TV, children fall into a deeply relaxed state in which their metabolism drops *below* its basal (resting) rate—an average decrease of 12 percent in normal-weight children (Klesges, Shelton, & Klesges, 1993). For obese children, metabolism drops 16 percent.

- *Activity level.* Because their metabolic rates are lower, inactive children burn fewer calories and are much more likely to be obese than are their more active counterparts. Children today are exercising less than in the past (Childstats, 2000). A child's activity level is influenced by many factors, including heredity, the availability of safe recreational areas, the activity levels modeled by the child's parents, and body weight itself, which is negatively correlated with exercise. Of these factors, the parents' exercise habits are particularly powerful influences on childhood weight—and even more so if the parents exercise with their children (Ross, Pate, Casperson, Domberg, & Svilar, 1987).

  Although school recreation programs have a well-documented beneficial effect on health, fitness, and the amount of exercise children seek outside of school (Brownell & Kay, 1982), financial woes have forced many schools to cut back on the programs that are the most beneficial to the majority of students. Instead, they emphasize the big money competitive sports that remain the most popular spectator sports in the community.

- *Food attitudes.* In some families, overeating is a common practice linked to celebrations and happiness. Some cultures, too, associate overeating with wealth, prosperity, and even the parents' love for their children. The implicit message is that "because I love you, I want you to eat. Because you love me, you will clean your plate."

Adolescence and Risk Taking

In most ways, the teenage years are also among the healthiest in the life span. There is a sharp decrease in the flus, colds, and other minor illnesses of childhood, as accumulated exposure to immunogens have strengthened the individual's immunity. Moreover, the leading causes of death during adulthood, including cardiovascular disease and cancer, are rare. A teenager's chance of succumbing to either a fatal heart attack or terminal cancer are only about one-third that of a 30-year-old adult and only one-hundredth that of a 70-year-old.

During adolescence, of course, individuals become more directly responsible for their own health, as they begin making their own decisions regarding whether to engage in health-enhancing or health-compromising behaviors. More than 50 percent of all cases of adolescent morbidity and mortality can be attributed to preventable risky behaviors, including poor eating habits, substance abuse, and risky sexual behavior (Eiser, 1997) (see also Chapters 7, 8, and 11, respectively).

Although most adolescents in developed countries are reasonably well nourished most of the time, it is also true that most teenagers are vulnerable to strange diets, food fads, and periods of overeating, undereating, and nutritional imbalance. Although poor eating habits are harmful at every age, they can be particularly damaging during the growth spurt of puberty, when the systems of the body must have adequate nourishment to reach their full growth potential. For girls in many industrialized nations, preoccupation with being thin is too often the precursor of a serious, potentially life-threatening eating disorder.

After a relatively long period of decline in the regular use of most drugs, the number of high school students admitting to drug use began to increase during the 1990s and continues to climb today (Jarvis & Sutherland, 2001). Particularly troublesome is the early onset of drug use. About half of all eighth graders in the United States have already had at least one drink and at least one cigarette. Nearly 20 percent have already tried marijuana, fully twice the percentage that admitted to doing so in 1991.

Many studies have shown that tobacco, alcohol, and marijuana often are *gateway drugs* for many teens, opening the door to other drugs and leading to serious drug- and alcohol-abuse problems later on (Gerstein & Green, 1993). Teenagers who begin to use tobacco, alcohol, or marijuana before the ninth grade are more likely to experiment with illegal drugs in high school and to have alcohol- and drug-abuse problems as adults. They are also more likely to engage in risky sexual behaviors, suffer poor physical health, and experience depression (Kandel & Davies, 1996).

Worldwide, more teenagers are becoming sexually active—and at a younger age—than ever before. In 1999, more than half of all American 16-year-olds had had sexual intercourse, as had 80 percent of 19-year-olds (National Center for Health Statistics). By their senior year of high school, an estimated 27 percent of American teenagers had already had four or more sexual partners. Teen intercourse rates are also high in Western Europe but are much lower in Asian and Arab countries (less than 3 percent of unmarried university students in China, for instance, report having had sexual intercourse) (McLaughlin, Chen, Greenberger, & Biermeier, 1997). Although data on younger teenagers are limited, at least one study of students in a poor New England city found that 19 percent of the 12-year-olds had already had sexual intercourse (Barone et al., 1996). In addition to unwanted pregnancy and interference with educational

■ **sexually transmitted diseases (STDs)** diseases such as gonorrhea, syphilis, chlamydia, genital herpes, and AIDS that are communicated through sexual contact

■ **invincibility fable** the mistaken belief of many adolescents that they are immune to the dangers of unprotected sex, drug abuse, or other risky behaviors

and vocational goals, the negative consequences of early sexual activity include a variety of **sexually transmitted diseases (STDs)**. In fact, sexually active adolescents have the highest rate of gonorrhea, genital herpes, syphilis, and chlamydia of all age groups (Maternal and Child Health Bureau, 2000). Moreover, as noted in Chapter 11, sexually active adolescents are more likely to engage in unsafe sex, dramatically increasing their risk of HIV.

Why is risk taking so common during adolescence? Christine Eiser (1997) offers three possible explanations.

1. Hormonal changes during puberty engender risk taking, causing those who mature earlier to be at greater health risk than adolescents who mature late or "on time." This is because their hormones cause them to desire sexual activity, but they are not psychologically mature enough to know how to protect themselves against possible unwanted consequences.

2. Sociodemographic factors promote risk taking. For example, children of alcohol abusers are more likely to drink excessively themselves.

3. Peer-conscious teens tend to behave in ways that will help them to be accepted by their peer group. Such behavior may be very different from behavior subject to their ordinary good common sense.

Eiser's explanations are all based on recognition that the typical teenager tends to have immature, if not faulty, reasoning skills, which are further limited by an **invincibility fable** ("it won't happen to me"). Risk taking during adolescence is also strongly influenced by a teen's personality. For example, rebelliousness, aggressiveness, and a general "deviance proneness" have been found to be strong predictors of substance abuse during adolescence (Eiser & Main, 2001). Teenagers who are emotionally detached from their families are also more likely to abuse drugs (Turner, Burciaga, Sussman, & Klein-Selski, 1993), in part because closeness to parents appears to predict choosing friends who are not drug users.

Interventions

What role does health psychology play in promoting well-being during childhood and adolescence? For a number of years, psychologists have been working with pediatricians and other physicians to prevent or to treat patients' health problems and to help parents deal with their child's illness or psychological problems (Drotar, 1995). Consider Chapel Hill Pediatrics, a private group practice serving approximately 20,000 patients in a small university town in North Carolina. Health psychologists have been involved with the practice since 1973, offering a wide range of services tailored to the needs of the patients and their parents. These services focus on prevention and early intervention, referred to as *well-child care.*

Interventions for Chronically Ill Children

Although childhood and adolescence are healthy periods of life, in 1997, 8 percent of U.S. children ages 5 to 17 were limited in their activities because of one or more chronic health conditions (Childstats, 2001). The most prevalent childhood chronic diseases are asthma, congenital heart disease, kidney disease, and childhood diabetes. These are generally not the same conditions that strike us in adulthood.

Children and adolescents who are diagnosed with chronic illnesses face a multitude of stressors. Many have to be hospitalized repeatedly, and many receive complicated sequences of uncomfortable treatments. The specific potential stresses associated with chronic childhood disease and hospitalization include (Melamed, Kaplan, & Fogel, 2001; Schmidt, 1997)

- separation from family.
- fantasies and anxieties about darkness, monsters, and other dangers associated with being in a strange situation.
- fears of disablement and death.
- pain, fear, and other complications of the illness or treatment.

These and other stresses may place chronically ill children at increased risk of a variety of psychological problems, including low self-esteem, feelings of helplessness, and depression (Holden, Chmielewski, Nelson, Kager, & Foltz, 1997).

Because adjustment to a child's chronic illness is influenced less by the severity of the condition than by psychological and environmental factors, health psychologists can play an important role in helping young people and their families cope with the strains of serious illness (Chaney, Mullins, Frank, & Peterson, 1997). Indeed, over the past 20 years, psychologists have been instrumental in improving the situation of children in most hospitals (Schmidt, 1997). More liberal visiting hours, rooming-in privileges for parents, shorter hospital stays, and thorough psychological preparation of children and family members prior to treatment or hospitalization are among the many initiatives that have produced this improved state of affairs. In addition, many pediatric floors offer play groups, activity rooms, and staff who are much better prepared to meet children's special needs. Thus, stimulation and nurturance have today superseded earlier inhumane conditions for hospitalized children.

How Children Respond to Illness

Christine Eiser (1990) identified three influences on how children respond to chronic illnesses. The first has to do with the extent to which the disease is life-threatening and disrupts the child's normal routine. As with other childhood stresses, such as divorce, illness evokes increasingly adverse reactions in the child as its impact disrupts the child's normal routine. In one study, 108 young students rated 28 health impairments in terms of three criteria: quality of life perceived to be possible, the extent to which the state was perceived as a fate better or worse than death, and the extent to which the state was perceived to interfere with the ability to engage in valued activities (Ditto, Druley, Moore, Danks, & Smucker, 1996). For any given health condition, the more it was perceived by individuals as likely to interfere with their most valued daily activities, the more negatively it was rated.

The second factor in children's ability to adjust is how they understand and interpret their illness and treatment (see Diversity and Healthy Living). In general, children who are older, more mature, and able to make realistic attributions for their condition are more likely to adjust positively to the disease. In one study (Bearison, Sadow, Granowetter, & Winckel, 1993), researchers explored the kinds of attributions that children with cancer make about the dis-

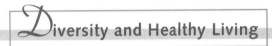

Diversity and Healthy Living

Children's Perceptions of Disease and Death

Almost all children need to understand the reasons for disease and death before they reach puberty. For the approximately 10 percent or so who develop a chronic or life-threatening condition themselves, the need arises through their struggle to understand why they feel bad, have a changed physical appearance, or need painful treatments. Others need to understand so they can cope with the sickness or death of a friend or relative and develop empathy for others who are struggling with a health problem. Probably most important, many psychologists believe that children should understand how to prevent diseases, such as heart disease, as early in life as is realistically possible (Sigelman, Maddock, Epstein, & Carpenter, 1993).

Many researchers have followed Jean Piaget's enormously influential stage theory of cognitive development. According to this model, thinking during the *preoperational stage* (2 to 6 years) is viewed as being quite limited in logical reasoning ability. Children at this age also are believed to be highly *egocentric,* that is, unable to see things from another individual's point of view.

Preoperational children often profess beliefs about illness that are superstitious, vague, and fraught with fear. Asked why people get colds, preoperational children have offered explanations such as "from kissing old ladies" and "they just do" (Bibace & Walsh, 1981). And like our ancestors, many children believe that illness (and its often unpleasant cures) is a form of punishment. Many preoper-

ational children also believe that death can be avoided or undone, making it difficult for them to understand the finality and irreversibility of death. And their egocentric thinking causes many preoperational children to feel somehow personally responsible when a friend or relative dies unexpectedly.

Because even very young children may experience death—from the death of a grandparent to the death of an adored pet—from an early age, they begin to reason and ask questions about this final stage of the life span. In her studies of children aged 3 to 10, Maria Nagy (1948) found evidence of three separate stages in understanding death. Very young children, up to about 5 years of age, tend to view death as a temporary separation, similar to being asleep, from which the individual is fully expected to return. Children in the second stage, up to about 9 years of age, understand that death is final but don't believe that they, themselves, will ever die. Finally, at age 10 or so, children reach the final stage of adultlike understanding, in which death is understood to be permanent, irreversible, and universal.

By about 6 or 7 years of age, according to Piaget, children enter the stage of *concrete operations,* during which they begin to think more logically—at least about tangible objects and events. At this time their thinking becomes more specific, and they begin to realize that illness and death have biological causes. By the end of this stage, they accept the reality and finality of death and understand that everyone—including themselves—will eventually die.

ease to determine whether attributional style predicted coping and adjustment. They found that children who avoided making self-blaming, internal attributions for the illness coped significantly better with the stresses of treatment than did those who made internal attributions or who made no attributions.

In Chapter 5, we drew a distinction between healthy *active coping* strategies such as cognitive reappraisal and potentially harmful *repressive coping* strategies such as denial. Researchers have found that these different strategies can be observed even in very young children. For example, Sean Phipps and Deo Srivastava (1997) found that compared with healthy children, children with cancer reported greater use of both **blunting** and avoidant coping (Phipps, Fairclough, & Mulhern, 1995). Blunting is a coping strategy that limits thoughts about threatening or distressing stimuli, thus reducing emotional distress and possibly protecting the child from full awareness of threats to his

blunting a coping strategy that limits threatening thoughts in an effort to reduce emotional stress

As their thinking becomes more sophisticated and rational during the *formal operational* stage (beginning at about age 12), children's understanding is refined even more, especially in terms of the relationship between biological and psychological health. While studies have shown that children generally know a great deal about the risks associated with some behaviors (such as sexual contact and shared drug needles), they remain confused about others, including the possible dangers of donating blood and kissing (Brown, Nassau, & Barone, 1990). In addition, their reasoning tends to be clouded by illusions of invincibility and a tendency to focus only on immediate concerns rather than on the long-term consequences of their actions.

Piaget's stage theory is controversial. One frequent criticism is that children's beliefs about sickness and death are much more variable than the theory would predict, given its tendency to underestimate the importance of social and cultural factors in development. Children who have some knowledge of a relative's illness, for example, have a more accurate understanding of *that* particular disease but not necessarily of others (Eiser, 1997). Similarly, children who have direct contact with a sick or dying person (such as when a relative is cared for at home) generally have a better understanding—and acceptance—than do children who have been kept away from the sick or dying person (Lauer, Mulhern, Wallskig, & Camitta, 1983).

An alternative approach stresses that how children organize their knowledge about illness and death deter-

mines their understanding and beliefs. Younger children often think about disease in terms of what they generally know about people and behavior (Carey, 1985). For example, based on their own experiences, they reason that being sent to bed must mean you're sick. As their reasoning matures, older children come to realize that symptoms, not behavior, define illness. In support of this hypothesis, Julie Hergenrather and Mitchell Rabinowitz (1991) found that, when younger children were asked to sort pictures depicting various causes, symptoms, and treatments of illness, they based their sorting decisions on general knowledge about how adults behave when a child is sick. Older children used disease-specific information such as sneezing, headaches, and other symptoms to guide their decisions.

Other researchers maintain that children's understanding of illness and death depends on the kinds of information to which they are most frequently exposed. In partial support of this hypothesis, some researchers have reported a recent cohort effect in health beliefs. During most of the twentieth century, young children were most often exposed to information about acute illnesses such as colds and influenza. It was only natural that they would generalize from these experiences and assume that all illnesses are contagious and readily transmitted through casual contact with others. During the past decade, children have increasingly been exposed to information about diseases such as cancer and AIDS, and so their views of illness may be undergoing a dramatic change (Eiser, 1997).

or her health. Although blunting is an avoidant strategy, it is conceptualized as a conscious, effortful response to a stressor; repression, on the other hand, is a defensive, automatic reaction, which normally occurs outside of conscious awareness. For this reason, children who blunt are able to alter their coping strategy in response to changing health conditions; repressors cannot.

A third factor in how children adjust to chronic illness relates to the characteristics of the child's family. Families that are close-knit, with good communication and problem-solving skills, tend to provide the social support that children need to make a healthy adjustment to *any* stressful circumstance, including serious illness. As we have seen throughout this book, people who perceive the presence of a strong, supportive network of family and friends generally have better health outcomes than do those who feel isolated or alienated from others. Sadly, some chronically ill children fear that they must endure their struggle alone and that friends will view them as outcasts at the time when they most need their support. As a result, some children "quarantine" themselves, refusing to see visitors and pleading with their parents to be allowed to stay away from school.

Health psychologists have found that social-skills training can improve the ability of children newly diagnosed with cancer to cope with this crisis. In one study, 5- to 13-year-old children were randomly assigned to either a social-skills training group or to a control school reintegration treatment group (Varni, Katz, Colegrove, & Dolgin, 1994). Children who received social-skills training reported significantly greater peer and teacher social support at a 9-month follow-up. In addition, parents of children in this experimental group reported significantly fewer behavior problems and an increase in school competence in their children, as compared to those in the control group.

In another investigation, James Varni and Ernest Katz (1997) evaluated 8- to 13-year-old cancer patients for symptoms of depression and social anxiety, level of self-esteem, and amount of perceived social support. Perceived peer, parent, and teacher social support was strongly correlated with lower psychological distress and higher self-esteem. Furthermore, perceived support of classmates was the strongest predictor of the child's overall adjustment to the treatment regimen.

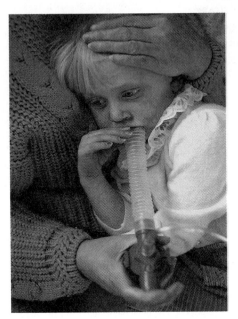

Asthma

Particularly important to a young child with a chronic condition such as asthma, as shown here, is family love and support. Knowing that her parents will help her through the difficult times ahead improves this 2-year-old girl's ability to cope with the strain of illness.

© Kent Meireis / The Image Works

Helping Children Cope with Stressful Medical Procedures

Health psychologists also promote health in children by helping them to cope with stressful medical procedures and to prepare for an upcoming treatment or hospital stay. Hospital tours, informational videos, relaxation training, and modeling sessions have helped many children (and their families) cope with a variety of medical procedures, including chemotherapy, radiotherapy, and surgery (Rudolph, Dennig, & Weisz, 1995).

One of the most stressful procedures to which children with cancer are frequently subjected is venipuncture (drawing blood). In one study, researchers at Memorial Sloan-Kettering Cancer Center developed a behavioral intervention that incorporated parent coaching, attentional distraction, and the use of positive reinforcement to control the children's distress during venipuncture (Memorial Sloan-Kettering Cancer Center, 2001). Children who formerly had required physical restraint were randomly assigned to either the behavioral intervention group or an attention-control group. Based on several measures of child distress, including self-reports and observational data gathered by parents and nurses, children in the behavioral intervention group exhibited significantly lower levels of distress than control children did. Moreover, the use of physical restraint to manage treatment was also reduced significantly.

Primary Prevention

Another area of intervention concerns efforts to help young people develop healthy attitudes and lifestyle behaviors. Many lifelong health attitudes and habits—which are viewed by many as risk factors for the later development of chronic diseases—are established at an early age (Gortmaker, Must, Perrin, & Sobol, 1993). Although young people who have poor eating habits, engage in early and unprotected sex, take drugs, and drive recklessly are not doomed to do so throughout their adult lives, changing unhealthy behaviors is often difficult once they are established. For this reason, most health psychologists emphasize the development of health-enhancing behaviors early in life. Fortunately, some risky behaviors (such as alcohol abuse) are often self-limiting and tend to decline with marriage, the birth of children, and the newly found responsibilities of early adulthood (Eiser, 1997).

Because many of these risk factors appear to be linked to a lack of knowledge about basic nutrition, an obvious solution would be to design nutrition education programs for children most likely to have unhealthy eating habits. As we have noted throughout this book, many health interventions—especially those tailored to young people—focus on primary prevention in the form of educational programs. Despite the widespread belief among health experts that sound decision making depends on a foundation of information, educational programs for adolescents do not always meet with approval. School instruction regarding a healthy diet is one thing; safe sex and drug education for teenagers, however, is quite another. Too often, parents and educators fear that a little knowledge will remove anxieties about drug use or sexual activity and trigger more permissive attitudes and experimentation with risky behaviors.

Most educational programs derive from either the traditional rational model of health education or the social influences–based models. The

ageism attitudes of prejudice and negative stereotypes against older people

rational model focuses on increasing teens' factual knowledge about risky behaviors; the social influences approach aims to help teens implement that knowledge in social contexts (Evans, 2001). Rational model programs tend to fail because, although they are generally effective in increasing knowledge, they are less effective in changing attitudes or behavior (Bruvold & Rundall, 1988). Social norms and immediate concerns often are more important factors in determining a teen's behavior in a given situation than knowledge about possible health consequences.

Social influences approaches tend to be more effective and are being more widely implemented today. However, their effectiveness depends heavily on the skills and approach of the teacher or group leader. In addition, some educators object to them because they generally are more time-consuming and are difficult to fit into an already jam-packed curriculum (Eiser, 1997).

Adulthood and Aging

Although gerontologists and psychologists once viewed adulthood as one long plateau between adolescence and the decline of old age, they now know that it is harder to generalize about stages of adult development than it is about development during childhood and adolescence. If you know that Carla is 3 years old and Rachel is 12, you probably could make a number of general statements about differences in their abilities, interests, and physical characteristics. Although Herman at 50 and David at 59 differ in age by the same number of years, you would be hard-pressed to generalize about their differences. Stated another way, during adulthood, age is only weakly correlated with people's biological, psychological, and social traits.

Consider older relatives, neighbors, celebrities, and others you may know. Why can 80-year-old Walt Stack still run 17 miles a day and compete in the Iron Man Triathlon, while your 60-year-old neighbor, 20 years his junior, needs a walker to creep down the block? Why could Leopold Stokowski sign a 6-year recording contract at age 94 and George Bernard Shaw produce some of his most brilliant writing at age 91, while some 50-year-olds find a simple crossword puzzle maddening? This is one of psychology's most fundamental "truisms": *at every age, but especially during adulthood, individual differences are far greater than differences between groups.* It is for this reason that **ageism**—categorizing people solely on the basis of their age—is so destructive. Ageism affects people of every age. Teenagers, for example, are often stereotyped as being lazy, irresponsible, and self-centered; older adults are seen as frail, in poor health, and mentally rigid. Ageism is most damaging, however, when it encourages stereotypes that isolate older adults from society and makes it difficult for younger people to see elderly people as individuals.

Fortunately, ageist stereotypes are weakening, in part because of the growing body of research in **gerontology,** the scientific study of old age, and **geriatric health psychology,** a branch of health psychology that focuses on the health needs of older people.

To call attention to the variety of trajectories in aging, gerontologists distinguish among the *young-old,* the *old-old,* and the *oldest-old*—a distinction that encompasses all the dimensions of aging (Zarit, 1996). The young-old who despite popular ageist stereotypes make up the majority of older people are, in general, physically vigorous and healthy, financially secure, and socially integrated into the lives of friends, family members, and the community at large. In contrast, the old-old suffer from one or more debilitating physical, psychological, or social deficits and require supportive health care. Finally, the oldest-old, who make up a small minority of elderly adults, are dependent on other people for almost everything. Although age is an unreliable predictor, generally speaking, the young-old are those under age 75, the old-old are generally over age 75, and the oldest old are generally over age 85.

Following the biopsychosocial model, a person's "true age" is more than chronological age; it is the sum of biological, psychological, and social factors that bring him or her to this point in the life cycle. Biological aging, or maturation, brings with it age-related changes in appearance, sharpness of vision, physical agility, and strength. Psychological aging involves several dimensions. One is adjusting to the physical changes that accompany aging. Another is coming to terms with annoying lapses of memory, not-so-speedy reaction times, and somewhat slower information processing. At the same time, as noted earlier, aging can stimulate personal growth, the development of new skills and abilities, and, especially, the wisdom of older age.

The social aspects of aging are equally complex, as our self-concepts change through the seasons of life from being "young" to "middle-aged" to "old." These concepts reflect cultural beliefs and changing social values. At other times in our nation's history, older adults were held in much higher esteem than they are by today's society, with its ageist stereotypes of older people. So too, in other cultures elderly adults are revered for their experience and wisdom.

As with other aspects of health, the three dimensions of aging interact with and influence one another. Occupation and lifestyle, for example, both influence and are influenced by biological aging. People who work at physically demanding jobs, as well as those who exercise regularly, typically maintain muscular strength and organ reserve until much later in life compared to those who work at desk jobs and are sedentary. Social factors such as a strong, loving

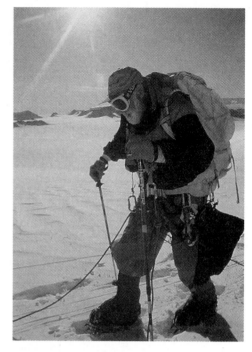

Old Age Doesn't Stop Him
An 88-year-old man takes his first steps on Mt. Vaughan. He was the first person to ascend the mountain in the Antarctic. © Gordon Wiltsie / Peter Arnold, Inc.

■ **gerontology** the scientific study of old age

■ **geriatric health psychology** the branch of health psychology devoted to the special needs of older adults

■ **primary aging** the inevitable and universal physical changes that accompany aging

■ **secondary aging** the specific diseases or health conditions that tend to be more common among older adults, but that are caused by lifestyle choices, genetic vulnerability, and other factors rather than aging itself

network of family and friends can affect psychological functioning, leading, for example, to a feeling of well-being and optimism for the future. And, as we have seen throughout the course of this book, psychological functioning can, in turn, influence our physical well-being, which influences both the psychological and social dimensions of aging.

Geriatric health psychologists distinguish between **primary aging,** which encompasses the universal and irreversible physical changes that all people experience with the passage of time, and **secondary aging,** which refers to the physical changes that are the by-products of illnesses or conditions that become more common with age. We will first discuss elements of primary aging, such as appearance, senses, perception, and physical vitality, then secondary aging, or the diseases that sometimes hinder the quality of the aging process.

Appearance

Despite the claims of cosmetic manufacturers who promise a fountain of youth in a tube or a bottle, for each of us there comes a time when the physical signs of aging can no longer be concealed. Regardless of age, most adults fear looking "old." Fortunately, although some manifestations of aging are inevitable, many more aspects of biological aging *can* be modified. More important, the most easily changed factors seem to be the ones that people generally consider most important to their well-being. Among these are memory, physical vitality, and risk of cancer, arthritis, cardiovascular disease, and other chronic conditions.

One of the most obvious changes in appearance occurs in the body's skin, hair, and fingernails and toenails. For example, as we age the hair becomes thinner and skin becomes less elastic, dry, and marked by wrinkling and increased prominence of blood vessels and darkened "age spots." As we saw in Chapter 10, photoaging speeds up the aging of the skin, giving older sun worshippers a leathery appearance that could have been slowed, if not prevented, by avoiding sun exposure and using UV-ray protecting sunscreens.

Hair begins to turn gray as the body's ability to produce *melanin,* the pigment that colors hair, is reduced. Of all the biological aspects of aging, loss of melanin and the graying of the hair correlate most accurately with a person's chronological age, far more accurately than changes in the skin, senses, muscular strength, or cardiorespiratory capacity (Balin, 1994).

Many older adults also lose an inch or so in height and several pounds in body weight. This latter change occurs in response to the loss of muscle tissue and a decline in bone calcium that occurs at the rate of about 1 to 2 percent a year after menopause in women and after age 55 in men.

Changes in physical appearance can lead to psychological and social consequences, particularly where appearing old is a social handicap. When older adults link their appearance with who they are or rely on the reactions of other people to bolster their egos, aging can be an unhappy time. Most older adults, however, take changes in physical appearance in stride, as they consider their attitudes, personalities, values, and identities to be the same as they were when they were younger (Troll & Skaff, 1997). This is especially true of older adults who are aging optimally in the psychological and social dimensions.

Sensory-Perceptual Changes

Ask elderly people what concerns them most about aging and most of them will not cite gray hair or looking old. Of much greater concern is their fear of becoming dependent on others due to mental decline and increasing isolation and loneliness—a clear expression of our lifelong needs to remain intellectually vigorous and to stay socially connected to others. These needs depend not only on the obvious social and psychological dimensions of health but also to a large extent on the healthy functioning of the eyes, ears, and other senses. Sensory and perceptual losses are among the unalterable manifestations of age, mostly as a result of the accumulation of irreversible scar tissue in our organs (Fries, 1999).

The Senses

Vision As we age, the eye's pupil becomes smaller and the lens becomes cloudier, decreasing the amount of light that falls upon a 65-year-old person's retina by nearly two-thirds the amount received by the retina of a 20-year-old person (Kline & Schieber, 1985). Older adults also may suffer from *cataracts,* which reduce the transparency of the lens, or *glaucoma,* an inherited vision-threatening eye disease that involves a buildup of fluid pressure inside the eyeball and occurs primarily in older adults. Decreased vision at night and seeing halos around lights in dim-light conditions are often the first signs of these problems. About six times as many African-Americans as white Americans develop glaucoma (Sommer et al., 1991). Rates are also higher among people with diabetes. There is no cure for glaucoma, but it can be managed through oral medication, laser treatment, eye drops, and surgery.

Hearing The eardrum and delicate bones of the middle ear become stiffer with age, causing gradual loss of hearing in older adults. One in four adults between the ages of 50 and 80 experiences a significant hearing problem that impairs the person's ability to hear conversation, detect the direction of a sound, and understand digitized speech, such as that heard on many voice mail systems (Thornton, 1989). In addition, a declining ability to hear high frequency sounds, called **presbycusis** (*"old hearing"*), affects about one in three persons after age 65. Presbycusis is due to a reduced supply of nutrients to the inner ear, causing a degeneration of sensitive receptor cells in the cochlea. Speech often becomes unintelligible, especially when background noise is present.

presbycusis literally "old hearing," a term that refers to the age-related loss in sensitivity to sounds—especially those in the high-frequency range

■ **senescence** a general term for all age-related declines in physical and psychological functions

Loss of hearing makes communication much more difficult for older adults. Equally devastating is the disruption of sensory inputs that older adults need to maintain their memories and reasoning skills. Many problems that are written off as "senility" are, in fact, side effects of age-related losses in hearing.

The Other Senses Although there has been much less research on the other senses than on vision and hearing, we do know that smell and taste sensitivities also decline with age. A person's sense of smell at age 70, for example, is only one-tenth of what it was at its peak during adolescence. Similarly, the number of taste buds in our tongue and mouth decreases from about 250 during our college years to about 100 at age 70. This decrease in taste sensitivity has been linked to malnutrition among the elderly. Foods simply don't taste as good when we are older.

Although there is no known way to prevent cataracts, shrinking pupils, and stiffening eardrums, many of the normal visual and hearing losses that accompany aging can be corrected or reduced with hearing aids and glasses. Even so, these changes require adjustment on the part of the older person, as well as family members and friends. As in responding to all health conditions, optimal adjustment is an active process in which the individual preserves a sense of control over his or her physical condition, rather than passively accepting an inevitable decline.

Perception and Reaction Time

Distance perception and reaction time also decline with age, which explains why it takes older people longer to avoid hazards while driving. Reaction time decreases as a direct result of the loss of neurons involved in coordinating muscular reactions to incoming sights and sounds. Still, not until about age 75 do these changes so impair driving ability that the rate of car accidents reaches the rate of fatal accidents of those in the 16- to 19-year-old age group (Stock, 1995).

Physical Vitality

In general, humans reach their overall physical peak around age 30. After that, muscular strength, reaction time, sensory acuity, and cardiovascular strength begin a gradual decline—a process called **senescence**—the rate and extent of which depend on the particular biological system as well as the individual's genetic legacy and health habits. Among the age-related signs of senescence are the following:

■ *Reduced lung capacity.* From age 20 to age 70, breathing capacity may decrease by as much as 40 percent.

■ *Increased body mass index (BMI).* Lean body mass declines with age. Beginning at about age 20, people lose approximately 7 pounds of muscle tissue with each decade, with the rate of loss increasing after the age of 45. As fat replaces muscle, BMI rises.

- *Loss of muscle strength.* Muscle fibers shrink in number and in size as you grow older, while fat increases. Muscle tissue also becomes less responsive to messages from the central nervous system. Together, these factors contribute to decreases in strength, balance, and coordination.

- *Decreased metabolism.* As muscle tissue declines and fat tissue increases, the body's *basal metabolic rate (BMR)* (see Chapter 7) also declines. Recall that fat requires fewer calories, pound for pound, to maintain than muscle tissue. As BMR drops by approximately 2 percent per decade beginning at age 20, we need fewer and fewer calories to maintain our fattier weight as we age.

The good news, as you'll soon see, is that our physical vitality is one of the most modifiable manifestations of aging. First, however, let's take a closer look at one of the most feared aspects of growing older—succumbing to a disabling or life-threatening chronic disease.

Disease

Secondary aging is the result of health habits, disease, and other factors that generally *accompany* aging but are not inevitable (Siegler, Bastian, & Bosworth, 2001). The message is clear: Whether a particular older adult has a serious illness, or is free of disease, depends less on his or her age than on his or her genetic vulnerabilities and strengths and on past and current health habits. Psychological factors, such as the person's optimism and perceived sense of control over his or her health, and social factors, such as social support and financial security, also have a substantial impact on how a person ages.

Aging and disease do not necessarily go hand in hand. In fact, research has shown that most older adults, most of the time, believe their health to be good or excellent. When surveyed, fewer than 15 percent of older adults report that their health limits their activities to a significant extent (Herzog, 1991). As a group, older people tend to be *less* susceptible to short-term illnesses, such as upper respiratory infections, due to accumulated antibodies.

Still, it is an unavoidable fact that four out of five people over the age of 70 have at least one chronic health condition *(Older Americans 2000)*. Many of these, such as cataracts, chronic sinusitis, and varicose veins, don't pose serious threats to health. Others, such as heart disease, cancer, and other irreversible *chronic illnesses,* are often fatal. Figure 15.2 (page 658) shows the top ten chronic afflictions—and their prevalence—among elderly Americans.

Older people are more likely to get sick in part because they have accumulated a number of risk factors for one or more chronic diseases. A key section in most tests to predict longevity asks about the number of years of smoking, excessive alcohol consumption, and sedentary living—all of which increase the risk of heart disease, cancer, osteoporosis, and other serious conditions.

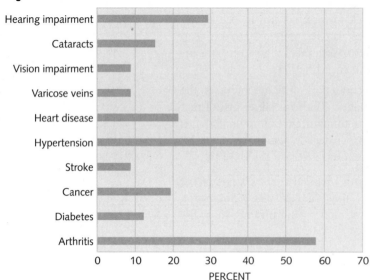

Most Prevalent Chronic Conditions among the Elderly

Four of five people over the age of 70 have at least one chronic health condition. Fortunately, many of these conditions don't pose serious threats to health. However, chronic conditions such as arthritis, diabetes, and heart disease can adversely affect quality of life and contribute to declines in functioning. Five of the six leading causes of death among older Americans are chronic diseases.

Source: *Older Americans, 2000: Key Indicators of Well-Being.* Washington, DC: Federal Interagency Forum on Aging-Related Statistics.

The link between aging and disease is also due in part to the weakening of the body's disease-fighting immune system. This deficiency, which is an example of primary aging, means that older persons are more susceptible to disease, take longer to recover from illness, and are more likely to die when disease does strike. In fact, the death rate from the eight leading causes of death is significantly higher for elderly people than for younger people. Even influenza, from which younger people recover within a few days, can kill an elderly person.

The three biggest killers of Americans aged 65 and older are heart disease, cancer, and stroke, which together account for nearly 70 percent of all deaths among older Americans. The most common form of heart disease among older adults is coronary artery disease resulting from the buildup of artery-blocking atherosclerotic plaques (see Chapter 9). The high rate of cancer deaths is due to the immune system's reduced ability to defend the aging body against precancerous and cancerous cells (see Chapter 10). Many older adults are not screened for malignant cells, nor are they treated as aggressively for them as are younger patients (Podolsky & Silberner, 1993). This *elder bias* in diagnosis and treatment prevents many older patients, especially those who are not assertive or financially secure, from receiving quality health care.

Memory and Intelligence

Racing through the store to pick up groceries for dinner, we find ourselves delayed by the painfully slow senior shopper ahead of us as she fumbles for her checkbook, then her pen, only to have forgotten the amount of the bill. Are these mental lapses typical of older adults as a group? How does aging really affect the mind?

Memory

With age, neural processing speed slows; older adults require more time to register and process information (Fry & Hale, 1996). In many cases, due to the vision and hearing losses that accompany aging, some information is simply never attended to. This is especially true when older adults work at complex tasks that require attending to several channels of information at the same time (Poon, 1987). In addition, areas of the brain devoted to storing memories begin to atrophy (Schacter, 1996); this, along with a small, gradual loss of brain cells causing a 5 to 7 percent reduction in the overall weight of the brain by age 80, may result in some memory losses. However, these small losses are more than compensated for by the proliferation of new neural connections, especially among older adults who remain physically and mentally active and socially connected (Coleman & Flood, 1986).

When age-related memory declines do occur, they mostly involve conscious, short-term memory. In most cases, however, this disruption is merely a minor nuisance and involves information such as telephone numbers and names of people we meet for the first time. And even these losses may be more the result of disuse and poor strategies of attention, memorization, and retrieval than the result of aging per se. When older persons are taught more efficient memorization and recall techniques, they often are able to use them effectively (Perlmutter, Kaplan, & Nyquist, 1990).

Another reason memory seems poorer in old age is that many older adults overestimate their memories when they were younger, and therefore perceive their current memory deficits to be much greater than they actually are. This may, in turn, reduce their motivation to succeed on memory tests—and lack of motivation often leads to poor performance.

A third explanation has to do with physical health. Because cognitive functioning is strongly correlated with good physical health, adults with arteriosclerosis, cardiovascular disease, diabetes, and untreated hypertension score more poorly on tests of cognitive functioning than do their healthier counterparts, perhaps as a result of reduced flow of blood and oxygen to the brain (Zelinski, Crimmins, Reynolds, & Seeman, 1998).

Intelligence

The popular misconception that intelligence inevitably declines with age is both a myth and an artifact of earlier experimental designs (see Chapter 2). Today, using a *cross-sequential* research design, in which the same group of people is periodically tested and retested (longitudinal research) and a new sample is added at each testing (cross-sectional research), researchers have discovered that the overall intellectual functioning of people in their 60s is not

fluid intelligence a person's basic ability to think quickly and efficiently and to reason abstractly; tends to decrease during later adulthood

crystallized intelligence a person's accumulation of facts, information, and learning and memory strategies that comes with experience and education; tends to increase with age

dementia a pathological loss of intellectual functioning with age; the symptoms include memory loss, rambling conversation, confusion about place and time, and changes in personality

Figure 15.3

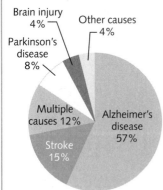

Causes of Dementia
Although dementia has many possible causes, Alzheimer's disease is the leading (and most feared) cause.

Brain injury 4%
Other causes 4%
Parkinson's disease 8%
Multiple causes 12%
Alzheimer's disease 57%
Stroke 15%

Source: Data from *Dementia and Aging: Ethics, Values, and Policy Choices,* by R. H. Binstock, S. G. Post, and P. J. Whitehouse, 1992. Baltimore, MD: Johns Hopkins University Press.

significantly different from that of people in their 50s. For most people in their 60s, the saying "use it or lose it" becomes an accurate description of intellectual change. Often, because they may be retired, people over 60 lose their career-related skills. Regular mental exercise, like physical activity, can stem the cognitive declines of aging (Schaie, 1994). This means that there are wide individual differences in intellectual functioning among people in their 60s, 70s, 80s, and beyond.

Another problem is the types of intelligence tests used. Intelligence tests tend to place older adults at a disadvantage because they focus on measures of **fluid intelligence,** such as the person's ability to reason speedily and abstractly. As we noted earlier, older adults' neural processing speed—and thus their reaction time—*does* decrease with age, but slower thinking is not necessarily less intelligent thinking. On measures of **crystallized intelligence,** which assess a person's accumulated knowledge, general vocabulary, and ability to integrate information, older adults do as well as or better than younger adults—at least well into their 70s (Baltes, 1999).

Alzheimer's Disease

A small percentage of adults experience **dementia,** a dramatic deterioration in reasoning ability and memory, caused by strokes, tumors, brain infections such as meningitis, abuse of alcohol, or **Alzheimer's disease (AD)** (see Figure 15.3). Although these traumas, which cause a substantial loss of brain cells, increase dramatically with age, they are not inevitable consequences of normal aging. AD strikes roughly 3 percent of the world's population by age 75 and claims the lives of more than 100,000 Americans each year (Dartiques & Letenneur, 2000).

The symptoms of AD begin with subtle cognitive changes, especially in short-term memory. Formerly routine tasks, such as using a telephone or remembering driving directions, become harder and harder to carry out. In the second stage, AD victims typically suffer impairment in a number of higher mental functions such as reading, writing, and the ability to do mental arithmetic. In the third stage, seizures and striking changes in language use are common. Although the speech of AD patients often sounds perfectly normal from a grammatical standpoint, closer listening reveals that it is often confused, as AD patients struggle to find the right word to express their thoughts. This disruption, called **aphasia,** is one of two major symptoms used to diagnose AD. The other is **apraxia,** which refers to the loss of memory for muscular movements to carry out basic daily tasks, such as those involved in personal hygiene, feeding, and food preparation. Unfortunately, there is presently no definitive physiological test for AD in living people. A diagnosis of AD can be confirmed only during an autopsy, where clumps of degenerative nerve cells called *neuritic plaques* and *neurofibrillary tangles* are easily seen. Together, these plaques and tangles appear in brain tissues that produce the neurotransmitter *acetylcholine*

(Ach), which is found in reduced levels in people with AD (Barinaga, 1995; Plomin, 1995). The neurons become tangled because of a process called **cross-linking,** in which cell proteins bind to one another, stiffening *collagen*—the connective tissue that supports tendons, cartilage, and bone (Yan et al., 1996). When plaques and tangles occur in the *hippocampus*—a brain region that plays a crucial role in the consolidation of recent memories—the brain struggles to consolidate memory, and reasoning skills deteriorate. As you'll later learn, some experts believe that cross-linking plays a fundamental role in all aspects of aging.

As in many chronic health conditions, genetic vulnerability appears to be a factor in the development of AD and other forms of dementia (Plomin, DeFries, McClearn, & McGuffin, 2001). People who inherit a particular form of the gene *APOe,* which directs production of the protein *apolipoprotein E,* stand a greater than average chance of developing the disease. Although how it works is not yet completely known, APOe appears to promote the development of neuritic plaques via its role in transporting cholesterol through the bloodstream (Weiner et al., 1999). Another piece of genetic evidence comes from studies of families with histories of AD, who seem to have a defect in chromosome 21, which is also implicated in Down syndrome, a disorder usually characterized by mental retardation.

Treatment for persons suspected of having AD focuses on drugs such as *Tacrine,* which slow the rate of AD-related decline by increasing the neural activity in remaining healthy Ach neurons (Davis, 1992). Focusing on prevention of AD symptoms, other researchers have reported that regular use of anti-inflammatory medications such as ibuprofen may ward off AD by preventing brain inflammation (Thal, 2000).

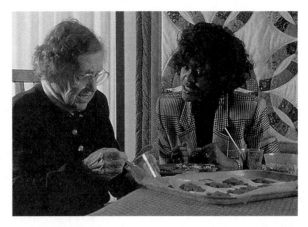

Alzheimer's Disease
Alzheimer's, a devastating disease that robs some older people of the ability to think, speak, or even perform basic daily activities. Interventions in which psychologists and other specialists work with patients help to forestall or at least temporarily halt some of the effects on mental functioning. © Will & Deni McIntyre/Photo Researchers

Depression

At every age, people report similar degrees of well-being, happiness, and satisfaction with life (Inglehart, 1990). The elderly, however, are slightly more likely to exhibit symptoms of depression and mild generalized anxiety disorder, which is characterized by persistent tension and worry. According to the National Institute on Aging, one in six adults 65 years of age and older suffers significant depression, often related to grief over the loss of loved ones, or due to dementia disorders such as AD or chronic illnesses such as heart disease or cancer. Those who are poor or lack social support and the residents of nursing homes are among those most likely to be depressed (Blazer, Burchett, Service,

■ **Alzheimer's disease (AD)** a degenerative disease of the brain that leads to dementia and a dramatic deterioration of thinking, memory, and reasoning

■ **aphasia** a distinctive speech disorder in which speech sounds normal but is lacking in content words; characteristic symptom of Alzheimer's disease

■ **apraxia** a loss of memory for motor movements, often apparent in later stages of Alzheimer's disease

■ **cross-linking** a tangling of brain neurons due to the stiffening of cell proteins and connective tissue; believed to be implicated in all aspects of aging

& George, 1991). Depression among the elderly often goes undetected and/or untreated for a combination of reasons: Its symptoms are often overshadowed by other physical complaints, it is often mistaken as a natural component of aging, and many proud older adults are loath to admit to depression (Goleman, 1995). This is doubly unfortunate today because, at least in its milder forms (which are most common among the elderly), depression is one of the most treatable mental illnesses.

On the positive side, depression can be avoided. Social support acts as a buffer against depression for most older adults, helping them to cope with the challenges of aging through shared experiences. Similarly, a recent multiethnic study has shown that high levels of emotional well-being correlate negatively with the risk of stroke (Ostir, Markides, Peek, & Goodwin, 2001).

Left untreated, depression can lead to a host of other problems. For example, depression produces a nearly threefold increase in the incidence of stroke among older adults with hypertension (Goleman, 1995). It can also lead to suicide, which tends to occur at a higher rate among those over age 60 than for any other age group. In most cases, an older person takes his or her own life following a social loss, such as widowhood or retirement (Canetto, 1992). Another common precipitating event for suicide in the elderly is being diagnosed with a serious illness, especially one like Alzheimer's disease, which impairs mental functioning.

The association between advancing age and depression is a clear example of the interaction among the dimensions of aging. Physical problems may lead to psychological and social problems, but positive psychological and social factors may ameliorate or even prevent physical problems.

Theories of Aging

Various theories have been proposed to explain the aging process. Among these are theories that view aging as the result of damage to the body's cells and biological systems and those that point to evidence that the moment of death is determined by heredity or the ticking of a biological "clock." Each theory has its strong points and each may be flawed, as you will see. In all likelihood, each of the theories accounts for some aspects of aging.

Damage Theories of Aging

Damage theories center around the idea that internal bodily changes and external environmental assaults damage cells and bodily systems, causing them to malfunction and leading to death.

The Wear-and-Tear Theory

The oldest damage theory of aging, the **wear-and-tear theory,** suggests that over the years our bodies are like machines whose parts eventually wear out through use. For some lower species of animals, this theory appears to make sense. For example, fruit flies living in confined quarters that limit their activity levels (and metabolic rates) live much longer than their counterparts who are allowed to fly freely.

Despite its commonsense appeal, there is, in fact, little evidence that the human body fails as a result of overuse. This is, in fact, one of the most common myths of aging. As we'll see, many older adults avoid exercise because they fear that it will accelerate aging. In fact, our bodies are far more likely to "rust out" with disuse than they are to wear out from exercise and a vigorous lifestyle.

Cellular Accidents

Another damage theory focuses on biochemical processes that might contribute to aging. The **free-radical theory** attributes aging to damage caused to body cells by the gradual accumulation of molecules called free radicals. These highly unstable molecules are produced in the mitochondria of cells as byproducts of *oxidative metabolism.* As they form, free radicals rob electrons from other cells, damaging cell membranes and DNA, which may cause us to age faster and become more vulnerable to age-related diseases such as cancer, cardiovascular disease, diabetes, and arthritis. Exposure to environmental hazards such as ultraviolet rays, pesticides, and pollution may also produce free radicals.

The healthy body, however, is not helpless against free radical attacks. Enzymes called *antioxidants* naturally destroy most free radicals. The body itself makes some antioxidants; others, like vitamins C, E, and beta-carotene, are contained in the foods we eat. As we age, the body produces fewer of its own antioxidants. For this reason, people who eat foods rich in antioxidants may be less likely to develop heart disease and cancer.

Interestingly, scientists have identified several genes that appear to extend the life span of certain laboratory species by detoxifying DNA-damaging free radicals. When these genes are made inactive via an experimental mutation in the fruit fly, its life span is reduced by 80 to 90 percent (Rogina, Reenan, Nilsen, & Helfand, 2000). Reversing the process by inserting into fruit fly DNA a "designer gene" that enhances oxygen detoxification has been shown to nearly double the life span of a fruit fly.

Cross-Linking Theory

As noted earlier, the neural damage that accompanies Alzheimer's disease appears to be caused by cross-links of cellular proteins that bind together, causing stiffening of bodily tissues. According to **cross-linking theory,** aging occurs because this process of stiffening causes all bodily processes to break

wear-and-tear theory a discredited theory of aging that states that the human body wears out with the passage of time

free-radical theory a damage theory that attributes aging to damage caused to body cells by the gradual accumulation of unstable molecules called free radicals

cross-linking theory a damage theory that attributes aging to the stiffening of body tissues that appears to be caused by cross-links of cellular proteins that bind together

■ **Hayflick limit** the number of times a human cell is capable of reproducing itself before it dies. Estimated to be approximately 50 divisions for most cells, this limit is believed by some experts to be the basis of the "genetic clock" that determines life span

■ **telomere** the end structure of DNA, which is gradually depleted each time the cell divides, until the cell can divide no more and dies; its shortening is believed to be the mechanism that underlies the Hayflick limit

down. The most visible example of cross-linking is the changed appearance of the skin as aging progresses. As collagen becomes cross-linked, laugh lines and fine furrows appear around the eyes and mouth as the skin begins to lose its elasticity. At a later age, wrinkles, crow's feet, and other facial lines appear. Still later, the skin becomes rougher and loses its uniform color.

The immune system's ability to battle cross-linking along with free radical damage decreases with primary aging. Although for many years researchers believed that once fibers became cross-linked, nothing could be done to break them apart, scientists are currently experimenting with a synthetic drug that shows some promise (Cleveland Clinic Heart Advisor, 2000).

Genetic Clock Theories

Some experts believe that aging is caused by a genetic program, or "clock," that is set at the moment of conception. At the heart of such theories is the idea that genes control the various biochemical processes that influence longevity. Support comes from family and twin studies showing, for example, that the age of death is much closer among monozygotic twins than it is among dizygotic twins (McGue, Vaupel, Holm, & Harvald, 1993).

Further support comes from laboratory studies of cellular aging, which show that most cells of the body are able to divide only a finite number of times before damage to DNA, or errors in protein synthesis, cause the cell to age and then die. This theoretical limit is called the **Hayflick limit,** after Leonard Hayflick, who discovered the phenomenon. After dividing about 50 times, normal human cells cease dividing and eventually die. Scientists suspect that the shortening of the **telomeres**—the end structures of DNA—are responsible for this. Telomeres become eroded each time a cell divides. As aging progresses and the telomeres become shorter, the chromosomes can become unstable and prone to damage.

Several research studies provide evidence for the Hayflick limit. For example, cells from longer-lived species divide more times before dying than do cells from shorter-lived species: Cells from newborn chickens, which normally live about 12 years, divide about 25 times, while cells from the Galapagos tortoise, which lives as long as 175 years, divide about 100 times (Hayflick, 1994). Further evidence comes from laboratory studies showing that when the nucleus of a younger cell is transplanted into an older cell, the cell divides more times. In fact, with just a few genetic alterations, scientists have created worms and flies with life spans twice the norm and that die healthy (Kolata, 1999). Reversing the process, Dolly, the 3-year-old Finn Dorset sheep cloned from a 6-year-old sheep, may have a less-than-average life span.

Aging and Natural Selection

The possibility of a genetic clock raises a puzzling question: Why should any species carry self-destructive genes? Why shouldn't all species have evolved to carry genes that enable them to live forever? Geneticists believe that the answer has to do with how each species has evolved to balance two fundamental needs: repair and ensuring the survival of the species. The human body is constantly under repair, even when we are asleep. The most visible example of this repair process is the healing of a fresh skin cut. But regular repair also takes place in each cell of the body. Aging occurs when the repair process slows down.

What causes the repair process to slow down? A good analogy is what happens to a car. If you had enough money to pay for endless repairs, you could probably keep your car running forever. But at some point it simply makes better sense to save up for a new car. The same is true of our bodies. At some point it makes more "sense"—that is, it is more adaptive for our species—to invest more energy in offspring, to ensure that our genes will survive into the next generation. As a compromise, we invest less in self-repair, and we age.

The rate of aging, and therefore each species' average life span, varies with the size of its "repair budget." Jared Diamond (1992) believes that we humans live twice as long as gorillas, chimpanzees, and other primate cousins because our species puts more biological energy into cellular repair. Diamond attributes this to the development of stone tools, axes, and other weapons about 5 million years ago, which dramatically increased our ancestors' ability to survive attacks from predators. With greater safety came less pressure to reproduce quickly, and our ancestors began to age more slowly.

Support for the *cellular repair hypothesis* comes from a recent Scripps Research Institute study comparing cells and genes from healthy people between 9 and 90 years of age with those from children suffering from **Hutchinson-Gilford progeria,** a rare disease that makes children age so rapidly that by 5 their hair begins falling out, their skin has the wrinkled appearance of a septuagenarian, and cardiovascular disease almost inevitably causes death by about age 12 (Ly, Lockhart, Lerner, & Schultz, 2000). The genes were put into four groups: normal young, normal middle-aged, normal old, and progeria. The results indicated the greatest (and most similar) impairment in the oldest cells and the progeria cells. Put simply, cells contain "checkpoint genes" that decide whether a newly divided cell is good enough to live or not. If the checkpoint genes work properly, genetic errors are stopped immediately. But when the checkpoints fail—as in the case of old cells and progeria cells—flawed cells make new cells with the same genetic mistakes. These genetic impairments could produce the typical changes of aging—gray hair, wrinkled skin, weaker muscles, and brittle bones.

Is Aging Just Genes?

As recently as 20 years ago, most doctors believed that as soon as science understood genetics, we would understand most of the basic medical problems. They felt that youth, health, and longevity were

■ **Hutchinson-Gilford progeria**
a rare genetic disease that causes young children to age at an extremely rapid rate and to die, usually by age 12

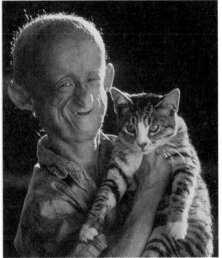

Progeria
Young children with Hutchinson-Gilford progeria age very rapidly, taking on the characteristics of septuagenarians by age 5. Unfortunately, there is no cure for this rare disease, which always leads to death at an early age. © Mark Wexler / Woodfin Camp & Associates

BYLINE HEALTH

Hispanics Live Longer
Diana A. Terry-Azios

The fountain of youth may be in Florida after all, says David E. Hayes-Bautista—or in any other location with a large Latino population. "The habits of the Latino heart—family and diet, religion, work, and culture—make for a profile that results in healthier and longer life," says Hayes-Bautista, executive director of the Center for the Study of Latino Health at UCLA School of Medicine.

As a possible solution to the economic crisis aging baby-boomers face, Hayes-Bautista recommends a look into the Latino lifestyle, particularly the Mexican American lifestyle, for secrets to living healthy past retirement age. Even though the median age of the Latino population averages 10 years younger than Anglos, the elderly are increasingly Latino, according to Hayes-Bautista.

Their life expectancy is also almost 4 years longer, based on Los Angeles County figures. In addition, the death rate for elderly Latinos from heart disease, cancer, stroke, pneumonia, homicide, suicide, and cirrhosis is 40 percent lower than Anglo rates in the county.

Hayes-Bautista attributes the astounding figures to traits prevalent in Latino culture, like work and religious ethics and the importance of community and family. Latinos remain in the workforce longer than Anglos and beyond retirement age; however, while 88 percent of elderly Anglos receive Social Security benefits, only 54 percent of senior Latinos do. To make up the difference in Social Security and other public services, Latinos rely on family. Hispanic adult children provide for 21 percent of senior Latinos in Los Angeles county; only 2 percent of Anglo adult children provide for their parents. Working hard and investing in their children assures future security for aging Latinos, speculates Hayes-Bautista.

A religious ethic as strong as the work ethic also contributes to longer life by reducing stress through a sense of well-being and belonging. Elderly Latinos are twice as likely as Anglos to belong to an organized church (particularly Roman Catholic) and to attend church services at least every 2 weeks. A Hebrew University study comparing the health of religious and secular kibbutz members showed that religious

activity lowered death rates and positively affected social, mental, and physical health.

Also benefiting Latinos' physical health is their traditional diet, says Hayes-Bautista. While Anglos tend to know more about what makes good diet and nutrition, Mexican American consumption typically includes more vegetables, legumes, and leaner meats.

All this combined equals a formula for a longer, healthier life that requires less medical care in old age, says Hayes-Bautista. It may also be a helpful model for the rest of the population.

Source: Terry-Azios, D. A. (2000, May). Hispanics live longer. *Hispanic, 13,* 66–67.

Exercises

1. How do Latino American morbidity rates and average life expectancy compare with those of Anglo Americans?

2. What aspects of Latino culture may account for these differences?

3. Do aspects of your cultural background compare favorably to the longevity-promoting aspects of Latino culture? Which ones?

all determined from the moment of conception and there was little a person could do about it. "It's all in the genes," was the word of the day. Much to their surprise, the more science has discovered about genetics, the more it has learned just how much the environment, and a person's interactions with it, make a difference in how genes affect us. Stated another way, we all have the genes we were born with, but how we age is primarily up to us.

Today, scientists estimate that genes account for less than 30 percent of all aging effects (Roizen, 1999) and that genes matter less and less the older you are. By the age of 80, lifestyle choices may account almost entirely for a person's overall health and longevity. As longevity and aging expert Michael Roizen notes, "People who are still able to live young even when their calendar age is old weren't necessarily born with 'good' genes nearly so much as they have made 'good' choices. They exercise, eat lots of fruits and vegetables, keep their minds engaged."

An obvious implication of many aging theories is that if damage is minimized or prevented, aging may be slowed or stopped altogether. This brings us to the subject of lifestyle and aging.

Lifestyle and Aging

The "fountain of youth" myth is present in the histories of nearly every culture and finds its current expression in the allegedly rejuvenating elixirs, creams, and gadgets that are hawked in infomercials, alternative medicine Web sites, and drugstore displays. Claims that people will soon live to be 200 years old because of megadoses of antioxidants, vitamins, herbs, or some other "magic bullet" have resulted in confusion about *longevity*. For decades, scientists have systematically investigated people's claims of having vastly exceeded the normal life span, and in every instance these claims could not be verified.

Even without a magic bullet, people today can expect to live much longer than previous cohorts. The major diseases of our ancestors, such as polio, smallpox, tetanus, diphtheria, and rheumatic fever, have been almost completely eradicated. Today's *average life expectancy* is about 76 years (up from about 47 years in the early twentieth century). Individual life expectancy in the United States varies considerably—from 65 years for African-American males to 79 years for white women. When other parts of the world are considered, the variation is even greater. In developing countries in sub-Saharan Africa and Southeast Asia, for example, life expectancy is only about 45 to 62 years for men and 48 to 64 years for women (World Health Organization, 2000). Ethiopia has the shortest life expectancy in the world: A male child can expect to live only to age 41, and a female baby to 43 years. To put these numbers in perspective, Ethiopians have a life expectancy even shorter than the average for people living in the United States in 1840.

Wherever we live, however, many of us do *not* reach our biological potential and "die before our time." Michael Roizen (1999), a preventive gerontologist and proponent of the concept of *RealAge*, notes that while an individual's chronological age is fixed, his or her biological age may be years older, depending on a combination of factors. The concept of RealAge calculates the aging effect of more than 100 different health behaviors—ranging from diet to stress control and chronic smoking. The good news is that a person's biological age can also be younger than his or her chronological age; in such cases, the person's rate of aging would be the same physiologically as that of a person who is younger in calendar years.

■ **quality-adjusted life years (QALYs)** a measure of aging that focuses on biological age rather than chronological age

■ **compression of morbidity** efforts to limit the time an older person spends ill or disabled

At the heart of the RealAge concept is an emphasis on optimal versus usual or impaired aging. This has led to a new measure of health that combines longevity with quality of life. **Quality-adjusted life years (QALYs)** is an index of an individual's biological age rather than his or her chronological age. By focusing on aerobic capacity, muscle strength, and other *biomarkers* that decline with age and disuse, QALYs represents a radical departure from traditional measures of longevity that focused only on mortality and morbidity rates. In 1999, the number of quality-adjusted life years for the population of adults in the United States was approximately 64. Stated differently, the average person lives about 12 years past the point of physical well-being. For African-Americans, the QALY is even lower—56 years.

In focusing on the individual's quality-adjusted life years, the goal of health psychologists and others is a **compression of morbidity,** a shortening of the amount of time older people spend disabled, ill, or in pain. To illustrate, consider twin brothers who, although genetically identical and exposed to the same health hazards while growing up, have had very different health experiences since adolescence. The first brother smokes two packs of cigarettes a day, has an obesity-indicating BMI of 30.2, never exercises, has an angry and pessimistic outlook on life, and eats foods containing excessive amounts of animal fat and sugar. The second brother pursues a much healthier lifestyle, avoiding tobacco and excessive stress, exercising regularly, watching his diet, and enjoying the social support of a close-knit circle of family and friends. As Figure 15.4 shows, although the two brothers have the same genetic vulnerabilities to

Figure 15.4

Compression of Morbidity
In focusing on the individual's quality-adjusted life years, health psychologists seek to limit the time a person spends ill or infirm, as illustrated in this diagram of the illnesses and eventual deaths of identical twin brothers. Although the brothers carry the same disease vulnerabilities and life span-limiting genetic clocks, the healthy lifestyle of one (b) keeps disease and disability at bay until primary aging is well advanced. In contrast, the unhealthy lifestyle of his brother (a) takes its toll at a much younger age.

Source: *Living Well: Taking Care of Your Health in the Middle and Later Years,* by J. F. Fries, 1994. Reading, MA: Addison-Wesley.

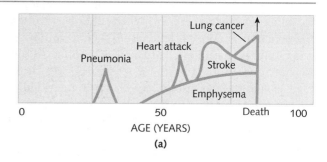

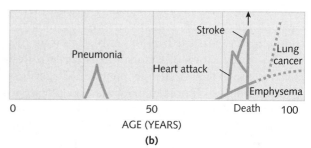

lung, circulatory, and cardiovascular disease, the unhealthy lifestyle of the first brother dooms him to an extended period of adulthood morbidity beginning at about age 45. In contrast, the healthier brother's lifestyle postpones disease until much later in life. If he does contract any of the illnesses, they are likely to be less severe and recovery will be quicker. In some cases, the illness, such as lung cancer, may be "postponed" right out of his life.

This compression of morbidity is one of the crowning achievements of science, allowing older adults to live with less pain, better senses, and clearer thinking and to be much more vigorous than age cohorts that came before (Bunker, Frazer, & Mosteller, 1995).

Exercise

Exercise becomes even more important as people age, and may help slow down or even reverse many of the effects of aging (Fries, 1999). Most important to maintaining physical vitality is *aerobic exercise,* in which the heart speeds up in order to pump larger amounts of blood, breathing is deeper and more frequent, and the cells of the body develop the ability to extract increasing amounts of oxygen from the blood. In addition, weight-bearing aerobic exercises such as walking, jogging, and racquetball help preserve muscular strength and maintain bone density.

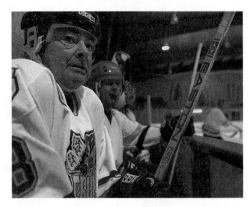

Exercise Is Good at Every Age
The Gray Wolves Hockey League in Syracuse, New York, accepts only players who are 65 years or older. These men obviously understand the benefits of exercise, although their form of exercise is probably well above what is needed.
© Dennis Nett/Syracuse Newspapers/The Image Works

The American College of Sports Medicine's fitness guidelines also now recommend weight training (also called *resistance training*) for people over 50. Weight training is particularly useful in enabling older people to maintain their independence by keeping them strong enough to do routine tasks. One University of Alabama study reported that older women who lifted weights regularly were able to carry bags of groceries with 36 percent less effort and to get up from their chairs with 40 percent less stress on their leg muscles than prior to the training (Mayo Health, 2001).

Exercise has been demonstrated to protect against *osteoporosis,* a disorder characterized by declining bone density due to calcium loss. Although osteoporosis is most common in postmenopausal women, it also occurs in men, as does the protective effect of exercise. Roughly one woman in four over age 60 has osteoporosis, with white and Asian women being at higher risk than African-American women. Osteoporosis results in more than 1 million bone fractures a year in the United States alone, the most debilitating of which are hip fractures. In one retrospective study, older men and women were asked to describe their level of exercise as adolescents, again at age 30, and again at age 50 (Greendale, Barrett-Connor, Edelstein, Ingles, & Halle, 1995). Both men and women with the highest reported activity levels had significantly greater bone mineral density than their more sedentary counterparts.

In addition to increasing physical strength and maintaining bone density, regular exercise reduces an older person's risk for two of the most common chronic illnesses of adulthood: cardiovascular disease and cancer. In one study, researchers investigated coronary risk factors in elderly men, aged 65 to 84 (Caspersen, Bloemberg, Saris, Merritt, & Kromhout, 1991). Even moderate exercise, such as gardening and walking, resulted in significant increases in HDL—the so-called *good cholesterol*—and decreased total serum cholesterol. Regular exercise is also linked to lower triglycerides, which have been implicated in the formation of atherosclerotic plaques (Lakka & Salonen, 1992). Focusing on walking, bicycling, running, swimming, tennis, and golf, Goya Wannamethee and his colleagues (1993) found an inverse relationship between the level of physical activity and deaths from all types of cancer.

However, during late adulthood, the intensity of exercise must be adjusted to reflect declines in cardiovascular and respiratory functioning. For some adults this means that walking replaces jogging; for others, such as former world-class marathoner Bill Rodgers, this means training at a 6-minute per mile pace rather than a 5-minute pace. As a guideline, *Healthy People 2000* recommends 150 minutes of total exercise each week, of which at least 60 minutes involve continuous, rhythmic aerobic activity. For many adults, turning off the TV helps promote exercise and better health. A recent study found that people who watched just 2 extra hours of TV per day were less likely to engage in active leisure activities and had higher body mass indexes (and other coronary risk factors) than people who watched less TV (Kronenberg et al., 2000).

Is It Ever Too Late to Begin Exercising?

No. In one study, frail nursing-home residents aged 72 to 98 participated in a 10-week program of muscle-strengthening resistance training three times a week (Raloff, 1996). After 10 weeks, those in the exercise group more than doubled their muscular strength and increased their stair-climbing power by 28 percent. In another study, Maria Fiatarone and her colleagues (1993) randomly assigned 100 subjects, who averaged 87 years of age, to one of four groups. Subjects in the first group engaged in regular resistance training exercises. Subjects in the second group took a daily multivitamin supplement. Subjects in the third group took the supplement and participated in the resistance training. Finally, subjects in the fourth group were permitted to engage in three activities of their choice (including aerobic exercise) but could not engage in resistance training. Over the course of the study, muscle strength more than doubled in the resistance groups, with an average increase of 113 percent, compared to a miniscule 3 percent increase in subjects in the second group. Interestingly, the group that exercised and took the supplement showed no greater improvement than the group that exercised alone.

Further evidence that it is never too late to start exercising comes from studies demonstrating that exercise even late in life may still help prevent or reduce the rate of loss in bone density. As compared to a control group of sedentary women, 50- to 70-year-old women who had been sedentary but were assigned to an exercise group showed significantly reduced loss in bone mineral content (Nelson et al., 1994). As added benefits, women in the exercise group increased their muscle mass and strength.

Why Don't More Older Adults Exercise?

Despite the well-documented benefits of lifelong exercise, the percentage of people who exercise regularly declines with age (Phillips, Kiernan & King, 2001). Why? For one thing, some older adults are reluctant, even fearful, of exercising too much, largely due to a number of myths associated with exercise. Among these myths are that exercise can accelerate the loss of bone density, lead to arthritis, and even increase the risk of dying from a heart attack. As noted earlier, in fact, the body is far more likely to rust out than it is to wear out. As the saying goes, "Use it or lose it!"

Exercising is also related to an individual's beliefs regarding its health benefits, confidence in his or her ability to correctly perform certain physical skills (*exercise self-efficacy*), and self-motivation. Believing that exercise will help one to live a longer, healthier life is a strong stimulus for initiating exercise. Many older people may lack basic information about the benefits of appropriate exercise and might view exercise as difficult, useless, or unsafe (Lee, 1993). Or they may feel that it is too late to improve their health through exercise because they think declines in health are inevitable and irreversible with increased age (O'Brien & Vertinsky, 1991).

There are several reasons that older adults might lack exercise self-efficacy. For one, they typically have less experience with exercise and have fewer exercising role models than other age groups. Older people are also faced with ageist stereotypes about what constitutes appropriate behavior; vigorous exercise, especially for women, is contrary to stereotypes of old age.

Finally, self-motivation is less common among older adults than younger adults. Too often, older adults view old age as a time of rest and relaxation, and so they lack the motivation necessary to initiate and maintain regular exercise.

To further explore why some adults choose to exercise, while others do not, Sara Wilcox and Martha Storandt of Washington University (1996) surveyed a random sample of 121 women aged 20 to 85, focusing on three psychological variables: exercise self-efficacy, self-motivation, and attitudes toward exercise. The sample consisted of two groups: *exercisers* and *nonexercisers*. Women in the exercise group had engaged in aerobic exercise for at least 20 minutes three or more times per week for at least 4 months prior to the study. Nonexercisers reported engaging in little or no aerobic exercise (less than two times per month) over the preceding 4 months.

The findings revealed that desire and willingness to exercise has less to do with age than with attitudes about exercise; the belief that exercise would be enjoyable and beneficial decreased with increasing age, but only among nonexercisers.

Those who continued to exercise throughout adulthood were significantly more self-motivated, had greater exercise self-efficacy, and had more positive attitudes toward exercise than did nonexercisers. These results suggest that education stressing the benefits and the required frequency, duration, and intensity of exercise needed to reach these benefits must be a key component in exercise interventions with older adults. In addition, stereotypes of old age as a time of inevitable decline need to be challenged. Finally, older adults will be less likely to begin an exercise regimen if they believe they are unable to do even basic exercises.

Nutrition

Nutrition is an especially important, yet often overlooked, aspect of a healthy lifestyle for older people. Ensuring good nutrition becomes more complex with aging. The need for vitamins, minerals, and other micronutrients *increases* with age because the body's ability to metabolize food and fully extract its nutrients decreases, due to the growing inefficiency of the digestive system (Reyes, 1999). Among the micronutrients that are essential for good health (and reducing the risk of morbidity) in later years are the following:

- Iron, which can help prevent anemia, can help correct memory deficits, and is believed to boost the immune system.
- Zinc, which enhances immunity, reduces the risk of respiratory infections, and may restore age-impaired sensory processes, such as taste and smell.
- Magnesium, which can help prevent cardiovascular disease and assists in maintaining the balance of calcium and potassium in the body.
- Copper, which is believed to help reduce the risk of cardiovascular disease, osteoporosis, and anemia.

Nutritional deficits are especially damaging during late adulthood. As we have seen, one of the key effects of inadequate nutrition is almost certainly faster aging (Chapter 6). In addition, several studies have suggested that older adults whose diets are deficient in B vitamins, particularly folic acid and B12, are more likely to have memory deficits than older adults with adequate intake of these nutrients (Wahlin, Hill, Winblad, & Backman, 1996).

Good nutrition can also help control blood triglycerides and cholesterol levels, both of which tend to increase with age, potentially accelerating the development of cardiovascular disease, cancer, and other chronic illnesses (Sacco et al., 2001). Recent data indicate that postmenopausal women whose diets are rich in whole grains have a 17 percent lower mortality rate than women who consume predominantly refined grain fiber (Jacobs, Pereira, Meyer, & Kushi, 2000). Older adults often need to monitor their diet to ensure that their intake of fats, particularly saturated and animal fats, is kept to a minimum. But they have to be careful. As was true at an earlier age, cutting fats too severely can be unhealthy, since fats help the body absorb vitamins A, D, E, and K and other fat-soluble nutrients.

Eating a healthy diet and getting the extra needed nutrients is not so easy for older adults. For one thing, it is complicated by the fact that while the vitamin and mineral needs remain the same as in the 20s and 30s, the daily number of calories needed to maintain body weight drops by about 100 calories per decade after age 45. This means that the average 70-year-old person needs 10 percent fewer calories per day than he or she did at middle age (Blumberg, 1996). This makes it all the more important that older adults consume a varied, nutrient-dense diet that emphasizes fresh vegetables and fruits, complex carbohydrates in the form of grains and cereals, fish, and lean protein.

Other physical changes also conspire against good nutrition. For one, the senses of taste and smell diminish with age, making everyday foods far less appealing to older adults. Second, dental problems such as *tooth loss* and gum disease make chewing hard foods more difficult, and so many older people substitute softer foods that are easier to chew. Third, as the digestive system loses efficiency, the esophageal sphincter often does not close properly, causing heartburn, gastritis, and a general nausea that makes eating far less pleasant than at a younger age.

As at every age, the biological domain is influenced by external social and economic factors. High-quality, nutritionally rich foods are, generally speaking, costlier, meaning that many older adults on fixed incomes find optimal nutrition to be out of reach financially. And proper nutrition is made all the more difficult when an older person lives alone, since those who eat alone (at any age) are more likely to eat quick, irregular meals.

Further complicating the picture is that many older adults take a variety of prescription and over-the-counter drugs that alter their nutritional needs. For example, a daily dose of aspirin, taken by many older adults to relieve the pain and inflammation of rheumatoid arthritis, increases the need for vitamin C. Cholestyramine, used by many older adults to lower blood cholesterol, can reduce iron absorption; long-term use of antacids can cause copper deficiency; antibiotics decrease the body's ability to absorb protein; and many laxatives deplete vitamins A and D (Russell, 2000).

Medication, Health Supplements, and Drug Use

Because of their greater susceptibility to chronic illnesses and the greater occurrence of major diseases, older adults are more likely than any other group to be taking a variety of prescription and over-the-counter drugs. Also, the media's promotion of various health supplements has led many who are otherwise healthy to take large doses of vitamins, minerals, and other supplements. In many cases, drugs are useful and necessary for keeping older people alive and functioning. However, drug use may lead to unintentional drug abuse, a major health hazard for many older adults. Although people over age 65 make up only 12 percent of the U.S. population, they account for more than one-third of all the prescriptions written each year and consume about 50 percent of all

polypharmacy the
dangerous practice of taking
several medications
simultaneously

over-the-counter drugs (Beizer, 1994). To make matters worse, in many instances older adults are taking several different medications for a variety of health complaints. This **polypharmacy** can result in dangerous drug interactions that can produce symptoms ranging from confusion to dementia to psychoses. In addition, as the liver's ability to metabolize drugs declines along with other body systems, some drugs may build up in the body and produce serious adverse effects. Because prescription drugs are usually tested on much younger people, their effects on the elderly are too often unknown, as is the proper dosage for this group. In the worst case, the appropriate dosage for a 20- or 30-year-old person may be an overdose for a 60-year-old, with declining liver functioning. Is it any wonder that adverse drug reactions are three to five times as prevalent among adults over age 60 as they are in younger adults (Higbee, 1994)?

A recent cause for concern is the excessive use of supplements by health-conscious older adults, often in response to recommendations from well-meaning friends, relatives, and even health care providers. Older adults need to be especially cautious in taking vitamins and minerals as supplements, since their digestive and excretory systems tend to be less efficient. Some vitamins, such as vitamin A, are toxic in large doses. And megadoses of others, even if not toxic, may still upset the person's natural nutritional balance, resulting in deficiencies in other needed elements.

An added problem among the elderly is alcohol use. Although 4 out of every 10 older Americans abstain completely from alcohol use, between 10 and 15 percent abuse alcohol (Forster, Pollow, & Stoller, 1993). In many cases, excessive drinking goes unnoticed among the elderly because it generally takes the form of steady, maintenance drinking rather than the binge drinking that is more common in early adulthood. More significantly, some may mistakenly interpret slurred speech, unsteady moments, and memory lapses as signs of aging. And for those older adults who live alone and have limited social contacts, there's no one even to notice.

As with many other drugs, alcohol has a much greater impact on elderly persons than it does on younger adults. Ounce for ounce, alcohol produces a much greater disruption in memory, reaction time, and reasoning ability in older adults than it does in younger adults. When these cognitive functions are already compromised as a result of aging, the added impairment due to excessive drinking is potentially catastrophic. In addition to its other damaging effects, excessive alcohol intake seriously damages nutrition, depleting B vitamins, calcium, magnesium, and vitamin C.

Psychosocial Factors, Aging, and Quality of Life

Although the positive effects of psychosocial variables on healthy aging have not been heavily researched, studies indicate that curiosity, social support, optimism, and a sense of control over one's life contribute strongly to successful aging (Ory, Abeles, & Lipman, 1992). Let's examine each of these factors.

Curiosity

Curiosity refers to a person's orientation or attraction to novel stimuli. Research suggests that curiosity in older people is associated with maintaining the health of the aging central nervous system. In examining the relationship between curiosity in older men and women and survival rates, researchers have found that, after 5 years, those with the highest levels of curiosity survived longer than those with lower levels (Swan & Carmelli, 1996). It's important to note, however, that this correlational evidence does not indicate that curiosity will automatically increase an older person's chances of survival; it may simply be a sign that his or her central nervous system is operating properly. Nevertheless, it is interesting to speculate as to why higher levels of curiosity might be related to better survival in older adults. One possible explanation is that in some individuals age-related declines in curiosity reflect declining mental functioning. In partial support of this hypothesis, one study reported decreased curiosity (measured as reduced exploratory eye movements to novel visual stimuli) in individuals with serious central nervous system disease, as compared with age-matched normal controls (Daffner, Scinto, Weintraub, Guinessey, & Mesulam, 1994). Because certain brain structures known to be involved in Alzheimer's disease are also involved in directed attention and novelty-seeking behavior, diminished curiosity may be one of the earliest signs of abnormal aging of the central nervous system.

Assuming that the person is a normal, healthy adult, curiosity may enhance healthy aging because it enables older adults to successfully meet daily environmental and physical challenges. Thus, the curious older adult uses active coping strategies (see Chapter 5) to approach potential problems and impediments and in this way manages to reduce the strain on his or her physical and mental resources. It seems that such an individual stands a better chance of being physically and mentally healthy in the later years (Ory & Cox, 1994).

Perceived Control and Self-Efficacy

In one major prospective study of personality traits and health, researchers interviewed 8,723 late-middle-aged and older persons living independently or in adapted housing for elderly people in the Netherlands (Kempen, Jelicic, & Ormel, 1997). Three measures of personality were investigated: mastery or personal control, general self-efficacy, and neuroticism (emotional instability). *Mastery* concerns the extent to which one regards one's own life changes as being under one's own control in contrast to being fatalistically ruled. *Self-efficacy* refers to the belief that one can successfully perform specific behaviors. *Neuroticism* is related to a constant preoccupation with things that might go wrong and a strong emotional reaction of anxiety to these thoughts. Research participants with lower levels of neuroticism and higher levels of mastery and self-efficacy perceived significantly higher levels of functioning and well-being.

Why should a sense of control and mastery improve health? Both behavioral and physiological factors are viable possibilities. Those who have a greater sense of control are more likely to take action, to engage in health-promoting behaviors, and to avoid health-damaging behaviors (Rodin, 1986). Because individuals with a high sense of control believe that what they do makes a difference, they behave in healthier ways (Lachman, Ziff, & Spiro, 1994). In contrast, those who feel helpless and fail to see a relationship between actions and outcomes are more prone to illness and disease (Peterson & Stunkard, 1989), perhaps because they fail to engage in health-promoting practices or because they tend toward health-compromising behaviors ("I could get lung cancer no matter what I do, so I might as well smoke").

Having a sense of control also seems to show physiological effects. Research has shown that people with a high sense of control have lower cortisol levels and return more quickly to baseline levels after stress (Seeman & Lewis, 1995). They also have stronger immune systems, as evidenced by their ability to fight off disease (Rodin, 1986).

Additional evidence for the relationship between a strong sense of control and good health comes from research involving people at different socioeconomic levels. Margie Lachman and Suzanne Weaver of Brandeis University (1998) examined three large national samples of 25- to 75-year-old men and women of various social classes and found that for all income groups, higher perceived control was related to better health, greater life satisfaction, and fewer negative emotions. Although the results showed that on average, those with lower income had lower perceived control, as well as poorer health, control beliefs played a moderating role, and participants in the lowest-income group with a high sense of control showed levels of health and well-being comparable with those of the higher-income groups. The results provide some evidence that psychosocial variables such as sense of control may be useful in understanding social-class differences in health.

Can a Sense of Control Have Negative Effects? Some research findings suggest that in some circumstances a strong sense of control may be damaging. For instance, a strong sense of control may be detrimental to the health of older adults in stressful circumstances. Those who view the world as controllable and predictable may be particularly vulnerable when faced with an uncontrollable event, such as widowhood. In one study, widows who had the strongest need for control had a more difficult time coping with the loss of their spouse than those with a lower sense of control (Wortman, Sheedy, Gluhoski, & Kessler, 1992). Why should this be the case? Perhaps those with a strong sense of control would be more likely to feel some sense of guilt over the death of a spouse—I didn't give him/her enough of the right foods. I didn't take him/her to the doctor soon enough, and so on. An alternative explanation is that those with a strong belief in control would have difficulty understanding that there are some things beyond their control.

A strong sense of control may also result in psychological problems for people with severe physical symptoms (Affleck, Tennen, Pfeiffer, & Fifield, 1987). This may be so because a strong sense of control in the face of serious physical limitations may lead to feelings of personal defeat (Reich & Zautra, 1995).

Similarly, a strong sense of control may cause psychological problems among those who require regular assistance with daily functioning (Newsom & Schulz, 1998). These people are accustomed to having control over their lives. Without it, they feel emotionally distressed and inadequate—their self-esteem suffers.

Maintaining Independence

Many gerontologists and geriatric health psychologists have emphasized that the key to healthy aging is *maintaining independence.* Independence doesn't mean that those who age successfully don't need other people. On the contrary, all of us, at every age, are dependent on others. Independence has to do with continuing to be able to make choices in life. The healthy older adult is able to make choices that influence his or her future well-being.

Highlighting this theme of independence, wellness expert James Fries (1999) has identified five key psychological structures for better health as we grow older. Among these structures are the following:

- *Avoiding learned helplessness.* As we discussed in Chapter 5, helplessness is passive behavior learned in a vicious cycle: Exposure to uncontrollable aversive events or continued failure lead to a passive, resigned attitude in which individuals eventually stop striving to succeed. People who are exposed to chronic aversive events that seem uncontrollable, such as chronic illness, may develop symptoms of helplessness. When their efforts to improve their health are not rewarded with success, some give up and drift into depression, passivity, and poorer health.

    The key to avoiding helplessness is to maintain a realistic, hopeful, and self-affirming *explanatory style.* People who age successfully keep things in perspective.

- *Developing self-efficacy.* Obviously, people who have a sense of self-efficacy, who believe that their lifestyle choices can have an effect on their health, are more likely to choose healthy activities and to maintain the effort needed to succeed. And people who strive and meet with success are reinforced for their efforts, which enhances their self-efficacy and helps prevent the vicious cycle by which helplessness develops. For example, arthritis patients who are taught to use exercise, relaxation, and pain-management techniques to manage their symptoms have been shown to feel less pain and disability than control subjects who use only medication (Fries, 1999).

- *Choosing healthy coping strategies.* Throughout this book we have cited research studies investigating the impact of stressful life events on health.

■ **selective optimization with compensation (SOC)** the theory that healthy aging involves assessing abilities realistically, choosing meaningful goals, and devising effective strategies to accomplish them, despite the limits associated with aging

Whether we are talking about divorce, illness, job loss, or the death of a loved one, studies have consistently revealed that it is how people cope with these crises, rather than the crises themselves, that most accurately predict their health.

Like all of life's problems, there are many ways of coping with aging. You can deny that it is happening, become bitter and angry, or abuse alcohol—and so hasten the rate of aging and jeopardize your health. Or you can accept the inevitable changes, use some of them as a stimulus for improvement in areas that matter most to your sense of well-being, and look to the future with a sense of hope and humor.

■ *Learning to choose one's battles.* Researcher Paul Baltes has suggested that older adults can choose to cope with the inevitable declines associated with aging through **selective optimization with compensation (SOC)** (Baltes & Carstensen, 1996). This concept derives from two observations of how people age. First, as we get older, it takes us longer to do certain things. Second, growth and improvement in most important skills—including physical strength, memory, and intellectual functioning—can be improved until very late in life. The paradox of aging is that because things take longer as we get older, there simply is not enough time to focus on all of them simultaneously. Healthy aging involves assessing one's abilities realistically, choosing meaningful goals, and then devising effective strategies to accomplish them, despite the limits associated with aging.

The SOC model provides a useful framework for understanding resilience throughout the life span. It builds on the assumption that throughout life people encounter certain opportunities (education, for example) as well as constraints (such as illness) that can be mastered adaptively by the interplay of three components: selection, optimization, and compensation. *Selection* refers to limiting goals because not all opportunities can be pursued. *Optimization* refers to allocating resources to achieve higher levels of functioning in selected goals. Finally, *compensation* refers to the substitution of activities in order to maintain a given level of functioning in the targeted domain. Those who age gracefully are *selective* in choosing those activities and areas they want to *optimize*.

Several research studies have reported that older adults who use SOC life-management strategies feel better about how they are aging than those who do not.

■ *Capitalize on the seasons of life.* In every culture, people have used the seasons of the calendar as a metaphor to mark life's transitions and to help understand the purpose and meaning of the journey through life. Increasingly, developmental psychologists are realizing that each season of life has its own problems, challenges, pains, and opportunities. Despite the declines of late adulthood, positive changes occur as well, as older adults have more time to approach things in greater depth, years of accumulated experience, and a wealth of *personal wisdom.* Many older adults become more responsive to nature, more appreciative of the arts, more philosophical, and more spiritual. Some psychologists refer to the **interiority** of the older adult: an increased tendency toward introspection, reflection, and putting life into perspective—to connect one's own life with that of future generations as well as those of the past (Kotre & Hall, 1990). These are powerful attributes: They shift the view of older adulthood from one of lost functioning to one of tremendous personal growth.

■ **interiority** an increased tendency toward introspection, reflection, and putting life into perspective that often accompanies aging

Conclusion

The central theme of this section has been that healthy habits pay huge dividends in terms of a longer and better life. But do people with healthy lifestyles— those who do not smoke or drink excessively; who remain physically, psychologically, and socially active; who maintain a healthy weight—actually live longer? Indeed they do. In one study, University of California researchers followed over 7,000 women and men for more than two decades. They found that men with healthier habits lived an average of 11 years longer than those who took more chances with their health. Among women, the longevity difference was slightly smaller but still highly significant. In another study, people with the healthiest lifestyles had the fewest chronic health problems. It's a lot like saving money for a rainy day. Investing early (and often) in good lifestyle habits is the best way to ensure living a long, healthy, and happy life.

Summing Up

Childhood and Adolescence

1. Compared to other states of the life span, the years of childhood are—for most children—uneventful in terms of overall health. Children are at an important formative stage for developing health-enhancing or health-compromising habits that may last a lifetime.

2. Between 20 and 30 percent of American children are obese. Although genes may predispose a body type that is vulnerable to obesity, activity level and food attitudes play important roles in promoting this health hazard. Another factor is excessive television viewing, which bombards children with unhealthy food commercials, lowers metabolic rate, and reduces the amount of time available for healthier activities.

3. In most ways, the teenage years are among the healthiest in the entire life span. More than 50 percent of all cases

of morbidity and mortality in adolescents can be accounted for by preventable risk behaviors, including poor eating habits, substance abuse, and risky sexual behavior.

4. Children with chronic illnesses are at increased risk for a variety of psychological problems, including low self-esteem, feelings of helplessness, and depression. In addition to the assistance they can give children and their families in dealing with these problems, health psychologists can play an important role in helping children cope with hospitalization and stressful medical procedures.

5. How a child responds to a chronic illness is influenced by several factors. Among these are the extent to which the illness is life-threatening and disrupts the child's normal routine, the child's age and maturity, and social support. Families that are close-knit, with good

communication and problem-solving skills, tend to provide the social support that children need to cope with stressful health outcomes.

Adulthood and Aging

6. American culture is characterized by an *ageist* philosophy that tends to emphasize youthfulness. Biological aging affects nearly every facet of health. Changes in appearance, muscle strength, endurance, and oxygen uptake reduce mobility and work capacity and become a social handicap. Sensory losses can interfere with communication, driving, and other activities of daily life.

7. Aging is not synonymous with disease. *Primary aging* is a lifelong process that includes biological, psychological, and social changes. Among the age-related signs of biological senescence are reduced lung capacity, increased body mass index, loss of muscle strength, and decreased metabolism. *Secondary aging* involves age-related changes caused by illness and other conditions rather than by the passing of time.

8. Despite the losses in *fluid intelligence* that accompany aging, there are gains in *crystallized intelligence* and wisdom as a result of accumulated education and experience. In addition, many adults become more philosophical and reflective as they grow older.

9. A small percentage of older adults suffer some form of dementia involving a dramatic deterioration in reasoning ability and memory, as a result of strokes, tumors, or Alzheimer's disease. One in six adults 65 years of age and older suffers significant depression, often related to grief over the loss of loved ones, dementia, or chronic disease.

Theories of Aging

10. One biomedical theory of aging proposes that our bodies wear out with the passage of time. Another proposes that cellular damage due to the accumulation of free radicals promotes disease and hastens aging. A third holds that each cell contains a genetic "clock" that limits the number of times it is able to divide and thereby fixes the maximum human life span.

Lifestyle and Aging

11. Older adults benefit more than any other age group from regular exercise, nutritious eating, and other healthy habits. Aerobic exercise and weight training improve older people's risk profile for the most common chronic illnesses of adulthood, including cardiovascular disease, cancer, and osteoporosis. Despite these benefits, too often older adults avoid exercise.

12. Although changes in metabolism, taste, and smell affect the overall desire and caloric need for food in older adults, the need for vitamins, minerals, and other micronutrients increases with age. Inadequate nutrition can accelerate aging, increase the risk of many chronic illnesses, and produce cognitive deficits.

13. Higher levels of curiosity have been linked to better health and increased longevity in older adults. Other psychological dimensions that have been linked to successful aging are maintaining a sense of mastery and control over one's life, avoiding learned helplessness, choosing healthy coping strategies, and being selective about the activities and areas of life in which to optimize one's abilities.

Key Terms and Concepts

sexually transmitted disease (STD), p. 646
invincibility fable, p. 646
blunting, p. 649
ageism, p. 652
gerontology, p. 653
geriatric health psychology, p. 653
primary aging, p. 654
secondary aging, p. 654
presbycusis, p. 655

senescence, p. 656
fluid intelligence, p. 660
crystallized intelligence, p. 660
dementia, p. 660
Alzheimer's disease (AD), p. 660
aphasia, p. 660
apraxia, p. 660
cross-linking, p. 661
wear-and-tear theory, p. 663
free-radical theory, p. 663

cross-linking theory, p. 663
Hayflick limit, p. 664
telomere, p. 664
Hutchinson-Gilford progeria, p. 665
quality-adjusted life years (QALYs), p. 668
compression of morbidity, p. 668
polypharmacy, p. 674
selective optimization with compensation (SOC), p. 678
interiority, p. 679

Health Psychology on the World Wide Web

Web Address	Description
http://childstats.gov	Child Health USA 2000, a complete report on the health status of American children published by the Maternal and Child Health Bureau of the U.S. Department of Health and Human Services.
http://www.nih.gov/nia/	The National Institute on Aging (NIA), which promotes healthy aging by conducting and supporting biomedical, social, and behavioral research and public education.
http://aging.ufl.edu/apadiv20/apadiv20.htm	Division 20 (Adult Development and Aging) of the American Psychological Association.
http://www.sportsci.org/	The Encyclopedia of Sports Medicine and Science, including many excellent articles on aging and exercise.

Critical Thinking Exercise

Aging and Health

Now that you have read and reviewed Chapter 15, take your learning a step further by testing your critical thinking skills on the following creative problem-solving exercise.

A major theme of this chapter is that age-related changes in health, and aging itself, are determined by many factors, including genetic and biological processes, personal health habits, and social and personality characteristics. Another is that most people's perceptions of aging are inaccurate and reflect ageist stereotypes of physical development in late adulthood. These stereotypes stem from our preoccupation with physical decline that is more the result of *secondary aging* than it is of *primary aging.*

To help you make meaningful connections between these themes and your own life, prepare answers to the following questions.

1. Several studies have found that early-maturing adolescents are more likely than their "on-time" counterparts to take health risks, including engaging in early and unprotected sex; using tobacco, alcohol, and other drugs; and driving dangerously. Think back to your own physical development when you were in the eighth or ninth grade—when you were 14 or 15 years old. Compared to your friends, were you an average-maturing, early-maturing, or late-maturing individual? What impact do you feel the timing of your own physical maturation had on your overall health, and health-related beliefs and behaviors, at the time? Were you, for example, a victim of the invincibility fable? In what ways do these beliefs and behaviors affect your health today?

2. How long a person lives is also influenced by factors in each of the three domains of health: biological, psychological, and social. For each domain, decide whether the choices you have made, or your inherited legacy, are likely to extend or shorten your own longevity. Be specific in identifying those habits or characteristic traits that are likely to extend your life and those that might shorten your life.

3. Think of two older adults whom you know: one who fits the description of a *young-old* and one who fits the description of an *old-old* person, as defined in the chapter. Briefly describe each person, focusing on his or her health, personality, and lifestyle, and explain why you have classified the person as young-old or old-old. Next, speculate as to why each person developed as she or he did. For example, what losses or other life experiences might the old-old person have experienced?

4. How would you explain the death of a grandparent to a 6-year-old child? A 10-year-old child? (Be aware of age-related differences in the understanding of death.)

Epilogue

Health Psychology Today and Tomorrow

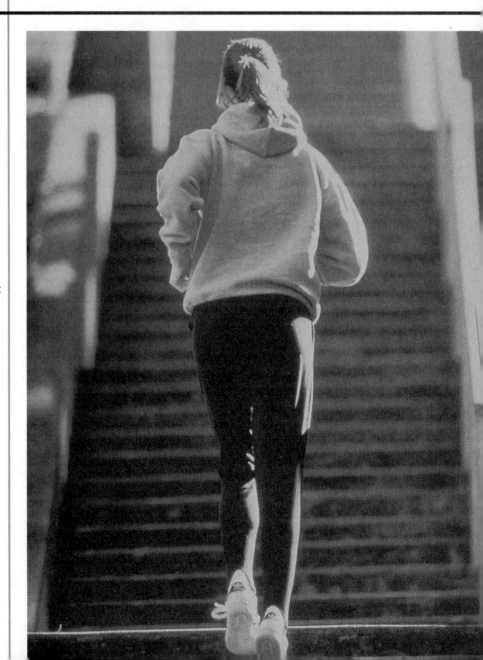

Health psychology has traveled a long way since the American Psychological Association first recognized it in 1978. Our goal in this Epilogue is to look back—to review what has been accomplished along the way—and to look ahead to the most pressing challenges of the future. Although we will focus on health psychologists' contributions to various health-related goals, it is important to remember that they clearly are not working alone. The medical profession and others in the health care industries all work together to achieve these ends.

Health Psychology's Goals

At the beginning of this text, you learned that the overall goal of health psychology is the enhancement of health and the prevention and treatment of illness. To achieve this goal, health psychology has four specific subgoals:

1. To pinpoint psychological, behavioral, and social factors in disease
2. To promote and maintain health
3. To prevent and treat illness
4. To improve the health care system and health care policy

Now that we're at the end of our journey through health psychology's major research findings, theoretical models, and clinical interventions, it is fair to ask whether these goals have been achieved.

Goal 1: To Pinpoint Psychological, Behavioral, and Social Factors in Disease

In the pre-antibiotic era of the early 1900s, the leading causes of death were acute infectious diseases such as tuberculosis, influenza, and pneumonia. Today, however, heart disease, cancer, and stroke account for two-thirds of all deaths in the United States. Unlike infectious diseases, these chronic conditions are in part "lifestyle diseases," often rooted in negative emotions, unhealthy behaviors, social alienation, and poor stress management. As we have seen, negative emotions can start a vicious cycle of low self-esteem, self-blaming, and hostility, which may lead to unhealthy behaviors such as drinking, social alienation, and poor stress management.

Unhealthy Behaviors and Social Alienation
The evidence is clear: Unhealthy behaviors such as smoking, alcohol use, poor nutrition, and inactivity lead to or at least accelerate the occurrence of illness

and disease. For example, extensive research has eliminated any doubt that smoking is causally related to lung cancer and that alcohol use is related both to diseases of the liver and to traffic fatalities. Similarly, a low-fiber, high-fat diet increases a person's risk of developing cardiovascular disease and some forms of cancer. And, of course, a sedentary life increases the risk of cardiovascular disease and certain kinds of cancer and results in poorer immune functioning.

Numerous studies suggest that psychosocial factors can also affect the development and progression of diseases ranging from a simple cold to chronic conditions such as cardiovascular disease, cancer, and AIDS. Among the psychosocial factors that affect cardiovascular health are socioeconomic status, gender, race, employment, acute and chronic stress, social support versus isolation, anger, and depression (Booth et al., 2001). The impact of these factors often equals or exceeds that of more traditional risk factors such as hypertension, diabetes, and even smoking (Ickovics, Viscoli, & Horwitz, 1997).

Psychosocial factors are also linked to life expectancy. As a specific example, prospective studies demonstrate that social support reduces the risk of mortality, independent of other factors, such as gender and ethnicity. Lisa Berkman and Leonard Syme (1994) investigated a sample of 4,725 residents in the western United States, obtaining a social integration score for each participant based on marital status, contacts with friends and relatives, church membership, and other group memberships. Over a 9-year follow-up, men with low social integration scores had a 2.3 greater risk of dying than did men with high scores; for women the rate was 2.8. This finding has been replicated in several other major studies (House, Robbins, & Metzner, 1982; Wills, 1997).

Researchers cannot yet unequivocally state exactly why social integration is protective against chronic disease. However, they can speculate. So far, the most valid hypotheses proposed include the following: Social support may buffer the effects of stress on the body; social support may positively influence health behaviors associated with disease (such as diet and exercise); and social support may directly affect underlying physical mechanisms associated with disease (Cohen, Kaplan, & Mauck, 1994). Conversely, social alienation is related to slower and poorer recovery from several chronic illnesses, including insulin-dependent diabetes (Littlefield, Rodin, Murray, & Craven, 1990), cardiovascular disease (Berkman, Vaccarino, & Seeman, 1993), and metastatic breast cancer (Spiegel, Bloom, Kraemer, & Gottheil, 1989).

Stress and Health

Since the pioneering stress research of Hans Selye (see Chapter 4), there has been mounting evidence that poor stress management can take a negative toll on health, increasing the risk of many chronic diseases, altering the progression of those diseases, and undermining the effectiveness of treatment (Booth et al., 2001; Matthews et al., 1997). Over the past 25 years, health psychologists have delineated the various possible consequences of how a person responds to daily hassles, occupational demands, environmental stressors, and other challenging events and situations. Even more important, they now understand many of the physiological mechanisms by which stress adversely affects health and increases the likelihood of illness. For example, poorly managed stress can result in elevated blood pressure and serum cholesterol (Baum & Posluzny, 1999).

Some of health psychology's most dramatic findings have focused on immune function (Miller & Cohen, 2001). For example, temporary psychological stress, including exam taking or daily hassles, can decrease immune function (Stone et al., 1994), especially in people who have poor coping skills and in those who magnify the impact of potential stressors and appraise them as uncontrollable. In addition, chronic stress, such as that arising from natural disasters or caring for a spouse with Alzheimer's disease, can reduce immunocompetence (Kiecolt-Glaser & Glaser, 1995). Furthermore, stress can increase the development and progression of cardiovascular diseases by increasing arrhythmias, blood clotting speed, and the heart's demand for oxygen while narrowing arteries that would normally dilate to provide more oxygenated blood (Mittleman et al., 1995). Figure E.1 charts the direct effects of stress on health along with a number of the indirect ways in which stress promotes disease, including increasing tobacco and alcohol use and decreasing compliance with medical treatment regimens.

One of health psychology's most important contributions in the area of stress and health has been the resolution of the controversy regarding whether stress is external or internal. Research has clearly revealed that it is both: Stress

Figure E.1

Direct and Indirect Effects of Stress on the Disease Process

Stress affects health directly by elevating blood pressure and serum cholesterol and by decreasing immunity. The indirect effects of stress include reducing compliance with treatment instructions and increasing smoking and a variety of other unhealthy behaviors.

Source: *Behavioral, Biological, and Environmental Interactions in Disease Processes,* by A. Baum, 1994. Washington, DC: NIH Publications.

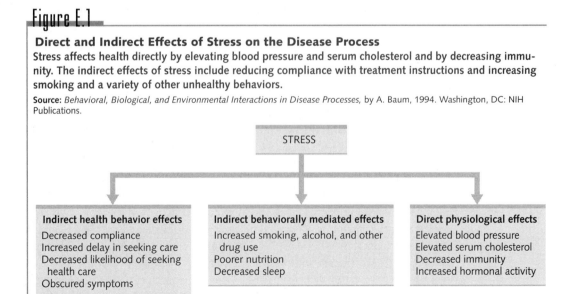

| STRESS |

Indirect health behavior effects	Indirect behaviorally mediated effects	Direct physiological effects
Decreased compliance Increased delay in seeking care Decreased likelihood of seeking health care Obscured symptoms	Increased smoking, alcohol, and other drug use Poorer nutrition Decreased sleep	Elevated blood pressure Elevated serum cholesterol Decreased immunity Increased hormonal activity

is a *transaction* in which each person must continually adjust to daily challenges. To this end, each person's psychological appraisal of potentially stressful events or situations plays an important role in determining the toll that daily hassles, job demands, and other stressors take on his or her well-being. Research has also shown that certain situations and events are more likely to be stressful than others, including those that are uncontrollable and unpredictable and those in which the person has few coping resources.

Goal 2: To Promote and Maintain Health

Promoting and maintaining health have been the mainstays of research and intervention in health psychology. We have seen that psychologists' efforts to change lifestyle behaviors, such as eating habits, tobacco use, and exercising, have focused primarily on cognitive and behavioral approaches. Have these measures been effective?

In 1998, a midcourse review of progress toward the goals of *Healthy People 2000* demonstrated that about 8 percent of the goals had been met or exceeded and that progress had occurred for 41 percent of the other goals. This progress included the following:

- A decline in the three leading causes of death (heart disease, cancer, and stroke). Although this improvement was due in part to improved medical care, it also reflected a national decline in health-compromising behaviors and an increase in health-enhancing behaviors.
- A decrease in the number of alcohol-related automobile deaths from 9.8 per 100,000 people to 6.8 per 100,000 people.
- A decrease in the number of suicides and work-related deaths.
- An increase in the percentage of Americans using seat belts, from 49.7 percent to 76 percent.
- A decline in marijuana and alcohol use among youth aged 12 to 17.
- A decline in the birth rate for unmarried women.
- Continued decline in the infant mortality rate.
- Continued increase in life expectancy.
- A leveling off in the death rate from AIDS.

Clearly, Americans have made fairly dramatic gains in improving their health habits. Many people have successfully quit using tobacco: Only 23 percent of adults smoked in 2000, well below the 42 percent rate in 1965 (Centers for Disease Control, 2001). Americans also moderated their intake of saturated fat and increased the amount of time they spent exercising. Worldwide, however, the picture is not so bright. Every year there are approximately 3 million tobacco-related deaths, and this number is growing. If present trends continue, according to a 1999 World Health Organization report, the annual mortality total will soon reach 10 million, meaning that *half a billion* people alive today will eventually die from tobacco-related causes (Lopez, 1999).

We saw earlier that diseases of the heart currently account for approximately 31 percent of all deaths in the United States, compared to about 23 percent for all forms of cancer, 7 percent for stroke, 5 percent for chronic lung disease, and 4 percent for accidents (National Center for Health Statistics, 2000). During its first quarter century, research in health psychology has reflected this discrepancy, as substantially more attention has been paid to understanding cardiovascular disease (CVD) and to developing interventions designed to prevent it than has been paid to interventions for other chronic illnesses. Health psychologists have focused intensively on the increased risk of CVD related to Type A behavior and hostility and have developed a variety of cognitive-behavioral interventions for lowering blood pressure and serum cholesterol, encouraging exercise, promoting a heart-healthy diet, and modifying negative emotions.

Although these efforts have paid off—death rates for cardiovascular disease have declined steadily over the past 25 years—health psychology has not yet fully met this goal. Alcohol consumption patterns haven't changed much, and obesity continues to increase among certain groups, such as young people. And while cardiovascular disease mortality has decreased, cancer deaths have crept steadily upward.

As the focus of health psychology research has broadened to devote more attention to cancer and other chronic diseases, researchers have begun to make some strides in promoting health by encouraging people to minimize their cancer-risk profile. Still, much more work needs to be done in identifying the psychological and behavioral correlates of cancer and in intervening to encourage people to change behaviors linked with this deadly disease.

Another reason health psychology has not fully met this goal is that behavioral relapse continues to be a critical problem. It has become quite clear that unhealthy lifestyles are much harder to change than to prevent in the first place. Although lifestyle interventions often meet with initial success, too many people "fall off the wagon." Ex-smokers, former heavy drinkers, and those who are new to exercise programs too often fall back into their old bad habits, a problem that must continue to be a focus for future health psychologists.

Goal 3: To Prevent and Treat Illness

The number and variety of health psychology interventions to help people cope with pain, anxiety, depression, and other by-products of chronic illness and other serious medical conditions are increasing every year. Twenty years ago, if you found a psychologist in a hospital or pain clinic, odds are that he or she was there only to evaluate a patient's emotional or psychological functioning by administering a personality test. Today, however, health psychologists perform a much wider range of activities, including training future doctors and nurses on the importance of psychosocial factors in patient compliance and recovery, and directly intervening to assist patients who are facing difficult procedures and adjusting to chronic illness (Table E.1).

Treatment interventions cover every domain of health (Belar & Deardorff, 1996; Redd & Jacobsen, 2001). In the biological domain, treatment is designed to directly change specific physiological responses involved in the illness. Examples include relaxation to reduce hypertension, hypnosis to alleviate pain, and systematic desensitization to reduce the nausea that often occurs in anticipation of chemotherapy. In the psychological domain, health psychologists have applied both cognitive and behavioral interventions. Cognitive interventions include stress inoculation to decrease anxiety about an upcoming medical procedure, cognitive-behavioral treatment for depression, and anger management for hostile cardiovascular disease patients. Behavioral interventions include teaching skills to improve patient–provider communication, to develop a behavior-change program to modify unhealthy habits, and to help train patients in self-management skills such as daily injections of insulin. Social interventions include establishing support groups for those suffering from chronic illness, providing counseling for families of the terminally ill, and conducting role-playing exercises with young children to socially "inoculate" them against being pressured by peers into risky behaviors.

Any fair assessment of health psychology's success in promoting health and treating illness must include a cautionary note. In the face of growing enthusiasm for health psychology's prospects in promoting health, Robert Kaplan (2000) has cautioned that health psychology must not promise more than is supported by the data. Although data support most of health psychology's assumptions (that behaviors increase the risk of certain diseases, that changes in

Table E.1

Examples of Health Psychology's Treatment Interventions

1. Desensitization of fears of medical and dental treatments, including needles, anesthesia, childbirth, or magnetic resonance imaging (MRI) procedures.
2. Treatment to enhance coping with or control over pain, including chronic back pain, headache, or severe burns.
3. Interventions to control symptoms such as vomiting with chemotherapy, scratching with neurodermatitis, or diarrhea with irritable bowel syndrome.
4. Support groups for chronic illness, cardiac rehabilitation, HIV-positive patients, or families of the terminally ill.
5. Training to overcome physical handicaps after trauma, cognitive retraining after stroke, or training to use prosthetic devices effectively.
6. Consultations and program development regarding patient compliance (e.g., special aids for the elderly or inpatient units for insulin-dependent diabetic children).

Source: Adapted from *Clinical Health Psychology in Medical Settings: A Practitioner's Guidebook,* by C. E. Belar and W. W. Deardorff, 1996. Washington, DC: American Psychological Association.

behaviors can reduce the probability of risk of certain diseases, that behavior can be changed easily, and that behavioral interventions are cost effective), the strength of the support is weaker than is assumed by many psychologists.

Kaplan's cautionary note was not intended to discourage health psychologists but rather to recognize that progress is likely to be slow and made in small steps. For example, influencing health behavior is not as easy as some clinical health psychologists seem to believe. In controlled smoking cessation studies, for example, the probability of influencing a smoker to stop is a meager 20 to 30 percent. And as we have seen, most programs are effective only in the short run, with very few achieving long-term abstinence.

Goal 4: To Improve the Health Care System and Health Care Policy

Among the goals of *Healthy People 2000* was a reduction in health care disparities between groups and an increase in access to preventive health services for all Americans. The clear message was that social and environmental factors such as poverty, culture, housing, access to health care, and exposure to racism are important aspects of the context in which health care is delivered.

Unfortunately, health care reform is still little more than a goal for the future. The most recent reports show that reform is slow in coming. As noted in Chapter 12, health care in the United States faces three fundamental problems: It is far too expensive; not all citizens have equal access to high-quality health care; and its services are often used inappropriately. For a variety of reasons, many people who need health care do not seek it; moreover, in 1998, 44.3 million Americans (16.3% of the entire population) were uninsured (National Center for Health Statistics, 1999), a situation that at worst completely blocked their access to health care and at best seriously reduced it. At the same time, health care in this country continues to focus much more on expensive inpatient care (and other efforts at secondary prevention) than on cost-effective primary prevention and health promotion (Kaplan, 2000).

To improve health care while cutting costs is among the most pressing of needs. One of health psychology's most fundamental messages is that prevention and health promotion or maintenance must be made as important in the health care system as disease treatment is now. To this end, health care must be defined more broadly, so that it doesn't focus solely on the services provided by doctors, nurses, clinicians, and hospitals. Many health psychologists believe that in the future, health care should recognize that patients have a central responsibility for their own well-being while also recognizing the important roles played by the individual's family, friends, and community. On this latter point, health care must recognize that schools, places of worship, and workplaces are important sites for promoting health and must become part of the network of interconnected services in the nation's health care system.

The Bottom Line

Any fair assessment of health psychology must recognize that the science is still in its infancy and its contributions are still unfolding. Thus, although impressive progress has been made in some goal areas, much work remains to be done. Implicit within each of the four goals are several principles that virtually all health psychologists agree on—in effect, "lessons" of the past three decades of research that all of us should heed. In the next section, we briefly review the most important of these lessons.

Health Psychology's Most Important Lessons

Health will always be one of our most important assets. In this book, we have described the way in which psychological and social factors, along with biological influences, affect health. You have been introduced to the elements of a healthy lifestyle, including good nutrition, exercise, and stress management. You have learned that your thoughts, attitudes, emotions, and behaviors are intimately connected and that all can influence health. Four lessons have emerged throughout the course of this book's discussion.

Lesson 1: Health and Illness Are Not Merely Matters of Genetics and Biology

As we have seen, for many diseases, heredity plays little or no role whatsoever. Even when genetic vulnerability *does* play a role, not every person with the same genetic vulnerability eventually develops the disease. Bacteria, viruses, and other microorganisms cause some diseases, but being exposed doesn't guarantee that a person will become ill. Stress, negative emotions, coping resources, healthy behaviors, and a number of other factors can make a person more or less susceptible to disease and can influence the progression of disease and how quickly (if at all) he or she recovers.

Stated another way, there is substantial evidence that behavior, mental processes, and health are intimately connected. This is, of course, the fundamental message of the *biopsychosocial (mind–body) model* of health. Even those among us with "hardy" genes and healthy immune systems can become ill if we engage in risky health behaviors, live in unhealthy social and physical environments, and develop a negative emotional style. Earlier, we summarized the links between behavior and health, but this last point—highlighting the emerging field of *psychoneuroimmunology*—is worth underscoring: When we have a calm sense of being in control, we tend to have a comparable emotional and physiological reaction. When we become angry or fearful or feel hopeless because we believe a situation is out of our control, we tend to become emotionally aroused, and consequently our physiological response is more dramatic. Because we know that reactions such as these, if repeated and chronic, can promote illness, it is important for us to learn to manage our thoughts and emotional reactions.

Lesson 2: Our Health Is Largely Our Own Responsibility

As people have become increasingly health conscious, a major shift has occurred in where they place the responsibility for their physical, social, and psychological well-being. More of us realize that the responsibility for our health does not rest solely in the hands of health care professionals but that we ourselves have a major role to play in determining our overall well-being.

As a nation, for example, Americans have become well informed about the hazards of smoking, substance abuse, poor dietary practices, and sedentary living. We know too, that stress, our emotional temperament, the quality of interpersonal relationships, and coping resources are important factors in health. We have learned about the importance of having regular checkups, adhering to our prescribed treatment, and seeking early detection screening for various chronic illnesses, especially if our age, gender, race, or ethnicity places us in the "high-risk" group for these conditions.

Although this awareness doesn't guarantee that people will follow through on what they know to be the healthiest course of action, American citizens have achieved a number of dramatic advances over the past three decades. Fewer people are using tobacco, alcohol consumption has decreased somewhat, and dietary patterns for many of us have shifted to favor more fruits and vegetables, nonanimal sources of protein, and less saturated fat. These healthy behavioral changes are reflected in declining mortality rates for heart disease, cancer, stroke, and homicide (National Center for Health Statistics, 2000).

The point is obvious: *Become an active participant in your health care!*

> I used to tell all the campaign staff: "If you will just let me get sleep and exercise, I can keep going, but if I start cheating on either one of those, then it will have its consequences."
> —Senator Bill Nelson (D), Florida (Krupin, 2001)

Lesson 3: Unhealthy Lifestyles Are Harder to Change than to Prevent

Take a survey of former heavy smokers, those who have lost substantial amounts of weight, or those who are struggling to stick with a new exercise regimen and the message will be clear: It's tough to undo a lifetime of poor health habits. Decades after quitting cigarettes, for example, many smokers continue to "worship at the altar of St. Nicotine." And most people who do quit eventually relapse, often within 6 months or less.

Good nutrition, fitness, responsible drinking, and healthy management of body weight, stress, and social relationships are lifelong challenges that are best begun at a young age. Most smokers, for example, take up the habit during adolescence, usually before they graduate from high school. But as we have seen, because of the *gradient of reinforcement* (see Chapter 6), preventing smoking, like preventing certain risky sexual activities, is a daunting challenge. Many people, especially young people, are more heavily influenced by the immediate "rewards" of smoking—the stimulating "kick" from nicotine, the self-image of doing something that seems mature or perhaps rebellious—than by worries about long-term health consequences.

Preventing poor health habits from developing in the first place will continue to be a high priority for health psychology. New research will investigate the most effective and efficient interventions for reaching the largest number of people in the workplace, schools and universities, and the community. The use of *behavioral immunization programs,* such as those targeting adolescents most likely to engage in risky sex, smoking, drug abuse, and under- or overeating, will also continue to grow. For some health behaviors, interventions will probably need to target even younger "at-risk" individuals. Among these are pediatric "well-parent/well-child" programs designed to teach new parents how to minimize the risks of accidents in the home and automobile and how to start their youngsters off on a lifetime of healthy eating and cardiopulmonary fitness.

Lesson 4: Stress Is in the Eye of the Beholder

As we have seen, learning to manage the stress we encounter is crucial to our physical, psychological, and emotional well-being. The goal of stress management is not to eliminate stress altogether but rather to learn to manage the stressors we encounter and to cope with their effects more adaptively. To this end, research has revealed the benefits of many specific strategies: keeping stress at manageable levels; preserving your physical resources by following a balanced diet, exercising, and drinking responsibly; establishing a stress-busting social network; increasing your psychological hardiness; disclosing your feelings when something is bothering you; cultivating a sense of humor; reducing hostile behaviors and negative emotions; and learning to relax.

And last, but certainly not least, learning to change stressful thoughts into stress-busting ones will go a long way toward cutting stress off before it gets a firm grip on you. As we learned in Chapters 4 and 5, each of life's events can be appraised as a stressor but also as a challenge or as an opportunity. You may not have asked for this "opportunity," but it is nevertheless here to be faced. How you view it will in large measure determine the impact it has on your health.

Health Psychology's Future Challenges

Most of health psychology's challenges stem from two major research agendas. The first is the Department of Health and Human Services report *Healthy People 2000,* which, as we have seen, outlined the nation's highest priorities for promoting health and preventing disease among all Americans. The report was based on the best judgments of a large group of health experts from the scientific community, professional health organizations, and the corporate world. The report set 300 specific health objectives to be achieved by the year 2000. These were organized in three broad categories: *increasing the span of healthy life, reducing health disparities among various socioeconomic and ethnic groups,* and *increasing access to preventive health services.*

The second research agenda, produced by the American Psychological Association in collaboration with the National Institutes of Health and 21 other professional societies, focuses more specifically on health psychology's role in health care reform. Published in 1995, *Doing the Right Thing: A Research Plan for Healthy Living* identified four research tasks in the new millennium (listed below), out of which emerge five challenges that we'll discuss in this section.

- Accelerating research related to health promotion and disease prevention.
- Extending research and health care to *traditionally underrepresented groups* such as women and minorities.
- Increasing the focus on the basic behavioral processes in the prevention, development, and treatment of chronic disease.
- Reshaping the health care system to meet tomorrow's needs.

Challenge 1: To Increase the Span of Healthy Life for All People

The rapid aging of the population draws our attention to a crucial challenge: developing effective interventions that will enable older adults to maintain the highest possible level of functioning, or to improve it, for the most number of years.

As you learned in Chapter 2, healthy life is a combination of average life expectancy and quality of life. The challenge for health psychology is to increase the number of *quality-adjusted life years (QALYs),* or "well years"—an index of a person's biological age rather than his or her chronological age—along with a *compression of morbidity*—which refers to a shortening of the amount of time older people spend disabled, ill, or in pain (see Chapter 15).

Some success has been achieved. But there is room for much additional improvement. Although life expectancy at birth currently is 79.7 years for women and 73.8 for men born in the United States, the number of well years is only 72.6 years for women and 67.5 years for men (World Health Report, 2000). This discrepancy between life expectancy and well years is even larger when we compare various socioeconomic groups and other countries of the world. Lower socioeconomic status is associated with shorter average life expectancy *and* fewer well years. Thus, separating life expectancy into years in good health and years lived with disability widens rather than narrows the difference in health status between richer and poorer populations. Around the world, the percentage of life expectancy lost to disability ranges from less than 9 percent in the healthiest regions to more than 14 percent in the least healthy. Recall from Chapter 6 that health psychologists use *disability-adjusted life expectancy (DALE)* as an index of the number of well years a person can expect.

Challenge 2: To Reduce Health Discrepancies and Increase Knowledge of Understudied Groups

Historically, several measures of health have shown substantial differences among various ethnic and sociodemographic groups, as well as between the genders. For example, in 1999, average life expectancy was 74.3 years for white males but only 67.2 years for African-American males, and 79.9 years for white females but only 74.7 years for African-American females (Centers for Disease Control and Prevention, 2000). Asking people about their health reveals even greater differences by ethnic group, as shown in Figure E.2. The reasons for these discrepancies are undoubtedly complex but may include unequal access to health care, genetic susceptibility to specific diseases, and lifestyle differences.

Health psychologists could not pinpoint the reasons for the discrepancies because until recently, what they knew about health and disease derived from research disproportionately concentrated on young, relatively healthy, white, male subjects. Although the theoretical basis of health psychology is drawn from many fields, early in its history, the field suffered from a fairly narrow view of the factors in health and disease, simply because of this bias in sampling. For example, in many major studies women and members of ethnic minorities were either excluded or included in insufficient numbers to adequately assess the effects of various variables on their health (Matthews et al., 1997). Similarly, although people over 65 are far more likely to develop chronic illnesses and to suffer from chronic pain, health psychology has only recently devoted much attention to the special health issues of the elderly (see Chapter 15).

Realizing this problem, health psychologists have begun to widen the scope of their research to include a more diverse pool of research participants or—

Figure E.2

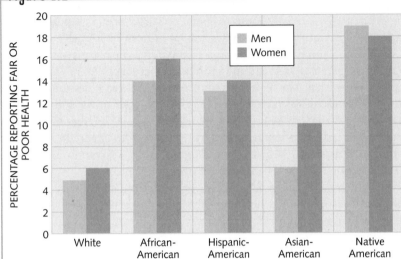

Quality of Health by Ethnic Group and Gender
When asked to describe their health, a surprisingly high percentage of all ethnic groups used "fair or poor." Except among Native Americans, women are more likely than men to describe their health in negative terms. Even more telling are the differences between ethnic groups, with whites having the most positive view of their health and Native Americans being least positive.

Source: *Healthy People 2000 Review,* by National Center for Health Statistics, 1999. Hyattsville, MD: Public Health Service.

even better—to focus specifically on understudied groups. For example, they have found that women and men have very different psychological, social, and biological characteristics and vulnerabilities and that they therefore differ in their susceptibility to various diseases and in their coping reactions to stress. The same seems to be true of many different ethnic and racial groups. For instance, research has demonstrated that disadvantaged women are at increased risk for early mortality and chronic disease (Adler, Boyce, Chesney, Folkman, & Syme, 1993). In addition, women are more likely to exhibit eating disorders than are men, minorities account for a disproportionate number of cases of AIDS in the United States, and the rates of smoking, sedentary living, and poor eating habits among women and men across various ethnic groups are different (Landrine & Klonoffl, 2001).

The negative effects of ethnicity and poverty on health may be the result of factors such as poor nutrition, crowded and unsanitary environments, inadequate medical care, stressful life events, and subjective perceptions that environmental stressors are beyond one's ability to cope. Another factor is less effective use of health screening among certain groups. For example, African-American women delay longer than white women in seeking care for breast symptoms, and older women, who frequently are at increased risk of breast cancer, are less likely to seek preventive care.

However, ethnic group disparities in health are not completely attributable to the social conditions in which people live. For example, Hispanic-Americans generally fare as well as or better than European Americans on most measures of health, actually having a lower death rate than European

Americans from heart disease, lung cancer, and stroke (USDHHS, 2001). This is paradoxical, given the high rates of hypertension, obesity, and tobacco use among Hispanic-Americans. Some researchers believe that this puzzling fact reflects a lag in acculturation, since the same trend can be found in all immigrant groups: as immigrants adopt an American lifestyle, they eventually develop the same patterns of illness and mortality (Marwick, 1991).

Another factor that may be important is education. Regardless of ethnicity, people who have achieved higher levels of education live longer and have better overall health than those with less education, most likely because people with fewer years of education generally are more likely to engage in unhealthy behaviors such as smoking and eating a high-fat diet than those with more years of education (Macera, Armstead, & Anderson, 2001).

Clearly, much more research is needed before health psychologists can confidently explain why there are health discrepancies among traditionally understudied groups. One attempt to fill the void is being provided by the *Women's Health Initiative (WHI)*, a long-term national health study focusing on the prevention of heart disease, breast and colorectal cancer, and osteoporosis in postmenopausal women (Matthews et al., 1997). WHI, which focuses on the effects of the social environment and individual characteristics on health (Figure E.3), includes three components: a randomized, controlled clinical trial of 64,500 women testing the impact of a low-fat diet, hormone replacement therapy, and calcium-vitamin D supplementation; an observational study of another 100,000 women, examining the biological and psychological determinants of these chronic diseases in women; and a massive study evaluating eight different model education/prevention programs in communities throughout the United States. Health psychologists have played an important role in the WHI study by suggesting key hypotheses to test and explaining how to design the interventions, how to recruit and retain women in the study, and how to increase treatment adherence.

Challenge 3: To Achieve Equal Access to Preventive Health Care Services for All People

As we have seen throughout this book, many minorities and impoverished Americans of every ethnicity and race have limited access to preventive health care. For this reason they tend to suffer disproportionately more health problems and have a higher mortality rate. More than 44 million working Americans have no health insurance, making every day, in effect, a roll of the dice with respect to their health. Health psychology faces the continuing challenge of understanding and removing barriers that limit access to health care in these groups.

The United States does a poorer job than any other industrialized nation in making health care available to all its citizens. Although the United States has the

Figure E.3

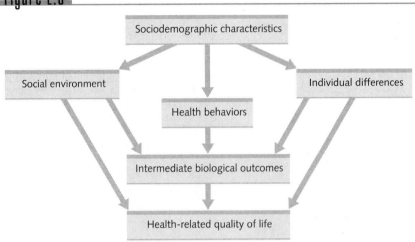

Sociodemographic Characteristics and Health-Related Quality of Life in Women

One goal of the Women's Health Initiative (WHI) is to understand the factors that contribute to the health of postmenopausal women and to evaluate the efficacy of practical interventions in preventing the major causes of morbidity and mortality in older women. They hope to accomplish this in part by testing the model depicted here, which suggests that the effects of the social environment and individual dispositions influence a woman's health through her health-related behaviors and intermediate biological outcomes.

Source: "Women's Health Initiative: Why Now? What Is It? What's New?" by K. A. Matthews, S. A. Shumaker, D. J. Bowen, R. D. Langer, J. R. Hunt, R. M. Kaplan, R. C. Klesges, and C. Ritenbaugh, *American Psychologist,* 1997, 52, pp. 101–116.

most costly health care system in the world, it is not necessarily the best (see Figure E.4 on page 698). For example, the United States ranks only twenty-first in the world in infant mortality, sixteenth in life expectancy for women, and seventeenth in life expectancy for men. In terms of its overall performance on eight measures of health, the U.S. health care system ranks thirty-seventh out of the member states of the World Health Organization (WHO, 2000). As we have seen, one reason for these low rankings is the tremendous disparity in the environmental conditions in which Americans live (Taylor, Repetti, & Seeman, 1997).

Underscoring the impact of this disparity in environmental conditions, the National School Boards Association recently issued its report *Ten Critical Threats to America's Children: Warning Signs for the Next Millennium* (1999). The threats included poverty, lack of health care, substance abuse, crime and dangers in the environment, abuse and neglect at home, inadequate child care, poor schools, teen pregnancy, and absent parents. It is obvious that each of these threats, either directly or indirectly, can have a powerful impact on children's health.

Figure E.4

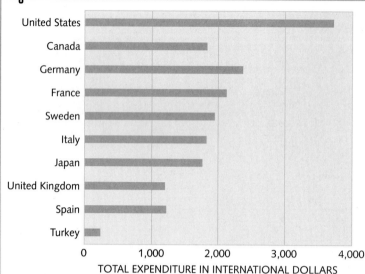

Health Care Costs around the World
This bar chart shows that the United States has the most costly health care system in the world. However, it is not necessarily the best system. For instance, the United Kingdom and Canada—both of which have socialized medicine—rank above the United States in the overall quality of their health care system but spend less money annually. Thus, improving health care while cutting costs is one of our most pressing challenges as a nation.
Source: Data from *Health Systems: Improving Performance,* by World Health Report, 2000, June 2000 (Annex Table 1, pp. 152–155). Geneva, Switzerland: World Health Organization.

Social and economic factors—including differences in education, income, occupational status, and racial and ethnic background—undoubtedly play a role. In this country, African-Americans, Hispanic-Americans, and Native Americans generally have a lower average income and less education than do Asian-Americans and European Americans. Most poor European Americans live in areas that are not classified as poverty areas, whereas only a small minority of poor African-Americans lives *outside* such areas. Thus, there is a disproportionate concentration of certain minority groups in unhealthy neighborhoods (Anderson & Armstead, 1995).

As long as socioeconomic differences allow some people to have access to quality health care while others have none, we will have a two-tiered health care system in this country: state of the art, high-tech care for those who can afford it and substandard care (or no care) for everyone else. Health care reform remains a continuing challenge—for health psychology as well as for the national political agenda.

Challenge 4: To Adjust the Focus of Research and Intervention to Maximize Health Promotion

In the past, health psychology followed biomedicine's lead in focusing on mortality rather than morbidity. Even when prevention was stressed, health psychologists tended to focus on those chronic diseases that were the leading causes of death (Kaplan, 2000). While reducing mortality will continue to be a priority, health psychology also must devote greater attention toward conditions such as arthritis, which have a minimal impact on mortality rates but a dramatic impact on wellness among the elderly.

A related challenge is to place more emphasis on health-enhancing behaviors and factors that may delay mortality and reduce morbidity. As we have seen, health psychologists have devoted the largest measure of their research to risk factors for chronic disease, and a substantially smaller amount of time to health-promoting aspects that seem to inoculate people from developing illness. To this end, greater attention to how hardy, or resilient, people self-manage stress, maintain a strong sense of control over their lives, and keep an upbeat, optimistic attitude—and whether these traits can be taught to others—will be an exciting challenge for future health psychologists.

A continuing challenge for health psychology is thorough documentation of the effectiveness of its interventions. This issue has been brought into sharp focus recently as debate continues over the extent to which psychological interventions should be covered by managed health insurance. Backed only by weak or poorly conducted research studies, even the most exciting new intervention is likely to meet with the same skeptical reaction from health care professionals as have many complementary and alternative therapies (see Chapter 14). Complicating the research picture, true primary prevention studies often take decades to complete and require expensive, long-term funding. Fortunately, the Centers for Disease Control and Prevention have shown considerable interest in continuing behavioral intervention research (Snider & Satcher, 1997).

Translating Knowledge into Behavior

Despite health psychology's successes, much remains to be done before the goals of *Healthy People 2000* are fully met. While the recently updated report (*Healthy People 2010*) continues to focus on eliminating health disparities among various sociocultural groups, emphasis has been shifted away from targeting special groups in favor of improved health for all Americans. The report also notes that use (and abuse) of certain drugs is once again on the rise, and nearly 1 million deaths in this country each year are preventable. On this last point, it is estimated that

- Control of underage and excess use of alcohol could prevent 100,000 deaths from automobile accidents and other alcohol-related injuries.
- Eliminating public possession of firearms could prevent 35,000 deaths.
- Eliminating all forms of tobacco use could prevent 400,000 deaths from cancer, stroke, and heart disease.
- Better nutrition and exercise programs could prevent 300,000 deaths from heart disease, diabetes, cancer, and stroke.

- Reducing risky sexual behaviors could prevent 30,000 deaths from sexually transmitted diseases.

- Providing full access to immunizations for infectious diseases could prevent 100,000 deaths.

Despite the clear health benefits of early detection and screening procedures in minimizing the impact of chronic disease, the use of such procedures is substantially less than it ought to be. We have seen that many people who are at high risk for HIV infection, various cancers, and hypertension avoid screening procedures and/or delay in seeking medical evaluation and treatment for symptoms. A related problem is why patients do not fully comply with treatment once a chronic disease or health condition has been diagnosed.

Research has revealed many psychological and behavioral barriers to early detection and adherence to treatment regimens. Among these are depression, anxiety disorders, pain, and the quality of the patient–provider relationship. A continuing challenge for health psychology is to find the most effective ways to counteract the human tendency to avoid screening procedures and treatment.

Avoiding Reductionism

As we have learned, health psychology's foundation was, in part, based on the limitations of the reductionist approach of traditional biomedicine, which dissociates the mind and body and almost never examines the larger psychological and social contexts in which illness occurs. Although the biomedical community is beginning to make a conceptual shift toward the biopsychosocial model, biological explanations continue to dominate most medical research.

Paradoxically, health psychology may also be subject to the criticism of being too reductionistic. Although health psychologists have developed increasingly sophisticated models of the impact of psychosocial factors on health and illness, they rarely include biological measures necessary to test proposed biological mechanisms. Even those research studies that attempt to integrate biological, psychological, and sociocultural factors in disease rarely test for interactions among biological and psychosocial factors (Fremont & Bird, 1999).

Consider once again the issue of gender in health. Health psychologists have examined the effects of gender inequality in the home and workplace on psychological stress, but few studies have assessed physical health consequences. For example, women's multiple roles frequently produce sustained high levels of stress hormones throughout the day and well into the evening, whereas men's stress hormone levels peak during the day but decline in the evening (Frankenhaeuser, Lundberg, Fredrikson, & Melin, 1989). And although health psychologists are now paying a great deal of attention to the need to include women in medical research, they are just beginning to realize that interventions may work differently in women and men due to differences in the types of stressors they experience (Matthews et al., 1997).

Challenge 5: To Assist in Health Care Reform

For well over a decade, researchers have been predicting a major revolution in the U.S. health care system. Many experts believe that the revolution is well under way. Among the issues pacing this revolution are universal access to health care, comprehensive mandated health benefits, cost containment, quality, accountability, and a shift in emphasis from secondary prevention to primary prevention (Belar & Deardorff, 1996; Kaplan, 2000). Although the dust has not yet settled, it is generally accepted as inevitable that health care reform will occur. How will health psychology fare in this new world of reformed health care?

The important role of psychologists in improving physical health through enhancing treatment outcomes has now been firmly established. This has led to a significant increase in the number of psychologists working in general health care settings (Groth-Marnat & Edkins, 1996; Winefield, 2001). Unfortunately, however, recent efforts to reduce health care costs threaten this trend. Listen to any discussion of health care on the floor of Congress, for example, and you will realize that psychosocial issues, primary health prevention, and the merits of psychological interventions are mentioned as an afterthought, if at all. And among hospital administrators, primary prevention and psychological services too often are viewed as optional services or even a frill. No wonder that primary prevention and psychological services are easy targets for hospital administrators seeking to contain costs.

As Robert Kaplan (2000) has noted, current health policy clearly places greater emphasis on preventing *further* episodes of disease in those who are already sick (secondary prevention) than on preventing the onset of disease in the first place (primary prevention). This is understandable, since secondary prevention is based on the traditional biomedical (disease) model and usually involves medical diagnosis, medication, surgery, and other procedures that are covered by health insurance. In contrast, primary prevention is based on a behavioral rather than a disease model and typically does not involve diagnosis because there is no disease to diagnose.

This is not only unfortunate but also counterproductive, since secondary prevention programs are often expensive and may produce few, if any, measurable benefits (Kaplan, 2000). One way to estimate the benefits of preventive actions is with combined measures of life expectancy and quality of life. For instance, across the general population, PSA prostate cancer screening for 70-year-old men extends life expectancy by an average of only about 5 hours (Krahn et al., 1994). Similarly, annual mammography screening for women between 40 and 50 extends the life expectancy by only 2.5 days (Lindfors & Rosenquist, 1995. (There is little debate, however, about the value of regular mammography for women 50 to 69 years of age.) For many individuals, these modest benefits may be overshadowed by the discomfort of the procedures, which reduce the overall quality of life. Stated in these terms, these common secondary prevention procedures are harmful rather than helpful for some people. In contrast, many primary prevention efforts and psychosocial interventions save money while producing equal or greater health benefit. For instance, regular exercise starting at age 35 extends average life expectancy 186 days, while smoking cessation may add as many as 1,800 days (Hatziandreu, Koplan, Weinstein, Caspersen, & Warner, 1988).

QALYs can be used to calculate the cost effectiveness of various primary and secondary prevention efforts. For example, a pharmaceutical treatment, medical screening procedure, or behavior intervention that improves the quality of life by half (0.5) for two people will result in the equivalent of 1 QALY over a period of 1 year. Researchers estimated that the small benefit of regular mammography among women 40 to 49 years of age (increasing life expectancy by only 2.5 days at a cost of $676 per woman) amounts to a cost of $100,000 for 1 full QALY (Salzmann, Kerlikowske, & Phillips, 1997). As a comparison, researchers have found that regular exercise produces 1 QALY for $11,313—a much more modest expenditure relative to many biomedical secondary prevention interventions (Hatziandreu et al., 1988).

Psychosocial Interventions

Psychosocial interventions for those who are sick also yield significant cost savings, particularly when used to prepare patients for surgery and other anxiety-producing medical procedures (Groth-Marnat & Schumaker, 1995). Patients who are overly anxious when facing hospitalization and invasive procedures such as surgery often experience a disintegration of normal coping skills (Horne, Vatmanidis, & Careri, 1994). Relaxation training, postsurgical exercises, distraction techniques, and control-enhancing techniques can reduce the length of hospitalization and the need for pain-relieving medication and help prevent disruptive patient behavior (Blankfield, 1991; Disbrow, Owings, & Bennett, 1993).

The challenge of cost-containment is likely to continue, since cardiovascular disease and cancer—chronic, age-related diseases that are extraordinarily costly to treat—will probably remain the leading causes of death for some time to come. And it is possible that escalating health care costs may actually boost health psychology's role, since one of the best ways to contain these costs is to help people improve their health behaviors and help those who become sick to recover as quickly as possible. For a variety of illnesses and conditions, psychosocial interventions can be effective in both situations. For example, a study by Mary Olbrisch (1981) reported a savings of 1.2 hospital days on average in adult surgical patients who received preoperative psychological services. Similarly, Durand Jacobs (1988) found a 72 percent reduction in the length of hospital stays among surgical patients who received biofeedback relaxation training. The strongest evidence comes from a meta-analysis of 49 controlled experiments using interventions designed to increase infor-mation control (see Chapter 12) prior to surgery. Averaged across all studies, patients in the intervention group required an average of 1.31 fewer days in the hospital compared to those who received standard hospital treatment (Devine & Cook, 1983).

Blended (Interdisciplinary) Care

As further testimony to health psychology's future role in helping the health care system's efforts to contain costs, the *Human Capital Initiative* has called for greater use of *blended care* (also called collaborative care; see Chapter 12). This interdisciplinary model, in which treatment teams approach diseases from bio-logical, psychological, and sociocultural perspectives, shows great promise in improving treatment while simultaneously cutting costs (Table E.2).

The success of blended, or interdisciplinary, care reflects health psychology's growing acceptance by traditional biomedicine over the past 25 years—a trend that is likely to continue into the future (Daw, 2001). One sign of this ac-ceptance is the dramatic increase in the number of psychologists working in medical school settings. Between 1960 and the late 1990s, psychology has grown from averaging about 2 psychologists per medical school to nearly 30 psychologists per medical school (Sheridan, 1999). Another sign is the growing role of nurses in delivering psychological services. An increasing number of nurses are obtaining advanced degrees in psychology, and nursing has estab-lished the *National Institute for Nursing Research (NINR),* which focuses on controlled studies of psychological variables in nursing.

Paradoxically, as medical care has grown more specialized and more com-plex, it has also begun to broaden its scope, incorporating more comple-mentary and alternative aspects of healing. Relaxation training, imagery, and some of the spiritual aspects of non-Western healing traditions are increas-ingly being welcomed by managed-care programs because these methods are

Table E.2

Reduction in Treatment Frequency with Blended Care

Total ambulatory care visits	− 17 %
Visits for minor illnesses	− 35 %
Pediatric acute illness visits	− 25 %
Office visits for acute asthma	− 49 %
Office visits by arthritis patients	− 40 %
Average length of stay in hospital for surgical patients	−1.5 days
Cesarean sections	− 56 %
Epidural anesthesia during labor and delivery	− 85 %

Source: *Doing the Right Thing: The Human Capital Initiative Strategy* (report). American Psychological Association, 1994, p. 16.

typically inexpensive and yet often effective in helping patients cope with a variety of stress-related symptoms. With today's rising medical costs, the *cost-effectiveness ratio* of such interventions can't be ignored.

International Reform

As we have seen, there is great variability in the prevalence of specific diseases throughout the world. Poverty, lack of health care, and ignorance generally contribute to a higher incidence of infectious diseases in developing countries than in developed countries. Just as smoking continues to decline in this country, its prevalence is increasing in developing parts of the world. So too, as Americans are becoming fitter through more exercise, many developing countries are becoming less fit as their modernization is accompanied by an increase in sedentary living.

Health psychology can take the lead in carrying the messages of the thousands of research studies to other parts of the world in which similar health problems are just beginning to emerge. This role is underscored by the central role of the sociocultural perspective in health psychology. Like other social and behavioral scientists, health psychologists are more likely than researchers in some areas to understand the importance of cultural factors in health care practices and behaviors.

But the transmission of information can flow in both directions. Health psychologists can help reform the U.S. health care system by helping policymakers understand those things that other countries actually do *better* than we do. For example, all Canadian citizens are covered through one government-subsidized health insurance provider. Although physicians work as independent service providers in private offices and clinics, much like those in the United States, their fees are fixed through regular negotiations with the government of the province in which they practice. Thus, physicians cannot charge more for their services than the agreed-upon price.

As another example, consider one aspect of the Australian system: well woman/well man clinics. The aim of these clinics is to promote the health of the total woman and man, focusing on wellness rather than only on disease. The National Woman's Health Policy, funded with a $33.5 million grant, focused on several initiatives: reproductive health and sexuality, emotional and mental health, violence against women, occupational health and safety, and the health effects of sex role stereotyping.

The free wellness clinics, which are staffed by nurse practitioners, are found throughout the country and focus on education, assessment, and nonmedicinal management of personal and family stress problems. All the clinics provide free breast examination and cervical smears, together with training in breast self-examination. Many also offer pregnancy testing and seminars, workshops, and educational information on nutrition, weight control and body image, menopause, and hormone replacement therapy.

Conclusion

Health psychology's outlook as a profession is bright. The field has made impressive advances in its brief history, but there is much more to learn and many challenges that face future health psychologists. As recently as March 2000, an American Psychological Association conference on the future of health psychology failed to reach consensus on a unified definition or vision of the field (Revenson & Baum, 2001). We have only scratched the surface of the many ways in which the study of psychology can bring good health to you as an individual, to the health care system, and to society. It is my hope that this book has sparked your interest in the field of health psychology and that you will pursue further study.

Critical Thinking Exercise

Revising a Textbook

Now that you have completed the Epilogue, take your learning a step further by testing your critical thinking skills on this creative problem-solving exercise.

Throughout the text you have read that no aspect of health can be fully understood without considering all three domains of health—*physical, psychological,* and *social*—as emphasized in the *biopsychosocial (BPS) model.* This means that important health-promoting and health-damaging behaviors—such as exercising and eating a nutritious diet versus drinking excessively and smoking—as well as chronic diseases and other medical conditions, cannot be easily characterized as falling within any single domain. For instance, although leukemia clearly is a physical disease, it greatly affects psychological and social health as well.

This exercise is designed to help consolidate your understanding of the three domains of health, and the BPS model, by asking you to imagine that you are an editor responsible for revising this text. You are attending an editorial committee meeting to plan the next edition.

1. Stress, pain, and healthy behavior are now each discussed in separate chapters. One editor suggests moving them together into a chapter on "psychological factors" in health. Do you agree with this change? Why or why not?

2. Cardiovascular disease, cancer, and AIDS are now each discussed in separate chapters. A reviewer suggests moving them into a single chapter on chronic diseases. Are there any advantages to this idea? Do you agree with this change? Why or why not?

3. In the current edition, many life-span issues are discussed throughout the text, but several major life-span topics are discussed in a separate chapter. One reviewer suggests that the chapter should be removed and *all* life-span information spread throughout the text. Are there any advantages to this idea? Do you agree with this change? Why or why not?

4. Ethnic and cultural issues in health and disease are currently discussed throughout the text. One instructor using the book believes that these issues should be collected together into a separate chapter. Are there any advantages to this idea? Do you agree with this change? Why or why not?

Glossary

acculturation the process in which a member of one ethnic or racial group adopts the values, customs, and behaviors of another

acupuncture a component of traditional Oriental medicine in which fine needles are inserted into the skin in order to relieve pain, treat addiction and illness, and promote health

acute pain sharp, stinging pain that is short-lived and usually related to tissue damage

adipocytes collapsible body cells that store fat

adrenal glands lying above the kidneys, the pair of endocrine glands that secrete epinephrine, norepinephrine, and cortisol, hormones that arouse the body during moments of stress

ageism attitudes of prejudice and negative stereotypes against older people

agonist a drug that attaches to a receptor and produces neural actions that mimic or enhance those of a naturally occurring neurotransmitter

AIDS (acquired immunodeficiency syndrome) a life-threatening disease caused by the human immunodeficiency virus in which the body's CD4 lymphocytes are destroyed, leaving the victim vulnerable to opportunistic diseases

AIDS dementia complex an AIDS-related syndrome involving memory loss, confusion, and personality changes

alcohol abuse a maladaptive drinking pattern in which drinking interferes with role obligations

alcohol dependence a state in which the use of alcohol is required for a person to function normally

alcohol expectancies individuals' beliefs about the effects of alcohol consumption on behavior, their own as well as that of other people

Alzheimer's disease a degenerative disease of the brain that leads to dementia and a dramatic deterioration of thinking, memory, and reasoning

amygdala two clusters of neurons in the limbic system that are linked to emotion, especially aggression

anabolism the constructive form of metabolism in a plant or animal by which food is converted into living tissue

anatomical theory the theory that the origins of specific diseases are found in the internal organs, musculature, and skeletal system of the human body

anecdotal evidence research evidence based on informal case histories, in which there is little or no objective documentation regarding a patient's diagnosis or the effectiveness of a treatment

angina pectoris a condition of extreme chest pain caused by a restriction of the blood supply to the heart

anorexia nervosa an eating disorder characterized by self-starvation, a distorted body image, and, in females, amenorrhea

antagonist a drug that blocks the action of a naturally occurring neurotransmitter or agonist

antigen a foreign substance that stimulates an immune response

aphasia a distinctive speech disorder in which speech sounds normal but is lacking in content words; characteristic symptom of Alzheimer's disease

apraxia a loss of memory for motor movements, often apparent in later stages of Alzheimer's disease

arteries blood vessels that carry blood away from the heart to other organs and tissues. A small artery is called an arteriole

arteriosclerosis also called "hardening of the artèries," a disease in which blood vessels lose their elasticity

association cortex areas of the cerebral cortex not directly involved in sensory or motor functions; rather, they integrate multisensory information and higher mental functions such as thinking and speaking

atherosclerosis a chronic disease in which cholesterol and other fats are deposited on the inner walls of the coronary arteries, reducing circulation to heart tissue

attentional focus a person's characteristic style of monitoring bodily symptoms, emotions, and overall well-being

autogenic training a relaxation-promoting form of self-hypnosis involving a series of exercises that induce feelings of heaviness and warmth in the body's limbs

average life expectancy the number of years the average child born in a given year is likely to live

aversion therapy a behavioral therapy that pairs an unpleasant stimulus (such as a nauseating drug) with an undesirable behavior (such as drinking or smoking), causing the patient to avoid the behavior

basal metabolic rate (BMR) the minimum number of calories the body needs to maintain bodily functions while at rest

behavioral disinhibition the false sense of confidence and freedom from social restraints that results from alcohol consumption

behavioral immunogen a health-enhancing behavior or habit

behavioral intention (BI) in theories of health behavior, the rational decision to engage in a health-related behavior or to refrain from engaging in the behavior

behavioral medicine an interdisciplinary field that integrates behavioral and biomedical science in promoting health and treating disease

behavioral pathogen a health-compromising behavior or habit

behavioral undercontrol a general personality syndrome linked to alcohol dependence and characterized by aggressiveness, unconventionality, and impulsiveness; also called deviance proneness

behavioral willingness (BW) in theories of health behavior, the reactive, unplanned motivation involved in the decision to engage in risky behavior

belief bias a form of faulty reasoning in which our expectations prevent us from seeing alternative explanations for our observations

biofeedback a system that provides audible or visible feedback information regarding involuntary physiological states

biolectrical impedance analysis a method of determining the percentage of body fat by analyzing the electrical resistance as an imperceptible electric current is passed through the body

biomedical model the dominant view of twentieth-century medicine that maintains that illness always has a physical cause

biopsychosocial (mind–body) perspective the viewpoint that health and other behaviors are determined by the interaction of biological mechanisms, psychological processes, and social influences

birth cohort a group of people who, because they were born at about the same time, experience similar historical and social conditions

blood alcohol level (BAL) the amount of alcohol in the blood, measured in grams per 100 milliliters

blood-brain barrier the network of tightly packed capillary cells that separates the blood and the brain

blunting a coping strategy that limits threatening thoughts in an effort to reduce emotional stress

body mass index (BMI) a measure of obesity calculated by dividing body weight by the square of a person's height

brainstem the oldest and most central region of the brain; includes the medulla, pons, and reticular formation

bronchi the pair of respiratory tubes that branch into progressively smaller passageways, the bronchioles, culminating in the air sacs within the right and left lungs (alveoli)

buffering hypothesis theory that social support produces its stress-busting effects indirectly, by helping the individual cope more effectively

bulimia nervosa an eating disorder characterized by alternating cycles of binge eating and purging through such techniques as vomiting or laxative abuse

burden of disease a measure of a population's health that indicates the percentage of all DALYs lost due to all causes accounted for by a particular disease or disability

burnout a job-related state of physical and psychological exhaustion

calorie a measure of food energy equivalent to the amount of energy needed to raise the temperature of 1 gram of water 1 degree Celsius

cancer a set of diseases in which abnormal body cells multiply and spread in uncontrolled fashion forming a tissue mass called a tumor

carcinogen a cancer-causing agent such as tobacco, ultraviolet radiation, or environmental toxin

carcinoma cancer of the epithelial cells that line the outer and inner surfaces of the body; includes breast, prostate, lung, and skin cancer

cardiovascular disease (CVD) disorders of the heart and blood vessel system, including stroke and coronary heart disease (CHD)

cardiovascular reactivity (CVR) an individual's characteristic reaction to stress, including changes in heart rate, blood pressure, and hormones

carotenoids light-absorbing pigments that give carrots, tomatoes, and other foods their color and are rich sources of antioxidant vitamins

carrier in genetics, a person who carries both a normal and a mutant version of a gene; a carrier may pass on a mutation that may lead to a disease in his or her offspring, even though the disease is not present in the carrier

case study a descriptive study in which one person is studied in depth in the hope of revealing general principles

catabolism the destructive form of metabolism in which living tissue is broken down for energy

cellular theory formulated in the nineteenth century, the theory that disease is the result of abnormalities in body cells

central nervous system the brain and spinal cord

cerebellum located at the rear of the brain, this brain structure coordinates voluntary movement and balance

cerebral cortex the thin layer of cells that covers the cerebrum; the seat of conscious sensation and information processing

chronic fatigue syndrome (CFS) a puzzling disorder of uncertain causes in which a person experiences headaches, infections of unknown origins, extreme tiredness, and difficulties with concentration and memory

chronic pain dull, burning pain that is long lasting

cilia the tiny hairs that line the air passageways in the nose, mouth, and trachea; moving in wavelike fashion, the cilia trap germs and force them out of the respiratory system

clinical pain pain that requires some form of medical treatment

cognitive-behavioral therapy (CBT) a multidisciplinary pain-management program that combines cognitive, physical, and emotional interventions

cognitive dissonance the psychological tension we experience when our behavior conflicts with our beliefs or attitudes regarding that behavior

cognitive reappraisal the process by which potentially stressful events are constantly reevaluated

cognitive therapy the category of treatments that teach people healthier ways of thinking

cohort differences differences between comparison groups due to the impact of members having been born and raised at different moments in history

collaborative care a cooperative form of health care in which physicians, psychologists, and other health care providers join forces to improve patient care

combative coping a reactive problem-focused coping strategy in which a person reacts to, or attempts to escape from, a stressor that cannot be avoided

comorbidity the simultaneous occurrence of two or more physical and/or psychological disorders or symptoms

complementary and alternative medicine (CAM) the use and practice of therapies or diagnostic techniques that fall outside of conventional biomedicine

compliance a patient's willingness to follow a prescribed regimen of treatment and success in actually doing so

compression of morbidity efforts to limit the time an older person spends ill or disabled

concordance rate the rate of agreement between a pair of twins for a given trait; a pair of twins is concordant for the trait if both of them have it or if neither has it

coping the cognitive, behavioral, and emotional ways in which people manage stressful situations

coronary angiography a diagnostic test for coronary heart disease in which dye is injected so that x-rays can reveal any obstructions in the coronary arteries

coronary angioplasty cardiac surgery in which an inflatable catheter is used to open a blocked coronary artery

coronary artery bypass graft (CABG) cardiac surgery in which a small piece of a healthy vein from elsewhere in the body is grafted around a blocked coronary artery, allowing blood to flow more freely to a portion of the heart

coronary heart disease (CHD) a chronic disease in which the arteries that supply the heart become narrowed or clogged; results from either atherosclerosis or arteriosclerosis

correlation coefficient a statistical measure of the strength and direction of the relationship between two variables, and thus of how well one predicts the other

corticosteroids hormones produced by the adrenal cortex that fight inflammation, promote healing, and trigger the release of stored energy

counterirritation analgesia in which one pain (for example, a pulled muscle) is relieved by creating another, counteracting stimulus (such as rubbing the site of the injury)

cross-linking a tangling of brain neurons due to the stiffening of cell proteins and connective tissue; believed to be implicated in all aspects of aging

cross-linking theory a damage theory that attributes aging to the stiffening of body tissues that appears to be caused by cross-links of cellular proteins that bind together

cross-sectional study a study comparing representative groups of people of various ages on a particular dependent variable

cross-sequential study a life-span research design that combines longitudinal and cross-sectional methods by studying groups of people of different ages over time

crystallized intelligence a person's accumulation of facts, information, and learning and memory strategies that comes with experience and education; tends to increase with age

delay behavior the tendency to avoid seeking medical care because symptoms go unnoticed *(appraisal delay)*, sickness seems unlikely *(illness delay)*, professional help is deemed unnecessary *(behavioral delay)*, the individual procrastinates in making an appointment *(scheduling delay)*, or the perceived benefits of treatment do not outweigh the perceived costs *(treatment delay)*

delirium tremens (DTs) a neurological state induced by excessive and prolonged use of alcohol and characterized by sweating, trembling, anxiety, and hallucinations; a symptom of alcohol withdrawal

dementia a pathological loss of intellectual functioning with age; the symptoms include memory loss, rambling conversation, confusion about place and time, and changes in personality

dependent variable the behavior or mental process in an experiment that may change in response to manipulations of the independent variable

descriptive study research method in which researchers observe and record participants' behaviors, often forming hypotheses that are later tested more systematically; includes case studies, interviews and surveys, and observational studies

detection behaviors behaviors designed to identify symptoms of sickness, such as health screening

diabetes mellitus a disorder of the endocrine system in which the body is unable to produce insulin (Type I) or is unable to properly utilize this pancreatic hormone (Type II)

diathesis-stress model the model that proposes that two interacting factors determine an individual's susceptibility to stress and illness: predisposing factors in the person (such as genetic vulnerability) and precipitating factors from the environment (such as traumatic experiences)

direct effect hypothesis theory that social support produces its beneficial effects during both stressful and nonstressful times by enhancing the body's physical responses to challenging situations

disability-adjusted life expectancy (DALE) the number of years of life that a person can expect to spend free from disease or disability

disability-adjusted life years (DALYs) a measure of a population's health that indicates how many years of full vitality are lost to a particular disease or disability

disinhibition overeating triggered by an event, emotion, or behavior that causes a restrained eater to abandon his or her restraint

dissociation a division in consciousness that presumably allows some thoughts and behaviors to occur simultaneously with others

dizygotic (DZ) twins fraternal twins who develop from separate fertilized eggs

double-blind study a technique designed to prevent observer- and participant-expectancy effects in which neither the researcher nor the subjects know the true purpose of the study or which subject is in which condition

drug abuse the use of a drug to the extent that it impairs the user's biological, psychological, or social well-being

drug addiction a pattern of behavior characterized by physical as well as possible psychological dependence on a drug as well as the development of tolerance

drug potentiation the effect of one drug to increase the effects of another

drug tolerance a state of progressively decreasing responsiveness to a frequently used drug

drug use the ingestion of a drug, regardless of the amount or effect of ingestion

electrocardiogram (ECG or EKG) a measure of the electrical discharges that emanate from the heart

emotion-focused coping coping strategy in which the person tries to control his or her emotional response to a stressor

enkephalins endogenous opioids found in nerve endings of cells in the brain and spinal cord that bind to opioid receptors

epidemic literally, *among the people;* an epidemic disease that spreads rapidly among many individuals in a community at the same time. A *pandemic* disease affects people over a large geographical area

epidemiology the scientific study of the frequency, distribution, and causes of a particular disease or other health outcome in a population

etiology the scientific study of the causes or origins of specific diseases

explanatory style a person's general propensity to attribute outcomes always to positive causes or always to negative causes, such as personality, luck, or another person's actions

ex post facto design a study in which the comparison groups differ on the variable of interest at the outset of the study

exposure-response prevention a behavioral treatment of bulimia nervosa that attempts to prevent purging (and therefore, reinforcement) following binge eating

fast nerve fibers large, myelinated nerve fibers that transmit sharp, stinging pain

female pattern obesity the "pear-shaped" body of women who carry excess weight on their thighs and hips

fetal alcohol syndrome (FAS) a cluster of birth defects that include facial abnormalities, low intelligence, and retarded body growth caused by the mother's use of alcohol during pregnancy

fluid intelligence a person's basic ability to think quickly and efficiently and to reason abstractly; tends to decrease during later adulthood

free nerve endings sensory receptors found throughout the body that respond to temperature, pressure, and painful stimuli

free radical theory a damage theory that attributes aging to damage caused to body cells by the gradual accumulation of unstable molecules called free radicals

gain-framed message a health message that focuses on attaining positive outcomes, or avoiding undesirable ones, by adopting a health-promoting behavior

galvanic skin response (GSR) a measure of the skin's resistance to electricity. Experiencing stress, a person may begin to perspire, causing a measurable increase in the electrical conductivity of the skin

gastrointestinal system the body's system for digesting food; includes the digestive tract, salivary glands, pancreas, liver, and gallbladder

gastroplasty a radical treatment for obesity in which a portion of the stomach is removed or stapled shut

gate control theory the idea that there is a neural "gate" in the spinal cord that regulates the experience of pain

gateway drug a drug that serves as a stepping-stone to the use of other, usually more dangerous, drugs

gender perspective theoretical perspective that focuses on gender-specific health problems and gender barriers to health care

general adaptation syndrome (GAS) Selye's term for the body's reaction to stress, which consists of three stages: alarm, resistance, and exhaustion

genetic linkage a statistical measure of the proximity of two or more genes on a chromosome; the stronger (closer together) the linkage between the genes, the greater the probability that they will be inherited together

genome all of the DNA information for an organism; the human genome consists of approximately 3 billion DNA sequences

genotype the sum total of all the genes present in an individual

geriatric health psychology the branch of health psychology devoted to the special needs of older adults

germ theory the theory that disease is caused by viruses, bacteria, and other microorganisms that invade body cells

gerontology the scientific study of old age

gradient of reinforcement the principle that immediate rewards and punishments are much more effective than delayed ones

guided imagery the use of one or more external devices to assist in relaxation and the formation of clear, strong, positive images

hardiness a cluster of stress-buffering traits consisting of commitment, challenges, and control

Hawthorne effect the phenomenon in which patients improve on their own simply because they think someone is doing something for them

Hayflick limit the number of times a human cell is capable of reproducing itself before it dies. Estimated to be approximately 50 divisions for most cells, this limit is believed by some experts to be the basis of the "genetic clock" that determines life span

health a state of complete physical, mental, and social well-being

health belief model (HBM) non-stage theory that identifies three beliefs that influence decision making regarding health behavior: perceived susceptibility to a health threat, perceived severity of the disease or condition, and perceived benefits of and barriers to the behavior

health education any planned intervention involving communication that promotes the learning of healthier behavior

health psychology the application of psychological principles and research to the enhancement of health, and the prevention and treatment of illness

hemophilia a genetic disease in which the blood fails to clot quickly enough, causing uncontrollable bleeding from even the smallest cut

heritability the amount of variation in a trait among individuals that can be attributed to genes

hippocampus a structure in the brain's limbic system linked to memory

HIV (human immunodeficiency virus) the retrovirus that causes AIDS; it injects its genome into lymphocytes, so that it reproduces when the cells are activated

holistic medicine an approach to medicine that considers not only physical health but also the emotional, spiritual, social, and psychological well-being of the person

homeostasis the tendency to maintain a balanced or constant internal state; the regulation of any aspect of body chemistry, such as the level of glucose in the blood, around a particular set point

hormones chemical messengers, released into the bloodstream by endocrine glands, that have an effect on distant organs

humoral theory a concept of health proposed by Hippocrates that considered wellness a state of perfect equilibrium among four basic body fluids, called humors. Sickness was believed to be the result of disturbances in the balance of humors

Hutchinson-Gilford progeria a rare genetic disease that causes young children to age at an extremely rapid rate and to die, usually by age 12

hydrostatic weighing a method of determining the percentage of body fat by comparing a person's weight underwater with his or her dry weight

hyperalgesia a condition in which a chronic pain sufferer becomes more sensitive to pain over time

hypercholesterolemia a genetic disease in which people have a chronically elevated level of cholesterol in their bloodstream

hypertension a sustained elevation of diastolic and systolic blood pressure (exceeding 140/90)

hypnosis a social interaction in which one person (the hypnotist) suggests to another that certain thoughts, feelings, perceptions, or behaviors will occur

hypochondriasis the condition of experiencing abnormal anxiety over one's health, often including imaginary symptoms

hypothalamic-pituitary-adrenocortical (HPAC) system the body's delayed response to stress, involving the secretion of corticosteroid hormones from the adrenal cortex

hypothalamus lying just below the thalamus, the region of the brain that influences hunger, thirst, body temperature, and sexual behavior; helps govern the endocrine system via the pituitary gland

hysterical epidemic the widespread attributing of bodily symptoms of stress to a particular disease that has become culturally fashionable

illness behavior people's responses to physical symptoms, including their recognition and interpretation of the symptoms

illness intrusiveness the extent to which a chronic illness disrupts an individual's life by interfering with valued activities and interests and reducing perceptions of personal control, self-efficacy, and self-esteem

illness representation how a person views a particular illness, including its label and symptoms, perceived causes, timeline, consequences, and controllability

immune surveillance theory the theory that cells of the immune system play a monitoring function in searching for and destroying abnormal cells such as those that form tumors

immunocompetence the overall ability of the immune system, at any given time, to defend the body against the harmful effects of foreign agents

immunotherapy chemotherapy in which medications are used to support or enhance the immune system's ability to selectively target cancer cells

incidence the number of new cases of a disease or condition that occur in a specific population within a defined time interval

independent variable the factor in an experiment that an experimenter manipulates; the variable whose effect is being studied

interiority an increased tendency toward introspection, reflection, and putting life into perspective that often accompanies aging

invincibility fable the irrational belief, common in adolescents, that one is immune to the dangers of engaging in risky behaviors

Kaposi's sarcoma a rare cancer of blood vessels serving the skin, mucous membranes, and other glands in the body

kilocalorie a measure of food energy equal to 1,000 calories

Korsakoff's syndrome an alcohol-induced neurological disorder characterized by the inability to store new memories

kwashiorkor a childhood disease resulting from protein-calorie deficiency

Lamaze training natural childbirth preparation designed to prepare prospective parents by enhancing their informational, cognitive, and behavioral control over the procedure

lay referral system an informal network of family members, friends, and other nonprofessionals who offer their own impressions, experiences, and recommendations regarding a set of bodily symptoms

learned helplessness the passive, hopeless resignation of a person or animal in the face of persistent uncontrollable stress

leptin the weight-signaling hormone monitored by the hypothalamus as an index of body fat

leukemia cancer of the blood and blood-producing system

life-course perspective theoretical perspective that focuses on age-related aspects of health and illness

life span the oldest age that members of a particular species live under ideal circumstances. In humans, this age is estimated to be between 110 and 113 years

limbic system a network of neurons surrounding the central core of the brain; associated with emotions such as fear and aggression; includes the hypothalamus, amygdala, and hippocampus

liposuction a radical form of cosmetic surgery in which fat tissue is suctioned from the body

longitudinal study a study in which a single group of people is observed over a long span of time

loss-framed message a health message that focuses on a negative outcome from failing to perform a health-promoting behavior

lymphocytes white blood cells produced in the bone marrow that fight antigens

lymphoma cancer of the body's lymph system; includes Hodgkin's disease and non-Hodgkin's lymphoma

male pattern obesity the "apple-shaped" body of men who carry excess weight around their upper body and abdomens

malingering making believe one is ill in order to benefit from sick role behavior

managed care health care that seeks to control costs by eliminating waste and unnecessary procedures and by providing economically sound treatment guidelines to hospitals and physicians

marasmus a growth-inhibiting disease of infancy caused by severe protein-calorie malnutrition

medulla the brainstem region that controls heartbeat and breathing

melanoma a potentially deadly form of cancer that strikes the melatonin-containing cells of the skin

meta-analysis a quantitative technique that combines the results of many studies examining the same effect or phenomenon

metastasis the process by which malignant body cells proliferate in number and spread to surrounding body tissues

mind–body dualism the philosophical viewpoint that mind and body are separate entities that do not interact

modeling learning by observing (and imitating) a role model

monozygotic (MZ) twins genetically identical twins who develop from a single fertilized egg that splits in two

morbidity disease; as a measure of health, the number of cases of a specific illness, injury, or disability in a given group of people at a given time

mortality death; as a measure of health, the number of deaths due to a specific cause in a given group of people at a given time

motor cortex lying at the rear of the frontal lobes, the region of the cerebral cortex that controls voluntary movements

mutagen a substance such as a carcinogen that causes mutations in a cell's genetic code

myocardial infarction (MI) a heart attack; the permanent death of heart tissue in response to an interruption of blood supply to the myocardium

naloxone an opioid antagonist that binds to opioid receptors in the body to block the effects of natural opiates and painkillers

naturopathic medicine the system that aims to provide holistic health care by drawing from several traditional healing systems, including homeopathy, herbal remedies, and traditional Oriental medicine

negative emotionality a state of alcohol abuse characterized by depression and anxiety

neuron a nerve cell, including the cell body, dendrites, and axon (which is sometimes insulated by a myelin sheath).

There are three types: sensory neurons, interneurons, and motor neurons

neurotransmitters chemical messengers released by a neuron at synapses that diffuse across the synaptic cleft and alter the electrical state of a receiving neuron

nicotine-titration model the theory that smokers who are physically dependent on nicotine regulate their smoking to maintain a steady level of the drug in their bodies

nociceptor (no-chi-SEP-tur) a specialized neuron that responds to painful stimuli

nonsteroidal anti-inflammatory drugs (NSAIDs) aspirin, ibuprofen, acetaminophen, and other analgesic drugs that relieve pain and reduce inflammation at the site of injured tissue

ob gene a gene that controls several physiological systems involved in obesity. Animals with a defective ob gene become hugely obese

obesity excessive accumulation of body fat

observational study a nonexperimental research method in which a researcher observes and records the behavior of a research participant

observer-expectancy effect the outcome of an investigation is influenced by the researcher's expectations

oncogenes genes that stimulate cellular growth and division

optimistic bias the tendency of some people to believe that they are less likely to become ill than other adults of their own age and gender

optimum level of arousal hypothesis the idea that there is an optimal level of arousal, or behavioral activation, at which behavior and mental processes are most efficient

overweight body weight that exceeds the desirable weight for a person of a given height, age, and body shape

palliative care health care that focuses on easing pain and providing comfort, especially at the end of life

pandemic a worldwide epidemic such as AIDS

participant-expectancy effect the behavior of study participants is affected by their expectations, which influences the outcome of the study

pathogen a virus, bacterium, or some other microorganism that causes a particular disease

periacqueductal gray (PAG) a region of the midbrain that plays an important role in the perception of pain; electrical stimulation in this region activates a descending neural pathway that produces analgesia by "closing the pain gate"

peripheral nervous system all the neurons outside the central nervous system; consists of both the somatic nervous system and the autonomic nervous system, which includes the sympathetic and parasympathetic nervous systems

personal control the belief that we make our own decisions and determine what we do or what others do to us

phantom limb pain following amputation of a limb, false pain sensations that appear to originate in the missing limb

phenotype a person's observable characteristics; determined by the interaction of the individual's genotype with the environment

physical dependence a state in which the use of a drug is required for a person to function normally

pituitary gland the master endocrine gland controlled by the hypothalamus; releases a variety of hormones that act on other glands throughout the body

placebo effect the power of a person's belief in the efficacy of a treatment to actually influence the treatment's effectiveness

polygraph often called a *lie detector,* a machine that measures several of the physiological responses that accompany stress and other emotional states

polypharmacy the dangerous practice of taking several medications simultaneously

population density a measure of crowding based on the total number of people living in an area of limited size

post-traumatic stress disorder (PTSD) a psychological disorder triggered by exposure to an extreme traumatic stressor, such as combat or a natural disaster. Symptoms of PTSD include haunting memories and nightmares of the traumatic event, extreme mental distress, and unwanted flashbacks

precaution adoption process model (PAPM) a stage model theory based on the assumption that people pass through seven discrete stages on their way to adopting precautionary health behaviors

presbycusis literally "old hearing," a term that refers to the age-related loss in sensitivity to sounds—especially those in the high-frequency range

prevalence the total number of diagnosed cases of a disease or condition that exist at a given time

prevention behaviors behaviors designed to stave off sickness, such as wearing sun block

primary aging the inevitable and universal physical changes that accompany aging

primary appraisal a person's initial determination of an event's meaning, whether irrelevant, benign-positive, or threatening

primary prevention health-enhancing efforts to prevent disease or injury from occurring

proactive coping a type of problem-focused coping in which people attempt to anticipate or detect potential stressors and act in advance to prevent them or to mute their impact

problem-focused coping coping strategy for dealing directly with a stressor, in which the person either reduces the stressor's demands or increases his or her resources for meeting its demands

progressive muscle relaxation a form of relaxation training that reduces muscle tension through a series of tensing and relaxing exercises involving the body's major muscle groups

prospective study a longitudinal study that begins with a healthy group of subjects and follows the development of a particular disease in that sample

prostaglandin the chemical substance responsible for localized pain and inflammation; prostaglandin also causes free nerve endings to become more and more sensitized as time passes

prototype/willingness theory (P/W) a decision-making theory that assumes that health behavior is a function of a person's motivation to engage in that behavior (behavioral willingness) and the social image associated with that behavior (social prototype)

psychneuroimmunology (PNI) the field of research that emphasizes the interaction of psychological, neural, and immunological processes in stress and illness

psychoactive drugs drugs that affect mood, behavior, and thought processes by altering the functioning of neurons in the brain; they include stimulants, depressants, and hallucinogens

psychological dependence an emotional and cognitive compulsion to use a drug

psychosomatic medicine an outdated branch of medicine that focused on the diagnosis and treatment of physical diseases caused by faulty psychological processes

quality-adjusted life years (QALYs) a measure of aging that focuses on biological age rather than chronological age

random assignment assigning research participants to groups by chance, thus minimizing preexisting differences among the groups

randomized clinical trial a true experiment testing the effects of one independent variable on individuals (single-subject design) or on groups of individuals (community field trials).

rational-emotive therapy (RET) a confrontational form of cognitive therapy, developed by Albert Ellis, which challenges people's irrational ideas and attitudes

reactance the tendency of some patients to respond to the depersonalization and helplessness of hospitalization with anger and efforts to assert themselves

referred pain pain manifested in an area of the body that is sensitive to pain but caused by disease or injury in an area of the body that has few pain receptors

regulatory control the various ways in which people modulate their thinking, emotions, and behavior over time and across changing circumstances

relative risk a statistical indicator of the likelihood of a causal relationship between a particular health risk factor and a health outcome; computed as the ratio of the incidence (or prevalence) of a health condition in a group exposed to the risk factor to its incidence (or prevalence) in a group not exposed to the risk factor

relaxation response a meditative state of relaxation in which metabolism slows and blood pressure lowers

reliability a measure of the degree to which a psychometric test yields dependably consistent results

representative sample an unbiased subset of research subjects that accurately reflects the population of individuals under investigation

repressive coping an emotion-focused coping style in which people attempt to inhibit their emotional responses, especially in social situations, so they can view themselves as imperturbable

repressors people who cope with health problems and other aversive events by ignoring or distancing themselves from stressful information

research bias the outcome of an experiment is influenced by some extraneous factor other than the independent variable

resilience the quality of some children to bounce or spring back from environmental stressors that might otherwise disrupt their development

restraint theory the theory that heightened sensitivity to norms for body weight triggers a pattern of eating that vacillates between strict dieting and binge eating

reticular formation a network of neurons running through the brainstem involved with alertness and arousal

retrospective study a "backward-looking" study in which a group of people who have a certain disease or condition are compared with a group of people who are free of the disease or condition, with the purpose of identifying background risk factors that may have contributed to the disease or condition

retrovirus a virus that copies its genetic information onto the DNA of a host cell

rumination repetitive focusing on the causes, meanings, and consequences of stressful experiences

sarcoma cancer that strikes muscles, bones, and cartilage

satiation a form of aversion therapy in which a smoker is forced to increase his or her smoking until an unpleasant state of "fullness" is reached

scatterplot a graphed cluster of data points, each of which represents the values of two variables in a descriptive study

secondary aging the specific diseases or health conditions that tend to be more common among older adults, but that are caused by lifestyle choices, genetic vulnerability, and other factors rather than aging itself

secondary appraisal a person's determination of whether his or her own resources and abilities are sufficient to meet the demands of an event that is appraised as potentially threatening or challenging

secondary gains the "rewards" associated with sick role behavior, including increased attention, the ability to rest, freedom from responsibility, and so forth

secondary prevention actions taken to identify and treat an illness or disability early in its course

selective optimization with compensation (SOC) the theory that healthy aging involves assessing abilities realistically, choosing meaningful goals, and devising effective strategies to accomplish them, despite the limits associated with aging

senescence a general term for all age-related declines in physical and psychological functions

sensitizers people who cope with health problems and other aversive events by closely scanning their bodies and environments for information

sensory cortex lying at the front of the parietal lobes, the region of the cerebral cortex that processes body sensations such as touch

seropositive the state of testing HIV-positive, indicating infection by the AIDS virus

set-point hypothesis the theory that each person's body weight is genetically set within a given range, or set point, that the body works hard to maintain

sexually transmitted diseases (STDs) diseases such as gonorrhea, syphilis, chlamydia, genital herpes, and AIDS that are communicated through sexual contact

sick role behavior people's responses to being diagnosed with a particular disease or health condition

slow nerve fibers small, unmyelinated nerve fibers that carry dull, aching pain

social influence theory the idea that hypnosis is a social phenomenon in which a highly suggestible person merely acts out a role

social prototype the predominant social image an individual associates with a particular group of people

social support companionship from others that conveys emotional concern, material assistance, or honest feedback about a situation

sociocultural perspective theoretical perspective that focuses on how social and cultural factors contribute to health and disease

somatization the translation of emotional distress into physical symptoms when there is no apparent biological cause for these symptoms

stamina the quality of some elderly adults to remain positive and upbeat in the face of adversity

standardization the process of establishing group norms on a psychometric test that serve as a source of comparison for evaluating an individual's performance

strain the physical and emotional wear and tear reaction of a person attempting to cope with a stressor

stratified sample a representative sample in which particular subgroups (or "strata") within a population are equally represented

stress the process by which we perceive and respond to events, called stressors, that are perceived as harmful, threatening, or challenging

stress-induced analgesia (SIA) a stress-related increase in tolerance to pain, presumably mediated by the body's endorphin system

stress inoculation training a form of cognitive therapy that helps people to confront stressful events with a variety of coping strategies that can be used before the event becomes overwhelming

stress management the various psychological methods designed to reduce the impact of potentially stressful experiences

stressor any event or situation that triggers coping adjustments

stroke a cerebrovascular accident that results in damage to the brain due to lack of oxygen; usually caused by atherosclerosis or arteriosclerosis

subjective norm an individual's interpretation of the views of other people regarding a particular health-related behavior

substance P a neurotransmitter secreted by pain fibers in the spinal cord that stimulates the transmission cells to send pain signals to the brain

substantia gelatinosa the dorsal region of the spinal cord where both fast and slow pain fibers synapse with sensory nerves on their way to the brain

suppressor genes genes that prevent the proliferation of malignant cells by acting as a brake on cellular growth and division

survey a questionnaire used to ascertain the self-reported attitudes or behaviors of a group of people

sympathoadreno-medullary (SAM) system the body's initial, rapid-acting response to stress, involving the release of epinephrine and norepinephrine from the adrenal medulla under the direction of the sympathetic nervous system

synapse the junction between one neuron's axon and the dendrites of an adjoining neuron, across which a nerve impulse may be transmitted

systematic desensitization a form of behavior therapy, commonly used for overcoming phobias, in which the person is exposed to a series of increasingly fearful situations while remaining deeply relaxed

systems theory the viewpoint that nature is best understood as a hierarchy of systems, in which each system is simultaneously composed of smaller subsystems and larger, interrelated systems

tai chi a form of "moving meditation" that blends exercise, dance, and concentration and is a component of traditional Oriental medicine

telomere the end structure of DNA, which is gradually depleted each time the cell divides, until the cell can divide no more and dies; its shortening is believed to be the mechanism that underlies the Hayflick limit

tension-reduction hypothesis an explanation of drinking behavior that proposes that alcohol is reinforcing because it reduces stress and tension

teratogens drugs, chemicals, and environmental agents that can damage the developing person during fetal development

tertiary prevention actions taken to contain damage once a disease or disability has progressed beyond its early stages

thalamus the brain's sensory switchboard. Located on top of the brainstem, it routes messages to the cerebral cortex

theory of planned behavior (TPB) a theory that predicts health behavior on the basis of three factors: personal attitude toward the behavior, the subjective norm regarding the behavior, and perceived degree of control over the behavior

theory of reasoned action (TRA) the theory that decision making regarding healthy behavior is shaped by a person's attitude toward the behavior and his or her motivation to comply with the views of others regarding the behavior in question

threshold the minimum change in electrical activity required to trigger an action potential in a neuron

token economy an operant conditioning procedure in which desired behavior is rewarded with tokens that can be exchanged for various types of reward

traditional Oriental medicine an ancient, integrated herb- and acupuncture-based system of healing founded on the principle that internal harmony is essential for good health

transactional model Lazarus' theory that the experience of stress depends as much on the individual's cognitive appraisal of a potential stressor's impact as it does on the event or situation itself

transcutaneous electrical nerve stimulation (TENS) a counterirritation form of analgesia involving electrically stimulating spinal nerves near a painful area

transtheoretical model (TTM) a widely used stage theory that contends that people pass through five stages in altering health-related behavior: precontemplation, contemplation, preparation, action, and maintenance

Type A Friedman and Rosenman's term for competitive, hurried, hostile people who may be at increased risk for developing cardiovascular disease

Type B Friedman and Rosenman's term for more relaxed people who are not pressured by time considerations and thus tend to be coronary-disease resistant

Type C (cancer-prone) personality a passive, uncomplaining person who tends to repress emotions and may be prone to developing cancer

validity a measure of the degree to which a test actually measures what it is supposed to measure (content validity), predicts a future behavior or condition (predictive validity), or measures a particular construct that cannot be directly observed (construct validity)

veins blood vessels that carry blood back to the heart from the capillaries

vitalism the concept of a general life force, popular in some varieties of complementary and alternative medicine

wear-and-tear theory a discredited theory of aging that states that the human body wears out with the passage of time

weight cycling repeated weight gains and losses through repeated dieting

well year a year of life that is free of any serious health-related problem

withdrawal the unpleasant physical and psychological symptoms that occur when a person abruptly ceases using certain drugs

X chromosome the sex chromosome found in males and females. Females have two X chromosomes; males have one

Y chromosome the sex chromosome found only in males; contains a gene that triggers the testes to begin producing testosterone

yoga a movement-based form of relaxation and meditation that combines diet, physical postures, and breathing to promote physical and spiritual well-being

zidovudine (AZT) the first anti-AIDS drug

zygote a fertilized egg cell

References

Abbey, A., McAuslan, P., & Ross, L. T. (1998). Sexual assault perpetration by college men: The role of alcohol, misperception of sexual intent, and sexual beliefs and experiences. *Journal of Social and Clinical Psychology, 17,* 167–195.

Abbey, A., Zawacki, T., & McAuslan, P. (2000). Alcohol's effects on sexual perception. *Journal of Studies on Alcohol, 61,* 688–697.

Abenhaim, L., Moride, Y., Brenot, F., Rich, S., Benichou, J., Kurz, X., Higenbottam, T., Oakley, C., Wouters, E., Aubier, M., Simonneau, G., & Begaud, B. (1996). Appetite-suppressant drugs and the risk of primary pulmonary hypertension. *New England Journal of Medicine, 335,* 609–616.

Ablashi, D. V., Eastman, H. B., Owen, C. B., Roman, M. M., Friedman, J., Zabriskie, J. B., Peterson, D. L., Pearson, G. R., & Whitman, J. E. (2000). Frequent HHV-6 reactivation in multiple sclerosis (MS) and chronic fatigue syndrome (CFS) patients. *Journal of Clinical Virology, 16,* 179–191.

Abood, D. A., & Chandler, S. B. (1997). Race and the role of weight, weight change, and body dissatisfaction in eating disorders. *American Journal of Health Behavior, 21,* 21–25.

Abraham, C., & Sheeran, P. (1994). Modeling and modifying young heterosexuals' HIV-preventive behaviour: A review of theories, findings and educational implications. *Patient Education and Counseling, 23,* 173–186.

Abraham, C., Sheeran, P., Spears, R., & Abrams, D. (1992). Health beliefs and promotion of HIV-preventive intentions among teenagers: A Scottish perspective. *Health Psychology, 11,* 363–370.

Abraido-Lanza, A. F., Dohrenwend, B. P., Ng-Mak, D. S., & Turner, J.B. (1999). The Latino mortality paradox: A test of the "salmon bias" and healthy migrant hypotheses. *American Journal of Public Health, 89,* 1543–1548.

Abrams, D. B., & Wilson, G. T. (1983). Alcohol, sexual arousal, and self-control. *Journal of Personality and Social Psychology, 45,* 188–198.

Ackerman, B. P., Kogos, J., Youngstrom, E., Schoff, K., & Izard, C. (1999). Family instability and the problem behaviors of children from economically disadvantaged families. *Developmental Psychology, 35,* 258–268.

Adams, P., & Mylander, M. (1998). *Gesundheit! Bringing good health to you, the medical system, and society through physician service, contemporary therapies, humor, and joy.* Rochester, NY: Inner Traditions International.

Ader, R., & Cohen, N. (1985). CNS-immune system interactions: Conditioning phenomena. *Behavioral and Brain Sciences, 8,* 379–394.

Ader, R., Felten, D. L., & Cohen, N. (2001). *Psychoneuroimmunology. Part IV: Behavioral effects on immunity* (3rd ed.). San Diego: Academic Press.

Adler, N. E., Boyce, W. T., Chesney, M. A., Folkman, S., & Syme, S. L. (1993). Socioeconomic inequalities in health: No easy solution. *Journal of the American Medical Association, 269,* 3140–3145.

Adler, N., & Matthews, K. (1994). Health psychology: Why do some people get sick and some stay well? *Annual Review of Psychology, 45,* 229–259.

Affleck, G., Tennen, H., Pfeiffer, C., & Fifield, J. (1987). Appraisals of control and predictability in adapting to a chronic disease. *Journal of Personality and Social Psychology, 53,* 273–279.

Agars, J., & McMurray, A. (1993). An evaluation of comparative strategies for teaching breast self-examination. *Journal of Advanced Nursing, 18,* 1595–1603.

Agras, W. S. (1993). Short-term psychological treatments for binge eating. In C. G. Fairburn & G. T. Wilson (Eds.), *Binge eating: Nature, assessment, and treatment* (pp. 270–286). New York: Guilford.

AHA. (2001). *Fast facts on U.S. hospitals.* American Hospital Association (www.aha.org).

Ajzen, I. (1991). The theory of planned behavior. *Organizational Behavior and Human Decision Processes, 50,* 179–211.

Ajzen, I., & Fishbein, M. (1980). *Understanding attitudes and predicting social behavior.* Englewood Cliffs, NJ: Prentice Hall.

Akiyama, H., Elliott, K., & Antonucci, T. C. (1996). Same-sex and cross-sex relationships. *Journal of Gerontology,* Series B: *Psychological Sciences and Social Sciences, 51B,* 374–382.

Albarracin, D., McNatt, P. S., Williams, W. R., Howworth, T., Zenilman, J., Ho, R. M., Rhodes, F., Malotte, C. K., Bolan, G. A., & Iatesta, M. (2000). Structure of outcome beliefs in condom use. *Health Psychology, 19,* 458–468.

Alexander, C. N., Langer, E. J., Newman, R. I., Chandler, H. M., & Davies, J. L. (1989). Transcendental meditation, mindfulness, and longevity: An experimental study with the elderly. *Journal of Personality and Social Psychology, 57,* 950–964.

Alexander, E. (1950). *Psychosomatic medicine.* New York: Norton.

Alexander, F. (1939). Psychological aspects of medicine. *Psychosomatic Medicine, 1,* 7–18.

Allen, J. R., & Setlow, V. P. (1991). Heterosexual transmission of HIV: A view of the future. *Journal of the American Medical Association, 266,* 1695–1696.

Altman, D. G. (1995). Sustaining interventions in community systems: On the relationship between researchers and communities. *Health Psychology, 14,* 526–536.

Altshuler, J. L., & Ruble, D. N. (1989). Developmental changes in children's awareness of strategies for coping with uncontrollable stress. *Child Development, 60,* 1337–1349.

Alzheimer's Association. (2000). Alzheimer's disease fact sheet. http://alzheimersdc-md.org/alzfacts.html.

Amanzio, M., & Benedetti, F. (1999). Neuropharmacological dissection of placebo analgesia: Expectation-activated opioid systems versus conditioning-activated specific subsystems. *Journal of Neuroscience, 19*, 484–494.

American Cancer Society (ACS). (2001). *Cancer facts and figures—2001.* Atlanta: American Cancer Society.

American Chiropractic Association. (1999). *American Chiropractic Association online: Insurance and managed care information* (http://www.americhiro.org/).

American Diabetes Association (ADA). (1997). National standards for diabetes self-management education programs and American Diabetes Association review criteria. *Diabetes Care, 20,* S67–S70.

American Diabetes Association (ADA). (2000). Diabetes facts and figures. www.diabetes.org/ada/facts.asp.

American Heart Association (AHA). (1999). *Heart and stroke facts.* www.americanheart.org.

American Medical Association (AMA) (1973). *Proceedings of the House of Delegates.* New York.

American Medical Association (AMA) (1995). *Proceedings of the House of Delegates.* Chicago.

American Psychiatric Association (APA). (1994). *Diagnostic and statistic manual of mental disorders* (3rd ed.). Washington, DC: Author.

American Psychiatric Association (APA). (1997). *Diagnostic and statistical manual of mental disorders* (4th ed.). Washington, DC: Author.

American Society of Health-System Pharmacists (2001, January 31). *USA Today,* p. 1B.

Amigo, I., Buceta, J. M., Becona, E., & Bueno, A. M. (1991). Cognitive behavioral treatment for essential hypertension: A controlled study. *Stress Medicine, 7,* 103–108.

Amundsen, D. W. (1996). *Medicine, society, and faith in the ancient and medieval worlds.* Baltimore: Johns Hopkins University Press.

Anastasi, A. (1997). *Psychological testing* (7th ed.). New York: Prentice Hall.

Anda, R., Williamson, D., Jones, D., Macera, C., Eaker, E., Glassman, A., & Marks, J. (1993). Depressed affect, hopelessness, and the risk of ischemic heart disease in a cohort of U.S. adults. *Epidemiology, 4,* 285–294.

Andersen, B., Ho, J., Brackett, J., Finkelstein, D., & Laffel, L. (1997). Parental involvement in diabetes management tasks: Relationships to blood glucose monitoring adherence and metabolic control in young adolescents with insulin-dependent diabetes mellitus. *Journal of Pediatrics, 130,* 257–265.

Andersen, B. L., Cacioppo, J. T., & Roberts, D. C. (1995). Delay in seeking a cancer diagnosis: Delay stages and psychophysiological comparison processes. *British Journal of Social Psychology, 34,* 33–52.

Andersen, B. L., & Golden-Kreutz, D. M. (2001). Cancer. In D. W. Johnston & M. Johnston (Eds.), *Health psychology* (pp. 217–236). Amsterdam: Elsevier.

Anderson, E. A., Balon, T. W., Hoffman, R. P., Sinkey, C. A., & Mark, A. L. (1992). Insulin increases sympathetic activity but not blood pressure in borderline hypertensive humans. *Hypertension, 6,* 621–627.

Anderson, N. B. (1995). Behavioral and sociocultural perspectives on ethnicity and health. *Health Psychology, 14*(7), 589–591.

Anderson, N. B., & Armstead, C. A. (1995). Toward understanding the association of socioeconomic status and health: A new challenge for the biopsychosocial approach. *Psychosomatic Medicine, 57,* 213–225.

Anderson, R., Meeker, W. C., & Wirick, B. E. (1992). A meta-analysis of clinical trials of spinal manipulation. *Journal of Manipulative and Physiological Therapeutics, 15,* 181–194.

Anderson, R. A., Baron, R. S., & Logan, H. (1991). Distraction, control, and dental stress. *Journal of Applied Social Psychology, 21,* 156–171.

Andrasik, F., & Attanasio, V. (1985). Biofeedback in pediatrics: Current status and appraisal. *Advances in Developmental and Behavioral Pediatrics, 6,* 241–286.

Andrasik, F., Blanchard, E. B., Arena, J. G., Teders, S. J., Teevan, R. C., & Rodichok, L. D. (1982). Psychological functioning in headache sufferers. *Psychosomatic Medicine, 44,* 171–182.

Anton, R. F., & Kranzler, H. R. (1994). *The pharmacology of alcohol abuse.* New York: Springer-Verlag.

Antoni, M. H., Cruess, D. G., Cruess, S., Lutgendorf, S., Kumar, M., Ironson, G., Kliomas, N., Fletcher, M. A., & Schneiderman, N. (2000). Cognitive-behavioral stress management intervention effects on anxiety, 24-hour urinary norepinephrine output, and T-cytotoxic/suppressor cells over time among symptomatic HIV-infected gay men. *Journal of Consulting & Clinical Psychology, 68,* 31–45.

Antoni, M. H., & Schneiderman, N. (2001). HIV and AIDS. In D. W. Johnston & M. Johnston (Eds.), *Health psychology: Comprehensive clinical psychology* (Vol. 8, pp. 237–275). Amsterdam: Elsevier.

Antonovsky, A. (1990). Personality and health: Testing the sense of coherence model. In H.S. Friedman (Ed.), *Personality and disease* (pp. 155–177). New York: Wiley.

Antony, V. B., Godbey, S. W., Hott, J. W., & Queener, S. F. (1993). Alcohol-induced inhibition of alveolar macrophage oxidant release in vivo and in vitro. *Alcoholism, Clinical and Experimental Research, 17,* 389–393.

Ardell, D. B. (1985). *The history and future of wellness.* Dubuque, IA: Kendall/Hunt.

Argyle, M. (1992). Benefits produced by supportive social relationships. In H. Veiel & U. Baumann (Eds.), *The meaning and measurement of social support* (pp. 13–32). New York: Hemisphere Publishing Group.

Armstead, C. A., Lawler, K. A., Gorden, G., Cross, J., & Gibbons, J. (1989). Relationship of racial stressors to blood pressure responses and anger expression in black college students. *Health Psychology, 8,* 541–556.

Arnow, B., Kenardy, J., & Agraw, S. W. (1992). Binge eating among the obese: A descriptive study. *Journal of Behavioral Medicine, 15,* 155–170.

Aron, A., Norman, C. C., Aron, E. N., McKenna, C., & Heyman, R. E. (2000). Couples' shared participation in novel and arousing activities and experienced relationship quality. *Journal of Personality and Social Psychology, 78,* 273–284.

Aronoff, J., Stollak, G. E., & Woike, B. A. (1994). Affect regulation and the breadth of interpersonal engagement. *Journal of Personality and Social Psychology, 67,* 105–114.

Aspinwall, L. G., Kemeny, M. E., Taylor, S. E., Schneider, S. G., & Dudley, J. P. (1991). Psychosocial predictors of gay men's AIDS risk-reduction behavior. *Health Psychology, 10,* 432–444.

Aspinwall, L. G., & Taylor, S. E. (1997). A stitch in time: Self-regulation and proactive coping. *Psychological Bulletin, 121,* 417–436.

Astin, J. A., Harkness, E., & Ernst, E. (2000). The efficacy of "distant healing": A systematic review of randomized trials. *Annals of Internal Medicine, 132,* 903–910.

Avants, S. K., Margolin, A., Holford, T. R., & Kosten, T. R. (2000). A randomized controlled trial of auricular acupuncture for cocaine dependence. *Archives of Internal Medicine, 160,* 2305–2312.

Ayanian, J. Z., & Epstein, A. M. (1991). Differences in the use of procedures between women and men hospitalized for coronary heart disease. *The New England Journal of Medicine, 325,* 221–225.

Ayanian, J. Z., & Epstein, A. M. (1997). Attitudes about treatment of coronary heart disease among women and men presenting for exercise testing. *Journal of General Internal Medicine, 12,* 311–314.

Azar, B. (1998). Psychosocial factors provide clues to pain. *Monitor of the American Psychological Association* (www.apa.org).

Azar, B. (1999). Antismoking ads that curb teen smoking. *American Psychological Association Monitor, 30,* 14.

Azar, B. (1999, June). Probing links between stress, cancer. *American Psychological Association Monitor, 30,* 13–15.

Bachen, E. A., Cohen, S., & Marsland, A. L. (1997). Psychoimmunology. In A. Baum, S. Newman, J. Weinman, R. West, & C. McManus (Eds.), *Cambridge handbook of psychology, health and medicine* (pp. 35–39). Cambridge, UK: Cambridge University Press.

Baer, J. S., Kivlahan, D. R., Fromme, K., & Marlatt, G. A. (1994). Secondary prevention of alcohol abuse with college populations: A skills-training approach. In G. S. Howard & P. E. Nathan (Eds.). *Alcohol use and misuse by young adults* (pp. 83–108). Notre Dame, IN: University of Notre Dame Press.

Bagley, S. P., Angel, R., Dilworth-Anderson, P., Liu, W., & Schinke, S. (1995). Adaptive health behaviors among ethnic minorities. *Health Psychology, 14*(7), 632–640.

Bagozzi, R. P. (1981). Attitudes, intentions, and behavior: A test of some key hypotheses. *Journal of Personality and Social Psychology, 41,* 607–627.

Bahra, A., Matharu, M. S., Buchel, C., Frackowiak, R. S. J., & Goadsby, P. J. (2001). Brainstem activation specific to migraine headache. *The Lancet, 357,* 1016–1017.

Bahrke, M. S., & Morgan, W. P. (1978). Anxiety reduction following exercise and meditation. *Cognitive Therapy and Research, 2,* 323–333.

Baillie, R. (2001, June). Teen drinking more dangerous than previously thought. *Monitor on Psychology* (Special issue on substance abuse), *32,* 12.

Baird, A. A., Gruber, S. A., Fein, D. A., Maas, L. C., Steingard, R. J., Renshaw, P. F., Cohen, B. M., & Yurgelun-Todd, D. A. (1999). Functional magnetic resonance imaging of facial affect recognition in children and adolescents. *Journal of the American Academy of Child and Adolescent Psychiatry, 38,* 195–199.

Baker, R., & Kirschenbaum, D. S. (1998). Weight control during the holidays: Highly consistent self-monitoring as a potentially useful coping mechanism. *Health Psychology, 17,* 367–370.

Balfour, L., White, R., Schiffrin, A., Dougherty, G., & Dufresne, J. (1993). Dietary disinhibition, perceived stress, and glucose control in young, type 1 diabetic women. *Health Psychology, 12,* 33–38.

Balin, A. K. (1994). Testimony in support of biomedical aging research. *Journal of the American Aging Association, 17,* 152–161.

Ballie, S. T. (1986). Housing- and neighborhood-related stress of female heads of single-parent households. *Dissertation Abstracts International, 47,* 2401.

Balter, M. (1996). New hope in HIV disease. *Science, 274,* 1988–1989.

Baltes, M. M., & Carstensen, L. L. (1996). The process of successful aging. *Aging and Society, 16,* 397–422.

Baltes, P. B. (1999). Age and aging as incomplete architecture of human ontogenesis. *Zeitschrift für Gerontologie und Geriatrie, 32,* 433–448.

Bandura, A. (1977). Self-efficacy: Toward a unifying theory of behavioral change. *Psychological Review, 84,* 191–215.

Bandura, A. (1992). Self-efficacy mechanism in psychobiologic functioning. In R. Schwarzer (Ed.), *Self-efficacy: Thought control of action* (pp. 255–394). Washington, DC: Hemisphere Publishing Group.

Bandura, A. (1997). *Self-efficacy: The exercise of control.* New York: Freeman.

Bandura, A., Cioffi, D., Taylor, C. B., & Brouillard, M. E. (1988). Perceived self-efficacy in coping with cognitive stressors and opioid activation. *Journal of Personality and Social Psychology, 55,* 479–488.

Banks, B. A., Silverman, R. A., Schwartz, R. H., & Tunnessen, W. W. (1992). Attitudes of teenagers toward sun exposure and sunscreen use. *Pediatrics, 89,* 40–42.

Banks, S. M., Salovey, P., Greener, S., Rothman, A. J., Moyer, A., Beauvais, J., & Spel, E. (1995). The effects of message framing on mammography utilization. *Health Psychology, 14,* 178–184.

Barber, T. (1977). Rapid induction analgesia: A clinical report. *American Journal of Clinical Hypnosis, 19,* 138–147.

Barber, T. (1996). A brief introduction to hypnotic analgesia. In J. Barber (Ed.), *Hypnosis and suggestion in the treatment of pain: A clinical guide* (pp. 3–32). New York: Norton.

Barefoot, J. C., Larsen, S., von der Lieth, L., & Schroll, M. (1995). Hostility, incidence of acute myocardial infarction, and mortality in a sample of older Danish men and women. *American Journal of Epidemiology, 142,* 477–484.

Barinaga, M. (1995). New Alzheimer's gene found. *Science, 268,* 1845–1846.

Barnard, N. D., & Kaufman, S. R. (1997). Animal research is wasteful and misleading. *Scientific American, 276*(2), 80–82.

Barnier, A. J., & McConkey, K. M. (1992). Reports of real and false memories: The relevance of hypnosis, hypnotizability, and context of memory test. *Journal of Abnormal Psychology, 101,* 521–527.

Barone, C., Ickovics, J. R., Ayers, T. S., Katz, S. M., Voyce, C. M., & Weissberg, R. P. (1996). High-risk sexual behavior among young urban students. *Family Planning Perspectives, 28,* 69–74.

Barrett, D. (2001, January/February). The power of hypnosis. *Psychology Today,* 58–65.

Bartlett, J. G., & Moore, R. D. (1998). Improving HIV therapy. *Scientific American* (www.sciam.com).

Baruch, G.K., & Barnett, R.C. (1986). Consequences of fathers' participation in family work: Parents' role strain and well-being. *Journal of Personality and Social Psychology, 51,* 983–992.

Basbaum, A. I., & Fields, H. L. (1984). Endogenous pain control systems: Brainstem spinal pathways and endorphin circuitry. *Annual Review of Neuroscience, 7,* 309–338.

Bates, M. E., & Labouvie, E. W. (1995). Personality-environment constellations and alcohol use: A process-oriented study of intraindividual change during adolescence. *Psychology of Addictive Behaviors, 9,* 23–35.

Bates, M. S., Rankin-Hill, L., & Sanchez-Ayendez, M. (1997). The effects of the cultural context of health care on treatment of and response to chronic pain and illness. *Social Science and Medicine, 45,* 1433–1477.

Baum, A., Davidson, L. M., Singer, J. E., & Street, S. W. (1987). Stress as a psychophysiological process. In A. Baum & J. E. Singer (Eds.), *Handbook of psychology and health, Vol. 5. Stress* (pp. 1–24). Hillsdale, NJ: Erlbaum.

Baum, A., & Fleming, I. (1993). Implications of psychological research on stress and technological accidents. *American Psychologist, 48,* 665–672.

Baum, A., & Grunberg, N. E. (1991). Gender, stress, and health. *Health Psychology, 10,* 80–85.

Baum, A., & Posluzny, D. M. (1999). Health psychology: Mapping biobehavioral contributions to health and illness. *Annual Review of Psychology, 50,* 137–163.

Baum, A., & Spencer, S. (1997). Post-traumatic stress disorder. In A. Baum, S. Newman, J. Weinman, R. West, & C. McManus (Eds.) *Cambridge handbook of psychology, health and medicine* (pp. 550–555). Cambridge, UK: Cambridge University Press.

Baumann, L. J., Cameron, L.D., Zimmerman, R. S., & Leventhal, H. (1989). Illness representations and matching labels with symptoms. *Health Psychology, 8,* 449–469.

Baumeister, R. F. (1997). Esteem threat, self-regulatory breakdown, and emotional stress as factors in self-defeating behavior. *Review of General Psychology, 1,* 147–174.

Bausell, R. B. (1986). Health-seeking behavior among the elderly. *The Gerontologist, 26,* 556–559.

Beaglehole, R., Bonita, R., & Kjellstrom, T. (1993) *Basic epidemiology.* Geneva: World Health Organization.

Bearison, D. J., Sadow, A. J., Granowetter, L., & Winckel, G. (1993). Patients' and parents' causal attributions for childhood cancer. *Journal of Psychosocial Oncology, 11,* 47–61.

Bechara, A., Dolan, S., Denburg, N., Hindes, A., Anderson, S. W., & Nathan, P. E. (2001). Decision-making deficits, linked to a dysfunctional ventromedial prefrontal cortex, revealed in alcohol and stimulant abusers. *Neuropsychologia, 39,* 376–389.

Beck, K. H., & Frankel, A. (1981). A conceptualization of threat communications and protective health behavior. *Social Psychology Quarterly, 44,* 204–217.

Becker, M. H., Kaback, M. M., Rosenstock, I. M., & Ruth, M. V. (1975). Some influences on public participation in a genetic screening program. *Journal of Community Health, 1,* 3–14.

Beckman, H. B., & Frankel, R. M. (1984). The effect of physician behavior on the collection of data. *Annals of Internal Medicine, 101,* 692–696.

Bedimo, A. L., Bennett, M., Kissinger, P., & Clark, R. A. (1998). Understanding barriers to condom use among HIV infected African-American women. *Journal of the Association of Nursing Care, 9,* 48–58.

Begley, S. (2001, June 11). AIDS at 20. *Newsweek,* 34–37.

Beizer, J. L. (1994). Medications and the aging body: Alteration as a function of age. *Journal of the Western Gerontological Society, 18,* 13–22.

Belar, C. D., & Deardorff, W. W. (1996). *Clinical health psychology in medical settings: A practitioner's guidebook.* Washington, DC: American Psychological Association.

Bellack, J. P., Graber, D. R., O'Neil, E. H., Musham, C., & Lancaster, C. (1999). Curriculum trends in nurse practitioner programs: Current and ideal. *Journal of Professional Nursing, 15,* 15–27.

Bender, R., Trautner, C., Spraul, M., & Berger, M. (1998). Assessment of excess mortality in obesity. *American Journal of Epidemiology, 147,* 42–48.

Ben-Eliyahu, S., Yirmiya, R., Liebeskind, J. C., Taylor, A. N., & Gale, R. P. (1991). Stress increases metastatic spread of mammary tumor in rats. Evidence for mediation by the immune system. *Brain, Behavior, and Immunity, 5,* 193–205.

Benight, C. C., Antoni, M. H., Kilbourn, K., Ironson, G., Kumar, M. A., Fletcher, M. A., Redwine, L., Baum, A., & Schneiderman, N. (1997). Coping self-efficacy buffers psychological and physiological disturbances in HIV-infected men following a natural disaster. *Health Psychology, 16,* 248–255.

Benishek, L. A. (1996). Evaluation of the factor structure underlying two measures of hardiness. *Assessment, 3,* 423–435.

Benishek, L. A., & Lopez, F. G. (1997). Critical evaluation of hardiness theory: Gender differences, perception of life events, and neuroticism. *Work and Stress, 11,* 33–45.

Bennett, H. L., Benson, D. R., & Kuiken, D. A. (1986). Preoperative instructions for decreased bleeding during spine surgery. *Anesthesiology, 65,* A245.

Bennett, H. L., & Disbrow, E. A. (1996). Preparing for surgery and medical procedures. In D. Goleman & J. Gurin (Eds.), *Mind-body medicine: How to use your mind for better health* (pp. 401–427). Yonkers, NY: Consumer Reports Books.

Bennett, P., & Carroll, D. (1997). Coronary heart disease: Impact. In A. Baum, S. Newman, J. Weinman, R. West, & C. McManus (Eds.), *Cambridge handbook of psychology, health and medicine* (pp. 419–421). Cambridge, UK: Cambridge University Press.

Benson, H. (1993). The relaxation response. In D. Goleman & J. Gurin (Eds.), *Mind-body medicine: How to use your mind for better health* (pp. 233–257). New York: Consumer Reports Books.

Benson, H. (1996). *Timeless healing: The power and biology of belief.* New York: Scribner.

Benyamini, Y., Leventhal, E. A., & Leventhal, H. (1997). Attributions and health. In A. Baum, S. Newman, J. Weinman, R. West, & C. McManus (Eds.), *Cambridge handbook of psychology, health and medicine* (pp. 72–77). Cambridge, UK: Cambridge University Press.

Ben-Zur, H., & Zeidner, M. (1996). Gender differences in coping reactions under community crisis and daily routine conditions. *Journal of Personality and Individual Differences, 20,* 331–340.

Berge K. G. (1998). Herbal remedies: There's no magic. *Mayo Clinic Health Oasis* (www.mayohealth.org/mayo/9703/htm/herbs.htm).

Berkman, L. F., & Syme, L. S. (1994). Social networks, host resistance, and mortality: A nine year follow-up study of Alameda County residents. In A. Steptoe & J. Wardle (Eds.), *Psychosocial processes and health: A reader* (pp. 43–67). Cambridge, UK: Cambridge University Press.

Berkman, L. F., Vaccarino, V., & Seeman, T. (1993). Gender differences in cardiovascular morbidity and mortality: The contributions of social networks and support. *Annals of Behavioral Medicine, 15,* 112–118.

Bernhardt, P. C., Dabbs, J. M., Fielden, J. A., & Lutter, C. D. (1998). Testosterone changes during vicarious experiences of winning and losing among fans at sporting events. *Physiology and Behavior, 65,* 59–62.

Berry, J. W. (1997). Immigration, acculturation, and adaptation. *Applied Psychology: An International Review, 46,* 5–34.

Bibace, R., & Walsh, M. E. (1979). Developmental stages in children's conceptions of illness. In G. C. Stone, F. Cohen, & N. E. Adler (Eds.), *Health psychology—A handbook* (pp. 285–301). San Francisco: Jossey-Bass.

Bibace, R., & Walsh, M. E. (1981). *Children's conceptions of health, illness, and bodily functions.* San Francisco: Jossey-Bass.

Biener, L., & Heaton, A. (1995). Women dieters of normal weight: Their motives, goals, and risks. *American Journal of Public Health, 85,* 714–717.

Billings, A. G., & Moos, R. H. (1981). The role of coping responses and social resources in attenuating the stress of life events. *Journal of Behavioral Medicine, 4,* 139–157.

Black, J. S., Sefcik, T., & Kapoor, W. (1990). Health promotion and disease prevention in the elderly: Comparison of house staff and attending physician attitudes and practices. *Archives of Internal Medicine, 150,* 389–393.

Blackburn, G. (1995). Effect of degree of weight loss on health benefits. *Obesity Research, 2,* 211s–216s.

Blair, S. N., Kohl, H. W., Paffenbarger, R. S., Clark, D. C., Cooper, K. H., & Gibbons, L. W. (1989). Physical fitness and all-cause mortality: A prospective study of healthy men and women. *Journal of the American Medical Association, 262,* 2395–2401.

Blakeslee, S. (1998, October 13). Placebos prove so powerful even experts are surprised. *The New York Times,* pp. D1, D4.

Blalock, S. J., DeVellis, R. F., Giorgino, K. B., DeVellis, B. M., Gold, D. T., Dooley, M. A., Anderson, J.J.B., & Smith, S. L. (1996). Osteoporosis prevention in premenopausal women: Using a stage model approach to examine the predictors of behavior. *Health Psychology, 15,* 84–93.

Blanchard, E. B., & Hickling, E. J. (1997). *After the crash: Assessment and treatment of motor vehicle accident survivors.* Washington, DC: American Psychological Association.

Blankfield, R. P. (1991). Suggestion, relaxation, and hypnosis as adjuncts in the care of surgery patients: A review of the literature. *American Journal of Clinical Hypnosis, 33,* 172–186.

Blanton, H., Gibbons, F. X., Gerrard, M., Congder, K. & Smith, G. E. (1997). Role of family and peers in the development of prototypes associated with substance use. *Journal of Family Psychology, 11,* 271–288.

Blazer, D., Burchett, B., Service, C., & George, L. K. (1991). The association of age and depression among the elderly: An epidemiologic exploration. *Journal of Gerontology, 46,* 210–215.

Block, L. G., & Keller, P. A. (1995). When to accentuate the negative: The effects of perceived efficacy and message framing on intentions to perform a health-related behavior. *Journal of Marketing Research, 32,* 192–203.

Blumberg, J. B. (1996). Status and functional impact of nutrition in older adults. In E. L. Schneider & J. U. W. Rowe (Eds.), *Handbook of the biology of aging* (4th ed.). San Diego: Academic Press.

Bondi, N. (1997, March 19). Stressed out? Holding it in may be deadly. *The Detroit News,* p. A1.

Bonebright, C. A., Clay, D. L., & Ankenmann, R. D. (2000, October). The relationship of workaholism with work-life conflict, life satisfaction, and purpose in life. *Journal of Counseling Psychology, 47,* 469–477.

Bonica, J. J. (1990). Evolution and current status of pain programs. *Journal of Pain and Symptom Management, 5,* 368–374.

Booth, R. J., Cohen, S., Cunningham, A., Dossey, L., Dreher, H., Kiecolt-Glaser, J. K., Glaser, R., Mehal-Madrona, L., Ornish, D., Payne, D., Pincus, T., Schwartz, G. E. R., Russek, L. G. S., Smith, R. C., Solomon, G. F., Spiegel, D., Cordova, M., Stone, A. A., Broderick, J. E., Targ, E., Taylor, S. E., Theorel, T., Williams, R. B., Woike, B., & Druk, J. (2001). The state of the science: The best evidence for the involvement of thoughts and feelings in physical health. *Advances in Mind-Body Medicine, 17,* 2–59.

Bor, R. (1997). AIDS. In A. Baum, S. Newman, J. Weinman, R. West, & C. McManus (Eds.), *Cambridge handbook of psychology, health and medicine* (pp. 343–347). Cambridge, UK: Cambridge University Press.

Bor, R., & Elford, J. (1994). *The family and HIV.* London: Cassell.

Borland, R., Owen, N., & Hocking, B. (1991). Changes in smoking behaviour after a total workplace smoking ban. *Australian Journal of Public Health, 15,* 130–134.

Borum, M. L. (2000). A comparison of smoking cessation efforts in African Americans by resident physicians in a traditional and primary care internal medicine residency. *Journal of the American Medical Association, 92,* 131–135.

Bosma, H., Stansfeld, S. A., & Marmot, M. G. (1998). Job control, personal characteristics, and heart disease. *Journal of Occupational Health Psychology, 3,* 402–409.

Botvin, G. J. (1980). A comprehensive school-based smoking prevention program. *Journal of School Health, 50,* 209–213.

Bowen, A. M., & Trotter, R. (1995). HIV risk in intravenous drug users and crack cocaine smokers: Predicting stage of change for condom use. *Journal of Consulting and Clinical Psychology, 63,* 238–248.

Bower, J. E., Kemeny, M. E., Taylor, S. E., & Fahey, J. L. (1998). Cognitive processing, discovery of meaning, CD4 decline, and AIDS-related mortality among bereaved HIV-seropositive men. *Journal of Consulting and Clinical Psychology, 66,* 979–986.

Bowers, K. S., & LeBaron, S. (1986). Hypnosis and hypnotizability: Implications for clinical intervention. *Hospital and Community Psychiatry, 37,* 457–467.

Boyles, S., Ness, R. B., Grisson, J. A., Markovic, N., Bromberger, J., & Cifelli, D. (2000). Life event stress and the association with spontaneous abortion in gravid women at an urban emergency department. *Health Psychology, 19,* 510–514.

Bradley, C. (1997). Diabetes mellitus. In A. Baum, S. Newman, J. Weinman, R. West, & C. McManus (Eds.), *Cambridge handbook of psychology, health and medicine* (pp. 432–436). Cambridge, UK: Cambridge University Press.

Bradley, L. A. (1993). Pain measurement in arthritis. *Arthritis Care and Research, 6,* 178–186.

Brand, P., & Yancey, P. (1994). And God created pain. *Christianity Today, 38,* 18–25.

Bratman, S. (1997). *The alternative medicine sourcebook: A realistic evaluation of alternative healing methods.* Los Angeles: Lowell House.

Brattberg, G. (1983). Acupuncture therapy for tennis elbow. *Pain, 16,* 285–288.

Bray, G. A. (1969). Effect of caloric restriction on energy expenditure in obese patients. *Lancet, 2,* 397–398.

Brehm, J. W. (1966). *A theory of psychological reactance.* New York: Academic Press.

Brems, C., & Johnson, M. E. (1989). Problem-solving appraisal and coping style: The influence of sex-role orientation and gender. *Journal of Psychology, 123,* 187–194.

Brennan, A. F., Walfish, S., & AuBuchon, P. (1986). Alcohol use and abuse in college students: A review of individual and personality correlates. *International Journal of the Addictions, 21,* 449–474.

Breslau, N., & Rasmussen, B. K. (2001). The impact of migraine: Epidemiology, risk factors, and co-morbidities. *Neurology* (Special Issue: Headache-related disability in the management of migraine), *56,* S4–S12.

Breslow, L., & Breslow, N. (1993). Health practices and disability: Some evidence from Alameda County. *Preventive Medicine, 22*(1), 86–95.

Brett, J. F., Brief, A. P., Burke, M. J., George, J. M., & Webster, J. (1990). Negative affectivity and the reporting of stressful life events. *Health Psychology, 9,* 57–68.

Brewer, B. W., & Karoly, P. (1992). Recurrent pain in college students. *Journal of American College Health, 41,* 67–69.

Brink, S. (1998, July 27). The hospitalist. *U.S. News & World Report, 125,* 48–52.

Brink, S. (1998, September 7). Unlocking the heart's secrets: Heart disease. *U.S. News and World Report, 125,* 58–65.

Brody, H. (2000a, July/August). Mind over medicine. *Psychology Today,* 60–67.

Brody, H. (2000b) *The placebo response.* New York: HarperCollins.

Brody, J. (1995, January 11). A closer look at the actual health effects of eggs. *The New York Times,* pp. C1, C11.

Brody, J. (1996a, February 28). Good habits outweigh genes as key to a healthy old age. *The New York Times,* p. B11.

Brody, J. (1996b, November 20). Personal health: Controlling anger is good medicine for the heart. *The New York Times,* pp. C15–C20.

Brody, J. (1998a, May 5). Taking stock of the mysteries of medicine. *The New York Times* (www.nytimes.com).

Brody, J. (1998b, May 12). A fatal shift in cancer's gender gap. *The New York Times* (www.nytimes.com).

Brody, J. (1998c, November 30). Diet is not a panacea, but it cuts risk of cancer. *The New York Times* (www.nytimes.com).

Brody, J. (1999a, March 16). When illness is real, but symptoms are unseen. *The New York Times* (www.nytimes.com).

Brody, J. (1999b, August 17). Choosing to test for cancer's genetic link. *The New York Times* (www.nytimes.com).

Brody, J. (1999c, August 24). Bad news, well delivered: A prescription for doctors. *The New York Times* (www.nytimes.com).

Broman, C. (1993). Social relationships and health-related behavior. *Journal of Behavioral Medicine, 16,* 335–350.

Bronzaft, A. L., & McCarthy, D. P. (1975). The effect of elevated train noise on reading ability. *Environment and Behavior, 7,* 517–527.

Brook, J., Cohen, P., Whiteman, M., & Gordon, A. S. (1992). Psychosocial risk factors in the transition from moderate to heavy use or abuse of drugs. In M. D. Glantz & R. W. Pickens (Eds.), *Vulnerability to drug abuse* (pp. 359–388). Washington, DC: American Psychological Association.

Brooke, J. (2000). Canada proposes scaring smokers with pictures on the pack. *The New York Times* (www.nytimes.com).

Brown, D. D., Mucci, W. G., Hetzler, R. K., & Knowlton, R. G. (1989). Cardiovascular and ventilatory responses during formalized T'ai Chi Chuan exercise. *Research Quarterly for Exercise and Sport, 60,* 246–250.

Brown, J. D. (1991). Staying fit and staying well: Physical fitness as a moderator of life stress. *Journal of Personality and Social Psychology, 60,* 555–561.

Brown, J. D., & Siegel, J. M. (1988). Exercise as a buffer of life stress: A prospective study of adolescent health. *Health Psychology, 7,* 341–353.

Brown, L. K., Nassau, J. H., & Barone, V. J. (1990). Differences in AIDS knowledge and attitudes by grade level. *The Journal of School Health, 60,* 270–275.

Brown, L. R., Kane, H., & Ayres, E. (1993). *Vital signs 1993: The trends that are shaping our future.* New York: Norton.

Brown, S. A., Myers, M. G., Mott, M. A., & Vik, P. W. (1994). Correlates of success following treatment for adolescent substance abuse. *Applied and Preventive Psychology, 3,* 61–73.

Brown, S. S., & Eisenberg, L. (1995). *The best intentions: Unintended pregnancy and the well-being of children and families.* Washington, DC: National Academy Press.

Brownell, K. D., & Kaye, F. S. (1982). A school-based behavior modification, nutrition education, and physical activity program for obese children. *The American Journal of Clinical Nutrition, 35,* 277–283.

Brownell, K. D., & Rodin, J. (1994). The dieting maelstrom: Is it possible and advisable to lose weight? *American Psychologist, 49,* 781–791.

Brownell, K. D., & Wadden, T. A. (1991). The heterogeneity of obesity: Fitting treatments to individuals. *Behavior Therapy, 22,* 153–177.

Brownell, K. D., & Wadden, T. A. (1992). Etiology and treatment of obesity: Understanding a serious, prevalent, and refractory disorder. *Journal of Consulting and Clinical Psychology, 60,* 505–517.

Brownlee, S. (1995, October 2). The route of phantom pain. *U.S. News & World Report, 119,* 76.

Brownlee, S., & Shute, N. (1998, May 18). Killing cancer. *U.S. News & World Report, 124*(19), 56, 58, 63–65, 67.

Brubaker, R. G., & Fowler, C. (1990). Encouraging college males to perform testicular self-examination: Evaluation of a persuasive message based on the revised theory of reasoned action. *Journal of Applied Social Psychology, 20,* 1411–1422.

Brubaker, R. G., & Wickersham, D. (1990). Encouraging the practice of testicular self-examination: A field application of the theory of reasoned action. *Health Psychology, 9,* 154–163.

Bruch, H. (1982). Anorexia nervosa: Therapy and theory. *American Journal of Psychiatry, 139,* 1531–1538.

Bruvold, W. H., & Rundall, T. G. (1988). A meta-analysis and theoretical review of school based tobacco and alcohol intervention programs. *Psychology and Health, 2,* 53–78.

Buckley, T. C., Blanchard, E. B., & Hickling, E. J. (1998). A confirmatory factor analysis of posttraumatic stress symptoms. *Behaviour Research and Therapy, 36,* 1091–1099.

Budzynski, T. H., Stoyva, J. M., Adler, C. S., & Mullaney, D. J. (1973). EMG biofeedback and tension headache: A controlled outcome study. *Psychosomatic Medicine, 35,* 484–496.

Bullock, M. L., Culliton, P. D., & Olander, R. T. (1989). Controlled trial of acupuncture for severe recidivist alcoholism. *Lancet, 1989,* 1435–1438.

Bullock, M. L., Kiresuk, T. J., & Pheley, A. M. (1999). Auricular acupuncture in the treatment of cocaine abuse. A study of efficacy and dosing. *Journal of Substance Abuse Treatment, 16,* 31–38.

Bullock, M. L., Umen, A. J., Culliton, P. D., & Olander, R. T. (1987). Acupuncture treatment of alcoholic recidivism: A pilot study. *Alcoholism: Clinical and Experimental Research, 11,* 292–295.

Bundy, C., Carroll, D., Wallace, L., & Nagle, R. (1998). Stress management and exercise training in chronic stable angina pectoris. *Psychology and Health, 13,* 147–155.

Bungener, N., Marchand-Gonod, N., & Jouvent, R. (2000). African and European HIV-positive women: Psychological and psychosocial differences. *AIDS Care, 12,* 541–548.

Bunker, J. P., Frazer, H. S., & Mosteller, F. (1995). The role of medical care in determining health: Creating an inventory of benefits. In B. C. Amick, S. Levine, A. R. Tarlov, & D. C. Walsh (Eds.), *Society and health.* New York: Oxford University Press.

Burack, J. H., Barrett, D. C., Stall, R. D., Chesney, M. A., Ekstrand, M. L., & Coates, T. J. (1993). Depressive symptoms and CD4 lymphocyte decline among HIV-infected men. *Journal of the American Medical Association, 270,* 2568–2573.

Burbach, D. J., & Peterson, L. (1986). Children's concepts of physical illness: A review and critique of the cognitive-developmental literature. *Health Psychology, 5,* 307–325.

Burd, S. (1994). NIH issues rules requiring women and minorities in clinical trials. *The Chronicle of Higher Education, 40,* p. A50.

Burg, M. M., & Seeman, T. E. (1994). Families and health: The negative side of social ties. *Annals of Behavioral Medicine, 16,* 109–115.

Burks, N., & Martin, B. (1985). Everyday problems and life change events: Ongoing versus acute sources of stress. *Journal of Human Stress, 1985, 11,* 27–35.

Burnam, M. A., Timbers, D. M., & Hough, R. L. (1984). Two measures of psychological distress among Mexican Americans, Mexicans, and Anglos. *Journal of Health and Social Behavior, 25,* 24–33.

Burrows, G. D., Elton, D., & Stanley, G. V. (1979). The relationship between psychophysical and perceptual variables and chronic pain. *British Journal of Social and Clinical Psychology, 18,* 425–430.

Bush, C., Ditto, B., & Feuerstein, M. (1985). A controlled evaluation of paraspinal EMG biofeedback in the treatment of chronic low back pain. *Health Psychology 4,* 307–321.

Byrd, J. C. (1992). Environmental tobacco smoke: Medical and legal issues. *The Medical Clinics of North America, 76,* 377–398.

Byrd, R. C. (1988). Positive therapeutic effects of intercessory prayer in a coronary care unit population. *Southern Medical Journal, 81,* 826–829.

Byrnes, D. M., Antoni, M. H., Goodkin, K., Efantis-Potter, J., Asthana, D., Simon, T., Munajj, J., Ironson, G., & Fletcher, M. A. (1998). Stressful events, pessimism, natural killer cell cytotoxicity, and cytotoxic/suppressor T cells in HIV+ black women at risk for cervical cancer. *Psychosomatic Medicine, 60,* 714–722.

Cabrera, N. J., Tamis-LeMonda, C. S., Bradley, R. H., Hofferth, S., & Lamb, M. E. (2000). Fatherhood in the twenty-first century. *Child Development, 71,* 127–136.

Cacioppo, J. T., Andersen, B. L., Turnquist, D. C., & Petty, R. E. (1986). Psychophysiological comparison processes: Interpreting cancer symptoms. In B. Andersen (Ed.), *Women with cancer: Psychological perspectives.* New York: Springer–Verlag.

Caetano, R. (1987). Acculturation and drinking patterns among U.S. Hispanics. *British Journal of Addictions, 82,* 789–799.

Cairns, R. B., & Cairns, B. D. (1994). *Lifelines and risks: Pathways of youth in our time.* Cambridge, UK: Cambridge University Press.

Calam, R., Waller, G., Slade, P. D., & Newton, T. (1990). Eating disorders and perceived relationships with parents. *International Journal of Eating Disorders, 9,* 479–485.

Calhoun, J. B. (1970). Space and the strategy of life. *Ekistics, 29,* 425–437.

Calle, E. E., Miracle-McMahill, H. L., Thun, M. J., & Heath, C.W. (1994). Cigarette smoking and risk of fatal breast cancer. *American Journal of Epidemiology, 139*(10), 1001–1007.

Cameron, L., Leventhal, E. A., & Leventhal, H. (1993). Symptom representations and affect as determinants of care seeking in a community-dwelling, adult sample population. *Health Psychology, 12,* 171–179.

Cameron, L., Leventhal, E. A., & Leventhal, H. (1995). Seeking medical care in response to symptoms and life stress. *Psychosomatic Medicine, 57,* 37–47.

Cameron, L. D., & Nicholls, G. (1998). Expression of stressful experiences through writing: Effects of a self-regulation manipulation for pessimists and optimists. *Health Psychology, 17,* 84–92.

Camp, D. E., Klesges, R. C., & Relyea, G. (1993). The relationship between body weight concerns and adolescent smoking. *Health Psychology, 12,* 24–32.

Canetto, S. S. (1992). Gender and suicide in the elderly. *Suicide and Life-threatening Behavior, 22,* 80–97.

Cannistra, L. B., Davis, S. M., & Bauman, A. G. (1997). Valvular heart disease associated with dexfenfluramine. *New England Journal of Medicine, 337,* 636.

Cannon, W. (1932). *The wisdom of the body.* New York: Norton.

Caplan, R. D., & Jones, K. W. (1975). Effects of work load, role ambiguity, and Type A personality on anxiety, depression, and heart rate. *Journal of Applied Psychology, 60,* 713–719.

Carey, S. (1985). *Conceptual change in childhood.* Boston: MIT Press.

Carlson, C. R., & Hoyle, R. H. (1993). Efficacy of abbreviated progressive muscle relaxation training: A quantitative review of behavioral medicine research. *Journal of Consulting and Clinical Psychology, 61,* 1059–1067.

Carmel, S., Shani, E., & Rosenberg, L. (1994). The role of age and an expanded Health Belief Model on predicting skin cancer protective behavior. *Health Education Research, 9,* 433–447.

Carmody, T. P. (1985). Co-concurrent use of cigarettes, alcohol, and coffee in healthy, community-living men and women. *Health Psychology, 4*(4), 323–335.

Carney, R. M., Freedland, K. E., Eisen, S. A., Rich, M. W., & Jaffe, A. S. (1995). Major depression and medical adherence in elderly patients with coronary artery disease. *Health Psychology, 14,* 88–90.

Carpenter, K. M., Hasin, D. S., Allison, D. B., & Faith, M. S. (2000). Relationships between obesity and DSM-IV major depressive disorder, suicide ideation, and suicide attempts: Results from a general population study. *American Journal of Public Health, 90,* 251–257.

Carpenter, S. (2001, June). Cognition is central to drug addiction. *Monitor on Psychology,* Special Issue on Substance Abuse, *32,* 34–35.

Carson, R. L. (1962). *Silent spring.* New York: Houghton Mifflin.

Carter, J. C., & Fairburn, C. G. (1998). Cognitive-behavioral self-help for binge eating disorder: A controlled effectiveness study. *Journal of Consulting and Clinical Psychology, 66,* 616–623.

Cartwright, F. F. (1972). *Disease and history.* New York: Crowell.

Carvajal, S. C., Garner, R. L., & Evans, R. I. (1998). Dispositional optimism as a protective factor in resisting HIV exposure in sexually active inner-city minority adolescents. *Journal of Applied Social Psychology, 28,* 2196–2211.

Carver, C. S., & Glass, D. C. (1978). Coronary-prone behavior pattern and interpersonal aggression. *Journal of Personality & Social Psychology, 36,* 361–366.

Carver, C. S., Pozo, C., Harris, S. D., Noriega, V., & Scheier, M. F. (1993). How coping mediates the effect of optimism on distress: A study of women with early stage breast cancer. *Journal of Personality and Social Psychology, 65,* 375–390.

Carver, C. S., Scheier, M. F., & Weintraub, J. K. (1989). Assessing coping strategies: A theoretically based approach. *Journal of Personality and Social Psychology, 56,* 267–283.

Case, R. B., Moss, A. J., Case, N., McDermott, M., & Eberly, S. (1992). Living alone after myocardial infarction. *Journal of the American Medical Association, 267,* 515–519.

Cash, T. F., & Henry, P. E. (1995). Women's body images: The results of a national survey in the U.S.A. *Sex Roles, 33,* 19–28.

Caspersen, C. J., Bloemberg, B. P., Saris, W. H., Merritt, R. K., & Kromhout, D. (1991). The prevalence of selected physical activities and their relation with coronary heart disease risk factors in elderly men: The Zutphen Study, 1985. *American Journal of Epidemiology, 133,* 1078–1092.

Casscells, W., Hennekens, C. H., Evans, D., Rosener, B., DeSilva, R. A., Lown, B., Davies, J. E., & Jesse, M. J. (1980). Retirement and coronary mortality. *Lancet, 1,* 1288–1289.

Catalano, R. A., Rook, K., & Dooley, D. (1986). Labor markets and help-seeking: A test of the employment security hypothesis. *Journal of Health and Social Behavior, 27,* 277–287.

Catania, J. A., Binson, D., Dolcini, M. M., Moskowitz, J. T., & van der Straten, A. (2001). Frontiers in the behavioral epidemiology of HIV/STDs. In A. Baum, T. A. Revenson, & J. E. Singer (Eds.), *Handbook of health psychology* (pp. 777–799). Mahwah, NJ: Erlbaum.

Catania, J. A., Coates, T. J., Stall, R., Turner, H., Peterson, J., Hearst, N., Dolcini, M. M., Hudes, E., Gagnon, J., & Wiley, J. (1992). Prevalence of AIDS-related risk factors and condom use in the United States. *Science, 258,* 1101–1106.

Causey, D. L., & Dubow, E. F. (1992). Development of a self-report coping measure for elementary school children. *Journal of Clinical Child Psychology, 21,* 47–59.

Centers for Disease Control and Prevention (CDC). (1998). *National and international HIV seroprevalence surveys—Summary of results.* Atlanta, GA: Department of Health and Human Services.

Centers for Disease Control and Prevention (CDC). (1999). Condoms and their use in preventing HIV infection and other STDs. www.cdc.gov/hiv/pubs/facts/condoms.htm.

Centers for Disease Control and Prevention (CDC). (2000). *Reducing tobacco use: A report of the surgeon general.* U.S. Department of Health and Human Services, www.cdc.gov/tobacco.

Centers for Disease Control and Prevention, (CDC). (2001). *HIV/AIDS Surveillance Supplemental Report, 2001, 7. Characteristics of persons living with AIDS at the end of 1999.* Atlanta, GA: Department of Health and Human Services.

Centers for Disease Control and Prevention (CDC). (2001). Mortality from coronary heart disease and acute myocardial infarction—United States, 1998. *Morbidity and Mortality Weekly Report, 50,* 90–93.

Centers for Disease Control and Prevention (CDC). (2001). Tobacco use prevention program *Tobacco Information and Prevention Source* (http://www.cdc.gov/tobacco).

Cervero, F. (2000). Visceral hyperalgesia revisited. *The Lancet, 9236,* 1127–1135.

Chamberlin, J. (2001, June). NIAAA to release findings of student drinking study. *Monitor on Psychology* (Special issue on substance abuse), *32,* 13.

Champion, V. L. (1994). Strategies to increase mammography utilization. *Medical Care, 32,* 118–129.

Chaney, J. M., Mullins, L. L., Frank, R. G., & Peterson, L. (1997). Transactional patterns of child, mother, and father adjustment in insulin-dependent diabetes mellitus: A prospective study. *Journal of Pediatric Psychology, 22,* 229–244.

Chapman, C. R. (1984). New directions in the understanding and management of pain. *Social Science and Medicine Special Issue: Chronic Pain, 19,* 1261–1277.

Chartrand, L. J., & Seidman, E. G. (1996). Celiac disease is a lifelong disorder. *Clinical and Investigative Medicine, 19,* 357–361.

Chassin, L., Presson, C. C., Sherman, S. J., & McGrew, J. (1987). The changing smoking environment for middle and high school students: 1980–1983. *Journal of Behavioral Medicine, 10*(6), 581–593.

Chassin, L., Presson, C. C., Todd, M., Rose, J. S., & Sherman, S. J. (1998). Maternal socialization of adolescent smoking: The intergenerational transmission of parenting and smoking. *Developmental Psychology, 34,* 1189–1201.

Chaves, J. F., & Barber, T. X. (1974). Cognitive strategies, experimenter modeling, and expectation in the attenuation of pain. *Journal of Abnormal Psychology, 83,* 356–363.

Chen, M. S. (1994). Behavioral and psychosocial cancer research in the underserved: An agenda for the future. *Cancer, 74,* 1503–1508.

Cherkin, D. C., Deyo, R. A., Battie, M., Street, J., & Barlow, W. (1998). A comparison of physical therapy, chiropractic manipulation, and provision of an educational booklet for the treatment of patients with low back pain. *New England Journal of Medicine, 339,* 1021–1029.

Chermack, S. T., & Giancola, P. R. (1997). The relation between alcohol and aggression: An integrated biopsychosocial conceptualization. *Clinical Psychology Review, 17,* 621–649.

Cherny, N. I. (1996). The problem of inadequately relieved suffering. *Journal of Social Issues, 52,* 13–30.

Childstats. (2001). Federal Interagency Forum on Child and Family Statistics. http://childstats.gov.

Chopra, D., (1993). *Ageless body, timeless mind.* New York: Harmony Books.

Christeff, N., Lortholary, O., Casassus, P., Thobie, N., Veyssier, P., Torri, O., Guillevin, L., & Nunez, E. A. (1996). Relationship between sex steroid hormone levels and CD4 lymphocytes in HIV infected men. *Experimental and Clinical Endocrinology and Diabetes, 104,* 130–136.

Christensen, A. (1996). *The American yoga association wellness book.* New York: Kensington.

Christensen, B., Iuhl, I., & Vilbeck, H. (1992). Acupuncture treatment of severe knee osteoarthritis: A long-term study. *Acta Anaesthesiology Scandinavia, 36,* 519.

Christiano, D. (2000, January). The best health news for women. *Woman's Day, 63,* 50–53.

Christoffel, K. K., & Ariza, A. (1998). The epidemiology of overweight in children: Relevance for Clinical care. *Pediatrics, 101,* 103–105.

Christophersen, R. R., & Gyulay, J. (1981). Parental compliance with car seat usage: A positive approach with long-term follow-up. *Journal of Pediatric Psychology, 6,* 301–312.

Chung, C. S. (1986). A Report on the Hawaii Behavioral Risk Factor Surveillance System for 1986. Honolulu: School of Public Health, University of Hawaii.

Ciechanowski, P. S., Katon, W. J., Russon, J. E., & Walker, E. A. (2001). The patient–provider relationship: Attachment theory and adherence to treatment in diabetes. *American Journal of Psychiatry, 158,* 29–35.

Ciesielski, C. (1992). Transmission of human immunodeficiency virus in a dental practice. *Annals of Internal Medicine, 116,* 798–805.

Cinciripini, P. M., Cinciripini, L. G., Wallfisch, A., Hague, W., & Van Vunakis, H. (1996). Behavior therapy and the transdermal nicotine patch: Effects on cessation outcome, affect, and coping. *Journal of Consulting and Clinical Psychology, 64,* 314–323.

Clark, W. C., & Mehl, L. (1971). Thermal pain: A sensory decision theory analysis of the effect of age and sex on d', various response criteria, and 50% pain threshold. *Journal of Abnormal Psychology, 78,* 202–212.

Clay, R. A. (1999, January). Drug prevention focus should be on families. *American Psychological Association Monitor, 30,* 14.

Clayton, R. R., & Ritter, C. (1985). The epidemiology of alcohol and drug abuse among adolescents. *Advances in Alcohol and Substance Abuse, 4,* 69–97.

Cleveland Clinic Heart Advisor Staff. (2000, November). New research examines best use of "super aspirins." *Cleveland Clinic Heart Advisor, 11,* 4–5.

Cloninger, C. R. (1987). Neurogenetic adaptive mechanisms in alcoholism. *Science, 236,* 410–416.

Cloninger, C. R., Bohman, M., Sigvardsson, S., & von Knorring, A. L. (1985). Psychopathology in adopted-out children of alcoholics. The Stockholm Adoption Study. *Recent Developments in Alcoholism, 3,* 37–51.

Coan, R. M., Wong, G., & Coan, P. L. (1980). The acupuncture treatment of low back pain: A randomized controlled study. *American Journal of Chinese Medicine, 8,* 181–189.

Coates, T. J., Stall, R. D., & Hoff, C. C. (1990). Changes in sexual behavior among gay and bisexual men since the beginning of the AIDS epidemic. In L. Temoshok & A. Baum (Eds.), *Psychosocial perspectives on AIDS: Etiology, prevention, and treatment* (pp. 103–137). Hillsdale, NJ: Erlbaum.

Cochran, S. D., & Mays, V. M. (1990). Sex, lies, and HIV. *New England Journal of Medicine, 322,* 774–775.

Codori, A., Petersen, G. M., Miglioretti, D. L., Larkin, E. K., Bushey, M. T., Young, C., Brensinger, J. D., Johnson, K., Bacon, J. A., & Booker, S. V. (1999). Attitudes toward colon cancer gene testing: Factors predicting test uptake. *Cancer Epidemiology, Biomarkers and Prevention, 8,* 345–352.

Cohen, S., Frank, E., Doyle, W. J., Skoner, D. P., Rabin, B. S. & Gwaltney, J. M. (1998). Types of stressors that increase susceptibility to the common cold in healthy adults. *Health Psychology, 17,* 214–223.

Cohen, S., Glass, D. C., & Singer, J. E. (1973). Apartment noise, auditory discrimination, and reading ability in children. *Journal of Experimental Social Psychology, 9,* 407–422.

Cohen, S., & Herbert, T. B. (1996). Health psychology: Psychological factors and physical disease from the perspective of human psychoneuroimmunology. *Annual Review of Psychology, 47,* 113–132.

Cohen, S., Kaplan, J. R., & Mauck, S. B. (1994). Social support and coronary heart disease: Underlying psychological and biological mechanisms. In S. A. Shumaker, & S. M. Czajkowski (Eds.), *Social support and cardiovascular disease.* New York: Plenum Press.

Cohen, S., & McKay, G. (1984). Social support, stress, and the buffering hypothesis: A theoretical analysis. In A. Baum, S. E. Taylor, & J. E. Singer (Eds.), *Handbook of psychology and health* (pp. 253–268). Hillsdale, NJ: Erlbaum.

Cohen, S., & Rodriguez, M. S. (1995). Pathways linking affective disturbances and physical disorders. *Health Psychology, 14,* 374–380.

Cohen, S., Sherrod, D. R., & Clark, M. S. (1986). Social skills and the stress-protective role of social support. *Journal of Personality and Social Psychology, 50,* 963–973.

Cohen, S., & Wills, T. A. (1985). Stress, social support, and the buffering hypothesis. *Psychological Bulletin, 93,* 310–357.

Colditz, G. A., Willett, W. C., Hunter, D. J., Stampfer, M. J., Manson, J. E., Hennekens, C. H., & Rosner, B. A. (1993). Family history, age, and risk of breast cancer. Prospective data from the Nurses' Health Study. *Journal of the American Medical Association, 270,* 338–343.

Cole, S. W., Kemeny, M. E., Taylor, S. E., Visscher, B. R., & Fahey, J. L. (1996). Accelerated course of human immunodeficiency virus infection in gay men who conceal their homosexual identity. *Psychosomatic Medicine, 58,* 219–231.

Coleman, J. (1997, June 30). Cigarette industry thriving in Japan. *Grand Rapids Press,* p. A14.

Coleman, L. M., Fowler, L. L., & Williams, M. E. (1995). Use of unproven therapies by people with Alzheimer's disease. *Journal of the American Geriatrics Society, 43,* 747–750.

Coleman, P. D., & Flood, D. G. (1986). Dendritic proliferation in the aging brain as a compensatory repair mechanism. *Progress in Brain Research, 70,* 227–237.

Colerick, E. J. (1985). Stamina in later life. *Social Science and Medicine, 21,* 997–1006.

Colligan, R. C., & Offord, K. P. (1988). The risky use of the MMPI hostility scale in assessing risk for coronary heart disease. *Psychosomatics, 29,* 188–196.

Collins, N. L., Dunkel-Schetter, C., Lobel, M., & Scrimshaw, S. C. (1993). Social support in pregnancy: Psychosocial correlates of birth outcomes and postpartum depression. *Journal of Personality and Social Psychology, 65,* 1243–1258.

Comarow, A. (2000, March 13). Healing the heart. *U. S. News & World Report, 128,* 54–57, 61–62, 64.

Compas, B. E., Haaga, D. A., Keefe, F. J., Leitenberg, H., & Williams, D. A. (1998). Sampling of empirically supported psychological treatments from health psychology: Smoking, chronic pain, cancer, and bulimia nervosa. *Journal of Consulting and Clinical Psychology, 66,* 89–112.

Connell, C. M., & D'Augelli, A. R. (1990). The contribution of personality characteristics to the relationship between social support and perceived physical health. *Health Psychology, 9,* 192–207.

Conner, M., & Sparks, P. (1996). The theory of planned behaviour and health behaviours. In M. Conner & P. Normal (Eds.), *Predicting health behavior: Research and practice with social cognition models* (pp. 121–162). Buckingham, UK: Open University Press, 121–162.

Connolly, H. M., Crary, J. L., McGoon, M. D., Hensrud, D. D., Edwards, B. S., Edwards, W. D., & Schaff, H. V. (1997). Valvular heart disease associated with fenfluramine-phentermine. *New England Journal of Medicine, 337,* 581–588.

Conrad, C. D., Magarinos, A. M., LeDoux, J. E., & McEwen, B. S. (1999). Repeated restrain stress facilitates fear conditioning independently of causing hippocampal CA3 dendritic atrophy. *Behavioral Neuroscience, 13,* 902–913.

Considine, R. V., & Caro, J. F. (1996). Leptin in humans: Current progress and future directions. *Clinical Chemistry, 6,* 843–844.

Constantini, A., Solano, L., DiNapoli, R., & Bosco, A. (1997). Relationship between hardiness and risk of burnout in a sample of 92 nurses working in oncology and AIDS wards. *Psychotherapy and Psychosomatics, 66,* 78–82.

Cook, E. H., Stein, M. A., Krasowski, M. D., Cox, N. J., Olkon, D. M., Kieffer, J. E., & Leventhal, B. L. (1995). Association of attention-deficit disorder and the dopamine transporter gene. *American Journal of Human Genetics, 56,* 993–998.

Cooper, M. L., Pierce, R. S., & Tidwell, M. O. (1995). Parental drinking problems and adolescent offspring substance use: Moderating effects of demographic and familial factors. *Psychology of Addictive Behaviors, 9,* 36–52.

Cooper, R. A., & Stoflet, S. J. (1996). Trends in the education and practice of alternative medicine clinicians. *Health Affairs, 15,* 226–238.

Cooper, R. S., Rotimi, C. N., & Ward, R. (1999). The puzzle of hypertension in African-Americans. *Scientific American, 280*(2), 56–63.

Costa, P. T., & McCrae, R. R. (1985). Hypochondriasis, neuroticism, and aging. When are somatic complaints unfounded? *American Psychologist, 40,* 19–28.

Cottington, E. M., Matthews, K. A., Talbott, E., & Kuller, L. H. (1986). Occupational stress, suppressed anger, and hypertension. *Psychosomatic Medicine, 48,* 249–260.

Cousins, N. (1976). Anatomy of an illness: As perceived by the patient. *New England Journal of Medicine, 295,* 1458–1463.

Cousins, N. (1979). *Anatomy of an illness as perceived by the patient: Reflections on healing and regeneration* (p. 695). New York: Norton.

Cox, D. J., Gonder-Frederick, L., Julian, D. M., & Clarke, W. (1994). Long-term follow-up evaluation of blood glucose awareness training. *Diabetes Care, 17,* 1–5.

Cox, S. (1997). Counting the uncountable? *Social Psychiatry and Psychiatric Epidemiology, 32,* 19–23.

Cramer, J. A., Mattson, R. H., Prevey, M. L., Scheyer, R. D., & Ouellette, V. L. (1989). How often is medication taken as prescribed? *Journal of the American Medical Association, 261,* 3273–3277.

Crawford, J. P., Hickson, G. S., & Wiles, M. R. (1986). The management of hypertensive disease: A review of spinal manipulation and the efficacy of conservative therapeusis. *Journal of Manipulative and Physiological Therapeutics, 9,* 27–32.

Crepaz, N., & Marks, G. (2001). Are negative affective states associated with HIV sexual risk behaviors? A meta-analytic review. *Health Psychology, 20,* 291–299.

Crowell, N. A., & Burgess, A. W. (1996). *Understanding violence against women.* Washington, DC: National Academy Press.

Croyle, R. T., & Uretsky, M. B. (1987). Effects of mood on self-appraisal of health status. *Health Psychology, 6,* 239–253.

Cruess, D. G., Antoni, M. H., Schneiderman, N., Ironson, G., McCabe, P., Fernandez, J. B., Cruess, S. E., Klimas, N., & Kumar, M. (2000). Cognitive-behavioral stress management increases free testosterone and decreases psychological distress in HIV-seropositive men. *Health Psychology, 19,* 12–20.

Culliton, P. D., Boucher, T. A., & Bullock, M. L. (1999). Complementary/alternative therapies in the treatment of alcohol and other addictions. In J. W. Spencer & J. J. Jacobs (Eds.), *Complementary/alternative medicine: An evidence-based approach.* St Louis, MO: Mosby.

Cummings, N. A. (1991). The somatizing patient. In C. S. Austad & W. H. Berman (Eds.), *Psychotherapy in managed health care: The optimal use of time and resources* (pp. 234–247). Washington, DC: American Psychological Association.

Cummings, P., & Psaty, B. M. (1994). The association between cholesterol and death from injury. *Annals of Internal Medicine, 120,* 848–855.

Curb, J. D., & Marcus, E. B. (1991). Body fat and obesity in Japanese Americans. *American Journal of Clinical Nutrition, 53,* 1552s–1555s.

D'Amico, E. J., & Fromme, K. (1997). Health risk behaviors of adolescent and young adult siblings. *Health Psychology, 16*(5), 426–432.

Daffner, K. R., Scinto, L. F., Weintraub, S., Guinessey, J., & Mesulam, M. M. (1994). The impact of aging on curiosity as measured by exploratory eye movements. *Archives of Neurology, 51,* 368–376.

Dahl, J., Melin, L., & Lund, L. (1987). Effects of a contingent relaxation treatment program on adults with refractory epileptic seizures. *Epilepsia, 28,* 125–132.

Daley, S. (1998). Dead zones: The burden of shame. *The New York Times* (www.nytimes.com).

Dartiques, J. F., & Letenneur, L. (2000). Genetic epidemiology of Alzheimer's disease. *Current Opinion in Neurology, 13,* 385–389.

Dattore, P. J., Shontz, F. C., & Coyne, L. (1980). Premorbid personality differentiation of cancer and non-cancer groups: A list of the hypotheses of cancer proneness. *Journal of Consulting and Clinical Psychology, 48,* 388–394.

Davis, K. L. (1992). A double-blind, placebo-controlled multicenter study of Tacrine for Alzheimer's disease. *New England Journal of Medicine, 327,* 1253–1257.

Davison, G. C. (1997). Behaviour therapy. In A. Baum, S. Newman, J. Weinman, R. West, & C. McManus (Eds.), *Cambridge handbook of psychology, health and medicine* (pp. 195–196). Cambridge, UK: Cambridge University Press.

Daw, J. (2001a, April). New rule will change the psychologist/physician relationship. *Monitor on Psychology* (www.apa.org/monitor/apr01).

Daw, J. (2001b, May). Academic medicine welcomes psychology. *Monitor on Psychology, 5* (www.apa.org/monitor/may.oq).

Dawber, T. R. (1980). *The Framingham study: The epidemiology of atherosclerotic disease.* Cambridge, MA: Harvard University Press.

DeAngelis, T. (1995, October). Primary care collaborations growing. *American Psychological Association Monitor,* p. 22.

Deeks, S. G, Smith, M., Holodniy, M., & Kahn, J. O. (1997). HIV-1 protease inhibitors. *Journal of the American Medical Association, 277,* 145–153.

Deffenbacher, J. L., & Stark, R. S. (1992). Relaxation and cognitive-relaxation treatments of general anger. *Journal of Counseling Psychology, 39,* 158–167.

Dejong, W. (1980). The stigma of obesity: The consequences of naïve assumptions concerning the causes of physical deviance. *Journal of Health and Social Behavior, 1,* 75–87.

Delahanty, D. L. & Baum, A. (2001). Stress and breast cancer. In A. Baum, T. A. Revenson, & J. E. Singer (Eds.), *Handbook of health psychology* (pp. 747–756). Mahwah, NJ: Erlbaum.

Denissenko, M. F., Pao, A., Tang, M., & Pfeifer, G. P. (1996). Preferential formation of benzoapyrene adducts at lung cancer mutational hotspots in P53. *Science, 274,* 430–432.

DeRosa, C. J., & Marks, G. (1998). Preventive counseling of HIV-positive men and self-disclosure of serostatus to sex partners: New opportunities for prevention. *Health Psychology, 17,* 224–231.

Detweiler, J. B., Bedell, B. T., Salovey, P., Pronin, E., & Rothman, A. J. (1999). Message framing and sunscreen use: Gain-framed messages motivate beach-goers. *Health Psychology, 18,* 189–196.

Devine, E. C., & Cook, T. D. (1983). A meta-analytic analysis of effects of psychoeducational interventions on length of postsurgical hospital stay. *Nursing Research, 32,* 267–274.

Devins, G. M., Hunsley, J., Mandin, H., Taub, K. J., & Paul, L. C. (1997). The marital context of end-stage renal disease: Illness intrusiveness and perceived changes in family environment. *Annals of Behavioral Medicine, 19,* 325–332.

Devor, E. J. (1994). A developmental-genetic model of alcoholism: Implications for genetic research. *Journal of Consulting and Clinical Psychology, 62,* 1108–1115.

De Vries, H., & Backbier, E. (1994). Self-efficacy as an important determinant of quitting among pregnant women who smoke: The o-pattern. *Preventive Medicine, 23,* 167–174.

Diamond, J. (1992). Evolutionary physiology: The red flag of optimality. *Nature, 355,* 204–205.

Dickens, E., & Lewith, G. (1989). A single-blind controlled and randomized clinical trial to evaluate the effect of acupuncture in the treatment of trapezio-metacarpal osteoarthritis. *Complementary Medical Research, 3,* 33–40.

DiClemente, R. J. (1991). Predictors of HIV-preventive sexual behavior in a high-risk adolescent population: The influence of perceived peer norms and sexual communication on incarcerated adolescents' consistent use of condoms. *Journal of Adolescent Health, 12,* 385–390.

Diehr, P., Bild, D. E., Harris, T. B., Duxbury, A., Siscovick, D., & Rossi, M. (1998). Body mass index and mortality in nonsmoking older adults: The Cardiovascular Health Study. *American Journal of Public Health, 88,* 623–629.

Diez-Ruiz, A., Tilz, G. P., Gutierrez-Gea, F., Gil-Extremerak, B., Murr, C., Wachter, H., & Fuchs, D. (1995). Neopterin and soluble tumor necrosis factor receptor type 1 in alcohol-induced cirrhosis. *Heptalogy, 21,* 976–978.

DiMatteo, M. R. (1993). Expectations in the physician-patient relationship: Implications for patient adherence to medical treatment recommendations. In P. D. Blanck (Ed.), *Interpersonal expectations: Theory, research, and applications* (pp. 296–315). New York: Cambridge University Press.

DiMatteo, M. R. (1994). Enhancing patient adherence to medical recommendations. *Journal of the American Medical Association, 271,* 79–83.

Dimsdale, J. E., Alper, B. S., & Schneiderman, N. (1986). Exercise as a modulator of cardiovascular reactivity. In K. A. Matthews, S. M. Weiss, T. Detre, T. M. Dembroski, B. Falkner, S. B. Mauck, & R. B. Williams (Eds.), *Handbook of stress, reactivity, and cardiovascular disease.* New York: Wiley.

Disbrow, E. A., Owings, J. T., & Bennett, H. L. (1993). Respond. *Western Journal of Medicine, 159,* 31–35.

Ditto, P. H., Druley, J. A., Moore, K. A., Danks, J. H., & Smucker, W. D. (1996). Fates worse than death: The role of valued life activities in health-state evaluations. *Health Psychology, 15,* 332–343.

Divekar, M. V., Bhat, M., & Mulla, A. (1998). Effect of Yoga therapy in diabetes and obesity. *Journal of the Diabests Association of India, 28,* 1331–1338.

Doherty, W. J., Schrott, H. G., Metcalf, L., & Iasiello-Vailas, L. (1983). Effect of spouse support and health beliefs on medication adherence. *Journal of Family Practice, 17,* 837–841.

Dohrenwend, B. P., & Shrout, P. E. (1985). "Hassles" in the conceptualization and measurement of life stress variables. *American Psychologist, 40,* 780–785.

Dolan, B., & Ford, K. (1991). Binge eating and dietary restraint: A cross-cultural analysis. *International Journal of Eating Disorders, 10,* 345–353.

Doll, J., & Ajzen, I. (1992). Accessibility and stability of predictors in the theory of planned behavior. *Journal of Personality and Social Psychology, 63,* 754–765.

Doll, R., & Peto, R. (1981). *The causes of cancer.* New York: Oxford University Press.

Domino, E. F. (1996). Estimating exposure to environmental tobacco smoke. *Journal of the American Medical Association, 276,* 603.

Donovan, J. E., Jessor, R., & Costa, F. M. (1988). Syndrome of problem behavior in adolescence: A replication. *Journal of Consulting and Clinical Psychology, 56*, 762–765.

Dossey, L. (1993). *Healing words: The power of prayer and the practice of medicine.* San Francisco: HarperCollins.

Dougall, A. L., & Baum, A. (2001). Stress, health, and illness. In A. Baum, T. A. Revenson, & J. E. Singer (Eds.), *Handbook of health psychology* (pp. 321–337). Mahwah, NJ: Erlbaum.

Downey, G., Silver, R. C., & Wortman, C. B. (1990). Reconsidering the attribution-adjustment relation following a major negative event: Coping with the loss of a child. *Journal of Personality and Social Psychology, 59*, 925–940.

Dowson, D. I., Lewith, G. T., & Machin, D. (1985). The effects of acupuncture versus placebo in the treatment of headache. *Pain, 21*, 35–42.

Driskell, J. E., Salas, E., & Johnston, J. (1999). Does stress lead to a loss of team perspective? *Group Dynamics, 3*, 291–302.

Drory, Y., Florian, V., & Kravetz, S. (1991). Sense of coherence: Sociodemographic variables and perceived psychological and physical health. *Psychologia: Israel Journal of Psychology, 2*, 119–125.

Drotar, D. (1995). *Consulting with pediatricians: Psychological perspectives.* New York: Plenum Press.

Druckman, D. E., & Bjork, R. A. (1994). *Learning, remembering, believing: Enhancing human performance.* Washington, DC: USA National Academy Press.

Druss, B. G., & Rosenheck, R. A. (1999). Association between use of unconventional therapies and conventional medical services. *Journal of the American Medical Association, 282*, 651–656.

Dubbert, P. M. (1992). Exercise in behavioral medicine. *Journal of Consulting and Clinical Psychology, 60*, 613–618.

Dunn, A. L., Reigle, T. G., Youngstedt, S. D., Armstrong, R. B., & Dishman, J. (1996). Brain norepinephrine and metabolites after treadmill training and wheel running in rats. *Medicine and Science in Sports and Exercise, 28*, 204–209.

Duquette, A., Kerouac, S., Sandhu, B. K., Ducharme, F., & Saulnier, C. F. (1995). Psychosocial determinants of burnout in geriatric nursing. *International Journal of Nursing Studies, 32*, 443–456.

Durazo-Arvizu, R. A., McGee, D. L., Cooper, R. S., Liao, Y., & Luke, A. (1998). Mortality and optimal body mass index in a sample of the U.S. population. *American Journal of Epidemiology, 147*, 739–749.

Eccleston, C. (1995). The attentional control of pain: Methodological and theoretical concerns. *Pain, 63*, 3–10.

Eckenrode, J. (1984). Impact of chronic and acute stressors on daily reports of mood. *Journal of Personality and Social Psychology, 46*, 907–918.

Edelman, B. (1999). *Centenarians: The story of the 20th century by the Americans who lived it.* New York: Farrar, Straus & Giroux.

Edgar, L., Rossberger, Z., & Nowlis, D. (1992). Coping with cancer during the first year after diagnosis: Assessment and intervention. *Cancer, Diagnosis, Treatment, Research, 69*, 817–828.

Egbert, L. D., Battit, C. E., Welch, C. E., & Bartlett, M. K. (1964). Reduction of postoperative pain by encouragement and instruction of patients. A study of doctor-patient rapport. *New England Journal of Medicine, 75*, 1008–1023.

Eifert, G. H., Hodson, S. E., Tracey, D. R., Seville, J. L., & Gunawardane, K. (1996). Heart-focused anxiety, illness beliefs, and behavioral impairment: Comparing healthy heart-anxious patients with cardiac and surgical inpatients. *Journal of Behavioral Medicine, 19*, 385–399.

Eisenberg, D. M. (1997). Advising patients who use alternative medical therapies. *Annals of Internal Medicine, 127*, 61–69.

Eisenberg, D. M., Davis, R. B., Ettner, S. L., Appel, S., Wilkey, S., Van Rompay, M., & Kessler, R. C. (1998). Trends in alternative medicine use in the United States, 1990–1997: Results of a follow–up national survey. *Journal of the American Medical Association, 280*, 1569–1575.

Eisenberg, D. M., Kessler, R. C., Foster, C., Norlock, F. E., Calkins, D. R., & Delbanco, T. L. (1993). Unconventional medicine in the United States: Prevalence, costs, and patterns of use. *New England Journal of Medicine, 328*, 246–252.

Eiser, C. (1990). Psychological effects of chronic disease. *Journal of Child Psychology and Psychiatry and Allied Disciplines, 31*, 85–98.

Eiser, C. (1997). Children's perceptions of illness and death. In A. Baum, S. Newman, J. Weinman, R. West, & C. McManus (Eds.), *Cambridge handbook of psychology, health and medicine* (pp. 81–83). Cambridge, UK: Cambridge University Press.

Eiser, C., & Main, N. (2001). Child health psychology. In D. W. Johnston & M. Johnston (Eds.), *Health psychology: Comprehensive clinical psychology* (pp. 617–643). Oxford, UK: Elsevier.

Eitel, P., Hatchett, L., Friend, R., & Griffin, K. W. (1995). Burden of self-care in seriously ill patients: Impact on adjustment. *Health Psychology, 14*, 457–463.

Elkins, P. D., & Roberts, M. C. (1983). Psychological preparation for pediatric hospitalization. *Clinical Psychology Review, 3*, 275–295.

Ellenberg, S. S., & Chen, R. T. (1997). The complicated task of monitoring vaccine safety. *Public Health Reports, 112*, 10–20.

Ellenhorst-Ryan, J. M. (1997). The nature of cancer. In C. Varricchio, M. Pierce, C. Walker, & T. B. Ads (Eds.), *A cancer source book for nurses* (7th ed., pp. 27–34). Atlanta: American Cancer Society.

Ellerbrock, T. V., Lieb, S., Harrington, P. E., Bush, T. J., Schoenfisch, S. A., Oxtoby, M. J., Howell, J. T., Rogers, M. F., & Witte, J. J. (1992). Heterosexually transmitted human immunodeficiency virus infection among pregnant women in a rural Florida community. *New England Journal of Medicine, 327*, 1704–1709.

Ellis, A. (1962). *Reason and emotion in psychotherapy.* Secaucus, NY: Citadel Press.

Elton, D., Stanley, G. V., & Burrows, G. D. (1983). *Psychological control of pain.* Sydney, Australia: Grune & Stratton.

Emery, C. F., Hauck, E. R., & Blumenthal, J. A. (1992). Exercise adherence or maintenance among older adults: 1-year follow-up study. *Psychology and Aging, 7*, 466–470.

Emmons, C. A., Joseph, J. G., Kessler, R. C., Wortman, C. B., Montgomery, S. B., & Ostrow, D. G. (1986). Psychosocial predictors of reported behavior change in homosexual men at risk for AIDS. *Health Education Quarterly, 13,* 331–345.

Endler, N. S., & Parker, J. D. (1990). State and trait anxiety, depression and coping styles. *Australian Journal of Psychology, 42,* 207–220.

English, E. H., & Baker, T. B. (1983). Relaxation training and cardiovascular response to experimental stressors. *Health Psychology, 2,* 239–259.

English, J. A., & Bauman, K. A. (1997). Evidence-based management of upper respiratory infection in a family practice teaching clinic. *Family Medicine, 29,* 38–41.

Enright, M. F., Resnick, R., DeLeon, P. H., Sciara, A. D., & Tanney, F. (1990). The practice of psychology in hospital settings. *American Psychologist, 45*(9), 1059–1065.

Epping-Jordan, J. E., Compas, B. E., & Howell, D. C. (1994). Predictors of cancer progression in young adult men and women: Avoidance, intrusive thoughts, and psychological symptoms. *Health Psychology, 13,* 539–547.

Epping-Jordan, J. E., Compas, B. E., Osowiecki, D. M., Oppedisano, G., Gerhardt, C., Primo, K., & Krag, D. N. (1999). Psychological adjustment in breast cancer: Processes of emotional distress. *Health Psychology, 18,* 315–326.

Epstein, A. M., Taylor, W. C., & Seage, G. R. (1985). Effects of patients' socioeconomic status and physicians' training and practice on patient-doctor communication. *American Journal of Medicine, 78,* 101–106.

Eriksson, S. V., Lundeberg, T., & Lundeberg, S. (1991). Interaction of diazepam and naloxone on acupuncture induced pain relief. *The American Journal of Chinese Medicine, 19,* 1–7.

Ernsberger, P., & Koletsky, R. J. (1999). Biomedical rationale for a wellness approach to obesity: An alternative to a focus on weight loss. *Journal of Social Issues, 55,* 221–259.

Ernst, E. (1996). *Complementary medicine: An objective appraisal.* Oxford, England: Butterworth–Heinemann.

Ernst, E., Resch, K. L., & White, A. R. (1995). Complementary medicine: What physicians think of it. *Archives of Internal Medicine, 155,* 2405–2408.

Escobedo, L. G., & Remington, P. L. (1989). Birth cohort analysis of prevalence of cigarette smoking among Hispanics in the United States. *Journal of the American Medical Association, 261,* 66–69.

Esplen, M. J., Toner, B., Hunter, J., Glendon, G., Butler, K., & Field, B. (1998). A group therapy approach to facilitate integration of risk information for women at risk for breast cancer. *Canadian Journal of Psychiatry, 43,* 375–380.

Esposito-Del Puente, A., Lillioja, S., Bogardus, C., McCubbin, J. A., Feinglos, M. N., Kuhn, C. M., & Surwit, R. S. (1994). Glycemic response to stress is altered in euglycemic Pima Indians. *International Journal of Obesity and Related Metabolic Disorders, 18,* 766–770.

Esterling, B. A., Kiecolt-Glaser, J. K., Bodnar, J. C., & Glaser, R. (1994). Chronic stress, social support, and persistent alterations in the natural killer cell response to cytokines in older adults. *Health Psychology, 13,* 291–298.

Evans, F. J. (1974). The placebo response in pain reduction. *Advances in Neurology, 4,* 289–234.

Evans, G. W., Hygge, S., & Bullinger, M. (1995). Chronic noise and psychological stress. *Psychological Science, 6,* 333–338.

Evans, R. I. (2001). Social influences in etiology and prevention of smoking and other health-threatening behaviors in children and adolescents. In A. Baum, T. A. Revenson, & J. E. Singer (Eds.), *Handbook of health psychology* (pp. 459–468). Mahwah, NJ: Erlbaum.

Evans, R. I., Rozell, R. M., Maxwell, S. E., Raines, B. E., Dill, C. A., Guthrie, T. J., Henderson, A. H., & Hill, D. C. (1981). Social modeling films to deter smoking in adolescents: Results of a three-year field investigation. *Journal of Applied Psychology, 66,* 399–414.

Eveleth, P. B., & Tanner, J. M. (1991). *Worldwide variation in human growth* (2nd ed.). Cambridge, England: Cambridge University Press.

Everall, I. P., Luthert, P. J., & Lantos, P. L. (1991). Neuronal loss in the frontal cortex in HIV infection. *Lancet, 337,* 1119–1121.

Everhart, J., & Wright, D. (1995). Diabetes mellitus as a risk factor for pancreatic cancer: A meta-analysis. *Journal of the American Medical Association, 273,* 1605–1609.

Everson, S. A., Goldberg, D. E., Kaplan, G. A., & Cohen, R. D. (1996). Hopelessness and risk of mortality and incidence of myocardial infarction and cancer. *Psychosomatic Medicine, 58,* 113–121.

Eysenck, H. J., Grossarth-Maticek, R., & Everitt, B. (1991). Personality, stress, smoking, and genetic predisposition as synergistic risk factors for cancer and coronary heart disease. *The Pavlovian Journal of Biological Science, 26,* 309–322.

Fabes, R. A., & Eisenberg, N. (1997). Regulatory control and adults' stress-related responses to daily life events. *Journal of Personality and Social Psychology, 73*(5), 1107–1117.

Fabes, R. A., Eisenberg, N., Karbon, M., Troyer, D. & Switzer, J. (1994). The relations of children's emotion regulation to their vicarious emotional responses and comforting behaviors. *Child Development, 65,* 1678–1693.

Fabrega, H., & Tyma, S. (1976). Culture, language and the shaping of illness: An illustration based on pain. *Journal of Psychosomatic Research, 20,* 323–337.

Fairburn, C. G., & Wilson, G. T. (1993). Binge eating: Definition and classification. In C. G. Fairburn & G. T. Wilson (Eds.), *Binge eating: Nature, assessment, and treatment* (pp. 3–14). New York: Guilford.

Fallowfield, L. (1997). Breast cancer. In A. Baum, S. Newman, J. Weinman, R. West, & C. McManus (Eds.), *Cambridge handbook of psychology, health, and medicine* (pp. 385–390). Cambridge, UK: Cambridge University Press.

Fang, C. Y., & Myers, H. F. (2001). The effects of racial stressors and hostility on cardiovascular reactivity in African American and Causasian men. *Health Psychology, 20,* 64–70.

Farrell, P. A., Gates, W. K., Maksud, M. G., & Morgan, W. P. (1982). Increases in plasma beta-endorphin/beta-lipotropin immunoreactivity after treadmill running in humans. *Journal of Applied Physiology, 52,* 1245–1249.

Farrington, J. (1999, January). What it means when you hurt. *Current Health, 5,* 166–168.

Farzadegan, H., Hoover, D. R., Astemborski, J., Lyles, C. M., Margolick, J. B., Markham, R. B., Quinn, T. C., & Vlahov, D. (1998). Sex differences in HIV-1 viral load and progression to AIDS. *Lancet, 352,* 1510–1514.

Faucett, J., Gordon, N., & Levine, J. (1994). Differences in postoperative pain severity among four ethnic groups. *Journal of Pain and Symptom Management, 9,* 383–389.

Fava, M., Copeland, P. M., Schweiger, U., & Herzog, D. B. (1989). Neurochemical abnormalities of anorexia nervosa and bulimia nervosa. *American Journal of Psychiatry, 146,* 963–971.

Fawzy, F. I., Fawzy, N. W., Hyun, C. S., Elashoff, R., Guthrie, D., Fahley, J. L., & Morton, D. L. (1993). Malignant melanoma: Effects of an early structured psychiatric intervention, coping, and affective state on recurrence and survival 6 years later. *Archives of General Psychiatry, 50,* 681–689.

Feifer, C., & Tansman, M. (1999). Promoting psychology in diabetes primary care. *Professional Psychology: Research and Practice, 30,* 14–21.

Feingold, A., & Mazzella, R. (1996). Gender differences in body image are increasing. *Psychological Science, 9,* 190–195.

Ferroli, C. (1996, January). Anger could be a fatal fault. *The Saturday Evening Post, 268,* p. 18.

Festinger, L. (1957). *A theory of cognitive dissonance.* Stanford, CA: Stanford University Press.

Feuerstein, M., & Beattie, P. (1995). Biobehavioral factors affecting pain and disability in low back pain: Mechanisms and assessment. *Physical Therapy, 75,* 267–280.

Feuerstein, M., Burrell, L. M., Miller, V. I., Lincoln, A., Huang, G. D., & Berger, R. (1999). Clinical management of carpal tunnel syndrome: A 12-year review of outcomes. *American Journal of Industrial Medicine, 35,* 232–245.

Fiatarone, M. A., O'Neill, E. F., Doyle, N., Clements, K. M., Roberts, S. B., Kehayias, J. J., Lipsitz, L. A., & Evans, W. J. (1993). The Boston FICSIT study: The effects of resistance training and nutritional supplementation on physical frailty in the oldest old. *Journal of the American Geriatrics Society, 41,* 333–337.

Fillingim, R. B. (2000). Sex, gender, and pain: Women and men really are different. *Current Review of Pain, 4,* 24–30.

Fiore, M. C., Smith, S. S., Jorenby, D. E., & Baker, T. B. (1994). The effectiveness of the nicotine patch for smoking cessation: A meta-analysis. *Journal of the American Medical Association, 271,* 1940–1947.

Fireman, P. (1993). Pathophysiology and pharmacotherapy of common upper respiratory disease. *Pharmacotherapy, 13,* 101–143.

Firth-Cozens, J. (1997). Stress in health professionals. In A. Baum, S. Newman, J. Weinman, R. West, & C. McManus (Eds.), *Cambridge handbook of psychology, health and medicine* (pp. 319–322). Cambridge, UK: Cambridge University Press.

Firth-Cozens, J., & Morrison, L. M. (1989). Sources of stress and ways of coping in junior house officers. *Stress Medicine, 5,* 121-126.

Fischman, J. (2000, March 13). The "man's illness" can be deadlier to women who don't spot cardiac trouble. *U. S. News & World Report, 128,* pp. 67–68.

Fishbein, H. D. (1982). The identified patient and stage of family development. *Journal of Marital and Family Therapy, 8,* 57–61.

Fisher, L. & Feldman, S. S. (1998). Familial antecedents of young adult health risk behavior: A longitudinal study. *Journal of Family Psychology, 12*(1), 66–80.

Fisher, P., & Ward, A. (1994). Complementary medicine in Europe. *British Medical Journal, 309,* 107–113.

Fisher, W. A., Fisher, J. D., & Rye, B. J. (1995). Understanding and promoting AIDS-preventive behavior. Insights from the theory of reasoned action. *Health Psychology, 14,* 255–264.

Flack, J. M., Amaro, H., Jenkins, W., Kunitz, S., Levy, J., Mixon, M., & Yu, E. (1995). Epidemiology of minority health. *Health Psychology, 14*(7), 592–600.

Flay, B. R. (1985). Psychosocial approaches to smoking prevention: A review of findings. *Health Psychology, 4,* 448–488.

Fleishman, J. A., & Fogel, B. (1994). Coping and depressive symptoms among people with AIDS. *Health Psychology, 13,* 156–169.

Fleming, R., Baum, A., Gisriel, M. M., & Gatchel, R. J. (1982). Mediating influences of social support on stress at Three Mile Island. *Journal of Human Stress, 8,* 14–22.

Flett, G. L., Hewitt, P. L., Blankstein, K. R., & Mosher, S. W. (1995). Perfectionism, life events, and depressive symptoms: A test of a diathesis-stress model. *Current Psychology: Developmental, Learning, Personality, Social, 14,* 112–137.

Flor, H., & Birbaumer, N. (1993). Comparison of the efficacy of electromyographic biofeedback, cognitive-behavioral therapy, and conservative medical interventions in the treatment of chronic musculoskeletal pain. *Journal of Consulting and Clinical Psychology, 61,* 653–658.

Florian, V., Mikulincer, M., & Taubman, O. (1995). Does hardiness contribute to mental health during a stressful real-life situation? The roles of appraisal and coping. *Journal of Personality and Social Psychology, 68,* 687–695.

Florio, G. A., Donnelly, J. P., & Zevon, M. A. (1998). The structure of work-related stress and coping among oncology nurses in high-stress medical settings: A transactional analysis. *Journal of Occupational Health Psychology, 3,* 227-242.

Foa, E. B., Riggs, D. S., & Gershuny, B. S. (1995). Arousal, numbing, and intrusion: Symptom structure of PTSD following assault. *American Journal of Psychiatry, 152,* 116–120.

Folsom, V., Krahn, D. D., Naim, K., & Gold, L. (1993). The impact of sexual and physical abuse on eating disordered and psychiatric symptoms: A comparison of eating disordered and psychiatric inpatients. *International Journal of Eating Disorders, 13,* 249–257.

Fondacaro, M. R., & Heller, K. (1983). Social support factors and drinking among college student males. *Journal of Youth and Adolescence, 12*, 285–299.

Fordyce, W. E. (1976). *Behavioral methods in chronic pain and illness.* St. Louis: Mosby.

Fordyce, W. E. (1988). Pain and suffering. A reappraisal. *The American Psychologist, 43*, 276–283.

Forster, L. E., Pollow, R., & Stoller, E. P. (1993). Alcohol use and potential risk for alcohol-related adverse drug reactions among community-based elderly. *Journal of Community Health, 18*, 225–239.

Foster, G. (1997). What is a reasonable weight loss? Patients' expectations and evaluations of obesity treatment outcomes. *Journal of Consulting and Clinical Psychology, 65*, 79–85.

Fowles, D. C. (1992). Schizophrenia: Diathesis-stress revisited. *Annual Review of Psychology, 43*, 303–336.

Foxhall, K. (2001, June). Preventing relapse. *Monitor on Psychology* (Special issue on substance abuse), *32*, 46–47.

Frank, E., Sperling, L., & Wu, K. (2000). Aspirin use among women physicians in the United States. *The American Journal of Cardiology, 86*, 465–466.

Frankenhaeuser, M. (1975). Sympathetic-adreno-medullary activity behavior and the psychosocial environment. In P. H. Venables & M. J. Christie (Eds.), *Research in psychophysiology* (pp. 71–94). New York: Wiley.

Frankenhaeuser, M. (1991). The psychophysiology of workload, stress, and health: Comparison between the sexes. *Annals of Behavioral Medicine, 13*, 197–204.

Frankenhaeuser, M., & Gardell, B. (1976). Underload and overload in working life: Outline of a multidisciplinary approach. *Journal of Human Stress, 2*, 35-46.

Frankenhaeuser, M., Lundberg, U., Fredrikson, M., & Melin, B. (1989). Stress on and off the job as related to sex and occupational status in white-collar workers. *Journal of Organizational Behavior, 10*, 321–346.

Fraser, G. E. (1991). Epidemiologic studies of Adventists. *Scope, 27*, 50–55.

Frasure-Smith, N., Lesperance, F., Juneau, M., Talajic, M., & Bourassa, M. G. (1999). Gender, depression, and one-year prognosis after myocardial infarction. *Psychosomatic Medicine, 61*, 26–37.

Frasure-Smith, N., Lesperance, F., & Talajic, M. (1995). The impact of negative emotions on prognosis following myocardial infarction: Is it more than depression. *Health Psychology, 14*, 388–398.

Frasure-Smith, N., & Prince, R. (1989). Long-term follow-up of the Ischemic Heart Disease Life Stress Monitoring Program. *Psychosomatic Medicine, 51*, 485–513.

Frederickson, B. L. (2001). The role of positive emotions in positive psychology: The broaden-and-build theory of positive emotions. *American Psychologist, 56*, 218–226.

Freedman, J. L. (1975). *Crowding and behavior.* New York: Freeman.

Fremont, A. M., & Bird, C. E. (1999). Integrating sociological and biological models. *Journal of Health and Social Behavior, 40*, 126–129.

French, S. A., Story, M., Downes, B., Resnick, M. D., & Blum, R. W. (1995). Frequent dieting among adolescents: Psychosocial and health behavior correlates. *American Journal of Public Health, 85*, 695–701.

Frerichs, R. R. (2000). *John Snow: A portrait.* UCLA Department of Epidemiology (http://www.ph.ucla.edu/epi/snow.html).

Friedman, E. (1992). Fact, fallacy and fairness: The ethics of health care reform. *California Hospitals, 6*, 19–20.

Friedman, H. S., & Booth-Kewley, S. (1987). The "disease-prone personality": A meta-analytic view of the construct. *American Psychologist, 42*(6), 539–555.

Friedman, H. S., Tucker, J. S., Schwartz, J. E., Martin, L. R., Tomlinson-Keasey, C., Wingard, D. L., & Criqui, M. H. (1995a). Childhood conscientiousness and longevity: Health behaviors and cause of death. *Journal of Personality and Social Psychology, 68*, 696–703.

Friedman, H. S., Tucker, J. S., Schwartz, J. E., Martin, L. R., Tomlinson-Keasey, C., Wingard, D. L., & Criqui, M. H. (1995b). Psychosocial and behavioral predictors of longevity: The aging and death of the "termites." *American Psychologist, 50*, 69–78.

Friedman, H. S., Tucker, J. S., Tomlinson-Keasey, C., Schwartz, J. E., Wingard, D. L., & Criqui, M. H. (1993). Does childhood personality predict longevity? *Journal of Personality and Social Psychology, 65*, 176–185.

Friedman, M., & Rosenman, R. H. (1959). Association of specific overt pattern with blood and cardiovascular findings. *Journal of the American Medical Association, 169*, 1286–1296.

Friedman, M., Thoresen, C., & Gill, J. (1986). Alteration of Type A behavior and its effects on cardiac recurrences in post myocardial infarction patients: Summary results of the recurrent coronary prevention project. *American Heart Journal, 112*, 653–665.

Friedman, M. A., & Brownell, K. D. (1995). Psychological correlates of obesity: Moving to the next research generation. *Psychological Bulletin, 117*, 3–20.

Fries, J. F. (1999). *Living well: Taking care of your health in the middle and later years.* Cambridge: Perseus Publishing.

Friese, K. H., Kruse, S., & Moeller, H. (1996). Acute otitis media in children: Comparison between conventional and homeopathic therapy. *HNO, 44*, 462–466.

Fritschi, L., Green, A., & Solomon, P. J. (1992). Sun exposure in Australian adolescents. *Journal of the American Academy of Dermatology, 27*, 25–28.

Froehle, R. M. (1996). Ear infection: A retrospective study examining improvement from chiropractic care and analyzing for influencing factors. *Journal of Manipulative and Physiological Therapeutics, 19*, 169–177.

Fry, A. F., & Hale, S. (1996). Processing speed, working memory, and fluid intelligence: Evidence for a developmental cascade. *Psychological Science, 7*, 237–241.

Fugh-Berman, A. (1997). *Alternative medicine: What works.* Baltimore: Williams & Wilkins.

Fugh-Berman, A. (2000). Herb-drug interactions. *Lancet, 355*, 134–138.

Fuller, T. D., Edwards, J. N., Sermsri, S., & Vorakitphokatorn, S. (1993). Gender and health: Some Asian evidence. *Journal of Health and Social Behavior, 34,* 252–271.

Fulton, J. R., Buechner, J. S., Scott, H., DeBuono, B. A., Feldman, J. P., Smith, R. A., & Kovenock, D. (1991). A study guided by the health belief model of the predictors of breast cancer screening of women ages 40 and older. *Public Health Reports, 106,* 410–419.

Furnham, A., & Baguma, P. (1994). Cross-cultural differences in the evaluation of male and female body shapes. *International Journal of Eating Disorders, 15,* 81–89.

Furukawa, T. (1994). Weight changes and eating attitudes of Japanese adolescents under acculturative stresses: A prospective study. *International Journal of Eating Disorders, 15,* 71–79.

Gailani, M. R., Leffell, D. J., Ziegler, A., Gross, E. G., Brash, D. E., & Bale, A. E. (1996). Relationship between sunlight exposure and a key genetic alteration in basal cell carcinoma. *Journal of the National Cancer Institute, 88,* 349–354.

Gainetdinov, R. R., & Caron, M. G. (1999). Genetic models in pharmacology: Present status and future. *Pharmacological Research, 39,* 403–404.

Galewitz, P. (1999, October 29). AMA joins health information Internet game. New York: Associated Press (wire.ap.org/).

Gallucci, W. T., Baum, A., & Laue, L. (1993). Sex differences in sensitivity of the hypothalamic-pituitary-adrenal axis. *Health Psychology, 12,* 420–425.

Gammon, M. D., John, E. M., & Britton, J. A. (1998). Recreational and occupational physical activities and risk of breast cancer. *Journal of the National Cancer Institute, 90,* 100–117.

Gao, F., Bailes, E., Robertson, D. L., Chen, Y., Rodenburg, C. M., Michael, S. F., Cummins, L. B., Arthur, L. O., Peeters, M., Shaw, G. M., Sharp, P. M., & Hahn, B. H. (1999). Origin of HIV-1 in the chimpanzee Pan troglodytes. *Nature, 397,* 436–441.

Garbarino, J. (1991). The context of child abuse and neglect assessment. In J. C. Westman (Ed.), *Who speaks for the children? The handbook of individual and class child advocacy* (pp. 183–203). Sarasota, FL: Professional Resource Exchange.

Garfinkel, M. S., Schumacher, H. R., & Husain, A. (1994). Evaluation of a yoga based regimen for treatment of osteoarthritis of the hands. *The Journal of Rheumatology, 21,* 2341–2343.

Garfinkel, P. E., & Garner, D. M. (1984). Bulimia in anorexia nervosa. In R. C. Hawkins, II, W. J. Remouw, & P. F. Clement (Eds.), *The binge-purge syndrome: Diagnosis, treatment and research* (pp. 442–446). New York: Springer.

Garmezy, N. (1993). Children in poverty: Resilience despite risk. *Interpersonal and Biological Processes* (Special Issue: *Children and Violence*), *56,* 127–136.

Garner, D. M., & Wolley, S. C. (1991). Confronting the failure of behavioral and dietary treatments for obesity. *Clinical Psychology Review, 11,* 729–780.

Gatchel, R. J. (1993). Psychophysiological disorders: Past and present perspectives. In R. J. Gatchel & E. B. Blanchard (Eds.), *Psychophysiological disorders: Research and clinical applications* (pp. 1–21). Washington, DC: American Psychological Association.

Gatchel, R. J. (1997). Biofeedback. In A. Baum, S. Newman, J. Weinman, R. West, & C. McManus (Eds.), *Cambridge handbook of psychology, health and medicine* (pp. 197–199). Cambridge, England: Cambridge University Press.

Gatchel, R. J. (2001). Biofeedback and self-regulation of physiological activity: A major adjunctive treatment modality in health psychology. In A. Baum, T. A. Revenson, & J. E. Singer (Eds.), *Handbook of health psychology* (pp. 95–103). Mahwah, NJ: Erlbaum.

Gavard, J. A., Lustman, P. J., & Clouse, R. E. (1993). Prevalence of depression in adults with diabetes: An epidemiological evaluation. *Diabetes Care, 16,* 1167–1178.

Gear, R. W., Miaskowski, C., Gordon, N. C., Paul, S. J., Heller, P. H., & Levine, J. D. (1996). Kappa-opioids produce significantly greater analgesia in women than in men. *Nature Medicine, 2,* 1248–1250.

Genuis, M. L. (1995). The use of hypnosis in helping cancer patients control anxiety, pain, and emesis: A review of recent empirical studies. *American Journal of Clinical Hypnosis, 37,* 316–326.

Gerrard, M., Gibbons, F. X., Benthin, A. C., & Hessling, R. M. (1996). A longitudinal study of the reciprocal nature of risk behaviors and cognitions in adolescents: What you do shapes what you think, and vice versa. *Health Psychology, 15,* 344–354.

Gerrard, M., & Luus, C. A. E. (1995). Judgments of vulnerability to pregnancy: The role of risk factors and individual differences. *Personality and Social Psychology Bulletin, 21*(2), 160–171.

Gerstein, D. R., & Green, L. W. (Eds.) (1993). *Preventing drug abuse: What do we know?* Washington, DC: National Academy Press.

Gessner, P. K., & Gessner, T. (1992). *Disulfiram and its metabolite, dithiocarb: Pharmacology and status in the treatment of alcoholism, human immunodeficiency virus infections and heavy metal intoxication.* New York: Chapman & Hall.

Giannini, A. J., & Miller, N. S. (1989). Drug abuse: A biopsychiatric model. *American Family Physician, 40,* 173–182.

Gibbons, F. X., & Gerrard, M. (1995). Predicting young adults' health risk behavior. *Journal of Personality and Social Psychology, 69,* 505–517.

Gibbons, F. X., Gerrard, M., Blanton, H., & Russell, D. W. (1998). Reasoned action and social reaction: Willingness and intention as independent predictors of health risk. *Journal of Personality and Social Psychology, 74,* 1164–1180.

Gibbs, W. W. (1996). Gaining on fat. *Scientific American, 275,* 88–95.

Giedt, J. F. (1997). A psychoneuroimmunological intervention in holistic nursing practice. *Journal of Holistic Nursing, 15,* 112–127.

Gilada, I. S. (1991). AIDS in Asia. *AIDS Care, 3,* 391–394.

Gillcrest A. (1998). Complementary and Alternative Medicine at the NIH. Office of Alternative Medicine. (www.altmed.od.nih.gov/oam).

Gillespie, C., & Gillespie, V. (1986). Reading the danger signs. *Nursing Times, 30,* 24–27.

Gillum, R. F., Mussolino, M. E., & Madans, J. H. (1998). Body fat distribution and hypertension incidence in women and men. The NHANES I epidemiologic follow-up study. *International Journal of Obesity and Related Metabolic Disorders, 22,* 127–134.

Glanz, K., Patterson, R. E., Kristal, A. R., & DiClemente, C. C. (1994). Stages of change in adopting healthy diets: Fat, fiber, and correlates of nutrient intake. *Health Education Quarterly, 21,* 499–519.

Glaser, R., Kiecolt-Glaser, J. K., Speicher, C. E., & Holliday, J. E. (1985). Stress, loneliness, and changes in herpes virus latency. *Journal of Behavioral Medicine, 8,* 249–260.

Glaser, R., Kiecolt-Glaser, J. K., Stout, J. C., Tarr, K. L., Speicher, C. E., & Holliday, J. E. (1985). Stress-related impairments in cellular immunity. *Psychiatry Research, 16,* 233–239.

Glass, D. C. , & Singer, J. E. (1972). *Urban stress: Experiments on noise and social stressors.* New York: Academic Press.

Glauert, H. P., Beaty, M. M., Clark, T. D., Greenwell, W. S., & Chow, C. K. (1990). The effect of dietary selenium on the induction of altered hepatic foci and hepatic tumors by the perosisome proliferator ciprofibrate. *Nutrition and Cancer, 14,* 261–272.

Godin, G., Valois, P., & Lepage, L. (1993). The pattern of influence of perceived behavioral control upon exercising behavior: An application of Ajzen's theory of planned behavior. *Journal of Behavioral Medicine, 16,* 81–102.

Godin, G., Valois, P., Lepage, L., & Desharnais, R. (1992). Predictors of smoking behavior: An application of Ajzen's theory of planned behaviour. *British Journal of Addiction, 87,* 1335–1343.

Goffman, E. (1961). *Asylums.* Garden City, NY: Doubleday.

Gold, P. W., Goodwin, F. K., & Chrousous, G. P. (1988). Clinical and biochemical manifestations of depression: Relation to the neurobiology of stress. *New England Journal of Medicine, 319,* 413–420.

Goldenhar, L. M., Swanson, N. G., Hurrell, J. J., Ruder, A., & Deddens, J. (1998). Stressors and adverse outcomes for female construction workers. *Journal of Occupational Health Psychology, 3,* 19–32.

Goldstein, M. S. (1999). *Alternative health care: Medicine, miracle, or mirage?* Philadelphia: Temple University Press.

Goleman, D. (1995). *Emotional intelligence.* New York: Bantam.

Goleman, D., & Gurin, J. (Eds.). (1993). *Mind-body medicine: How to use your mnd for better health.* New York: Consumer Reports Books.

Gonder-Frederick, L. A., Cox, D. J., Bobbitt, S. A., & Pennebaker, J. W. (1989). Mood changes associated with blood glucose fluctuations in insulin-dependent diabetes mellitus. *Health Psychology, 8,* 45–59.

Goodall, T. A., & Halford, W. K. (1991). Self-management of diabetes mellitus: A critical review. *Health Psychology, 10,* 1–8.

Gordon, C. M., & Carey, M. P. (1996). Alcohol's effects on requisites for sexual risk reduction in men: An initial experimental investigation. *Health Psychology, 15,* 56–60.

Gortmaker, S. L., Must, A., Perrin, J. M., & Sobol, A. M. (1993). Social and economic consequences of overweight in adolescence and young adulthood. *New England Journal of Medicine, 329,* 1008–1012.

Gottesman, D., & Lewis, M. S. (1982). Differences in crisis reactions among cancer and surgery patients. *Journal of Consulting and Clinical Psychology, 50,* 381–388.

Gottlieb, A. M., Killen, J. D., Marlatt, G. A., & Taylor, C. B. (1987). Psychological and pharmacological influences in cigarette smoking withdrawal: Effects of nicotine gum and expectancy on smoking withdrawal symptoms and relapse. *Journal of Consulting and Clinical Psychology, 55,* 606–608.

Gottlieb, B. H. (1996). Theories and practices of mobilizing support in stressful circumstances. In C. L. Cooper (Ed.), *Handbook of stress, medicine, and health* (pp. 339–356). Boca Raton, FL: CRC Press.

Gottlieb, M. S. (1997). Conservative management of spinal osteoarthritis with glucosamine sulfate and chiropractic treatment. *Journal of Manipulative and Physiological Therapeutics, 20,* 400–414.

Graber, J. A., Brooks-Gunn, J., Paikoff, R. L., & Warren, M. P. (1994). Prediction of eating problems: An 8-year study of adolescent girls. *Developmental Psychology, 30,* 823–834.

Graham, J. W., Marks, G., & Hansen, W. B. (1991). Social influence processes affecting adolescent substance use. *Journal of Applied Psychology, 76,* 291–298.

Gramling, S. E., Clawson, E. P., & McDonald, M. K. (1996). Perceptual and cognitive abnormality model of hypochondriasis: Amplification and physiological reactivity in women. *Psychosomatic Medicine, 58,* 423–431.

Grant, L. D., & Haverkamp, B. E. (1995). A cognitive-behavioral approach to chronic pain management. *Journal of Counseling & Development, 74,* 25–32.

Grant, S., Contoreggi, C., & London, E. D. (2000). Drug abusers show impaired performance in a laboratory test of decision-making. *Neuropsychologia, 38,* 1180–1187.

Gray, D. (1985). The treatment strategies of arthritis sufferers. *Social Science and Medicine, 21,* 507–515.

Gray, J. J., Ford, K., & Kelly, L. M. (1987). The prevalence of bulimia in a Black college population. *International Journal of Eating Disorders, 6,* 733–740.

Green, L. W., & Kreuter, M. W. (1990). Health promotion as a public health strategy for the 1990s. *Annual Review of Public Health, 11,* 319–334.

Green, L. W., & McAlister, A. L. (1984). Macro-intervention to support health behavior: Some theoretical perspectives and practical reflections. *Health Education Quarterly, 11,* 323–339.

Greendale, G. A., Barrett-Connor, E., Edelstein, S., Ingles, S., & Halle, R. (1995). Lifetime leisure exercise and osteoporosis: The Rancho Bernardo Study. *American Journal of Epidemiology, 141,* 951–959.

Greenfield, S., & Kaplan, S. (1985). Expanding patient involvement in care: Effects on patient outcomes. *Annals of Internal Medicine, 102,* 520–528.

Greenfield, S., Kaplan, S. H., Ware, J. E., Yano, E. M., & Frank, H. J. (1988). Patients' participation in medical care: Effects on blood sugar control and quality of life in diabetes. *Journal of General Internal Medicine, 3,* 448–457.

Greenglass, E. R., & Noguchi, K. (1996, August). *Longevity, gender and health: A psychocultural perspective.* Paper presented at the meeting of the International Society of Health Psychology, Montreal, CA.

Greenhill, L. L. (1992). Pharmacologic treatment of attention deficit hyperactivity disorder. *Psychiatric Clinics of North America, 15,* 1–27.

Greenlee, R. T., Hill-Harmon, M. B., Murray, T., & Thun, M. (2001). Cancer statistics, 2001. *CA: A Cancer Journal for Clinicians, 51,* 15–36.

Greenwood, D., Szapocnik, J., McIntosh, S., & Antoni, M. (1996). African American women, their families, and HIV/AIDS. In R. J. Resnick & R. H. Rozensky (Eds.), *Health psychology through the life span: Practice and research opportunities* (pp. 349–359). Washington, DC: American Psychological Association.

Greer, S. (1991). Psychological response to cancer and survival. *Psychological Medicine, 21,* 43–49.

Greiger-Zanlungo, P. (2001). HIV and women: An update. *Female Patient, 26,* 12–16.

Griffith, J. (1983). Relationship between acculturation and psychological impairment in adult Mexican Americans. *Hispanic Journal of Behavioral Sciences, 5,* 431–459.

Grilo, C. M., & Pogue-Geile, M. F. (1991). The nature of environmental influences on weight and obesity: A behavior genetic analysis. *Psychological Bulletin, 110*(3), 520–537.

Grob, G. N. (1983). Historical origins of deinstitutionalization. *New Directions for Mental Health Services, 17,* 15–29.

Gross, J. J. (1998). The emerging field of emotion regulation: An integrative review. *Review of General Psychology, 2,* 271–299.

Gross, J. J., & Levenson, R. W. (1997). Emotional suppression: Physiology, self-report, and expressive behavior. *Journal of Personality and Social Psychology, 64,* 970–986.

Grossarth-Maticek, R., Eysenck, H. J., Pfeifer, A., Schmidt, P., & Koppel, G. (1997). The specific action of different personality risk factors on cancer of the breast, cervix, corpus uteri and other types of cancer: A prospective investigation. *Personality and Individual Differences, 23,* 949–960.

Grossman, M., & Wood, W. (1993). Sex differences in intensity of emotional experience: A social role interpretation. *Journal of Personality and Social Psychology, 65,* 1010–1022.

Groth-Marnat, G., & Edkins, G. (1996). Professional psychologists in general health care settings: A review of the financial efficacy of direct treatment interventions. *Professional Psychology: Research and Practice, 27,* 161–174.

Groth-Marnat, G., & Schumaker, J. (1995). Psychologists in disease prevention and health promotion: A review of the cost effectiveness literature. *Psychology, 32,* 1–9.

Grunberg, N. E. (1986). Nicotine as a psychoactive drug: Appetite regulation. *Psychopharmacology Bulletin, 22,* 875–881.

Grunberg, N. E., Brown, K. J., & Klein, L. C. (1997). Tobacco smoking. In A. Baum, S. Newman, J. Weinman, R. West, & C. McManus (Eds.), *Cambridge handbook of psychology, health and medicine* (pp. 606–611). Cambridge, England: Cambridge University Press.

Grunberg, N. E., Faraday, M. M., & Rahman, M. A. (2001). The psychobiology of nicotine self-administration. In A. Baum, T. A. Revenson, & J. E. Singer (Eds.), *Handbook of Health Psychology* (pp. 249–261). Mahwah, NJ: Erlbaum.

Grunberg, N. E., & Straub, R. O. (1992). The role of gender and taste class in the effects of stress on eating. *Health Psychology, 11,* 97–100.

Gullette, E. C., Blumenthal, J. A., Babyak, M., & Jiang, W. (1997). Effects of mental stress on myocardial ischemia during daily life. *Journal of the American Medical Association, 277,* 1521–1526.

Gump, B. B., & Matthews, K. A. (2000). Are vacations good for your health? The 9-year mortality experience after the multiple risk factor intervention trial. *Psychosomatic Medicine, 62,* 608–612.

Gura, T. (1997). Obesity sheds its secrets. *Science, 275,* 751–753.

Gylling, H., & Miettinen, T. A. (1997). Cholesterol absorption, synthesis, and LDL metabolism in NIDDM. *Diabetes Care, 20,* 90–95.

Hackman, R. M. (1998, September). Flavonoids and the French Paradox: Unhealthy-living French have low rate of heart attacks. *USA Today Magazine, 127,* p. 58.

Halaas, J. L., Gajiwala, K. S., Maffei, M., Cohen, S. L., Chait, B. T., Rabinowitz, D., Lallone, R. L., Burley, S. K., & Friedman, J. M. (1995). Weight-reducing effects of the plasma protein encoded by the obese gene. *Science, 269,* 543–545.

Hall, J. A., Irish, J. T., Roter, D. L., Ehrlich, C. M., & Miller, L. H. (1994). Gender in medical encounters: An analysis of physician and patient communication in a primary care setting. *Health Psychology, 13,* 384–392.

Hall, S. M., Herning, R. I., Jones, R. T., Benowitz, N. L., & Jacob, P. (1984). Blood cotinine levels as indicators of smoking treatment outcome. *Clinical Pharmacology and Therapeutics, 35,* 810–814.

Hamila, H. (1996, July). Vitamin C supplementation and common cold symptoms: Problems with inaccurate reviews. *Nutrition, 12,* 804–810.

Hamila, H. (1997). Vitamin C intake and susceptibility to the common cold. *British Journal of Nutrition, 77,* 59.

Hammarstrom, A. (1994). Health consequences of youth unemployment—review from a gender perspective. *Social Science and Medicine, 38,* 699–709.

Hammer, G. P. (1997). *Hepatitis B vaccine acceptance among nursing home workers.* Unpublished doctoral dissertation, Department of Health Policy and Management, Johns Hopkins University, Baltimore.

Haney, D. Q. (2001, April 29). New AIDS research gives sad answer: A cure is unlikely. *Cleveland Plain Dealer*, p. 11-A.

Hanna, E., Defour, M. C., Elliott, S., Stinson, F., & Harford, T. C. (1992). Dying to be equal: Women, alcohol, and cardiovascular disease. *British Journal of Addiction, 87,* 1593–1597.

Harburg, E., Erfurt, J. C., Havenstein, L. S., Chape, C., Schull, W. J., & Schork, M. A. (1973). Socioecological stress, suppressed hostility, skin color, and black-white male blood pressure: Detroit. *Psychosomatic Medicine, 35,* 276–-296.

Hardy, J. D., & Smith, T. W. (1988). Cynical hostility and vulnerability to disease: Social support, life stress, and physiological response to conflict. *Health Psychology, 7,* 447–459.

Harman, D. (1993). Free radical involvement in aging. *Drugs and Aging, 3,* 60–80.

Harris, D. J., & Kuba, S. A. (1997). Ethnocultural identity and eating disorders in women of color. *Professional Psychology: Research and Practice, 28,* 341–347.

Harris, M. A., & Lustman, P. J. (1998). The psychologist in diabetes care. *Clinical Diabetes, 16,* 91–93.

Harris, M. B., Walters, L. C., & Waschull, S. (1991). Gender and ethnic differences in obesity-related behaviors and attitudes in a college sample. *Journal of Applied Social Psychology, 21,* 1545–1566.

Harrison, J. A., Mullen, P. D., & Green, L. W. (1992). A meta-analysis of studies of the health belief model with adults. *Health Education Research, 7,* 107–116.

Hart, S. (1997). Old age and health behaviour. In A. Baum, S. Newman, J. Weinman, R. West, & C. McManus (Eds.), *Cambridge handbook of psychology, health and medicine* (pp. 143–146). Cambridge, UK: Cambridge University Press.

Hartung, B. D. (1987). Acculturation and family variables in substance abuse: An investigation with Mexican American high school males. *Dissertation Abstracts International, 48,* 264.

Haskell, W. L., Luskin, F. M., & Marvasti, F. F. (1999). Complementary/alternative therapies in general medicine: Cardiovascular disease. In J. W. Spencer & J. J. Jacobs (Eds.), *Complementary/alternative medicine: An evidence–based approach* (pp. 90–106). St. Louis, MO: Mosby.

Haslam, R. H., Dalby, J. T., & Rademaker, A. W. (1984). Effects of megavitamin therapy on children with attention deficit disorders. *Pediatrics, 74,* 103–111.

Hatziandreu, E. I., Koplan, J. P., Weinstein, M. C., Caspersen, C. J., & Warner, K. E. (1988). A cost-effectiveness analysis of exercise as a health promotion activity. *American Journal of Public Health, 78,* 1417–1421.

Haug, M. R. (1994). Elderly patients, caregivers, and physicians: Theory and research on health care trends. *Journal of Health and Social Behavior, 35,* 1–12.

Haug, M. R., & Ory, M. G. (1987). Issues in elderly patient-provider interactions. *Research on Aging, 9,* 3–44.

Hawkins, J. D., Catalano, R. F., & Miller, J. Y. (1992). Risk and protective factors for alcohol and other drug problems in adolescence and early adulthood: Implications for substance abuse prevention. *Psychological Bulletin, 112,* 64–105.

Hawkins, W. E. (1992). Problem behaviors and health-enhancing practices of adolescents: A multivariate analysis. *Health Values, 16*(4), 46–54.

Hawley, D. J. (1984). Nontraditional treatment of arthritis, *Clinical Nursing in North America, 19,* 663–667.

Hayflick, L. (1994). *How and why we age.* New York: Ballantine Books.

Haynes, S. G., Feinleib, M., & Kannel, W. B. (1980). The relationship of psycho-social factors in coronary heart disease in the Framingham Study III: Eight year incidence of coronary heart disease. *American Journal of Epidemiology, 111,* 37–58.

Hays, R. B., Turner, H., & Coates, T. J. (1992). Social support, AIDS-related symptoms, and depression among gay men. *Journal of Consulting and Clinical Psychology, 60,* 463–469.

Hazuda, H. P., Mitchell, B. D., Haffner, S. M., & Stern, M. P. (1991). Obesity in Mexican-American subgroups: Findings from the San Antonio Heart Study. *The American Journal of Clinical Nutrition, 53,* 1529S–1534S.

Healthink, 2001. Passive smoke exposure nearly doubles women's risk of heart attack. http://content.health.msn.com/content/article/1758. 52825

Heath, A. C., & Madden, P. A. (1995). Genetic influences on smoking behavior. In J. R. Turner & L. R. Cardon (Eds.), *Behavior genetic approaches in behavioral medicine* (pp. 45–66). New York: Plenum Press.

Heatherton, T. F., Mahamedi, F., Striepe, M., & Field, A. E. (1997). A 10-year longitudinal study of body weight, dieting, and eating disorder symptoms. *Journal of Abnormal Psychology, 106,* 117–125.

Heatherton, T. F., Nichols, P., Mahamedi, F., & Keel, P. (1995). Body weight, dieting, and eating disorder symptoms among college students, 1982 to 1992. *American Journal of Psychiatry, 152,* 1623–1629.

Hebb, D. O. (1955). Drives and the conceptual nervous system. *Psychological Review, 62,* 243–253.

Heckmann, S. M., Heckmann, J. G., Hilz, M. J., Popp, M., Marthol, H., Neundoerfer, B., & Hummel, T. (2001). Oral mucosal blood flow in patients with burning mouth syndrome. *Pain, 90,* 281–286.

Heinrich, R. L., Cohen, M. J., Naliboff, B. D., Collins, G. A., & Bonnebakker, A. D. (1985). Comparing physical and behavior therapy for chronic low back pain on physical abilities, psychological distress, and patients' perceptions. *Journal of Behavioral Medicine, 8,* 61–78.

Heller, K., King, C. M., Arroyo, A. M., & Polk, D. E. (1997). Community-based interventions. In A. Baum, S. Newman, J. Weinman, R. West, & C. McManus (Eds.), *Cambridge handbook of psychology, health and medicine* (pp. 203–206). Cambridge, UK: Cambridge University Press.

Helmrich, S. P., Ragland, D. R., Leung, R. W., & Paffenbarger, R. S. (1991). Physical activity and reduced occurrence of non-insulin-dependent diabetes mellitus. *New England Journal of Medicine, 325,* 147–152.

Helms, J. E. (1995). An update of Helm's white and people of color racial identity models. In J. G. Ponterotto, & M. J. Casas (Eds.), *Handbook of multicultural counseling*. Thousand Oaks, CA: Sage, 181–198.

Helms, J. M. (1987). Acupuncture for the management of primary dysmenorrhea. *Obstetrics and Gynecology, 69*, 51–56.

Helmstetter, F. J., & Bellgowan, P. S. (1994). Hypoalgesia in response to sensitization during acute noise stress. *Behavioral Neuroscience, 108*, 177–185.

Helsing, K. J., Szklo, M., & Comstock, G. W. (1981). Factors associated with mortality after widowhood. *American Journal of Public Health, 71*, 802–809.

Helzer, J. E., Robins, L. N., & McEvoy, L. (1987). Post-traumatic stress disorder in the general population: Findings of the Epidemiologic Catchment Area survey. *New England Journal of Medicine, 317*, 1630–1634.

Henderson, M. M., Kushi, L. H., Thompson, D. J., Gorbach, S. L., Clifford, C. K., Insull, W., Moskowitz, M., & Thompson, R. S. (1990). Feasibility of a randomized trial of a low-fat diet for the prevention of breast cancer: Dietary compliance in the Women's Health Trial Vanguard Study. *Preventive Medicine, 19*, 115–121.

Hennekens, C. H., Buring, J. E., Manson, J. E., Stampfer, M., Rosner, B., Cook, N. R., Belanger, C., LaMotte, F., Gaziano, J. M., Ridker, P. M., Willett, W., & Peto, R. (1996). Lack of effect of long-term supplementation with beta carotene on the incidence of malignant neoplasms and cardiovascular disease. *New England Journal of Medicine, 334*, 1145–1149.

Henningfield, J. E., Cohen, C., & Pickworth, W. B. (1993). Psychopharmacology of nicotine. In C. T. Orleans & J. D. Slade (Eds.), *Nicotine addiction: Principles and management* (pp. 24–45). New York: Oxford University Press.

Herbert, T. B., & Cohen, S. (1993). Stress and immunity in humans: A meta-analytic review. *Psychosomatic Medicine, 55*, 364–379.

Herbert, T. B., & Cohen, S. (1994). Stress and illness. In V. S. Ramachandran (Ed.), *Encyclopedia of human behavior* (vol. 4, pp. 325–332). San Diego, CA: Academic Press.

Herek, G. M., & Capitanio, J. P. (1997). AIDS stigma and contact with persons with AIDS: Effects of direct and vicarious contact. *Journal of Applied Social Psychology, 27*, 1–36.

Hergenrather, J. R., & Rabinowitz, M. (1991). Age-related differences in the organization of children's knowledge of illness. *Developmental Psychology, 27*, 952–959.

Herman, C. P., & Polivy, J. (1975). Anxiety, restraint, and eating behavior. *Journal of Abnormal Psychology, 84*, 666–672.

Herman, C. P., & Polivy, J. (1980). Restrained eating. In A. J. Stunkard (Ed.), *Obesity* (pp. 593–607). Philadelphia: Saunders.

Hermann, C., Kim, M., & Blanchard, E. B. (1995). Behavioral and prophylactic pharmacological intervention studies of pediatric migraine: An exploratory meta-analysis. *Pain, 60*, 239–255.

Herrnstein, R. J. (1990). Rational choice theory: Necessary but not sufficient. *American Psychologist, 45*, 356–367.

Herzog, A. R. (1991). Measurement of vitality in the Americans' changing lives study. *Vital and Health Statistics, Series 5, Comparative International Vital and Health Statistics Reports, 229*, 223–231.

Herzog, A. R., House, J. D., & Morgan, J. N. (1991). Relation of work and retirement to health and well-being in older age. *Psychology and Aging, 6*, 202–211.

Hewison, J. & Dowswell, T. (1994). *Child health care and the working mother*. London: Chapman & Hall.

Higbee, M. D. (1994). Consumer guidelines for using medications wisely. *Generations, 18*, 43–48.

Higgins, E. M., & duVivier, A. W. P. (1994). Alcohol abuse and treatment resistance in skin disease. *Journal of the American Academy of Dermatology, 30*, 1048–1054.

Hilbert, G. A. (1994). Cardiac patients and spouses: Family functioning and emotions. *Clinical Nursing Research, 3*, 243–252.

Hilgard, E. R. (1965). *Hypnotic susceptibility*. New York: Harcourt Brace & World.

Hilgard, E. R. (1992). Dissociation and theories of hypnosis. In E. Fromm & M. R. Nash (Eds.), *Contemporary hypnosis research*. New York: Guilford.

Hill, C. S. (1995). When will adequate pain treatment be the norm? *Journal of the American Medical Association, 274*, 1881–1882.

Hinds, G. M. F., & McCluskey, D. R. (1993). A retrospective study of the chronic fatigue syndrome. *Proceedings of the Royal College of Physicians, 23*, 10–12.

Hinkle, J. S. (1992). Aerobic running behavior and psycho-therapeutics: Implications for sports counseling and psychology. *Journal of Sport Behavior, 15*, 263–277.

Hobfoll, S. E., Jackson, A. P., Lavin, J., Britton, P. J., & Shepherd, J. B. (1993). Safer sex knowledge, behavior, and attitudes of inner-city women. *Health Psychology, 12*, 481–488.

Hochschild, A. R. (1997). *The time bind: When work becomes home, and home becomes work*. New York: Metropolitan Books.

Hoebel, B. G., & Teitelbaum, P. (1966). Effects of forcefeeding and starvation on food intake and body weight in a rat with ventromedial hypothalamic lesions. *Journal of Comparative and Physiological Psychology, 61*, 189–193.

Hofferberth, B. (1994). The effect of Egb 761 in patients with senile dementia of the Alzheimer's type: A double-blind placebo-controlled study on different levels of investigation. *Psychopharmacologia, 9*, 215.

Hoffman, R. M. (2000). Vitamin E supplementation and cardiovascular events in high-risk patients. *New England Journal of Medicine, 342*, 154–160.

Holahan, C. J., Holahan, C. K., Moos, R. H., & Brennan, P. L. (1997). Psychosocial adjustment in patients reporting cardiac illness. *Psychology and Health, 12*, 345–359.

Holahan, C. J., & Moos, R. H. (1982). Social support and adjustment: Predictive benefits of social climate indices. *American Journal of Community Psychology, 10*, 403–415.

Holden, C. (1996). Bright spots in a bleak Russian landscape. *Science, 283*, 1621.

Holden, E. W., Chmielewski, D., Nelson, C., Kager, V. A., & Foltz, L. (1997). Controlling for general and disease-specific effects in child and family adjustment to chronic childhood illness. *Journal of Pediatric Psychology, 22,* 15–28.

Holland, J. C., & Lewis, S. (1996). Emotions and cancer: What do we really know? In D. Goleman & J. Gurin (Eds.), *Mind/body medicine: How to use your mind for better health* (pp. 85–109). Yonkers, NY: Consumer Reports Books.

Holmes, D. S. (1984). Meditation and somatic arousal reduction: A review of the experimental evidence. *American Psychologist, 39,* 1–10.

Holmes, T. H., & Rahe, R. H. (1967). The Social Readjustment Rating Scale. *Journal of Psychosomatic Research, 11,* 213–218.

Holroyd, K. A., France, J. L., Cordingley, G. E., Rokicki, L. A., Kvaal, S. A., Lipchik, G. L., & McCool, H. R. (1995). Enhancing the effectiveness of relaxation-thermal biofeedback training with propranolol hydrochloride. *Journal of Consulting and Clinical Psychology, 63,* 327–330.

Holroyd, K. A., & Penzien, D. B. (1986). Client variables and the behavioral treatment of recurrent tension headache: A meta-analytic review. *Journal of Behavioral Medicine, 9,* 515–536.

Horan, J. J., Laying, F. C., & Pursell, C. H. (1976). Preliminary study of effects of "in vivo" emotive imagery on dental discomfort. *Perceptual and Motor Skills, 42,* 105–106.

Horne, D. J., Vatmanidis, P., & Careri, A. (1994). Preparing patients for invasive medical and surgical procedures. 1: Adding behavioral and cognitive interventions. *Behavioral Medicine, 20,* 5–13.

Hough, E. E., Lewis, F. M., & Woods, N. F. (1991). Family response to mother's chronic illness: Case studies of well- and poorly adjusted families. *Western Journal of Nursing Research, 13,* 568–596.

House, J. S., Lepkowski, K. D., Williams, R., Mero, R. P., Lantz, P. M., Robert, S. A., & Chen, J. (2000). Excess mortality among urban residents: How much, for whom, and why? *American Journal of Public Health* (http://www.apha.org/journal/).

House, J. S., Robbins, C., & Metzner, H. L. (1982). The association of social relationships and activities with mortality: Prospective evidence from the Tecumseh Community Health Study. *American Journal of Epidemiology, 116,* 123–140.

Hrobjartsson, A., & Gotzche, P. C. (2001). Is the placebo powerless? An analysis of clinical trials comparing placebo with no treatment. *New England Journal of Medicine, 344,* 1594–1602.

Hsieh, K. H. (1996). Evaluation of efficacy of traditional Chinese medicines in the treatment of childhood bronchial asthma: Clinical trial, immunological tests and animal study. *Pediatric Allergy and Immunology, 7,* 130–140.

Hsu, L. K. G. (1990). *Eating disorders.* New York: Guilford.

Hughes, J. R. (1993). Treatment of smoking cessation in smokers with past alcohol/drug problems. *Journal of Substance Abuse Treatment, 2,* 181–187.

Hughes, T. A., Ross, H. F., Musa, S., Bhattacherjee, S., Nathan, R. N., Mindham, R. H. S., & Spokes, E. G. S. (2000). A 10-year study of the incidence of and factors predicting dementia in Parkinson's disease. *Neurology, 54*(8), 1596–1602.

Hui, K. S., Liu, J., Makris, N., Gollub, R. L., Chen, A. J. W., Moore, C. I., Kennedy, D. N., Rosen, B. R., & Kwong, K. K. (2000). Acupuncture modulates the limbic system and subcortical gray structures of the human brain: Evidence from fMRI studies in normal subjects. *Human Brain Mapping, 9,* 13–25.

Hull, J. G. (1987). Self-awareness model. In H. T. Blane & K. E. Leonard (Eds.), *Psychological theories of drinking and alcoholism* (pp. 272–304). New York: Guilford.

Hummer, R. A., Rogers, R. G., Nam, C. B., & Ellison, C. G. (1999). Religious involvement and U. S. adult mortality. *Demography, 36,* 273–285.

Humphrey, L. (1987). Comparison of bulimic-anorexic and nondistressed families using structural analysis of social behavior. *Journal of the American Academy of Child and Adolescent Psychiatry, 26,* 248–255.

Hunt, M. E. (1997). A comparison of family of origin factors between children of alcoholics and children of non-alcoholics in a longitudinal panel. *American Journal of Drug and Alcohol Abuse, 23,* 597–613.

Huston, P. (1997). Cardiovascular disease burden shifts. *Lancet, 350,* 121.

Hutchinson, K. E., Collins, F. L., Tassey, J., & Rosenberg, E. (1996). Stress, naltrexone, and the reinforcement value of nicotine. *Experimental and Clinical Psychopharmacology, 4,* 431–437.

Hwang, M. Y., & Molter, R. M. (1998). Alternative choices: What it means to use nonconventional medical therapy. *Journal of the American Medical Association, 280,* 1640.

Hygge, S. (1997). Noise: Effects on health. In A. Baum, S. Newman, J. Weinman, R. West, & C. McManus (Eds.), *Cambridge handbook of psychology, health and medicine* (pp. 139–143). Cambridge, UK: Cambridge University Press.

Hyman, R. B., Baker, S., Ephraim, R., Moadel, A., & Philip, J. (1994). Health Belief Model variables as predictors of screening mammography utilization. *Journal of Behavior Medicine, 17,* 391–406.

Ickovics, J. R., Grigorenko, E., Beren, S. E., Druley, J. A., Morrill, A. C., & Rodin, J. (1998). Long-term effects of HIV counseling and testing for women: Behavioral and psychological consequences are limited at 18 months posttest. *Health Psychology, 17,* 395–402.

Ickovics, J. R., Thayaparan, B., & Ethier, K. A. (2001). Women and AIDS: A contextual analysis. In A. Baum, T. A. Revenson, & J. E. Singer (Eds.), *Handbook of health psychology* (pp. 817–839). Mahwah, NJ: Erlbaum.

Ickovics, J. R., Viscoli, C. M., & Horwitz, R. I. (1997). Functional recovery after myocardial infarction in men: The independent effects of social class. *Annals of Internal Medicine, 127,* 518–525.

Ingham, R., Woodcock, A., & Stenner, S. (1991). Getting to know you: Young people's knowledge of their partners at first intercourse. *Journal of Community and Applied Social Psychology* (Special issue: Social dimensions of AIDS), *1,* 117–132.

Ingledew, D. K., Hardy, L., & Cooper, C. L. (1997). Do resources bolster coping and does coping buffer stress? An organizational study with longitudinal aspect and control for negative affectivity. *Journal of Occupational Health Psychology, 2,* 118–133.

Inglehart, R. (1990). *Culture shift in advanced industrial society.* Princeton, NJ: Princeton University Press.

Ironson, G., Schneiderman, H., Kumar, M., & Antoni, M. H. (1994). Psychosocial stress, endocrine and immune response in HIV-1 disease. *Homeostasis in Health & Disease, 35,* 137–148.

Ishibe, N., Hankinson, S. E., Colditz, G. A., Spiegelman, D., Willett, W. C., Speizer, F. E., Kelsey, K. T., & Hunter, D. J. (1998). Cigarette smoking, cytochrome P450 1A1 polymorphisms, and breast cancer risk in the Nurses' Health Study. *Cancer Research, 58,* 667–671.

Itil, T., & Martorano, D. (1995). Natural substances in psychiatry (ginkgo biloba in dementia). *Psychopharmacology Bulletin, 31,* 147–158.

Jablon, S., Hrubec, Z., & Boice, J. D. (1991). Cancer in populations living near nuclear facilities. A survey of mortality nationwide and incidence in two states. *Journal of the American Medical Association, 265,* 1403–1408.

Jacchia, G. E., Butler, U. P., Innocenti, M., & Capone, A. (1994). Low-back pain in athletes: Pathogenetic mechanisms and therapy. *La Chirurgia degli organi di movimento, 79,* 47–53.

Jackson, J. S. (1996). A life-course perspective on physical and psychological health. In R. J. Resnick & R. H. Rozensky (Eds.), *Health psychology through the lifespan* (pp. 39–57). Washington, DC: American Psychological Association.

Jackson, K. M., & Aiken, L. S. (2000). A psychosocial model of sun protection and sunbathing in young women: The impact of health beliefs, attitudes, norms, and self-efficacy for sun protection. *Health Psychology, 19,* 469–478.

Jackson, R. L., Maier, S. F., & Coon, D. J. (1979). Long-term analgesic effects of inescapable shock and learned helplessness. *Science, 206,* 91–93.

Jacobs, A. L., Kurtz, R. M., & Strube, M. J. (1995). Hypnotic analgesia, expectancy effects, and choice of design: A reexamination. *International Journal of Clinical and Experimental Hypnosis, 43,* 55–69.

Jacobs, B. L. (1994). Serotonin, motor activity, and depression-related disorders. *American Scientist, 82,* 456–463.

Jacobs, D. F. (1988). Marketing psychological services in the public sector. *Psychotherapy: Theory, Research, Practice, Training. Special Issue: Psychotherapy and the New Health Care System, 25,* 377–386.

Jacobs, D. R., Muldoon, M. F., & Rastam, L. (1995). Invited commentary: Low blood cholesterol, nonillness mortality, and other nonatherosclerotic disease mortality: A search for causes and confounders. *American Journal of Epidemiology, 141,* 518–522.

Jacobs, D. R., Pereira, M. A., Meyer, K. A., & Kushi, L.H. (2000). Fiber from whole grains, but not refined grains, is inversely associated with all-cause mortality in older women: The Iowa Women's Health Study. *Journal of the American College of Nutrition, 19,* 326S–330S.

Jacobs, J. J. (1999). Looking ahead: Complementary/alternative medicine in the twenty-first century. In J. W. Spencer & J. J. Jacobs (Eds.), *Complementary/alternative medicine: An evidence-based approach* (pp. 411–420). St. Louis, MO: Mosby.

Jacobson, A. M. (1996). The psychological care of patients with insulin-dependent diabetes mellitus. *New England Journal of Medicine, 334,* 1249–1253.

Jacobson, E. (1938). *Progressive relaxation.* Chicago: University of Chicago Press.

Jahoda, M. (1979). The impact of unemployment in the 1930s and the 1970s. *Bulletin of the British Psychological Society, 32,* 309–314.

James, F. R., Large, R. G., Bushnell, J. A., & Wells, J. E. (1991). Epidemiology of pain in New Zealand. *Pain, 44,* 279–283.

Janis, I. L. (1958). *Psychological stress.* New York: Wiley.

Janis, I. L., & Feshbach, S. (1953). Effects of fear-arousing communications. *Journal of Abnormal and Social Psychology, 48,* 78–92.

Janz, N. K., & Becker, M. H. (1984). The Health Belief Model: A decade later. *Health Education Quarterly, 11,* 1–47.

Jargowsky, P. A. (1997). Metropolitan restructuring and urban policy. *Stanford Law and Policy Review, 8,* 47–56.

Jarvis, M. J., & Sutherland, G. (2001). Tobacco smoking. In D. W. Johnston & M. Johnson (Eds.), *Health Psychology* (pp. 645–674). Amsterdam: Elsevier

Jarvis, S. (1994). *Drug prevention with youth.* Tulsa, OK: National Resource Center for Youth Services.

Jeffery, R. W., Forster, S. A., French, S. H., Kelder, H. A., Lando, H. A., McGovern, D. R., Jacobs, D. R., & Baxter, J. E. (1993). The healthy worker project: A worksite intervention for weight control and smoking cessation. *American Journal of Public Health, 83,* 395–401.

Jemmott, J. B., Croyle, R. T., & Ditto, P. H. (1988). Commonsense epidemiology: Self-based judgments from laypersons and physicians. *Health Psychology, 7,* 55–73.

Jemmott, J. B., & Jemmott, L. S. (2000), HIV behavioral interventions for adolescents in community settings. In J. L. Peterson & R. J. DiClemente (Eds.), *Handbook of HIV prevention* (pp. 337–356). New York: Kluwer Academic/Plenum.

Jemmott, J. B., Jemmott, L. S., & Fong, G. T. (1992). Reductions in HIV risk-associated sexual behaviors among black male adolescents: Effects of an AIDS prevention intervention. *American Journal of Public Health, 82,* 372–377.

Jemmott, J. B., Jemmott, L. W., Spears, H., Hewitt, N., & Cruz-Collins, M. (1992). Self-efficacy, hedonistic expectancies, and condom-use intentions among inner-city black adolescent women: A social cognitive approach to AIDS risk behavior. *Journal of Adolescent Health, 13,* 512–519.

Jemmott, J. B., & Locke, S. E. (1984). Psychosocial factors, immunologic mediation, and human susceptibility to infectious disease: How much do we know? *Psychological Bulletin, 95,* 78–108.

Jencks, C. (1994). *The homeless*. Cambridge, MA: Harvard University Press.

Jennings, G., Nelson, L., Nestel, P., Esler, M., Korner, P., Burton, D., & Bazelmans, J. (1986). The effects of changes in physical activity on major cardiovascular risk factors, hemodynamics, sympathetic function, and glucose utilization in man: A controlled study of four levels of activity. *Circulation, 73,* 30–40.

Jensen, M. P., & Karoly, P. (1991). Coping beliefs, coping efforts, and adjustment to chronic pain. *Journal of Consulting and Clinical Psychology, 59,* 431–438.

Jensen, M. P., & McFarland, C. A. (1993). Increasing the reliability and validity of pain intensity measurement in chronic pain patients. *Pain, 55,* 195–203.

Jessor, R. (1987). Problem-behavior theory, psychosocial development, and adolescent problem drinking. *British Journal of Addiction,* Special Issue: Psychology and addiction, *82,* 331–342.

Jessor, R. (1992). Risk behavior in adolescence: A psychosocial framework for understanding and action. *Developmental Review, 12*(4), 374–390.

Jin, P. (1992). Efficacy of T'ai Chi, brisk walking, meditation, and reading in reducing mental and emotional stress. *Journal of Psychosomatic Research, 36,* 361–370.

Johnson, K. W., Anderson, N. B., Bastida, E., Kramer, B. J., Williams, D., & Wong, M. (1995). Macrosocial and environmental influences on minority health. *Health Psychology, 14*(7), 601–612.

Johnson, M., & Vogele, C. (1993). Benefits of psychological preparation for surgery: A meta-analysis. *Annals of Behavioral Medicine, 15,* 245–256.

Johnston, L. D. (1996, December 19) Monitoring the future study of drug use. Ann Arbor: News and Information Services, University of Michigan.

Johnston, L. D., Bachman, J. G., & O'Malley, P. M. (1999, December 17.) *Drug trends in 1999 among American teens are mixed* (pp. 275–281). Ann Arbor: News and Information Services, University of Michigan.

Johnston, M., & Vogele, C. (1993). Benefits of psychological preparation for surgery: A meta-analysis. *Annals of Behavioral Medicine, 15,* 245–256.

Jonas, J. M., & Gold, M. S. (1988). The use of opiate antagonists in treating bulimia: A study of low-dose versus high-dose naltrexone. *Psychiatry Research, 24,* 195–199.

Jonas, W. (1996). Safety in complementary medicine. In E. Ernst (Ed.), *Complementary medicine: An objective appraisal,* Oxford, England: Butterworth-Heinemann.

Jones, A., Johnson, Z. C., Robinson, J. D., & Ybarra, M. A. (1998). Cholesterol and aggression: An ethnocultural perspective. *Journal of Clinical Psychology in Medical Settings, 5,* 249–258.

Jones, J. L., & Leary, M. R. (1994). Effects of appearance-based admonitions against sun exposure on tanning intentions in young adults. *Health Psychology, 13,* 86–90.

Jones, R. T. (1992). What have we learned from nicotine, cocaine, and marijuana about addiction? In C. P. O'Brien & J. H. Jaffe (Eds.), *Addictive states* (pp. 109–122). New York: Raven Press.

Jorgensen, R. S., Johnson, B. T., Kolodziej, M. E., & Schreer, G. E. (1996). Elevated blood pressure and personality: A meta-analytic review. *Psychological Bulletin, 120,* 293–320.

Julien, R. M. (2001). *A primer of drug action* (9th ed.). New York: Worth.

Kabakian-Khasholian, T., Campbell, O., Shediac-Rizkaliah, M., & Ghorayeb, F. (2000). Women's experiences of maternity care: Satisfaction or passivity? *Social Science and Medicine, 51,* 103–113.

Kabat-Zinn, J. (1982). An outpatient program in behavioral medicine for chronic pain patients based on the practice of mindfulness meditation: Theoretical considerations and preliminary results. *General Hospital Psychiatry, 4,* 33–47.

Kaiser Foundation. (2000, March). *Uninsured in America: Key facts.* The Kaiser Commission on Medicaid and the uninsured. www.kff.org/content/2000.

Kalichman, S. C. (1998). *Understanding AIDS: Advances in research and treatment* (2nd ed.). Washington, DC: American Psychological Association.

Kalichman, S. C., Carey, M. P., & Johnson, B. T. (1996). Prevention of sexually transmitted HIV infection: A meta-analytic review of the behavioral outcome literature. *Annals of Behavioral Medicine, 18,* 6–15.

Kalichman, S. C., & Coley, B. (1995). Context framing to enhance HIV-antibody-testing messages targeted to African American women. *Health Psychology, 14,* 247–254.

Kalichman, S. C., & Hospers, H. J. (1997). Efficacy of behavioral-skills enhancement HIV risk-reduction interventions in community settings. *AIDS, 11* (supplement A), S191–S199.

Kalichman, S. C., Kelly, J. A., Hunter, T. L., Murphy, D. A., & Tyler, R. (1993). Culturally tailored HIV-AIDS risk-reduction messages targeted to African-American urban women: Impact on risk sensitization and risk reduction. *Journal of Consulting and Clinical Psychology, 61,* 291–295.

Kalichman, S. C., Nachimson, D., Cherry, C., & Williams, E. (1998). AIDS treatment advances and behavioral prevention setbacks: Preliminary assessment of reduced perceived threat of HIV-AIDS. *Health Psychology, 17,* 546–550.

Kalichman, S. C., Roffman, R. A., Picciano, J. F., & Bolan, M. (1998). Risk for HIV infection among bisexual men seeking HIV-prevention services and risks posed to their female partners. *Health Psychology, 17,* 320–327.

Kamarck, T. W., & Lichtenstein, E. (1985). Current trends in clinic-based smoking control. *Annals of Behavioral Medicine, 7,* 19–23.

Kamarck, T. W., & Lichtenstein, E. (1998). Program adherence and coping strategies as predictors of success in a smoking treatment program. *Health Psychology, 7,* 557–574.

Kaminski, P. L., & McNamara, K. (1996). A treatment for college women at risk for bulimia: A controlled evaluation. *Journal of Counseling and Development, 74,* 288–374.

Kandel, D. B., & Davies, M. (1996). High school students who use crack and other drugs. *Archives of General Psychiatry, 53,* 71–80.

Kane, R. L., Olsen, D., & Leymaster, C. (1974). Manipulating the patient: A comparison of the effectiveness of physician and chiropractor care. *Lancet,* 1333–1336.

Kanner, A. D., Coyne, J. C., Schaefer, C., & Lazarus, R. S. (1981). Comparison of two modes of stress measurement: Daily hassles and uplifts versus major life events. *Journal of Behavioral Medicine, 4,* 1–39.

Kanowski, S., Hermann, W. M., Stephan, K., Wierich, W., & Hoerr, R. (1996). Proof of efficacy of the ginkbo biloba special extract Egb 761 in outpatients suffering from mild to moderate primary degenerative dementia of the Alzheimer type or multi-infarct dementia. *Pharmacopsychiatry, 29,* 47–56.

Kaplan, G. A., & Keil, J. E. (1993). Socioeconomic factors and cardiovascular disease: A review of the literature. *Circulation, 88,* 1973–1998.

Kaplan, G. A., & Reynolds, P. (1988). Depression and cancer mortality and morbidity: Prospective evidence from the Alameda County study. *Journal of Behavioral Medicine, 11,* 1–13.

Kaplan, G. A., Salonen, J. T., Cohen, R. D., Brand, R. J., Syme, S. L., & Puska, P. (1988). Social connections and mortality from all causes and from cardiovascular disease: Prospective evidence from eastern Finland. *American Journal of Epidemiology, 128,* 370–380.

Kaplan, H. B., & Johnson, R. J. (1992). Relationships between circumstances surrounding initial illicit drug use and escalation of drug use: Moderating effects of gender and early adolescent experiences. In M. D. Glantz & R. W. Pickens (Eds.), *Vulnerability to drug abuse* (pp. 299–358). Washington, DC: American Psychological Association.

Kaplan, R. M. (1993). *The Hippocratic predicament: Affordability, access, and accountability in American medicine.* San Diego: Academic Press.

Kaplan, R. M. (2000). Two pathways to prevention. *American Psychologist, 55*(4), 382–396.

Kaplan, R. M., & Bush, J. W. (1982). Health-related quality of life measurement for evaluation research and policy analysis. *Health Psychology, 1,* 61–80.

Kark, J. D., Shemi, G., Friedlander, Y., Martin, O., Manor, O., & Blondheim, S. H.(1996). Does religious observance promote health? Mortality in secular vs. religious kibbutzim in Israel. *American Journal of Public Health, 86,* 341–346.

Karoly, P. (1988). Pain assessment in children I: Concepts and measurement strategies. In P. Karoly (Ed.), *Handbook of child health assessment: Biopsychosocial perspectives* (pp. 357–386). New York: Wiley.

Kasl, S. V. (1997). Unemployment and health. In A. Baum, S. Newman, J. Weinman, R. West, & C. McManus (Eds.), *Cambridge handbook of psychology, health and medicine* (pp. 186–189). Cambridge, UK: Cambridge University Press.

Kasl, S. V., & Cobb, S. (1966). Health behavior, illness behavior, and sick-role behavior. *Archives of Environmental Health, 12,* 531–541.

Kassirer, J. P. (2000, November/December). Patients, physicians, and the Internet. *Health Affairs, 19,* 115–123.

Katon, W., & Sullivan, M. D. (1990). Depression and chronic medical illness. *Journal of Clinical Psychiatry, 51,* 12–14.

Katzmarzyk, P. T., Mahaney, M. C., Blangero, J., Quek, J. J., & Malina, R. M. (1999). Potential effects of ethnicity in genetic and environmental sources of variability in the stature, mass, and body index of children. *Human Biology, 71,* 977–987.

Kawachi, I., Colditz, G. A., Stampfer, M. J., Willett, W. C., Manson, J. E., Rosner, B., Speizer, F. E., & Hennekens, C. H. (1994). Smoking cessation and time course of decreased risks of coronary heart disease in middle-aged women. *Archives of Internal Medicine, 154,* 169–175.

Keane, T. M., & Wolfe, J. (1990). Comorbidity in post-traumatic stress disorder: An analysis of community and clinical studies. *Journal of Applied Social Psychology, 20,* 1776–1788.

Keefe, F. J. (1982). Behavioral assessment and treatment of chronic pain: Current status and future directions. *Journal of Consulting and Clinical Psychology, 50,* 896–911.

Keefe, F. J., Dunsmore, J., & Burnett, R. (1992). Behavioral and cognitive-behavioral approaches to chronic pain: Recent advances and future directions. *Journal of Consulting and Clinical Psychology, 60,* 528–536.

Keesey, R. E., & Corbett, S. W. (1983). Metabolic defense of the body weight set-point. In A. J. Stunkard & E. Stellar (Eds.), *Eating and its disorders* (pp. 327–331). New York: Raven Press.

Keesling, B., & Friedman, H. S. (1987). Psychosocial factors in sunbathing and sunscreen use. *Health Psychology, 6,* 477–493.

Kelley, J. A., & Kalichman, S. C. (1998). Reinforcement value of unsafe sex as a predictor of condom use and continued HIV/AIDS risk behavior among gay and bisexual men. *Health Psychology, 17,* 328–325.

Kelly, E. L., & Conley, J. J. (1987). Personality and compatibility: A prospective analysis of marital stability and marital satisfaction. *Journal of Personality and Social Psychology, 52,* 27–40.

Keltner, D., Ellsworth, P. C., & Edwards, K. (1993). Beyond simple pessimism: Effects of sadness and anger on social perception. *Journal of Personality and Social Psychology, 64,* 740–752.

Kemeny, M., Weiner, H., Taylor, S. E., & Schneider, S. (1994). Repeated bereavement, depressed mood, and immune parameters in HIV seropositive and seronegative gay men. *Health Psychology, 13,* 14–24.

Kempen, G. I., Jelicic, M., & Ormel, J. (1997). Personality, chronic medical morbidity, and health-related quality of life among older persons. *Health Psychology, 16,* 539–546.

Kendler, K. S., Neale, M., Kessler, R., Heath, A., & Eaves, L. (1993). A twin study of recent life events and difficulties. *Archives of General Psychiatry, 50,* 789–796.

Kendler, K. S., Preschott, C. A., Neale, M. C., & Pedersen, N. L. (1997). Temperance Board registration for alcohol abuse in a national sample of Swedish male twins, born 1902 to 1949. *Archives of General Psychiatry, 54,* 178–184.

Kessler, R. C., Foster, C., Joseph, J., Ostrow, D., Wortman, C., Phair, J., & Chmiel, J. (1991). Stressful life events and symptom onset in HIV infection. *American Journal of Psychiatry, 148,* 733–738.

Keys, A., Brozek, J., Henschel, A., Mickelsen, O., & Taylor, H. L. (1950). *The biology of human starvation.* Minneapolis: University of Minnesota Press.

Kiecolt-Glaser, J. K., Dura, J. R., Speicher, C. E., Trask, O. J., & Glaser, R. (1991). Spousal caregivers of dementia victims: Longitudinal changes in immunity and health. *Psychosomatic Medicine, 53,* 345–362.

Kiecolt-Glaser, J. K., Fisher, L., Ogrocki, P., Stout, J. C., Speicher, C. E., & Glaser, R. (1987). Marital quality, marital disruption, and immune function. *Psychosomatic Medicine, 49,* 13–34.

Kiecolt-Glaser, J. K., Garner, W., Speicher, C. E., Penn, G. M., Holliday, J. E., & Glaser, R. (1984). Psychosocial modifiers of immunocompetence in medical students. *Psychosomatic Medicine, 46,* 7–14.

Kiecolt-Glaser, J. K., & Glaser, R. (1989). Psychoneuroimmunology: Past, present, and future. *Health Psychology, 8,* 677–682.

Kiecolt-Glaser, J. K., & Glaser, R. (1995). Psychoneuroimmunology and health consequences: Data and shared mechanisms. *Psychosomatic Medicine, 57,* 269–274.

Kiecolt-Glaser, J. K., Glaser, R., Gravenstein, S., Malarkey, W. B., & Sheridan, J. (1996). Chronic stress alters the immune response to influenza virus vaccine in older adults. *Proceedings of the National Academy of Science, 93,* 3043–3047.

Kiecolt-Glaser, J. K., Glaser, R., Strain, E., Stout, J., Tarr, K., Holliday, J., & Speicher, C. (1986). Modulation of cellular immunity in medical students. *Journal of Behavioral Medicine, 9,* 5–21.

Kiecolt-Glaser, J. K., Glaser, R., & Williger, D. (1985). Psychosocial enhancement of immunocompetence in a geriatric population. *Health Psychology, 4,* 25–41.

Kiecolt-Glaser, J. K., Malarkey, W. B., Cacioppo, J. T., & Glaser, R. (1994). Stressful personal relationships: Immune and endocrine function. In R. Glaser & J. K. Kiecolt-Glaser (Eds.), *Handbook of human stress and immunity* (pp. 321–339). San Diego, CA: Academic Press.

Kiecolt-Glaser, J. K., Newton, T., Cacioppo, J. T., MacCallum, R. C., Glaser, R., & Malarkey, W. B. (1997). Marital conflict and endocrine function: Are men really more physiologically affected than women? *Journal of Consulting and Clinical Psychology, 64,* 324–332.

Kiecolt-Glaser, J. K., Page, G. G., Marucha, P. T., MacCallum, R. C., & Glaser, R. (1998). Psychological influences on surgical recovery: Perspectives from psychoneuroimmunology. *American Psychologist, 53,* 1209–1218.

Kiecolt-Glaser, J. K., & Williams, D. A. (1987). Self-blame, compliance, and distress among burn patients. *Journal of Personality and Social Psychology, 53,* 187–193.

Kien, C. L. (1990). Current controversies in nutrition. *Current Problems in Pediatrics, 20,* 349–408.

Kihlstrom, J. F. (1985). Hypnosis. *Annual Review of Psychology, 36,* 385–418.

Kilbourne, J. (1994). Still killing us softly: Advertising and the obsession with thinness. In P. Fallon, M. A. Katzman, & S. C. Wolley (Eds.), *Feminist perspectives on eating disorders* (pp. 395–418). New York: Guilford.

Killen, J. D., Fortmann, S. P., Kraemer, H. C., & Varady, A. (1992). Who will relapse? Symptoms of nicotine dependence predict long-term relapse after smoking cessation. *Journal of Consulting and Clinical Psychology, 60,* 797–801.

Kim, E. L., Larimer, M. E., Walker, D. D., & Marlatt, G. A. (1997). Relationship of alcohol use to other health behaviors among college students. *Psychology of Addictive Behaviors, 11,* 166–173.

Kim, J., & Dellon, A. L. (2001). Pain at the site of tarsal tunnel incision due to neuroma of the posterior branch of the saphenous nerve. *Journal of the American Podiatric Medical Association, 91,* 109–114.

King, D. A., Peragallo-Dittko, V., Polonsky, W. H., Prochaska, J. O., & Vinicor, F. (1998). Strategies for improving self-care. *Patient Care, 32,* 91–111.

Kinloch-de Loes, S., Hirschel, B. J., Hoen, B., Cooper, D. A., Tindal, B., Carr, A., Saurat, J. H., Clumeck, N., Lazzarin, A., & Mathiesen, L. (1995). A controlled trial of zidovudine in primary human immunodeficiency virus infection. *The New England Journal of Medicine, 333,* 408–413.

Kinney, R. K., Gatchel, R. J., Polatin, P. B., Fogarty, W. , & Mayer, T. (1993). Prevalence of psychopathology in acute and chronic low back pain patients. *Journal of Occupational Rehabilitation, 3,* 95–103.

Kiyak, H. A., Vitaliano, P. P., & Crinean, J. (1988). Patients' expectations as predictors of orthographic surgery outcomes. *Health Psychology, 7,* 251–268.

Klag, M. J., Ford, D. E., Mead, L. A., He, J., Whelton, P. K., Liang, K. Y., & Levine, D. M. (1993). Serum cholesterol in young men and subsequent cardiovascular disease. *New England Journal of Medicine, 328,* 313–318.

Klesges, R. C., Shelton, M. L., & Klesges, L. M. (1993). Effects of television on metabolic rate: Potential implications for childhood obesity. *Pediatrics, 91,* 281–286.

Kliewer, W. (1991). Coping in middle childhood: Relations to competence, Type A behavior, monitoring, blunting, and locus of control. *Developmental Psychology, 27,* 689–697.

Kline, A., & Strickler, J. (1993). Perceptions of risk for AIDS among women in drug treatment. *Health Psychology, 12,* 313–323.

Kline, A., & VanLandingham, M. (1994). HIV-infected women and sexual risk reduction: The relevance of existing models of behavior change. *AIDS Education and Prevention, 6,* 390–402.

Kline, D. W., & Schieber, F. (1985). Vision and aging. In J. E. Birren & K. W. Schaie (Eds.), *Handbook of the psychology of aging* (2nd ed., pp. 296–331*).* New York: Van Nostrand Reinhold.

Klonoff, E. A., & Landrine, H. (1993). Appraisal and response to pain may be a function of its bodily location. *Journal of Psychosomatic Research, 37,* 661–670.

Klonoff, E. A., & Landrine, H. (1994). Culture and gender diversity in commonsense beliefs about the causes of six illnesses. *Journal of Behavioral Medicine, 17,* 407–418.

Kluver, H., & Bucy, P. C. (1939). Preliminary analysis of functions of the temporal lobes in monkeys. *Archives of Neurology and Psychiatry, 42,* 979–1000.

Knipschild, P. (1994). Systematic reviews: Some examples. *British Medical Journal, 309,* 719–721.

Kobasa, S. C., Maddi, S. R., & Kahn, S. (1982). Hardiness and health: A prospective study. *Journal of Personality and Social Psychology, 42(1),* 168–277.

Kobasa, S. C., Maddi, S. R., Puccetti, M. C., & Zola, M. A. (1985). Effectiveness of hardiness, exercise and social support as resources against illness. *Journal of Psychosomatic Research, 29,* 525–533.

Koenig, H. G., & Larson, D. B. (1998). Use of hospital services, religious attendance, and religious affiliation. *Southern Medical Journal, 91,* 925–932.

Kohn, P. M., Lafreniere, K., & Gurevich, M. (1991). Hassles, health, and personality. *Journal of Personality and Social Psychology, 61,* 478–482.

Kok, G. (1997). Health education. In A. Baum, S. Newman, J. Weinman, R. West, & C. McManus (Eds.), *Cambridge handbook of psychology, health and medicine* (pp. 216–219). Cambridge, UK: Cambridge University Press.

Kolata, G. (1998). For unlucky few, gene sends HIV on wild stampede. *The New York Times* (www.nytimes.com).

Kolata, G. (1999, March 9). Pushing limits of the human life span. *The New York Times* (www.nytimes.com/library/national/science).

Kolb, B., & Wishaw, I. Q. (2001). *Introduction to brain and behavior.* New York: Worth.

Komaroff, A. L., & Buchwald, D. (1991). Symptoms and signs of chronic fatigue syndrome. *Reviews of Infectious Diseases, 13,* Supplement 1: S8–11.

Kop, W. J., Gottdiener, J. S., & Krantz, D. S. (2001). Stress and silent ischemia. In A. Baum, T. A. Revenson, & J. E. Singer (Eds.), *Handbook of health psychology* (pp. 669–682). Mahwah, NJ: Erlbaum.

Kop, W. J., & Krantz, D. S. (1997). Type A behaviour, hostility and coronary artery disease. In A. Baum, S. Newman, J. Weinman, R. West, & C. McManus (Eds.), *Cambridge handbook of psychology, health and medicine* (pp. 183–186). Cambridge, UK: Cambridge University Press.

Koriat, A., Melkman, R., Averill, J. R., & Lazarus, R. S. (1972). The self-control of emotional reactions to a stressful film. *Journal of Personality, 40,* 601–619.

Kotre, J., & Hall, E. (1990). *Seasons of life: Our dramatic journey from birth to death.* Boston, MA: Little, Brown.

Kottke, T. E., Puska, P., Salonen, J. T., Tuomilehto, J., & Nissinen, A. (1984). Changes in perceived heart disease risk and health during a community-based heart disease prevention program: The North Karelia project. *American Journal of Public Health, 74,* 1404–1405.

Kozlowski, L. T., Appel, C. P., Fredcker, R. C., & Khouw, W. (1982). Nicotine, a prescribable drug available without prescription. *Lancet, 6,* 334.

Krahn, M. D., Mahoney, J. E., Eckman, M. H., Trachtenberg, J., Pauker, S. G., & Detsky, A. S. (1994). Screening for prostate cancer. A decision analytic view. *Journal of the American Medical Association, 272,* 773–780.

Kral, J. G. (1992). Overview of surgical techniques for treating obesity. *American Journal of Clinical Nutrition, 55,* 552–555.

Krantz, D. S., Glass, D. G., & Snyder, M. L. (1974). Helplessness, stress level, and the coronary-prone behavior pattern. *Journal of Experimental Social Psychology, 10,* 284–300.

Krantz, D. S., & Manuck, S. B. (1984). Acute psychophysiologic reactivity and risk of cardiovascular disease: A review and methodologic critique. *Psychological Bulletin, 96,* 435–464.

Krieger, N., Rowley, D. L., Herman, A. A., Avery, B., & Phillips, M. T. (1993). Racism, sexism, and social class: Implications for studies of health, disease, and well-being. *American Journal of Preventive Medicine, 9,* 82–122.

Krieger, N., & Sidney, S. (1996). Racial discrimination and blood pressure: The CARDIA study of young black and white adults. *American Journal of Public Health, 86,* 1370–1378.

Krieger, N., Sidney, S., & Coakley, E. (1998). Racial discrimination and skin color in the CARDIA study: Implications for public health research. *American Journal of Public Health, 88,* 1308–1313.

Kroening, R. J., & Oleson, T. D. (1985). Rapid narcotic detoxification in chronic pain patients treated with auricular electroacupuncture and naloxone. *The International Journal of the Addictions, 20,* 1347–1360.

Kronenberg, F., Pereira, M. A., Schmitz, M. K., Arnett, D. K., Evenson, K. R., Crapo, R. O., Jensen, R. L., Burke, G. L., Sholinsky, P., Ellison, R. C., & Hunt, S. C. (2000). Influence of leisure time physical activity and television watching on atherosclerosis risk factors in the NHLBI Family Heart Study. *Atherosclerosis, 153,* 433–443.

Kroner-Herwig, B., Jakle, C., Frettloh, J., Peters, K., Seemann, H., Franz, C., & Basler, H. (1996). Predicting subjective disability in chronic pain patients. *International Journal of Behavioral Medicine, 3,* 30–41.

Kronmal, R. A., Cain, K. C., Ye, Z., & Omenn, G. (1993). Total serum cholesterol levels and mortality risk as a function of age: A report based on the Framingham data. *Archives of Internal Medicine, 153,* 1065–1073.

Krupin, S. (2001, August 14). No mere political exercise: Fitness key to success for some lawmakers. *The Palm Beach Post,* p. 1A.

Kulik, J. A., & Mahler, H. I. M. (1993). Emotional support as a moderator of adjustment and compliance after coronary artery bypass surgery: A longitudinal study. *Journal of Behavioral Medicine, 26,* 48–63.

Kulkarni, R. R., Patki, P. S., Jog, V. P., Gandage, S. G., & Patwardhan, B. (1991). Treatment of osteoarthritis with a herbomineral formulation: A double-blind, placebo-controlled, crossover study. *Journal of Ethnopharmacology, 33,* 91–95.

Lacayo, R. (1995, June 12). Violent reaction. *Time,* 25–39.

Lachman, M. E., & Weaver, S. L. (1998). The sense of control as a moderator of social class differences in health and well-being. *Journal of Personality and Social Psychology, 74,* 763–773.

Lachman, M. E., Ziff, M. A., & Spiro, A. (1994). Maintaining a sense of control in later life. In R. P. Abeles & H. C. Gift (Eds.), *Aging and quality of life.* New York: Springer.

LaCroix, A. Z., & Haynes, S. (1987). Gender differences in the health effects of workplace roles. In R. C. Barnett & L. Biener (Eds.), *Gender and stress* (pp. 96–121). New York: Free Press.

Laforge, R. G., Greene, G. W., & Prochaska, J. O. (1994). Psychosocial factors influencing low fruit and vegetable consumption. *Journal of Behavioural Medicine, 17,* 361–374.

Lai, J. S., Lan, C., Wong, K. H., & Teng, S. H. (1995). Two-year trends in cardiorespiratory function among older T'ai Chi Chuan practitioners and sedentary subjects. *Journal of the American Geriatric Society, 43,* 1222–1227.

Lakka, T. A., & Salonen, J. T. (1992). Physical activity and serum lipids: A cross-sectional population study in Eastern Finnish men. *American Journal of Epidemiology, 136,* 806–818.

Lammers, C., Ireland, M., Resnick, M., & Blum, R. (2000). Influences on adolescents' decision to postpone onset of sexual intercourse: A survival analysis of virginity among youths aged 13 to 18 years. *Journal of Adolescent Health, 26,* 42–48.

Landis, B., Jovanovic, L., Landis, E., Peterson, C. M., Groshen, S., Johnson, K., & Miller, N. E. (1985). Effects of stress on reduction of daily glucose range in previously stabilized insulin-dependent diabetic patients. *Diabetes Care, 8,* 624–626.

Lando, H. A. (1986). Long-term modification of chronic smoking behavior: A paradigmatic approach. *Bulletin of the Society of Psychologists in Addictive Behaviors, 5,* 5–17.

Landrine, H., & Klonoff, E. A. (1994). Cultural diversity in causal attributions for illness: The role of the supernatural. *Journal of Behavioral Medicine, 17,* 181–193.

Landrine, H., & Klonoff, E. A. (2001). Cultural diversity and health psychology. In A. Baum, T. Revenson, & J. E. Singer (Eds.), *Handbook of health psychology* (pp. 851–891). Mahwah, NJ: Erlbaum.

Landro, L. (2001, February 2). Health groups push 'information therapy' to help treat patients. *The Wall Street Journal,* BI.

Lange de Klerk, E. S., Blommers, J., Kuik, D. J., & Bezemer, P. D. (1994). Effect of homeopathic medicines on daily burden of symptoms in children with recurrent upper respiratory tract infections. *British Medical Journal, 309,* 1329–1332.

Langer, E. J. (1983). *The psychology of control.* Beverly Hills, CA: Sage.

Langer, E. J., Janis, I. L., & Wolfer, J. A. (1975). Reduction of psychological stress in surgical patients. *Journal of Experimental Social Psychology, 11,* 155–165.

Langer, E. J., & Rodin, J. (1976). The effects of choice and enhanced personal responsibility for the aged: A field experiment in an institutional setting. *Journal of Personality and Social Psychology, 34,* 191–198.

Langner, T., & Michael, S. (1960). *Life stress and mental health.* New York: Free Press.

LaPerriere, A. R., Antoni, M. H., Schneiderman, N., Ironson, G., Klimas, N., Caralis, P., & Fletcher, M. A. (1990). Exercise intervention attenuates emotional distress and natural killer cell decrements following notification of positive serologic status for HIV-1. *Biofeedback and Self Regulation, 15,* 229–242.

Larimer, M. (1992). Alcohol abuse and the Greek system: An exploration of fraternity and sorority drinking. *Dissertation Abstracts International, 53,* 757.

Larsen, R. J. (1992). Neuroticism and selective encoding and recall of symptoms: Evidence from a combined concurrent-retrospective study. *Journal of Personality and Social Psychology, 62,* 480–488.

Lauer, M., Mulhern, R., Wallskig, J., & Camitta, B. (1983). A comparison study of parental adaptation following a child's death at home or in hospital. *Pediatrics, 71,* 107–111.

Launer, L. J., & Kalmijn, S. (1998). Anti-oxidants and cognitive function: A review of clinical and epidemiologic studies. *Journal of Neural Transmission, 53,* 1–8.

Law, A., Logan, H., & Baron, R. S. (1994). Desire for control, felt control, and stress inoculation training through dental treatment. *Journal of Personality and Social Psychology, 67,* 926–936.

Lawlis, G. F., Selby, D., Hinnant, D., & McCoy, C. E. (1985). Reduction of postoperative pain parameters by presurgical relaxation instructions for spinal pain patients. *Spine, 10,* 649–651.

Lazarus, R. S. (1984). On the primacy of cognition. *American Psychologist, 39,* 124–129.

Lazarus, R. S. (1990). Stress, coping and illness. In H. S. Friedman (Ed.), *Personality and disease* (pp. 97–120). New York: Wiley.

Lazarus, R. S. (1993). From psychological stress to the emotions: A history of changing outlooks. *Annual Review of Psychology, 44,* 1–21.

Lazarus, R. S., & Folkman, S. (1984). *Stress, appraisal, and coping.* New York: Springer.

Lazarus, R. S., & Launier, R. (1978). Stress-related transactions between person and environment. In L.A. Pervin & M. Lewis (Eds.), *Internal and external determinants of behavior* (pp. 287–327). New York: Plenum.

Leary, M. R., & Jones, J. L. (1993). The social psychology of tanning and sunscreen use: Self-presentational motives as a predictor of health risk. *Journal of Applied Social Psychology, 23,* 1390–1406.

Leary, M. R., Tchividjian, L. R., & Kraxberger, B. E. (1994). Self-presentation can be hazardous to your health: Impression management and health risk. *Health Psychology, 13,* 461–470.

Leclere, F. B., Rogers, R. G., & Peters, K. (1998). Neighborhood social context and racial differences in women's heart disease mortality. *Journal of Health and Social Behavior, 39,* 91–107.

Lee, C. (1993). Attitudes, knowledge, and stages of change: A survey of exercise patterns in older Australian women. *Health Psychology, 12,* 476–480.

Lee, I. M., & Paffenbarger, R. S. (1992). Change in body weight and longevity. *Journal of the American Medical Association, 268,* 2045–2049.

Leedham, B., Meyerowitz, B. E., Muirhead, J., & Frist, W. H. (1995). Positive expectations predict health after heart transplantation. *Health psychology, 14,* 74–79.

Leffell, D. J., & Brash, D. E. (1996). Sunlight and skin cancer. *Scientific American, 275,* 38–43.

Lehman, C. D., Rodin, J., McEwen, B., & Brinton, R. (1991). Impact of environmental stress on the expression of insulin-dependent diabetes mellitus. *Behavioral Neuroscience, 105,* 241–245.

Lehrer, P. M., Carr, R., Sargunaraj, D., & Woolfolk, R. L. (1994). Stress management techniques: Are they all equivalent, or do they have specific effects? *Biofeedback and Self Regulation, 19,* 353–401.

Leibel, R. L., Rosenbaum, M., & Hirsch, J. (1995). Changes in energy expenditure resulting from altered body weight. *New England Journal of Medicine, 332,* 621–629.

Leigh, B. C. (1989). Attitudes and expectancies as predictors of drinking habits: A comparison of three scales. *Journal of Studies on Alcohol, 50,* 432–440.

Leiss, J. K., & Savitz, D. A. (1995). Home pesticide use and childhood cancer: A case-control study. *American Journal of Public Health, 85,* 249–257.

Lemley, B. (1999, August). Alternative medicine man: Why so many doctors hate Andrew Weil. *Discover,* 56–63.

Leproult, R., Copinschi, G., Buxton, O., & Van Cauter, E. (1997). Sleep loss results in an elevation of cortisol levels the next evening. *Sleep, 20,* 865–870.

LeResche, L. (2000). Epidemiologic perspectives on sex differences in pain. In R.B. Fillingim (Ed.), *Sex, gender, and pain* (pp. 233–249). Seattle, WA: IASP Press.

Lerman, C., Hughes, C., Benkendorf, J. L., Biesecker, B., Kerner, J., Willison, J., Eads, N., Hadley, D., & Lynch, J. (1999). Racial differences in testing motivation and psychological distress following pretest education for BRCA1 gene testing. *Cancer Epidemiology, Biomarkers and Prevention, 8,* 361–368.

Lerman, C., & Rimer, B. K. (1995). Psychosocial impact of cancer screening. In R. T. Croyle (Ed.), *Psychosocial effects of screening for disease prevention and detection* (pp. 65–81). New York: Oxford University Press.

Lerman, C., Schwartz, M. D., Miller, S. M., Daly, M., Sands, C., & Rimer, B. K. (1996). A randomized trial of breast cancer risk counseling: Interacting effects of counseling, educational level, and coping style. *Health Psychology, 15,* 75–83.

Lescano, C. M., & Rodrigue, J. R. (1997). Skin cancer prevention behaviors among parents of young children. *Children's Health Care, 26,* 107–114.

Leserman, J., Perkins, D. O., & Evans, D. L. (1992). Coping with the threat of AIDS: The role of social support. *American Journal of Psychiatry, 149,* 1514–1520.

Leserman, J., Petitto, J. M., Golden, R. N., Gaynes, B. N., Gu, H., Perkins, D. O., Silva, S. G., Folds, J. D., & Evans, D. L. (2000). Impact of stressful life events, depression, social support, coping, and cortisol on progression to AIDS. *American Journal of Psychiatry, 157,* 1221–1228.

Leshner, A. I. (2001). What does it mean that addiction is a brain disease? *Monitor on Psychology,* Special Issue on Substance Abuse, *32,* 19.

Lester, T., & Petrie, T. A. (1998). Physical, psychological, and societal correlates of bulimic symptomatology among African American college women. *Journal of Counseling Psychology, 3,* 315–321.

Letzel, H., Haan, J., & Feil, W. B. (1996). Nootropics: Efficacy and tolerability of products from three active substance classes. *Journal of Drug Development and Clinical Practice, 8,* 77–83.

Leutwyler, K. (1995, April). The price of prevention. *Scientific American, 272,* 124–129.

Leventhal, E. A., Hansell, S., Diefenbach, M., Leventhal, H. & Glass, D. C. (1996). Negative affect and self-report of physical symptoms: Two longitudinal studies of older adults. *Health Psychology, 15,* 193–199.

Leventhal, E. A., & Prohaska, T. R. (1986). Age, symptom interpretation, and health behavior. *Journal of the American Geriatrics Society, 34,* 185–191.

Leventhal, H., Benyamini, Y., Brownlee, S., Diefenbach, M., Leventhal, E. A., Patrick-Miller, L., & Robitaille, C. (1997). Illness representations: Theoretical foundations. In K. J. Petrie & J. A. Weinman (Eds.), *Perceptions of health and illness: Current research and applications* (pp. 19–45). Singapore: Harwood Academic Publishers.

Leventhal, H., & Cleary, P. D. (1980). The smoking problem: A review of the research and theory in behavioral risk modification. *Psychological Bulletin, 88,* 370–405.

Leventhal, H., & Diefenbach, M. (1991). The active side of illness cognition. In J. A. Skelton & R. T. Croyle (Eds.). *Mental representation in health and illness* (pp. 247–272). New York: Springer–Verlag.

Levesque, D. A., Prochaska, J. M., & Prochaska, J. O. (1999). Stages of change and integrated service delivery. *Consulting Psychology Journal: Practice and Research, 51,* 226–241.

Levi, L. (1974). Psychosocial stress and disease: A conceptual model. In E. K. E. Gunderson & R. H. Rahe (Eds.), *Life stress and illness* (pp. 8–33). Springfield, IL: Thomas.

Levin, J. S., & Vanderpool, H. Y. (1987). Is frequent religious attendance really conducive to better health? *Social Science and Medicine, 24,* 589–600.

Levine, F. M., & DeSimone, L. L. (1991). The effect of experimenter gender on pain report in male and female subjects. *Pain, 44,* 69–72.

Levine, J. D., Gordon, N. C., & Fields, H. L. (1978). The mechanism of placebo analgesia. *The Lancet, 8091,* 654–657.

Levy, S. M. (1985). Prognostic risk assessment in primary breast cancer by behavioral and immunological parameters. *Health Psychology, 4,* 99–113.

Lewis, V. J. (1997). Weight control. In A. Baum, S. Newman, J. Weinman, R. West, & C. McManus (Eds.), *Cambridge handbook of psychology, health and medicine* (pp. 189–192). Cambridge, UK: Cambridge University Press.

Lewitt, E. M., & Kerrebrock, N. (1998). Child indicators: Dental health. *The Future of Children: Protecting Children from Abuse and Neglect, 8,* 4–22.

Ley, P. (1988). *Communicating with patients.* London: Chapman and Hall.

Ley, P. (1997). Recall by patients. In A. Baum, S. Newman, J. Weinman, R. West, & C. McManus (Eds.), *Cambridge handbook of psychology, health and medicine* (pp. 315–317). Cambridge, UK: Cambridge University Press.

Liaw, F. & & Brooks-Gunn, J. (1993). Patterns of low-birth-weight children's cognitive development. *Developmental Psychology, 29*(6), 1024–1035.

Lichstein, K. L. (1988). *Clinical relaxation strategies.* New York: Wiley.

Lichtenstein, A. H., Kennedy, E., Barrier, P., Danford, D., Ernst, N. D., Grundy, S. M., Leveille, G. A., Van Horn, L., Williams, C. L., & Booth, S. L. (1998). Dietary fat consumption and health. *Nutrition Review, 56,* S3–S19.

Lichtenstein, E., & Glasgow, R. E. (1992). Smoking cessation: What have we learned over the past decade? *Journal of Consulting and Clinical Psychology, 4,* 518–527.

Lichtenstein, E., & Glasgow, R. E. (1997). A pragmatic framework for smoking cessation: Implications for clinical and public health programs. *Psychology of Addictive Behaviors, 11,* 142–151.

Lichtman, S. W., Pisarska, K., Berman, E. R., & Prestone, M. (1992). Discrepancy between self-reported and actual caloric intake and exercise in obese subjects. *New England Journal of Medicine, 327,* 1893–1898.

Lieberman, M. A. (1982). The effects of social supports on responses to stress. In L. Goldberger & L. Breznitz (Eds.), *Handbook of stress.* New York: Free Press.

Lierman, L. M., Kasprzyk, D., & Benoliel, J. Q. (1991). Understanding adherence to breast self-examination in older women. *Western Journal of Nursing Research, 13,* 46–66.

Liese, B. S., & Franz, R. A. (1996). Treating substance use disorders with cognitive therapy: Lessons learned and implications for the future. In P. M. Salkoviskis (Ed.), *Frontiers of cognitive therapy* (pp. 470–508). New York: Guilford.

Lightfoot, C. (1997). *The culture of adolescent risk-taking.* New York: Guilford.

Lin, E. H., & Peterson, C. (1990). Pessimistic explanatory style and response to illness. *Behaviour Research and Therapy, 28,* 243–248.

Lindfors, K. K., & Rosenquist, C. J. (1995). The cost-effectiveness of mammographic screening strategies. *Journal of the American Medical Association, 274,* 881–884.

Lindsted, K. D., & Singh, P. N. (1997). Body mass and 26-year risk of mortality among women who never smoked: Findings from the Adventist Mortality Study. *American Journal of Epidemiology, 146,* 1–11.

Linkins, R. W., & Comstock, G. W. (1988). Depressed mood and development of cancer. *American Journal of Epidemiology, 128* (Abstract), 894.

Lipton, J. A., & Marbach, J. J. (1984). Ethnicity and the pain experience. *Social Science and Medicine, 19,* 1279–1298.

Littlefield, C. H., Craven, J. L., Rodin, G. M., Daneman, D., Murray, M. A., & Rydall, A. C. (1992). Relationship of self-efficacy and binging to adherence to diabetes regimen among adolescents. *Diabetes Care, 15,* 90–94.

Littlefield, C. H., Rodin, G. M., Murray, M. A., & Craven, J. L. (1990). Influence of functional impairment and social support on depressive symptoms in persons with diabetes. *Health Psychology, 9,* 737–749.

Liu, S., Siegel, P. Z., Brewer, R. D., Mokdad, A. H., Sleet, D. A., & Serdula, M. (1997). Prevalence of alcohol-impaired driving: Results from a national self-reported survey of health behaviors. *Journal of the American Medical Association, 277,* 122–125.

Long, B. C., & van Stavel, R. (1995). Effects of exercise training on anxiety: A meta-analysis. *Journal of Applied Sport Psychology, 7,* 167–189.

Loo, M. (1999). Complementary/alternative therapies in select populations: Children. In J. W. Spencer & J. J. Jacobs (Eds.), *Complementary/alternative medicine: An evidence–based approach* (pp. 371–390). St. Louis, MO: Mosby.

Loo, M., Naeser, M. A., Hinshaw, S., & Bay, R. B. (1998). *Laser acupuncture treatment for ADHD.* Presented at annual American Academy of Medical Acupuncture (AAMA) Symposium. San Diego, CA.

Lopez, A. D. (1999). Measuring the health hazards of tobacco: Commentary. *Bulletin of the World Health Organization, 77,* 82–83.

Lorber, J. (1975). Good patients and problem patients: Conformity and deviance in a general hospital. *Journal of Health and Social Behavior, 16,* 213–225.

Lovallo, W. R., & Pishkin, V. (1980). A psychophysiological comparison of type A and B men exposed to failure and uncontrollable noise. *Psychophysiology, 17,* 29–36.

Low, A. W., & Peck, C. L. (1987). The MMPI and psychological factors in chronic low back pain: A review. *Pain, 28,* 1–12.

Lowe, M. R. (1993). The effects of dieting on eating behavior: A three-factor model. *Psychological Bulletin, 114,* 100–121.

Lowrey, G. H. (1986). *Growth and development of children* (8th ed.). Chicago: Year Book Medical Publishers.

Lowry, R., Holtzman, D., Truman, B., Kann, L., Collins, J. L., & Kolbe, L. J. (1994). Substance use and HIV-related sexual behaviors among U.S. high school students: Are they related? *American Journal of Public Health, 84,* 1116–1120.

Lox, C. L., McAuley, E., & Tucker, R. S. (1996). Physical training effects on acute exercise-induced feeling states in HIV-1 positive individuals. *Journal of Health Psychology, 1,* 235–240.

Luks, D., & Anderson, M. R. (1996). Antihistamines and the common cold: A review and critique of the literature. *Journal of General Internal Medicine, 11*, 240–244.

Lundberg, U., & Frankenhaeuser, M. (1999). Stress and workload of men and women in high-ranking positions. *Journal of Occupational Health Psychology, 4*, 142–151.

Lundberg, U., Mardberg, B., & Frankenhaeuser, M. (1994). The total workload of male and female white collar workers as related to age, occupational level, and number of children. *Scandinavian Journal of Psychology, 35*, 315–327.

Lupien, S. J., de Leon, M., De Santi, S., Convit, A., Tarshish, C., Nair, N. P. V., Thakur, M., McEwen, B. S., Hauger, R. L., & Meaney, M. J. (1998). Cortisol levels during human aging predict hippocampal atrophy and memory deficits. *Nature Neuroscience, 1*, 69–73.

Luskin, F. M., Newell, K. A., Griffith, M., Holmes, M., Telles, S., Dinucci, E., Marvasti, F. F., Hill, M., Pelletier, K. R., & Haskell, W. L. (2000). A review of mind/body therapies in the treatment of musculoskeletal disorders with implications for the elderly. *Alternative Therapies, 6*, 46–56.

Ly, D. H., Lockhart, D. J., Lerner, R. A., & Schultz, P. G. (2000). Mitotic misregulation and human aging. *Science, 287*, 2486–2492.

Lynch, B. S., Bonnie, R. J., & Nelson, D. E. (1995). Growing up tobacco free. *Journal of Public Health Policy, 16*, 492–493.

Lynch, D. J., Birk, T. J., Weaver, M. T., Gohara, A. F., Leighton, R. F., Repka, F. J., & Walsh, M. E. (1992). Adherence to exercise interventions in the treatment of hypercholesterolemia. *Journal of Behavioral Medicine, 15*, 365–378.

Lyness, S. A. (1993). Predictors of differences between Type A and B individuals in heart rate and blood pressure reactivity. *Psychological Bulletin, 114*, 266–295.

Lynne, S. (1999, April 5). Pregnant women should avoid unsafe herbs. *The University Record, 54*, 10.

Lyons, A. S., & Petrucelli, J. R. (1978). *Medicine: An illustrated history.* New York: Harry N. Abrams.

Lytle, C. D. (1993). *An overview of acupuncture.* Rockville, MD: United States Public Health Service, Center for Devices and Radiological health, Food and Drug Administration.

Lyubomirsky, S., Caldwell, N. D., & Nolen-Hoeksema, S. (1998). Effects of ruminative and distracting responses to depressed mood on retrieval of autobiographical memories. *Journal of Personality and Social Psychology, 75*, 166–177.

Lyubomirsky, S., & Nolen-Hoeksema, S. (1995). Effects of self-focused rumination on negative thinking and interpersonal problem solving. *Journal of Personality and Social Psychology, 69*, s176–190.

Lyvers, M. (1998). Drug addiction as a physical disease: The role of physical dependence and other chronic drug-induced neurophysiological changes in compulsive drug self-administration. *Experimental and Clinical Psychopharmacology, 6*, 107–125.

MacDonald, T., Zanna, M. P., & Fong, G. T. (1996). Why common sense goes out the window: Effects of alcohol on intentions to use condoms. *Personality and Social Psychology Bulletin, 22*, 763–775.

MacDorman, M. F., & Atkinson, J. O. (1999). Infant mortality statistics from the 1997 period linked birth/infant death data set. *National Vital Statistics Reports, 47*, 1–23.

Macera, C. A., Armstead, C. A., & Anderson, N. B. (2001). Sociocultural influences on health. In A. Baum, T. A. Revenson, & J. E. Singer (Eds.) *Handbook of health psychology* (pp. 427-440). Mahwah, NJ: Erlbaum.

Macklin, M. L., Metzger, L. J., Litz, B. T., McNally, R. J., Lasko, N. B., Orr, S. P., & Pitman, R. K. (1998). Lower precombat intelligence is a risk factor for posttraumatic stress disorder. *Journal of Consulting and Clinical Psychology, 66*, 323–326.

Madden, T. J., Ellen, P. S., & Ajzen, I. (1992). A comparison of the theory of planned behavior and the theory of reasoned action. *Personality and Social Psychology Bulletin, 18*, 3–9.

Maddi, S. R., & Kobasa, S. C. (1991). The development of hardiness. In A. Monat & R. Lazarus (Eds.), *Stress and coping: An anthology* (pp. 245–257). New York: Columbia University Press.

Maes, H. M., Neale, M. C., & Eaves, L. J. (1997). Genetic and environmental factors in relative body weight and human adiposity [Special Issue: The genetics of obesity]. *Behavioral Genetics, 27*, 325–351.

Magni, G., Silvestro, A., Tamiello, M., Zanesco, L., & Carl, B. (1988). An integrated approach to the assessment of family adjustment to acute lymphocytic leukemia in children. *Acta Psychiatrica Scandinavica, 78*, 639–642.

Maher, V. M., Brown, B. G. Marcovina, S. M., Hillger, L. A., & Zhao, X. (1995). Effects of lowering elevated LDL cholesterol on the cardiovascular risk of lipoprotein. *Journal of the American Medical Association, 22*, 1771–1774.

Mahler, H. I., Fitzpatrick, B., Parker, P., & Lapin, A. (1997). The relative effects of a health-based versus an appearance-based intervention designed to increase sunscreen use. *American Journal of Health Promotion, 11*, 426–429.

Mairs, D. A. (1995). Hypnosis and pain in childbirth. *Contemporary Hypnosis, 12*, 111–118.

Malarkey, W. B., Kiecolt-Glaser, J. K., Pearl, D., & Glaser, R. (1994). Hostile behavior during marital conflict alters pituitary and adrenal hormones. *Psychosomatic Medicine, 56*, 41–51.

Maldonado, R., Saiardi, A., Valverde, O., Samad, T. A., Rogues, B. P., & Borrell, E. (1997). Absence of opiate rewarding effects in mice lacking dopamine D2 receptors. *Nature, 388*, 586–589.

Malt, U. F., Nerdrum., P., Oppedal, B., Gundersen, R., Holte, M., & Lone, J. (1997). Physical and mental problems attributed to dental amalgam fillings: A descriptive study of 99 self-referred patients compared with 272 controls. *Psychosomatic Medicine, 59*, 32–41.

Manjer, J., Berglund, G., Bondesson, L., Garne, J. P., Janzon, L., Lindgren, A., Malina, J., & Matson, S. (2000). Intra-urban differences in breast cancer mortality: A study from the city of Malmö in Sweden. *Journal of Epidemiology and Community Health, 54*(4), 279–285.

Mann, T., Nolen-Hoeksema, S., Huang, K., & Burgard, D. (1997). Are two interventions worse than none? Joint primary and secondary prevention of eating disorders in college females. *Health Psychology, 16*, 215–225.

Manne, S. L., & Zautra, A. J. (1990). Couples coping with chronic illness: Women with rheumatoid arthritis and their healthy husbands. *Journal of Behavioral Medicine, 13*, 327–342.

Mansergh, G., Marks, G., & Simoni, J. M. (1995). Self-disclosure of HIV infection among men who vary in time since seropositive diagnosis and symptomatic status. *AIDS, 9*, 639–644.

Manyande, A., Berg, S., Gettins, D., Stanford, S. C., Mazhero, S., Marks, D. F., & Salmon, P. (1995). Preoperative rehearsal of active coping imagery influences subjective and hormonal responses to abdominal surgery. *Psychosomatic Medicine, 57*, 177–182.

Marin, B. V., & Gomez, C. A. (1992). Predictors of condom accessibility among Hispanics in San Francisco. *American Journal of Public Health, 82*, 592–595.

Marin, B. V., Gomez, C. A., Tschann, J. M., & Gregorich, S. E. (1997). Condom use in unmarried Latino men: A test of cultural constructs. *Health Psychology, 16*, 458–467.

Marin, L., Rodriguez Kauth, A., & Ottaviano, L. (1993). A methodological contribution to psychosocial alienation. *Acta Psiquiatricay Psicologica de Americalatina, 39*, 246–253.

Markovitz, J. H., Matthews, K. A., Kannel, W. B., Cobb, J. L., & D'Agostino, R. B. (1993). Psychological predictors of hypertension in the Framingham Study. Is there tension in hypertension? *Journal of the American Medical Association, 270*, 2439–2443.

Marlatt, G. A., Baer, J. S., & Larimer, M. (1995). Preventing alcohol abuse in college students: A harm-reduction approach. In G. M. Boyd & J. Howard (Eds.), *Alcohol problems among adolescents: Current directions in prevention research* (pp. 147–172). Hillsdale, NJ: Erlbaum.

Marlatt, G. A., & Gordon, A. (1985). Abstinence and controlled drinking: Alternative treatment goals for alcoholism and problem drinking? *Bulletin of the Society of Psychologists in Addictive Behaviors, 4*, 123–150.

Martin, J. L., & Dean, L. (1993). Bereavement following death from AIDS: Unique problems, reactions, and special needs. In M. S. Stroebe & W. Stroebe (Eds.), *Handbook of bereavement: Theory, research, and intervention* (pp. 317–330). New York: Cambridge University Press.

Martin, L. L., & Tesser, A. (1989). Toward a motivational and structural theory of ruminative thought. In J. S. Uleman & J. A. Bargh (Eds.), *Unintended thought* (pp. 306–326). New York: Guilford.

Martin, R. A., & Lefcourt, H. M. (1983). Sense of humor as a moderator of the relation between stressors and moods. *Journal of Personality and Social Psychology, 45*, 1313–1324.

Marucah, P. T., Kiecolt-Glaser, J. K., & Favagehi, M. (1998). Mucosal wound healing is impaired by examination stress. *Psychosomatic Medicine, 60*, 362–365.

Maruta, T., Colligan, R. C., Malinchoc, M., & Offord, K. P. (2000). Optimists vs. pessimists: Survival rate among medical patients over a 30-year period. *Mayo Clinic Proceedings, 75*, 140–143.

Marvan, M. L., & Cortes-Iniestra, C. (2001). Women's beliefs about the prevalence of premenstrual syndrome and biases in recall of premenstrual changes. *Health Psychology, 20*, 276–280.

Marwick, C. (1991). Hispanic HANES takes a long look at Latino health. *Journal of the American Medical Association, 265*, 177, 181.

Maslach, C. (1986). Stress, burnout, and workaholism. In R. R. Kilburg & P. E. Nathan, *Professionals in distress: Issues, syndromes, and solutions in psychology* (pp. 53–75). Washington, DC: American Psychological Association.

Mason, J. W. (1975). A historical view of the stress field. *Journal of Human Stress, 1*, 22–36.

Mason, J. W., Kosten, T. R., Southwick, S. M. , & Giller, E. L. (1990). The use of psychoendocrine strategies in post-traumatic stress disorder. *Journal of Applied Social Psychology, 20*, 1822–1846.

Massey, C. V., Hupp, C. H., Kreisberg, M., Alpert, M. A., & Hoff, C. (2000). Estrogen replacement therapy is underutilized among postmenopausal women at high risk for coronary heart disease. *American Journal of the Medical Sciences, 320*, 124–127.

Masten, A. S. (2001). Ordinary magic: Resilience processes in development. *American Psychologist, 56*, 218–226.

Matarazzo, J. D. (1984). Behavioral immunogens and pathogens in health and illness. In B. L. Hammonds & J. C. Scheirer (Eds.), *Psychology and health* (pp. 9–43). Washington, DC: American Psychological Association.

Maternal and Child Health Bureau. (2000). *Child Health USA, 2000.* Washington, DC: U. S. Department of Health and Human Services.

Matthews, D. A. (1997). Religion and spirituality in primary care. *Mind/Body Medicine, 2*, 9–19.

Matthews, K. A., Owens, J. F., Allen, M. T., & Stoney, C. M. (1992). Do cardiovascular responses to laboratory stress relate to ambulatory blood pressure levels? Yes, in some of the people, some of the time. *Psychosomatic Medicine, 54*, 686–697.

Matthews, K. A., Shumaker, S. A., Bowen, D. J., Langer, R. D., Hunt, J. R., Kaplan, R. M., Klesges, R. C., & Ritenbaugh, C. (1997). Women's Health Initiative: Why now? What is it? What's new? *American Psychologist, 52*, 101–116.

Matthews, K. A., Siegel, J. M., Kuller, L. H., Thompson, M., & Varat, M. (1983). Determinants of decisions to seek medical treatment by patients with acute myocardial infarction symptoms. *Journal of Personality and Social Psychology, 44*, 1144–1156.

Mayday PainLink Report (2000). http://www.edc.org/PainLink/index.html.

Mayer, D. J., & Price, D. D. (1976). Central nervous system mechanisms of analgesia. *Pain, 2*, 379–404.

Mayer, J. A., & Frederiksen, L. W. (1986). Encouraging long-term compliance with breast self-examination: The evaluation of prompting strategies. *Journal of Behavioral Medicine, 9*, 179–190.

Mayne, T. J., Acree, M., Chesney, M. A., & Folkman, S. (1998). HIV sexual risk behavior following bereavement in gay men. *Health Psychology, 17,* 403–411.

Mayo Clinic (1996, May 22). Facts about calories. www.mayohealth.org.

Mayo Clinic (2001, January 25). Do you need to lose weight? www.mayohealth.org.

Mayo Clinic Health Oasis. (2000). Breast cancer gene testing: Is it right for you? www.mayohealth.org/home?id=HQ00350.

Mayo Health (2001). Everyone active: Exercise for healthy aging. www.mayohealth.org.

Mays, V. M., So, B. T., Cochran, S. D., Detels, R., Benjamin, R., Allen, E., & Kwon, S. (2001). HIV disease in ethnic minorities: Implications of racial/ethnic differences in disease susceptibility and drug dosage response for HIV infection and treatment. In A. Baum, T. A. Revenson, & J. E. Singer (Eds.), *Handbook of health psychology* (pp. 801–816). Mahwah, NJ: Erlbaum.

Mazurk, P. M., Tierney, H., Tarfidd, K., Gross, E. M., Morgan, E. G., Hsu, M. A., & Mann, J. G. (1988). Increased risk of suicide in persons with AIDS. *Journal of the American Medical Association, 259,* 1332–1333.

McAuliffe, K. (1997). Surprising ways the seasons affect your body—and your mind. *Redbook, 188,* 55–56, 98.

McCann, I. L., & Holmes, D. S. (1984). Influence of aerobic exercise on depression. *Journal of Personality and Social Psychology, 46,* 1142–1147.

McCarthy, J. (2001, May). Superfoods or superfrauds? *Shape, 20,* 104–106.

McCaul, K. D., Branstetter, A. D., Schroeder, D. M., & Glascow, R. E. (1996). What is the relationship between breast cancer risk and mammography screening? A meta-analytic review. *Health Psychology, 15,* 423–429.

McCracken, L. M., Zayfert, C., & Gross, R. T. (1992). The Pain Anxiety Symptoms Scale: Development and validation of a scale to measure fear of pain. *Pain, 50,* 67–73.

McCullough, M. E., Hoyt, W. T., Larson, D. B., Koenig, H. G., & Thoresen, C. (2000). Religious involvement and mortality: A meta-analytic review. *Health Psychology, 19,* 211–222.

McEwen, B. S., & Magarinos, A. M. (1997). Stress effects on morphology and function of the hippocampus. In R. Yehuda & A. C. McFarlane (Eds.), *Psychobiology of posttraumatic stress disorder* (pp. 271–284). New York: New York Academy of Sciences.

McGrady, A. (1994). Effects of group relaxation training and thermal biofeedback on blood pressure and related physiological and psychological variables in essential hypertension. *Biofeedback and Self-Regulation, 19,* 51–66.

McGrady, A., & Horner, J. (1999). Role of mood in outcome of biofeedback assisted relaxation therapy in insulin dependent diabetes mellitus. *Applied Psychophysiology and Biofeedback, 24,* 79–88.

McGue, M. (2000). *Behavioral genetic models of alcoholism and drinking.* New York: Guilford.

McGue, M., Vaupel, J. W., Holm, M., & Harvald, B. (1993). Longevity is moderately heritable in a sample of Danish twins born 1870–1880. *Journal of Gerontology, 48,* B237–B244.

McGuire, P. A. (1999, June) Psychology and medicine connecting in war on cancer. *American Psychological Association Monitor, 30*(6), 8–9.

McKenna, M. C., Zevon, M. A., Corn, B., & Rounds, J. (1999). Psychosocial factors and the development of breast cancer: A meta-analysis. *Health Psychology, 18,* 520–531.

McLaughlin, C. S., Chen, C., Greenberger, E., & Biermeier, C. (1997). Family, peer, and individual correlates of sexual experience among Caucasian and Asian American late adolescents. *Journal of Research on Adolescence, 7,* 33–53.

Mclellan, A. T., Grossman, D. S., Blaine, J. D., & Haverkos, H. W. (1993). Acupuncture treatment for drug abuse. A technical review. *Journal of Substance Abuse Treatment, 10,* 569–575.

McMillen, D. L., Smith, S. M., & Wells-Parker, E. (1989). The effects of alcohol, expectancy, and sensation seeking on driving risk taking. *Addictive Behaviors, 14,* 477–483.

McMurtrie, B. (1994, July 19). Overweight fatten ranks. *New York Newsday,* p. A26.

McNeilly, M. D., Anderson, N. B., Armstead, C. A., Clark, R., Corbett, M., Robinson, E. L., Pieper, C. F., & Lepisto, E. M. (1996). The perceived racism scale: A multidimensional assessment of the experience of white racism among African Americans. *Ethnicity and Disease, 6,* 154–166.

McVeigh, C. (1999, October 1). Medical schools offering spirituality and medicine courses. Rockville, MD: National Institute for Healthcare Research (www.nihr.org).

Mechanic, D. (1978). *Medical sociology.* New York: Free Press.

Mechanic, D., & Angel, R. J. (1987). Some factors associated with the report and evaluation of back pain. *Journal of Health and Social Behavior, 28,* 131–139.

Meichenbaum, D. (1985). *Stress inoculation training.* New York: Pergamon.

Meichenbaum, D. (1997). Cognitive behavior therapy. In A. Baum, S. Newman, J. Weinman, R. West, & C. McManus (Eds.), *Cambridge handbook of psychology, health and medicine* (pp. 200–203). Cambridge, UK: Cambridge University Press.

Melamed, B. G., Kaplan, B., & Fogel, J. (2001). Childhood health issues across the life span. In A. Baum, T. A., Revenson, & J. E. Singer (Eds.), *Handbook of health psychology* (pp. 449–457). Mahwah, NJ: Erlbaum.

Melamed, B. G., & Siegel, L. J. (1975). Reduction of anxiety in children facing hospitalization and surgery by filmed modeling. *Journal of Consulting and Clinical Psychology, 43,* 511–521.

Melchart, D., Linde, K., Worku, F., Sarkady, L., Holzmann, M., Jurcic, K., & Wagner, H. (1995). Results of five randomized studies on the immunomodulatory activity of preparations of Echinacea. *Journal of Alternative and Complementary Medicine, 1,* 145–160.

Melzack, R. (1993). Pain: Past, present, and future. *Canadian Journal of Experimental Psychology, 47,* 615–629.

Melzack, R., & Torgerson, W. S. (1971). On the language of pain. *Anesthesiology, 34,* 50–59.

Melzack, R., & Wall, P. D. (1965). Pain mechanisms: A new theory. *Science, 150,* 971–979.

Melzack, R., & Wall, P. D. (1988). *The challenge of pain.* New York: Basic Books.

Memorial Sloan-Kettering Cancer Center. (2001, June 16). Our approach to cancer treatment. www.mskcc.org/pediatric_cancer_care/.

Merriman, J. (1999, May 13). These pounds aren't sterling. www.abcnews.go.com.

Metzler, C. W., Noell, J., Biglan, A., & Ary, D. (1994). The social context for risky sexual behavior among adolescents. *Journal of Behavioral Medicine, 17*(4), 419–438.

Meyer, D., Leventhal, H., & Gutmann, M. (1985). Common-sense models of illness: The example of hypertension. *Health Psychology, 4,* 115–135.

Meyer, J. M., & Stunkard, A. J. (1994). Twin studies of human obesity. In C. Bouchard (Ed.), *The genetics of obesity* (pp. 63–78). Boca Raton, FL: CRC Press.

Meyerowitz, B. E., Richardson, J., Hudson, S., & Leedham, B. (1998). Ethnicity and cancer outcomes: Behavioral and psychosocial considerations. *Psychological Bulletin, 123,* 47–70.

Meyerowitz, B. E., Wilson, D. K., & Chaiken, S. (1991, June). *Loss-framed messages increase breast self-examination for women who perceive risk.* Paper presented at the annual convention of the American Psychological Society, Washington, DC.

Michie, S., Marteau, T. M., & Kidd, J. (1992). Predicting antenatal class attendance: Attitudes of self and others. *Psychology and Health, 7,* 225–234.

Milberger, S., Biederman, J., Faraone, S. V., Chen, L., & Jones, J. (1996). Is maternal smoking during pregnancy a risk factor for attention deficit hyperactivity disorder in children? *American Journal of Psychiatry, 153,* 1138–1142.

Milkie, M. A., & Peltola, P. (1999). Playing all the roles: Gender and the work-family balancing act. *Journal of Marriage and the Family, 61,* 476–490.

Millar, M. G., & Millar, K. (1995). Negative affective consequences of thinking about disease detection behaviors. *Health Psychology, 14,* 141–146.

Miller, D. A., McCluskey-Fawcett, K., & Irving, L. M. (1993). The relationship between childhood sexual abuse and subsequent onset of bulimia nervosa. *Child Abuse & Neglect, 17,* 305–314.

Miller, G. A., & Nuessle, W. (1978). Characteristics of the emotional responsiveness of sensitizers and repressors to social stimuli. *Journal of Consulting and Clinical Psychology, 46,* 339–340.

Miller, G. E., & Cohen, S. (2001). Psychological interventions and the immune system: A meta-analytic review and critique. *Health Psychology, 20,* 47–63.

Miller, J. J., Fletcher, K., & Kabat-Zinn, J. (1995). Three-year follow-up and clinical implications of a mindfulness meditation-based stress reduction intervention in the treatment of anxiety disorders. *General Hospital Psychiatry, 17,* 192–200.

Miller, L., & Smith, A. D. (1998) Your personal stress action plan. *The Executive Female, 16,* 29–30.

Miller, L. C., Bettencourt, B. A., DeBro, S., & Hoffman, V. (1993). Negotiating safer sex: Interpersonal dynamics. In J. B. Pryor & G. D. Reeder (Eds.). *The social psychology of HIV infection* (pp. 85–123). Hillsdale, NJ: Erlbaum.

Miller, L. J., Holicky, E. L., Ulrich, C. D., & Wieben, E. D. (1995). Abnormal processing of the human cholecystokinin receptor gene in association with gallstones and obesity. *Gastroenterology, 109,* 1375–1380.

Miller, M. F., Barabasz, A. F., & Barabasz, M. (1991). Effects of active alert and relaxation hypnotic inductions on cold pressor pain. *Journal of Abnormal Psychology, 100,* 223–226.

Miller, N. S., & Giannini, A. J. (1990). The disease model of addiction: A biopsychiatrist's view. *Journal of Psychoactive Drugs, 22,* 83–85.

Miller, R. H., & Luft, H. S. (1994). Managed care plans: Characteristics, growth, and premium performance. *Annual Review of Public Health, 15,* 437–459.

Miller, S. M., & Mangan, C. E. (1983). Interacting effects of information and coping style in adapting to gynecologic stress: Should the doctor tell all? *Journal of Personality and Social Psychology, 45,* 223–236.

Miller, T. Q., Smith, T. W., Turner, C. W., Guijarro, M. L., & Hallet, A. J. (1996). A meta-analytic review of research on hostility and physical health. *Psychological Bulletin, 119,* 322–348.

Miller, W. C. (1999). Fitness and fatness in relation to health: Implications for a paradigm shift. *Journal of Social Issues, 55,* 207–220.

Miller, W. R., Westerberg, V. S., Harris, R. J., & Tonigan, J. S. (1996). What predicts relapse? Prospective testing of antecedent models. *Addiction, 91,* S155–172.

Mills, J. K., & Adrianopoulos, G. D. (1993). The relationship between childhood onset obesity and psychopathology in adulthood. *Journal of Psychology, 127,* 547–551.

Millstein, S. G. (1996). Utility of the theories of reasoned action and planned behavior for predicting physician behavior: A prospective analysis. *Health Psychology, 15,* 398–402.

Mintz, L. B., & Kashubeck, S. (1999). Body image and disordered eating among Asian American and Caucasian college students: An examination of race and gender differences. *Psychology of Women Quarterly, 23,* 781–796.

Mintz, L. B., Kashubeck, S., & Tracy, L.S. (1995). Relations among parental alcoholism, eating disorders, and substance abuse in nonclinical college women: Additional evidence against the uniformity myth. *Journal of Counseling Psychology, 42,* 65–70.

Minuchin, S., Rosman, B. L., & Baker, L. (1978). *Psychosomatic families: Anorexia nervosa in context.* Cambridge, MA: Harvard University Press.

Miranda, J. A., Perez-Stable, E. J., Munoz, R., Hargreaves, W., & Henke, C. J. (1991). Somatization, psychiatric disorder, and stress in utilization of ambulatory medical services. *Health Psychology, 10,* 46–51.

Mirin, S. M., & Weiss, R. D. (1989). Genetic factors in the development of alcoholism. *Psychiatric Annals, 19*(5), 239–242.

Mittleman, M. A., Maclure, M., Sherwood, J. B., Mulry, R. P., Tofler, G. H., Jacobs, S. C., Friedman, R., Benson, H., & Muller, J. E. (1995). Triggering of acute myocardial infarction onset by episodes of anger. Determinants of Myocardial Infarction Onset Study Investigators. *Circulation, 92,* 1720–1725.

Moen, P., & Yu, Y. (1999). Having it all: Overall work/life success in two-earner families. In T. Parcel (Ed.), *Research in the sociology of work,* vol. 7 (pp. 109–139). Greenwich, CT: JAI Press.

Monitoring the Future (2000). *National survey results on drug use from the Monitoring the Future Study: Secondary school students.* Washington, DC: National Institute on Drug Abuse.

Monroe, S. M., & Simons, A. D. (1991). Diathesis-stress theories in the context of life stress research: Implications for the depressive disorders. *Psychological Bulletin, 110,* 406–425.

Montano, D. E., Thompson, B., Taylor, V. M., & Mahloch, J. (1997). Understanding mammography intention and utilization among women in an inner city public hospital clinic. *Preventive Medicine, 26,* 817–824.

Montgomery, G., & Kirsch, I. (1996). Mechanisms of placebo pain reduction: An empirical investigation. *Psychological Science, 7,* 174–176.

Monti, P. M., Rohsenow, D. J., Rubonis, A. V., & Niaura, R. S. (1993). Cue exposure with coping skills treatment for male alcoholics: A preliminary investigation. *Journal of Consulting and Clinical Psychology, 61,* 1011–1019.

Moore, J. S. (1993). *Chiropractic in America.* Baltimore: Johns Hopkins University Press.

Moos, R. H., Brennan, P. L., Fondacaro, M. R., & Moos, B. S. (1990). Approach and avoidance coping responses among older problem and nonproblem drinkers. *Psychology and Aging, 5,* 31–40.

Moos, R. H., & Schaefer, J. A. (1987). Evaluating health care work settings: A holistic conceptual framework. *Psychology and Health, 1,* 97–122.

Moret, V., Forster, A., Laverriere, M. C., & Lambert, H. (1991). Mechanism of analgesia induced by hypnosis and acupuncture: Is there a difference? *Pain, 45,* 135–140.

Morey, S. S. (1998). NIH issues consensus statement on acupuncture. *American Family Physician, 57,* 2545–2546.

Morgan, R. E., Palinkas, L. A., Barrett-Connor, E. L., & Wingard, D. L. (1993). Plasma cholesterol and depressive symptoms in older men. *Lancet, 341,* 75–79.

Morley, S. (1997). Pain management. In A. Baum, S. Newman, J. Weinman, R. West, & C. McManus (Eds.), *Cambridge handbook of psychology, health and medicine* (pp. 234–237). Cambridge, England: Cambridge University Press.

Morojele, N. K., & Stephenson, G. M. (1994). Addictive behaviours: Predictors of abstinence intentions and expectations in the theory of planned behavior. In D.R. Rutter & L. Quine (Eds.), *Social psychology and health: European perspectives* (pp. 47–70). Aldershot, England: Avebury.

Morokoff, P. J., Holmes, E., & Weisse, C. S. (1987). A psychoeducational program for HIV seropositive persons. *Patient Education & Counseling, 10,* 287–300.

Morrill, A. C., Ickovics, J. R., Golubchikov, V. V., Beren, S. E. & Rodin, J. (1996). Safer sex: Social and psychological predictors of behavioral maintenance and change among heterosexual women. *Journal of Consulting & Clinical Psychology, 64,* 819–828.

Morris, D. L., Kritchevsky, S. B., & Davis, C. E. (1994). Serum carotenoids and coronary heart disease. The Lipid Research Clinics Coronary Primary Prevention Trial and Follow-up Study. *Journal of the American Medical Association, 272,* 1439–1441.

Morris, R. D., & Rimm, A. A. (1991). Association of waist to hip ratio and family history with the prevalence of NIDDM among 25,272 adult, white females. *American Journal of Public Health, 81,* 507–509.

Morrow, G. R., Asbury, R., Hammon, S., & Dobkin, P. (1992). Comparing the effectiveness of behavioral treatment for chemotherapy-induced nausea and vomiting when administered by oncologists, oncology nurses, and clinical psychologists. *Health Psychology, 11,* 250–256.

Moskowitz, J. T., Folkman, S., Collette, L., & Vittinghoff, E. (1996). Coping and mood during AIDS-related caregiving and bereavement. *Annals of Behavioral Medicine, 18,* 49–57.

Moss, A. J., Allen, K. F., Giovino, G. A., & Mills, S. L. (1992). Recent trends in adolescent smoking, smoking-update correlates, and expectations about the future. *Advance Data* No. 221 (Vital and Health Statistics of the Centers for Disease Control and Prevention).

Moss-Morris, R., & Petrie, K. J. (1997). Cognitive distortions of somatic experiences: Revision and validation of a measure. *Journal of Psychosomatic Research, 43,* 293–306.

Muellersdorf, M., & Soederback, I. (2000). The actual state of the effects, treatment and incidence of disabling pain in a gender perspective—A Swedish study. *Disability and Rehabilitation, 22,* 840–854.

Mulder, C. L., de Vroome, E. M., van Griensven, G. J., Antoni, M. H., & Sandfort, T. G. (1999). Avoidance as a predictor of the biological course of HIV infection over a 7-year period in gay men. *Health Psychology, 18,* 107–113.

Muraven, M., Tice, D. M., & Baumeister, R. F. (1998). Self-control as a limited resource: Regulatory depletion patterns. *Journal of Personality and Social Psychology, 74,* 774–789.

Murphy, L. R. (1996). Stress management in work settings: A critical review of the health effects. *American Journal of Health Promotion, 11,* 112–135.

Murray, B. (1999, June). Customized appeals may increase cancer screening. *American Psychological Association Monitor, 30,* 35–36.

Murray, D. M., Richards, P. S., Luepker, R. V., & Johnson, C. A. (1987). The prevention of cigarette smoking in children: Two- and three-year follow-up comparisons of four prevention strategies. *Journal of Behavioral Medicine, 10,* 595–611.

Murray, M., & Chamberlain, K. (1999). *Qualitative health psychology: Theories and methods.* London: Sage.

Myers, H. F., Kagawa-Singer, M., Kumanika, S. K., Lex, B. W., & Markides, K. S. (1995). Panel III: Behavioral risk factors related to chronic diseases in ethnic minorities. *Health Psychology, 14,* 613–621.

Myers, L., Coughlin, S. S., Webber, L. S., Srinivasan, S. R., & Berenson, G. S. (1995). Prediction of adult cardiovascular multifactorial risk factors from childhood risk factor levels: The Bogalusa Heart Study. *American Journal of Epidemiology, 142,* 918–924.

Nagasawa, R., Qian, Z., & Wong, P. (2000). Social control theory as a theory of conformity: The case of Asian/Pacific drug and alcohol nonuse. *Sociological Perspectives, 43,* 581–603.

Nagy, M. (1948). The child's theories concerning death. *Journal of Genetic Psychology, 73,* 3–27.

Nakamura, M., Tanaka, M., Kinukawa, N., Abe, S., Itoh, K., Imai, K., Masuda, T., & Nakao, H. (2000). Association between basal serum and leptin levels and changes in abdominal fat distribution during weight loss. *Journal of Atherosclerosis and Thrombosis, 6,* 28–32.

Nakao, M., Nomura, S., Shimosawa, T., Yoshiuchi, K., Kumano, H., Kuboki, T., Suematsu, H., & Fujita, T. (1997). Clinical effects of blood pressure biofeedback treatment on hypertension by auto-shaping. *Psychosomatic Medicine, 59,* 331–338.

Naliboff, B. D., Heitkemper, M., Chang, L., & Mayer, E. A. (2000). Sex and gender in irritable bowel syndrome. In R. B. Fillingim (Ed.), *Sex, gender, and pain* (pp. 327–353). Seattle, WA: IASP Press.

Naparstek, B. (1994). *Staying well with guided imagery.* New York: Warner Books.

Nasser, M. (1997). *Culture and weight consciousness.* New York: Routledge.

Nathan, P. E., & O'Brien, J. S. (1971). An experimental analysis of the behavior of alcoholics and nonalcoholics during prolonged experimental drinking: A necessary precursor of behavior therapy? *Behavior Therapy, 2,* 455–476.

National Center for Complementary and Alternative Medicine (NCCAM) (2001). *Considering complementary and alternative medicine therapies?* Washington, DC: National Institutes of Health (http://nccam.nih.gov//).

National Center for Health Statistics. (1997). *Health, United States, 1996.* Hyattsville, MD: U. S. Public Health Service.

National Center for Health Statistics. (1999). *Deaths: Final data for 1998.* Hyattsville, MD: U.S. Department of Health and Human Services.

National Center for Health Statistics. (1999). Health insurance coverage, 1998. www.census.gov/hhes/hlthins/hlthin98/hlt98asc.html.

National Center for Health Statistics. (1999). *Health, United States, 1999: With health and aging chartbook.* Hyattsville, MD: U. S. Government Printing Office.

National Center for Health Statistics. (2000). *Health, United States, 2000.* www.cdc.gov/nchs.

National Center for Health Statistics. (2000). *National Vital Statistics Reports, 2000, 48* (p. 5). Hyattsville, MD: Department of Health and Human Services.

National Center for Health Statistics. (2001). *National hospital discharge survey.* Washington, DC: Centers for Disease Control and Prevention.

National Center for Health Statistics, National Health and Nutrition Examination Surveys. (2000). Prevalence of overweight and obesity among adults: United States. Washington, DC: U.S. Government Printing Office.

National Institute on Alcohol Abuse and Alcoholism (NIAAA). (2001, March). *Quick Facts.* Bethesda, MD: National Institutes of Health (www.niaaa.nih.gov/databases).

National Institutes of Health (NIH). (1998). Technology Assessment Statement: *Acupuncture.* Washington, DC: National Institutes of Health.

National School Boards Association (NSBA). (1999). *Ten critical threats to America's children: Warning signs for the next millennium.* www.nsba.org/highlights/ten_threats.htm.

National Cholesterol Education Program (NCEP). (2001). Executive Summary of the Third Report of the National Cholesterol Education Program Expert Panel on Detection, Evaluation, and Treatment of High Blood Cholesterol in Adults. *Journal of the American Medical Association* (http://jama.ama-assn.org/issues/v285n19).

Neergaard, L. (1999, June 18). Six deadliest diseases are cheap to prevent. *The Tribune,* p. A3.

Nelson, M. E., Fiatarone, M. A., Morganti, C. M., Trice, I., Greenberg, R. A., & Evans, W. J. (1994). Effects of high-intensity strength training on multiple risk factors for osteoporotic fractures. A randomized controlled trial. *Journal of the American Medical Association, 272,* 1909–1914.

Nemeroff, C. J. (1995). Magical thinking about illness virulence: Conceptions of germs from "safe" versus "dangerous" others. *Health Psychology, 14,* 147–151.

Nespor, K., & Csemy, L. (1994). Alcohol and drugs in Central Europe—Problems and possible solutions. *Casopis LekaruCeskych, 133,* 483.

Nesse, R. M., & Williams, G. C. (1998). Evolution and the origins of disease. *Scientific American* (www.sciam.com).

Nevid, J. S. (1996). Smoking cessation with ethnic minorities: Themes and approaches. *Journal of Social Distress and the Homeless, 5,* 39–54.

Nevid, J. S., Javier, R. A., & Moulton, J. (1996). Factors predicting participant attrition in a community-based culturally-specific smoking cessation program for Hispanic smokers. *Health Psychology, 15,* 226–229.

Nevid, J. S., Rathus, S. A., & Rubenstein, H. R. (1998). *Health in the new millennium.* New York: Worth.

Newcomb, P. A., & Carbone, P. P. (1992). The health consequences of smoking. Cancer. *Medical Clinics of North America, 76,* 305–331.

Newsom, J. T., & Schulz, R. (1998). Caregiving from the patient's perspective: Negative reactions to being helped. *Health Psychology, 17,* 172–181.

Newton, T. L., & Contrada, R. J. (1992). Repressive coping and verbal autonomic response dissociation: The influence of social context. *Journal of Personality and Social Psychology, 62,* 159–167.

Nezu, A. M., Nezu, C. M., & Blissett, S. E. (1988). Sense of humor as a moderator of the relation between stressful events and psychological distress: A prospective analysis. *Journal of Personality and Social Psychology, 54,* 520–525.

Nicholson, P. W., & Harland, S. J. (1995). Inheritance and testicular cancer. *The British Journal of Cancer, 71* (abstract), 421.

Nikiforov, S. V., & Mamaev, V. B. (1998). The development of sex differences in cardiovascular disease mortality: A historical perspective. *American Journal of Public Health, 88,* 1348–1353.

Nivision, M. E., & Endresen, I. M. (1993). An analysis of relationships among environmental noise, annoyance and sensitivity to noise, and the consequences for health and sleep. *Journal of Behavior Medicine, 16,* 257–276.

Nolen-Hoeksema, S., & Davis, C. G. (1999). "Thanks for sharing that: Ruminators and their social support networks." *Journal of Personality and Social Psychology, 77,* 801–814.

Nolen-Hoeksema, S., Parker, L. E., & Larson, J. (1994). Ruminative coping with depressed mood following loss. *Journal of Personality and Social Psychology, 67,* 92–104.

Norris, J., Nurius, P. S., & Dimeff, L. A. (1996). Through her eyes: Factors affecting women's perception of and resistance to acquaintance sexual aggression threat. *Psychology of Women Quarterly, 20,* 123–145.

Norvell, N., & Belles, D. (1993). Psychological and physical benefits of circuit weight training in law enforcement personnel. *Journal of Consulting and Clinical Psychology, 61,* 520–527.

Nowak, R. (1994). Nicotine research. Key study unveiled—11 years late. *Science, 264,* 196–197.

Nuclear Energy Agency (1995). Chernobyl ten years on: Radiological and health impact. www.nea.fr/html/rp/chernobyl.

Nutrition Action Newsletter, 2001. *The best and worst breakfasts.* www.cspinet.org/nah/index.htm.

Nyamathi, A., Stein, J. A., & Brecht, M. (1995). Psychosocial predictors of AIDS risk behavior and drug use behavior in homeless and drug addicted women of color. *Health Psychology, 14,* 265–273.

Nyiendo, J., & Olsen, E. (1988). Visit characteristics of 217 children attending a chiropractic college teaching clinic. *Journal of Manipulative and Physiological Therapeutics, 11,* 78–84.

O'Brien, S. J., & Vertinsky, P. A. (1991). Unfit survivors: Exercise as a resource for aging women. *The Gerontologist, 31,* 347–357.

O'Callaghan, F. V., Chang, D. C., Callan, V. J., & Baglioni, A. (1997). Models of alcohol use by young adults: An examination of various attitude-behavior theories. *Journal of Studies on Alcohol, 5,* 502–507.

O'Connor, E. (2001, April). The integrative approach to cancer care. *Monitor on Psychology* (www.apa.org/monitor/apr01).

Ogletree, S. M., Williams, S. W., Raffeld, P., Mason, B., & Fricke, K. (1990). Female attractiveness and eating disorders: Do children's television commercials play a role? *Sex Roles, 22,* 11–12.

Ohlund, C., Lindstrom, I., Areskoug, B., Eek, C., Peterson, L. E., & Nachemson, A. (1994). Pain behavior in industrial subacute low back pain. *Pain, 58,* 201–209.

Olbrisch, M. E. (1981). Evaluation of a stress management program for high utilizers of a prepaid university health service. *Medical Care, 19,* 153–159.

Older Americans 2000: Key indicators of well-being. Federal Interagency Forum on Aging Related Statistics (www.agingstats.gov/chartbook2000/olderamericans2000).

Oldridge, N. B., (1988). Cardiac rehabilitation exercise programme. Compliance and compliance-enhancing strategies. *Sports Medicine, 6,* 42–55.

Olds, J., & Milner, P. (1954). Positive reinforcement produced by electrical stimulation of the septal area and other regions of rat brain. *Journal of Comparative and Physiological Psychology, 47,* 419–427.

Olness, K. (1993). Hypnosis: The power of attention. In D. Goleman & J. Gurin (Eds.), *Mind-body medicine: How to use your mind for better health* (pp. 277–290). New York: Consumer Reports Books.

O'Neill, J. (1998, August 11). A leg up for the heart. *The New York Times* (www.nytimes.com).

Onishi, N. (2001, February 21). In Africa, Rubensesque rules: Women use animal feed, steroids for beauty ideal. *Anchorage Daily News,* A-1, A-5.

Orne, M. T. (1980). Hypnotic control of pain: Toward a clarification of the different psychological processes involved. In J. J. Bonica (Ed.), *Pain* (pp. 155–172). New York: Raven Press.

Ornish, D., Brown, S. E., Scherwitz, L. W., Billings, J. H., Armstrong, W. T., Ports, T. A., McLanahan, S. M., Kirkeeide, R. L., Brand, R. J., & Gould, K. L. (1990). Can lifestyle changes reverse coronary heart disease? The Lifestyle Heart Trial. *Lancet, 336,* 129–133.

Orth-Gomer, K., Rosengren, A., & Wilhelmsen, L. (1993). Lack of social support and incidence of coronary heart disease in middle-aged Swedish men. *Psychosomatic Medicine, 55,* 37–43.

Ory, M. G., Abeles, R. P., & Lipman, P. D. (1992). *Aging, health, and behavior.* Thousand Oaks, CA: Sage Publications.

Ory, M. G., & Cox, D. M. (1994). Forging ahead: Linking health and behavior to improve quality of life in older people. *Social Indicators Research, 33,* 89–120.

Oster, G., Thompson, D., Edelsberg, J., Bird, A. P., & Colditz, G. A. (1999). Lifetime health and economic benefits of weight loss among obese persons. *American Journal of Public Health, 89,* 1536–1542.

Ostir, G. V., Markides, K. S., Black, S. A., & Goodwin, J. S. (2000). Emotional well-being predicts subsequent functional independence and survival. *Journal of the American Geriatrics Society, 48,* 473–478.

Ostir, G. V., Markides, K. S., Peek, M. K., & Goodwin, J. S. (2001). The association between emotional well-being and the incidence of stroke in older adults. *Psychosomatic Medicine, 63,* 210–215.

Overmier, J. B., & Gahtan, E. (1998). Psychoneuroimmunology: The final hurdle. *Integrative Physiological and Behavioral Science, 33,* 137–140.

Owen, N., & Vita, P. (1997). Physical activity and health. In A. Baum, S. Newman, J. Weinman, R. West, & C. McManus (Eds.), *Cambridge handbook of psychology, health and medicine* (pp. 154–157). Cambridge, England: Cambridge University Press.

Oxman, T. E., Berkman, L. F., Kasl, S., Freeman, D. H., & Barrett, J. (1992). Social support and depressive symptoms in the elderly. *American Journal of Epidemiology, 135,* 356–368.

Pall, M. L. (2000). Elevated, sustained peroxynitrite levels as the cause of chronic fatigue syndrome. *Medical Hypotheses, 54,* 115–125.

Papas, C. A. (1999, June 15). Unlike women, many men avoid doctor even when feeling pain. *USA Today,* p. 11D.

Paramore, L. C. (1997). Use of alternative therapies: Estimates from the 1994 Robert Wood Johnson Foundation National Access to Care Survey. *Journal of Pain and Symptom Management, 13,* 83–89.

Paran, E., Amir, M., & Yaniv, N. (1996). Evaluating the response of mild hypertensives to biofeedback-assisted relaxation using a mental stress test. *Journal of Behavior Therapy and Experimental Psychiatry, 27,* 157–167.

Parker, D., Manstead, A. S., Stradling, S. G., & Reason, J. T. (1992). Intention to commit driving violations: An application of the theory of planned behavior. *Journal of Applied Psychology, 77,* 94–101.

Parker, P. A., & Kulik, J. A. (1995). Burnout, self- and supervisor-rated job performance, and absenteeism among nurses. *Journal of Behavioral Medicine, 18,* 581–599.

Parker, R. (2000). Health literacy: A challenge for American patients and their health care providers. *Health Promotion International, 15,* 277–283.

Parrott, A. C. (1999). Does cigarette smoking cause stress? *American Psychologist, 54,* 817–820.

Pate, J. E., Pumariega, A. J., Hester, C., & Garner, D. M. (1992). Cross-cultural patterns in eating disorders: A review. *Journal of the American Academy of Child and Adolescent Psychiatry, 31,* 802–809.

Patel, M. (1987). Problems in the evaluation of alternative medicine. *Social Science and Medicine, 25,* 669–675.

Patel, M., Gutzwiller, F., Paccaud, F., & Marazzi, A. (1989). A meta-analysis of acupuncture for chronic pain. *International Journal of Epidemiology, 18,* 900–906.

Patenaude, A. F., Hirsch, D., Breyer, J., & Astbury, J. (1990). Psychosocial effects of transfusion-related HIV infection in pediatric cancer patients. *Journal of Psychosocial Oncology, 8,* 41–58.

Paton, D. (1992). Disaster research: The Scottish dimension. *The Psychologist: Bulletin of the British Psychological Society, 5,* 535–538.

Patterson, T. L., Shaw, W. S., Semple, S. J., & Cherner, M. (1996). Relationship of psychosocial factors to HIV disease progression. *Annals of Behavioral Medicine, 18,* 30–39.

Pauls, D. L., Morton, L. A., & Egeland, J. A. (1992). Risks of affective illness among first-degree relatives of bipolar I old-order Amish probands. *Archives of General Psychiatry, 49,* 703–708.

Peat, G. M., Moores, L., Goldingay, S., & Hunter, M. (2001). Pain management program follow-ups. A national survey of current practice in the United Kingdom. *Journal of Pain and Symptom Management, 21,* 218–226.

Pechmann, C., & Shih, C. F. (1999). Smoking scenes in movies and antismoking advertisements before movies: Effects on youth. *Journal of Marketing, 63,* 1–13.

Pender, N. J., Walker, S. N., Sechrist, K. R., & Frank-Stromborg, M. (1990). Predicting health-promoting lifestyles in the workplace. *Nursing Research, 39,* 326–332.

Pennebaker, J. W. (1980). Perceptual and environmental determinants of coughing. *Basic and Applied Social Psychology, 1,* 83–91.

Pennebaker, J. W. (1982). *The psychology of physical symptoms.* New York: Springer-Verlag.

Pennebaker, J. W. (1992). Inhibition as the linchpin of health. In H. S. Friedman (Ed.), *Hostility, coping, & health* (pp. 127–139). Washington, DC: American Psychological Association.

Pennebaker, J. W., Burnam, M. A., Schaeffer, M. A., & Harper, D. C. (1977). Lack of control as a determinant of perceived physical symptoms. *Journal of Personality and Social Psychology, 35,* 167–174.

Pennebaker, J. W., & Epstein, D. (1983). Implicit psychophysiology: Effects of common beliefs and idiosyncratic physiological responses on symptom reporting. *Journal of Personality, 51,* 468–496.

Pennebaker, J. W., & Francis, M. E. (1996). Cognitive, emotional, and language processes in disclosure. *Cognition & Emotion, 10,* 601–626.

Pennebaker, J. W., Mayne, T. J., & Francis, M. E. (1997). Linguistic predictors of adaptive bereavement. *Journal of Personality and Social Psychology, 72,* 863–871.

Penninx, B. W., Guralnik, J. M., Pahor, M., Ferrucci, L., Cerhan, J. R., Wallace, R. B., & Havlik, R. J. (1998). Chronically depressed mood and cancer risk in older persons. *Journal of the National Cancer Institute, 90,* 1888–1893.

Penninx, B. W., van Tilburg, T., Boeke, A. J., Deeg, D. J., Kriegsman, D. M., & van Eijk, J. T. (1998). Effects of social support and personal coping resources on depressive symptoms: Different for various chronic diseases? *Health Psychology, 17,* 551–558.

Perkins, K. A., Dubbert, P. M., Martin, J. E., Faulstich, M. E., & Harris, J. K. (1986). Cardiovascular reactivity to psychological stress in aerobically trained versus untrained mild hypertensives and normotensives. *Health Psychology, 5,* 407–421.

Perlick, D., & Silverstein, B. (1994). Faces of female discontent: Depression, disordered eating, and changing gender roles. In P. Fallon & M. A. Katzman (Eds.), *Feminist perspectives on eating disorders* (pp. 77–93). New York: Guilford.

Perlmutter, M., Kaplan, M., & Nyquist, L. (1990). Development of adaptive competence in adulthood. *Human Development, 33,* 185–197.

Perls, T. T., & Fretts, R. C. (1998). Why women live longer than men. *Scientific American* (www.sciam.com).

Perri, M. G. (1998). The maintenance of treatment effects in the long-term management of obesity. *Clinical Psychology: Science and Practice, 5,* 526–543.

Persky, V. W., Kempthrone-Rawson, J., & Shekelle, R. B. (1987) Personality and risk of cancer: 20-year follow-up of the Western Electric Study. *Psychosomatic Medicine, 49,* 435–439.

Pert, C. B., Dreher, H. E., & Ruff, M. R. (1998). The psychosomatic network: Foundations of mind–body medicine. *Alternative Therapies in Health and Medicine, 4,* 30–41.

Perz, C. A., DiClemente, C. C., & Carbonari, J. P. (1996). Doing the right thing at the right time? The interaction of stages and processes of change in successful smoking cessation. *Health Psychology, 15,* 462–468.

Peterson, A. V., Kealey, K. A., Mann, S. L., Marek, P. M., & Sarason, I. G. (2000). Hutchinson Smoking Prevention Project: Long-term randomized trial in school-based tobacco use prevention—results on smoking. *Journal of the National Cancer Institute, 92,* 1979–1991.

Peterson, C. (2000). The future of optimism. *American Psychologist, 55*(1), 44–55.

Peterson, C., & Bossio, L. M. (1991). *Health and optimism.* New York: Free Press.

Peterson, C., Seligman, M. E. P., Yurko, K. H., Martin, L. R., & Friedman, H. S. (1998). Catastrophizing and untimely death. *Psychological Science, 9,* 127–130.

Peterson, C., & Stunkard, A. J. (1989). Personal control and health promotion. *Social Science and Medicine, 28,* 819–828.

Peterson, K. (1997). Success in the face of adversity: Six stories of minority career achievement. In H. S. Farmer (Ed.), *Diversity and women's career development: From adolescence to adulthood* (pp. 172–186). Thousand Oaks, CA: Sage Publications.

Peterson, L., Crowson, J., Saldana, L., & Holdridge, S. (1999). Of needles and skinned knees: Children's coping with medical procedures and minor injuries for self and other. *Health Psychology, 18,* 197–200.

Peto, R., Lopez, A. D., Boreham, J., Thun, M., Heath, C., & Doll, R. (1996). Mortality from smoking worldwide. *British Medical Bulletin, 52,* 12–21.

Petrie, K. J., Booth, R. J., & Davison, K. P. (1995). Repression, disclosure, and immune function: Recent findings and methodological issues. In J. W. Pennebaker (Ed.), *Emotion, disclosure, and health* (pp. 223–237). Washington, DC: American Psychological Association.

Petrie, K. J., Booth, R. J. & Pennebaker, J. W. (1998). The immunological effects of thought suppression. *Journal of Personality and Social Psychology, 75*(5), 1264–1272.

Philips, H. C. (1988). Changing chronic pain experience. *Pain, 32,* 165–172.

Phillips, W. T., Kiernan, M., & King, A. C. (2001). The effects of physical activity on physical and psychological health. In A.

Baum, T. A. Revenson, & J. E. Singer (Eds.), *Handbook of health Psychology* (pp. 627–657). Mahwah, NJ: Erlbaum.

Phipps, S., Fairclough, D., & Mulhern, R. K. (1995). Avoidant coping in children with cancer. *Journal of Pediatric Psychology, 20,* 217–232.

Phipps, S., & Srivastava, D. K. (1997). Repressive adaptation in children with cancer. *Health Psychology, 16,* 521–528.

Pichichero, M. E. (2000, April 15). Acute otitis media: Treatment in an era of increasing antibiotic resistance. *American Family Physician, 61,* 2410–2416.

Pike, K. M., & Rodin, J. (1991). Mothers, daughters, and disordered eating. *Journal of Abnormal Psychology, 100,* 1–7.

Pilisuk, M., Boylan, R., & Acredolo, C. (1987). Social support, life stress, and subsequent medical care utilization. *Health Psychology, 6,* 273–288.

Pingitore, R., Dugoni, B. L., Tindale, R. S., & Spring, B. (1994). Bias against overweight job applicants in a simulated employment interview. *Journal of Applied Psychology, 79,* 909–917.

Piscitelli, S. C., Burstein, A. H., Chaitt, D., Alfaro, R. M., & Falloon, J. (2000). Indinavir concentrations and St. John's wort. *Lancet, 355,* 547–548.

Pistrang, N., & Barker, C. (1995). The partner relationship in psychological response to breast cancer. *Social Science and Medicine, 40,* 689–697.

Pitskhelauri, G. Z. (1982). *The long-living of Soviet Georgia.* New York: Human Sciences Press.

Place, M. (1984). Hypnosis and the child. *Journal of Child Psychology and Psychiatry and Allied Disciplines, 25,* 339–347.

Plomin, R. (1995). Molecular genetics and psychology. *Current Directions in Psychological Science, 4,* 114–117.

Plomin, R. (1997). Identifying genes for cognitive abilities and disabilities. In R. J. Sternberg, E. L. Grigorenkon, et al. (Eds.), *Intelligence, heredity, and environment* (pp. 89–104). New York: Cambridge University Press.

Plomin, R., DeFries, J. C., McClearn, G. E., & McGuffin, P. (2001). *Behavioral genetics* (4th ed.). New York: Worth.

Podolsky, D., & Silberner, J. (1993). How medicine mistreats the elderly. *U.S. News & World Report,* January 18, 72–79.

Polivy, J. (1996). Psychological consequences of food restriction. *Journal of the American Dietetic Association, 96,* 589–594.

Polivy, J., & Herman, C. P. (1987). Diagnosis and treatment of normal eating. *Journal of Consulting and Clinical Psychology, 55,* 635–644.

Pollock, S. E. (1986). Human responses to chronic illness: Physiologic and psychosocial adaptation. *Nursing Research, 35,* 90–95.

Poon, L. W. (1987). *Myths and truisms: Beyond extant analyses of speed of behavior and age.* Address to the Eastern Psychological Association.

Porges, S. W., Doussard-Roosevelt, J. A., & Maiti, A. K. (1994). Vagal tone and the physiological regulation of emotion. *Monographs of the Society for Research in Child Development, 59,* 167–186.

Potter, J. D. (1997). Hazards and benefits of alcohol. *New England Journal of Medicine, 337,* 1763–1764.

Prentice, D. A., & Miller, D. T. (1993). Pluralistic ignorance and alcohol use on campus: Some consequences of misperceiving the social norm. *Journal of Personality and Social Psychology, 64*, 243–256.

Prescott, E., Osler, M., Hein, H. O., Borch-Johnsen, K., Schnohr, P., & Vestbo, J. (1998). Life expectancy in Danish women and men related to smoking habits: Smoking may affect women more. *Journal of Epidemiology and Community Health, 52*(2), 131–132.

Price, D. D. (1999). *Psychological mechanism of pain and analgesia.* Seattle, WA: IASP Press.

Primack, A., & Spencer, J. (1996). *The collection and evaluation of clinical research data relevant to alternative medicine and cancer.* Bethesda, MD: Office of Alternative Medicine, National Institutes of Health.

Prochaska, J. O. (1996a). Revolution in health promotion: Smoking cessation as a case study. In R. J. Resnick & R. H. Rozensky (Eds.), *Health psychology through the life span: Practice and research opportunities* (pp. 361–375). Washington, DC: American Psychological Association.

Prochaska, J. O. (1996b). A stage paradigm for integrating clinical and public health approaches to smoking cessation. *Addictive Behaviors, 21*, 721–732.

Prochaska, J. O., & DiClemente, C. C. (1984). *The transtheoretical approach: Crossing traditional boundaries of therapy.* Chicago: Dow Jones/Irwin.

Prochaska, J. O., Redding, C. A., Harlow, L. L., Rossi, J. S., & Velicer, W. F. (1994). The transtheoretical model of change and HIV prevention: A review. *Health Education Quarterly, 21*, 471–486.

Prochaska, J. O., Velicer, W. F., Fava, J., & Laforge, R. (1995). Toward disease-state management for smoking: Stage-matched expert systems for a total managed care population of smokers. (Manuscript submitted for publication.)

Ptacek, J. T., & Eberhardt, T. L. (1996). Breaking bad news. A review of the literature. *Journal of the American Medical Association, 276*, 496–502.

Ptacek, J. T., Smith, R. E., & Zanas, J. (1992). Gender, appraisal, and coping: A longitudinal analysis. *Journal of Personality, 60*, 747–770.

Pumariega, A. J. (1986). Acculturation and eating attitudes in adolescent girls: A comparative and correlational study. *Journal of the American Academy of Child Psychiatry, 25*, 276–279.

Purves, W., Sadava, D., Orians, G., Heller, C. (2001). *Life: The science of biology* (6th ed.). New York: W. H. Freeman.

Quick, J. C., & Quick, J. D. (1984). *Organizational stress and preventive management.* New York: McGraw-Hill.

Quigley, L. A., & Marlatt, G. A. (1996). Drinking among young adults: Prevalence, patterns and consequences. *Alcohol Health and Research World, 20*, 185–191.

Quill, T. E. (1985). Somatization disorder. One of medicine's blind spots. *Journal of the American Medical Association, 254*, 3075–3079.

Rabasca, L. (1999, June). Psychosocial support is lacking for cancer patients, finds IOM report. *American Psychological Association Monitor, 30*, 10.

Rabasca, L. (1999, November). Imagery, massage and relaxation recognized as ways to manage pain. *American Psychological Association Monitor, 30*, 9.

Rahe, R. H., Mahan, J. L., & Arthur, R. J. (1970). Prediction of near-future health changes from subjects' preceding life changes. *Journal of Psychosomatic Research, 14*, 401–406.

Rakowski, W., Fulton, J. P., & Feldman, J. P. (1993). Women's decision making about mammography: A replication of the relationship between stages of adoption and decision balance. *Health Psychology, 12*, 209–214.

Raloff, J. (1996). Vanishing flesh: Muscle loss in the elderly finally gets some respect. *Science News, 150*, 90–91.

Ramachandran, V.S., & Rogers-Ramachandran, D. (2000). Phantom limbs and neural plasticity. *Archives of Neurology, 57*, 317-320.

Ranadive, U. (1997). Phantom limbs and rewired brains. *Technology Review, 100*, 17–18.

Rand, C. S., & Kuldau, J. M. (1990). The epidemiology of obesity and self-defined weight problem in the general population: Gender, race, age, and social class. *International Journal of Eating Disorders, 9*, 329–343.

Rawlins, W. K. (1995). Friendships in later life. In J. F. Nussbaum & J. Coupland (Eds.), *Handbook of communication and aging research* (pp. 227–257). Mahwah, NJ: Erlbaum.

Ray, C. (1997). Chronic fatigue syndrome. In A. Baum, S. Newman, J. Weinman, R. West, & C. McManus (Eds.), *Cambridge handbook of psychology, health and medicine* (pp. 408–409). Cambridge, UK: Cambridge University Press.

Read, J. P., Kahler, C. W., & Stevenson, J. F. (2001). Bridging the gap between alcoholism treatment research and practice: Identifying what works and why. *Professional Psychology: Research and Practice, 32*, 22–238.

Redd, W. H., & Jacobsen, P. (2001). Behavioral intervention in comprehensive cancer care. In A. Baum, T. A. Revenson, & J. E. Singer (Eds.), *Handbook of health psychology* (pp. 757–776). Mahwah, NJ: Erlbaum.

Reed, D., McGee, D., Yano, K., & Feinleib, M. (1983). Social Networks and coronary heart disease among Japanese men in Hawaii. *American Journal of Epidemiology, 117*, 384–396.

Reed, G. M., Kemeny, M. E., Taylor, S. E., Wang, H. Y., & Visscher, B. R. (1994). Realistic acceptance as a predictor of decreased survival time in gay men with AIDS. *Health Psychology, 13*, 299–307.

Reich, J. W., & Zautra, A. J. (1995). Spouse encouragement of self-reliance and other-reliance in rheumatoid arthritis couples. *Journal of Behavioral Medicine, 18*, 249–260.

Reiff, M., Zakut, H., & Weingarten, M. A. (1999). Illness and treatment perceptions of Ethiopian immigrants and their doctors in Israel. *American Journal of Public Health, 89*, 1814–1818.

Relman, A. S. (1998, December 14). A trip to stonesville. *The New Republic Online.* (http://www.tnr.com/archive/1298/121498/relman121498.html).

Repetti, R. L. (1993). Short-term effects of occupational stressors on daily mood and health complaints. *Health Psychology, 12,* 125–131.

Resnick, H. S., Kilpatrick, D. G., Best, C. L., & Kramer, T. L. (1992). Vulnerability-stress factors in development of posttraumatic stress disorder. *Journal of Nervous and Mental Disease, 180,* 424–430.

Revenson, T. A., & Baum, A. (2001). Introduction. In A. Baum, T. Revenson, & J. E. Singer (Eds.), *Handbook of health psychology* (pp. xv–xx). Mahwah, NJ: Erlbaum.

Rexrode, K. M., Carey, V. J., Hennekens, C. H., Walters, E. E., Colditz, G. A., Stampfer, M. J., Willett, W. C., & Manson, J. E. (1998). Abdominal adiposity and coronary heart disease in women. *Journal of the American Medical Association, 280,* 1843–1848.

Reyes, A. (1999, April 19). Striking a healthy dietary balance for the elderly. *The University Record,* p. 24.

Reynolds, D. V. (1969). Surgery in the rat during electrical analgesia induced by focal brain stimulation. *Science, 164,* 444–445.

Reynolds, P., & Kaplan, G. A. (1990). Social connections and risk for cancer: Prospective evidence from the Alameda County Study. *Behavioral Medicine, 16,* 101–110.

Richards, M. H., Boxer, A. M., Petersen, A. C., & Albrecht, R. (1990). Relation of weight to body image in pubertal girls and boys from two communities. *Developmental Psychology, 26,* 313–321.

Richardson, P. H. (1994). Placebo effects in pain management. *Pain Reviews, 1,* 15–32.

Richardson, P. H. (1997). Placebos. In A. Baum, S. Newman, J. Weinman, R. West, & C. McManus (Eds.), *Cambridge handbook of psychology, health and medicine* (pp. 237–241). Cambridge, UK: Cambridge University Press.

Richardson, P. H., & Vincent, C. A. (1986). Acupuncture for the treatment of pain: A review of evaluative research. *Pain, 24,* 15–40.

Richardson, S. A. (1971). Children's values and friendships: A study of physical disability. *Journal of Health and Social Behavior, 12,* 253–258.

Ries, L. A., Wingo, P. A., Miller, D. S., Howe, H. L., Weir, H. K., Rosenberg, H. M., Vernon, S. W., Cronin, K., & Edwards, B. K. (2000). The annual report to the nation on the status of cancer, 1973–1997, with a special section on colorectal cancer. *Cancer, 88,* 2398–2424.

Rigotti, N. A., Lee, J. E., & Wechsler, H. (2000). US college students' use of tobacco products: Results of a national survey. *Journal of the American Medical Association, 284,* 699–705.

Riley, J. L., Robinson, M. E., Wise, E. A., Myers, C. D., & Fillingim, R. B. (1998). Sex differences in the perception of noxious experimental stimuli: A meta-analysis. *Pain, 74,* 181–187.

Robberson, M. R., & Rogers, R. W. (1988). Beyond fear appeals: Negative and positive persuasive appeals to health and self-esteem. *Journal of Applied Social Psychology, 18,* 277–287.

Robbins, A. (1993). The children's vaccine initiative. *American Journal of Diseases of Children, 147,* 152–157.

Robert Wood Johnson Foundation (2001). *Substance Abuse: The Nation's Number One Health Problem.* www.rwjf.org.

Roberts, S. S. (1998). Working toward a world without Type I diabetes. *Diabetes Forecast, 51,* 85–87.

Robinson, T. E., & Berridge, K. C. (2000). The psychology and neurobiology of addiction: An incentive-sensitization view. *Addiction, 95,* S91–S117.

Rockhill, B., Willett, W. C., Hunter, D. J., Manson, J. E., Hankinson, S. E., & Colditz, G. A. (1999). A prospective study of recreational physical activity and breast cancer risk. *Archives of Internal Medicine, 159,* 2290–2296.

Rodin, J. (1981). Current status of the internal-external hypothesis for obesity: What went wrong? *American Psychologist, 36,* 361–372.

Rodin, J. (1986). Aging and health: Effects of the sense of control. *Science, 233,* 1271–1276.

Roehling, M. V., & Winters, D. (2000). Job security rights: The effects of specific policies and practices on the evaluation of employers. *Employee Responsibilities and Rights Journal, 12,* 25–38.

Roethlisberger, F. J., & Dickson, W. J. (1939). Management and the worker. Cambridge, MA: Harvard University Press.

Rogina, B., Reenan, R. A., Nilsen, S. P., & Helfand, S. L. (2000). Extended life-span conferred by cotransporter gene mutations in Drosophila. *Science, 290,* 2137–2140.

Roizen, M. F. (1999). *Real age: Are you as young as you can be?* New York: Cliff Street Books.

Ronis, D. L. (1992). Conditional health threats: Health beliefs, decisions, and behaviors among adults. *Health Psychology, 11,* 127–134.

Root, M. P. (1990). Disordered eating in women of color [Special issue: Gender and ethnicity: Perspectives on dual status]. *Sex Roles, 227,* 525–536.

Root-Bernstein, R., & Root-Bernstein, M. (1997). *Honey, mud, maggots and other medical marvels.* New York: Houghton Mifflin.

Rosario, M., Shinn, M., Morch, H., & Huckabee, C. (1988). Gender differences in coping and social supports: Testing socialization and role constraint theories. *Journal of Community Psychology* (Special Issue: *Women in the Community*), *16,* 55–69.

Rosch, E. (1978). Principles of categorization. In E. Rosch & B. L. Lloyd (Eds.), *Cognition and categorization* (pp. 132–147). Hillsdale, NJ: Erlbaum.

Rosen, J. C., & Leitenberg, H. (1982). Bulimia nervosa: Treatment with exposure and response prevention. *Behavior Therapy, 13,* 117–124.

Rosen, M., Nystrom, L., & Wall, S. (1988). Diet and cancer mortality in the counties of Sweden. *American Journal of Epidemiology, 127,* 42–49.

Rosenberg, E. L., Ekman, P., & Blumenthal, J. A. (1998). Facial expression and the affective component of cynical hostility in male coronary heart disease patients. *Health Psychology, 17,* 376–380.

Rosenbloom, A. L., Joe, J. R., Young, R. S., & Winter, W. E. (1999). Emerging epidemic of type 2 diabetes in youth. *Diabetes Care, 22,* 345–354.

Rosenfield, S. (1992). The costs of sharing: Wives' employment and husbands' mental health. *Journal of Health and Social Behavior, 33,* 213–225.

Rosenman, R. H., Brand, R. J., Jenkins, C. D., Friedman, M., Straus, R., & Wurm, M. (1975). Coronary heart disease in the Western Collaborative Group Study: Final follow-up experience of 8 1/2 years. *Journal of the American Medical Association, 233,* 872–877.

Rosenstock, I., Strecher, V. J., & Becker, M. H. (1994). The health belief model and HIV risk behavior change. In R. J. DiClemente & J. L. Peterson (Eds.), *Preventing AIDS: Theories and methods of behavioral interventions* (pp. 5–24). New York: Plenum.

Rosenthal, E. (1993, October 13). Does fragmented medicine harm the health of women? *New York Times,* pp. A1, B7.

Ross, J. G., Pate, R. R., Casperson, C. J., Domberg, C. L., & Svilar, M. (1987). Home and community in children's exercise habits. *Journal of Physical Education, Recreation, and Dance, 58,* 85–92.

Roth, D. L., & Holmes, D. S. (1985). Influence of physical fitness in deterring the impact of stressful events on physical and psychologic health. *Psychosomatic Medicine, 47,* 164–173.

Roth, O. (1979). *Heart attack: A question and answer book.* New York: Macmillan.

Roth, S., & Cohen, S. (1986). Approach, avoidance, and coping with stress. *American Psychologist, 41,* 813–819.

Rotheram-Borus, M. J., Murphy, D. A., Reid, H. M., & Coleman, C. L. (1996). Correlates of emotional distress among HIV+ youths: Health status, stress, and personal resources. *Annals of Behavioral Medicine, 18,* 16–23.

Rothman, A. J., & Salovey, P. (1997). Shaping perceptions to motivate healthy behavior: The role of message framing. *Psychological Bulletin, 121,* 3–19.

Rothman, A. J., Salovey, P., Antone, C., & Keough, K. (1993). The influence of message framing on intentions to perform health behaviors. *Journal of Experimental Social Psychology, 29,* 408–433.

Rowe, M. (1997). Hardiness, stress, temperament, coping, and burnout in health professionals. *American Journal of Health Behavior, 21,* 163–171.

Ruberman, W., Weinblatt, E., Goldberg, J. D., & Chaudhary, B. S. (1984). Psychosocial influences on mortality after myocardial infarction. *New England Journal of Medicine, 311,* 552–559.

Ruble, D. (1972). Premenstrual symptoms: A reinterpretation. *Science, 197,* 291–292.

Rubonis, A. V., & Bickman, L. (1991). Psychological impairment in the wake of disaster: The disaster-psychopathology relationship. *Psychological Bulletin, 109,* 384–399.

Rudolph, K. D., Dennig, M. D., & Weisz, J. R. (1995). Determinants and consequences of children's coping in the medical setting: Conceptualization, review, and critique. *Psychological Bulletin, 118,* 328–357.

Ruffin, C. L. (1993). Stress and health—little hassles vs. major life events. *Australian Psychologist, 28,* 201–208.

Rundall, T. G., & Wheeler, J. R. C. (1979). The effect of income on use of preventive care: An evaluation of alternative explanations. *Journal of Health and Social Behavior, 20,* 297–406.

Rusell, R. M. (2000, August). The aging process as a modifier of metabolism. *American Journal of Clinical Nutrition, 72,* 529–532.

Russell, M. A. (1971). Cigarette dependence: Nature and classification. *British Medical Journal, 2,* 330–331.

Russell, R. G. (1979). Bulimia nervosa: An ominous variant of anorexia nervosa. *Psychological Medicine, 9,* 429–448.

Rutter, M. (1979). Protective factors in children's responses to stress and disadvantage. In W. M. Kent & J. E. Roll (Eds.), *Primary prevention of psychopathology,* vol. 3 (pp. 49–74). Hanover, NH: University Press of New England.

Rutz, D. (1998, September 22). Study tracks causes, treatment of perplexing chronic fatigue syndrome. www.cnn.com/health.

Ryff, C. D., Singer, B. H., Wing, E., & Love, G. D. (2001). Elective affinities and uninvited agonies: Mapping emotion with significant others onto health. In C. D. Ryff & B. H. Singer (Eds.), *Emotion, social relationships, and health* (pp. 133–175). New York: Oxford University Press.

Sacco, R. L., Benson, R. T., Kargman, D. E., Boden-Albala, B., Tuck, C., Lin, I. F., Cheng, J. F., Paik, M. C., Shea, S., & Berglund, L. (2001). High-density lipoprotein cholesterol and ischemic stroke in the elderly: The Northern Manhattan Stroke Study. *Journal of the American Medical Association, 285,* 2729–2735.

Sacks, M. H. (1990). Eating disorders and long-distance running: The ascetic condition. *Integrative Psychiatry, 5,* 205–206.

Saez, E., Tontonoz, P., Nelson, M. C., Alvarez, J. G., Baird, S. M., Thomazy, V. A., & Evans, R. M. (1998). Activators of the nuclear receptor PPARg enhance polyp formation. *Nature Medicine, 4,* 1058–1061.

Safer, M. A., Tharps, Q. J., Jackson, T. C., & Leventhal, H. (1979). Determinants of three stages of delay in seeking care at a medical clinic. *Medical Care, 17,* 11–29.

Salovey, P., O'Leary, A., Stretton, M. S., Fishkin, S. A., & Drake, C. A. (1991). Influence of mood on judgments about health and illness. In J. P. Firgas (Ed.), *Emotion and social judgments* (pp. 241–262). New York: Pergamon.

Salovey, P., Rothman, A. J., & Rodin, J. (1998). Health behavior. In D. T. Gilbert & S. T. Fiske (Eds.), *The handbook of social psychology* (4th ed., Vol. 2, pp. 633–683). New Haven, CT: Yale University Press.

Salzmann, P., Kerlikowske, K., & Phillips, K. (1997). Cost-effectiveness of extending screening mammography guidelines to include women 40 to 49 years of age. *Annals of Internal Medicine, 127,* 955–965.

Sanders, S. H., Brena, S. F., Spier, C. J., Beltrutti, D., McConnell, H., & Quintero, O. (1992). Chronic low back patients around the world: Cross-cultural similarities and differences. *The Clinical Journal of Pain, 8,* 317–323.

Sapadin, L. (1988). Friendship and gender: Perspectives of professional men and women. *Journal of Social and Personal Relationships, 5,* 387–403.

Sapolsky, R. M. (1996). Why stress is bad for your brain. *Science, 273,* 749–750.

Sarwer, D. B., Wadden, T. A., & Foster, G. D. (1998). Assessment of body image dissatisfaction in obese women: Specificity, severity, and clinical significance. *Journal of Consulting and Clinical Psychology, 66,* 651–654.

Sayette, M. A. (1993). An appraisal-disruption model of alcohol's effects on stress responses in social drinkers. *Psychological Bulletin, 114,* 459–476.

Sayette, M. A., & Hufford, M. R. (1997). Effects of smoking urge on generation of smoking-related information. *Journal of Applied Social Psychology, 27,* 1295–1405.

Scanlon, C. (1996). Euthanasia and nursing practice—right question, wrong answer. *New England Journal of Medicine, 334,* 1401–1402.

Schaalma, H. P., Kok, G., & Peters, L. (1993). Reactions among Dutch youth toward people with AIDS. *Journal of School Health, 63,* 182–187.

Schachter, S. (1971). Some extraordinary facts about obese humans and rats. *American Psychologist, 26,* 129–144.

Schachter, S. (1978). Pharmacological and psychological determinants of smoking. *Annals of Internal Medicine, 88,* 104–114.

Schachter, S., Silverstein, B., Kozlowski, L. T., Perlick, D., Herman, C. P., & Liebling, B. (1977). Studies of the interaction of psychological and pharmacological determinants of smoking. *Journal of Experimental Psychology General, 106,* 3–12.

Schacter, D. L. (1996). Illusory memories: A cognitive neuroscience analysis. *Proceedings of the National Academy of Sciences, 93,* 13527–13533.

Schaie, K. W. (1994). The course of adult intellectual development. *The American Psychologist, 49,* 304–313.

Schaie, K. W. (1996). *Intellectual development in adulthood: The Seattle Longitudinal Study.* Cambridge, UK: Cambridge University Press.

Schaubroeck, J., Ganster, D. C., & Kemmerer, B. E. (1994). Job complexity, "type A" behavior, and cardiovascular disorder: A prospective study. *Academy of Management Journal, 37,* 426–438.

Scheier, L. M., & Botvin, G. J. (1997). Expectancies as mediators of the effects of social influences and alcohol knowledge on adolescent alcohol use: A prospective analysis. *Psychology of Addictive Behaviors, 11,* 48–64.

Scheier, M. F., & Bridges, M. W. (1995). Person variables and health: Personality predispositions and acute psychological states as shared determinants for disease. *Psychosomatic Medicine, 57,* 255–268.

Scheier, M. F., & Carver, C. S. (1985). Optimism, coping, and health: Assessment and implications of generalized outcome expectancies. *Health Psychology, 4,* 219–247.

Scheier, M. F., Matthews, K. A., Owens, J. F., & Magovern, G. J. (1989). Dispositional optimism and recovery from coronary artery bypass surgery: The beneficial effects on physical and psychological well-being. *Journal of Personality and Social Psychology, 57,* 1024–1040.

Scheier, M. F., Weintraub, J. K., & Carver, C. S. (1986). Coping with stress: Divergent strategies of optimists and pessimists. *Journal of Personality and Social Psychology, 51,* 1257–1264.

Schell, F. J., Allolio, B., & Schonecke, O. W. (1994). Physiological and psychological effects of Hatha-Yoga exercise in healthy women. *International Journal of Psychosomatics, 41,* 46–52.

Scherwitz, L., Perkins, L., Chesney, M., & Hughes, G. (1991). Cook-Medley Hostility Scale and subsets: Relationship to demographic and psychosocial characteristics in young adults in the CARDIA study. *Psychosomatic Medicine, 53,* 36–49.

Scherwitz, L., & Rugulies, R. (1992). Life-style and hostility. In H. S. Friedman (Ed.), *Hostility, coping, and health* (pp. 77–98). Washington, DC: American Psychological Association.

Schifter, D. E., & Ajzen, I. (1985). Intention, perceived control, and weight loss: An application of the theory of planned behavior. *Journal of Personality and Social Psychology, 49,* 843–851.

Schlegel, R. P., D'Avernas, J. R., Zanna, M. P., & DeCourville, N. H. (1992). Problem drinking: A problem for the theory of reasoned action? *Journal of Applied Social Psychology, 22,* 358–385.

Schleifer, S. J., Keller, S. E., Camerino, M., Thorton, J. C., & Stein, M. (1983). Suppression of lymphocyte stimulation following bereavement. *Journal of the American Medical Association, 250,* 374–377.

Schmidt, L. (1997). Hospitalization in children. In A. Baum, S. Newman, J. Weinman, R. West, & C. McManus (Eds.), *Cambridge handbook of psychology, health, and medicine* (pp. 124–127). Cambridge, UK: Cambridge University Press.

Schmied, L. A., & Lawler, K. A. (1986). Hardiness, Type A behavior, and the stress-illness relation in working women. *Journal of Personality and Social Psychology, 51,* 1218–1223.

Schneider, B. E. (2001). Women, families, and HIV/AIDS: A sociological perspective on the epidemic in America. *Gender & Society, 15,* 155–156.

Schneider, W. J., & Nevid, J. S. (1993). Overcoming math anxiety: A comparison of stress inoculation training and systematic desensitization. *Journal of College Student Development, 34,* 283–288.

Schneiderman, N. E., McCabe, P., & Baum, A. (1992). *Stress and disease processes.* Hillsdale, NJ: Erlbaum.

Schreiber, G. B., Busch, M. P., Kleinman, S. H., & Korelitz, J. J. (1996). The risk of transfusion-transmitted viral infections. The retrovirus epidemiology donor study. *New England Journal of Medicine, 334,* 1685–1690.

Schuckit, M. A., & Smith, T. L. (1996). An 8-year follow-up of 450 sons of alcoholic and control subjects. *Archives of General Psychiatry, 53*(3), 202–210.

Schulenberg, J., Bachman, J. G., O'Malley, P. M., & Johnston, L. D. (1994). High school educational success and subsequent substance abuse. *Journal of Health and Social Behavior, 35*(1), 45–62.

Schulman, K. A., Berlin, J., Harless, W., Kerner, J. F., Sistrunk, S. H., Garish, B. J., Dubé, R., Taleghani, C. K., Burke, J. E., Williams, S., Eisenberg, J. M., & Escarce, J. (1999). The effect of race and sex on physicians' recommendations for cardiac catheterization. *New England Journal of Medicine, 340*(8), 618–625.

Schwartz, J. (1999, January 22). FDA warns against supplement. *Washington Post,* p. A02.

Schwartz, J., & Pomfret, J. (1998, November 20). Smoking-related deaths in China are up sharply. *Washington Post* (www.washingtonpost.com).

Schwartz, M. B., & Brownell, K. D. (1995). Matching individuals to weight loss treatments: A survey of obesity experts. *Journal of Consulting and Clinical Psychology, 63,* 149–153.

Schwartz, M. D., Lerman, C., Miller, S. M., Daly, M., & Masny, A. (1995). Coping disposition, perceived risk, and psychological distress among women at increased risk for ovarian cancer. *Health Psychology, 14,* 232–235.

Schwarzer, R., & Leppin, A. (1992). Possible impact of social ties and support on morbidity and mortality. In H. Veiel & U. Baumann (Eds.), *The meaning and measurement of social support.* New York: Hemisphere Publishing.

Scott, S. (1999, September 3). Wellness programs benefit bottom line, studies show. *Houston Business Journal* (www. bizjournals.com/houston/).

Scrimshaw, S. M., Engle, P. L., & Zambrana, R. E. (1983). *Prenatal anxiety and birth outcome in U. S. Latinas: Implications for psychosocial interventions.* Paper presented at the annual meeting of the American Psychological Association, Anaheim, CA.

Sears, S. F., Urizar, G. G., & Evans, G. D. (2000). Examining a stress-coping model of burnout and depression in extension agents. *Journal of Occupational Health Psychology, 5,* 56–62.

Sedlacek, K., & Taub, E. (1996). Biofeedback treatment of Raynaud's disease. *Professional Psychology: Research and Practice, 27,* 548–553.

Seeman, M., & Lewis, S. (1995). Powerlessness, health and mortality: A longitudinal study of older men and mature women. *Social Science and Medicine, 41,* 517–525.

Segerstrom, S. C., Taylor, S. E., Kemeny, M. E., & Fahey, J. (1998). Optimism is associated with mood, coping and immune change in response to stress. *Journal of Personality and Social Psychology, 74*(6), 1646–1655.

Segerstrom, S. C., Taylor, S. E., Kemeny, M. E., Reed, G. M., & Visscher, B. R. (1996). Causal attributions predict rate of immune decline in HIV-seropositive gay men. *Health Psychology, 15,* 485–493.

Seid, R. (1994). Too "close to the bone": The historical context for women's obsession with slenderness. In P. Fallon & M. A. Katzman (Eds.), *Feminist perspectives on eating disorders* (pp. 3–16). New York: Guilford.

Self, C. A., & Rogers, R. W. (1990). Coping with threats to health: Effects of persuasive appeals on depressed, normal, and antisocial personalities. *Journal of Behavioral Medicine, 13,* 343–358.

Self, D. W., & Nestler, E. J. (1995). Molecular mechanisms of drug reinforcement and addiction. *Annual Review of Neuroscience, 18,* 463–495.

Seligman, M. E. P. (1991). *Learned optimism.* New York: Knopf.

Seligman, M. E. P. (1995). The effectiveness of psychotherapy: The *Consumer Reports* study. *American Psychologist, 50*(12), 965–974.

Seligman, M. E. P., & Csikszentmihalyi, M. (2000). Positive psychology: An introduction. *American Psychologist, 55,* 5–14.

Seligman, M. E. P., & Maier, S. F. (1967). Failure to escape traumatic shock. *Journal of Experimental Psychology, 74,* 1–9.

Seligman, M. E. P., Reivich, K., Jaycox, L., & Gillham, J. (1995). *The optimistic child.* Boston, MA: Houghton Mifflin.

Selwyn, P. A. (1986). AIDS: What is now known. *Hospital Practice, 21,* 125–130.

Selye, H. (1974). *The stress of life.* New York: McGraw-Hill.

Senchak, M., Leonard, K. E., & Greene, B. W. (1998). Alcohol use among college students as a function of their typical social drinking context. *Psychology of Addictive Behaviors, 12,* 62–70.

Serdula, M. K., Collins, M. E., Williamson, D. F., Anda, R. F., Pamuk, E., & Byers, T. E. (1993). Weight control practices of U.S. adolescents and adults. *Annals of Internal Medicine, 119,* 667–671.

Serdula, M. K., Mokdad, A., Williamson, D. F., Galuska, D. A., Mendlein, J. M., & Heath, G. W. (1999). Prevalence of attempting weight loss and strategies for controlling weight. *Journal of the American Medical Association, 282,* 1353–1358.

Seto, M. C., & Barbaree, H. E. (1995). The role of alcohol in sexual aggression. *Clinical Psychology Review, 15,* 545–566.

Shannahoff-Khalsa, D. S., & Beckett, L. R. (1996). Clinical case report: Efficacy of yogic techniques in the treatment of obsessive compulsive disorders. *International Journal of Neuroscience, 85,* 1–17.

Shapiro, A. P. (2001). Nonpharmacological treatment of hypertension. In A. Baum, T. A. Revenson, & J. E. Singer (Eds.), *Handbook of health psychology* (pp. 697–708). Mahwah, NJ: Erlbaum.

Shapiro, D., Tursky, B., Gershon, E., & Stern, M. (1969). Effects of feedback and reinforcement on the control of human systolic blood pressure. *Science, 163,* 588–590.

Shapiro, J. A., Jacobs, E. J., & Thun, M. J. (2000). Cigar smoking in men and risk of death from tobacco-related cancers. *Journal of the National Cancer Institute, 92,* 333–337.

Shapiro, S. (1994). Meta-analysis/shmeta-analysis. *American Journal of Epidemiology, 140*(9), 771.

Sharpe, M., Hawton, K., Simkin, S., Surawy, C., Hackmann, A., Klimes, I., Peto, T., Warrell, D., & Seagroatt, V. (1996). Cognitive behaviour therapy for the chronic fatigue syndrome: A randomized clinical trial. *British Medical Journal, 312,* 22–26.

Shaywitz, B. A., Fletcher, J. M., & Shaywitz, S. E. (1997). Attention-deficit/hyperactivity disorder. *Advances in Pediatrics, 44,* 331–338.

Shekelle, P. G., Adams, A. H., & Chassin, M. R. (1992). Spinal manipulation for low-back pain. *Annals of Internal Medicine, 117,* 590–595.

Shekelle, P. G., & Brook, R. H. (1991). A community-based study of the use of chiropractic services. *American Journal of Public Health, 81,* 439–442.

Shekelle, R., B., Gale, M., Ostfield, A. M., & Paul, O. (1983). Hostility, risk of coronary heart disease and mortality. *Psychosomatic Medicine, 45,* 109–114.

Sheppard, B. H., Hartwick, J., & Warshaw, P. R. (1988). The theory of reasoned action: A meta-analysis of past research with recommendations for modifications and future research. *Journal of Consumer Research, 15,* 325–343.

Sher, K. J., Bartholow, B. D., & Nanda, S. (2001). Short- and long-term effects of fraternity and sorority membership on heavy drinking: A social norms perspective. *Psychology of Addictive Behaviors, 15,* 42–51.

Sherbourne, C. D., Hays, R. D., Ordway, L., DiMatteo, M. R., & Kravitz, R. L. (1992). Antecedents of adherence to medical recommendations: Results from the Medical Outcomes Study. *Journal of Behavioral Medicine, 15,* 447–468.

Sheridan, E. P. (1999). Psychology's future in medical schools and academic health care centers. *American Psychologist, 54,* 267–271.

Sherman, R. A., Sherman, C. J., & Parker, L. (1984). Chronic phantom and stump pain among American veterans: Results of a survey. *Pain, 18,* 83–95.

Sherwin, E. D., Elliott, T. R., Rybarczyk, B. D., & Frank, R. G. (1992). Negotiating the reality of caregiving: Hope, burnout and nursing. *Journal of Social & Clinical Psychology, 11,* 129–139.

Shilts, R. (1987). *And the band played on: Politics, people, and the AIDS epidemic.* New York: St. Martin's.

Shipley, R. H., Butt, J. H., Horwitz, B., & Farbry, J. E. (1979). Preparation for a stressful medical procedure: Effect of amount of stimulus preexposure and coping style. *Journal of Consulting and Clinical Psychology, 46,* 499–507.

Shoff, S. M., Newcomb, P. A., Trentham-Dietz, A., Remington, P. L., Mittendorf, R., Greenberg, E. R., & Willett, W. C. (2000). Early-life physical activity and postmenopausal breast cancer: Effect of body size and weight change. *Cancer Epidemiology, 9,* 591–595.

Showalter, E. (1999). *Hystories: Hysterical epidemics and modern culture.* New York: Columbia University Press.

Shumaker, S. A., & Hill, D. R. (1991). Gender differences in social support and physical health. *Health Psychology: Special Issue: Gender and Health, 10,* 102–111.

Siegel, J. M., Angulo, F. J., Detels, R., Wesch, J., & Mullen, A. (1999). AIDS diagnosis and depression in the Multicenter AIDS Cohort Study: The ameliorating impact of pet ownership. *AIDS Care, 11,* 157–170.

Siegel, K., & Krauss, B. J. (1991). Living with HIV infection: Adaptive tasks of seropositive gay men. *Journal of Health and Social Behavior, 32,* 17–32.

Siegel, K., Raveis, V. H., & Karus, D. (1997). Illness-related support and negative network interactions: Effects on HIV-infected men's depressive symptomatology. *American Journal of Community Psychology, 25,* 395–420.

Siegler, I. C., Bastian, L. A, & Bosworth, H. B. (2001). Health, behavior, and aging. In A. Baum, T. A. Revenson, & J. E. Singer (Eds.), *Handbook of health psychology* (pp. 469–476). Mahwah, NJ: Erlbaum.

Siegler, I. C., Peterson, B. L., Barefoot, J. C., & Williams, R. B. (1992). Hostility during late adolescence predicts coronary risk factors at mid-life. *American Journal of Epidemiology, 136,* 146–154.

Sigelman, C., Maddock, A., Epstein, J., & Carpenter, W. (1993). Age differences in understanding of disease causality: AIDS, colds, and cancer. *Child Development, 64,* 272–284.

Sigerist, H. E. (1958). *The great doctors.* New York: Doubleday Anchor Books.

Sigerist, H. E. (1971). *The great doctors: A biographical history of medicine.* Freeport, NY: Books for Libraries Press.

Sihvonen, M., Kayhko, K., & Kekki, P. (1989). Factors influencing the patient-provider relationship. *Vard i Norden, 9,* 4–9.

Silverman, M. M., Eichler, A., & Williams, G. D. (1987). Self-reported stress: Findings from the 1985 National Health Interview Survey. *Public Health Reports, 102,* 47–53.

Silverstein, P. (1992). Smoking and wound healing. *American Journal of Medicine, 93,* 1A–22S.

Simon, G., Gater, R., Kisely, S., & Piccinelli, M. (1996). Somatic symptoms of distress: An international primary care study. *Psychosomatic Medicine, 58,* 481–488.

Simpson, N., Lenton, S., & Randall, R. (1995). Parental refusal to have children immunized: Extent and reasons. *British Medical Journal, 310,* 227–230.

Singer, E. M. (1988). Delay behavior among women with breast symptoms. In T. Field, & P. M. McCabe (Eds.), *Stress and coping across development* (pp. 163–188). Hillsdale, NJ: Erlbaum.

Singer, J. E., Lundberg, U., & Frankenhaeuser, M. (1978). Stress on the train: A study of urban community. In A. Baum, J. E. Singer, & S. Valins (Eds.), *Advances in environmental psychology.* Hillsdale, NJ: Erlbaum.

Sjostrom, L.V. (1992). Morbidity of severely obese subjects. *American Journal of Clinical Nutrition, 55,* 508–515.

Skevington, S. M. (1995). *Psychology of pain.* Chichester, England: Wiley.

Sloan, R. P., Bagiella, E., & Powell, T. (1999). Religion, spirituality, and medicine. *Lancet, 353,* 664–667.

Sloman, R., Ahern, M., Wright, A., & Brown, L. (2001). Nurses' knowledge of pain in the elderly. *Journal of Pain and Symptom Management, 21,* 317–322.

Smith, D. (2001, June). Treatment of nonviolent drug offenders: A wave of the future? *Monitor on Psychology* (Special issue on substance abuse), *32,* 16, 51.

Smith, M. Y., Redd, W., DuHamel, K., Vickberg, S. J., & Ricketts, P. (1999). Validation of the PTSD checklist, civilian version, in survivors of bone marrow transplantation. *Journal of Traumatic Stress, 12,* 485–499.

Smith, T. J. (1998). Health service studies in the terminally ill patient. *Cancer Treatment and Research, 97,* 81–97.

Smith, T. W. (1994). Concepts and methods in the study of anger, hostility, and health. In A. W. Siegman & T. W. Smith (Eds.), *Anger, hostility, and the heart* (pp. 23–42). Hillsdale, NJ: Erlbaum.

Smith, T. W., & Gallo, L. C. (2001). Personality traits as risk factors for physical illness. In A. Baum, T. A. Revenson, & J. E. Singer (Eds.), *Handbook of health psychology* (pp. 139–173). Mahwah, NJ: Erlbaum.

Smyth, J. M., & Pennebaker, J. W. (2001). What are the health effects of disclosure? In A. Baum, T. A. Revenson, & J. E. Singer (Eds.), *Handbook of health psychology* (pp. 339–348). Mahwah, NJ: Erlbaum.

Snider, D. E., & Satcher, D. (1997). Behavioral and social sciences at the Centers for Disease Control and Prevention. Critical disciplines for public health. *American Psychologist, 52,* 40–42.

Sobal, J., & Stunkard, A. J. (1989). Socioeconomic status and obesity: A review of the literature. *Psychological Bulletin, 105,* 260–275.

Society for Women's Health Research (SAWHR). (1998). Just the facts: Gender-based biology. www.womens-health.org.

Solomon, G. F. (1991). Psychosocial factors, exercise, and immunity: Athletes, elderly persons, and AIDS patients. *International Journal of Sports Medicine, 12* (supplement 1), S50–S52.

Solomon, G. F., Segerstrom, S. C., Grohr, P., Kemeny, M., & Fahey, J. (1997). Shaking up immunity: Psychological and immunologic changes after a natural disaster. *Psychosomatic Medicine, 59,* 114–127.

Sommer, A., Tielsch, J. M., Katz, J., Quigley, H. A., Gottsch, J. D., Javitt, J. C., Martone, J. F., Royall, R. M., Witt, K. A., & Ezrine, S. (1991). Racial differences in the cause-specific prevalence of blindness in east Baltimore. *New England Journal of Medicine, 325,* 1412–1417.

Sorensen, G. (1985). Sex differences in the relationship between work and health: The Minnesota Heart Survey. *Journal of Health & Social Behavior, 26,* 379–394.

Spanos, N. P. (1991). A sociocognitive approach to hypnosis. In S. J. Lynn & J. W. Rhue (Eds.), *Theories of hypnosis: Current models and perspectives* (pp. 324–361). New York: Guilford.

Spanos, N. P. (1994). Multiple identity enactments and multiple personality disorder: A sociocognitive perspective. *Psychological Bulletin, 116,* 143–165.

Spanos, N. P. (1996). *Multiple identities and false memories: A sociocognitive perspective.* Washington, DC: American Psychological Association.

Spanos, N. P., & Coe, W. C. (1992). A social-psychological approach to hypnosis. In E. Fromm & M. R. Nash (Eds.), *Contemporary hypnosis research.* New York: Guilford.

Sparks, P., & Shepherd, R. (1992). Self-identity and the theory of planned behavior: Assessing the role of identification with "green consumerism." *Social Psychology Quarterly, 55,* 388–399.

Spasojevic, J., & Alloy, L. B. (2001). Rumination as a common mechanism relating depressive risk factors to depression. *Emotion, 1,* 25–37.

Spence, J. T., Losoff, M., & Robbins, A. S. (1991). Sexually aggressive tactics in dating relationships: Personality and attitudinal correlates. *Journal of Social and Clinical Psychology, 10,* 289–304.

Spencer, J., & Jonas, W. (1997). And now . . . alternative medicine. *Archives of Family Medicine, 6,* 155.

Spencer, J. W. (1999). Essential issues in complementary/alternative medicine. In J. W. Spencer & J. J. Jacobs (Eds.), *Complementary/alternative medicine: An evidence–based approach* (pp. 1–36). St. Louis, MO: Mosby.

Spencer, S. M., Lehman, J. M., Wynings, C., Arena, P., Carver, C. S., Antoni, M. H., Derhagopian, R. P., Ironson, G., & Love, N. (1999). Concerns about breast cancer and relations to psychosocial well-being in a multiethnic sample of early-stage patients. *Health Psychology, 18,* 159–168.

Spiegel, D., Bloom, J. R., Kraemer, H. C., & Gottheil, E. (1989). Effect of psychosocial treatment on survival of patients with metastatic breast cancer. *Lancet, 2,* 888–891.

Spiegelblatt, L. S. (1994). The use of alternative medicine by children. *Pediatrics, 94,* 811–820.

Spiegelblatt, L. S. (1995). Alternative medicine: Should it be used by children? *Current Problems in Pediatrics, 25,* 180–184.

Srivastava, K. C., & Mustafa, T. (1992). Ginger (*Zingiber officinale*) in rheumatism and musculoskeletal disorders. *Medical Hypotheses, 39,* 342–348.

St. Lawrence, J. (1993). African-American adolescents' knowledge, health-related attitudes, sexual behavior, and contraceptive decisions: Implications for the prevention of adolescent infection. *Journal of Consulting and Clinical Psychology, 61,* 104–112.

Stacy, A. W., Bentler, P. M., & Flay, B. R. (1994). Attitudes and health behavior in diverse populations: Drunk driving, alcohol use, binge eating, marijuana use, and cigarette use. *Health Psychology, 13,* 73–85.

Stalonas, P. M., Perri, M. G., & Kerzner, A. B. (1984). Do behavioral treatments of obesity last? A five-year follow-up investigation. *Addictive Behaviors, 9,* 175–183.

Stamler, J., Stamler, R., Neaton, J. D., Wentworth, D., Daviglus, M. L., Garside, D., Dyer, A. R., Liu, K., & Greenland, P. (1999). Low-risk factor profile and long-term cardiovascular and noncardiovascular mortality and life expectancy: Findings for 5 large cohorts of young adult and middle-aged men and women. *Journal of the American Medical Association, 282,* 2012–2018.

Stampfer, M. J., Rimm, E. B., & Walsh, D. C. (1993). Commentary: Alcohol, the heart, and public policy. *American Journal of Public Health, 83,* 801–804.

Stanovich, K. E., & West, R. F. (1998). Individual differences in rational thought. *Journal of Experimental Psychology: General, 127*(2), 161–188.

Stanton, A. L., Kirk, S. B., Cameron, C. L., & Danoff-Burg, S. (2000). Coping through emotional approach: Scale construction and validation. *Journal of Personality and Social Psychology, 78,* 1150, 1169.

Stanton, A. L., & Snider, P. R. (1993). Coping with a breast cancer diagnosis: A prospective study. *Health Psychology, 12,* 16–23.

Stanton, W. R., Mahalski, P. A., McGee, R., & Silva, P. A. (1993). Reasons for smoking or not smoking in early adolescence. *Addictive Behaviors, 18,* 321–329.

Stark, M. J., Tesselaar, H. M., O'Connell, A. A., Person, B., Galavotti, C., Cohen, A., & Walls, C. (1998). Psychosocial factors associated with the Stages of Change for condom use among women at risk for HIV and STDs: Implications for intervention development. *Journal of Consulting and Clinical Psychology, 66,* 967–978.

Starobrat-Hermelin, B., & Kozielec, T. (1997). The effects of magnesium physiological supplementation on hyperactivity in children with attention deficit hyperactivity disorder (ADHD). Positive response to magnesium oral loading test. *Magnesium Research, 10,* 149–156.

Statistics Canada (1999). *Statistical report on the health of Canadians.* Prepared by the Federal, Provincial and Territorial Advisory Committee on Population Health for the Meeting of Ministers of Health, Charlottetown, PEI, September 16–17.

Stein, J., & Nyamathi, A. (1999). Gender differences in behavioural and psychosocial predictors of HIV testing and return for test results in a high-risk population. *AIDS Care* Special Issue: AIDS Impact: 4th International Conference on the Biopsychosocial Aspects of HIV Infection, *12,* 343–356.

Steinglass, P., & Gerrity, E. (1990). Natural disasters and post-traumatic stress disorder: Short-term versus long-term recovery in two disaster-affected communities. *Journal of Applied Social Psychology, 20,* 1746–1765.

Steinmetz, K. A., Kushi, L. H., Bostick, R. M., Folsom, A. R., & Potter, J. D. (1994). Vegetables, fruit, and colon cancer in the Iowa Women's Health Study. *American Journal of Epidemiology, 139,* 1–15.

Steptoe, A. (1997). Stress and disease. In A. Baum, S. Newman, J. Weinman, R. West, & C. McManus (Eds.), *Cambridge handbook of psychology, health and medicine* (pp. 174–177). Cambridge, England: Cambridge University Press.

Steptoe, A., Fieldman, G., & Evans, O. (1993). An experimental study of the effects of control over work pace on cardiovascular responsivity. *Journal of Psychophysiology, 7,* 290–300.

Steptoe, A., Wardle, J., Pollard, T. M., & Canaan, L. (1996). Stress, social support and health-related behavior: A study of smoking, alcohol consumption and physical exercise. *Journal of Psychosomatic Research, 41,* 171–180.

Stern, M., Norman, S., & Komm, C. (1993). Medical students' differential use of coping strategies as a function of stressor type, year of training, and gender. *Behavioral Medicine, 18,* 173–180.

Sternbach, R. A. (1986). Pain and "hassles" in the United States: Findings of the Nuprin Pain Report. *Pain, 27,* 69–80.

Stice, E., Mazotti, L., Krebs, M., & Martin, S. (1998). Predictors of adolescent dieting behaviors: A longitudinal study. *Psychology of Addictive Behaviors, 12,* 195–205.

Stice, E., Myers, M. G., & Brown, S. A. (1998). Relations of delinquency to adolescent substance use and problem use: A prospective study. *Psychology of Addictive Behaviors, 12,* 136–146.

Stock, R. W. (1995, July 13). Reducing the risk for older drivers. *The New York Times,* p. C1.

Stone, A. A., Mezzacappa, E. S., Donatone, B. A., & Gonder, M. (1999). Psychosocial stress and social support are associated with prostate-specific antigen levels in men: Results from a community screening program. *Health Psychology, 18*(5), 482–486.

Stone, A. A., Neale, J. M., Cox, D. S., Napoli, A., Valdimarsdottir, H., & Kennedy-Moore, E. (1994). Daily events are associated with a secretory immune response to an oral antigen in men. *Health Psychology, 13,* 440–446.

Stone, G. C., Cohen, F., & Adler, N. (1979). *Health psychology—A handbook.* San Francisco: Jossey-Bass.

Stoney, C. M., Matthews, K. A., McDonald, R. H., & Johnson, C. A. (1988). Sex differences in lipid, lipoprotein, cardiovascular, and neuroendocrine responses to acute stress. *Psychophysiology, 25,* 645–656.

Story, M., & Faulkner, P. (1990). The prime time diet: Eating behavior and food messages in television program content commercials. *American Journal of Public Health, 80,* 738–740.

Stratton, J. F., Buckley, C. H., Lowe, D., & Ponder, B. A. (1999). Comparison of prophylactic oophorectomy specimens from carriers and noncarriers of a BRCA1 or BRCA2 gene mutation. *Journal of the National Cancer Institute, 91,* 626–628.

Straub, R. O., Grunberg, N. E., Street, S. W., & Singer, J. E. (1990). Dominance: Another facet of type A. *Journal of Applied Social Psychology, 20,* 1051–1062.

Straub, R. O., Singer, J. E., & Grunberg, N. E. (1986). Toward an animal model of Type A behavior. *Health Psychology 5*(1), 71–85.

Strawbridge, W. J., Wallhagen, M. I., & Shema, S. J. (2000). New NHLBI clinical guidelines for obesity and overweight: Will they promote health? *American Journal of Public Health, 90,* 340–343.

Strecher, V. J., & Rosenstock, I. M. (1997). The health belief model. In A. Baum, S. Newman, J. Weinman, R. West, & C. McManus (Eds.), *Cambridge handbook of psychology, health and medicine* (pp. 113–117). Cambridge, UK: Cambridge University Press.

Striegel-Moore, R. H., Silberstein, L. R., & Rodin, J. (1986). Toward an understanding of risk factors for bulimia. *American Psychologist, 41,* 246–263.

Striegel-Moore, R. H., Silberstein, L. R., & Rodin, J. (1993). The social self in bulimia nervosa: Public self-consciousness, social anxiety, and perceived fraudulence. *Journal of Abnormal Psychology, 102,* 297–303.

Strober, M., Morrell, W., Burroughs, J., Salkin, B., & Jacobs, C. (1985). A controlled family study of anorexia nervosa. *Journal of Psychiatric Research, 19,* 239–246.

Stuart, R. B. (1974). Teaching facts about drugs: Pushing or preventing. *Journal of Educational Psychology, 66,* 189–201.

Stuckey, S. J., Jacobs, A., & Goldfarb, J. (1986). EMG biofeedback training, relaxation training, and placebo for the relief of chronic back pain. *Perceptual and Motor Skills, 63,* 1023–1036.

Stunkard, A. J. (1979). Behavioral medicine and beyond: The example of obesity. In O. F. Pomerleau & J. P. Brady (Eds.), *Behavioral medicine: Theory and practice* (pp. 279–298). Baltimore, MD: Williams & Wilkins.

Stunkard, A. J., & Sorensen, T. I. (1993). Obesity and socioeconomic status—a complex relation. *New England Journal of Medicine, 329,* 1036–1037.

Suddendorf, R. F. (1989). Research on alcohol metabolism among Asians and its implications for understanding causes of alcoholism. *Public Health Reports, 104,* 615–620.

Sue, S., & Zane, N. (1995). The role of culture and cultural techniques in psychotherapy: A critique and reformulation. In N. R. Goldberger, N. Rule, & J. B. Veroff (Eds.), *The culture and psychology reader* (pp. 767–788). New York: New York University Press.

Sulfaro, F., Fasher, B., & Burgess, M. A. (1994). Homeopathic vaccination. What does it mean? *Medical Journal of Australia, 161,* 305–307.

Sullivan, M. J. L., Reesor, K., Mikail, S., & Fisher, R. (1992). The treatment of depression in chronic low back pain: Review and recommendations. *Pain, 50,* 5–13.

Sullivan, P. F., Bulik, C. M., Fear, J. L., & Pickering, A. (1998). Outcome of anorexia nervosa: A case-control study. *American Journal of Psychiatry, 155,* 939–946.

Suls, J., & Fletcher, B. (1985). The relative efficacy of avoidant and nonavoidant coping strategies: A meta-analysis. *Health Psychology, 4,* 249–288.

Sun, Y. (1994). Clinical observation and treatment of hyperkinesias in children by traditional Chinese medicine. *Journal of Traditional Chinese Medicine, 14,* 105–110.

Sundstrom, E. (1978). Crowding as a sequential process: Review of research on the effects of population density on humans. In A. Baum & Y. M. Epstein (Eds.), *Human response to crowding* (pp. 31–116). Hillsdale, NJ: Erlbaum.

Surwit, R. S., & Williams, P. G. (1996). Animal models provide insight into psychosomatic factors in diabetes. *Psychosomatic Medicine, 58,* 582–589.

Susser, M. (1995). The tribulations of trials—interventions in communities. *American Journal of Public Health, 85,* 156–158.

Sussman, S., Simon, T. R., & Stacy, A. W. (1999). The association of group self-identification and adolescent drug use in three samples varying in risk. *Journal of Applied Social Psychology, 29,* 1555–1581.

Sutton, S. R. (1989). Smoking attitudes and behavior: Applications of Fishbein and Ajzen's theory of reasoned action to predicting and understanding smoking decisions. In T. Ney & A. Gale (Eds.), *Smoking and human behavior* (pp. 289–312). Chichester, UK: Wiley.

Sutton, S. R. (1996). Can "stages of change" provide guidance in the treatment of addictions? A critical examination of Prochaska and DiClemente's model. In G. Edwards & C. Dare (Eds.), *Psychotherapy, psychological treatments, and the addictions* (pp. 189–205). Cambridge, UK: Cambridge University Press.

Sutton, S. R. (1997). Theory of planned behavior. The health belief model. In A. Baum, S. Newman, J. Weinman, R. West, & C. McManus (Eds.), *Cambridge handbook of psychology, health and medicine* (pp. 177–180). Cambridge, UK: Cambridge University Press.

Swan, G. E., & Carmelli, D. (1996). Curiosity and mortality in aging adults: A 5-year follow-up of the Western Collaborative Group Study. *Psychology and Aging, 11,* 449–453.

Swarr, A., & Richards, M. (1996). Longitudinal effects of adolescent girls' pubertal development, perceptions of pubertal timing, and parental relations on eating problems. *Developmental Psychology, 32,* 636–646.

Sweet, J. J., Rozensky, R. H., & Tovian, S. M. (Eds.). (1991). *Handbook of clinical psychology in medical settings.* New York: Plenum.

Swenson, R. M., & Vogel, W. H. (1983). Plasma catecholamine and corticosterone as well as brain catecholamine changes during coping in rats exposed to stressful footshock. *Pharmacology, Biochemistry and Behavior, 18,* 689–693.

Symister, P., & Friend, R. (1996). Quality of life and adjustment in renal disease: A health psychology perspective. In R. J. Resnick & R. H. Rozensky (Eds.), *Health psychology through the life span: Practice and research opportunities.* Washington, DC: American Psychological Association, 265–287.

Szasz, T. S., & Hollender, M. H. (1956). A contribution to the philosophy of medicine. *Archives of Internal Medicine, 97,* 585–592.

Talbot, F., Nouwen, A., Gingras, J., Belanger, A., & Audet, J. (1999). Relations of diabetes intrusiveness and personal control to symptoms of depression among adults with diabetes. *Health Psychology, 18,* 537–542.

Talbot, M. (2000, January 9). The placebo prescription. *New York Times Sunday Magazine,* 34–39; 44; 58–60.

Tashkin, D. P., Kroening, R. J., Bresler, D. E., Simmons, M., Coulson, A. H., & Kerschnar, H. (1985). A controlled trial of real and simulated acupuncture in the management of chronic asthma. *The Journal of Allergy and Clinical Immunology, 76,* 855–864.

Taylor, E. (1997). Shiftwork and health: In A. Baum, S. Newman, J. Weinman, R. West, & C. McManus (Eds.) *Cambridge handbook of psychology, health and medicine* (pp. 318–319). Cambridge, UK: Cambridge University Press.

Taylor, R. D., Roberts, D., & Jacobson, L. (1997). Stressful life events, psychological well-being, and parenting in African American mothers. *Journal of Family Psychology, 11,* 436–446.

Taylor, S. E. (1979). Hospital patient behavior: Reactance, helplessness, or control? *Journal of Social Issues, 35,* 156–184.

Taylor, S. E., Lichtman, R. R., & Wood, J. V. (1984). Compliance with chemotherapy among breast cancer patients. *Health Psychology, 3,* 553–562.

Taylor, S. E., Repetti, R. L., & Seeman, T. (1997). Health psychology: What is an unhealthy environment and how does it get under the skin? *Annual Review of Psychology, 48,* 411–447.

Telles, S., Nagarathna, R., Nagendra, H. R., & Desiraju, T. (1993). Physiological changes in sports teachers following 3 months of training in Yoga. *Indian Journal of Medical Sciences, 47,* 235–238.

ter-Kuile, M. M., Spinhoven, P., Linssen, A., Corry, G., Zitman, F. G., & Rooijmans, H. G. M. (1994). Autogenic training and cognitive self-hypnosis for the treatment of recurrent headaches in three different subject groups. *Pain, 58,* 331–340.

ter Riet, G., Kleijnen, J., & Knipschild, P. (1990). Acupuncture and chronic pain: A criteria-based meta-analysis. *Journal of Clinical Epidemiology, 43,* 191–199.

Thackwray, D. E., Smith, M. C., Bodfish, J. W., & Meyers, A. W. (1993). A comparison of behavioral and cognitive-behavioral interventions for bulimia nervosa. *Journal of Consulting and Clinical Psychology, 61,* 639–645.

Thal, L. J. (2000). Anti-inflammatory drugs and Alzheimer's disease. *Neurobiology of Aging, 21,* 449–450.

Thayer, R. E., Newman, J. R., & McClain, T. M. (1994). Self-regulation of mood: Strategies for changing a bad mood, raising energy, and reducing tension. *Journal of Personality and Social Psychology, 67,* 910–925.

Theorell, T., Blomkvist, V., Jonsson, H., Schulman, S., Berntorp, E., & Stigendal, L. (1995). Social support and the development of immune function in human immunodeficiency virus infection. *Psychosomatic Medicine, 57,* 32–36.

Thomas, M., Eriksson, S. V., & Lundeberg, T. (1991). A comparative study of diazepam and acupuncture in patients with osteoarthritis pain: A placebo controlled study. *The American Journal of Chinese Medicine, 19,* 95–100.

Thomas, W., White, C. M., Mah, J., Geisser, M. S., Church, T. R., & Mandel, J. S. (1995). Longitudinal compliance with annual screening for fecal occult blood. *American Journal of Epidemiology, 142,* 176–182.

Thomasson, H. R., & Li, T. (1993). How alcohol and aldehyde dehydrogenase genes modify alcohol drinking, alcohol flushing, and the risk for alcoholism. *Alcohol Health and Research World,* Special Issue: Alcohol, Aggression, and Injury, *17,* 167–172.

Thompson, F. E., & Dennison, B. A. (1994). Dietary sources of fats and cholesterol in U. S. children aged 2 through 5 years. *American Journal of Public Health, 84,* 799–806.

Thompson, L., Andersen, B. L., & DePetrillo, D. (1992). The psychological processes of recovery from gynecologic cancer. In M. Coppleson, P. Morrow, & M. Tattersal (Eds.), *Gynecologic Oncology.* Edinburgh: Churchill Livingstone.

Thompson, R. (2000). *The brain: A neuroscience primer* (3rd ed.). New York: Worth.

Thompson, S. M., Dahlquist, L. M., Koenning, G. M., & Bartholomew, L. K. (1995). Brief report: Adherence-facilitating behaviors of a multidisciplinary pediatric rheumatology staff. *Journal of Pediatric Psychology, 20,* 291–297.

Thornton, H. A. (1989). *A medical handbook for senior citizens and their families.* Dover, MA: Auburn House.

Tomkins, S. S. (1966). Psychological model for smoking behavior. *American Journal of Public Health and the Nation's Health, 56,* 17–20.

Tonnesen, P., Norregaard, J., Simonsen, K., & Sawe, U. (1991). A double-blind trial of a 16-hour transdermal nicotine patch in smoking cessation. *New England Journal of Medicine, 325,* 311–315.

Toribara, N. W., & Sleisenger, M. H. (1995). Screening for colorectal cancer. *New England Journal of Medicine, 332,* 861–867.

Trichopoulous, D., Li, F. P., & Hunter, D. J. (1996). What causes cancer? *Scientific American* (www.sciam.com/0996issue).

Trimble, J. E. (1996). Alcohol abuse in urban Indian adolescents and women: A longitudinal study for assessment and risk evaluation. *American Indian and Alaska Native Mental Health Research, 7,* 81–90.

Troll, L. E., & Skaff, M. M. (1997). Perceived continuity of self in very old age. *Psychology and Aging, 12,* 162–169.

Tsang, Y. C. (1938). Hunger motivation in gastrectomized rats. *Journal of Comparative Psychology, 26,* 1–17.

Tse, S. K., & Bailey, D. M. (1992). T'ai chi and postural control in the well elderly. *American Journal of Occupational Therapy, 46,* 295–300.

Tucker, J. S., Friedman, H. S., Wingard, D. L., & Schwartz, J. E. (1996). Marital history at midlife as a predictor of longevity: Alternative explanations to the protective effect of marriage. *Health Psychology, 15,* 94–101.

Turk, D. (2001). Physiological and psychological bases of pain. In A. Baum, T. A. Revenson, & J. E. Singer (Eds.), *Handbook of Health Psychology* (pp. 117–137). Mahwah, NJ: Erlbaum.

Turk, D. C., Litt, M. D., Salovey, P., & Walker, J. (1985). Seeking urgent pediatric treatment: Factors contributing to frequency, delay, and appropriateness. *Health Psychology, 4,* 43–59.

Turk, D. C., Meichenbaum, D. H., & Berman, W. H. (1979). Application of biofeedback for the regulation of pain: A critical review. *Psychological Bulletin, 86,* 1322–1338.

Turk, D. C., & Nash, J. M. (1996). Psychologic issues in chronic pain. *Contemporary Neurology Series, 48,* 323.

Turk, D. C., Zaki, H. S., & Rudy, T. E. (1993). Effects of intraoral appliance and biofeedback/stress management alone and in combination in treating pain and depression in patients with temporomandibular disorders. *The Journal of Prosthetic Dentistry, 70,* 158–164.

Turner, G. E., Burciaga, C., Sussman, S., & Klein-Selski, E. (1993). Which lesson components mediate refusal assertion skill improvement in school-based adolescent tobacco use prevention? *International Journal of the Addictions, 28,* 749–763.

Turner, H. A., Catania, J. A., & Gagnon, J. (1994). The prevalence of informal caregiving to persons with AIDS in the United States: Caregiver characteristics and their implications. *Social Science and Medicine, 38,* 1543–1552.

Turner, R. J., & Asvison, W. R. (1992). Innovations in the measurement of life stress: Crisis theory and the significance of event resolution. *Journal of Health and Social Behavior, 33,* 36–50.

Turnquist, D. C., Harvey, J. H., & Andersen, B. A. (1988). Attributions and adjustment to life-threatening illness. *British Journal of Clinical Psychology, 27,* 55–65.

Tyler, P., & Cushway, D. (1992). Stress, coping and mental well-being in hospital nurses. *Stress Medicine, 8,* 91–98.

Ulbrich, P. M., & Bradshjer, J. E. (1993). Perceived support, help seeking, and adaptation to stress among older black and white women living alone. *Journal of Aging and Health, 5,* 265–286.

Ulrich, R. E. (1991). Animal rights, animal wrongs and the question of balance. *Psychological Science, 2,* 197–201.

UNAIDS. (2000). Report on the global HIV/AIDS epidemic: June 2000.

U.S. Bureau of the Census (USBC). (1999). *Statistical abstract of the United States, 1999.* Washington, DC: U.S. Department of Commerce.

U.S. Bureau of the Census (USBC). (2000). *Statistical abstracts of the United States: 2000.* (120th ed.). Washington, DC: U.S. Government Printing Office.

U.S. Department of Health and Human Services (USDHHS). (1991). *Healthy people 2000: National health promotion and disease prevention objectives.* (PHS Publication NO. 91-50212). Washington, DC: U.S. Government Printing Office.

U.S. Department of Health and Human Services (USDHHS). (1995). *Healthy people 2000 review, 1994.* Washington, DC: U.S. Government Printing Office.

U.S. Department of Health and Human Services (USDHHS). (1997). *Ninth special report to the U.S. Congress on alcohol and health.* Washington, DC: U.S. Government Printing Office.

U.S. Department of Health and Human Services (USDHHS). (1998). *Health, United States, 1998.* Washington, DC: U.S. Government Printing Office.

U.S. Department of Health and Human Services (USDHHS), Office of Minority Health (2001). *Data/Statistics.* www.omhrc.gov/OMH/sidebar/datastats.htm.

Ussher, J. M. (1997). Gender issues and women's health. In A. Baum, S. Newman, J. Weinman, R. West, & C. McManus (Eds.), *Cambridge handbook of psychology, health, and medicine,* pp. 110–112. Cambridge, UK: Cambridge University Press.

Van der Velde, F. W., & Van der Pligt, J. (1991). AIDS-related health behavior: Coping, protection motivation, and previous behavior. *Journal of Behavioral Medicine, 14,* 429–451.

Varni, J. W., & Katz, E. R. (1997). Stress, social support and negative affectivity in children with newly diagnosed cancer: A prospective transactional analysis. *Psycho-oncology, 6,* 267–278.

Varni, J. W., Katz, E. R., Colegrove, R., & Dolgin, M. (1994). Perceived social support and adjustment of children with newly diagnosed cancer. *Journal of Developmental & Behavioral Pediatrics, 15,* 20–26.

Varni, J. W., Setoguchi, Y., Rappaport, L. R., & Talbot, D. (1992). Psychological adjustment and perceived social support in children with congenital/acquired limb deficiencies. *Journal of Behavioral Medicine, 15,* 31–44.

Vena, J. E., Graham, S., Zielezny, M., Swanson, M. K., Barnes, R. E., & Nolan, J. (1985). Lifetime occupational exercise and colon cancer. *American Journal of Epidemiology, 122,* 357–365.

Verbrugge, L. M., & Steiner, R. P. (1981). Physician treatment of men and women patients: Sex bias or appropriate care? *Medical Care, 19,* 609–632.

Vernon, D. T., Foley, J. M., Sipowicz, R. R., & Schulman, J. L. (1971). The psychological responses of children to hospitalization and illness. *The Japanese Journal of Nursing Research, 4,* 45–54.

Vincent, C. A. (1989). A controlled trial of the treatment of migraine by acupuncture. *Clinical Journal of Pain, 5,* 305–312.

Vincent, C., & Furnham, A. (1997). *Complementary medicine: A research perspective.* New York: Wiley.

Vinokur, A. D., Schul, Y., Vuori, J., & Price, R. H. (2000). Two years after a job loss: Long-term impact of the JOBS program on reemployment and mental health. *Journal of Occupational Health Psychology, 5,* 32–47.

Visser, A., & Herbert, C. P. (1999) Psychosocial factors in cancer. *Patient Education and Counseling, 37*(3), 197–200.

Von Korff, M., Galer, B. S., & Stang, P. (1995). Chronic use of symptomatic headache medications. *Pain, 62,* 179–286.

Wadden, T. A., & Anderton, C. H. (1982). The clinical use of hypnosis. *Psychological Bulletin, 91,* 215–243.

Wadden, T. A., Foster, G. D., & Letizia, K. A. (1994). One-year behavioral treatment of obesity: Comparison of moderate and severe caloric restriction and the effects of weight maintenance therapy. *Journal of Consulting & Clinical Psychology, 62,* 165–171.

Wadden, T. A., Steen, S. N., Wingate, B. J., & Foster, G. D. (1996). Psychosocial consequences of weight reduction: How much weight loss is enough? *American Journal of Clinical Nutrition, 63,* 461S–465S.

Wagner, D. R., & Heyward, V. H. (2000). Measures of body composition in blacks and whites: A comparative review. *American Journal of Clinical Nutrition, 71,* 1392–1402.

Wahlin, A., Hill, R. D., Winblad, B., & Backman, L. (1996). Effects of serum vitamin B12 and folate status on episodic memory performance in very old age: A population-based study. *Psychology and Aging, 11,* 487–496.

Wall, T. L., Garcia-Andrade, C., Thomasson, H. R., Carr, L. G., & Ehlers, C. L. (1997). Alcohol dehydrogenase polymorphisms in Native Americans: Identification of the ADH2*3 allele. *Alcohol and Alcoholism, 32,* 129–132.

Wallston, K. A., Wallston, B. S., Smith, S., & Dobbins, C. (1997). Perceived control and health. *Current Psychological Research and Reviews* (Special Issue: *Health Psychology*), *6,* 5–25.

Walters, E. E., & Kendler, K. S. (1995). Anorexia nervosa and anorexic-like syndromes in a population-based female sample. *American Journal of Psychiatry, 152,* 64–71.

Walters, G. D. (1996). Addiction and identity: Exploring the possibility of a relationship. *Psychology of Addictive Behaviors, 10,* 9–17.

Wannamethee, G., Shaper, A. G., & MacFarlane, P. W. (1993). Heart rate, physical activity, and mortality from cancer and other noncardiovascular diseases. *American Journal of Epidemiology, 137*, 735–748.

Wardle, J. (1995). Parental influence on children's diets. *Proceedings of the Nutrition Society, 54*, 747–758.

Wardle, J. (1997). Dieting. In A. Baum, S. Newman, J. Weinman, R. West, & C. McManus (Eds.), *Cambridge handbook of psychology, health and medicine* (pp. 436–437). Cambridge, UK: Cambridge University Press.

Wardle, J., & Beales, S. (1988). Control and loss of control over eating: An experimental investigation. *Journal of Abnormal Psychology, 97*, 35–40.

Wardle, J., Pernet, A., Collins, W., & Bourne, T. (1994). False positive results in ovarian cancer screening: One year follow-up of psychological status. *Psychology and Health, 10*, 33–40.

Warshofsky, F. (1999). *Stealing time: The new science of aging*. New York: TV Books.

Warwick-Evans, L. A., Masters, I. J., & Redstone, S. B. (1991). A double-blind placebo controlled evaluation of acupressure in the treatment of motion sickness. *Aviation, Space, and Environmental Medicine, 62*, 776–778.

Waterhouse, J. (1993). Circadian rhythms. *British Medical Journal, 306*, 448–451.

Weil, A. (1999). *Eight weeks to optimum health*. New York: Random House.

Weinberg, R. (1996). How cancer arises. *Scientific American, 275*, 62–70.

Weinberg, R. S., & Gould, D. (1995). *Foundations of sport and exercise psychology*. Champaign, IL: Human Kinetics.

Weinberger, D. A., Schwartz, G. E., & Davidson, R. J. (1979). Low-anxious, high-anxious, and repressive coping styles: Psychometric patterns and behavioral and physiological responses to stress. *Journal of Abnormal Psychology, 88*, 369–380.

Weinberger, M., Hiner, S. L., & Tierney, W. M. (1987). Assessing social support in elderly adults. *Social Science & Medicine, 25*, 1049-1055.

Weiner, M. F., Vega, G., Risser, R. C., Honig, L. S., Cullum, C. M., Crumpacker, D., & Rosenberg, D. M. (1999). Apolipoprotein E epsion 4, other risk factors, and course of Alzheimer's disease. *Biological Psychiatry, 45*, 633–638.

Weinman, J. (1997). Doctor-patient communication. In A. Baum, S. Newman, J. Weinman, R. West, & C. McManus (Eds.), *Cambridge handbook of psychology, health and medicine* (pp. 284–287). Cambridge, UK: Cambridge University Press.

Weinman, J. (2001). Health care. In M. Johnston & D. W. Johnston (Eds.), *Health psychology: Comprehensive clinical psychology* (vol. 8, pp. 79–112). Amsterdam: Elsevier.

Weinstein, N. D. (1982) Unrealistic optimism about susceptibility to health problems. *Journal of Behavioral Medicine, 5*(40), 441–460.

Weinstein, N. D., & Klein, W. M. (1996). Unrealistic optimism: Present and future. *Journal of Social and Clinical Psychology, 15*(1), 1–8.

Weinstein, N. D., Lyon, J. E., Rothman, A. J., & Cuite, C. L. (2000). Changes in perceived vulnerability following natural disaster. *Journal of Social & Clinical Psychology, 19*, 372–395.

Weinstein, N. D., Rothman, A. J., & Sutton, S. R. (1998). Stage theories of health behavior: Conceptual and methodological issues. *Health Psychology, 17*, 290–299.

Weinstein, N. D., & Sandman, P. M. (1992). A model of the precaution adoption process: Evidence from home radon testing. *Health Psychology, 11*, 170–180.

Weisner, C., Greenfield, T., & Room, R. (1995). Trends in the treatment of alcohol problems in the US general population, 1979 through 1990. *American Journal of Public Health, 85*, 55–60.

Weisse, C. S., Sorum, P. C., Sanders, K. N., & Syat, B. L. (2001). Do gender and race affect decisions about pain management? *Journal of General Internal Medicine, 16*, 211–217.

Weisz, J. R., McCabe, M. A., & Dennig, M. D. (1994). Primary and secondary control among children undergoing medical procedures: Adjustment as a function of coping style. *Journal of Consulting and Clinical Psychology, 62*, 324–332.

Wells, A. J. (1994). Passive smoking as a cause of heart disease. *Journal of the American College of Cardiology, 24*, 546–554.

Wenzlaff, R. M., Wegner, D. M., & Roper, D. W. (1988). Depression and mental control: The resurgence of unwanted negative thoughts. *Journal of Personality and Social Psychology, 55*, 882–892.

Werbach, M. R. (1994). *Healing with food: Two hundred eighty-one nutritional plans for common ailments*. New York: HarperCollins.

Werner, E. (1997). Endangered childhood in modern times: Protective factors. *Vierteljahresschrift für Heilpädagogik und ihre Nachbargebiete, 66*, 192–203.

West, R., & Rink, L. (1997). Osteoarthritis. In A. Baum, S. Newman, J. Weinman, R. West, & C. McManus (Eds.), *Cambridge handbook of psychology, health, and medicine* (pp. 543–544). Cambridge, UK: Cambridge University Press.

Wetter, D. W., Fiore, M. C., Baker, T. B., & Young, T. B. (1995). Tobacco withdrawal and nicotine replacement influence objective measures of sleep. *Journal of Consulting and Clinical Psychology, 63*, 658–667.

Wheelwright, J. (2001, March). Don't eat again until you read this. *Discover, 22*, 36–42.

Whitaker, L. C. (1989). Myths and heroes: Visions of the future. *Journal of College Student Psychotherapy, 4*, 13–33.

Whitaker, R. C., Wright, J. A., Pepe, M. S., Seidel, K. D., & Dietz, W. H. (1997). Predicting obesity in young adulthood from childhood and parental obesity. *New England Journal of Medicine, 337*, 869–873.

White, E., Jacobs, E. J., & Daling, J. R. (1996). Physical activity in relation to colon cancer in middle-aged men and women. *American Journal of Epidemiology, 144*, 42–50.

White, E., Urban, N., & Taylor, V. (1993). Mammography utilization, public health impact, and cost-effectiveness in the United States. *Annual Review of Public Health, 14*, 605–633.

White, K. (1999). Nurses' study disproves link of fat to breast cancer. *Journal of Women's Health and Gender Based Medicine, 8*, 437–438.

Whiteman, M. C., Fowkes, F. G., & Deary, I. J. (1997). Hostility and the heart. *British Medical Journal, 315,* 379–380.

Whittemore, A. S., Kolonel, L. N., Wu, A. H., John, E. M., Gallagher, R. P., Howe, G. R., Burch, J. D., Hankin, J., Dreon, D. M., & West, D. W. (1995). Prostate cancer in relation to diet, physical activity, and body size in blacks, whites, and Asians in the United States and Canada. *Journal of the National Cancer Institute, 86,* 652–660.

Wichstrom, L. (1994). Predictors of Norwegian adolescents' sunbathing and use of sunscreen. *Health Psychology, 13,* 412–420.

Wideman, M. V., & Singer, J. E. (1984). The role of psychological mechanisms in preparation for childbirth. *American Psychologist, 39,* 1357–1371.

Wiertelak, E. P., Smith, K. P., Furness, L., Mooney-Heiberger, K., Mayr, T., Maier, S. F., & Watkins, L. R. (1994). Acute and conditioned hyperalgesic responses to illness. *Pain, 56,* 227–234.

Wierzbicki, M., & Pekarik, G. (1993). A meta-analysis of psychotherapy dropout. *Professional Psychology: Research and Practice, 24,* 190–195.

Wight, R. G., LeBlanc, A. J., & Aneshensel, C. S. (1998). AIDS caregiving and health among midlife and older women. *Health Psychology, 17,* 130–137.

Wilcox, D., & Dowrick, P. W. (1992). Anger management with adolescents. *Residential Treatment for Children & Youth, 9,* 29–39.

Wilcox, S., & Storandt, M. (1996). Relations among age, exercise, and psychological variables in a community sample of women. *Health Psychology, 15,* 110–113.

Wilcox, V. L., Kasl, S. V., & Berkman, L. F. (1994). Social support and physical disability in older people after hospitalization: A prospective study. *Health Psychology, 13,* 170–179.

Wilfley, D. E., Schreiber, G. B., Pike, K. M., Striegel-Moore, R. H., Wright, D. J., & Rodin, J. (1996). Eating disturbance and body image: A comparison of a community sample of adult black and white women. *International Journal of Eating Disorders, 20,* 377–387.

Willett, W. C. (1994). Diet and health: What should we eat? *Science, 264,* 532–537.

Willett, W. C., Colditz, G. A., & Mueller, N. E. (1996). Strategies for minimizing cancer risk. *Scientific American, 275,* 88–95.

Williams, A. F., & Lund, A. K. (1992). Injury control: What psychologists can contribute. *American Psychologist, 47,* 1036–1039.

Williams, C. L., & Berry, J. W. (1991). Primary prevention of acculturative stress among refugees: Application of psychological theory and practice. *American Psychologist, 46,* 632–641.

Williams, D. A. (1996). Acute pain management. In R. Gatchel & D. C. Turk (Eds.), *Psychological approaches to pain management: A practitioner's handbook* (pp. 55–77). New York: Guilford.

Williams, J. E., Paton, C. C., Siegler, I. C., Eigenbrot, M. L., Nieto, F. J., & Tyroler, H. A. (2000). Clinical investigation and reports: Anger proneness predicts coronary heart disease risk: Prospective analysis from the Atherosclerosis Risk in Communities (ARIC) Study. *Circulation, 101,* 2034–2039.

Williams, K. J., Suls, J., Alliger, G. M., Learner, S. M., & Wan, C. K. (1991). Multiple role juggling and daily mood states in working mothers: An experience sampling study. *Journal of Applied Psychology, 76,* 664–674.

Williams, P. G., Wiebe, D. J., & Smith, T. W. (1992). Coping processes as mediators of the relationship between hardiness and health. *Journal of Behavioral Medicine, 15,* 237–255.

Williams, R. B. (1989). *The trusting heart: Great news about Type A behavior.* New York: Times Books.

Williams, R. B. (1996). Hostility and the heart. In D. Goleman & J. Gurin (Eds.), *Mind-body medicine* (pp. 65–83). New York: Consumer Reports Books.

Williams, R. B. (2001). Hostility (and other psychosocial risk factors): Effects on health and the potential for successful behavioral approaches to prevention and treatment. In A. Baum, T. A. Revenson, & J. E. Singer (Eds.), *Handbook of health psychology* (pp. 661–668). Mahwah, NJ: Erlbaum.

Williamson, D. F., Serdula, M. K., Anda, R. F., Levy, A., & Byers, W. (1992). Weight loss attempts in adults: Goals, duration, and rate of weight loss. *American Journal of Public Health, 82,* 1251–1257.

Willis, W. D. (1995). Neurobiology, cold, pain and the brain. *Nature, 373,* 19–20.

Wills, T. A. (1997). Social support and health. In A. Baum, S. Newman, J. Weinman, R. West, & C. McManus (Eds.), *Cambridge handbook of psychology, health, and medicine* (pp. 168–171). Cambridge, UK: Cambridge University Press.

Wills, T. A. (1998). Social support. In E. A. Blechman & K. D. Brownell (Eds.), *Behavioral medicine and women: A comprehensive handbook* (pp. 118–128). New York: Guilford.

Windle, M., & Windle, R. C. (2001). Depressive symptoms and cigarette smoking among middle adolescents: Prospective associations and intrapersonal and interpersonal influences. *Journal of Consulting and Clinical Psychology, 69,* 215–226.

Winefield, H. R. (2001). Teaching and training other health disciplines. In M. Johnston and D. W. Johnston (Eds.), *Health psychology: Comprehensive clinical psychology* (Vol. 8, pp. 171–187). Amsterdam: Elsevier.

Wing, R. R. (1993). Behavioural treatment of obesity: Its application to Type II diabetes. *Diabetes Care, 16,* 193–199.

Wing, R. R., & Polley, B. A. (2001). Obesity. In A. Baum, T. A. Revenson, & J. E. Singer (Eds.), *Handbook of health psychology* (pp. 263-279). Mahwah, NJ: Erlbaum.

Winkleby, M. A., Kraemer, H. C., Ahn, D. K., & Varady, A. N. (1998). Ethnic and socioeconomic differences in cardiovascular disease risk factors: Findings from women from the Third National Health and Nutrition Examination Survey, 1988–1994. *Journal of the American Medical Association, 280,* 356–362.

Winkleby, M. A., Robinson, T. N., Sundquist, J., & Kraemer, H. C. (1999). Ethnic variation in cardiovascular disease risk factors among children and young adults: Findings from the Third National Health and Nutrition Examination Survey, 1988–1994. *Journal of the American Medical Association, 281,* 1006–1013.

Winslow, R. W., Franzini, L. R., & Hwang, J. (1992). Perceived peer norms, casual sex, and AIDS risk prevention. *Journal of Applied Social Psychology, 22,* 1809–1827.

Withers, N. W., Pulvirent, L., Koob, G .F., & Gillin, J. C. (1995). Cocaine abuse and dependence. *Journal of Clinical Psychopharmacology, 15,* 63–78.

Wolfgan, L. (1997). Charting recent progress in alcohol research. *Ninth Special Report to the U.S. Congress on Alcohol and Health.* www.niaa.nih.gov.

Wolin, S. (1993). *The resilient self: How survivors of troubled families rise above adversity.* New York: Villard Books.

Wonderlich, S., Klein, M. H., & Council, J. R. (1996). Relationship of social perceptions and self-concept in bulimia nervosa. *Journal of Consulting and Clinical Psychology, 64,* 1231–1237.

Wong, M., & Kaloupek, D. G. (1986). Coping with dental treatment: The potential impact of situational demands. *Journal of Behavioral Medicine, 9,* 579–597.

Wood, M. D., Vinson, D. C., & Sher, K. J. (2001). Alcohol use and misuse. In A. Baum, T. A. Revenson, & J. E. Singer (Eds.), *Handbook of health psychology* (pp. 249–261). Mahwah, NJ: Erlbaum.

Woodrow, K. M., Friedman, G. D., Siegelaub, A. B., & Collen, M. F. (1972). Pain tolerance: Differences according to age, sex and race. *Psychosomatic Medicine, 34,* 548–556.

Wooley, O. W. (1994). . . . And man created "woman": Representations of women's bodies in Western culture. In P. Fallon & M. A. Katzman (Eds.), *Feminist perspectives on eating disorders* (pp. 17–52). New York: Guilford.

Worden, J., & Flynn, B. (1999). Multimedia-TV: Shock to stop? *British Medical Journal, 318,* 64.

Workman, E. A., & La Via, M. F. (1987). Immunological effects of psychological stressors: A review of the literature. *International Journal of Psychosomatics, 34,* 35–40.

World Health Organization (WHO). (1990). *Diet, nutrition and the prevention of chronic diseases* (WHO Technical Report Series, no. 997). Geneva, Switzerland: United Nations.

World Health Organization (WHO). (2000, June). *The world health report 2000: Health systems: Improving performance.* Geneva, Switzerland: United Nations.

Wortman, C. B., Sheedy, C., Gluhoski, V., & Kessler, R. C. (1992). Stress, coping, and health: Conceptual issues and directions for future research. In H. S. Friedman (Ed.), *Hostility, coping, and health* (pp. 227–256). Washington, DC: American Psychological Association.

Wulfert, E., & Wan, C. K. (1993). Condom use: A self-efficacy model. *Health Psychology, 12,* 346–353.

Wulfert, E., Wan, C. K., & Backus, C. A. (1996). Gay men's safer sex behavior: An integration of three models. *Journal of Behavioral Medicine, 19,* 345–366.

Wynder, E. L., Fujita, Y., & Harris, R. E. (1991). Comparative epidemiology of cancer between the United States and Japan. *Cancer, 67,* 746–763.

Yaari, S., & Goldbourt, U. (1998). Voluntary and involuntary weight loss: Associations with long-term mortality in 9,228 middle-aged and elderly men. *American Journal of Epidemiology, 148,* 546–555.

Yan, J. Y., Best, N., Zhang, J. Z., Ren, H. J., Jiang, R., Hou, J., & Dovichi, N. J. (1996). The limiting mobility of DNA sequencing fragments for both cross-linked and noncross-linked polymers in capillary electrophoresis: DNA sequencing at 1200 V cm-1. *Electrophoresis, 17,* 1037–1045.

Yankelovich Parners (1997, December 15). Ability of spirituality to help people who are sick. (Press release).

Yee, B., W. K., Castro, F. G., Hammond, W. R., John, R., Wyatt, G. E., & Yung, B. R. (1995). Risk-taking and abusive behaviors among ethnic minorities. *Health Psychology, 14*(7), 622–631.

Yee, P. L., Edmondson, B., Santoro, K. E., Begg, A. E., & Hunter, C. D. (1996). Cognitive effects of life stress and learned helplessness. *Anxiety, Stress, & Coping, 9,* 301–319.

Young, K., & Zane, N. (1995). Ethnocultural influences in evaluation and management. In P. M. Nicassio & T. W. Smith (Eds.), *Managing chronic illness: A biopsychosocial perspective.* Washington, DC: American Psychological Association.

Yzer, M. C., Fisher, J. D., Bakker, A. B., Siero, F. W., & Misovich, S. J. (1998). The effects of information about AIDS risk and self-efficacy on women's intentions to engage in AIDS preventive behavior. *Journal of Applied Social Psychology, 28,* 1837–1852.

Zabin, L. S. (1993). *Adolescent sexual behavior and childbearing.* Newbury Park, CA: Sage.

Zarit, S. H. (1996). Continuities and discontinuities in very late life. In V. L. Bengston (Ed.), *Adulthood and aging: Research on continuities and discontinuities.* New York: Springer.

Zastowny, T. R., Kirschenbaum, D. S., & Meng, A. L. (1986). Coping skills training for children: Effects on distress before, during, and after hospitalization for surgery. *Health Psychology, 5,* 231–247.

Zelinski, E. M., Crimmins, E., Reynolds, S., & Seeman, T. (1998). Do medical conditions affect cognition in older adults? *Health Psychology, 17,* 504–512.

Zhang, H., & Huang, J. (1990). Preliminary study of traditional Chinese medicine treatment of minimal brain dysfunction: Analysis of 100 cases. Cited in J. W. Spencer & J. J. Jacobs (Eds.), *Complementary/alternative medicine: An evidence-based approach* (pp. 371–390). St. Louis, MO: Mosby.

Zhang, S., Hunter, D. J., Forman, M. R., Rosner, B. A., Speizer, F. E., Colditz, G. A., Manson, J. E., Hankinson, S. E., & Willett, W. C. (1999). Dietary carotenoids and vitamins A, C, and E and risk of breast cancer. *Journal of the National Cancer Institute, 91,* 547–556.

Zhang, W. H., & Po, A. L. (1994). The effectiveness of topically applied capsaicin: A meta-analysis. *European Journal of Clinical Pharmacology, 46,* 517–528.

Zhang, Y., Proenca, R., Maffei, M., & Barone, M. (1994). Positional cloning of the mouse obese gene and its human analogue. *Nature, 372,* 425–432.

Zhuo, D., Shephard, R. J., Plyley, M. J., & Davis, G. M. (1984). Cardiorespiratory and metabolic response durng Tai chi chuan exercise. *Canadian Journal of Applied Sport Sciences, 9,* 7–10.

Ziment, I. (1988). Acetylcysteine: A drug that is much more than a mucokinetic. *Biomedicine and Pharmacotherapy, 42,* 513–519.

Zimmerman, D. C. (1979). Preplanning, surgical, and postoperative considerations in the removal of the difficult impaction. *Dental Clinics of North America, 517,* 451–459.

Zimmerman, R. S., & Olson, K. (1994). AIDS-related risk behavior and behavior change in a sexually active heterosexual sample: A test of three models of prevention. *AIDS Education and Prevention, 6,* 189–204.

Zisook, S., Shuchter, S. R., Irwin, M., Darko, D. F., Sledge, P., & Resovsky, K. (1994). Bereavement, depression, and immune function. *Psychiatry Research, 52,* 1–10.

Zonderman, A. B., Costa, P. T., & McCrae, R. R. (1989). Depression as a risk for cancer morbidity and mortality in a nationally representative sample. *Journal of the American Medical Association, 262,* 1191–1195.

Zubin, J., & Spring, B. (1977). Vulnerability—a new view of schizophrenia. *Journal of Abnormal Psychology, 86,* 103–127.

Zuckerman, D. M. (1989). Stress, self-esteem, and mental health: How does gender make a difference? *Sex Roles, 20,* 429–444.

Zuger, A. (1998, March 24). At the hospital, a new doctor is in. *The New York Times,* p. B19.

Zwolfer, W., Grubhofer, G., Cartellieri, M., & Sapcek, A. (1992). Acupuncture in gonarthrotic pain: "Bachmann's knee program." *The American Journal of Chinese Medicine, 20,* 325–329.

Name Index

Subject Index

Locators in **bold** indicate additional display material.